Spine Surgery

Bernhard Meyer • Michael Rauschmann
Editors

Spine Surgery

A Case-Based Approach

Springer

Editors
Bernhard Meyer
Department of Neurosurgery
Klinikum rechts der Isar
Technische Universität München
Munich
Germany

Michael Rauschmann
Department of Spine Surgery
Sana Klinikum Offenbach
Offenbach
Germany

ISBN 978-3-319-98874-0 ISBN 978-3-319-98875-7 (eBook)
https://doi.org/10.1007/978-3-319-98875-7

Library of Congress Control Number: 2018965410

This Springer imprint is published by the registered company Springer Nature Switzerland AG
The registered company address is: Gewerbestrasse 11, 6330 Cham, Switzerland

Preface

We are very excited to introduce this new book on spinal surgery, which follows the curriculum of the EUROSPINE basic and advanced diploma courses. The approach we take is a purely case-based one, in which each case illustrates the concepts surrounding the treatment of a given pathology, including the uncertainties and problems in decision-making. The readers will notice that in many instances a lack of evidence for a given treatment exists. So decisions taken are usually not a clearcut matter of black or white, but merely different shades of gray. Probably in a lot of cases, there is often more than one option to treat the patient. The authors were asked to convey this message to the reader, giving him a guidance as what would be accepted within the mainstream. In addition, the reader is provided with the most updated literature and evidence on the topic.

Most of the authors are teachers in the courses of EUROSPINE or other national societies with often vast clinical experience and have given their own perspective and reasoning.

We believe that the readers will profit very much from this variety and bandwidth of knowledge provided for them in the individual chapters. We have given the authors extensive liberty as to what they consider the best solution for their case. It is thus a representative picture of what is considered standard of care for spine pathologies in Europe.

We hope that this book will be an ideal complement for trainees to the courses they take.

Munich, Germany — Bernhard Meyer
Offenbach, Germany — Michael Rauschmann

Contents

Part VII Advanced Module 2: Complications and Management

Contributors

R. Emre Acaroglu Ankara Spine Center, Ankara, Turkey

Mohammad Arabmotlagh Spine Department, Academic University Hospital Sana Klinik Offenbach, Goethe University Frankfurt, Offenbach, Germany

Eleftherios Archavlis Department of Neurosurgery, Universitätsmedizin Mainz, Johannes Gutenberg Universität Mainz, Mainz, Germany

Alkinoos Athanasiou First Department of Neurosurgery, AHEPA University General Hospital, Aristotle University of Thessaloniki, Thessaloniki, Greece

Massimo Balsano UOC Ortopedia e Traumatologia, Regional Spinal Department, AOUI, Verona, Italy

Cédric Y. Barrey Department of Spine and Spinal Cord Surgery, University Hospital Pierre Wertheimer (GHE), Claude Bernard University of Lyon 1, Hospices Civils de Lyon, Lyon, France

Simon Bayerl Department of Neurosurgery, Charitè – Universitätsmedizin Berlin, Berlin, Germany

Lukas Bobinski Department of Orthopedics, Spine Unit, Umeå University Hospital, Umeå, Sweden

Etienne Bourassa-Moreau Oxford University Hospitals NHS Foundation Trust, Nuffield Orthopaedic Centre, Oxford, UK

Adrian T. H. Casey Victor Horsley Department of Neurosurgery, The National Hospital for Neurology and Neurosurgery, Queen Square, London, UK

Jens Castein Zentrum für Wirbelsäulenchirurgie und Neurotraumatologie, BG Unfallklinik Frankfurt am Main, Frankfurt am Main, Germany

Yann Philippe Charles Service de Chirurgie du Rachis, Hôpitaux Universitaires de Strasbourg, Strasbourg, France

Jens Conrad Department of Neurosurgery, Universitätsmedizin Mainz, Johannes Gutenberg Universität Mainz, Mainz, Germany

Marcus Czabanka Department of Neurosurgery, Charité – Universitätsmedizin Berlin, Berlin, Germany

Julius Dengler Department of Neurosurgery, Charitè – Universitätsmedizin Berlin, Berlin, Germany

Michael E. Doany Department of Orthopedics, Stony Brook University, Stony Brook, NY, USA

John M. Duff Department of Clinical Neurosciences, University Hospital of Lausanne, CHUV, Lausanne, Switzerland

A. El Rahal Department of Spine and Spinal Cord Surgery, University Hospital Pierre Wertheimer (GHE), Claude Bernard University of Lyon 1, Hospices Civils de Lyon, Lyon, France

V. Fiere Department of Spine Surgery, Mermoz Private Hospital, Lyon, France

Christoph Fleege Spine Department, Orthopaedic University Hospital Friedrichsheim, Frankfurt, Germany

Jörg Franke Department of Orthopedics, Klinikum Magdeburg, Magdeburg, Germany

Martin Gehrchen Spine Unit, Department of Orthopaedic Surgery Rigshospitalet, University of Copenhagen, Copenhagen, Denmark

Jens Gempt Department of Neurosurgery, Klinikum rechts der Isar, Technische Universität München, Munich, Germany

Angelika Gutenberg Department of Neurosurgery, Universitätsmedizin Mainz, Johannes Gutenberg Universität Mainz, Mainz, Germany

Sleiman Haddad Department of Orthopaedic Surgery, Spine Unit, University Hospital Vall d'Hebron, Barcelona, Spain

Spine Surgery, Hospital Universitari Vall d'Hebron, Spine Institute Hospital Quiron, Barcelona, Spain

Sebastian Hartmann Department of Neurosurgery, Medical University Innsbruck, Innsbruck, Austria

Nils Hecht Department of Neurosurgery, Charité – Universitätsmedizin Berlin, Berlin, Germany

Sebastian Ille Department of Neurosurgery, Klinikum rechts der Isar, Technische Universität München, Munich, Germany

Max Jägersberg Department of Neurosurgery, University Medical Center Mainz, Mainz, Germany

Dezsö Jeszenszky Department of Spine Surgery, Schulthess Klinik, Zürich, Switzerland

Frank Kandziora Zentrum für Wirbelsäulenchirurgie und Neurotraumatologie, Berufsgenossenschaftliche Unfallklinik Frankfurt am Main, Frankfurt am Main, Germany

Sven R. Kantelhardt Department of Neurosurgery, Universitätsmedizin Mainz, Johannes Gutenberg Universität Mainz, Mainz, Germany

David Kieser University of Otago, Department of Orthopaedic Surgery and Musculoskeletal Medicine, Christchurch School of Medicine, Christchurch, New Zealand

Esat Kiter Pamukkale University, Department of Orthopedics, Denizli, Turkey

Sandro M. Krieg Department of Neurosurgery, Klinikum rechts der Isar, Technische Universität München, Munich, Germany

Jesús Lafuente Servicio de Neurocirugía, Hospital del Mar, Universidad de Barcelona, Barcelona, Spain

Ulf Liljenqvist Department for Spine Surgery, St. Franziskus Hospital, Münster, Germany

Markus Loibl Department of Spine Surgery, Schulthess Klinik, Zürich, Switzerland

Rodolfo Maduri Department of Clinical Neurosciences, University Hospital of Lausanne, CHUV, Lausanne, Switzerland

Ioannis Magras First Department of Neurosurgery, AHEPA University General Hospital, Aristotle University of Thessaloniki, Thessaloniki, Greece

Vasiliki Magra Plastic Surgery Department, Lister Hospital, East & North Hertfordshire NHS Trust, Hertfordshire, UK

Antonia Matamalas Department of Orthopaedic Surgery, Spine Unit, University Hospital Vall d'Hebron, Barcelona, Spain

Bernhard Meyer Department of Neurosurgery, Klinikum rechts der Isar, Technische Universität München, Munich, Germany

Hanno S. Meyer Department of Neurosurgery, Klinikum rechts der Isar, Technische Universität München, Munich, Germany

S. Michalitsis Department of Orthopedics, Klinikum Magdeburg, Magdeburg, Germany

Wouter A. Moojen Haaglanden Medical Center, The Hague, The Netherlands

Haga Teaching Hospital, The Hague, The Netherlands

Leiden University Medical Center, Leiden, The Netherlands

Stefano Negri UOC Ortopedia e Traumatologia, Regional Spinal Department, AOUI, Verona, Italy

Susana Núñez-Pereira Spine Unit, Hospital Universitario Donostia, Donostia/San Sebastián, Spain

Nusret Ok Pamukkale University, Department of Orthopedics, Denizli, Turkey

Haiko Pape Department of Neurosurgery, Klinikum rechts der Isar, Technische Universität München, Munich, Germany

Juan D. Patino Neurosurgery Department, Hospital de la Santa Creu i Sant Pau, Barcelona, Spain

Ferran Pellisé Department of Orthopaedic Surgery, Spine Unit, University Hospital Vall d'Hebron, Barcelona, Spain

Andreas Pingel Zentrum für Wirbelsäulenchirurgie und Neurotraumatologie, BG Unfallklinik Frankfurt am Main, Frankfurt, Germany

George K. Prezerakos Victor Horsley Department of Neurosurgery, The National Hospital for Neurology and Neurosurgery, Queen Square, London, UK

Michael Rauschmann Department of Spine Surgery, Sana Klinikum Offenbach, Offenbach, Germany

Jeremy J. Reynolds Oxford University Hospitals NHS Foundation Trust, Nuffield Orthopaedic Centre, Oxford, UK

Marcus Richter Spine Center, St. Josefs-Hospital, Wiesbaden, Germany

Florian Ringel Department of Neurosurgery, Universitätsmedizin Mainz, Johannes Gutenberg Universität Mainz, Mainz, Germany

David Rodríguez-Rubio Servicio de Neurocirugía, Hospital del Mar, Universidad de Barcelona, Barcelona, Spain

Dominique A. Rothenfluh Oxford University Hospitals NHS Foundation Trust, Nuffield Orthopaedic Centre, Oxford, UK

Yu-Mi Ryang Department of Neurosurgery, Klinikum rechts der Isar, Technische Universität München, Munich, Germany

Philipp Schleicher Zentrum für Wirbelsäulenchirurgie und Neurotraumatologie, Berufsgenossenschaftliche Unfallklinik Frankfurt am Main, Frankfurt am Main, Germany

Matti Scholz Zentrum für Wirbelsäulenchirurgie und Neurotraumatologie, Berufsgenossenschaftliche Unfallklinik Frankfurt am Main, Frankfurt am Main, Germany

Alpaslan Senkoylu Gazi University, Ankara, Turkey

Ehab Shiban Department of Neurosurgery, Klinikum rechts der Isar, Technische Universität München, Munich, Germany

Andrei Slavici Department of Spine and Reconstructive Orthopedic Surgery, Sana Klinikum Offenbach, Offenbach am Main, Germany

F. Solla Department of Pediatrics Orthopedics, Lenval Hospital, Nice, France

Michael Stoffel Department of Neurosurgery, Helios Klinikum Krefeld, Krefeld, Germany

Enrico Tessitore Department of Neurosurgery, Faculty of Medicine, University of Geneva, Geneva, Switzerland

Claudius Thomé Department of Neurosurgery, Medical University Innsbruck, Innsbruck, Austria

Dimitri Tkatschenko Department of Neurosurgery, Charitè – Universitätsmedizin Berlin, Berlin, Germany

Aurélie Toquart Department of Spine and Spinal Cord Surgery, University Hospital Pierre Wertheimer (GHE), Claude Bernard University of Lyon 1, Hospices Civils de Lyon, Lyon, France

Sven Kevin Tschoeke Department of Spine Surgery, Klinikum Dortmund gGmbH, Dortmund, Germany

Anja Tschugg Department of Neurosurgery, Medical University Innsbruck, Innsbruck, Austria

Peter Vajkoczy Department of Neurosurgery, Charitè – Universitätsmedizin Berlin, Berlin, Germany

N. A. van der Gaag Haaglanden Medical Center, The Hague, The Netherlands

Haga Teaching Hospital, The Hague, The Netherlands

Lars Wessels Department of Neurosurgery, Charité Universitätsmedizin Berlin, Berlin, Germany

Maria Wostrack Department of Neurosurgery, Klinikum rechts der Isar, Technische Universität München, Munich, Germany

Ulas Yildiz Zentrum für Wirbelsäulenchirurgie und Neurotraumatologie, BG Unfallklinik Frankfurt am Main, Frankfurt, Germany

Caglar Yilgor Acibadem Mehmet Ali Aydinlar University School of Medicine, Department of Orthopedics and Traumatology, Istanbul, Turkey

Kimia Rahnama Zand Clinical Neurophysiology, Intraoperative Neuromonitoring, Hospital Universitari Vall d'Hebron, Spine Institute Hospital Quiron, Barcelona, Spain

Anna Zdunczyk Department of Neurosurgery, Charité Universitätsmedizin Berlin, Berlin, Germany

Part I

Basic Module 1: Conservative Therapy

1 Treatment for Acute, Subacute and Chronic Low Back Pain

Ehab Shiban and Bernhard Meyer

1.1 Introduction

Low back pain (LBP) has become the leading cause for living with disability in the world [3]. In an analysis of two national surveys in the United States one third of U.S adult reported having LBP at least for 1 day during the last 3 months [4]. In a national German survey 25% of women and 17% of men reported having LBP lasting for at least 3 months during the last year [5]. LBP causes also a great financial burden to the health care system with high direct costs related to treatment as well as indirect costs due to sick leave or diminished productivity.

In general LBP is classified and treated based on duration of symptoms, potential cause, presence or absence of radicular symptoms and corresponding radiological abnormalities [2]. Thereby specific LBP is to be distinguished from nonspecific LBP. Specific LBP has a detectable somatic cause and treatment thereof will probably lead to pain reduction (e.g. herniated disc, spinal canal stenosis, infection, vertebral metastasis etc.). On the other hand, in nonspecific LBP treatment is mainly symptomatic [1]. Acute LBP lasts less than 1 month, subacute LBP lasts between 1 and 3 months and chronic LBP lasts more than 3 months. In 2017 the German and North American national societies each published revised guidelines for the treatment of non-specific LBP [1, 2]. Thereby the initial evaluation, necessity of further laboratory or imaging evaluation as well as the efficacy of treatment modalities are discussed.

This chapter will outline these guidelines. Moreover, the different treatment modalities are discussed with regards to their efficacy and level of evidence. At the end of this chapter the readers should be able correctly manage patients with nonspecific LBP.

The aim of the presented case is to illustrate the management algorithms and treatment allocation for patients with chronic non-specific LBP.

1.2 Case Description

A 48 year-old female patient presented with a 3-day history of exacerbated LBP. Pain exacerbation was following lifting her 3 year-old son. The patient reported having episodic LBP for the last 18 months. She already had magnetic resonance imaging 6 months prior illustrating slight degenerative disc changes of the lower spine (Fig. 1.1). She already had acupuncture and massages that help reduce the pain intermittently. She also reported having facet joint

E. Shiban (✉) · B. Meyer
Department of Neurosurgery, Klinikum rechts der Isar, Technische Universität München, Munich, Germany
e-mail: Ehab.shiban@tum.de

B. Meyer, M. Rauschmann (eds.), *Spine Surgery*, https://doi.org/10.1007/978-3-319-98875-7_1

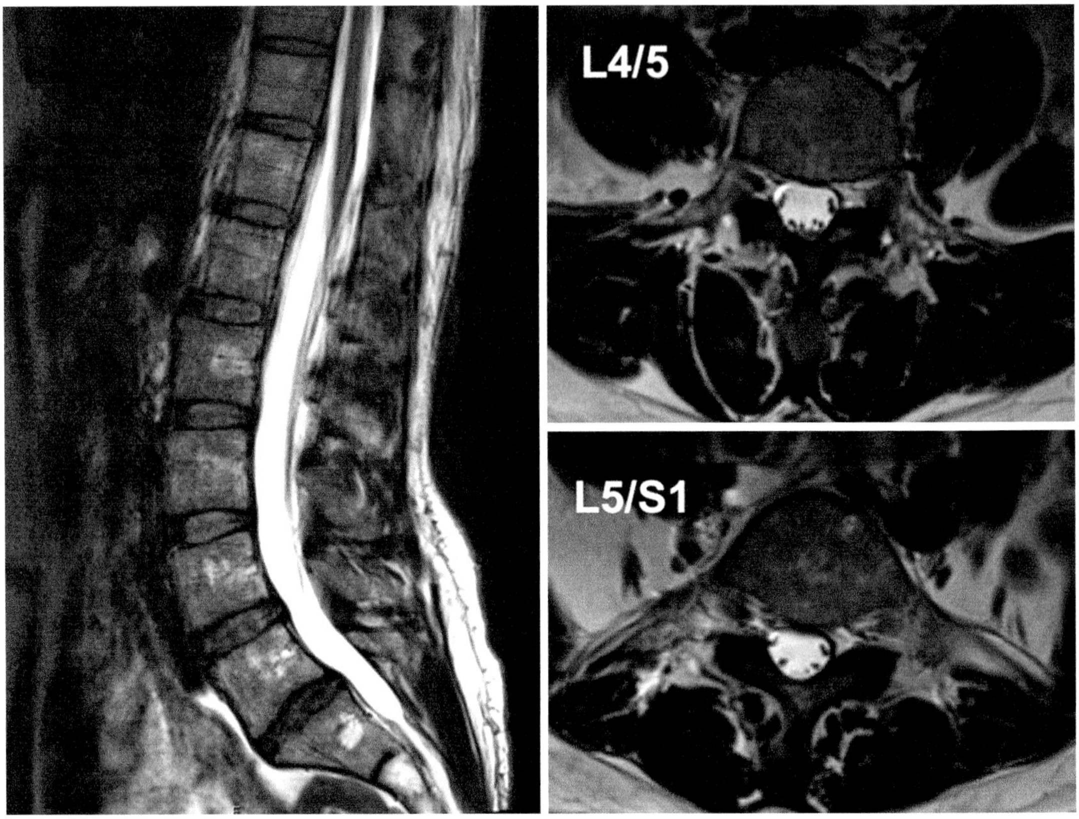

Fig. 1.1 Magnetic resonance imaging of the lumbar spine. Slight degenerative changes in L5/S1 are noted. No disc herniation or spinal canal stenosis

infiltration therapy 2 months prior to presentation that resulted in markedly reduced pain for 6 weeks. Upon presentation she was on 800 mg Ibuprofen twice daily for the last 6 months. Otherwise she was very healthy without any other preexisting conditions. She had a normal physical examination. The patient was initially managed with intravenous Piritramide and oral Metamizole. Because there were no new symptoms, there was no need for a new MRI. Dynamic radiographs ruled out apparent instability (Fig. 1.2). In order to facilitate pain relief bilateral facet joint infiltration to L4/5 and L5/S1 were performed. Thereafter the pain was markedly reduced and the intravenous pain medication was stopped. The patient was then discharged with oral Tramadol (50 mg) twice daily for 2 weeks and was referred to multidisciplinary biopsychosocial rehabilitation.

1.3 Discussion of the Case

1.3.1 Why Were Things Done This Way

The patient in the above mention clinical vignette was suffering form non-specific low back pain. MRI imaging 6 months prior to presentation not did show any specific pathologies and dynamic radiograph ruled out apparent instability. Because there were no "red flags" there was also no need for any new or further diagnostic imaging. Initial short-term intravenous opioids were given to facilitate rapid pain reduction. Because the patient already had positive experience with facet joint infiltration, we decided to repeat them and discharge the patient with a short period of oral opioids and referral to a multidisciplinary rehabilitation program.

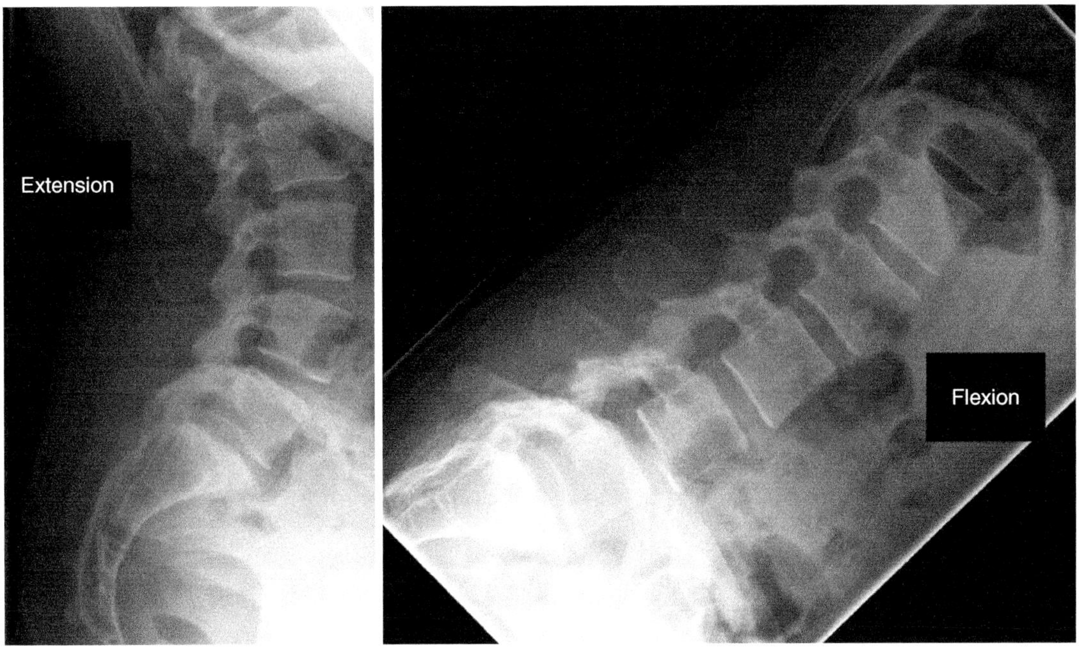

Fig. 1.2 Dynamic radiographs (Flexion/Extension) of the lumbar spine. No signs are apparent instability are noted

1.3.2 Were They in Accordance with the Literature Guidelines

In 2017 both the German [1] and the North American [2] national societies have each published a new version of the guidelines for the treatment of LBP. Both guidelines are very similar and recommend that for patients with acute or subacute LBP without any "red flags" (Table 1.1) clinicians should avoid unnecessary tests and treatments because in most cases the pain will resolved in time without a specific treatment.

Initially it is very important to explain to the patient that LBP is extremely common, the prognosis is generally very good and that pain does not necessarily mean organ damage. At first non-medical treatment with or without pain medication should be recommended. Although there are some general recommendations for medical treatment (Table 1.2), no clear recommendations can be made with regards to any specific treatment modality because the treatment effects are small and often show no clear benefit when compared to controls (Tables 1.3 and 1.4). If at this stage any psychosocial risk factors are identified or are already known, these risk factors need to be incorporated in the counseling and should be adequately addressed [8].

Table 1.1 "Red flags" in the assessment of low back pain

Fracture/osteoporosis: severe to moderate trauma cases; minimal trauma in the elderly; systemic steroid use
Infection: fever, shivering; i.v. Drug abuse; immunocompromised, recent infiltration therapy to the spine
Neurological compromise: cauda-equina syndrome; muscle weakness; genital hypoesthesia; micturition problems
Tumor/metastases: History of cancer; B-symptoms (fever, night sweats, and weight loss); pain exacerbation in prone position

After 12 weeks of pain and restrictions in daily activity despite treatment, a multidisciplinary assessment and treatment should be done. The goal is to empower patients through acceptance-based strategies to actively and consciously shape their lives despite the pain. Thereby multimodal behavioral therapy strategies seem to be most effective. In a Cochrane review of 41 studies and 6858 patients the

Table 1.2 General consideration for medical treatment of LBP

Non-opioid pain medication	
Non-steroidal antiphlogistics (NSAIDs)	1. No clinical superiority of any specific NSAIDs 2. No evidence for parental use, therefore oral application are recommended 3. Daily dose of 1.2 g of Ibuprofen, 100 mg of Diclofenac or 750 mg of Naproxen should not be exceeded. However if the effect is insufficient, the dose may be briefly increased to 2.4 g of Ibuprofen, 150 mg of Diclofenac or 1.25 g of Naproxen 4. Concomitant administration of Proton-pump Inhibitors is recommended
COX-2 inhibitors	1. If NSAIDs are contraindicated 2. Contraindicated in patients with coronary heart disease, stroke, hart failure or peripheral artery disease
Metamizole	1. If NSAIDs are contraindicated 2. Caution in patients with concomitant long-term Acetaminophen treatment (causes platelet aggregation inhibition) 3. Agranulocytosis is a rare but very severe adverse effect
Paracetamol	Two high level RCTs did not show any benefit compered to placebo, therefore administration is not recommended anymore [9]
Opioids	1. The opioid therapy should be regularly reevaluated, in acute LBP 4 weeks at the latest, in chronic LBP after 3 months at the latest 2. Opioids are to be used for the long-term treatment of chronic LBP only in the context of multimodal behavioral therapy strategies 3. Transdermal opioids should not be used to treat acute and subacute LBP
Muscle relaxants	Not recommended for LBP
Antidepressants	Only recommended in the presence of comorbid depression or sleep disorder
Antiepileptic drugs	Not recommended for LBP
Herbal medicine	1. Taking into account the side effects and contraindications (similar to those of the NSAIDs), a therapy trial with willow bark can be undertaken as part of an overall therapeutic concept 2. Due to the lower level of evidence for the use of devil's claw is not recommended.
Topical applications	1. Moderate level evidence exist for the use of capsaicin 2. Topical NSAIDs are not recommended
Intravenous, intramuscular or subcutaneous applications	Given the effectiveness of a wide range of oral analgesics the use of injections of painkillers, local anesthetics, etc. due to side effects and complications is not recommended for LBP

Table 1.3 Medical treatment vs. placebo (acute low back pain)

	Magnitude of effect	Strength of evidence
Acetaminophen	No effect	Low (1 RCT)
NSAIDs	Small	Moderate (5 RCTs)
Muscle relaxants	Small	Moderate (5 RCTs)
Systemic corticosteroids	No effect	Low (2 RCTs)

Modified from [2]

Table 1.4 Non-medical treatment vs. sham or usual treatment (acute & subacute low back pain)

Intervention	Magnitude of Effect	Strength of evidence
Heat wrap vs. placebo	Moderate	Moderate (4 RCTs)
Exercise vs. usual care	No effect	Low (6 RCTs)
Acupuncture vs. sham acupuncture	Small effect	Low (2 RCTs)
Massage vs. sham massage	1 week: Moderate 5 weeks: No effect	Low (2 RCTs)
Spinal manipulation vs. inert treatment	No effect	Low (3 RCTs)
Spinal manipulation vs. sham treatment	Small	Low (2 RCTs)

Modified from [2]

Table 1.5 Non-medical treatment vs. sham or usual treatment (chronic low back pain)

Intervention	Magnitude of effect	Strength of evidence
Exercise vs. no exercise	Small	Moderate (19 RCTs)
Exercise vs. usual care	Small	Moderate (18 RCTs)
Motor control exercise	Moderate	Low (2 RCTs)
Tai chi vs. wait-list or no tai chi	Moderate	Low (2 RCTs)
Yoga vs. usual care	Moderate	Low (1 RCTs)
Yoga vs. education	No effect	Low (5 RCTs)
Mindfulness-based stress reduction vs. usual care	Improved	Moderate (3 RCTs)
Progressive relaxation vs. wait list control	Moderate	Low (3 RCTs)
Electromyography biofeedback vs. wait-list control or placebo	Moderate	Low (3 RCTs)
Operant therapy vs. wait list	Small	Low (3 RCTs)
Cognitive behavioral therapy vs. wait-list control	Moderate	Low (3 RCTs)
Multidisciplinary rehabilitation vs. usual care	Small	Moderate (9 RCTs)
Multidisciplinary rehabilitation vs. no multidisciplinary rehabilitation	Moderate	Low (3 RCTs)
Acupuncture vs. sham acupuncture	Moderate	Low (9 RCTs)
Acupuncture vs. no acupuncture	Moderate	Moderate (4 RCTs)
Massage vs. usual care	No effect	Low (1RCT)
Spinal manipulation vs. sham treatment	No effect	Low (4 RCTs)
Spinal manipulation vs. inert treatment	Small	Low (7 RCTs)
Ultrasound vs. sham ultrasound	No effect	Low (5 RCTs)
Ultrasound vs. no ultrasound	No effect	Low (5 RCTs)
TENS vs. sham treatment	No effect	Low (4 RCTs)
Laser-therapy vs. sham laser	Small	Low (3 RCTs)
Kinesio taping vs. sham taping	No effect	Low (2 RCTs)

Modified from [2]

Table 1.6 Medical treatment vs. placebo (chronic low back pain)

Intervention	Magnitude of effect	Strength of evidence
NSAIDs	Small to moderate	Moderate (6 RCTs)
Strong opioids	Small	Moderate (10 RCTs)
Tramadol	Moderate	Moderate (7 RCTs)
Tetrazepam	Small	Low (2 RCTs)
Opioids: buprenorphine or sublingual	Small	Moderate (7 RCTs)
Antidepressants	No effect	Low (2 RCTs)
SSRI	No effect	Moderate (3 RCTS)
Duloxetine	Small	Moderate (3 RCTs)

Modified from [2]

superiority of multidisciplinary biopsychosocial rehabilitation compared to usual care and physical treatment was illustrated [7]. Otherwise like in acute and subacute LBP also in chronic LBP there are no clear recommendations for a specific medical or non-medical treatment modality because the treatment effects are small and often show no clear benefit when compared to controls (Tables 1.5 and 1.6).

1.3.3 Invasive Treatment Options

1.3.3.1 Percutaneous Therapy

There is insufficient evidence to support the use of injection therapy in subacute and chronic low-back pain [10]. However, the heterogeneity of the included patient groups, the small number of patients in the studies, the frequent lack of differentiation between specific and nonspecific causes of LBP, and inconsistent control interventions make the ability to identify specific subgroups that might benefit from a percutaneous procedure very difficult [6].

1.3.3.2 Surgery

Because most surgical studies are performed on patients with specific LBP, there are is no data available for the use of surgery in acute and chronic non-specific LBP.

Clinical Pearls

- Acute or subacute low back pain without any "red flags" need to be reassured that in most cases the pain will resolve in time and therefore potentially harmful and costly tests and treatments should be avoided
- Patients with acute, subacute or chronic low back pain should be advised to remain active as tolerated and not to avoid daily activity
- Both medical and non-medical treatment options show small improvement in pain and often fail to demonstrate clear benefits compared to controls
- There are almost no differences in recommended therapies when studied in head-to-head trials. Therefore, recommendations should primarily be guided by the patient's preferences taking into consideration to minimize harms, such as long-term opioids

Editorial Comment

The use of Facet Joint Infiltrations in this case was thus not in accordance with guidelines in a strict sense, but acceptable due to the rapid pain relief provided by the steroids.

References (Including EBM Level)

1. Bundesärztekammer (BÄK), Kassenärztliche Bundesvereinigung (KBV), Arbeitsgemeinschaft der Wissenschaftlichen Medizinischen Fachgesellschaften (AWMF). Nationale VersorgungsLeitlinie Nicht-spezifischer Kreuzschmerz – Langfassung, 2. Auflage. Version 1. 2017.
2. Qaseem A, Wilt TJ, McLean RM, Forciea MA. Clinical Guidelines Committee of the American College of Physicians.Noninvasive Treatments for Acute, Subacute, and Chronic Low Back Pain: A Clinical Practice Guideline From the American College of Physicians. Ann Intern Med. 2017;166(7):514–30.
3. GBD 2015 Disease and Injury Incidence and Prevalence Collaborators. Global, regional, and national incidence, prevalence, and years lived with disability for 310 diseases and injuries, 1990–2015: a systematic analysis for the Global Burden of Disease Study 2015. Lancet. 2016;388(10053):1545–602. **(EBM=2C)**.
4. Deyo RA, Mirza SK, Martin BI. Back pain prevalence and visit rates: estimates from U.S. national surveys, 2002. Spine (Phila Pa 1976). 2006;31(23):2724–7. **(EBM 2B)**.
5. Robert Koch Institut (RKI). Gesundheit in Deutschland. Gesundheitsberichterstattung des Bundes. Gemeinsam getragen von RKI und-Destatis. Berlin: RKI; 2015. http://www.rki.de/DE/Content/Gesundheitsmonitoring/Gesundheitsberichterstattung/GesInDtld/gesundheit_in_deutschland_2015.pdf. **(EBM 2B)**.
6. Henschke N, Kuijpers T, Rubinstein SM, van Middelkoop M, Ostelo R, Verhagen A, Koes BW, van Tulder MW. Injection therapy and denervation procedures for chronic low- back pain: a systematic review. Eur Spine J. 2010;19(9):1425–49. **(EBM=2A).**
7. Kamper SJ, Apeldoorn AT, Chiarotto A, Smeets RJ, Ostelo RW, Guzman J, van Tulder MW. Multidisciplinary biopsychosocial rehabilitation for chronic low back pain. Cochrane Database Syst Rev. 2014;9:CD000963. **(EBM=1A).**
8. Linton SJ, Nordin E. A 5-year follow-up evaluation of the health and economic consequences of an early cognitive behavioral intervention for back pain: a randomized, controlled trial. Spine. 2006;31(8):853–8. **(EBM=1B).**
9. Machado GC, Maher CG, Ferreira PH, et al. Efficacy and safety of paracetamol for spinal pain and osteoarthritis: systematic review and meta-analysis of randomised placebo controlled trials. BMJ. 2015;350:h1225. **(EBM=1A).**
10. Staal JB, de Bie RA, de Vet HC, Hildebrandt J, Nelemans P. Injection therapy for subacute and chronic low back pain: an updated Cochrane review. Spine (Phila Pa 1976). 2009;34(1):49–59. **(EBM=1A).**

2 Indications for Emergency Surgical Treatment

Max Jägersberg and Enrico Tessitore

2.1 Introduction

Indications for emergency surgical treatment in degenerative spinal conditions are limited to those where a delay in surgical management may lead to potentially catastrophic and irreversible sequelae. Indeed, those conditions are rarely encountered during clinical practice. The most typical scenarios in the thoraco-lumbar region are cauda equina syndrome (CES) and progressive radicular motor deficit (PRMD), both primarily caused by degenerative lumbar pathology. Early surgical treatment may influence the partial or full recovery and the long-term outcome of concerned patients.

CES is a rare condition where the majority of cauda equina nerve roots are suddenly compressed with sudden loss of motor function, of sensation in the saddle area, of sphincter (bladder and/or bowel) and sexual function [1]. PRMD is an analogous pathological condition where patients present with a progressive motor deficit in lower limbs, related to solitary or double nerve root involvement. The typically encountered clinical type of PRMD is *foot drop* due to L5 and/or L4 nerve root compression. The severity of motor deficit of PRMD is graded by means of the manual muscle testing (MMT) according to the Medical Research Council Scale (Table 2.1) [2].

In most of the cases, both CES and PRMD are caused by an acute disc prolapse compressing the nerve roots, especially if the onset of symptoms is sudden. Nevertheless, other degenerative disorders such as synovial cysts, lumbar stenosis, spondylolisthesis and other compressive pathology (e.g. infections, tumors) can cause the neurological deficit. MRI should be the radiologic imaging of choice since it can not only confirm compression of spinal nerve structures, but also define the underlying pathology. Additional radiographs, with dynamic flexion and extension images and CT might be added if the spinal morphology as encountered on MRI demands for this.

The aim of this chapter is to illustrate via two cases the surgical management of CES and PMRD patients, outlining indication and timing for surgery as well as discussing the evidences in the literature.

Table 2.1 Manual Muscle Testing (MMT) according to the Medical Research Council scale of muscle strength [2]

0	No contraction
1	Flicker or trace of contraction
2	Active movement, with gravity eliminated
3	Active movement against gravity
4	Active movement against gravity and resistance
5	Normal power

M. Jägersberg (✉)
Department of Neurosurgery, University Medical Center Mainz, Mainz, Germany
e mail: max.jaegersberg@unimedizin-mainz.de

E. Tessitore
Department of Neurosurgery, Faculty of Medicine, University of Geneva, Geneva, Switzerland

B. Meyer, M. Rauschmann (eds.), *Spine Surgery*, https://doi.org/10.1007/978-3-319-98875-7_2

2.2 Case Description

2.2.1 Case 1

A 39 years old male was admitted to a tertiary hospital complaining of right sciatic pain without neurological deficit for 10 days. A medical therapy with pain killers (NSAID drugs) was prescribed and the patient discharged. Five days later, he was admitted in our emergency department complaining of acute onset of bilateral foot distal weakness, associated with perineal loss of sensation, urinary retention and constipation.

The neurological exam showed a L4 paraplegia with bilateral L5-S1 weakness (MMT 1/5), sacral (S1-S5) hypoesthesia, and urinary retention. The patient was catheterized and sent to MRI. The MRI showed a L3-L4 disc prolapse in the context of a congenital and acquired multiple level lumbar stenosis. The herniation compressed the cauda equina and the canal sagittal diameter was dramatically reduced (Fig. 2.1).

The patient was immediately brought to OR for emergency surgical decompression. Surgery consisted of posterior midline approach with L3-L4 flavectomy, L4 right laminectomy and contralateral undercutting, sequestrectomy and microdiscectomy. Surgery was uneventful and the patient admitted to the recovery room.

Then, the patient was sent to a specialized center for rehabilitation. He underwent physical therapy, ergo-therapy, vector physical therapy, swimming, and he received psychological support. Sphincter deficits were treated with anticholinergic drugs, self-catheterization, and manual rectal clear. The patient was discharged after 2 months and ambulatory physical therapy was prescribed to him.

A one-year postoperative MRI (Fig. 2.2) showed no more disc herniation and a persistent congenital and acquired lumbar stenosis. The patient was able to walk 1 km with crutches. He was still performing self-catheterizations and manual rectal clear 2 times/day. Persistent neurogenic perineal pain was treated by pregabalin.

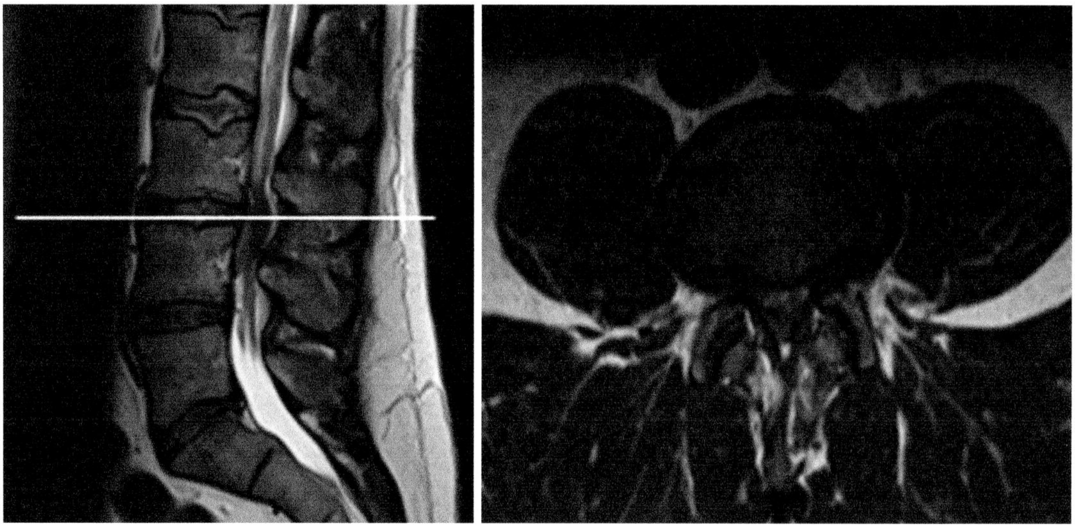

Fig. 2.1 Sagittal (left) and axial (right) MRI showing a large, median and downward migrated disc fragment at L3-L4 level, with cauda equina compression

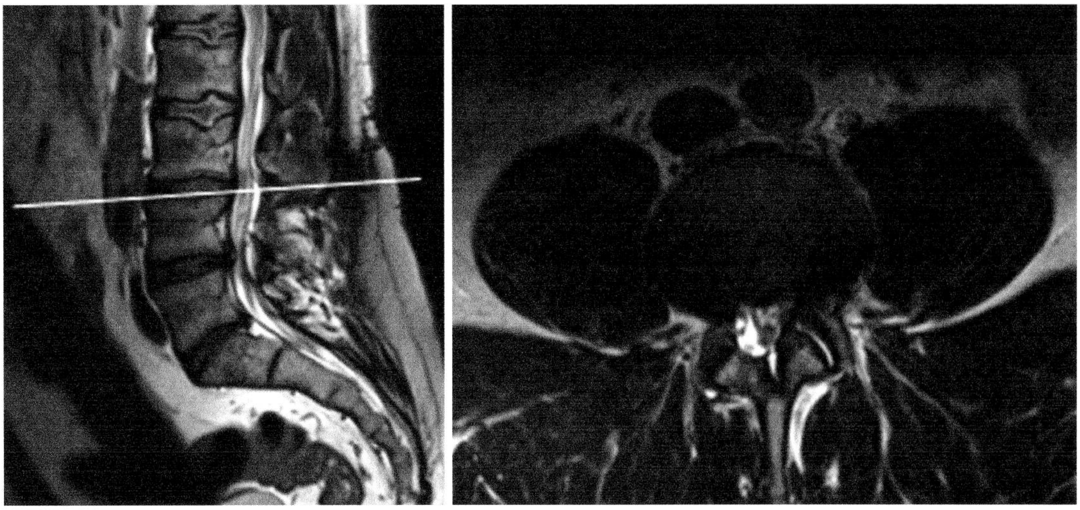

Fig. 2.2 Sagittal (left) and axial (right) 1 year post-operative MRI showing absence of recurrent disc herniation and a complete nerve roots' decompression

2.2.2 Case 2

A 62 years old male patient consulted with left irradiating leg pain into the foot and associated inability to dorsiflex the left ankle. Onset had been 3 months prior to presentation, without injury or brisk movement. No bladder or bowel problems were reported.

Clinical examination revealed a motor deficit MMT 3/5 of both extensor hallucis longus and tibialis anterior muscles. The patient showed the characteristic foot drop steppage gait. Straight leg test was negative. Mechanical back pain testing was low.

The clinical pattern was in line with the radiologic finding of compression of the left L4 and L5 nerve roots, caused by a synovial cyst of the left L4/5 zygoapophyseal joint and by spondylosis and grade I degenerative spondylolisthesis with consecutive stenosis of the L5 recess (Fig. 2.3).

Because no major instability criteria were evident, microsurgical decompressive surgery was advocated and carried out 10 days later. A left L5 hemilaminectomy, cyst removal, and L4 and L5 nerve root decompression were carried out without complications.

Following surgery, the patient was relieved from leg pain. However, he did not observe improvement of muscle strength. Postoperative MRI was carried out but did not show residual nerve root compression (Fig. 2.4). An ankle-foot orthosis was prescribed, but the patient did not see any functional benefit from it.

The surgical result (relief from leg pain, foot drop persistence, MMT 3/5) remained unchanged at follow-up at 3 months, 1 year and 2 years following surgery. Repeated electromyography and nerve conduction studies confirmed an L5 nerve root damage that appeared permanent.

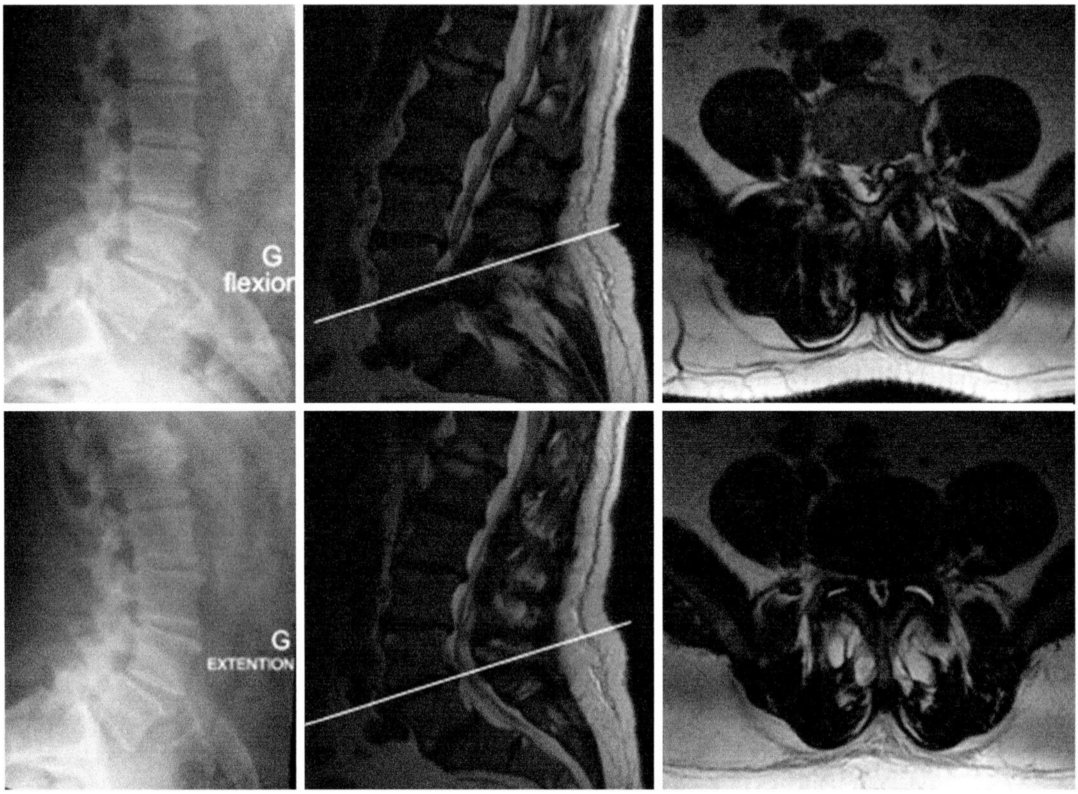

Fig. 2.3 Preoperative dynamic radiographs in flexion and extension, showing minor spondylolisthesis between L4/L5 and L5/S1, without dynamic component. T2-weighted MRI in sagittal and axial planes showing radiologic compression of the left L4 nerve root by synovial cyst formation, left L5 nerve root compression by spondylosis and spondylolisthesis with consecutive recess stenosis

2.3 Discussion of the Cases

2.3.1 Case 1

This case illustrates a typical clinical scenario of CES related to a disc prolapse.

In this particular case, symptoms started in form of severe sciatic pain few days before the installation of CES. The surgical decompression was immediately performed. Time to decompression is the best described outcome predictor in CES. Ahn *et al.* performed a meta-analysis to determine the correlation between timing of decompression and clinical outcome in 322 patients [3]. Significant differences were found in resolution of sensory and motor deficits as well as urinary and rectal function in patients treated within 48 h compared with those treated more than 48 h after onset of symptoms.

In that specific case, despite the fact that the treatment was performed according to the literature guidelines, the patient kept some sequelae of CES at 1 year time follow-up. This demonstrate how this condition may be disabling even though correctly managed.

Contrary to the well-known and studied prevalence and outcome of motor and sensitive sequelae, few data are available on the long-term outcome of micturition, defecation and sexual function after spinal surgery for CES. A study from a Dutch group clearly demonstrated that dysfunction of micturition, defecation and sexual functions are still highly prevalent in a large number of CES patients even years postoperatively [4].

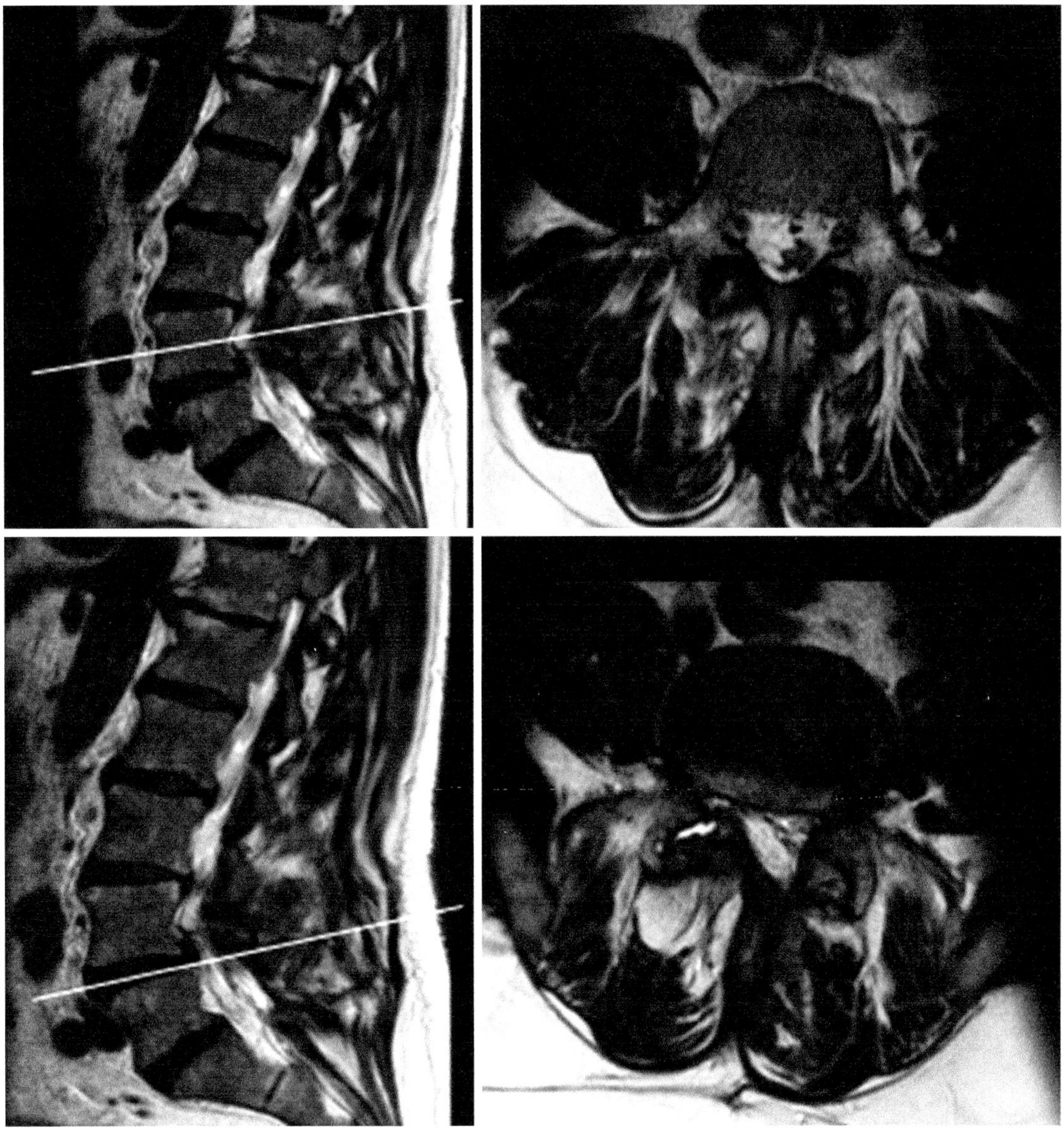

Fig. 2.4 Postoperative T2-weighted MRI in sagittal and axial planes showing effective decompression of both nerve roots by resection of the synovial cyst and recessotomy

2.3.2 Case 2

This chapter covers the emergency situation of severe motor deficit attributable to degenerative spinal disorders at the example of the descriptive symptom *foot drop*. The first step in the management of this scenario is to rule out alternative causes of foot drop (peroneal nerve palsy, brain lesions, spinal cord lesions, MS, polyneuropathy, etc.). A thorough clinical examination and radiologic workup will allow to determine if lumbar degenerative disorder can be responsible or not.

Assessment of motor deficit follows the manual muscle testing (MMT) according to the Medical Research Council Scale (Table 2.1) [2]. It should be mentioned that several studies define foot drop as MMT of less than 3 (i.e. 2, 1 or 0), and "good" recovery if a postoperative MMT of 3 is achieved. In contrast, our case presentation shows well that MMT 3 effectively remains a

Table 2.2 Probability estimates of postoperative motor recovery to strength ≥3 or ≥4 MMT according to Takenaka et al. [8]

	Predictors		Outcome	
Frequency (n_{total} = 102)	Pre tibialis anterior muscle strength	Duration (days)	Post tibialis anterior muscle strength ≥3	Post tibialis anterior muscle strength ≥4
31.4% (n = 32)	2 or 3–	≤ 30	96.9%(n = 31/32)	87.5% (n = 28/32)
33.3% (n = 34)	2 or 3–	> 30	61.7% (n = 21/34)	41.2% (n = 14/34)
14.7% (n = 15)	0 or 1	≤ 30	53.3% (n = 8/15)	46.7% (n = 7/15)
20.6% (n = 21)	0 or 1	> 30	14.3% (n = 3/21)	9.5% (n = 2/21)

foot drop, hence, it should not be considered a good recovery result.

Strong evidence of the superiority of decompressive surgery over conservative treatment for PRMD in the literature is sparse. One explanation for this is the difficulty to perform a randomized controlled trial on this issue – MMT3 or less or progressive deficit are considered absolute indications for surgery, [5] since deficits of this importance as potential final outcome render conservative strategies inappropriate for clinicians and patients. Foot drop is a severe handicap for daily live and the general paradigm to perform surgical decompression of neural structures to reduce ongoing compressive secondary damage has every reason to be applied here as long as no opposed evidence is published.

Overdevest *et al.* have published a subanalysis of 150 patients with sciatic pain and PRMD [6]. The data was taken from a formed subgroup of the prospective randomized controlled Sciatica Trial of Peul *et al.* – a study designed to analyze surgery versus prolonged conservative treatment for radicular pain, independent from PRMD [7]. The authors of the former found a significantly faster recovery of motor deficit following surgery, but no remaining difference between motor function recovery of the surgical and the conservative arms of the sub-group 1 year after randomization. The original study of Peul *et al.* had excluded patients with MMT less than 3 for the reason mentioned above, hence the collective of Overdevest *et al.* contained only patients with MMT 3 or 4, of which patients with MMT 4 showed better recovery. Even if the study did not show time to surgery as a factor for motor recovery, it must be mentioned that this interval was fairly long, 11 weeks in average due to the design of the original work, and it can be argued that faster surgery might have further improved the surgical results. This is strengthened by retrospective studies that focus on preoperative MMT and time to surgery as factors influencing recovery [8, 9]. Elder patient age and etiology other than soft disc hernia are also considered negative predictive factors [8]. On the basis of the analysis of their retrospective work on 102 patients with foot drop due to lumbar degenerative disorder, Takenaka *et al.* have published a decision support tool that indicates, with reference to the respective preoperative MMT and time to surgery, the potential of recovery following surgery (Table 2.2) [8].

The advantage of surgery might become more difficult to advocate when no nerve root pain is present upon presentation, since the absence of leg pain takes out the best reproducible effect of surgery, leg pain reduction. Significant improvement after surgery in painless cases was nonetheless observed in 65% of patients in one retrospective work dedicated to painless foot drop of 20 patients [10].

The available data point on the effect of surgery and furthermore on the importance of time to surgery. Hence, it is a logic approach to consider that the earlier the presentation to the surgeon, the higher the benefit from early or urgent surgery. That is, a patient with MMT 3 since 6 h is more urgent than a patient with MMT 2 since 3 months. In our institution, patients with acute onset of MMT 3 or less or progressive deficit are operated the same day.

2.4 Conclusions and Take-Home Messages

Early surgical decompression for CES or PRMD such as foot drop, if attributable to spinal disorder, remains the standard of care at date. Urgent surgery in less than 48 h should be advocated unless in exceptional cases. Even partial functional recovery will make a difference for every day life for these patients. Persistent sexual and urinary dysfunction should not be trivialized and will require close follow-up and neurorehabilitation counseling.

Pearls

- Sudden limb weakness or bladder or bowel dysfunction requires immediate clinical and radiological work-up
- Profound knowledge of nerve root patterns and a thorough clinical examination indicate the affected compressed nerve root or nerve roots
- PRMD and CES result in severe handicaps. Perform decompression surgery as early as possible to maximize recovery chances for your patient

Editorial Comment

It is the editors' strong belief, that a CES is always an immediate emergency situation and that there is no given time limit for surgery. A motor weakness grade 4 may be treated with prolonged conservative care, while a greater weakness should prompt urgent (<24h) surgery.

References

1. Fraser S, Roberts L, Murphy E. Cauda equina syndrome: a literature review of its definition and clinical presentation. Arch Phys Med Rehabil. 2009;90(11):1964–8.
2. Council MR. Aids to the examination of the peripheral nervous system Memorandum No. 45 (superseding War Memorandum No. 7). Her Majesty's stationary office. 1976.
3. Ahn UM, Ahn NU, Buchowski JM, Garrett ES, Sieber AN, Kostuik JP. Cauda equina syndrome secondary to lumbar disc herniation: a meta-analysis of surgical outcomes. Spine (Phila Pa 1976). 2000;25(12):1515–22.
4. Korse NS, Veldman AB, Peul WC, Vleggeert-Lankamp CLA. The long term outcome of micturition, defecation and sexual function after spinal surgery for cauda equina syndrome. PLoS One. 2017;12(4):e0175987.
5. Arts MP, Peul WC, Koes BW, Thomeer RT, Leiden-The Hague Spine Intervention Prognostic Study (SIPS) Group. Management of sciatica due to lumbar disc herniation in the Netherlands: a survey among spine surgeons. J Neurosurg Spine. 2008;9(1):32–9.
6. Overdevest GM, Vleggeert-Lankamp CL, Jacobs WC, Brand R, Koes BW, Peul WC, Leiden-The Hague Spine Intervention Prognostic Study Group. Recovery of motor deficit accompanying sciatica--subgroup analysis of a randomized controlled trial. Spine J. 2014;14(9):1817–24.
7. Peul WC, van Houwelingen HC, van den Hout WB, Brand R, Eekhof JA, Tans JT, et al. Surgery versus prolonged conservative treatment for sciatica. N Engl J Med. 2007;356(22):2245–56.
8. Takenaka S, Aono H. Prediction of postoperative clinical recovery of drop foot attributable to lumbar degenerative diseases, via a Bayesian network. Clin Orthop Relat Res. 2017;475(3):872–80.
9. Macki M, Syeda S, Kerezoudis P, Gokaslan ZL, Bydon A, Bydon M. Preoperative motor strength and time to surgery are the most important predictors of improvement in foot drop due to degenerative lumbar disease. J Neurol Sci. 2016;361:133–6.
10. Aono H, Nagamoto Y, Tobimatsu H, Takenaka S, Iwasaki M. Surgical outcomes for painless drop foot due to degenerative lumbar disorders. J Spinal Disord Tech. 2014;27(7):E258–61.

Part II

Basic Module 2: Surgical Treatment of Degenerative Cervical, Thoracic and Lumbar Spinal Pathologies

3 Anterior Cervical Subaxial Treatment (Fusion)

Florian Ringel and Sven R. Kantelhardt

3.1 Introduction

Cervical radiculopathy caused by a soft disc herniation or a foraminal stenosis is a common problem. While symptoms from soft disc herniations have high chances to recover after conservative therapy persisting radicular pain or a neurological deficit are accepted as an indication for surgical treatment though high class evidence for the best timing of surgery is not available.

The surgical technique regarded as gold standard for cervical radiculopathy in the subaxial cervical spine is an anterior cervical discectomy followed by fusion as described in the 1950ies independently by Smith/Robinson [26], and Cloward [7]. With slight modifications from its initial description the technique is one of the most commonly used in spine surgery at present for cervical radiculopathy as well as myelopathy, and non-degenerative pathologies. While Smith/Robinson and Cloward described the use of autologous iliac crest bone for segmental fusion after a discectomy, nowadays most surgeons do use PEEK or titanium interbody cages leading to similar high fusion rates [3, 11, 18, 24, 25] but avoiding the donor site morbidity of an iliac crest harvest [18, 29]. Regarding the necessity of plating there is still an ongoing and unsolved debate and many international differences exist [33].

However, alternatives to ACDF for radiculopathy and foraminal stenosis exist for certain indications with posterior foraminotomy [10, 23] and total disc replacement [8].

This chapter will outline the indications for anterior cervical discectomy, the clinical and radiographic results as well as the potential complications and secondary problems. At the end of this chapter the reader should have an understanding of the benfits and limitations of anterior cervical discectomy and fusion in the subaxial cervical spine for degenerative indications as soft disc herniations and foraminal stenoses.

3.2 Case Description

A 46 y/o female patient with fluctuating right sided brachialgia for 1 year. She presented with acute exacerbation of her right sided arm pain (VAS 8/10), neck pain and dysesthesia of the right arm. No motor weakness on exam (Figs. 3.1 and 3.2).

After another course of conservative therapy during which the patient initially improved, her symptoms relapsed and after failure of further conservative therapy there was a relative indication for surgery. The patient underwent anterior cervical discectomy and cage implantation without plating (Fig. 3.3).

F. Ringel (✉) · S. R. Kantelhardt
Department of Neurosurgery, Universitätsmedizin Mainz, Johannes Gutenberg Universität Mainz, Mainz, Germany
e-mail: florian.ringel@unimedizin-mainz.de

B. Meyer, M. Rauschmann (eds.), *Spine Surgery*, https://doi.org/10.1007/978-3-319-98875-7_3

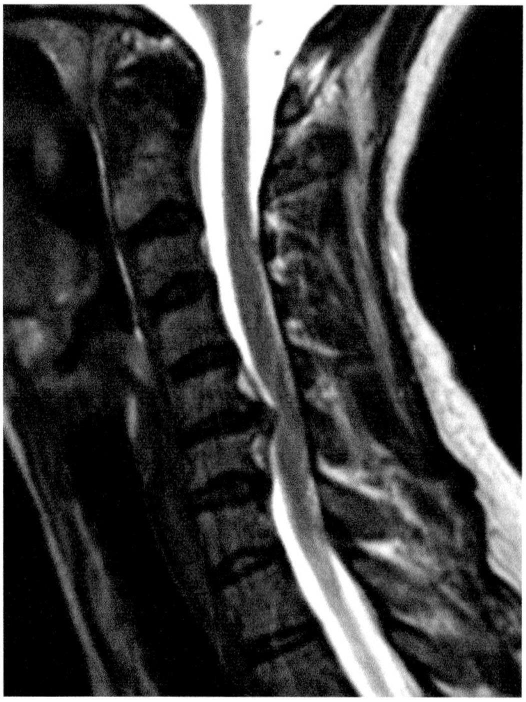

Fig. 3.1 The MRI scan of the cervical spine in the sagittal plane shows a large soft disc herniation at the level C5/6

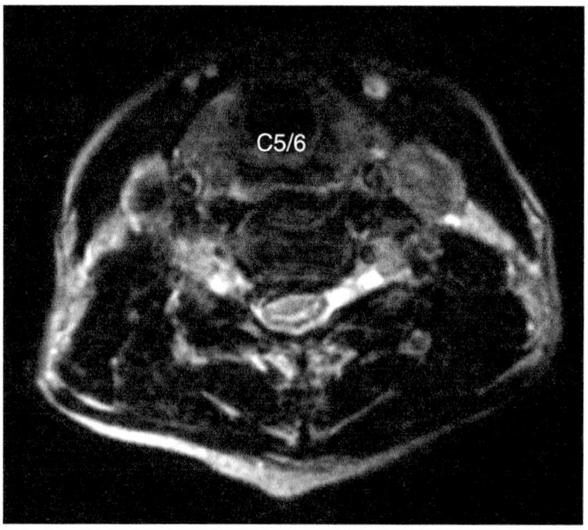

Fig. 3.2 The MRI scan of the cervical spine in axial cuts shows the broad based herniated disc reaching the foramen on the right side

3.3 Discussion of the Case

3.3.1 Indication

The patient described above suffered from radicular arm pain with sensory deficits but no motor deficit. She had a history of recurrent pain during conservative treatment with analgetics and physiotherapy for already 1 year.

Though the indication for surgery has not been proven unequivocally by large prospective randomized trials [16, 17], symptoms refractory to conservative therapy are accepted as an indication for surgery as well as motor deficits. So far, from few class II evidence and class III evidence the benefits of surgery in comparison to ongoing physiotherapy and analgetics have been shown [1, 5, 6, 19, 21, 22, 28].

The CASINO trial which randomizes ongoing conservative therapy versus surgery in patients with cervical radiculopathy is currently recruiting patients [32].

3.3.2 Choice of Surgical Technique

As surgical techniques an anterior cervical discectomy with fusion, a posterior cervical foraminotomy or an anterior cervical discectomy with total disc replacement are available to treat cervical soft disc herniations or foraminal stenoses.

However, the so called gold standard technique to treat a cervical soft disc herniation or a cervical foraminal stenosis is an anterior cervical discectomy and fusion. The surgical technique includes a standard anterior approach to the cervical spine, the disc is excised from anterior and completely removed, posteriorly to the posterior longitudinal ligament and laterally to the uncinate processes. After disc removal uncinate processes can be resected in order to decompress any bony foraminal stenosis. Finallly, the posterior longitudinal ligament is opened and resected to clear any disc material from the spinal canal and to visualize the exiting nerve roots. Following the decompression a fusion of the segment is usually performed originally by implantation of iliac crest bone but nowadays more commonly by implantation of a titanium or PEEK cage. Optionally an anterior plate is implanted to additionally stabilize the operated segment. However, the necessity of some of these surgical steps is questioned – as implantation of fusion material and plating – and will be discussed below.

In comparison to a posterior cervical foraminotomy and a total disc replacement an ACDF can be performed for almost any cervical anterior

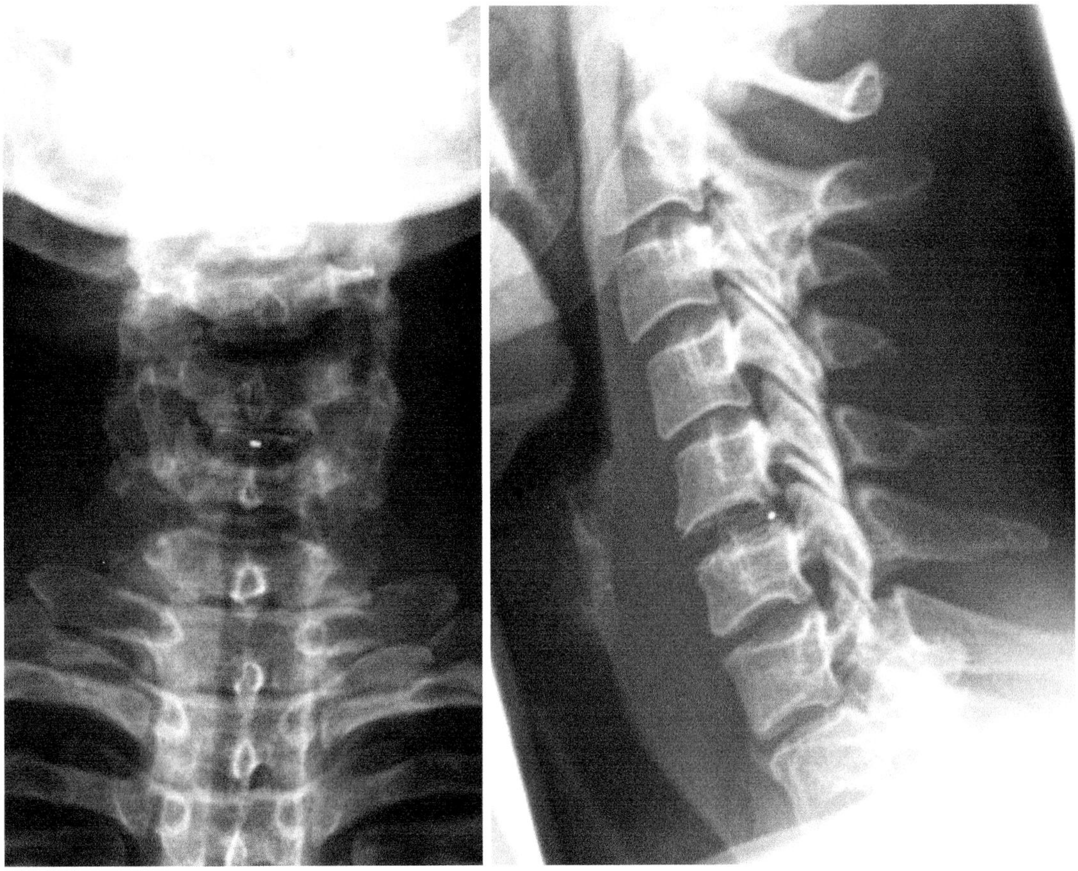

Fig. 3.3 Ap and lateral postoperative x-rays of the cervical spine. Postoperative x-ray images of the cervical spine demonstrate an adequate cage position and regular alignment of the cervical spine

degenerative pathology irrespective of mobility of the segment or extent of degenerative changes of the motion segment.

Clinical results of anterior cervical discectomy are excellent for soft disc herniations as well as for foraminal stenoses and show an excellent outcome with a decrease of the mean VAS-score by 2.5–5.4 points for radicular symptoms and 2.0–6.0 for neck pain [1, 5, 22, 28].

Fusion rates were found to be 85%, 80% and 65% in one, two and three level ACDFs, respectively as reported in a meta-analysis [9]. Fusion rates can be increased by the addition of anterior cervical plates to 92%, 95%, and 83% for one to three level ACDFs. However, clinical results do not necessarily depend on fusion rate. While the implantation of iliac crest bone graft was the initial standard for ACDF [7, 25, 26], since many years cage implantation of PEEK or titanium cages is regarded as standard [3, 11, 24, 25] as the donor site morbidity of the iliac crest graft is omitted. Alternatively, even the anterior cervical discectomy without grafting for fusion is popular at some institutions [13, 27]. So far, while differences in fusion rates occur with iliac crest grafts resulting in the highest fusion rates, studies failed to show any difference in clinical outcome [13]. Therefore, it seems even less justified to perform additional instrumentation by anterior plates as a clinical standard for ACDF, especially as most early reoperations after ACDF are due to plate/instrumentation problems [12, 14, 31]. Only, for cases with a high amount of instability requiring immediate stabilization anterior plating is mandatory.

Typical approach related complications include intermittand dysphagia occuring in 2–83% and esophageal injury in 0.02–1.52% of cases [12, 20] and intermittend recurrent laryngeal nerve palsy with or without hoarsness in 2.3–8.3 and 15.9–24.2%, respectively, which led to lasting vocal cord palsy in 0.16–2.5% [4, 14, 30]. In other studies this rate could be significantly reduced from initially 6.5 to 1.3% by variations of the surgical technique, such as left-sided approaches and deflation of the endotracheal tube cuff [15, 30]. The only relevant long term complication of an anterior discectomy and fusion is adjacent level degeneration resulting from fusion and increased adjacent segment motion and the resulting biomechanical forces. A recent meta-analysis which analyzed radiographic adjacent segment degeneration and adjacent segment disease reported 47.33% (16–96) and 11.99% (1.8–36) following 106.5 months (24–296) after ACDF [2]. Clinical sequelae however are infrequent.

Alternative techniques to preserve segmental motion are available for certain constellations of soft disc herniations or foraminal stenoses as presented in the following chapters.

3.3.3 Accordance with the Literature Guidelines

As discussed above, insufficient data is available for the indication of surgery. However, the indication for surgery is in accordance with the general accepted criteria for a surgical treatment of a cervical disc herniation as well as foraminal stenosis. ACDF is still the gold standard for treatment of a herniated disc or foraminal stenosis though alternative techniques are available. The cage is the present standard to achieve fusion, the necessity of additional instrumentation with an anterior plate under ongoing discussion. Though different fusion rates exist following fusion with iliac crest versus cage and with and without plate, the clinical outcome is not different.

3.4 Conclusions and Take Home Message

Anterior cervical discectomy is the gold standard for cervical radiculopathy from a soft disc herniation or foraminal stenosis. Clinical outcome is excellent ragarding arm and neck pain. ACDF is suitable for most anterior segmental degenerative pathologies with all grades of segmental degeneration and segmental motion. Typical early complications of ACDF include anterior approach related complications as dysphagia and recurrent laryngeal nerve palsies, late complications are adjacent segment degenerations.

Pearls

- ACDF as gold-standard for cervical soft disc herniation or foraminal stenosis
- Titanium or PEEK cage are the present standard for fusion
- Anterior plating is not mandatory on many cases
- Clinical outcome does not correlate closely with radiographic fusion and/or alignment

Editorial Comment

It is our opinion, that it is not worthwhile to further discuss the question whether a plate is necessary in every case or not. It should remain at the discretion of the individual surgeon. A pragmatic approach is to add plates in cases of more that 2 levels, in segmental instabilities as seen on flexion/extension films and with risk factors such as smoking, osteoporosis etc. Further it is unnecessary to fill cervical cages with any kind of material.

References

1. Buttermann GR. Anterior cervical discectomy and fusion outcomes over 10 years: a prospective study. Spine. 2018;43(3):207–14.
2. Carrier CS, Bono CM, Lebl DR. Evidence-based analysis of adjacent segment degeneration and disease after ACDF: a systematic review. Spine J. 2013;13(10):1370–8.
3. Cauthen JC, Kinard RE, Vogler JB, Jackson DE, DePaz OB, Hunter OL, Wasserburger LB, Williams VM. Outcome analysis of noninstrumented anterior cervical discectomy and interbody fusion in 348 patients. Spine. 1998;23(2):188–92.
4. Chen CC, Huang YC, Lee ST, Chen JF, Wu CT, Tu PH. Long-term result of vocal cord paralysis after anterior cervical disectomy. Eur Spine J. 2014;23(3):622–6.
5. Chotai S. Impact of old age on patient-report outcomes and cost utility for anterior cervical discectomy and fusion surgery for degenerative spine disease. Eur Spine J. 2017;26(4):1236–45.
6. Cien A, Lai DM, Wang SF, Hsu WL, Cheng CH, Wang JL. Comparison of cervical kinematics, pain, and functional disability between single- and two-level anterior cervical discectomy and fusion. Spine. 2016;41(15):E915–22.
7. Cloward RB. The anterior approach for removal of ruptured cervical disks. J Neurosurg. 1958;15(6):602–17.
8. Dong L, Xu Z, Chen X, Wang D, Li D, Liu T, Hao D. The change of adjacent segment after cervical disc arthroplasty compared with anterior cervical discectomy and fusion: a meta-analysis of randomized controlled trials. Spine J. 2017;17(10):1549–58.
9. Fraser JF, Härtl R. Anterior approaches to fusion of the cervical spine: a metaanalysis of fusion rates. J Neurosurg Spine. 2007;6(4):298–303.
10. Fehlings MG, Barry S, Kopjar B, Yoon ST, Arnold P, Massicotte EM, Vaccaro A, Brodke DS, Shaffrey C, Smith JS, Woodard E, Banco RJ, Chapman J, Janssen M, Bono C, Sasso R, Dekutoski M, Gokaslan ZL. Anterior versus posterior surgical approaches to treat cervical spondylotic myelopathy: outcomes of the prospective multicenter AOSpine North America CSM study in 264 patients. Spine. 2013;38(26):2247–52.
11. Hacker RJ, Cauthen JC, Gilbert TJ, Griffith SL. A prospective randomized multicenter clinical evaluation of an anterior cervical fusion cage. Spine. 2000;25:2646–54.
12. Halani SH, Baum GR, Riley JP, Pradilla G, Refai D, Rodts GE Jr, Ahmad FU. Esophageal perforation after anterior cervical spine surgery: a systematic review of the literature. J Neurosurg Spine. 2016;25(3):285–91.
13. Jacobs W, Willems PC, van Limbeek J, Bartels R, Pavlov P, Anderson PG, Oner C. Single or double-level anterior interbody fusion techniques for cervical degenerative disc disease. Cochrane Database Syst Rev. 2011;19(1):CD004958.
14. Jung A, Schramm J, Lehnerdt K, Herberhold C. Recurrent laryngeal nerve palsy during anterior cervical spine surgery: a prospective study. J Neurosurg Spine. 2005;2(2):123–7.
15. Jung A, Schramm J. How to reduce recurrent laryngeal nerve palsy in anterior cervical spine surgery: a prospective observational study. Neurosurgery. 2010;67(1):10–5.
16. Kadaňka Z, Mares M, Bednaník J, Smrcka V, Krbec K, Stejskal L, Chaloupka R, Surelová D, Novotný O, Urbánek I, Dusek L. Approaches to spondylotic cervical myelopathy: conservative versus surgical results in a 3-year follow-up study. Spine. 2002;27(20):2205–10.
17. Kadaňka Z, Bednařík J, Novotný O, Urbánek I, Dušek L. Cervical spondylotic myelopathy: conservative versus surgical treatment after 10 years. Eur Spine J. 2011;20(9):1533–8.
18. Lied B, Roenning PA, Sundseth J, Helseth E. Anterior cervical discectomy with fusion in patients with cervical disc degeneration: a prospective outcome study of 258 patients (181 fused with autologous bone graft and 77 fused with a PEEK cage). BMC Surg. 2010;10:10.
19. Matz PG, Holly LT, Groff MW, Vresilovic EJ, Anderso PA, Heary RF, Kaiser MG, Mummaneni PV, Ryken TC, Choudhri TF, Resnick DK, Joint Section on Disorders of the Spine and Peripheral Nerves of the American Association of Neurological Surgeons and Congress of Neurological Surgeons. Indications for anterior cervical decompression for the treatment of cervical degenerative radiculopathy. J Neurosurg Spine. 2009;11(2):174–82.
20. Min Y, Kim WS, Kang SS, Choi JM, Yeom JS, Paik NJ. Incidence of dysphagia and serial videofluoroscopic swallow study findings after anterior cervical discectomy and fusion: a prospective study. Clin Spine Surg. 2016;29(4):E177–81.
21. Nikolaidis I, Fouyas IP, Sandercock PA, Statham PF. Surgery for cervical radiculopathy or myelopathy. Cochrane Database Syst Rev. 2010;1(1):CD001466.
22. Persson LC, Moritz U, Brandt L, Carlsson CA. Cervical radiculopathy: pain, muscle weakness and sensory loss in patients with cervical radiculopathy treated with surgery, physiotherapy or cervical collar. A prospective, controlled study. Eur Spine J. 1997;6(4):256–66.
23. Rosomoff HL, Rossmann F. Treatment of cervical spondylosis by anterior cervical diskectomy and fusion. Arch Neurol. 1966;14(4):392–8.
24. Seaman S, Kerezoudis P, Bydon M, Torner JC, Hitchon PW. Titanium vs. polyetheretherketone (PEEK) interbody fusion: meta-analysis and review of the literature. J Clin Neurosci. 2017;44:23–9.
25. Siddiqui AA, Jackowski A. Cage versus tricortical graft for cervical interbody fusion. A prospective randomised study. J Bone Joint Surg Br. 2003;85(7):1019–25.

26. Smith GW, Robinson RA. The treatment of certain cervical-spine disorders by anterior removal of the intervertebral disc and interbody fusion. J Bone Joint Surg Am. 1958;40-A(3):607–24.
27. Sonntag VK, Klara P. Controversy in spine care. Is fusion necessary after anterior cervical discectomy? Spine. 1996;21(9):1111–3.
28. Suk KS, Lee SH, Park SY, Kim HS, Moon SH, Lee HM. Clinical outcome and changes of foraminal dimension in patients with foraminal stenosis after ACDF. J Spinal Disord Tech. 2015;28(8):E449–53.
29. Summers BN, Eisenstein SM. Donor site pain from the ilium. A complication of lumbar spine fusion. J Bone Joint Surg Br. 1989;71:677–80.
30. Tan TP, Govindarajulu AP, Massicotte EM, Venkatraghavan L. Vocal cord palsy after anterior cervical spine surgery: a qualitative systematic review. Spine J. 2014;14(7):1332–42.
31. Vaccaro AR, Falatyn SP, Scuderi GJ, Eismont FJ, McGuire RA, Singh K, Garfin SR. Early failure of long segment anterior cervical plate fixation. J Spinal Disord. 1998;11(5):410–5.
32. van Geest S, Kuijper B, Oterdoom M, van den Hout W, Brand R, Stijnen T, Assendelft P, Koes B, Jacobs W, Peul W, Vleggeert-Lankamp C. CASINO: surgical or nonsurgical treatment for cervical radiculopathy, a randomised controlled trial. BMC Musculoskelet Disord. 2014;15:129.
33. Wright IP, Eisenstein SM. Anterior cervical discectomy and fusion without instrumentation. Spine. 2007;32(7):772–4.

Cervical Motion Preserving Procedures (TDR)

4

Florian Ringel and Eleftherios Archavlis

4.1 Introduction

Symptomatic cervical degenerative disc disease leading to radiculopathy is a common problem with an incidence of 0.83–1.79 per 1.000 person years. While many episodes of radicular symptoms can be successfully managed by conservative therapy, patients with refractory symptoms or a significant paresis are candidates for a surgical treatment. However, different surgical techniques have been available to treat cervical degenerative disc disease for a long period, as anterior cervical discectomy without fusion, anterior cervical discectomy with fusion or posterior foraminotomy. Anterior cervical discectomy with fusion as described in the 1960's (Chap. 3) is currently regarded as the gold standard. Although ACDF provides excellent results with regard to relief of cervical radicular symptoms and neck pain, the loss of motion at the fused level might be associated with secondary problems. Loss of motion at a fused segment is typically compensated by a significant increase in the ROM of flexion/extension, lateral bending and rotation at adjacent levels [22] which can accelerate degeneration of these adjacent levels. Therefore, up to 25% of cervically fused patients develop symptomatic adjacent segment degeneration within 10 years after fusion surgery associated with a high rates of revision surgery [16]. In order to overcome this problem the motion preservation concept developed and cervical disc prostheses maintaining segmental motion became available in the 1990ies. From there on a large selection of different cervical disc prostheses became available which are well studied in comparison to anterior cervical discectomy and fusion in several prospective randomized trials.

This chapter aims to provide indications and contraindication for cervical disc prosthesis, technical surgical considerations and outcome data for cervical disc prosthesis.

4.2 Case Description

A 31 y/o female patient suffered from progressive pain of the left shoulder and neck with radiation along the lateral upper arm reaching into the elbow. Additionally she complained of some restriction of mobility of the left upper extremity over the last 2 weeks. One week after the onset of symptoms a reduction in strength of the left upper extremity developed with limitation of the elevation of the left arm above the horizontal plane. A MRI scan showed soft herniations of the discs C4/5 and C5/6 with spinal cord and radicular compression on the left side as well as a slight disc protrusion at the level C6/7 (Fig. 4.1).

F. Ringel (✉) · E. Archavlis
Department of Neurosurgery, Universitätsmedizin Mainz, Johannes Gutenberg Universität Mainz, Mainz, Germany
e-mail: florian.ringel@unimedizin-mainz.de

B. Meyer, M. Rauschmann (eds.), *Spine Surgery*, https://doi.org/10.1007/978-3-319-98875-7_4

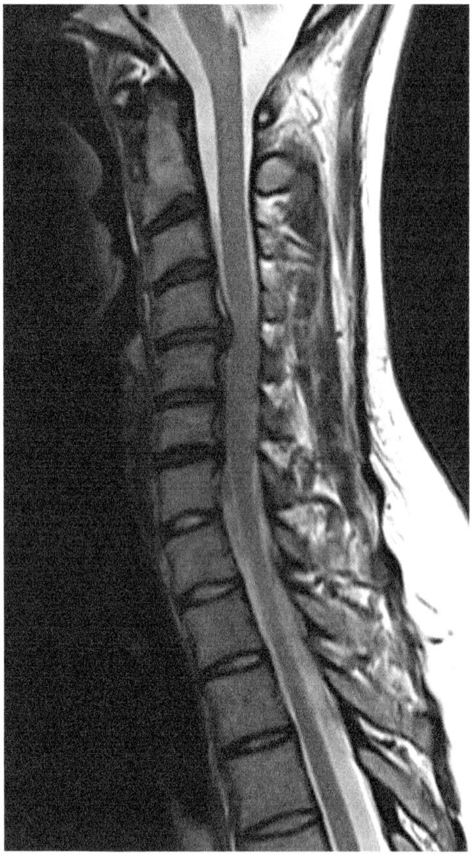

Fig. 4.1 MRI scan on outpatient visit. The MRI scan shows herniated discs in C4/5 and C5/6 and a minor protrusion in C6/7

No relevant further degenerative changes of the C-spine were seen. X-ray images in neutral position and flexion/extension of the C-spine revealed a proper lordotic alignment and regular motion of the affected segments (Fig. 4.2).

The patient was referred after MRI to our department. The neurological examination revealed a deltoid paresis 3/5 and a mild biceps paresis 4/5 on the left upper extremity. Due to the progression of symptoms during initial conservative management and the paresis there was a clear indication for surgical treatment. The patient was operated on the day after admission. The patient was operated in general anesthesia in supine position. The c-spine was positioned in neutral alignment any kyphotic or lordotic position was avoided. A standard anterior approach to the c-spine was performed followed by an anterior cervical discectomy at C4/5 and C5/6 with resection of the posterior longitudinal ligament and decompression of the spinal canal and nerve roots. After decompression artificial disc prostheses were implanted at both levels. Surgery was eventless.

Pain as well as the preoperative deltoid and biceps paresis of the left upper extremity completely recovered early after surgery. No new focal neurological deficits were detectable.

On the 2nd postoperative day, functional x ray images were taken and showed a correct position of the intervertebral disc prostheses and no abnormal segmental mobility (Fig. 4.3).

The patient was discharged on the 3rd postoperative day, she had an uneventful recovery without relevant neck pain.

4.3 Discussion of the Case

The patient described suffered from a cervical radiculopathy with pain and a motor deficit refractory to conservative therapy from cervical soft disc herniations involving two segments. This is a classical indication for a surgical treatment though not supported by prospective randomized studies which are not available, so far, but are currently recruiting patients [26].

The surgical gold standard for the treatment of a cervical disc pathology causing radiculopathy or myelopathy from a soft disc herniation or spondylosis would be an anterior cervical discectomy followed by fusion with or without segmental plating (see Chap. 3). While this technique is associated with excellent results with regard to the radicular symptoms and neck pain in more than 90% of patients, follow-up studies after ACDF could demonstrate a degeneration of adjacent segments mostly cranial to the fusion with increasing time after fusion [16]. Already in 1997 Hillibrand et al. reported a 2.9% revision rate per year after ACDF and predicted a 25% revision rate within 10 years for adjacent level degeneration [8]. In a systematic review the reported incidence of a radiographic adjacent segment degeneration ranges from 16-96% with a mean of 47.33% after 106 months of follow up, while 12% of patients developed a symptomatic

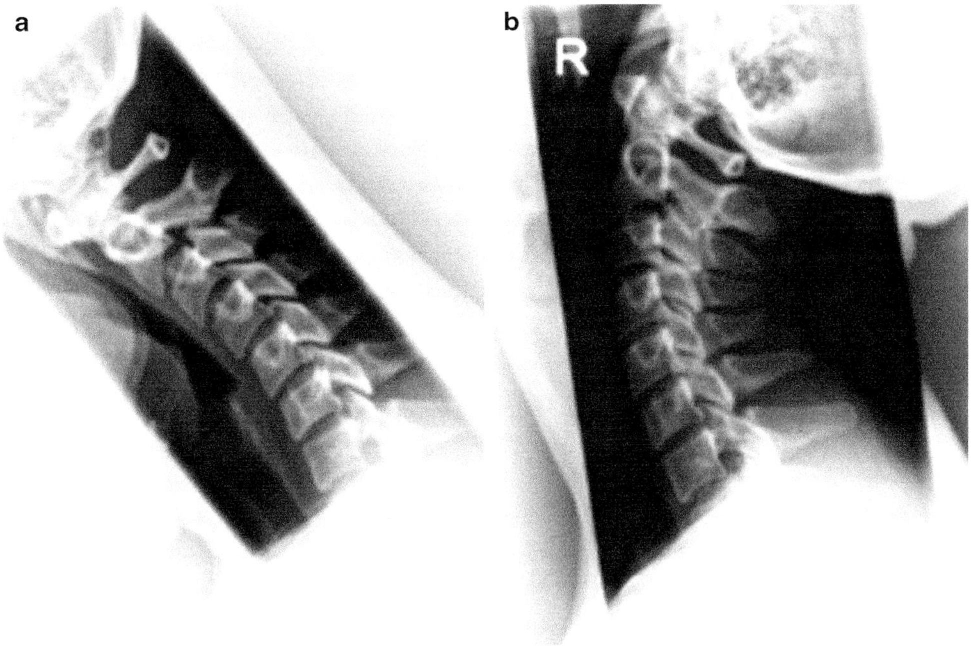

Fig. 4.2 Preoperative flexion/extension x-ray of the cervical spine. Flexion (**a**) and extension (**b**) x-rays demonstrate regular motion of the affected segments C4/5 and 5/6

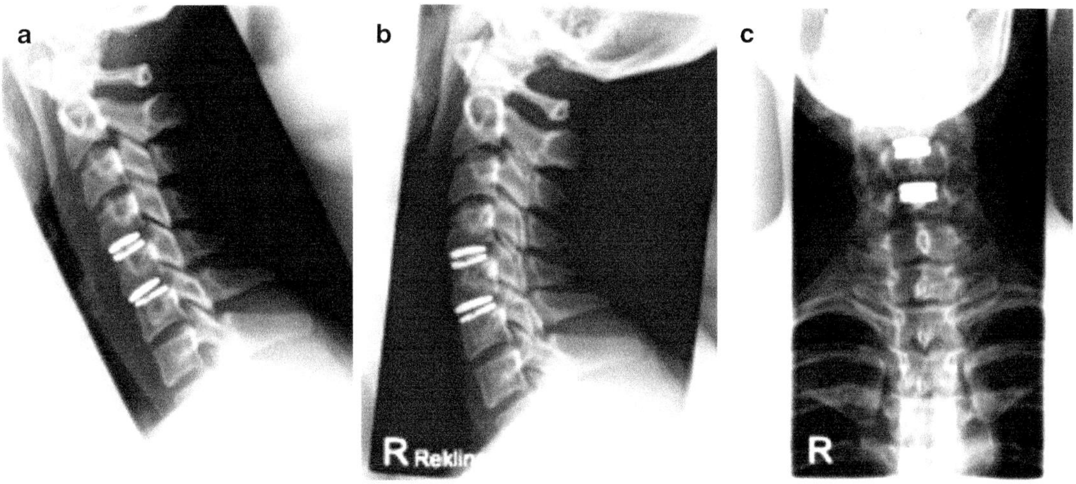

Fig. 4.3 Postoperative flexion (**a**), extension (**b**) and ap (**c**) x-ray of the cervical spine. The postoperative x-ray images show a regular position and function of the prostheses at C4/5 and C5/6

adjacent segment degeneration after fusion during the same follow-up [4]. Whether this is a natural progression of the underlying degenerative disease or a consequence of increased adjacent segment motion and biomechanical strains after fusion remains not fully elucidated at present [15]. However, in order to overcome this problem, the concept of motion preservation in contrast to fusion evolved to maintain mobility of the treated segment. Motion preserving total disc replacements or disc arthroplasty became available in the 1990ies and gained increasing importance [11]. Aim of total disc replacement (TDR) is the removal of the pain generating structure, restoration of disc height, maintenance of segmental kinematics, a natural balance of the segment and protection of the adjacent segment. Up to now, many different designs of disc prostheses are available and have been evaluated in large multicenter prospective randomized non-inferiority trials regarding the clinical and radiographic outcome in comparison to fusion.

4.3.1 Indications and Contraindications for Cervical TDR

The best established indication for total disc replacement is a soft disc herniation in a biologically young patient with preserved segmental motion and a straight or lordotic alignment of the cervical spine. While the most beneficial typical indication would be radiculopathy, patients with myelopathic symptoms have been included in the IDE studies as well showing beneficial results.

TDR is usually limited to a maximum of 2 segments, in exceptional cases 3 segments. Only minor facet joint degeneration as well as no muscular degeneration should be present as this might result in persisting neck pain after TDR. In addition to soft disc herniation a mild spondylotic stenosis is seen as a good indication for TDR and data support the use of TDR in adjacent level degeneration following ACDF as well.

However, a significant spondylotic degeneration, ossification of the longitudinal ligament, bridging osteophytes, segmental height loss >50%, kyphotic deformity, hypo- or hypermobility (>3.5 mm sagittal plane translation, >20° sagittal plane angulation) of the segment and osteopenia or osteoporosis are contraindications for motion preserving techniques as well as non-degenerative pathologies as tumors, infection or trauma.

4.3.2 TDR Outcome

So far, several prospective randomized trials designed as non-inferiority trials against ACDF as IDE studies assessed the outcome up to 7 years after single-level TDR using different types of prostheses with different designs and thereby different kinematic characteristics [5, 7, 14, 19, 25]. All studies could prove, that the motion of the index segment is preserved during follow-up in comparison to ACDF. The clinical outcome with regard to pain and function was slightly but statistically significantly superior following TDR to the results after ACDF irrespective of the type of prosthesis implanted. However, the difference is small and probably not clinically relevant. The frequency of secondary surgery for the index segment was lower after TDR than after ACDF. Furthermore, some studies could reveal a lower incidence of adjacent segment degeneration and a lower rate of adjacent segment surgery during follow-up in the TDR treated patient group providing evidence for adjacent segment protection by TDR [3, 9, 18]. Whether any prosthesis design and kinematics are superior in comparison to others has not been assessed, so far.

While all studies show slightly superior results of TDR in comparison to ACDF criticism arose that most studies are prone to bias for missing blinding leading to confirmation bias and potential conflict of interest since most larger studies are industry-sponsored [21].

While many high quality studies are available for single level TDR few studies assessed the results of two level TDR as well. In comparison to two level ACDF two level TDR resulted in improved results for NDI, SF-12 and overall success with a lower rate of secondary surgery and adjacent segment degeneration [6, 10, 20]. Furthermore, no difference was detected in outcome 4 years after one or two level TDR, with a satisfaction rate of 85% and 4% of secondary surgery after two level TDR [1].

Another potential indication for TDR would be an adjacent segment disease after cervical fusion. Studies with small patient numbers and short follow-up duration show no difference in outcome of primary TDR versus TDR for adjacent segment degeneration after previous fusion [17].

Assessing hybrid surgery (ACDF plus TDR) for multilevel degeneration yielded similar if not superior results in comparison to multilevel ACDF [12].

Therefore, TDR is an option for single or two level degeneration, for adjacent segment degeneration following fusion or as a hybrid concept with ACDF in multilevel degeneration if above mentioned exclusion criteria for ACDF are well considered.

4.3.3 Problems and Limitations of TDR

A common problem following cervical TDR is heterotopic ossification (HO) which is defined as an abnormal bone formation in extraskeletal tissue. HO can potentially reduce the extent of motion and is graded from 1–4 with 4 being a fusion of the segment [13]. Reported incidences of high grade HO (grade III: bridging ossification which still allows movement; grade IV:complete fusion) after 4 years ranges between 1.5 and 63% [2, 23, 24, 27]. However, a recent meta-analysis on the influence of HO on patient outcome could not reveal any significant influence [28]. The worst case of a grade 4 HO following TDR does lead to the same results as ACDF, i.e. fusion, without any adverse events by HO.

Further problems of TDR are implant failure and displacement which might occur as in all implants. But, reported numbers of implant-related problems are very low.

4.3.4 Accordance with the Literature Guidelines

The indication for treatment was given in the above described case. While ACDF would have been the gold standard for treatment TDR is an alternative supported by clinical data, as well as for two level indication.

Level of Evidence: I, Grade of Recommendation: A

The level of evidence available to date is high comprising several prospective randomized trials of TDR in comparison to ACDF.

4.4 Conclusions and Take Home Message

High quality data support the use of total disc replacement in single and two level mild to moderate cervical degeneration. TDR shows at least non-inferior clinical outcome in comparison to ACDF being superior in many studies. Furthermore, radiographic and symptomatic adjacent segment degeneration can be reduced by TDR in comparison to ACDF. The problem of heterotopic ossification which can lead to fusion of an artificial disc does not significantly influence clinical outcome.

Pearls

- Same/superior results as ACDF with prudent indication
- Maintained segmental motion, imitating the natural process of loss of ROM
- Reduced adjacent segment degeneration seen after long term follow up

Editorial Comment

A number of items in this chapter deserve a personal comment. Cervical TDR has partly fallen into disgrace, because an overuse with extended indications has taken place and 2 to 4 year follow up data in the cohorts of the above mentioned RCTs did not prove a significant reduction of ASD as compared to fusion, because the overall incidence was low. Only after 5 years and beyond a difference can be detected in favour of TDR. Thus cervical TDR has a place in the treatment of soft disc radiculopathy in biologically younger individuals, which will then give them a small but relevant advantage over ACDF in the long term. The key is to stick to a narrow indication to avoid the downsides such as HO, relevant persistent neck pain etc. It should be mentioned, that especially complex, i.e. 3-piece TDR constructs are more prone to produce significant morbidity due to implant failure, although this has not found its way into the literature. Several products had to be taken from the market, because of this with relevant liability sequelae.

References

1. Bae HW, Kim KD, Nunley PD, Jackson RJ, Hisey MS, Davis RJ, Hoffman GA, Gaede SE, Danielson GO, Peterson DL, Stokes JM, Araghi A. Comparison of clinical outcomes of 1-and 2-level total disc replacement. Spine. 2015;40(11):759–66.
2. Barbagallo GMV, Certo F, Visocchi M, Sciacca G, Albanese V. Double-level cervical total disc replacement for adjacent segment disease: is it a useful treatment? Description of late onset heterotopic ossification and review of the literature. Eur Rev Med Pharmacol Sci. 2014;18:15–23.
3. Burkus JK, Traynelis VC, Haid RW Jr, Mummaneni PV. Clinical and radiographic analysis of an artificial cervical disc: 7-year follow-up from the Prestige prospective randomized controlled clinical trial: clinical article. J Neurosurg Spine. 2014;21(4):516–28.
4. Carrier CS, Bono CM, Lebl DR. Evidence-based analysis of adjacent segment degeneration and disease after ACDF: a systematic review. Spine J. 2013;13(10):1370–8.
5. Coric D, Nunley PD, Guyer RD, Musante D, Carmody CN, Gordon CR, Lauryssen C, Ohnmeiss DD, Boltes MO. Prospective, randomized, multicenter study of cervical arthroplasty: 269 patients from the KineflexIC artificial disc investigational device exemption study with a minimum 2-year follow-up clinical article. J Neurosurg Spine. 2011;15(4):348–58.
6. Davis RJ, Nunley PD, Kim KD, Hisey MS, Jackson RJ, Bae HW, Hoffman GA, Gaede SE, Danielson GO, Gordon C, Stone MB. Two-level total disc replacement with Mobi-C cervical artificial disc versus anterior discectomy and fusion: a prospective, randomized, controlled multicenter clinical trial with 4-year follow-up results. J Neurosurg Spine. 2015;22(1):15–25.
7. Heller JG, Sasso RC, Papadopoulos SM, Anderson PA, Fessler RG, Hacker RJ, Coric D, Cauthen JC, Riew DK. Comparison of BRYAN cervical disc arthroplasty with anterior cervical decompression and fusion clinical and radiographic results of a randomized, controlled, clinical trial. Spine. 2009;34(2):101–7.
8. Hilibrand AS, Yoo JU, Carlson GD, Bohlman HH. The success of anterior cervical arthrodesis adjacent to a previous fusion. Spine. 1997;22(14):1574–9.
9. Jackson RJ, Davis RJ, Hoffman GA, Bae HW, Hisey MS, Kim KD, Gaede SE, Nunley PD. Subsequent surgery rates after cervical total disc replacement using a Mobi-C cervical disc prosthesis versus anterior cervical discectomy and fusion: a prospective randomized clinical trial with 5-year follow-up. J Neurosurg Spine. 2016;24(5):734–45.
10. Lanman TH, Burkus JK, Dryer RG, Gornet MF, McConnell J, Hodges SD. Long-term clinical and radiographic outcomes of the Prestige LP artificial cervical disc replacement at 2 levels: results from a prospective randomized controlled clinical trial. J Neurosurg Spine. 2017;27(1):7–19.
11. Le H, Thongtrangan I, Kim DH. Historical review of cervical arthroplasty. Neurosurg Focus. 2004;17(3):E1.
12. Lu VM, Zhang L, Scherman DB, Rao PJ, Mobbs RJ, Phan K. Treating multi-level cervical disc disease with hybrid surgery compared to anterior cervical discectomy and fusion: a systematic review and meta-analysis. Eur Spine J. 2017;26(2):546–57.
13. Mehren C, Suchomel P, Grochulla F, Barsa P, Sourkova P, Hradil J, Korge A, Mayer HM. Heterotopic ossification in total cervical artificial disc replacement. Spine. 2006;31(24):2802–6.
14. Murrey D, Janssen M, Delamarter R, Goldstein J, Zigler J, Tay B, Darden B. Results of the prospective, randomized, controlled multicenter food and drug Administration investigational, device exemption study of the ProDisc-C total disc replacement versus anterior discectomy and fusion for the treatment of 1-level symptomatic cervical disc disease. Spine J. 2009;9(4):275–86.
15. Park DK, Lin EL, Phillips FM. Index and adjacent level kinematics after cervical disc replacement and anterior fusion in vivo quantitative radiographic analysis. Spine. 2011;36(9):721–30.
16. Park JB, Cho YS, Riew KD. Development of adjacent-level ossification in patients with an anterior cervical plate. J Bone Joint Surg Am Vol. 2005;87a(3):558–63.
17. Phillips FM, Allen TR, Regan JJ, Albert TJ, Cappuccino A, Devine JG, Ahrens JE, Hipp JA, McAfee PC. Cervical disc replacement in patients with and without previous adjacent level fusion surgery a prospective study. Spine. 2009;34(6):556–65.
18. Phillips FM, Geisler FH, Gilder KM, Reah C, Howell KM, McAfee PC. Long-term outcomes of the US FDA IDE prospective, randomized controlled clinical trial comparing PCM cervical disc Arthroplasty with anterior cervical discectomy and fusion. Spine (Phila Pa 1976). 2015;40(10):674–83.
19. Phillips FM, Lee JYB, Geisler FH, Cappuccino A, Chaput CD, DeVine JG, Reah C, Gilder KM, Howell KM, McAfee PC. A prospective, randomized, controlled clinical investigation comparing PCM cervical disc Arthroplasty with anterior cervical discectomy and fusion 2-year results from the US FDA IDE clinical trial. Spine. 2013;38(15):E907–18.
20. Radcliff K, Coric D, Albert T. Five-year clinical results of cervical total disc replacement compared with anterior discectomy and fusion for treatment of 2-level symptomatic degenerative disc disease: a prospective, randomized, controlled, multicenter investigational device exemption clinical trial. J Neurosurg Spine. 2016;25(2):213–24.
21. Radcliff K, Siburn S, Murphy H, Woods B, Qureshi S. Bias in cervical total disc replacement trials. Curr Rev Muscoskelet Med. 2017;10(2):170–6.
22. Schwab JS, Diangelo DJ, Foley KT. Motion compensation associated with single-level cervical fusion:

where does the lost motion go? Spine (Phila Pa 1976). 2006;31(21):2439–48.
23. Suchomel P, Jurak L, Benes V, Brabec R, Bradac O, Elgawhary S. Clinical results and development of heterotopic ossification in total cervical disc replacement during a 4-year follow-up. Eur Spine J. 2010;19(2):307–15.
24. Tu TH, Wu JC, Huang WC, Wu CL, Ko CC, Cheng H. The effects of carpentry on heterotopic ossification and mobility in cervical arthroplasty: determination by computed tomography with a minimum 2-year follow-up: clinical article. J Neurosurg Spine. 2012;16(6):601–9.
25. Vaccaro A, Beutler W, Peppelman W, Marzluff JM, Highsmith J, Mugglin A, DeMuth G, Gudipally M, Baker KJ. Clinical outcomes with selectively constrained SECURE-C cervical disc Arthroplasty two-year results from a prospectivei, randomized, controlled, multicenter investigational device exemption study. Spine. 2013;38(26):2227–39.
26. van Geest S, Kuijper B, Oterdoom M, van den Hout W, Brand R, Stijnen T, Assendelft P, Koes B, Jacobs W, Peul W, Vleggeert-Lankamp C. CASINO: surgical or nonsurgical treatment for cervical radiculopathy, a randomised controlled trial. BMC Musculoskelet Disord. 2014;15:129.
27. Wu JC, Huang WC, Tsai TY, Fay LY, Ko CC, Tu TH, Wu CL, Cheng H. Multilevel arthroplasty for cervical spondylosis more heterotopic ossification at 3 years of follow-up. Spine. 2012;37(20):E1251–9.
28. Zhou HH, Qu Y, Dong RP, Kang MY, Zhao JW. Does heterotopic ossification affect the outcomes of cervical Total disc replacement? Spine. 2015;40(6):E332–40.

Posterior 'Motion Preserving' Procedures (Frykholm)

5

Florian Ringel and Angelika Gutenberg

5.1 Introduction

Cervical radiculopathy from degenerative disease is a common problem with an incidence of 0.83–1.79 per 1000 person years. It can be caused by a cervical disc herniation, bony foraminal stenosis or spinal canal stenosis.

Upon failure of conservative therapy or a significant motor deficit surgical treatment is indicated. The technique presently regarded as the gold standard of surgical treatment is an anterior cervical discectomy followed by fusion as already described in the 1950ies by Smith/Robinson and Cloward. However alternative surgical techniques are available for selected cases as total disc replacement (Chap. 4) or a posterior foraminotomy. Both techniques aim to preserve segmental motion by the avoidance of fusion. While total disc replacement evolved in the 1990ies, posterior foraminotomy was already described in 1951 by Ragnar Frykholm and still carries his name as Frykholm procedure. It describes a posterior approach to the cervical spine and posterior laminoforaminotomy to decompress cervical nerve roots from laterally localized disc herniations or foraminal stenoses.

This chapter will outline the indications and limitations of posterior cervical foraminotomies, briefly the surgical steps and the outcome.

At the end of this chapter the reader should be aware of the advantages and disadvantages of posterior foraminotomies to treat cervical radiculopathy.

5.2 Case Description

A 37 y/o female patient suffered from neck pain and right-sided brachialgia with acute onset. Pain distribution was according to the dermatome C7, her neurological examination revealed a right-sided paresis of elbow extension grade 4 out of 5. A MRI scan of the cervical spine showed a right-sided laterally located disc herniation at the C6/7 level (Fig. 5.1). A preoperative CT scan excluded a relevant bony foraminal stenosis or further degenerative osteophytic changes.

After diagnosis of the herniated disc a conservative therapy was initiated. However, as the conservative treatment could not control the patient's symptoms, surgical treatment was indicated. A posterior tubular transmuscular approach to the level C6/7 at the right side was performed. After reaching the bony spine the laminas of C6 an C7 and the joint C6/7 were identified. A partial laminotomy of C6 and 7 and partial facet joint resection was performed as illustrated in Fig. 5.2 and thereby creating a posterior foraminotomy at the

F. Ringel (✉) · A. Gutenberg
Department of Neurosurgery, Universitätsmedizin Mainz, Johannes Gutenberg Universität Mainz, Mainz, Germany
e-mail: florian.ringel@unimedizin-mainz.de

B. Meyer, M. Rauschmann (eds.), *Spine Surgery*, https://doi.org/10.1007/978-3-319-98875-7_5

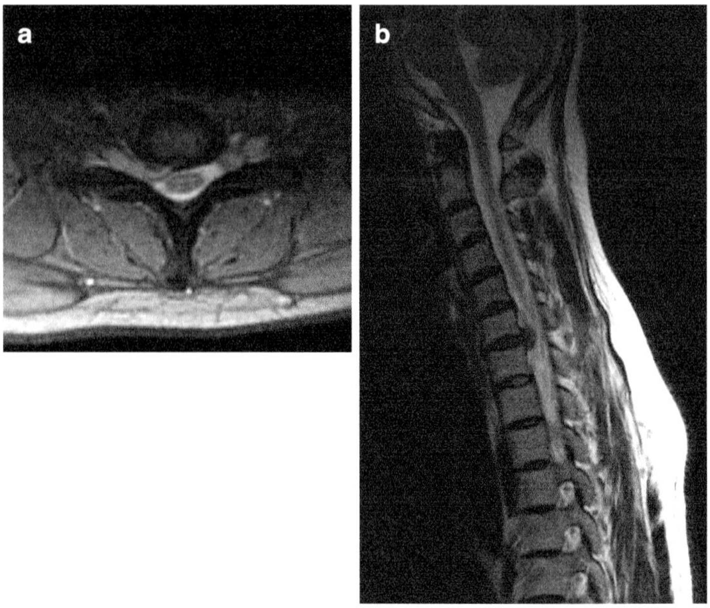

Fig. 5.1 Preoperative MRI scan of the cervical spine in an axial (**a**) and sagittal (**b**) orientation. The MRI scan shows a right-sided lateral C6/7 disc herniation causing C7 root compression. The herniated disc is laterally located i.e. the majority of the herniation is lateral to the spinal cord

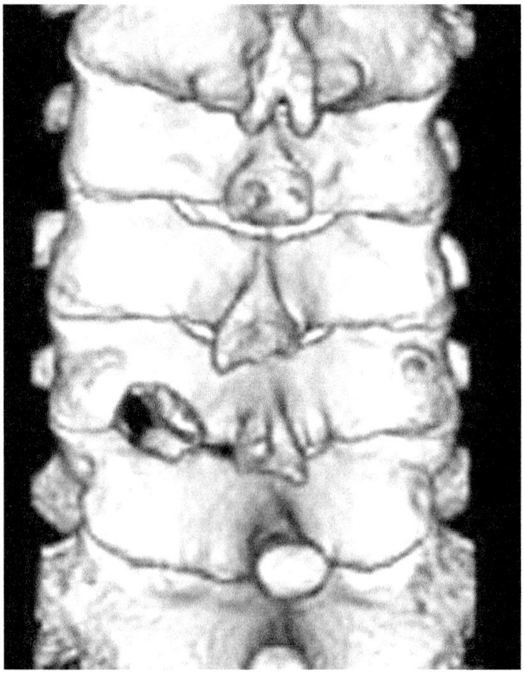

Fig. 5.2 Bony surgical access. A 3D reconstruction of a bony spine after a posterior foraminotomy is shown. The extent of the bony drilling necessary to achieve posterior access to the foramen is shown, the stability of the facet joint is maintained

level C6/7 (Fig. 5.2). The soft disc fragment was removed thus decompressing the nerve root.

Early after surgery the patient was pain-free regarding the radicular arm pain. The paresis recovered within a few days. The patient initially complained of some neck pain which recovered completely during follow-up.

5.3 Discussion of the Case

5.3.1 Indication for Surgery

The patient described in the case suffered from a cervical radiculopathy with pain and a mild paresis. The causative soft disc herniation was laterally localized at the segment C6/7.

Usually, cervical radiculopathies from soft disc herniations recover well under conservative therapy [3, 20], but symptoms refractory to conservative therapy as well as significant pareses are an indication for surgery. So far, no data from well-designed studies provide information on when and who to operate. Few smaller studies assessed the difference between ongoing conservative therapy and surgery providing contradictory results [8, 11, 16, 18]. The CASINO trial is currently examining the difference of conservative and operative therapy in a well-designed prospective randomized controlled study and is still recruiting patients [22].

Due to the lack of conclusive data the decision for surgery is mainly based on experience and can vary at different centers. A commonly accepted indication for surgery would be a persisting, quality of life reducing, radicular pain despite conservative therapy or a paresis of 3 out of 5 or worse.

However, the question remains which technique to choose for decompression, or – for this chapter – when is a posterior cervical foraminotomy an option and what are the potential advantages or disadvantages.

5.3.2 Surgical Technique

For a posterior foraminotomy (PF) the patient can be placed either in a prone concorde position or a semisitting position. Height localization is performed by intraoperative fluoroscopy which can be demanding in the lower cervical spine in short-necked patients where the shoulders overly the lower cervical spine. The approach is either by a medial incision and detachment of the muscles from the spine or, more commonly, a paramedian transmuscular approach. Endoscopic techniques for PF are available as well. Target at the bony spine is the junction between the laminae of the upper and lower vertebra and the facet joint laterally (Fig. 5.2). As a next step it is necessary to perform lateral partial laminotomy by removing 4–5 mm from the superior and inferior lamina using a high-speed drill to allow visibility of the dura [17]. The junction between the medial thecal sac and the exiting root is the medial border of the exposure, the root can be followed laterally as far as necessary. It is safe to remove up to 5 mm of the lateral mass (for most cases approximately 50% of the facet joint) to allow easy mobilization of the nerve root for sequestrectomy without producing instability [1, 4, 25]. After removing the bone usually brisk epidural bleeding from the venous plexus is experienced. A soft disc herniation is usually localized below the exiting nerve root and a sequestrectomy can be performed here.

5.3.3 Indication, Contraindications, Advantages, Disadvantages, Complications and Outcome of Posterior Foraminotomies

Pathologies which can be approached by a PF are unilateral and lateral to the spinal cord, as the cord cannot be displaced to get access to more medial pathologies. Therefore, a typical indication for a PF is a unilateral soft disc herniation with more than 2/3 of the disc herniation lateral to the spinal cord, or a bony foraminal stenosis. Paramedian or medially located disc herniations are not reachable by a posterior foraminotomy and would be a contraindication. Thus, a PF is suitable for a small subsets of patients with cervical radiculopathies only.

However, if patients are well selected, PF provides as beneficial long-term clinical results as the gold-standard ACDF with good to excellent success rates of up to 94% in most published series [7]. A recent meta-analysis found no differences in patients reported outcome measures following PF versus ACDF, a sufficient pain relief in 75–100% and a success rate of 85% [14].

But why prefer a PF in comparison to ACDF or TDR? Advantages of the PF are (i) the lack of implants and thereby the reduction of implant-related complications and costs, (ii) the non-fusion characteristic of the technique maintaining segmental motion and thereby potentially reducing adjacent segment degeneration and (iii) the avoidance of complications associated with the anterior approach as dysphagia, laryngeal nerve palsy and other soft tissue damage. From a health care economics perspective the lack of implants in PF generates 89% less costs than an ACDF [26]. Studies assessing the segmental motion after PF elucidate that PF was not associated with a reduction of segmental motion in most cases and furthermore was not associated with an increased adjacent segment motion as following an ACDF [6, 13, 19].

However, concerns associated with the technique of PF are regarding (i) a potential instability from a partial resection of the facet joint resulting in neck pain and potential deformity, (ii) persisting approach related neck pain from muscular damage, (iii) worse outcomes in bony foraminal stenoses and (iv) a higher reoperation rate compared to ACDF at the index level [19]. The complications reported with PF include nerve root injury (especially C5 palsy) and dural tear [5, 19].

Some controversies exist regarding the extent of facet joint resection associated with a segmental instability. While some studies report a higher incidence of instability after >50% of resection, other studies show sufficient stability of the cervical spine even after larger amounts of resection [12, 21, 25]. However, for most cases a facet joint resection of <50% seems sufficient which does not endanger stability [1, 4]. But, as a resection of posterior elements is necessary, a segmental kyphosis or cervical lordosis <10° is regarded as a contraindication for PF as a secondary progressive kyphosis may occur [12].

Faught and colleagues [9] showed an excellent long-time quality of life outcome equally for patient treated with PF for both soft disc or osteophyte disease. In contrast, excellent results for soft disc herniations treated by PF were found in 92.6% by Yoo et al., while cases with foraminal stenosis resulted in excellent results after PF in 55.0% of cases only [24]. The outcome of foraminal stenosis decompression with PF seems to depend on the shape and thereby the extent of stenosis [10]. While V-shaped stenoses, i.e. medial stenosis opening towards the lateral part of the foramen can be treated with good results with PF, parallel stenoses, i.e. extending to the lateral part of the foramen, are associated with potentially inferior results as a decompression far lateral is necessary [10]. Therefore, for medial foraminal stenoses a posterior decompression seems to be suitable. Non good candidates for PF are patients with anterior spurs and a foraminal stenosis extending far lateral. Overall, reoperation rate at the index level after PF receiving ACDF is low [23] Regarding reoperation rates after PF and ACDF a recent comparisons of propensity matched cohort of patients treated with PF versus ACDF revealed a reoperation rate of 6.4% versus 4.8% after PF versus ACDF, respectively, thus with no significant difference [15]. Patient lacking preoperative neck pain have the lowest rate of revision surgery after PF [2].

5.4 Conclusions and Take Home Message

The posterior cervical foraminotomy (PF) initially described by Frykholm is a surgical option for unilateral pathologies of cervical foramina, i.e. lateral disc herniations or medial bony foraminal stenoses. Surgical results in appropriately selected patients do not show significant differences to patients treated with ACDFs. An advantage of PF is the preservation of motion and the lack of necessary implants. Medial or mediolateral disc herniations or foraminal stenoses reaching far lateral should not be approached by a PF. Segmental instability after PF is a rare problem. Contraindications include radiographic evidence of a central compressive pathological entity, kyphosis, or a clinical presentation consistent with myelopathy.

Pearls

- The PF is primarily indicated for foraminal lesions and highly effective in treating cervical radiculopathy caused by a lateral disc herniation
- PF results in excellent quality-of-life outcome results of up to 93–96% of patients.
- PF is motion preserving without requiring additional instrumentation, making it both minimally invasive and cost-effective
- Contraindications for PF include radiographic evidence of a central compressive pathological entity, kyphosis, or a clinical presentation consistent with myelopathy.

References

1. Barakat M, Hussein Y. Anatomical study of the cervical nerve roots for posterior foraminotomy: cadaveric study. Eur Spine J. 2012;21(7):1383–8.
2. Bydon M, Mathios D, Macki M, de la Garza-Ramos R, Sciubba DM, Witham TF, Wolinsky JP, Gokaslan ZL, Bydon A. Long-term patient outcomes after

posterior cervical foraminotomy: an analysis of 151 cases. J Neurosurg Spine. 2014;21(5):727–31.
3. Carette S, Fehlings MG. Clinical practice. Cervical radiculopathy. N Engl J Med. 2005;353(4):392–9.
4. Chen BH, Natarajan RN, An HS, Andersson GB. Comparison of biomechanical response to surgical procedures used for cervical radiculopathy: posterior keyhole foraminotomy versus anterior foraminotomy and discectomy versus anterior discectomy with fusion. J Spinal Disord. 2001;14(1):17–20.
5. Choi KC, Ahn Y, Kang BU, Ahn ST, Lee SH. Motor palsy after posterior cervical foraminotomy: anatomical consideration. World Neurosurg. 2013;79(2):405 e401–4.
6. Clarke MJ, Ecker RD, Krauss WE, McClelland RL, Dekutoski MB. Same-segment and adjacent-segment disease following posterior cervical foraminotomy. J Neurosurg Spine. 2007;6(1):5–9.
7. Dohrmann GJ, Hsieh JC. Long-term results of anterior versus posterior operations for herniated cervical discs: analysis of 6,000 patients. Med Princ Pract. 2014;23(1):70–3.
8. Engquist M, Lofgren H, Oberg B, Holtz A, Peolsson A, Soderlund A, Vavruch L, Lind B. Surgery versus nonsurgical treatment of cervical radiculopathy: a prospective, randomized study comparing surgery plus physiotherapy with physiotherapy alone with a 2-year follow-up. Spine (Phila Pa 1976). 2013;38(20):1715–22.
9. Faught RW, Church EW, Halpern CH, Balmuri U, Attiah MA, Stein SC, Dante SJ, Welch WC, Simeone FA. Long-term quality of life after posterior cervical foraminotomy for radiculopathy. Clin Neurol Neurosurg. 2016;142:22–5.
10. Gu BS, Park JH, Seong HY, Jung SK, Roh SW. Feasibility of posterior cervical foraminotomy in cervical foraminal stenosis: prediction of surgical outcomes by the foraminal shape on preoperative computed tomography. Spine (Phila Pa 1976). 2017;42(5):E267–71.
11. Heckmann JG, Lang CJ, Zobelein I, Laumer R, Druschky A, Neundorfer B. Herniated cervical intervertebral discs with radiculopathy: an outcome study of conservatively or surgically treated patients. J Spinal Disord. 1999;12(5):396–401.
12. Jagannathan J, Sherman JH, Szabo T, Shaffrey CI, Jane JA. The posterior cervical foraminotomy in the treatment of cervical disc/osteophyte disease: a single-surgeon experience with a minimum of 5 years' clinical and radiographic follow-up. J Neurosurg Spine. 2009;10(4):347–56.
13. Lee SB, Cho KS. Cervical arthroplasty versus anterior cervical fusion for symptomatic adjacent segment disease after anterior cervical fusion surgery: review of treatment in 41 patients. Clin Neurol Neurosurg. 2017;162:59–66.
14. Liu WJ, Hu L, Chou PH, Wang JW, Kan WS. Comparison of anterior cervical discectomy and fusion versus posterior cervical foraminotomy in the treatment of cervical radiculopathy: a systematic review. Orthop Surg. 2016;8(4):425–31.
15. Lubelski D, Healy AT, Silverstein MP, Abdullah KG, Thompson NR, Riew KD, Steinmetz MP, Benzel EC, Mroz TE. Reoperation rates after anterior cervical discectomy and fusion versus posterior cervical foraminotomy: a propensity-matched analysis. Spine J. 2015;15(6):1277–83.
16. Persson LC, Carlsson CA, Carlsson JY. Long-lasting cervical radicular pain managed with surgery, physiotherapy, or a cervical collar. A prospective, randomized study. Spine (Phila Pa 1976). 1997;22(7):751–8.
17. Roh SW, Kim DH, Cardoso AC, Fessler RG. Endoscopic foraminotomy using MED system in cadaveric specimens. Spine (Phila Pa 1976). 2000;25(2):260–4.
18. Sampath P, Bendebba M, Davis JD, Ducker T. Outcome in patients with cervical radiculopathy. Prospective, multicenter study with independent clinical review. Spine (Phila Pa 1976). 1999;24(6):591–7.
19. Steinberg JA, German JW. The effect of minimally invasive posterior cervical approaches versus open anterior approaches on neck pain and disability. Int J Spine Surg. 2012;6:55–61.
20. Thoomes EJ, Scholten-Peeters W, Koes B, Falla D, Verhagen AP. The effectiveness of conservative treatment for patients with cervical radiculopathy: a systematic review. Clin J Pain. 2013;29(12):1073–86.
21. Ulrich C, Woersdoerfer O, Kalff R, Claes L, Wilke HJ. Biomechanics of fixation systems to the cervical spine. Spine (Phila Pa 1976). 1991;16(3 Suppl):S4–9.
22. van Geest S, Kuijper B, Oterdoom M, van den Hout W, Brand R, Stijnen T, Assendelft P, Koes B, Jacobs W, Peul W, Vleggeert-Lankamp C. CASINO: surgical or nonsurgical treatment for cervical radiculopathy, a randomised controlled trial. BMC Musculoskelet Disord. 2014;15:129.
23. Wang TY, Lubelski D, Abdullah KG, Steinmetz MP, Benzel EC, Mroz TE. Rates of anterior cervical discectomy and fusion after initial posterior cervical foraminotomy. Spine J. 2015;15(5):971–6.
24. Yoo HJ, Park JH, Seong HY, Roh SW. Comparison of surgical results between soft ruptured disc and foraminal stenosis patients in posterior cervical laminoforaminotomy. Korean J Neurotrauma. 2017;13(2):124–9.
25. Zdeblick TA, Zou D, Warden KE, McCabe R, Kunz D, Vanderby R. Cervical stability after foraminotomy. A biomechanical in vitro analysis. J Bone Joint Surg Am. 1992;74(1):22–7.
26. Mansfield HE, Canar WJ, Gerard CS, O'Toole JE. Single-level anterior cervical discectomy and fusion versus minimally invasive posterior cervicalforaminotomy for patients with cervical radiculopathy: a cost analysis. Neurosurg Focus. 2014;37(5):E9.

6 Cervical Myelopathy: Indication and Operative Procedure

Marcus Czabanka and Peter Vajkoczy

6.1 Introduction

The most common cause of spinal cord dysfunction is related to nontraumatic, noninfectious and nononcologic causes such as degenerative disc disease, hypertrophy of the ligamentum flavum, ossification of the posterior longitudinal ligament (OPLL) and progressive kyphosis [1, 2]. Cervical spinal cord dysfunction due to these pathologies is referred to as degenerative cervical myelopathy (DCM) leading to neurological deterioration and reduced quality of life [3, 4]. Treatment options for DCM range from non-surgical conservative approaches to surgical 360° reconstruction procedures of the cervical spine [5]. Optimal treatment requires thorough knowledge of the natural history of the disease, detailed expertise in surgical decision making, experience in anterior and posterior approaches to the cervical spine as well as medical expertise related to intra- and postoperative management of patients with (chronic) spinal cord injury [1, 5]. The following chapter outlines three different cases of DCM focusing on timing of treatment and treatment indication (Case 1), surgical decision making (anterior vs. posterior vs. combined technique, Case 2) and the special pathology of ossification of posterior longitudinal ligament (OPLL, Case 3). Rationale for surgical treatment derived from typical symptomatology and preoperative imaging/diagnostics is demonstrated. Surgical techniques, approaches and risks are discussed in relation to the pathoanatomical presentation of DCM based on three exemplary cases.

M. Czabanka (✉) · P. Vajkoczy
Department of Neurosurgery,
Charitè – Universitätsmedizin Berlin,
Berlin, Germany
e-mail: marcus.czabanka@charite.de

6.2 Case Descriptions

6.2.1 Mild Degenerative Myelopathy C5/6

A 45 year old male patient presented with persistent radicular pain for 3–6 months in the right arm corresponding to the C6 dermatome paralleled by dysesthesia. The patient did not experience changes in gait or fine motor movements of the hands. Furthermore no paresis was detected on physical exam. The patient has not performed specific therapeutic interventions except for pain medication that did not lead to permanent control of the radicular symptoms.

Physical exam: visual analogue scale (VAS) for radicular pain right arm: 6 points; modified Japanese Orthopaedic Association scale (mJOA): 17 points; NURICK scale grade 0 (Fig. 6.1).

Based on these findings the patient presents with a severe spinal canal stenosis and the presence of myelomalacia in MRI, yet without clinical signs of myelopathy. The radicular pain in the

B. Meyer, M. Rauschmann (eds.), *Spine Surgery*, https://doi.org/10.1007/978-3-319-98875-7_6

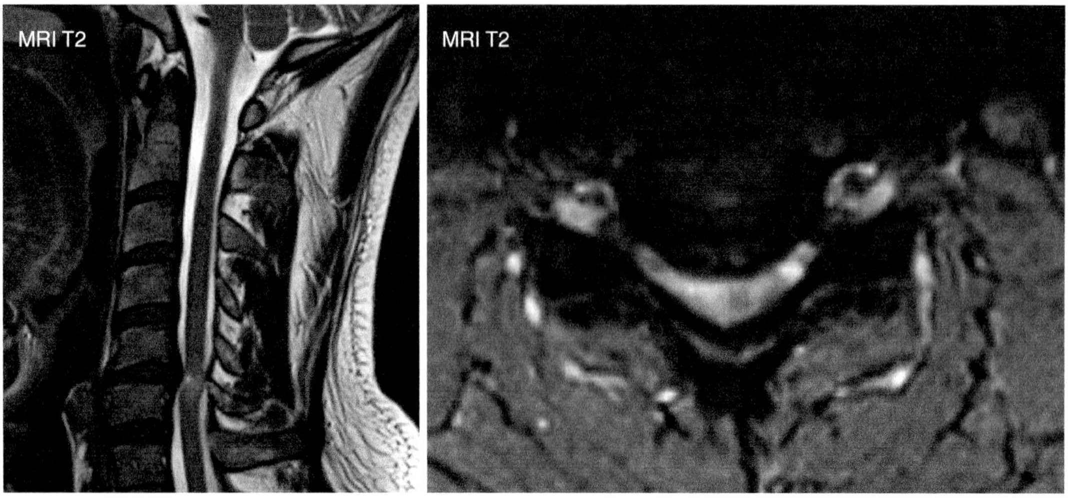

Fig. 6.1 MRI scan. The MRI scan demonstrates severe cervical spinal canal stenosis in C5/6 with corresponding signs of myelomalacia due to a broad based disc protrusion and bilateral foraminal stenosis

right C6 dermatome may be due to foraminal stenosis and / or to the presence of myelomalacia which may not be differentiated clinically. Results of the mJOA and Nurick scale underline the clinical diagnosis with very low scores. This clinically mild or almost non-present form of myelopathy is in clear contrast to the myelomalacia (T2 hyperintensity) demonstrated in MRI. In these cases, electrophysiological assessment adds important information beyond findings in physical examination (e.g. clinically non-detectable compromise of MEPs or SEPs). Therefore in order to further analyse the patients pathology flexion/extension x-ray of the cervical spine and electrophysiological analysis of somatosensory evoked (SEP) and motor evoked potentials (MEP) was performed. No deficits in SEP and MEP analysis were detected while x-ray imaging did reveal a non-moving segment C5/6. Additional CT imaging verified a soft disc protrusion causing the spinal canal stenosis (Fig. 6.2).

Due to persistent radicular pain and the presence of severe spinal canal stenosis the decision was made to operate the patient using an anterior cervical discectomy and fusion (ACDF) in order do decompress the spinal canal and the foraminal stenosis.

6.2.2 Severe Degenerative Multisegmental Myelopathy

A 44 year old female patient presented with progressive gait ataxia, persistent paresthesia in the left arm and left foot. Especially the gait disturbance has worsened over the last 12 months. The patient had received MRI with the diagnosis of a cervical spinal canal stenosis 4 years ago due to similar but less pronounced symptoms. The indication for surgical decompression was already seen at that time, however the patient declined surgical treatment due to tolerable symptoms and decided for conservative management.

Physical exam: mJOA 10 points, NURICK scale grade 3, VAS 5 points for neck pain (Fig. 6.3).

Additional electrophysiological analysis demonstrated a reduced response in SEPs from the upper extremity verifying spinal cord injury. Consequently surgical treatment was recommended for that patient. Due to cervical kyphosis and the compressive pathology restricted to the disc segment without signs of ossification, the decision was made to perform three-level ACDF in order to decompress the spinal cord and to correct the kyphotic deformity (Fig. 6.4).

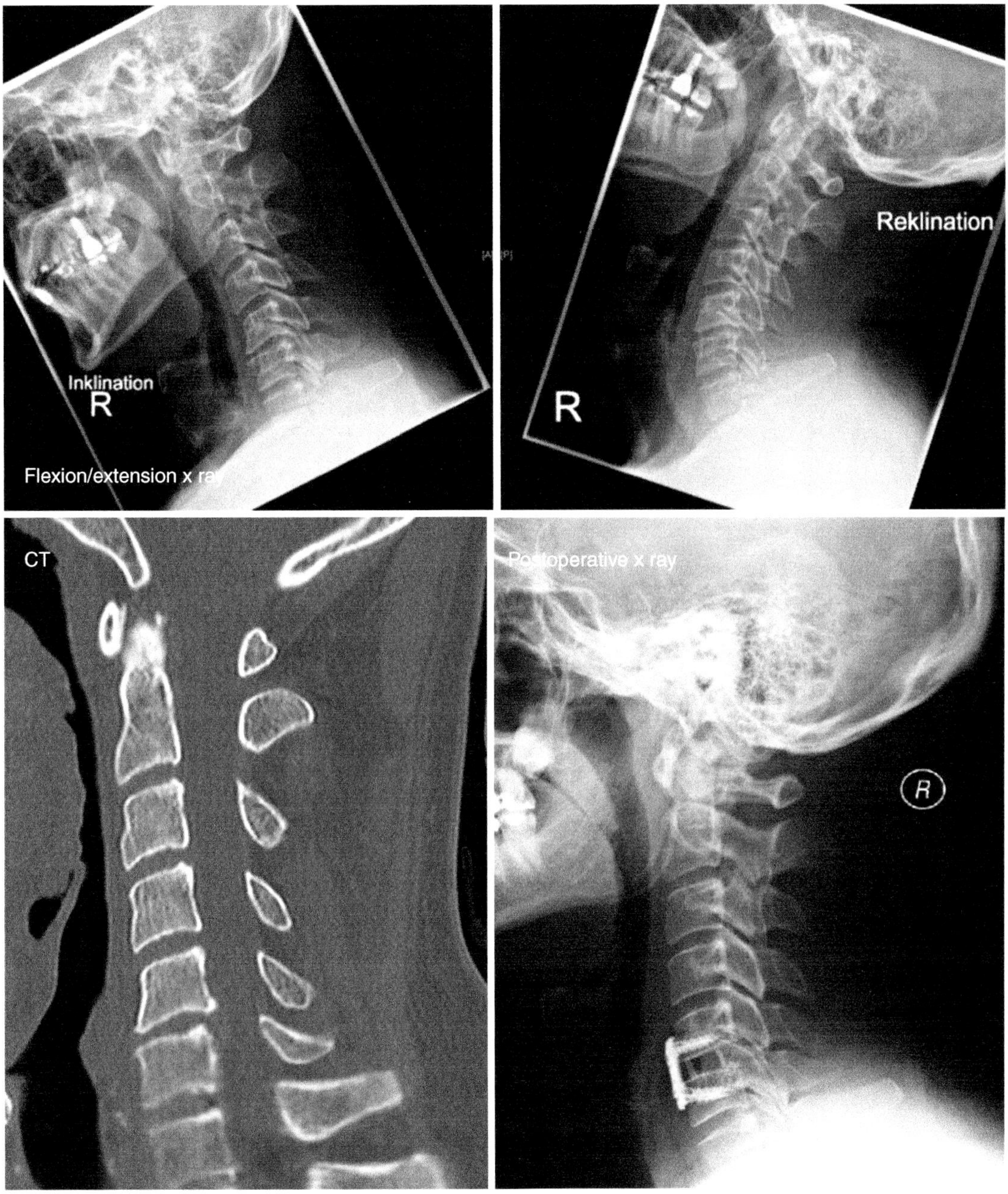

Fig. 6.2 x-ray and CT imaging of the cervical spine. Flexion/extension x-ray of the cervical spine shows a fixed C5/6 segment without signs of instability. CT imaging demonstrates a soft disc protrusion without signs of ossification in C5/6. A postoperative x-ray control verifies a three level discectomy and fusion from C3-6

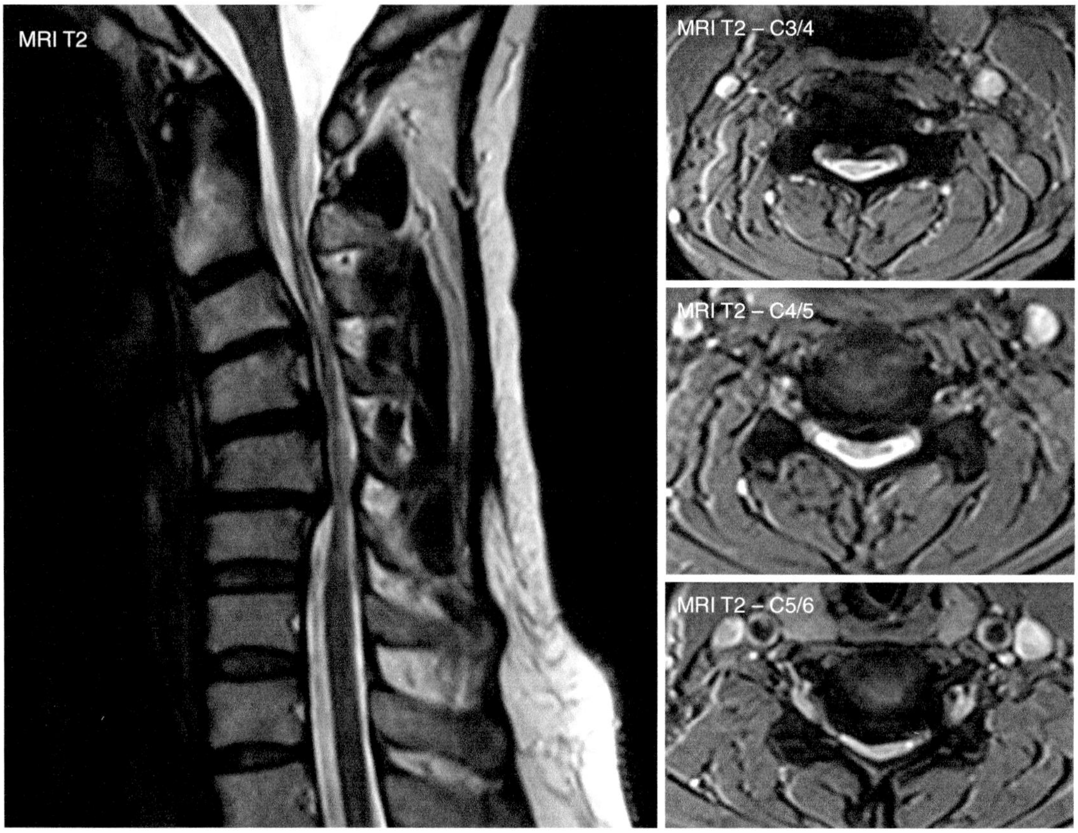

Fig. 6.3 Preoperative MRI. MRI demonstrates cervical degenerative kyphosis with severe spinal canal stenosis in segments C3/4, C4/5 and C5/6 and associated myelomalcia

6.2.3 Degenerative Myelopathy Due to Ossification of the Posterior Longitudinal Ligament

A 57 year old male patient presented with coordination problems and fine motor dysfunction of both hands especially when eating and manipulating small items. Additionally a gait disturbance has developed over the last 9 months resulting in 2 domestic falls while walking to the bathroom at night without turning the lights on. The patient had received MRI at an external institution demonstrating severe spinal canal stenosis with a maximum extension behind C4 and C5. A less pronounced spinal canal stenosis is shown in C5/6.

Physical exam: mJOA 13 points, NURICK scale grade 2 (Fig. 6.5).

Electrophysiological assessment showed delayed latencies in MEPs from the upper and lower extremity verifying spinal cord injury. Due to the unusual compressive pathology in MR imaging a CT scan was initiated which verified a broad based OPLL behind the vertebral bodies of C4 and C5. In the presence of OPLL surgical treatment was recommended using a posterior approach with wide laminectomy and posterior instrumentation using spinal navigation for the placement of cervical pedicle screws (Fig. 6.6).

6.3 Discussion of the Cases

6.3.1 Indication Case 1

The patient in case 1 represents a non-myelopathic patient with imaging evidence of cord compression and radiculopathy. Indication for surgical treatment is based upon natural history of the disease, rates of disease progression/myelopathy

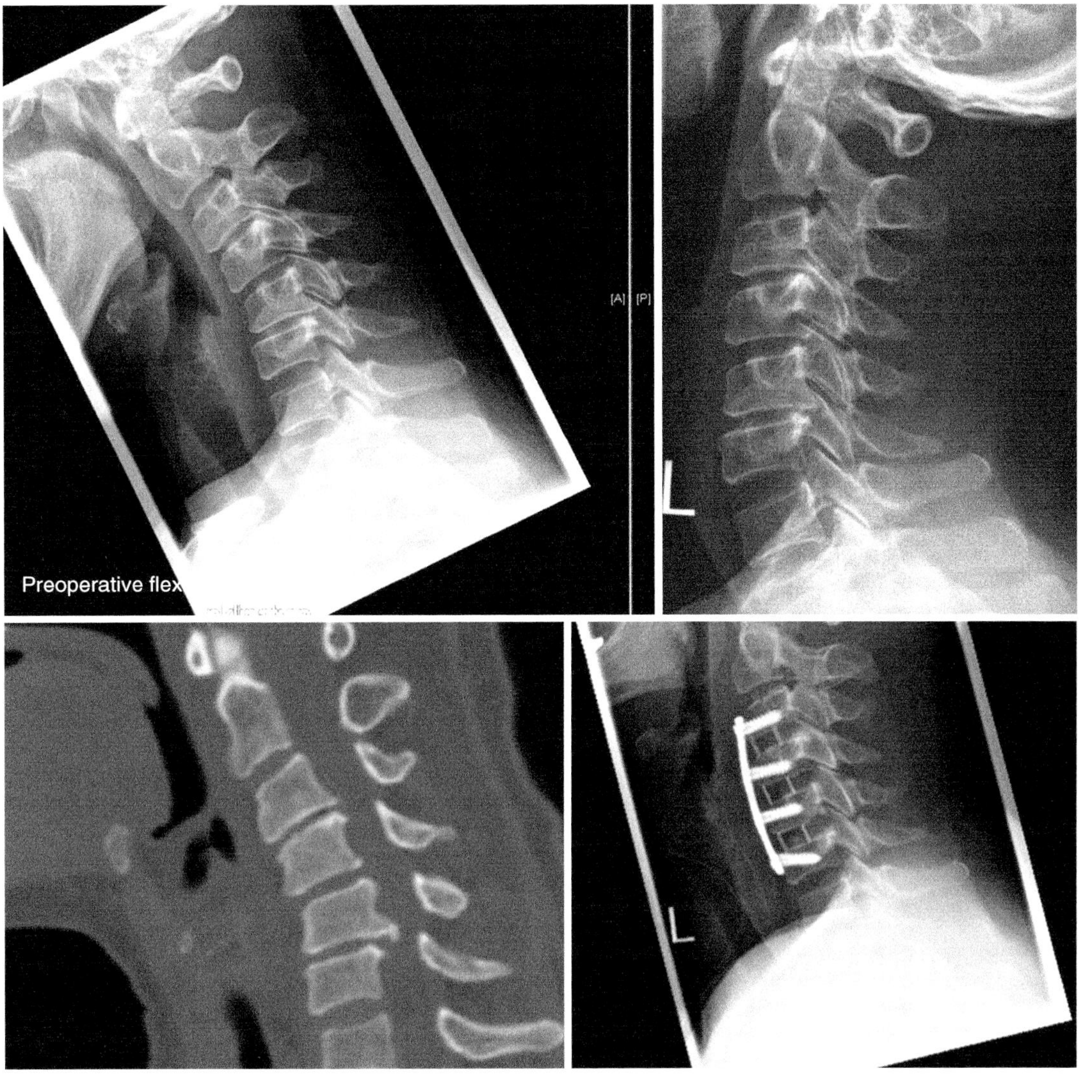

Fig. 6.4 CT and x-ray imaging. CT imaging verifies soft disc protrusions and dorsolateral spondylophytes as cord-compression pathology without signs of ossification. Flexion/extension x-ray demonstrates preserved motion in C2/3 and C6/7 while the degenerated segments are fixed. No signs of instability are demonstrated. Postoperative X-ray imaging demonstrates ventral discectomy and decompression in segments C3/4, C4/5 and C5/6 with ventral plating from C3-6 and correction of cervical kyphosis

development and risks of operative intervention [1]. Over an observation period of 44 months, 22.6% of patients with imaging evidence of cord compression/cervical spinal canal stenosis develop clinically manifest myelopathy [6]. In the case of OPLL, the rate may rise up to 61.5% of patients developing myelopathy. Presence of radiculopathy and electrophysiological compromise (prolonged SEPs and MEPs, evidence of anterior horn cell lesion) have been identified as distinct and independent risk factors favoring early myelopathy development within 12 months [6]. Clinical radiculopathy was found in 62.5% of patients which eventually developed myelopathy as compared to only 26.35% of patients without developing myelopathy [6]. Once myelopathic symptoms exist more than 50% of patients worsen at performing activities of daily living over a 10 year period and experience a significantly higher rate for spinal cord injury-related hospitalization [1, 7]. In contrast, non-operative treatment is not well-defined consisting of different treatment

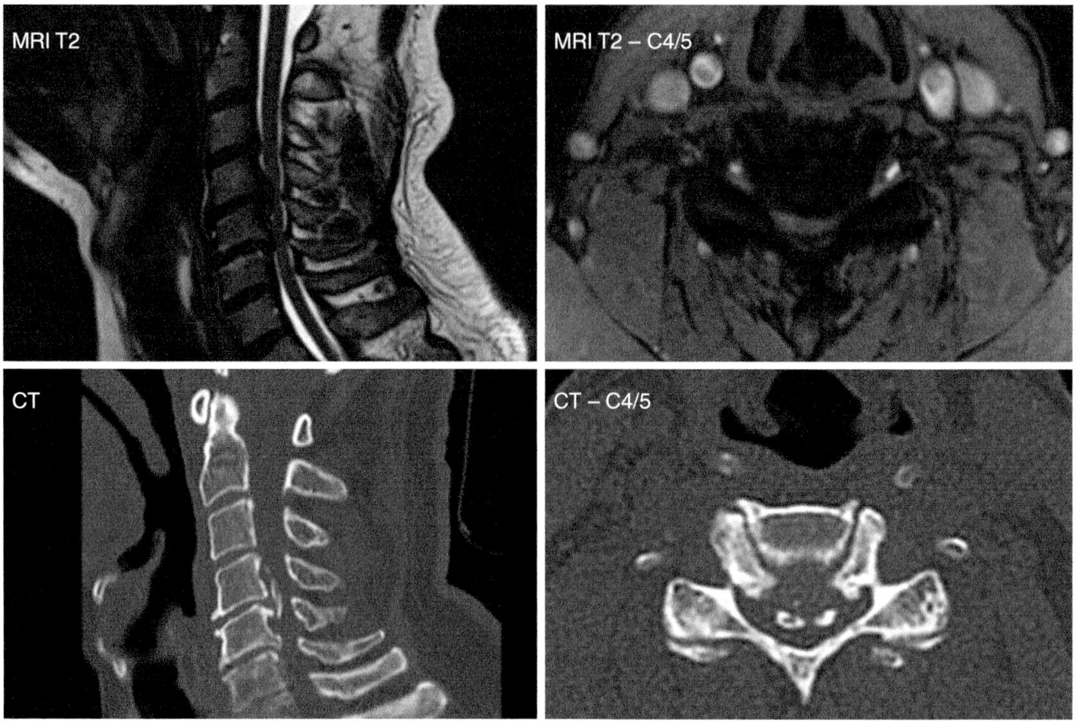

Fig. 6.5 MRI and CT. MRI demonstrates spinal canal stenosis and myelomalacia due to a cord compressing mass behind the vertebral bodies of C4 and C5 extending clearly beyond the disc segment. A moderate spinal canal stenosis is verified in C5/6 restricted to the disc segment. CT imaging demonstrates a long ossified mass located behind vertebral bodies C4 and C5 (continuous OPLL) leading to severe spinal canal stenosis in axial view

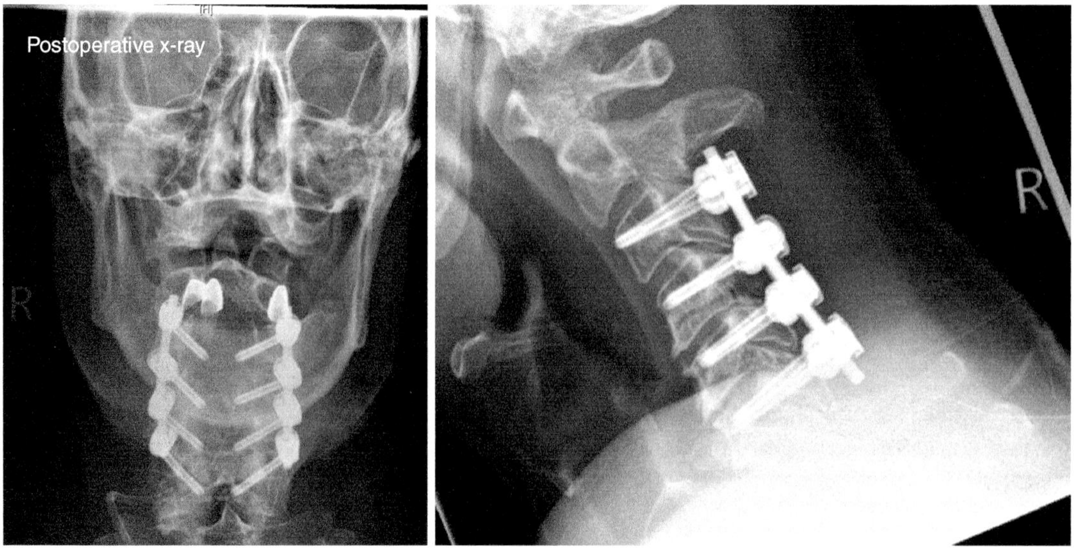

Fig. 6.6 Postoperative X-ray. Postoperative imaging verifies posterior decompression and fusion with cervical pedicle screws

algorithms including bed rest, cervical traction, cervical immobilization, thermal therapy, physical therapy and/or non-steroidal anti-inflammatory drugs [1, 3]. In the lack of clear evidence-base data, non-surgical treatment does not lead to a significant recovery of myelopathic patients with the exception for a specific subgroup of patients suffering from soft disc herniation and dynamic myelopathic symptoms [1]. Additionally, 23–54% of patients under non-surgical treatment eventually undergo surgical decompression due to conservative treatment failure [1, 8]. In contrast, the cumulative risk for complications after surgical treatment is low (overall complication rate 14.1%) with major complications ranging from 0.3% to 3.3% [1]. Based on these data, current treatment guidelines recommend either surgical treatment or a trial of structured non-operative treatment in non-melopathic patients with imaging evidence of spinal cord compression and a relevant risk profile for developing myelopathic symptoms [1]. A shared decision making process between the treating physician and the patient must be performed as the use of prophylactic surgery is likely costly and of limited benefit. Nevertheless, a structured conservative treatment protocol may be challenging beyond practicability of every day life. Yoshimatsu et al. proposed a conservative treatment protocol of cervical traction of 4 h per day for 3 months paralleled by immobilization of the cervical spine, exercise therapy, drug and thermal therapy [9]. Furthermore, if patients experience neurological deterioration during conservative treatment they should be advised to surgical treatment because a longer duration of myelopathic symptoms and a higher severity of symptoms reduce the patients` chances to recover to a non-myelopathic neurological state [1]. In case 1, the indication for surgical intervention was seen due to the patients risk profile for developing myelopathic symptoms and the long-standing severe radiculopathy that significantly reduced the patients quality of life.

6.3.2 Choice of Approach

DCM may be caused by compression of the spinal cord from either anteriorly located, posteriorly located or a combined localization of degenerative pathologies. Consequently both anterior and posterior approaches are available for the treatment of DCM. Following evidence based data, surgical decompression strategies utilizing both approaches have been demonstrated to effectively treat DCM [10]. Due to the scientific equiopoise concerning the superiority of both approaches current treatment guidelines recommend an individualized approach when treating patients with CSM accounting for pathoanatomical variations (ventral vs. dorsal, focal vs. diffuse, sagittal, dynamic instability) [5]. The usual recommendation points out that if the compression occurs from anterior a ventral approach should be performed, if it occurs from posterior a dorsal approach represents the strategy of choice. In case 1 we chose an anterior approach due to the fact that a broad based soft disc protrusion led to an anterior compression of the spinal cord and the neuroforamina. Decompression of the neuroforamina is more easily achieved via an anterior approach compared to a posterior approach. Moreover, the compressive pathology is restricted to the level of the cervical disc, which can be completely addressed by anterior discectomy and fusion (ACDF) and the segment shows a slight kyphotic alignment, which is better corrected by an anterior approach. Additionally, the risk profile for postoperative neck pain favours an anterior approach [5]. The risk for laryngeal nerve palsy and major complications like vessel injury, esophageal injury and tracheal injury is very low (<2%) [11]. The rate of transient postoperative dysphagia lies around 6% [12].

6.3.3 Accordance with the Literature Guidelines

The current guidelines for the treatment of cervical myelopathy were the basis for the presented cases and the discussion of indication and approach.

Level of Evidence: C
The level of evidence available to date is low by only consisting of metaanalysis based upon retrospective series, cohort studies and few prospective studies.

6.3.4 Indication Case 2

The patient in case 2 presents clinical symptoms of severe DCM in response to a three segmental compression of the spinal cord at the disc level as a result of a progressive degenerative process leading to kyphotic deformity of the cervical spine. There is strong recommendation for surgical treatment for patients suffering from severe myelopathy as defined by an mJOA score of 0–11 [1]. Surgical treatment has been shown to significantly improve patients symptoms assessed by JOA, mJOA, Neck Disability Index, VAS and Nurick scores over a follow-up period of up to 36 months [1]. The overall risk profile for surgical treatment is very favorable with 14.1% [1]. Based on the fact that myelopathic patients have a high risk for symptom progression (more than 50% of patients demonstrate a decline in symptoms over 10 years) and a decline in daily living activities paralleled by a high risk for spinal cord injury related hospitalization, surgical treatment may be regarded to be cost-effective for the health care system [1]. Special considerations have to be addressed when counseling patients about the effects of surgery in the presence of severe myelopathy: (1) the duration of symptoms negatively correlates with the odds to recover to a non-myelopathic neurologiocal state (mJOA >16) following surgery [13, 14]; (2) the odds to achieve a postoperative mJOA score >16 decline by 22% if the symptoms persist from a short to a long term duration (statistically every 3 months) [13, 15]; (3) clinical improvement compared to baseline level is greater in patients with severe DCM as compared to patients with mild DCM, however the minimal clinically important difference is greater in patients with severe DCM as compared to patients with mild DCM [1, 4].

This means that patients with severe myelopathic symptoms need to massively improve after surgery to experience a minimal clinically important difference (MCID) as compared to the preoperative state because their baseline level of symptoms is very low. This may be the result of long lasting myelon compression resulting in partially irreversible spinal cord injury. Patients suffering from mild myelopathic symptoms need small improvements to experience a MCID. The overall chances to achieve a clinically relevant benefit improve with a shorter duration of symptoms and a milder form of DCM. Therefore, surgery should be considered in a timely fashion and before symptoms progress to a severe form of the disease.

6.3.5 Choice of Approach

The patient demonstrates severe spinal cord compression with signs of myelomalacia in MRI on the disc level (C3/4, C4/5 and C5/6) with a regular width of the spinal canal behind the vertebral bodies (multisegmental, focal stenosis). Moreover, there is evidence of kyphotic deformity of the cervical spine with remaining mobility in flexion/extension in the adjacent segments. These two factors favor an anterior approach in order to decompress the spinal cord and to correct the deformity while maintaining posterior structures, which may beneficial for the development of postoperative neck pain and muscle atrophy. A posterior approach has the advantage of a superior widening of the spinal canal (especially behind the vertebral bodies; useful for diffuse multisegmental stenosis), yet suffers from reduced efficacy to correct the sagittal alignment and the higher rate of postoperative neck pain [5]. In this patient, widening of the spinal canal behind the vertebral bodies of less importance as the spinal cord compression is restricted to the disc level. Multisegmental anterior discectomies with plating have been shown to be superior in improvement of clinical outcomes and correction of the sagittal alignment compared to ventral corpectomies or hybrid discectomy-corpectomy strategies while maintaining a lower risk profile for postoperative C5 palsies (1–5%) and a comparative risk profile for postoperative dysphagia(<20%), infection(1–2%) and nonunion (1–18%) [16]. Consequently, we chose a three level discectomy strategy with ventral plating to decompress the spinal cord and to restore the sagittal profile.

6.3.6 Accordance with the Literature Guidelines

The current guideline for the treatment of cervical myelopathy were the basis for the presented cases and the discussion of indication and approach.

Level of Evidence: C
The level of evidence available to date is low by only consisting of metaanalysis based upon retrospective series, cohort studies and few prospective studies.

6.3.7 Indication Case 3

The patient in case 3 shows signs of moderate DCM in response to an OPLL induced compression of the spinal chord. MRI demonstrates a spinal canal stenosis which extends beyond the disc level of C4/C5. CT imaging demonstrates hallmarks of a continous OPLL from C4 to C5. Following current treatment guidelines, surgical decompression is recommended for the treatment of mild DCM [1]. The rationale for this indication is summarized in Cases 1 and 2. Despite the fact the OPLL represents a special cause of DCM, surgical treatment has proved to be equally effective in OPLL patients similar to patients suffering from other forms of DCM [17]. However, it must be mentioned that surgical decompression of OPLL may be associated with an increased complication risk of 21.8% [1, 17, 18].CSF leaks, C5 palsies and implant failure are among the most frequent complications following surgical decompression for OPLL [18]. In contrast, non-melopathic OPLL-patients should not receive prophylactic surgery [18]. The risk to develop myelopathy in response to OPLL is quite low with >70% of asymptomatic OPLL patients remaining without myelopathic symptoms over an observation period of 30 years [18]. The most important risk factor for potential development of myelopathy was spinal canal stenosis due to OPLL of >60% [18]. In these cases, surgical decompression is also recommended as 100% of patients with a spinal canal stenosis of more than 60% caused by the OPLL develop myelopathy [18].

6.3.8 Choice of Approach

The patient in Case 3 demonstrates severe spinal cord compression with signs of myelomalacia in MRI due to compression from a continuous OPLL. In order to achieve adequate decompression a posterior approach was chosen to release the myelon. Currently both anterior and posterior approaches have to be considered equally effective to treat OPLL induced DCM even though there seems to be a higher complication profile for anterior approaches [5, 17, 18]. CSF leaks, implant failure and dysphagia/hoarseness are associated with anterior approaches despite the fact that the anterior floating decompression technique is applied [18]. Usually multilevel corpectomies have to be performed to treat OPLL which predisposes to implant failure and non-union [18]. In contrast, posterior approaches are associated with a lower risk profile for CSF leak, yet they represent indirect decompression strategies with a higher risk for C5 palsies and axial neck pain [18]. Different posterior techniques are available like laminoplasty, laminectomy and laminectomy/fusion. Today, laminectomy is usually not recommended due to the risk of postoperative deformities [18]. Laminoplasty is described as a useful strategy to treat OPLL induced DCM, yet laminoplasty is associated with increased rate of postoperative neck pain and almost 70% of patients that received laminoplasty demonstrate signs of OPLL progression [19, 20]. Laminectomy and fusion is mostly associated with an increased rate of nerve root affections, yet it currently represents a useful tool to decompress the spinal cord with a low complication profile [18, 20]. In order to decide about the optimal approach the K-line may be used to differentiate K-line positive from K-line negative OPLL patients [18]. The K-line on the lateral radiographs connects the midpoints of the spinal canal at C2 and C7. In K-line positive cases, the OPLL is ventral to the line (recommendation posterior approach) and in K-line-negative cases, the OPLL is dorsal to the line (optional anterior or posterior approach) [18]. In cases of multisegmental anterior corpectomies (2 levels and more) an additional posterior instrumentation should be considered to reduce the risk of non-union and implant failure [18]. For posterior approaches decompression of the adjacent segments above and below the OPLL is recommended to avoid kinking of the myelon after dorsal decompression [18].

In our institution OPLL patients are usually treated by multisegmental posterior decompression and fusion except for patients with severe kyphotic deformity that require additional correction of cervical kyphosis. Consequently, the patient in Case 3 demonstrates adequate cervical lordosis with a K-line positive OPLL which was treated by posterior decompression and fusion.

6.3.9 Accordance with the Literature Guidelines

The current guideline for the treatment of cervical myelopathy were the basis for the presented cases and the discussion of indication and approach.

Level of Evidence: C
The level of evidence available to date is low by only consisting of metaanalysis based upon retrospective series, cohort studies and few prospective studies.

6.4 Conclusions and Take Home Message

Patients with DCM should be treated at an early time point before the symptoms progress and the chances of recovery to a non-myelopathic state decline. Treatment of choice is surgical decompression either from an anterior or posterior approach depending on the patients pathoanatomical characteristics. Non-myelopathic patients with imaging signs of spinal cord compression may also receive surgical treatment if risk factors for the development of myelopathy exist. In OPLL patients, the same rationale for surgical treatment as for the other forms of DCM exist. However OPLL patients may experience a higher complication profile as patients with other causes of DCM.

Pearls

- DCM represents a major cause of spinal cord injury and leads to severe impairment of daily living activities due to neurological deficits if left untreated
- Surgical decompression represents an an effective and cost-efficient treatment for DCM
- Anterior and posterior approaches for spinal decompression are equally effective and therefore pathoanatomical characteristics of the patient decide about individualized surgical strategies
- OPLL represents a special cause of DCM with a high rate of spinal cord injury related hospitalizations and a severe neurological decline if myelopathic symptoms exist requiring surgical decompression as treatment of choice

Editorial Comment

This is an excellent chapter on a very important topic. There is no level 1 evidence for timing or surgical technique in patients with CM, the most common treatable cause of chronic spinal cord injury. Since it will take a very long time -if at all- to accumulate better evidence, we encourage the readers to digest the authors' reasoning and line of arguments very closely, because they constitute the standard of care today.

References

1. Fehlings MG, et al. A clinical practice guideline for the management of patients with degenerative cervical myelopathy: recommendations for patients with mild, moderate, and severe disease and nonmyelopathic patients with evidence of cord compression. Global Spine J. 2017;7:70S–83S.
2. Nouri A, Tetreault L, Singh A, Karadimas SK, Fehlings MG. Degenerative cervical myelopathy: epidemiology, genetics, and pathogenesis. Spine (Phila Pa 1976). 2015;40:E675–93.

3. Tetreault LA, et al. Change in function, pain, and quality of life following structured nonoperative treatment in patients with degenerative cervical myelopathy: a systematic review. Global Spine J. 2017;7:42S–52S.
4. Tetreault L, Nouri A, Kopjar B, Côté P, Fehlings MG. The minimum clinically important difference of the modified Japanese Orthopaedic Association scale in patients with degenerative cervical myelopathy. Spine (Phila Pa 1976). 2015;40:1653–9.
5. Lawrence BD, et al. Anterior versus posterior approach for treatment of cervical spondylotic myelopathy: a systematic review. Spine (Phila Pa 1976). 2013;38:S173–82.
6. Wilson JR, et al. Frequency, timing, and predictors of neurological dysfunction in the nonmyelopathic patient with cervical spinal cord compression, canal stenosis, and/or ossification of the posterior longitudinal ligament. Spine (Phila Pa 1976). 2013;38:S37–54.
7. Tetreault LA, et al. The natural history of degenerative cervical myelopathy and the rate of hospitalization following spinal cord injury: an updated systematic review. Global Spine J. 2017;7:28S–34S.
8. Matsumoto M, et al. Relationships between outcomes of conservative treatment and magnetic resonance imaging findings in patients with mild cervical myelopathy caused by soft disc herniations. Spine (Phila Pa 1976). 2001;26:1592–8.
9. Yoshimatsu H, et al. Conservative treatment for cervical spondylotic myelopathy. Prediction of treatment effects by multivariate analysis. Spine J. 2001;1:269–73.
10. Kato S, et al. Comparison of anterior and posterior surgery for degenerative cervical myelopathy: an MRI-based propensity-score-matched analysis using data from the prospective multicenter AOSpine CSM North America and International Studies. J Bone Joint Surg Am. 2017;99:1013–21.
11. Tempel ZJ, et al. A multicenter review of superior laryngeal nerve injury following anterior cervical spine surgery. Global Spine J. 2017;7:7S–11S.
12. Nagoshi N, et al. Risk factors for and clinical outcomes of dysphagia after anterior cervical surgery for degenerative cervical myelopathy: results from the AOSpine International and North America Studies. J Bone Joint Surg Am. 2017;99:1069–77.
13. Tetreault LA, et al. A clinical prediction model to determine outcomes in patients with cervical spondylotic myelopathy undergoing surgical treatment: data from the prospective, multi-center AOSpine North America study. J Bone Joint Surg Am. 2013;95:1659–66.
14. Li FN, et al. The treatment of mild cervical spondylotic myelopathy with increased signal intensity on T2-weighted magnetic resonance imaging. Spinal Cord. 2014;52:348–53.
15. Fukui K, Kataoka O, Sho T, Sumi M. Pathomechanism, pathogenesis, and results of treatment in cervical spondylotic myelopathy caused by dynamic canal stenosis. Spine (Phila Pa 1976). 1990;15:1148–52.
16. Shamji MF, et al. Comparison of anterior surgical options for the treatment of multilevel cervical spondylotic myelopathy: a systematic review. Spine (Phila Pa 1976). 2013;38:S195–209.
17. Nakashima H, et al. Comparison of outcomes of surgical treatment for ossification of the posterior longitudinal ligament versus other forms of degenerative cervical myelopathy. J Bone Joint Surg. 2016;98:370–8.
18. Abiola R, Rubery P, Mesfin A. Ossification of the posterior longitudinal ligament: etiology, diagnosis, and outcomes of nonoperative and operative management. Global Spine J. 2016;6:195–204.
19. Iwasaki M, Kawaguchi Y, Kimura T, Yonenobu K. Long-term results of expansive laminoplasty for ossification of the posterior longitudinal ligament of the cervical spine: more than 10 years follow up. J Neurosurg Spine. 2002;96:180–9.
20. Fehlings MG, et al. Laminectomy and fusion versus laminoplasty for the treatment of degenerative cervical myelopathy: results from the AOSpine North America and International Prospective Multicenter Studies. Spine J. 2017;17:102–8.

7 Cervical Posterior Long Construct Stabilization

Lukas Bobinski

7.1 Introduction

The cervical spine has a widest range of motion in comparison to the rest of the spine. As part of the physiological global sagittal alignment it acts as a well-tuned adjustment instrument which sustain the horizontal gaze and supports the mass of the head. Due to this complex task, the cervical spine is particular susceptible to a variety of disorders that inevitably can warrant surgical consideration. Hence, the choice of surgical technique should recognize the importance of cervical sagittal alignment as a significant factor that prevents late complications like pseudarthrosis, adjacent segmental degeneration, pain and neurological deterioration.

The typical example of pathology that very often requires long posterior cervical instrumentation is the fracture/dislocation in ankylosing spondylitis (AS).

AS is a chronic inflammatory disease, causing ossification of the joints and ligaments with auto-fusion and widespread ankylosis, that secondary leads to atrophy of the surrounding muscles and osteoporosis. During this process, patients can develop fixed cervicothoracic deformity that leads to difficulty with forward gaze and social outlook. The global kyphotic sagittal imbalance with anterior displacement center of gravity makes patients with AS very prone toward fall trauma. The rigid, osteoporotic cervical spine in kyphotic position creates long lever arm, which is susceptible to distraction fractures in close relationship to junctional levels, even with a minor trauma. Furthermore, even slight displacement of these fractures can lead to a catastrophic neurologic deficit as they tend to be very unstable, and therefore demand a solid construct that withstand shearing forces across the fracture site similar to fixations technique used for long bone fractures.

The authors describe a case of highly unstable cervical fracture that preferably should be treated with a long posterior cervical screw and rod fixation. The preoperative radiological evaluation provides the reader with visualization of the problem to increase understanding of the clinical implications essential for surgical planning. Furthermore, the applied techniques are explained with highlighting their advantages.

This chapter's objective is to equip the reader in sufficient information to be able to plan long posterior screw and rod fixation in cervical spine in case of complex cervical pathology.

L. Bobinski (✉)
Department of Orthopedics, Spine Unit, Umeå University Hospital, Umeå, Sweden

B. Meyer, M. Rauschmann (eds.), *Spine Surgery*, https://doi.org/10.1007/978-3-319-98875-7_7

7.2 Case Description

A 66 y/o male with known AS was admitted to the local hospital after he fell at his home and suffered a low energy cervical trauma. The patient presented with severe pain in cervicothoracic region. The neurological exam according to ASIA score revealed signs of central-cord syndrome with motor weakness (3/5) distally in the upper and proximally in the lower extremities with preservation of sacral function (ASIA D). The initial radiological evaluation with computer tomography revealed a highly unstable, distraction fracture C7/T1: B3 displaced anteriorly (Fig. 7.1a–c) [1]. The left C7 pedicle was intact, however the fracture continued through the right C7 pedicle. Patient was urgently referred to our unit at university hospital, level 1 trauma center. The external immobilization was impossible due to severely advanced global kyphotic deformity. This was also the reason, why the radiological investigations were not completed with the MRI. The status at the admission was unchanged. As a result of this highly unstable fracture with serious risk of displacement, neurological deterioration and threat for free airways, the patient was scheduled for emergency surgery with long posterior cervical fixation bridging across cervicothoracic junction (CTJ). Unfortunately, the intraoperative neuromonitoring was not available in this case.

7.2.1 Surgery

After awake intubation, patient was gently log-rolled to prone position with his head secured in the head holder on the horse-shoe support with a slight traction (3 kg). The effort was made to keep the patient's abdomen completely free, with a support on the table on a padded chest plate and anterior iliac crest pads. After applying padded support to patient's feet, the table was put in reversed Trendelenburg position in order to minimize perioperative bleeding. Due to extreme kyphotic deformity, use of intraoperative fluoroscopy was impossible.

The exposure was carried out from C2 to T3. It was then confirmed, intraoperatively, the presence of subluxation at C7/T1 level. The cervical spine was completely fused. This created two long lever arms displaced against each other. Even slightest attempt on instrumenting cervical spine above the fracture caused eminent thread to further displacement. Moreover, the bone fragment of the right broken pedicle injured dura mater in close relationship to the C8 nerve root with CSF leak.

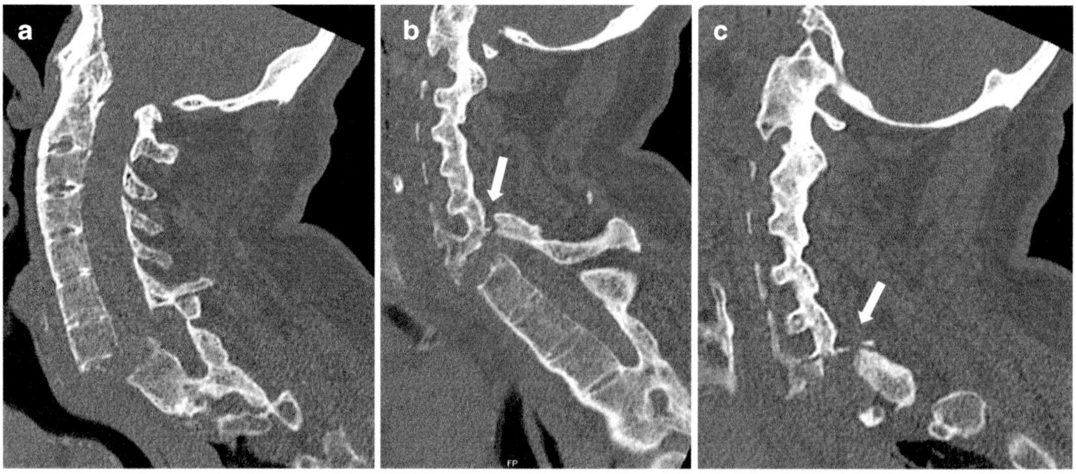

Fig. 7.1 CT scan on admission to primary hospital after the trauma. The CT scan shows an anteriorly displaced, luxated cervical fracture C7/T1: B3 according to AOSpine subaxial cervical spine injury classification fracture [1]. Typical characteristics of AS with "bamboo spine" appearance is clearly visible. Arrows point at three column disruption and fractured right C7 pedicle. (**a**) midline slice, (**b**) left side slice, (**c**) right side slice

Under direct visualization the short segment fixation was carried out on left side between C7 and T1. This maneuver allowed re-alignment of the column. On the right side the C7 pedicle was not suitable for instrumentation. This is the reason, C6 pedicle and T1 were used for another short instrumentation. This completed reposition of the fracture and provided with sufficient segmental stability for further instrumentation at the higher levels (Fig. 7.2). The Magerl technique was then used at C1/C2 vertebrae bilateral since they were already auto-fused. This created a solid cranial bone purchase. Lower subaxial segments were instrumented with use bi-cortical, lateral-mass screw technique. The caudal instrumentation was extended toward T3 due to of very poor bone quality. The four-rods (3.0 mm titanium each) technique was applied to connect and close the construct (Fig. 7.3a, b). The fixation was followed by laminectomy C6-T1 with suturing a dural tear and evacuation of minor intraspinal hematoma. No attempts were taken to correct the

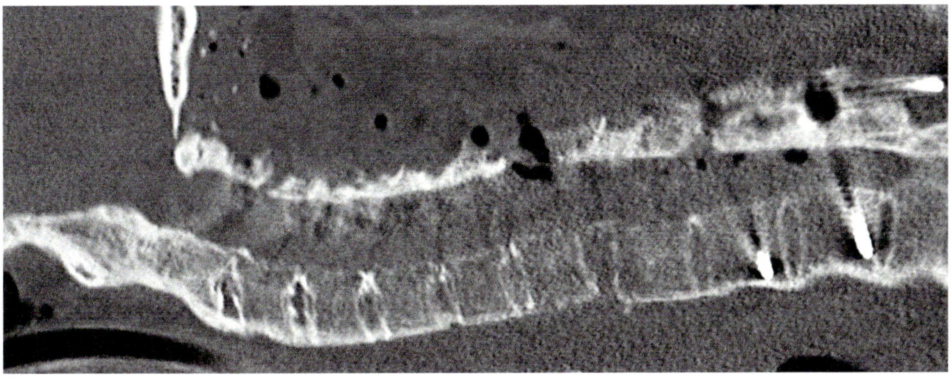

Fig. 7.2 Postoperative CT scan. The postoperative CT confirmed realignment of the cervical column with a long posterior screw and rod fixation crossing CTJ

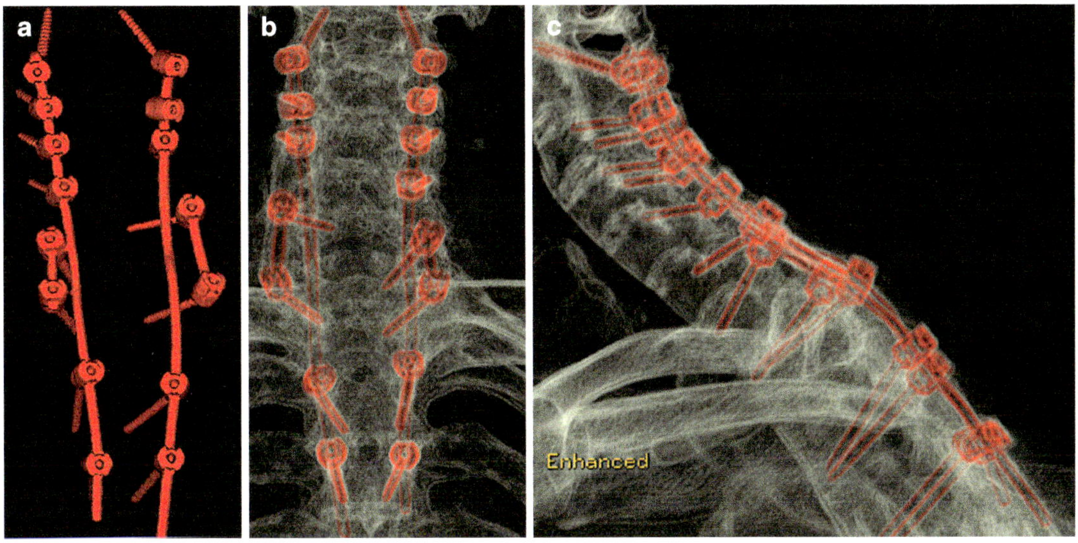

Fig. 7.3 Enhanced images of the construct. The construct consisted of: Magerl screws at most cranial C1/C2 segments bilateral, followed by lateral-mass screws and pedicle screws at levels T2 and T3. Additional two short segment fixations: right C6 pedicle screw to T1 pedicle screw and left C7 pedicle screw to T1 pedicle screw. (**a**) and (**b**) coronal and (**c**) sagittal view

kyphotic deformity because of the risk of further neurological deterioration.

The wound was closed in layers in regular fashion. No drain was used to in order to prevent development of CSF fistula.

Postoperatively patient presented with unchanged neurological status. He was discharged for rehabilitation after a few days at our unit.

7.2.2 Follow-Up

The patient presented a full recovery of his neurological deficit at the 3 months follow-up. He was also pain-free. The following radiological examination at 6 and 12 months showed complete fusion of the segment (Fig. 7.4a, b).

However, due to the global kyphotic deformity, the patient was scheduled for corrective surgery with PSO at the lumbar segments and instrumentation (Figs. 7.5 and 7.6).

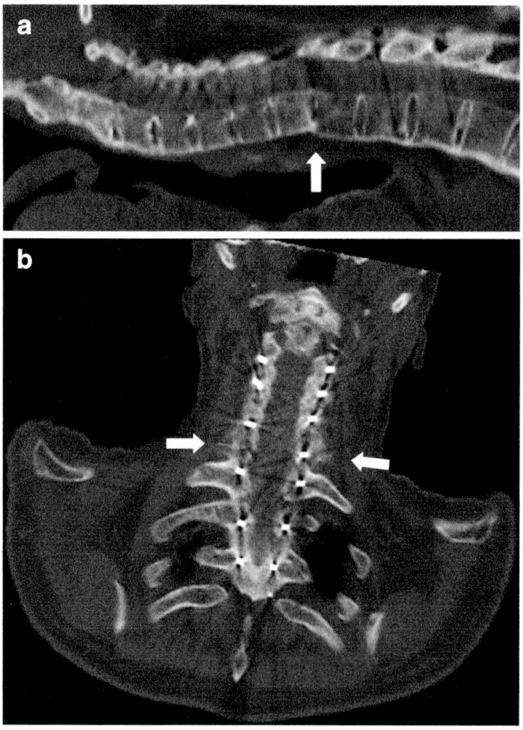

Fig. 7.4 CT scan at 12 months follow-up. This CT scan clearly shows solid, circumferential fusion at the previous broken and dislocated segment C7/T1. Images show: (**a**) sagittal and (**b**) coronal view. There are no signs of hardware failure

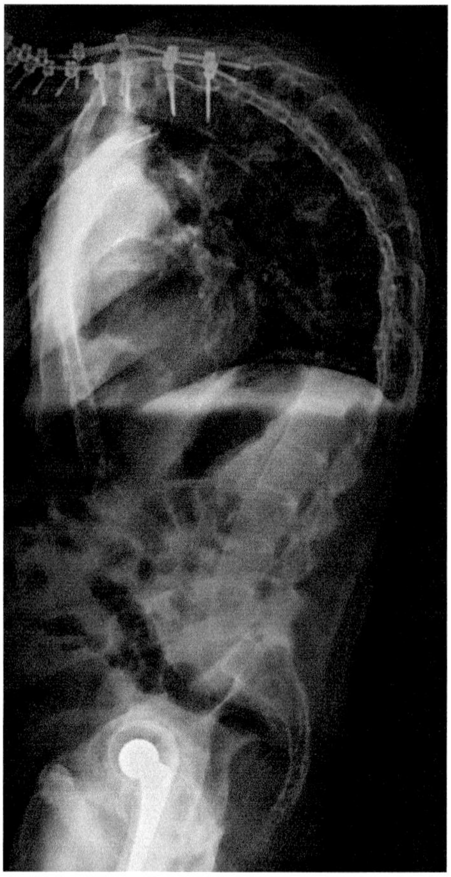

Fig. 7.5 Long, standing scoliosis X-ray film. The images show a global kyphotic deformity due to AS. Patient present with chin-on-chest deformity which impairs forward gaze

7.3 Discussion of the Case

7.3.1 Indications

This patient suffered from a minimal trauma to the neck. Complete ankylosis of the spinal column sk. "bamboo spine" creates a long lever arms that makes the fractures in AS patients extremely unstable. Additional kyphosis with almost chin-on-chest deformity makes external immobilization merely impossible. Patients with AS who sustained fracture due to low-energy

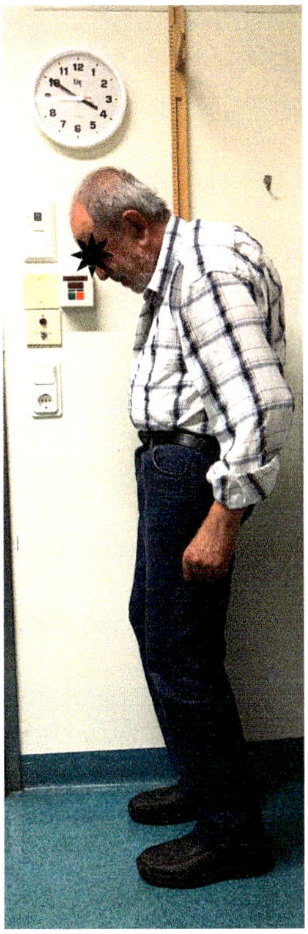

Fig. 7.6 Photography of the patient during the last follow-up. The image confirms a severe global spinal kyphotic deformity

trauma tend to deteriorate neurologically and have high morbidity and mortality rate [2, 3]. This advocates an urgent and aggressive surgical treatment. Although, conservative treatment has been described in the literature usually is reserved to non-displaced fractures without deformity [2].

In this case of a severely displaced, highly unstable fracture with a central cord syndrome (ASIA D) the surgical option was mandatory.

The neurophysiologic surveillance with evoked potentials is recommended because of the risk of displacement of the fracture during positioning and surgery.

7.3.2 Choice of Approach

There are three main approaches to cervical spine: anterior, posterior and combined. In general, there is no single gold standard which approach is the optimal one. Each approach has particular advantages and disadvantages thus, the decision is made on case to case basis. However, the access to CTJ, especially in case of distorted anatomy (tumor, displaced fracture, deformity), is very limited due to position of the sternum and close relationship to major vascular elements as well as lungs and structures of mediastinum. The approach, by itself, can theoretically, enhance the surgical morbidity. The CTJ is a complex anatomical region, where very flexible, lordotic cervical spine shifts into to a rigid, kyphotic thoracic spine. Therefore, surgery in cervical spine in close relationship to cervicothoracic junction (CTJ) requires meticulous surgical planning and a surgical approach that addresses these challenges. Moreover, the biomechanical investigation indicates that anterior stabilization can be insufficient to stabilize the CTJ [4].

On opposite to this, posterior stabilization with long construct crossing CTJ, reinforced with T1 or T2 pedicle screws, provides sufficient stabilization even in a case of multi-segmental failure of anterior column [5]. Clinical studies indicate that a risk for revision due to pseudarthrosis and hardware failure seems to be much higher with short posterior cervical fixations, which don't bridge over CTJ [6, 7].

Posterior instrumented stabilization and fusion is a well-established surgical procedure in cervical spine. It is a valid surgical option for the treatment of a wide variety of cervical pathologies like: cervical spondylotic myelopathy, spinal oncology, fractures, infections and deformities.

Lateral mass fixation is very popular and accepted technique for achieving stabilization and promoting fusion of the subaxial cervical spine [8].

Cervical pedicle screws technique remains controversial because of the potential risk of injuring vertebral arteries. However, cervical pedicle screws have twice as high pull-out resistance and can be particular useful for three column reconstruction, especially in case of cervical deformity or poor bone quality [9, 10]. This can be especially important in case of AS because of high rate of osteoporosis and high instability.

There are several technical issues to be addressed when planning for a long posterior cervical instrumentation:

- most often the CTJ is impossible to visualize with the side fluoroscopy
- surgeon should be familiar with cervical and thoracic junctional anatomy and be experienced in both lateral mass and thoracic pedicle screw instrumentation techniques
- in case of osteoporosis and ankylosis, most cranial instrumentation can be extended as high as to C1 in order to provide the high pull-out resistance
- the rule of thumb is that in case of AS the instrumentation should be extended minimal to 3 segments above and 3 segments below the fracture [3]
- in case of close relationship to CTJ, the instrumentation should always bridge across the junction (especially in case of AS)
- use of the image guidance is advocated especially when planning CTJ instrumentation and/or use of cervical pedicle screw technique [11]
- use of continuous intraoperative neurophysiological surveillance should be mandatory if available

Whether the instrumentation should cross the CTJ can be questioned since there are available studies demonstrating good results with constructs ending at C6 and C7 [12]. Nevertheless, the authors personal opinion is that thoracic instrumentation at T1 and T2 levels does not considerable prolong surgery but creates a solid foundation of the construct and protects the caudal anchorage. Therefore, we suggest that long posterior cervical fixation should not be stopped at CTJ and must always be considered as a valid option if there is a doubt regarding bone quality and instability.

7.3.3 Accordance with the Literature Guidelines

Unfortunately, there is insufficient power of evidence in the current literature to draw conclusions regarding use of long vs short posterior cervical fixations and the most caudal point of anchoring. Therefore, we cannot apply any general guidelines based on these data. However, there is informal agreement on indication for use of long cervical posterior instrumentation as well as the use of this surgical approach in close relation to CTJ.

Level of Evidence: C
Most available studies regarding this matter are larger retrospective single center cohorts and biomechanical cadaver studies. Publication by Truumees et al. [12] is the only cited retrospective multicenter study.

7.4 Conclusions and Take-Home Message

Although use of long posterior cervical fixation can be debatable, it is relatively straightforward technique and can be applied to the various spinal pathologies. It offers a strong and solid fixation but in the same time can be combined with other techniques like: laminectomy, foraminotomy and even osteotomy for corrective purposes.

Common consensus is that anterior column failure should be managed from anterior approach and complete disruption of the cervical column from 360° combined anterior and posterior approach. This can prolong surgical time and enhance surgical trauma. We advocate using only long posterior cervical fixation, which is sufficient to support and protect the cervical column especially when cervical pedicle and upper thoracic pedicle screw fixation has been used.

Pearls

- preoperative investigation with CT scan and MR images, including upper thoracic levels are mandatory
- long posterior cervical fixation constructs can be used as a posterior-only strategy even with multi-segmental failure of the anterior column
- in case of complete disruption of the spinal column at least 3 segments above and below should be instrumented
- CTJ should be crossed with instrumentation on the T1 and T2 pedicles if the pathology is close or embodies the junction
- image guided surgery should be used for cervical pedicle screws at least

Editorial Comment

The author has chosen a non-degenerative case to illustrate the technical principles and especially the potential of such constructs, which can obviously be applied to every other pathology as well. The development of these stable screw-rod constructs enabled surgeons to treat almost every cervical instabilty with a very high reliability regarding strength of instrumentation and versatilty in reducing complex 3D deformities while avoiding the need for any form of postoperative bracing. When cervical pedicle screws are applied the biomechanical properties allow for a posterior only strategy even in severe multicolumn instabilities. The use of navigation is highly recommended for this (see Chap. 18).

References

1. Vaccaro AR, Koerner JD, Radcliff KE, et al. AOSpine subaxial cervical spine injury classification system. Eur Spine J. 2016;25(7):2173–84.
2. Westerveld LA, van Bemmel JC, Dhert WJ, Oner FC, Verlaan JJ. Clinical outcome after traumatic spinal fractures in patients with ankylosing spinal disorders compared with control patients. Spine J. 2014;14(5):729–40.
3. Caron T, Bransford R, Nguyen Q, Agel J, Chapman J, Bellabarba C. Spine fractures in patients with ankylosing spinal disorders. Spine (Phila Pa 1976). 2010;35(11):E458–64.
4. Kirkpatrick JS, Levy JA, Carillo J, Moeini SR. Reconstruction after multilevel corpectomy in the cervical spine. A sagittal plane biomechanical study. Spine (Phila Pa 1976). 1999;24(12):1186–90; discussion 1191.
5. Singh K, Vaccaro AR, Kim J, Lorenz EP, Lim TH, An HS. Biomechanical comparison of cervical spine reconstructive techniques after a multilevel corpectomy of the cervical spine. Spine (Phila Pa 1976). 2003;28(20):2352–8; discussion 2358.
6. Schroeder GD, Kepler CK, Kurd MF, et al. Is it necessary to extend a multilevel posterior cervical decompression and fusion to the upper thoracic spine? Spine (Phila Pa 1976). 2016;41(23):1845–9.
7. Osterhoff G, Ryang YM, von Oelhafen J, Meyer B, Ringel F. Posterior multilevel instrumentation of the lower cervical spine: is bridging the cervicothoracic junction necessary? World Neurosurg. 2017;103:419–23.
8. Yoshihara H, Passias PG, Errico TJ. Screw-related complications in the subaxial cervical spine with the use of lateral mass versus cervical pedicle screws: a systematic review. J Neurosurg Spine. 2013;19(5):614–23.
9. Johnston TL, Karaikovic EE, Lautenschlager EP, Marcu D. Cervical pedicle screws vs. lateral mass screws: uniplanar fatigue analysis and residual pullout strengths. Spine J. 2006;6(6):667–72.
10. Abumi K, Ito M, Sudo H. Reconstruction of the subaxial cervical spine using pedicle screw instrumentation. Spine (Phila Pa 1976). 2012;37(5):E349–56.
11. Ito Y, Sugimoto Y, Tomioka M, Hasegawa Y, Nakago K, Yagata Y. Clinical accuracy of 3D fluoroscopy-assisted cervical pedicle screw insertion. J Neurosurg Spine. 2008;9(5):450–3.
12. Truumees E, Singh D, Geck MJ, Stokes JK. Should long-segment cervical fusions be routinely carried into the thoracic spine? A multicenter analysis. Spine J. 2018;18(5):782–7.

Thoracic Disc Herniation and Myelopathy

8

Bernhard Meyer and Sandro M. Krieg

8.1 Introduction

Thoracic disc herniation is a rare degenerative spine disease which only accounts for about 1% of surgically treated intervertebral disc pathologies [8].

Thus, even experienced spine surgeons only see a very limited number of these cases [5].

Typically, thoracic disc herniations cause a range of different unspecific symptoms and most patients already went through a variety of specialties and diagnostics until the proper diagnosis is made [1]. Its surgical therapy requires experience in indications and knowledge of 360° approaches in order to provide the optimal solution for each individual case.

This chapter will outline the specifics of thoracic disc herniation, its typical symptomatology, mandatory preoperative imaging and surgical approaches. Moreover, the rationale for the different surgical approaches is discussed.

At the end of this chapter the reader should be aware of the problems and pitfalls we face when treating thoracic disc herniation.

The aim of the presented case is therefore to emphasize these potential problems and lack of evidence in the diagnosis and treatment of this disease. Such specifics are:

- prolonged history until diagnosis
- difficult indication for surgery
- complex choice of the proper approach depending on the lesion location, size and consistency
- giant calcified disc as a unique problem

8.2 Case Description

A 71 y/o female patient suffered from thoracic and leg pain over the last years. Her neurological examination and evoked potentials were normal. She was finally referred to a neurologist who ordered a MRI scan. The scan showed a medial giant T8/9 disc causing severe spinal cord compression (Fig. 8.1). The initial CT scan shows calcification (Fig. 8.2).

She was then operated in another center via a posterior approach with instrumentation. An attempt to resect the disc herniation via a posterolateral access failed. The patient was left with a complete paraplegia and some sensory function preserved (ASIA B). In a second surgery on the same day another attempt was made to resect the large calcified disc via an anterolateral, transthoracic approach, again without success and change in neurological status (Fig. 8.3). The patient was referred to a specialized spinal cord injury rehabilitation unit for para- and tetraplegic patients, from which our department was contacted for further evaluation of the case.

B. Meyer · S. M. Krieg (✉)
Department of Neurosurgery, Klinikum rechts der Isar, Technische Universität München, Munich, Germany
e-mail: Sandro.Krieg@tum.de

B. Meyer, M. Rauschmann (eds.), *Spine Surgery*, https://doi.org/10.1007/978-3-319-98875-7_8

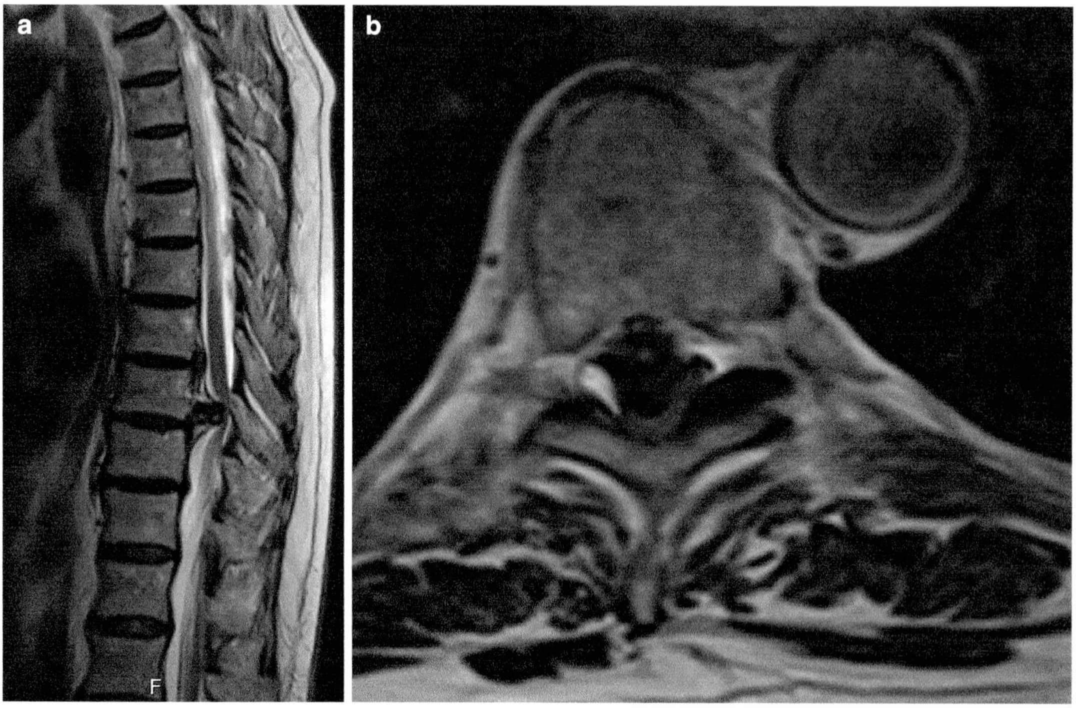

Fig. 8.1 MRI scan on outpatient visit. The MRI scan shows a giant T8/9 disc herniation causing severe ventral spinal cord compression. Sagittal **a** and, axial slices **b**

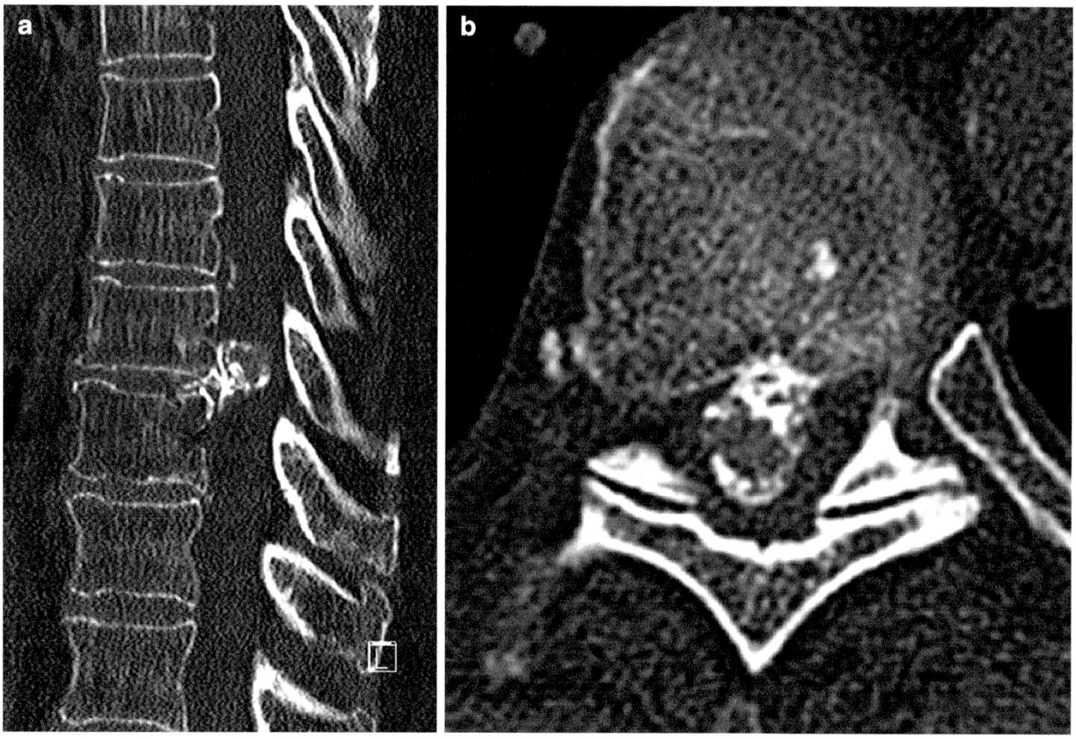

Fig. 8.2 Preoperative CT scan. The CT on sagittal (**a**) and axial (**b**) slices confirms the calcification in the center of the herniated disc as suspected in the MRI scan

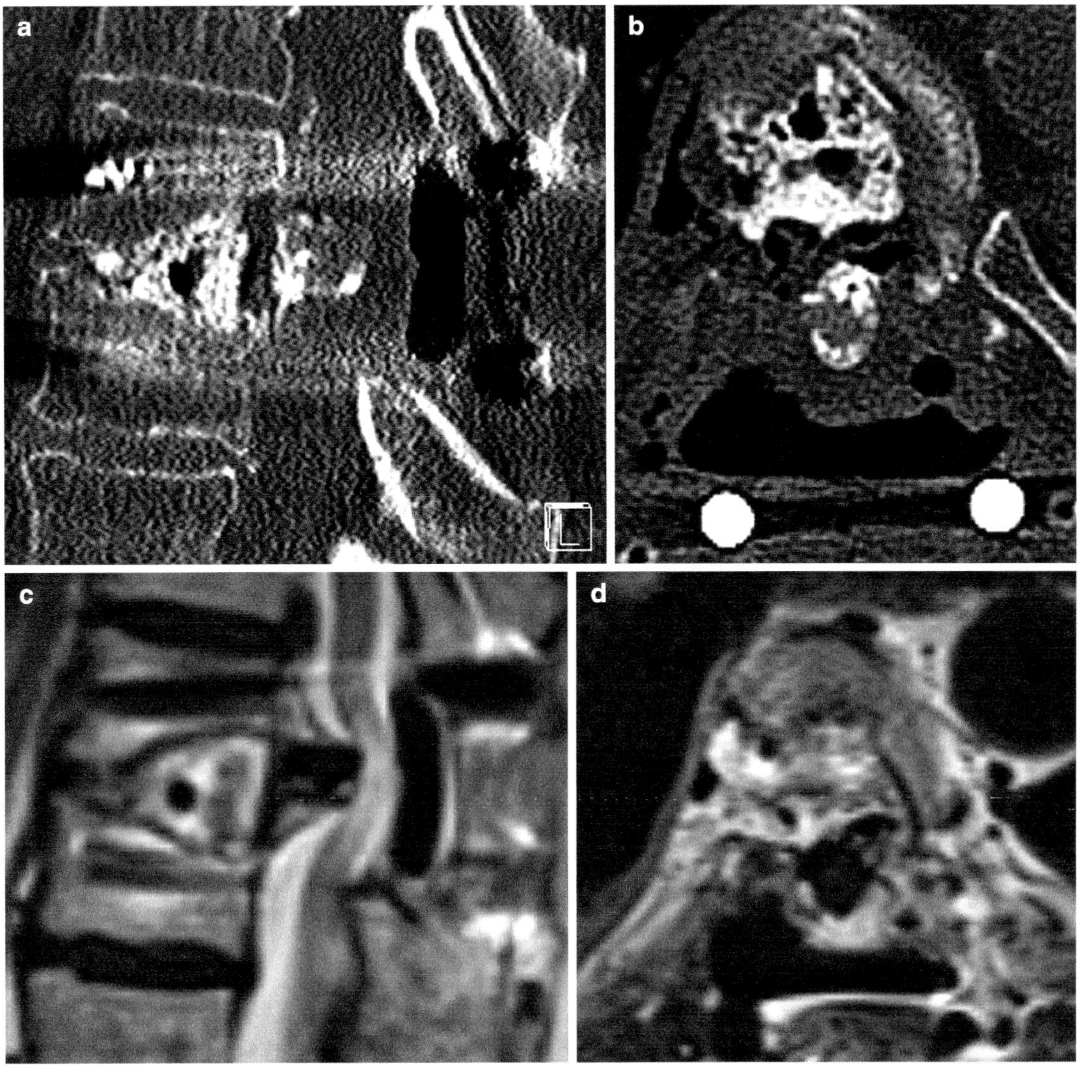

Fig. 8.3 CT and MRI scans after the first surgeries. The CT **a**, **b** still shows the GIANT calcified disc after the initial surgeries. MRI **c**, **d** shows still severe spinal cord compression

Due to the persistent space-occupying effect and small chance of improving the sensory deficit her doctors referred the patient to our department. Physical examination confirmed persisting incomplete spinal cord injury ASIA B at L1. The relative indication for surgery was discussed in detail with the patient and her family. A posterolateral transdural approach was finally chosen to resect the calcified disc (Fig. 8.4).

Surgery went without adverse events and the patient did not show further deterioration. Sufficient decompression was confirmed by postoperative CT scan on the first postoperative day (Fig. 8.5). The patient was transferred back to her rehabilitation unit and has no change in status 3 months after surgery.

8.3 Discussion of the Case

8.3.1 Indication

This patient only suffered from leg and back pain. Evoked potentials were normal as well as her clinical findings. Patients suffering from axial or radicular pain are usually not treated surgi-

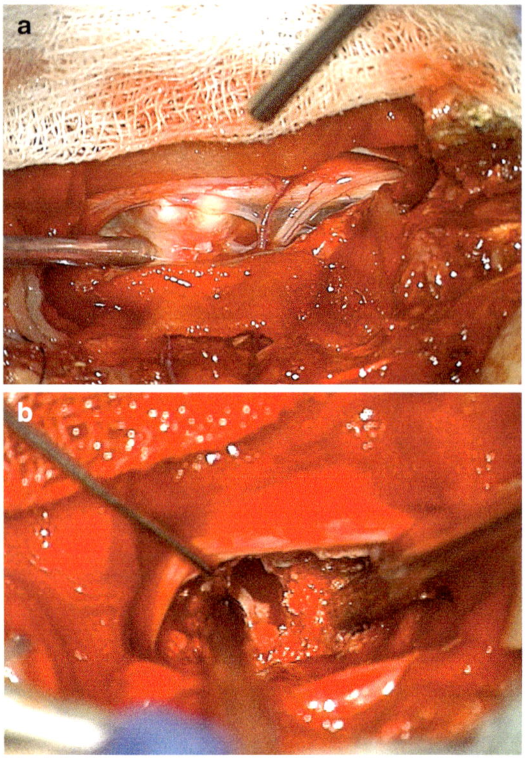

Fig. 8.4 Intraoperative exposure. This intraoperative picture shows the transdural posterolateral exposure of the disc herniation before **a** and after **b** resection. The spinal cord as the structure at risk can be visualized and therefore spared in an optimal way. Cutting the dentate ligaments or even a rootlet releases the spinal cord for careful rotational mobilization

cally. Conservative treatment by steroidal or non-steroidal anti-inflammatory drugs and physical therapy are frequently reported options [8]. Nonetheless, patient with severe complaints that do not improve by conservative therapy can be evaluated for surgery. The decision to operate is mainly influenced by size, localization, and consistency of the prolapse, i.e. a lateral soft prolapse harbors a much lower threshold for surgical treatment, because of a much lower risk profile of the procedure.

In this case of a giant calcified disc, the threshold would however be very high, because the complication rates for the surgical treatment of thoracic disc herniation, being reported to be up to 30% [7, 8].

Hence, there is no evidence whom, when, and how to operate on thoracic disc herniations because no larger series, let alone trials, exist; it is a rare disease. Yet, the natural history of thoracic disc herniation indicates that patients might remain asymptomatic for a long period of time and that it is unlikely that they develop any acute myelopathy [10].

In patients suffering from myelopathy and being diagnosed with a thoracic disc herniation, surgery should be discussed since up to 77% of patients show an improvement of myelopathic symptoms after surgery [7, 9]. In patients without

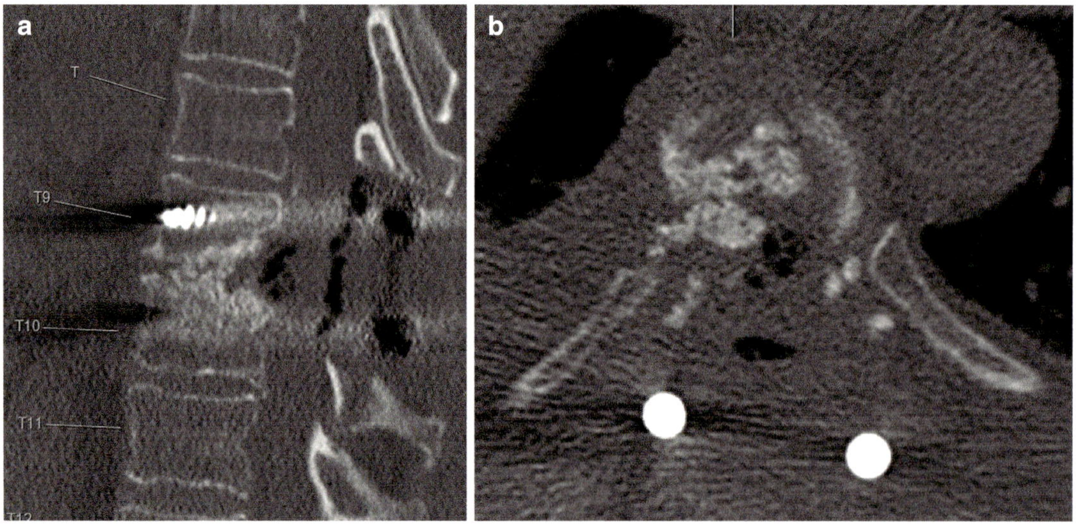

Fig. 8.5 Postoperative CT scan. The postoperative CT scan shows the resection of the calcified herniation on sagittal **a** and axial slices **b**

apparent symptoms, evoked potentials are recommended since these allow for early detection of clinically unapparent myelopathy. However, it is unclear in thoracic myelopathy whether impairment of evoked potentials might then be regarded as an indication for surgery.

8.3.2 Choice of Approach

Despite being a rare disease, there are a variety of reports describing a range of different approaches. In general, there is not one single gold standard approach for thoracic disc herniations and each approach has particular advantages and disadvantages for a given individual case [8]. The only common consensus is that a strictly posterior approach, i.e. a laminectomy is no longer considered an option, because of high risk for neurological injury [1, 4]. In general one can divide the approaches used today into posterolateral and anterolateral ones.

It is further commonly accepted that the former are well suited for lateral and mediolateral disc herniations and eventually for medial ones which are not calcified. [7, 8].

The latter are classically used for calcified larger medial discs, i.e. giant ones like the case described. Potential posterolateral variations are costotransversectomy, transpedicular, and transfacet pedicle-sparing approaches. Anterolateral approaches are transthoracic either endoscopic or mini-open and transpleural or retropleural approaches. For an orphan disease according to these authors a redundancy of minor variations.

A further debatable issue is which patient needs additional instrumented fusion. There is no clear guideline for this and left to the individual surgeon's preference [3, 6].

While some authors advocate for lateral (transfacet/transpedicular) approaches [11], most others agree on the necessity of anterior (transthoracic) approaches in cases of calcified large medial discs [2]. In the majority of articles published, posterolateral approaches are only recommended for soft and lateral calcified herniations.

On the presented case, the literature and our experience are quite clear and speak against laminectomy. A posterolateral approach to resect the lesion is also not considered the best choice nowadays by the majority of peers, since the exposure of the prolapse, especially if calcified is far from being easy and the risk for spinal cord injury is high, as evidenced by the outcome.

Whether an instrumented fusion would have been necessary at all is a matter of debate; to do so before resection of the space-occupying lesion, as it has been done here, is certainly very risky.

The majority of experienced spine surgeons would have used an anterolateral transthoracic approach for resection of this giant calcified disc provided it would have been symptomatic. The default method nowadays would be via a mini-open approach as opposed to an endoscopic one, which has been popular 10–15 years ago. Nowadays the majority of surgeons having used endoscopy have gone back to mini-open for this indication, due to the intrinsic surgical difficulties in handling this type of pathology with very long instruments without adequate 3D vision [7]. Specifically, the tight adherence of this pathology to the dura prohibits smooth and careful handling. As for now the additional use of instrumented fusion is up to the discretion of the surgeon and follows no clear recommendations.

An alternative to the above more commonly accepted solutions for initial surgery in a giant calcified disc would be according to us an initially counterintuitive concept: the posterior transdural approach as described by Coppes et al. in 2012 [3]. It has evoked quite a lot of resistance, but probably just because it is unusual and unknown especially for surgeons not used to treat intradural pathology [5]. However looking at it from a more sober perspective it applies very sound principles known from other fields of surgery, i.e. that the best way to protect a structure during surgery is to visualize it. Further this takes into account that giant calcified discs are probably a different entity than the normal disc and behave in an OPLL-like fashion being very adherent to the dura. In essence, these lesion can be resected similar to a ventrally located intradural meningioma.

8.3.3 Accordance with the Literature Guidelines

As discussed above, guidelines cannot be derived from the literature. However, the indication for treatment as well as the surgical approach were most probably not in accordance with the current common consensus of the majority of peers. Yet the same accounts for the authors´ preferred method.

Level of Evidence: C

The level of evidence available to date is poor by only consisting of larger retrospective single center cohorts. Only one series provides data on retrospective data on multiple centers [9].

Pearls

- the major factors in terms of surgery are calcification, location, and size
- preoperative CT scan of the segment is therefore mandatory
- large calcified cases should be regarded (and treated) as OPLL-like lesions and resected like intradural extramedullary pathologies

8.4 Conclusions and Take Home Message

Although being seen on MRI scans quiet frequently, symptomatic thoracic disc herniation is a very rare disease. These lesions can cause myelopathy or radicular pain and should only be treated when symptomatic. Common consensus is that symptomatic lateral soft disc herniations can be treated rather safely with posterolateral approaches alone. Anterolateral mini open approaches are the most widely used and safest options for large calcified lesions. However, they still have considerable morbidity. Therefore the future surgical treatment of the latter lesions should eventually be regarded in analogy to intradural extramedullary tumors.

References

1. Benson MK, Byrnes DP. The clinical syndromes and surgical treatment of thoracic intervertebral disc prolapse. J Bone Joint Surg Br. 1975;57(4):471–7.
2. Bilsky MH. Transpedicular approach for thoracic disc herniations. Neurosurg Focus. 2000;9(4):e3.
3. Coppes MH, Bakker NA, Metzemaekers JD, Groen RJ. Posterior transdural discectomy: a new approach for the removal of a central thoracic disc herniation. Eur Spine J. 2012;21(4):623–8. https://doi.org/10.1007/s00586-011-1990-4.
4. Logue V. Thoracic intervertebral disc prolapse with spinal cord compression. J Neurol Neurosurg Psychiatry. 1952;15(4):227–41.
5. Mehdian SM. Reviewer's comment concerning. Posterior transdural discectomy: a new approach for the removal of a central thoracic disc herniation. (https://doi.org/10.1007/s00586-011-1990-4 by H.M. Coppes et al.). Eur Spine J. 2012;21(4):629. https://doi.org/10.1007/s00586-011-1999-8.
6. Oppenlander ME, Clark JC, Kalyvas J, Dickman CA. Indications and techniques for spinal instrumentation in thoracic disk surgery. Clin Spine Surg. 2016;29(2):E99–E106. https://doi.org/10.1097/BSD.0000000000000110.
7. Quraishi NA, Khurana A, Tsegaye MM, Boszczyk BM, Mehdian SM. Calcified giant thoracic disc herniations: considerations and treatment strategies. Eur Spine J. 2014;23(Suppl 1):S76–83. https://doi.org/10.1007/s00586-014-3210-5.
8. Stillerman CB, Chen TC, Couldwell WT, Zhang W, Weiss MH. Experience in the surgical management of 82 symptomatic herniated thoracic discs and review of the literature. J Neurosurg. 1998;88(4):623–33. https://doi.org/10.3171/jns.1998.88.4.0623.
9. Uribe JS, Smith WD, Pimenta L, Hartl R, Dakwar E, Modhia UM, et al. Minimally invasive lateral approach for symptomatic thoracic disc herniation: initial multicenter clinical experience. J Neurosurg Spine. 2012;16(3):264–79. https://doi.org/10.3171/2011.10.SPINE11291.
10. Wood KB, Blair JM, Aepple DM, Schendel MJ, Garvey TA, Gundry CR, et al. The natural history of asymptomatic thoracic disc herniations. Spine (Phila Pa 1976). 1997;22(5):525–9; discussion 529–530.
11. Yoshihara H. Surgical treatment for thoracic disc herniation: an update. Spine (Phila Pa 1976). 2014;39(6):E406–12. https://doi.org/10.1097/BRS.0000000000000171.

9 Lumbar Disc Herniation, Nucleo- and Sequesterectomy

Timing and Technique

N. A. van der Gaag and Wouter A. Moojen

9.1 Introduction

The objective of this case is to provide an update based on the current highest level of evidence on several aspects of one the most commonly performed neurosurgical procedures, lumbar disc surgery for sciatica. Using a straightforward case we discuss the following issues: timing of surgery for sciatica, surgical approach of symptomatic disk herniation surgery (tube, transforaminal or microdiscektomy), and technique of removal (nucleo- and sequesterectomy).

9.2 Case Description

A 29-year-old female patient suffered from radiating leg pain for 6 months. The pain originated from the back to the lateral side of the upper left leg, lower leg to the instep. Bending, coughing and sneezing led to aggravation of the complaints. She did not have back pain. Over the months the course of the disease was progressively worse. Her medical history consisted only of asthma. To reduce current complaints of pain she was prescribed paracetamol and opioids. The patient could not fulfill her job as a secretary due to the severeness of the pain. She did not try any other conservative therapy such as physiotherapy.

At examination the straight leg raise test was positive at an angle of 45°. A hypesthesia of dermatome L5 was present, but she had no muscle weakness. Deep-tendon reflexes were not different between left and right side.

Magnetic Resonance Imaging (MRI) demonstrated a hypointense signal intensity of the nucleus pulposus on T2 sagittal images at the level of L4-5 (Fig. 9.1). Disc height was nearly normal without the presence of upper and lower vertebral endplate changes. Within the disc level a clear herniated disc was present. On axial slices the disc protrusion obliterated the left subarticular zone with clear compression of the left L5 root with flattening of the emerging root sheath (Fig. 9.2). All other disc levels had a normal disc contour and signal intensity.

For the duration of symptoms and progressive course surgery was proposed. The patient underwent removal of the symptomatic disk herniation through a minimal unilateral transflaval approach with magnification, with the patient under general anesthesia. An annular

N. A. van der Gaag (✉)
Haaglanden Medical Center, The Hague, The Netherlands

Haga Teaching Hospital, The Hague, The Netherlands
e-mail: n.vandergaag@hagaziekenhuis.nl

W. A. Moojen
Haaglanden Medical Center, The Hague, The Netherlands

Haga Teaching Hospital, The Hague, The Netherlands

Leiden University Medical Center, Leiden, The Netherlands

B. Meyer, M. Rauschmann (eds.), *Spine Surgery*, https://doi.org/10.1007/978-3-319-98875-7_9

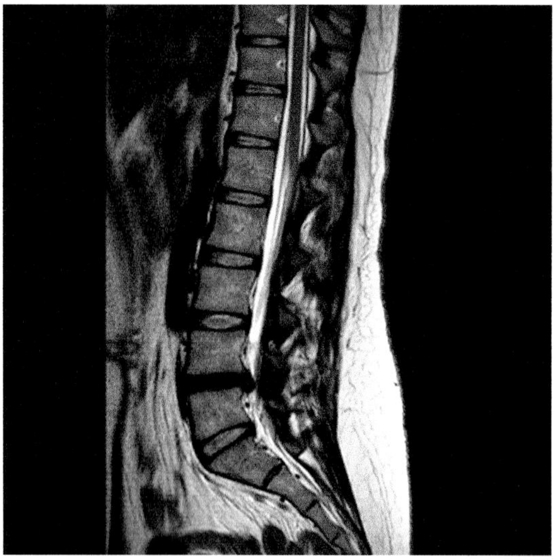

Fig. 9.1 Sagittal T2 sequence of the lumbar spine showing a disc herniation at the level L4-5

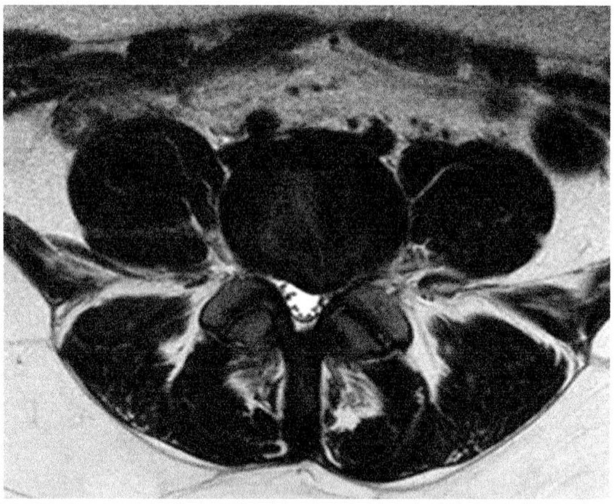

Fig. 9.2 Axial T2 sequence of a cross-section at the level L4-5 showing a paramedian herniated disc with compression of the left L5 root

fenestration was performed with curettage, and removal of loose degenerated disk material from the disk space with the use of a rongeur, without attempting to perform a (sub)total diskectomy.

She was discharged one day after the surgery in good condition. Complaints of pain had nearly completely resolved. At follow-up 2 months later the patient had a full recovery.

9.3 Discussion of the Case

Sciatica is defined as intense leg pain in an area served by one or more spinal nerve roots and can be accompanied by neurological deficit. The most common cause of sciatica is a herniated disc [1]. Lumbar-disk surgery is generally performed for patients with sciatica that does not resolve within 6–8 weeks. From the largest randomized controlled trial (RCT) on the subject it is demonstrated that surgery results in >80% improvement in pain and disability scores in the first weeks after surgery [1]. Early surgery provides relief of symptoms twice as fast compared to patients treated conservatively. However, compared to prolonged conservative care equal outcomes were observed at 1, 2 and even 5 years follow-up in this trial. It should be noted that, despite at least 6 months of conservative treatment, 46% of the conservatively allocated patients were treated surgically for persistent severe leg pain and disability [2]. Therefore, patients should be informed that prolonged conservative care gives them a good chance for resolution of pain and disability in the long run, without the need of a surgical intervention. This strategy carries a fair chance that waiting with pain still ends with surgery. Furthermore, an analysis of predictive factors demonstrated that, compared to patients with lower scores initially, those with more intense leg pain or higher disability scores were at higher risk to undergo delayed surgery.

Although it is generally presumed that late surgery is associated with less effectiveness and a higher chance of unsatisfactory outcome, due to more chronic changes around the disc protrusion or sequester, firm evidence is not (yet) available. From the RCT we found that early surgery resulted in a faster recovery of motor deficit accompanying sciatica compared with prolonged conservative treatment, but the difference was no longer significant during the final follow-up examination at 1 year [3]. Severe motor deficit at baseline (MRC grade 3) was a risk factor for persistent deficit at 1 year. A recent study suggest that immediate surgery resulted in higher recovery for severe paresis

(MRC gr 0–3) compared to delayed surgery [4]. In our presented case surgery was proposed for a 6-month period of pain without improvement without paresis, an example of an individual surgical decision process, complemented by patient preferences.

Magnetic resonance imaging (MRI) is considered the imaging procedure of choice for patients suspected of lumbar herniated discs. Both imaging and clinical findings determine the final decision of surgery. In a MRI study of the Sciatic cohort our group demonstrated that inter-observer agreement was excellent to predict the affected disc level (kappa range 0.81–0.86) and the nerve root (kappa range 0.86–0.89) [5]. However, generally moderate agreement was found regarding the characteristics of the impaired disc level and the herniated disc such as signal intensity of the nucleus pulposus, loss of disc height, absence of epidural fat adjacent to the dural sac or surrounding the nerve root sheath, flattening of the dural sac or the emerging root sheath, and nerve root thickness distal to the site of compression. Although the presented case is quite straightforward these study results prompt for a generally critical attitude towards this information normally enclosed in the radiology report. Therefore, to establish the indication for surgery requires clinical data and observation together with the necessary radiological information as only available to the clinician. Back pain, as discussed in the similar study mentioned above is not a prognostic indicator for good outcome after surgery neither did it correlate with the severeness of nerve rood compression. No significant differences existed in prevalence of Vertebral Endplate Signal Changes (Modic) between sciatica patients with and without disabling back pain (41% vs. 43%, P = 0.70). No significant size differences were seen on preoperative MR images between patients with and without disabling back pain on there. Large disc herniations (size >50% of spinal canal) were observed in an equal percentage (18%) between patients with and without disabling back pain. Also, no significant difference existed in extrusions between patients with and without disabling back pain (64% vs. 67%, P = 0.66).

With the introduction of magnification, the original laminectomy for lumbar-disk surgery as introduced in 1934 was refined into open microdiskectomy, to date the most common procedure. The minimally invasive technique of intralaminar, transmuscular tubular discectomy was introduced in 1997 with the rationale of replacing the conventional subperiosteal muscle dissection by the muscle-splitting transmuscular approach of tubular discectomy. This should lead to less tissue damage, resulting in a faster rate of recovery but with similar long-term outcomes. Patients are expected to have reduced postoperative back pain, thus allowing quicker mobilization and contributing to shorter hospitalization and faster resumption of work and daily activities. In a large multicenter double-blinded (RCT) 167 patients were assigned to tubular discectomy versus 161 patients to conventional microdiskectomy [6]. The primary outcome was functional assessment on the Roland-Morris Disability Questionnaire (RDQ) for sciatica (higher scores indicating worse functional status) at 8 weeks and 1 year after randomization. Secondary outcomes were scores on the visual analog scale (VAS) for leg pain and back pain. At 1 year follow-up statistically significant differences for RDQ and VAS leg and back pain were observed in favor for the conventional microdiskectomy, but the differences did not reach published minimal clinically important differences. However, a 10% higher proportion of patients reported a perceived a good recovery at the final evaluation point of 52 weeks in the conventional microdiskectomy group [79%]. Therefore, the minimally invasive technique of tubular diskectomy seems an attractive surgical method for treating sciatica, but these data do not support a higher rate of recovery when compared with conventional microdiskectomy. Furthermore, the conventional microdiskectomy had far lower recurrence rate (7%) compared with the tubular technique (11%).

The increase in minimally invasive techniques to access the disc or sequestered disc fragment have led to an alternative, transforaminal route, the percutaneous transforaminal endoscopic discectomy (PTED). For this technique a lateral percutaneous technique is used to access the herniated disc through a small working channel that runs through the foramen. A systematic review comparing the conventional microdiskectomy technique with PTED included 3 RCT's and three retrospective studies [7]. With respect to the key outcomes of back pain, leg pain, function and general improvement there was moderate to low quality evidence of no differences PTED and conventional microdiscectomy. This finding was not affected by length of follow-up or inclusion of non-randomised studies. However, the authors concluded that studies comparing PTED with conventional surgery with sufficient sample size and methodological robustness are lacking. In The Netherlands a pragmatic, multicenter, non-inferiority, randomised controlled trial is currently running to determine the effectiveness and cost-effectiveness of PTED versus open microdiscectomy. Until these results become available we consider PTED as an experimental treatment option.

Another aspect of lumbar-disk surgery addresses the technique of removal of disc fragments only, sequestrectomy, or the removal of the disc fragments and disc materials in disc space, in this context called conventional microdiscectomy. Sequestrectomy may be particularly suitable for patients with a small annular defect. A potential disadvantage of sequestrectomy versus conventional discectomy is a higher presumed risk of recurrent disc herniation, potential advantages are more preserved architecture of the spine and less back pain after surgery. A recent systematic review identified 5 studies (746 participants) of sequestrectomy versus microdiscectomy of which one study was a RCT, the other 4 were nonrandomized prospective comparisons [8]. Sequestrectomy and standard microdiscectomy were associated with similar effects on leg and back pain after surgery, and functional outcome. Also complications and recurrence rate within 2 years after surgery were not different. Possibly the sequestrectomy was associated with less postoperative analgesic consumption, with the reservation that all studies were assessed as being at a high risk of bias. The only RCT in this systematic review assessed health-related quality of life (QOL), which found sequestrectomy associated with higher (better) scores QOL scores. The authors suggest for this topic that well-designed randomized trials are needed to further clarify the effects of sequestrectomy versus microdiscectomy in patients in whom sequestrectomy is felt to be indicated. Studies with longer-term follow-up help to determine whether sequestrectomy is associated with an increased risk of recurrent herniation.

9.4 Conclusions and Take Home Message

To conclude, the abovementioned patient was treated with the (to-date) gold standard microdiskectomy technique with sequesterectomy only. PTED treatment is currently considered an experimental treatment option. Literature shows that prolonged conservative treatment is a valid option. Our patient was treated within six months because she initially preferred to treat her radicular pain conservatively. There is no clear scientific proof available which can help us physicians selecting the 'right' patient to go for surgery. Patients should therefore be closely involved to decide for the proper treatment.

Pearls

- early surgery provides relief of symptoms twice as fast compared to patients treated conservatively
- mild paresis (MRC grade 4) is not an indication for immediate surgery, for progressive and severe paresis (MRC grade 0–3) the option might be considered but amount of evidence is restricted
- back pain is not related to the severeness of the nerve root compression neither is

severe back pain prognostic for a good outcome after treatment
- sequestrectomy and standard microdiscectomy are associated with similar effects on leg and back pain after surgery, and functional outcome
- possibly sequestrectomy is associated with less postoperative analgesic consumption, with the reservation that available studies were considered high risk of bias
- tubular microdiskectomy is associated with a higher recurrence rate compared with conventional microdiskectomy and less treatment satisfaction
- PTED is an experimental option

Editorial Comment

This chapter summarizes in an excellent and sober fashion the state of the art knowledge regarding lumbar disc herniations in the year 2019. We strongly recommend to apply this knowledge outlined here in the counselling of patients with this common disease, especially because the level of evidence is extraordinarily high.

References

1. Peul WC, van Houwelingen HC, van den Hout WB, Brand R, Eekhof JA, Tans JT, Thomeer RT, Koes BW. Surgery versus prolonged conservative treatment for sciatica. N Engl J Med. 2007;356(22):2245–56.
2. Lequin MB, Verbaan D, Jacobs WC, Brand R, Bouma GJ, Vandertop WP, Peul WC, Leiden-The Hague Spine Intervention Prognostic Study Group, Peul WC, Koes BW, Thomeer RTWM, van den Hout WB, Brand R. Surgery versus prolonged conservative treatment for sciatica: 5-year results of a randomised controlled trial. BMJ Open. 2013;3(5):e002534.
3. Overdevest GM, Vleggeert-Lankamp CL, Jacobs WC, Brand R, Koes BW, Peul WC. Recovery of motor deficit accompanying sciatica--subgroup analysis of a randomized controlled trial. Spine J. 2014;14(9):1817–24. https://doi.org/10.1016/j.spinee.2013.07.456. Epub 2013 Nov 5.
4. Petr O, Glodny B, Brawanski K, Kerschbaumer J, Freyschlag C, Pinggera D, Rehwald R, Hartmann S, Ortler M, Thomé C. Immediate versus delayed surgical treatment of lumbar disc herniation for acute motor deficits: the impact of surgical timing on functional outcome. Spine (Phila Pa 1976). 2017. (Publish ahead of print)
5. EL Barzouhi A, Vleggeert-Lankamp CL, Lycklama À Nijeholt GJ, Van der Kallen BF, van den Hout WB, Verwoerd AJ, Koes BW, Peul WC. Magnetic resonance imaging interpretation in patients with sciatica who are potential candidates for lumbar disc surgery. Paul F, editor. PLoS One 2013;8(7):e68411–11.
6. Arts MP, Brand R, van den Akker ME, Koes BW, Bartels RH, Peul WC. Tubular diskectomy vs conventional microdiskectomy for sciatica: a randomized controlled trial. JAMA. 2009;302(2):149–58.
7. Kamper SJ, Ostelo RW, Rubinstein SM, Nellensteijn JM, Peul WC, Arts MP, van Tulder MW. Minimally invasive surgery for lumbar disc herniation: a systematic review and meta-analysis. Eur Spine J. 2014;23(5):1021–43.
8. Azarhomayoun A, Chou R, Shirdel S, Lakeh MM, Vaccaro AR, Rahimi-Movaghar V. Sequestrectomy versus conventional microdiscectomy for the treatment of a lumbar disc herniation: a systematic review. Spine (Phila Pa 1976). 2015;40(24):E1330–9.

10 Lumbar Spinal Stenosis Requiring Decompression and Fusion

Ioannis Magras, Alkinoos Athanasiou, and Vasiliki Magra

10.1 Introduction

Stenosis due to lumbar degenerative disease is a common condition associated with the aging process that can eventually cause compression of the neural elements in the lumbar canal [1]. The degenerative process is considered a reaction to pathological hypermobility that induces instability of the spine [2]. Conservative treatment is always considered the first line of approach but in certain cases, symptomatology persists, especially when it is partially due to the instability itself [2]. In cases where decision for operative treatment is made, then decompression alone is not always enough as it can deteriorate the balance of the lumbar spine, worsen listhesis if present and cause kyphoscoliosis [3]. This is the point of interest for lumbar instrumentation and fusion.

Although a lot of surgeons have increased the use of materials in lumbar degenerative disease and stenosis, performing fusion with screws and rods, the decision to fuse is not always applied consistently to cases where fusion is indicated [4]. Recent literature has limited the potential use of fusion material to cases that there is documented need for fusion and suggests differentiating them from cases that fusion can be omitted [5]. The reasons for this tendency lie not only with cost effectiveness and reduced morbidity but also with a series of publications that support no difference in outcomes when fusion is routinely performed [3, 6]. In reality, there are cases that show a documented need for fusion and those cases should be analyzed separately. While expert discussion has not yet clarified the exact indications for fusion treatment of lumbar degenerative disease, experience and recent evidence can help drawing solid conclusions at least on a case by case basis.

With this case, we would like to illustrate an overview of such important decision-making problems when treating lumbar stenosis and considering fusion for instability. We briefly present the ongoing discussion on the indications and the evidence in favor of fusion in cases where instability is manifest.

10.2 Case Description

Our case regards a 78-yo female patient, who presented at our department with neurological claudication for at least 12 months. During the neurological examination we performed, no neurological deficit was present. The patient was evaluated with lumbar x-rays (Fig. 10.1) and

I. Magras (✉) · A. Athanasiou
First Department of Neurosurgery, AHEPA University General Hospital, Aristotle University of Thessaloniki, Thessaloniki, Greece

V. Magra
Plastic Surgery Department, Lister Hospital, East & North Hertfordshire NHS Trust, Hertfordshire, UK

B. Meyer, M. Rauschmann (eds.), *Spine Surgery*, https://doi.org/10.1007/978-3-319-98875-7_10

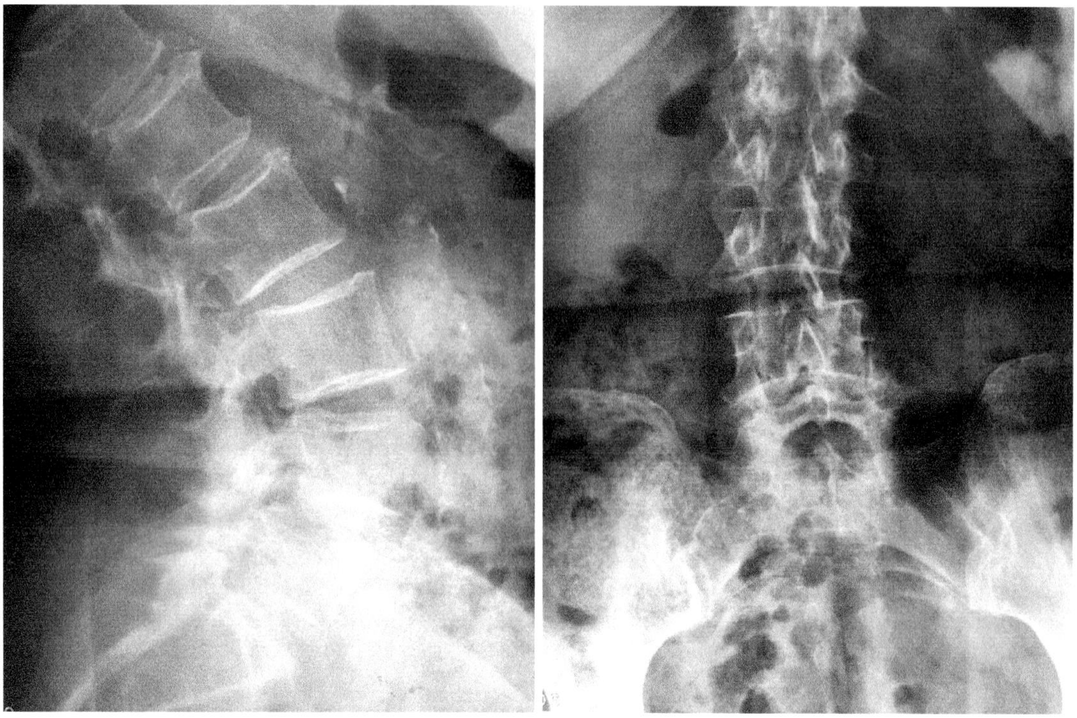

Fig. 10.1 Pre-op x-rays

MRI scan (Fig. 10.2). The pre-op x-rays revealed lumbar olisthesis at the level L4-L5 (Fig. 10.1). MRI scan illustrated severe stenosis due to hypertrophy of the ligamentum flavum and mild bulging of the disc at the L4-L5 level and also evidence of lumbar olisthesis at L4-L5 (Fig. 10.2).

The patient was operated using a laminectomy of L4, flavectomy and due to instability that was checked intraoperatively, also fusion L4-L5 with screws and rods. Although from the MRI scan there was an impression of disc fragment, no disc material was found at this level. Instead severe hypertrophy of the ligamentum flavum was detected descending bilaterally to the sac. After the flavectomy, both L5 nerve roots and the sac were decompressed. Post-operatively the patient gradually recovered and she was ambulatory without presenting claudication. At the routine post-op x-ray no further olisthesis was detected and the instrumentation material were properly placed (Fig. 10.3).

10.3 Discussion of the Case

Due to severe stenosis with instability, that was also checked by visual inspection of segmental mobility during the operation, the treatment decision was in favor of performing decompression with short segment fixation using pedicle screws and rods. Relevant literature has demonstrated that decompression while preserving facets minimizes the risk of postoperative instability and slip progression [7] but in cases where instrumentation is performed for fusion of the segment, then laminectomy can also be considered. In our case, laminectomy was a viable technique to offer decompression without causing further instability, as stabilization of the posterior elements at the L4-L5 would be offered by the instrumentation materials. Since no disc material was found at the level of laminectomy, no discectomy was performed.

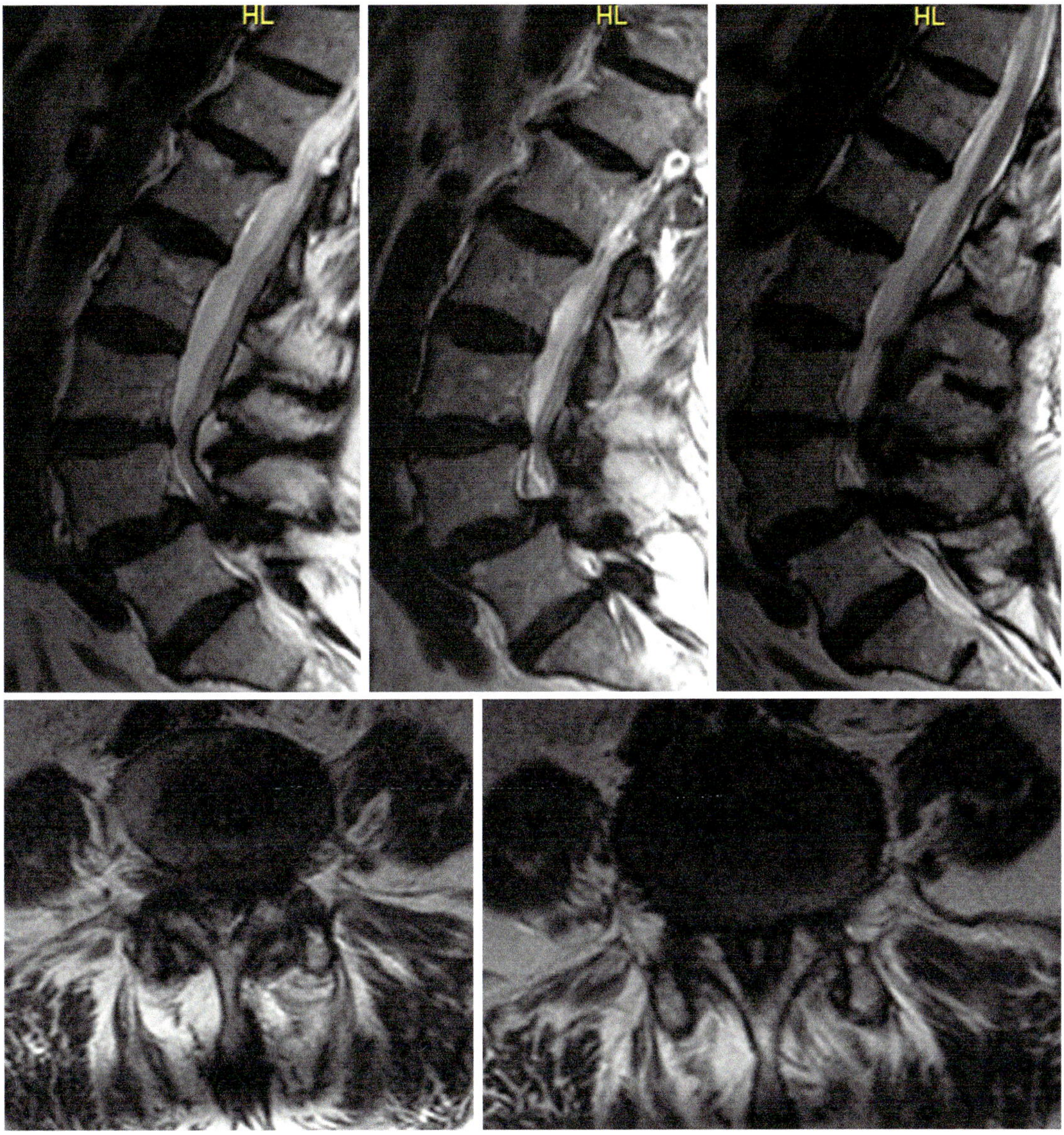

Fig. 10.2 Pre-op lumbar MRI imaging

Indeed stenosis due to degenerative disease has been argued that is caused by segmental instability [2]. Many authors suggest fusion when there is evidence of such instability, including spondilolisthesis of high degree, segmental pathological hypermobility or pain associated with the instability [8]. In cases where fusion is needed, routine 360° should avoided if possible, when the intevertebral disc is checked radiographically and intraoperatively to be relatively healthy. Evermore, it should be noted that currently there is an ongoing discussion on whether routine anterior column fusion produces superior results when the disc is healthy [9]. Nonetheless, iatrogenic hypolordosis can cause severe biomechanical sequelae and preservation of the "nor-

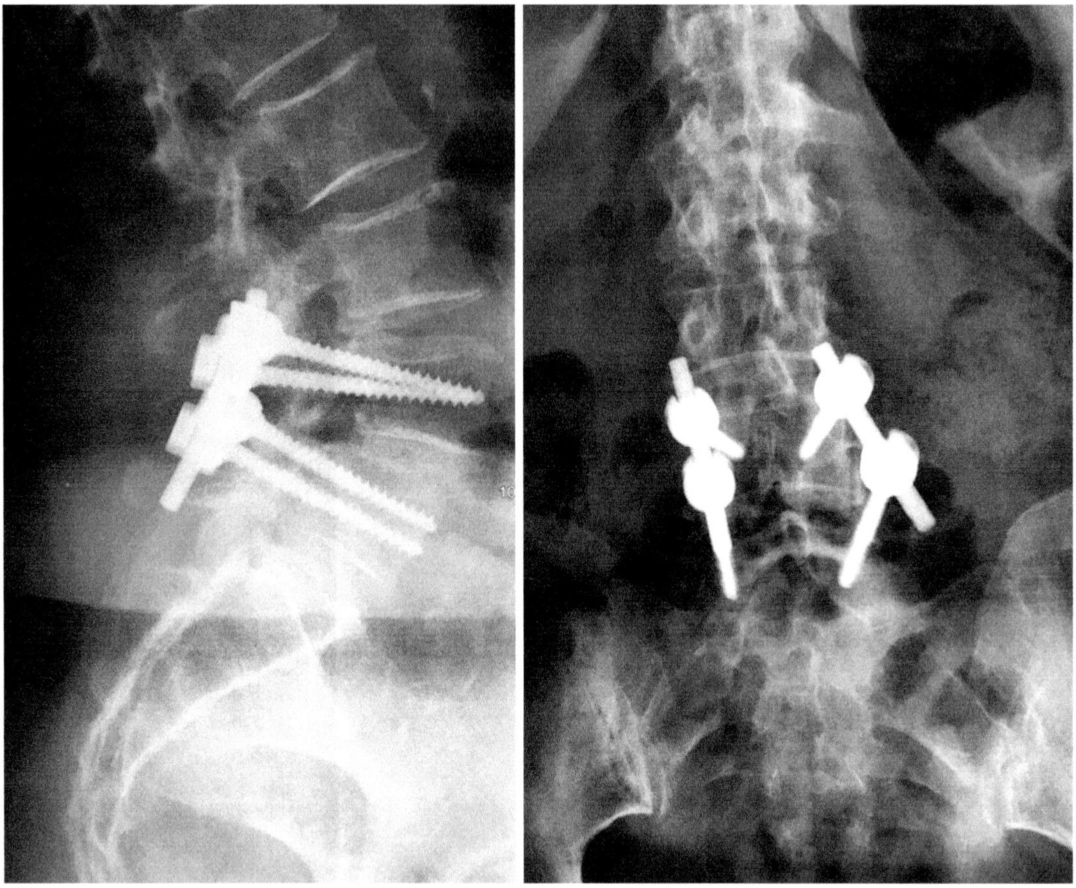

Fig. 10.3 Post-op lumbar x-ray

mal" sagittal balance parameters should be taken into account, especially in longer segment fusion operations [10]. In such cases, discectomy in moderately affected discs could be considered in order to perform ALIFF or TLIFF/PLIFF surgery, according to the angulation needed [9].

Fusion and instrumentation are important tools in the spine surgeons' arsenal and when applied carefully, under expertise and an evidence-based approach, they can offer clinical benefit to the patient. Recent literature suggests that the need for fusion should be evaluated on a case by case basis, taking into account manifestations of instability (serious spondylolisthesis, disruption of sagital balance, pathological hypermobility) and individual patient differences and needs [11].

10.4 Conclusions and Take Home Message

- When decompression alone is performed, preservation of the facet joints leads to better outcome and minimally invasive surgical techniques can be performed.
- If there is evidence for instability then fusion should be considered.
- When fusion is needed then wide laminectomy can be performed.

Pearls

- Pathological instability is the main indication for fusion
- Watch for clinical evidence of instability
- Fusion allows for wider decompression
- Check sagital balance parameters
- Evaluate for 360° fusion, do not perform routinely

Editorial Comment

The authors had the task to elaborate on a common, important and controversial topic, i.e. when to fuse or not in patients with spinal stenosis plus/minus low grade spondylolisthesis. The new level one evidence available in [3, 6] are somewhat game-changing for patients without clear instabilities in the sense that "if in doubt, do less" is the favourable approach. In a nutshell there is no difference in the rate of reoperation rates whether you fuse or not, but simple decompression is the faster and safer initial procedure.

References

1. Covaro A, Vilà-Canet G, de Frutos AG, et al. Management of degenerative lumbar spinal stenosis: an evidence-based review. EFORT Open Rev. 2017;1(7):267–74. https://doi.org/10.1302/2058-5241.1.000030.
2. Thomé C, Börm W, Meyer F. Degenerative lumbar spinal stenosis: current strategies in diagnosis and treatment. Dtsch Arztebl Int. 2008;105(20):373–9. https://doi.org/10.3238/arztebl.2008.0373.
3. Försth P, Ólafsson G, Carlsson T, et al. A randomized, controlled trial of fusion surgery for lumbar spinal stenosis. N Engl J Med. 374(15):1413–23. https://doi.org/10.1056/NEJMoa1513721.
4. Willems PC, Staal JB, Walenkamp GH, et al. Spinal fusion for chronic low back pain: systematic review on the accuracy of tests for patient selection. Spine J. 2013;13(2):99–109.
5. Kalff R, Ewald C, Waschke A, et al. Degenerative lumbar spinal stenosis in older people: current treatment options. Dtsch Arztebl Int. 2013;110(37):613–23 quiz 624. https://doi.org/10.3238/arztebl.2013.0613.
6. Ghogawala Z, Dziura J, Butler WE, et al. Laminectomy plus fusion versus laminectomy alone for lumbar spondylolisthesis. N Engl J Med. 2016;374(15):1424–34. https://doi.org/10.1056/NEJMoa1508788.
7. Rompe JD, Eysel P, Zöllner J, et al. Degenerative lumbar spinal stenosis. Long-term results after undercutting decompression compared with decompressive laminectomy alone or with instrumented fusion. Neurosurg Rev. 1999;22(2–3):102–6.
8. Resnick DK, Choudhri TF, Dailey AT, et al. Guidelines for the performance of fusion procedures for degenerative disease of the lumbar spine. Part 10: fusion following decompression in patients with stenosis without spondylolisthesis. J Neurosurg Spine. 2005;2(6):686–91.
9. Afathi M, Zairi F, Devos P, et al. Anterior lumbar sagittal alignment after anterior or lateral interbody fusion. Orthop Traumatol Surg Res. 2017;103(8):1245–50. https://doi.org/10.1016/j.otsr.2017.09.014.
10. Umehara S, Zindrick MR, Patwardhan AG, et al. The biomechanical effect of postoperative hypolordosis in instrumented lumbar fusion on instrumented and adjacent spinal segments. Spine (Phila Pa 1976). 2000;25(13):1617–24.
11. Watters WC 3rd, Bono CM, Gilbert TJ, et al. An evidence-based clinical guideline for the diagnosis and treatment of degenerative lumbar spondylolisthesis. Spine J. 2009;9(7):609–14. https://doi.org/10.1016/j.spinee.2009.03.016.

Lumbar Spinal Stenosis

11

Ioannis Magras, Alkinoos Athanasiou, and Vasiliki Magra

11.1 Introduction

Stenosis due to lumbar degenerative disease is a common condition associated with the aging process that can eventually cause compression of the neural elements in the lumbar canal [1]. Although lumbar stenosis does not always become symptomatic, symptoms may vary from focal pain to sciatica and neurogenic claudication [2]. When conservative therapy fails, decompression surgery is required for treatment and alleviation of the symptoms. Wide laminectomy, once a the standard approach for stenosis cases, has steadily been giving ground to more minimal procedures, such as fenestration and undercutting, that provide decompression while preserving bone structures and reduce morbidity and iatrogenic complications [3].

During the last two decades, a lot of spine surgeons became more familiar with instrumentation techniques and materials and subsequently increased the use of both for the treatment of lumbar degenerative disease/stenosis. Performing fixation with screws and rods at various lengths became a widely popular tool among spine surgeons and can now be even considered among the basic techniques of the craft [4].

Recent articles have attempted to limit the potential use of fusion materials, investigating outcomes and complications related to this practice and trying to set more concrete indications for the implementation of instrumentation [5].

Nowadays, an ongoing discussion, one where expert opinions clash more often than not, is held regarding the optimal treatment of patients with lumbar stenosis. Although this discussion is considered yet unresolved, accumulated experience and recent evidence can help drawing solid conclusions in many cases [6].

With this case, we would like to illustrate an overview of such important decision-making problems when treating lumbar stenosis. Those pertain to several questions on decompression, implementation of fusion/stabilization (or not) and the type thereof, as well as the indications of each approach. Regarding decompression one should always consider the benefits and drawbacks of each type (undercutting in our case), the need for discectomy and the absolute requirement to avoid causing further instability.

11.2 Case Description

Our case regards an 83-yo female patient, complaining of neurological claudication for 12 months who presented to our department with severe bilateral

I. Magras (✉) · A. Athanasiou
First Department of Neurosurgery, AHEPA University General Hospital, Aristotle University of Thessaloniki, Thessaloniki, Greece

V. Magra
Plastic Surgery Department, Lister Hospital, East & North Hertfordshire NHS Trust, Hertfordshire, UK

B. Meyer, M. Rauschmann (eds.), *Spine Surgery*, https://doi.org/10.1007/978-3-319-98875-7_11

paresis of L5 nerve roots since four weeks. Muscle strength of extensor hallucis longus and tibialis anterior was examined at 3/5 bilaterally while no sensory deficit was present. She was investigated with flexion-extension lumbar x-rays (Fig. 11.1) and an lumbar spine MRI scan (Fig. 11.2). The imaging revealed lumbar degenerative disease causing severe stenosis at the L4-L5 due to hypertrophy of the ligamentum flavum and mild bulging of the disc at the L5-S1 level (Fig. 11.2). The imaging also revealed 1st degree olisthesis at the level L4-L5 that remained unchanged in flexion and extention x-rays (Fig. 11.1).

The patient was operated using an undercutting technique and bilateral flavectomy at the level L4-L5 without performing short-segmental fusion. No disc material fragments were found so no discectomy was performed either. Immediatelly post-operatively the patient presented an almost complete neurological recovery. Examination of the affected muscles revealed a muscle strenght of 4/5 at the left side and 5/5 at the right side. At the routine post-op x-ray no further olisthesis was detected (Fig. 11.3).

11.3 Discussion of the Case

Severe motor weakness is an uncommon symptom of lumbar stenosis [7, 8]. Our decision for treatment was based on the following factors: (a) the patient's advanced age (83 y.o.) and osteoporosis, (b) the low degree of olisthesis that remained unchanged in flexion and extention x-ray imaging. Relevant literature has demonstrated that in older patients decompression while preserving facets, without fusion, minimizes the risk of postoperative instability and slip progression and also reduces morbidity associated with instrumentation.

Less invasive techniques are preferred over laminectomy since they are usually successful in adequately decompressing the neural elements that are stenosed due to hypertrophy of the ligamentum flavum and joint facets. Along these lines, undercutting technique has been shown to produce sufficient decompression and facet preservation. Moreover, although stenosis is evident of segmental instability [9], the extensive degenerative process itself has been shown to prevent

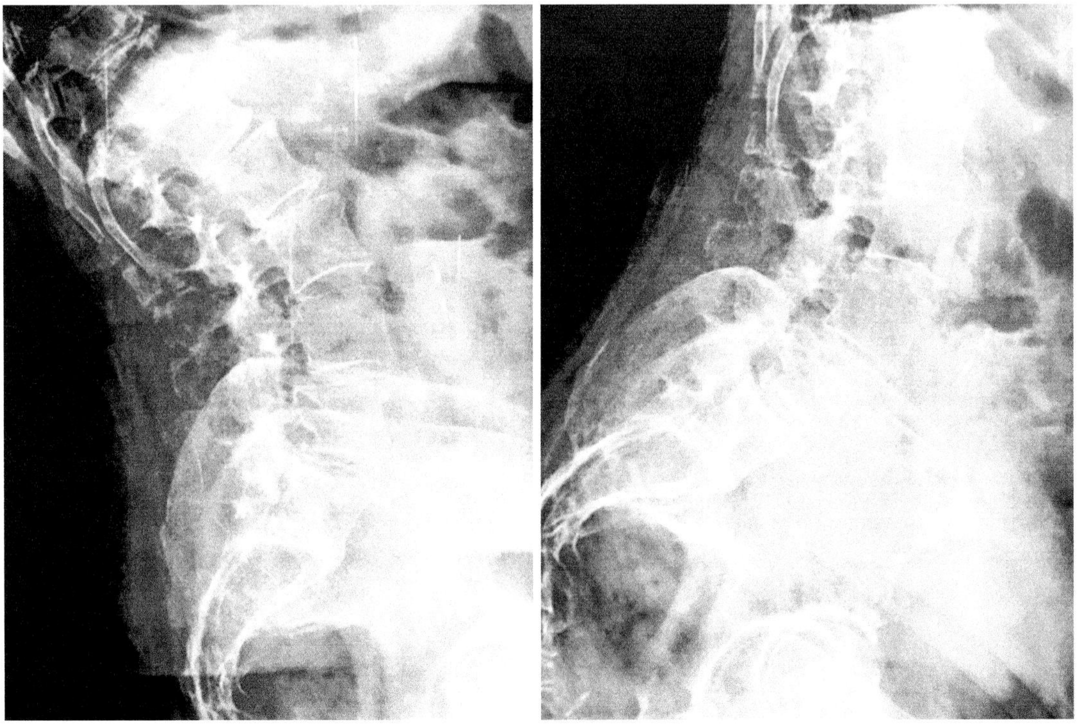

Fig. 11.1 Pre-op flexion-extension lumbar x-rays

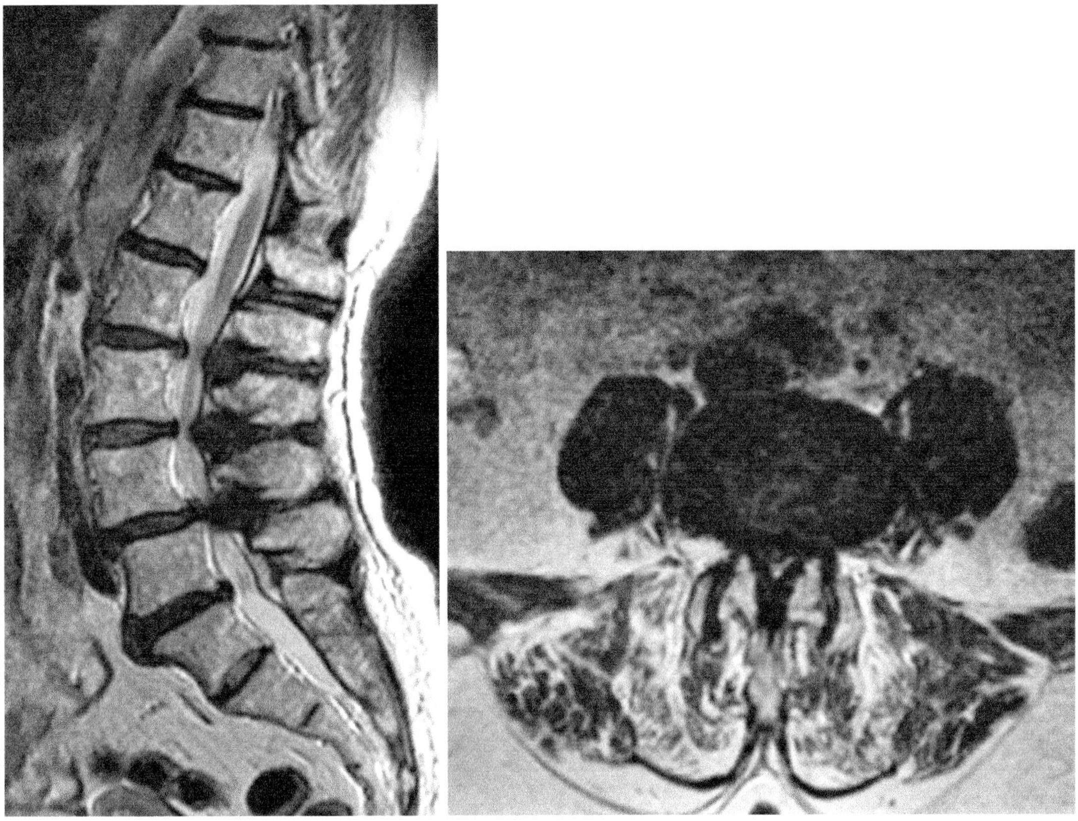

Fig. 11.2 Pre-op lumbar MRI imaging

progression of instability (increasing olisthesis in flexion/extention). Therefore, routine use of instrumentation, that is associated with moderate risk of added morbidity, does not always provide benefits over decompression alone and should not be performed without evidence of definite need for stabilization. Instead, recent literature suggests that the need for fusion should be evaluated on a case by case basis, taking into account manifestetions of instability (serious spondylolisthesis, disruption of saggital balance, pathological hypermobility) and individual patient differences and needs [10]. Thomé et al. [9] suggested a treatment algorithm for lumbar spinal stenosis that as a first general rule acknowledges indication for surgery in consistent clinical and radiological findings after three months of adequate conservative therapeutic treatment. Moreover, existing evidence-based clinical guidelines should be applied into clinical practice as they are helpful, and often mandatory, tools that help spine surgeons provide the best available treatment to lumbar spinal stenosis patients [10].

11.4 Conclusions and Take Home Message

- In patients with spinal stenosis and severe neurological deficits an adequate decompression is recommended.
- Undercutting provides excellent decompression without aggravating instability in most cases.
- If there is no disc protrusion no discectomy is necessary.
- If there is no severe instability in flexion-extension plain radiograph, fusion can be avoided initially in most patients.

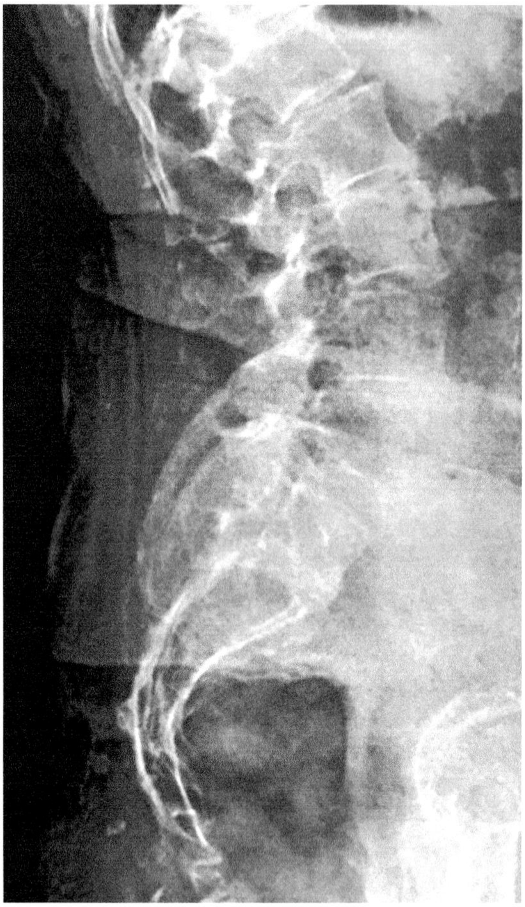

Fig. 11.3 Post-op lumbar x-ray

Pearls

- Stenosis in imaging and clinical findings should match
- Routine fusion should be avoided
- Decompression should not cause instability
- Preserve facets, consider undercutting technique

Editorial Comment

This chapter complements the arguments used in chapter 10. The principle "if in doubt, do less" was applied here and no fusion used. The question whether a less invasive decompression technique truly reduces the incidence of symptomatic iatrogenic instabilities is somewhat questioned by the editors, although it id often propagated by "experts". Nevertheless, unilateral laminotomy and undercutting is considered the best standard by us in the year 2019.

References

1. Covaro A, Vilà-Canet G, de Frutos AG, et al. Management of degenerative lumbar spinal stenosis: an evidence-based review. EFORT Open Rev. 2017;1(7):267–74. https://doi.org/10.1302/2058-5241.1.000030.
2. Kalff R, Ewald C, Waschke A, et al. Degenerative lumbar spinal stenosis in older people: current treatment options. Dtsch Arztebl Int. 2013;110(37):613–23 quiz 624. https://doi.org/10.3238/arztebl.2013.0613.
3. Rompe JD, Eysel P, Zöllner J, et al. Degenerative lumbar spinal stenosis. Long-term results after undercutting decompression compared with decompressive laminectomy alone or with instrumented fusion. Neurosurg Rev. 1999;22(2–3):102–6.
4. Resnick DK, Choudhri TF, Dailey AT, et al. Guidelines for the performance of fusion procedures for degenerative disease of the lumbar spine. Part 10: fusion following decompression in patients with stenosis without spondylolisthesis. J Neurosurg Spine. 2005;2(6):686–91.
5. Ghogawala Z, Dziura J, Butler WE, et al. Laminectomy plus fusion versus laminectomy alone for lumbar spondylolisthesis. N Engl J Med. 2016;374(15):1424–34. https://doi.org/10.1056/NEJMoa1508788.
6. Försth P, Ólafsson G, Carlsson T, et al. A randomized, controlled trial of fusion surgery for lumbar spinal stenosis. N Engl J Med. 2016;374(15):1413–23. https://doi.org/10.1056/NEJMoa1513721.
7. Guigui P, Delecourt C, Delhoume J, et al. Severe motor weakness associated with lumbar spinal stenosis. A retrospective study of a series of 61 patients. Rev Chir Orthop Reparatrice Appar Mot. 1997;83(7):622–8. [Article in French].
8. Jönsson B, Strömqvist B. Motor affliction of the L5 nerve root in lumbar nerve root compression syndromes. Spine (Phila Pa 1976). 1995;20(18):2012–5.
9. Thomé C, Börm W, Meyer F. Degenerative lumbar spinal stenosis: current strategies in diagnosis and treatment. Dtsch Arztebl Int. 2008;105(20):373–9. https://doi.org/10.3238/arztebl.2008.0373.
10. Watters WC 3rd, Bono CM, Gilbert TJ, et al. An evidence-based clinical guideline for the diagnosis and treatment of degenerative lumbar spondylolisthesis. Spine J. 2009;9(7):609–14. https://doi.org/10.1016/j.spinee.2009.03.016.

12 Degenerative Spondylolisthesis

Juan D. Patino and Jesús Lafuente

12.1 Introduction

Spondylolisthesis is described as the anterior translation of one vertebral body over another adjacent vertebra in the absence of a defect of the pars interarticularis. Patients with this condition can remain asymptomatic with only occasional back pain; chronic low back pain with or without radicular symptoms; radicular symptoms with or without neurologic deficit; and intermittent neurogenic claudication [1]. This condition can severely restrict function, walking ability, and quality of life.

Classification of spondylolisthesis is based in several features. Etiology of this condition is variated ranging from dysplastic anterolisthesis (type 1) resulting from congenital abnormalities. Isthmic anterolisthesis (type 2) caused by a defect in the pars interarticularis. Degenerative anterolisthesis (type 3) which develops as a result of degenerative changes of aging, such as intervertebral disc degeneration, ligamentous hypertrophy or buckling, and osteophyte proliferation. Traumatic anterolisthesis (type 4) resulting from acute fractures. Pathologic anterolisthesis (type 5) caused by either infection or a malignancy. Iatrogenic (type 6) due to complications after surgery [2]. Meyerding's classification, perhaps the most used in practice takes into account the degree of the displacement measured as percentage of the width of the vertebral body. Grade I (0–25%) and II (25–50%) are commonly seen in general practice, meanwhile grade III (50–75%), IV (75–100%), and V (greater than 100%) are less common.

Surgical treatment is offered to those patients with symptomatic spondylolisthesis who fail nonoperative treatment measures such as physical therapy and epidural steroid injections. Surgical techniques are variated, for those patients who do have spondylolisthesis and who also have significant mechanical back pain lumbar decompression with or without fusion may be offered [3]. An interesting topic is the relation between spondylolisthesis and lumbar stenosis, recently, conflicting studies have been published on the efficacy of decompression alone versus decompression with fusion [4, 5].

We present a prototypic case of a 65-year-old female patient with spondylolisthesis and radicular pain, which enlightens the common clinical features of this disease, she was treated with a combination of anterior/posterior fusion and left foramen decompression. Since this condition is very common, the purpose of this case is to

J. D. Patino
Neurosurgery Department,
Hospital de la Santa Creu i Sant Pau,
Barcelona, Spain

J. Lafuente (✉)
Servicio de Neurocirugía, Hospital del Mar,
Universidad de Barcelona, Barcelona, Spain

B. Meyer, M. Rauschmann (eds.), *Spine Surgery*, https://doi.org/10.1007/978-3-319-98875-7_12

highlight the general characteristics and nuances that can be found in daily neurosurgical practice with special emphasis on the modalities of treatment.

12.2 Case Description

A 65-year-old woman with no relevant past medical history presented in our department with low lumbar and bilateral radicular pain from approximately one year. After being treated with analgesics and injections no improvement was detected. The pain branched from the lower lumbar back through the hips and buttocks, and down each leg predominantly on the left side. Physical examination showed sciatic pain in the left side when leg was flexed at 45° (Lasègue sign), no motor or sensitivity deficits at lower extremities were detected with preservation of tone and reflexes.

A lumbar magnetic resonance imaging (MRI) showed a L4 degenerative anterolisthesis over L5 grade I associated with foraminal stenosis on the left side and bilateral facet subluxation (Fig. 12.1). Functional flexion/extension X-rays demonstrated increased listhesis at L4-L5 level within grade I range (Fig. 12.2). Finally, a computer tomography scan (CT-scan) completed the study which confirms the presence of the spondylolisthesis and the bilateral facet arthrosis (Fig. 12.3).

We perform a transforaminal lumbar interbody fusion (TLIF) in L4-L5 vertebrae level, using four transpedicular screws and one interbody cage with autologous bone graft, in order to perform maximum stability and fusion rate. Instrumentation was carried under intraoperative neurophysiological monitoring. We took special care in obtaining a complete decompression of left foramen since foraminal stenosis contributed significantly in the symptoms of the patient. Postoperative plain X-rays showed no complications related with position of the arthrodesis system (Fig. 12.4).

Patient underwent an uneventful postoperative recovery, she was mobilized on the first postoperative day without any peripheral neurological symptom and discharged on the third

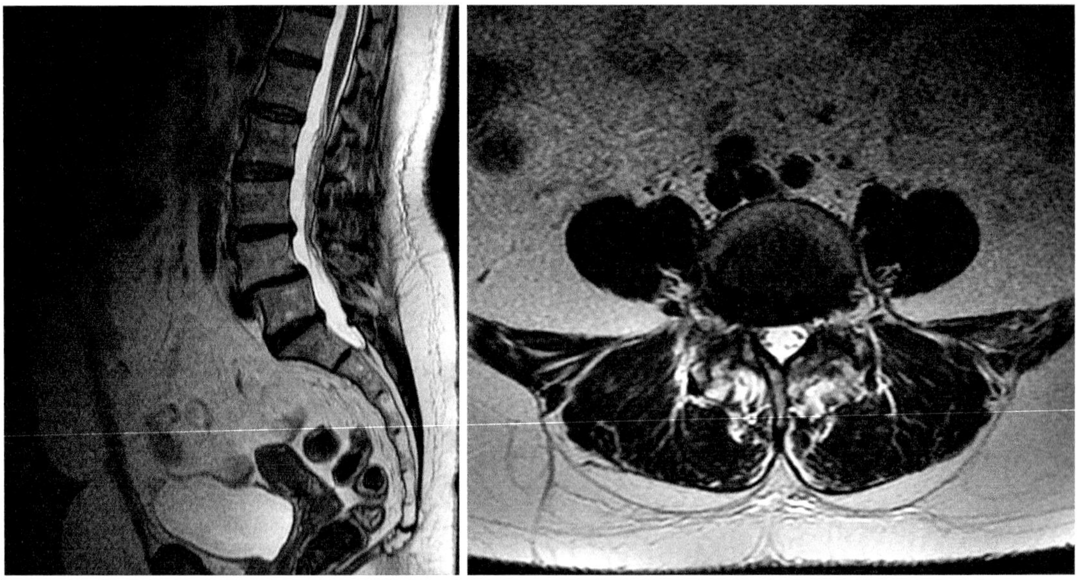

Fig. 12.1 T2 weighted images of the Lumbar spine sagittal (Left) and axial (Right) demonstrating L4-L5 degenerative spondylolisthesis grade I. Mild-moderate stenosis of the spinal canal at level L4-L5. Narrowing of bilateral and L4-L5 conjunction foramen, predominantly left

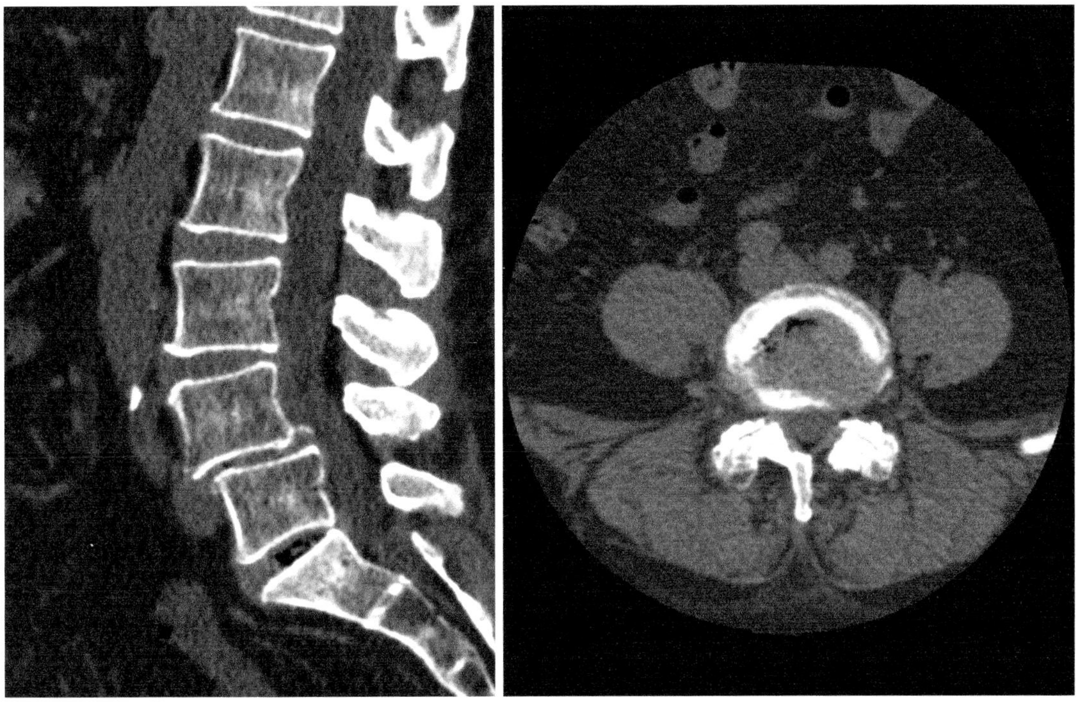

Fig. 12.2 Flexion (Left) and extension (Right) view of the lumbar vertebrae showed a grade I spondylolisthesis

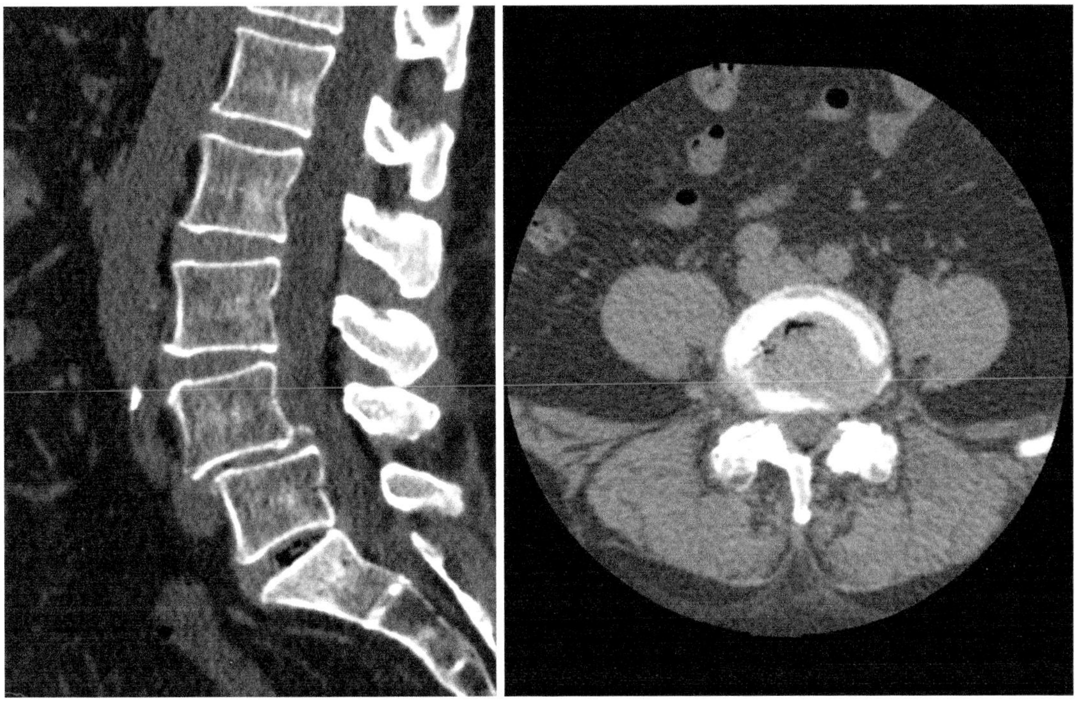

Fig. 12.3 CT-scan sagittal (Left) and axial (Right) shows the spondylolisthesis and marked facet arthrosis L4-L5

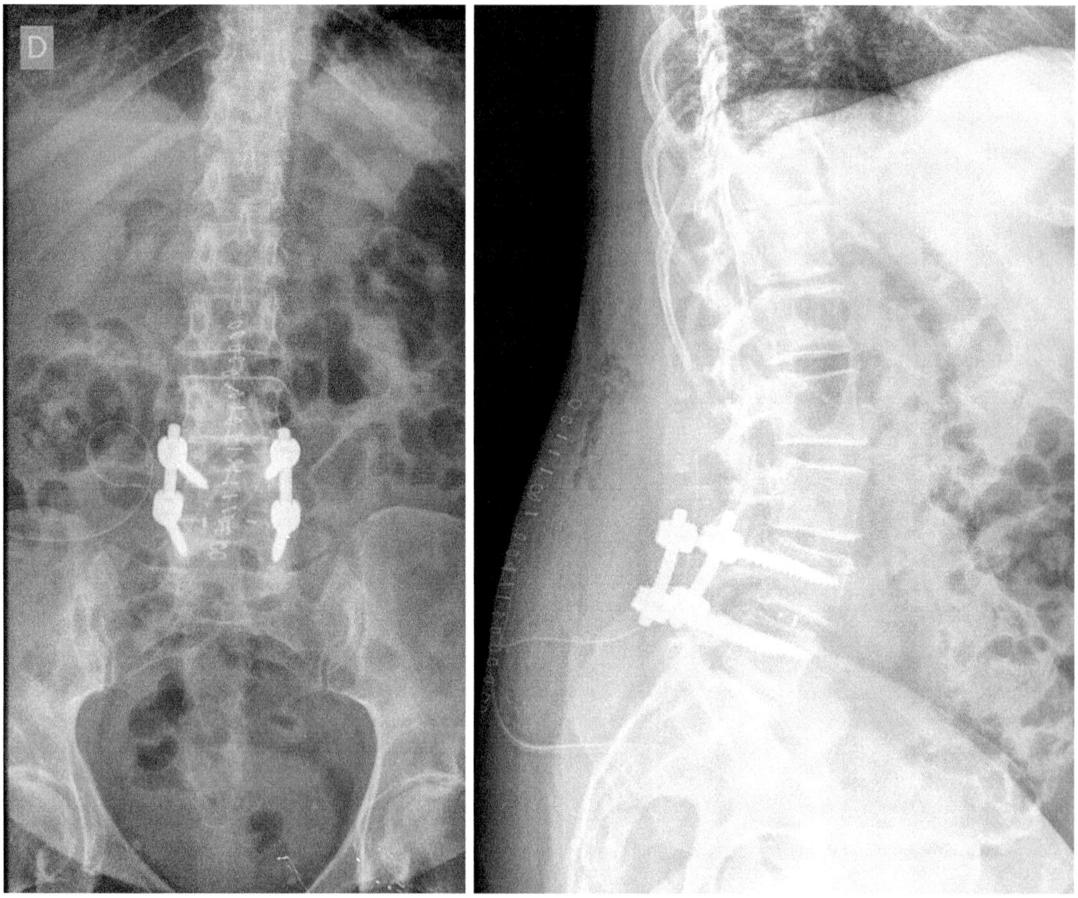

Fig. 12.4 Immediate postoperative anteroposterior (Left) and lateral (Right) X-rays showing L4–L5 instrumentation

day. Follow-up was carried at 1, 3, 6 months, flexion/extension X-rays revealed good alignment of the vertebral bodies. The patient was free of lumbar or leg pain, she started to work and return to his normal activities. A CT scan at one year as part of our routine F/U showed, maintenance of L4/5 alignment, with radiological signs of postero-lateral bony fusion.

12.3 Discussion

Spondylolisthesis can result from degenerative disease, current clinical guidelines establish that the first-line therapy when dealing with this condition are non-surgical measures, surgical treatment may be offered in the setting of intense back or leg pain unresponsive to nonsurgical measures, if neurological deficits develop, or if the listhesis is shown to be progressive [1]. In our case the patient receive a combination of analgesics and steroid-injections without any improvement. There is poor evidence about what patients had better responses to conservative measures. However, in the non-surgical cohort of the Spine Patient Outcomes Research Trial (SPORT), patients with grade I slip and hypermobile slip had better outcomes [6]. Therefore, in patients with mobile or low-grade spondylolisthesis, without neurological deficits, a trial of non-operative therapy is indicated and generally associated with good clinical outcomes.

In regard of the surgical treatment, several studies have been designed to compare treatment approaches [2]. A review from the data of the SPORT trial at 8 years shows that 7% were

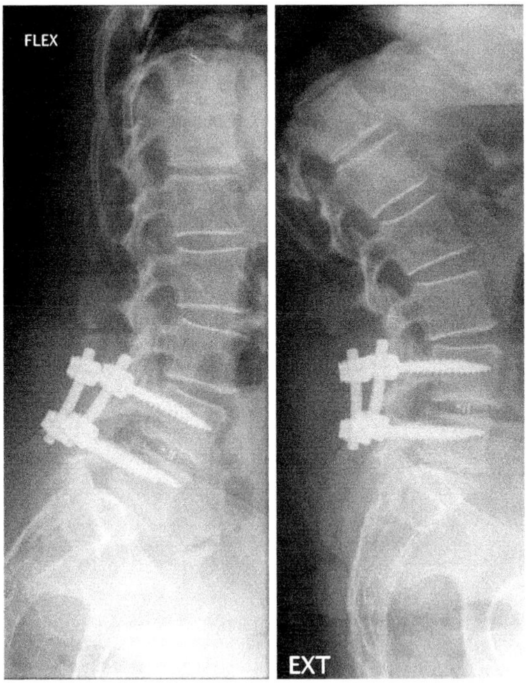

Fig. 12.5 Postoperative flexion (Left) and extension (Right) X-rays showing L4–L5 complete spondylolisthesis reduction at 1 month follow-up

treated with decompression alone, 21% were treated with non-instrumented fusion, and 71% were treated with fusion surgery. The reoperation rate is high at 22% at 8 years after initial surgery [7].

A systematic review about the specific surgical management of degenerative lumbar spondylolisthesis demonstrated that satisfactory outcomes were significantly more likely with fusion than with decompression alone. In addition, there was a significantly greater probability of achieving fusion with the use of instrumentation. However, use of instrumentation was not associated with a significant improvement in clinical outcome [8]. In the same line, in a more recent randomized controlled trial of 133 patients, spinal decompression versus fusion was compared. There was no significant difference in outcomes at 2 years except for lower operative time and hospital length of stay with decompression [4]. Currently, there is an intense debate in the community about the management of spondylolisthesis associated with lumbar spinal stenosis [2, 4, 9].

We decided to perform a TLIF in order to achieve greater fusion, better restoration of disc height, and indirect decompression of the exit foramina. Nonetheless, in spite of this theoretical benefits, there is insufficient evidence to make a clear recommendation at present time. In a recent systemic review [10], the authors concluded that there was not sufficient evidence to recommend for or against inter-body fusion in the treatment of spondylolisthesis. Although, it may play a role in cases deemed unstable or excessively mobile. The same recommendation was stated in the recent North American Spine Society (NASS) guidelines for the treatment of spondylolisthesis [1].

Another approaches like anterior lumbar interbody fusion (ALIF) has been proposed, when compared ALIF versus TLIF in a prospective study [11], both anterior and posterior methods improved overall patient satisfaction, and low back and leg pain. Low back pain was significantly improved in the ALIF group compared with those in the TLIF group; however, the periods of hospital stay and of bed rest were significantly longer.

Minimally invasive techniques (MIS) for spine surgery are increasingly being utilized to reduce surgical morbidity and maintain spine stability. As this new field grows, investigation of MIS techniques for treatment of spondylolisthesis has also been increasingly studied, nonetheless little high-quality evidence exists, making it difficult to draw definitive conclusions for the moment [1].

Controversy persists in detailing the best surgical option for degenerative spondylolisthesis and optimum techniques in certain clinical scenarios. Since current guidelines are weak and based on limited high-quality evidence [1], each case must be individualized, looking at the clinical and radiological features to decide the optimal treatment.

12.4 Conclusions

Current Evidence-Based Clinical Guidelines for treatment of spondylolisthesis support operative treatment of patients refractory to conservative measures. However, the optimal operative treatment remains poorly established. There is some moderate evidence that decompression alone may be a feasible treatment with lower surgical morbidity and similar outcomes to fusion when performed in a select population. Nonetheless, the optimal treatment approach remains an area of active study.

Pearls and Pitfalls

– Many patients will improve with a non-operative treatment course for some time. Surgical treatment should be individualized for each patient. Not all patients improve significantly after surgery. External factors such as overweight and harmful habits must be addressed. The future of minimally invasive treatment options will continue to perfect outcomes. Additional research will be directed towards optimizing treatment and predicting which patients will respond better to surgical measures.

Editorial Comment

This chapter complements chapters 10 and 11. It illustrates a patient with a mobile symptomatic degenerative lumbar spondylolisthesis, who was treated according to the present state of the art and evidence. There is level one evidence supporting surgery for patients with symptoms refarctory to conservative treatment, which has mostly an transient effect anyway. There is also very good evidence that these patients profit even more from surgery than patients with a spinal stenosis.

References

1. Matz P, Meagher R, Lamer T, Tontz W. NASS evidence-based clinical guidelines for multidisciplinary spine care: diagnosis and treatment of degenerative lumbar spondylolisthesis. 2nd ed; 2014. p. 121. Available: https://www.spine.org/Documents/ResearchClinicalCare/Guidelines/Spondylolisthesis.pdf.
2. Samuel AM, Moore HG, Cunningham ME. Treatment for degenerative lumbar spondylolisthesis: current concepts and new evidence. Curr Rev Musculoskelet Med. 2017:2–10. Available: http://link.springer.com/10.1007/s12178-017-9442-3.
3. Ghogawala Z, Resnick DK, Glassman SD, Dziura J, Shaffrey CI, Mummaneni PV. Achieving optimal outcome for degenerative lumbar spondylolisthesis: randomized controlled trial results. Neurosurgery. 2017;64:40–4. Available: http://academic.oup.com/neurosurgery/article/64/CN{_}suppl{_}1/40/4093178/Achieving-Optimal-Outcome-for-Degenerative-Lumbar.
4. Försth P, Ólafsson G, Carlsson T, Frost A, Borgström F, Fritzell P, et al. A randomized, controlled trial of fusion surgery for lumbar spinal stenosis. N Engl J Med. 2016;374:1413–23. Available: http://www.nejm.org/doi/10.1056/NEJMoa1513721.
5. Weinstein JN, Tosteson TD, Lurie JD, Tosteson ANA, Blood E, Hanscom B, et al. Surgical versus nonsurgical therapy for lumbar spinal stenosis. N Engl J Med. 2008;358:794–810. Available: https://www.ncbi.nlm.nih.gov/pubmed/18287602, http://www.nejm.org/doi/pdf/10.1056/NEJMoa0707136.
6. Pearson AM, Lurie JD, Blood EA, Frymoyer JW, Braeutigam H, An H, et al. Spine patient outcomes research trial: radiographic predictors of clinical outcomes after operative or nonoperative treatment of degenerative spondylolisthesis. Spine. 2008;33:2759–66.
7. Lurie JD, Tosteson TD, Tosteson A, Abdu WA, Zhao W, Morgan TS, et al. Long-term outcomes of lumbar spinal stenosis: eight-year results of the Spine Patient Outcomes Research Trial (SPORT) NIH Public Access. Spine. 2015;15:63–76.
8. Martin CR, Gruszczynski AT, Braunsfurth HA, Fallatah SM, O'Neil J, Wai EK. The surgical management of degenerative lumbar spondylolisthesis: a systematic review. Spine. 2007;32:1791–8. Available: http://www.ncbi.nlm.nih.gov/pubmed/17632401.
9. Ghogawala Z, Dziura J, Butler WE, Dai F, Terrin N, Magge SN, et al. Laminectomy plus fusion versus laminectomy alone for lumbar spondylolisthesis. N Engl J Med. 2016;374:1424–34. Available: http://www.nejm.org/doi/10.1056/NEJMoa1508788.
10. Baker JF, Errico TJ, Kim Y, Razi A. Degenerative spondylolisthesis: contemporary review of the role of interbody fusion. Eur J Orthop Surg Traumatol. 2017;27:169–80. Available: http://link.springer.com/10.1007/s00590-016-1885-5.
11. Ohtori S, Koshi T, Yamashita M, Takaso M, Yamauchi K, Inoue G, et al. Single-level instrumented posterolateral fusion versus non-instrumented anterior interbody fusion for lumbar spondylolisthesis: a prospective study with a 2-year follow-up. J Orthop Sci. 2011;16:352–8.

Basic Degenerative Lumbar Scoliosis

13

Sebastian Hartmann, Anja Tschugg, and Claudius Thomé

13.1 Introduction

Degenerative lumbar scoliosis (DLS) or "de novo scoliosis" represents a pathological condition associated with rotational subluxation and anteroposterior or lateral olisthesis leading to coronal deformity [22]. DLS is defined as a coronal Cobb angle of more than 10° but rarely exceeding 50° [1, 12]. The etiological progress is multifactorial and still unclear but starting with intervertebral disc degeneration, facet joint degeneration and changes in canal as well as pedicle morphology [15, 25]. The scoliotic curve typically develops in the fifth decade of life and is not based on idiopathic adolescent scoliosis (AIS). Life time prevalence is between 8–13% increasing with age, so that the prevalence in the sixth decade of life rises up to 60% with women being more frequently affected than men [3, 5, 7, 8, 26, 27]. In contrast to patients with AIS, the clinical symptomatology in DLS patients is usually characterized by low back pain, neurogenic claudication associated with neurological deficits in the lower extremities and rarely cauda equina syndrome. The spinal deformity shows a mean annual curvature progression in the coronal plain of 3–4°, although the progression does not translate linearly, so that the prognosis which curve is progressing cannot be reliably predicted [16]. Nevertheless, the literature provides evidence, that increased intervertebral disc degeneration, lateral translation >6 mm and an intercrest line through the L5 vertebra may be considered as progression factors of these coronal deformities [6]. The majority of DLS show an accompanied segmental kyphosis resulting in moderate or severe sagittal imbalance [5, 8, 26]. As a result, a classification system of degenerative disc disease based on the distribution of the diseased segments and the balance status of the spine has been generated to guide the treatment of DLS [2]. Therefore, the treatment of DLS patients is characterized by a wide variability of surgical options ranging from simple lumbar nerve root decompression to complex thoracolumbar fusions with sagittal deformity corrections. The surgical treatment is even more complex due to the accompanied comorbidities associated with the increased age in DLS patients.

This chapter will capture the essentials of degenerative lumbar scoliosis, the clinical presentation, the indications and the surgical approach.

13.2 Case Description

A 67 year-old female patient presented with severe back pain for years and she complained about new right-sided radicular pain in the lower

S. Hartmann (✉) · A. Tschugg · C. Thomé
Department of Neurosurgery, Medical University Innsbruck, Innsbruck, Austria
e-mail: sebastian.hartmann@i-med.ac.at

B. Meyer, M. Rauschmann (eds.), *Spine Surgery*, https://doi.org/10.1007/978-3-319-98875-7_13

extremities for about 4 months (NRS, Numeric rating scale 7/10). The patient suffered from neurogenic claudication with a walking distance of less than 300 metres. Conservative treatment including pain therapy, physical therapy as well as behavioural therapy was undertaken with only minimal and short-lasting improvement. Preoperative long-standing lateral and anteroposterior as well as conventional lumbar x-ray images revealed a degenerative left convex lumbar scoliosis with the apex at the L3/L4 motion segment (Fig. 13.1). The end vertebrae were identified at the levels L2 and L5 (Fig. 13.1). The coronal profile showed a Cobb angle of approximately 27° with an apical and segmental Cobb angle of the motion segment L3/L4 of approximately 17° accompanied with a rotatory subluxation (Fig. 13.1). A compensatory right thoracic curve was observed without any pain or discomfort at this region (Fig. 13.1). The sagittal profile was appropriately aligned with a lumbar lordosis (LL) of approximately 37°, a pelvic incidence (PI) of 45° with a corresponding pelvic tilt (PT) of 20° and a sagittal vertical axis (SVA) of <30 mm. According to the proposed classification systems to evaluate the sagittal profile, PI and LL did not differ much. Nevertheless, for patients with low PI the authors recommend a LL in the range of PI plus 10° (PI of 45°, type B or type 2 according to the classification system of LeHuec and Roussouly, respectively) [10, 17, 20]. The motion segment of the level L3/L4 showed a collapsed neuroforamen on the right side with L3 and L4 radicular pain without motor deficits caused by the right concave degenerative lumbar curve (Fig. 13.2). Magnetic resonance imaging (MRI) revealed central canal stenosis at the level L2/L3 and predominantly lateral recess stenosis at the level L3/L4 (Fig. 13.3). Adequate decompression followed by dorsal pedicle screw

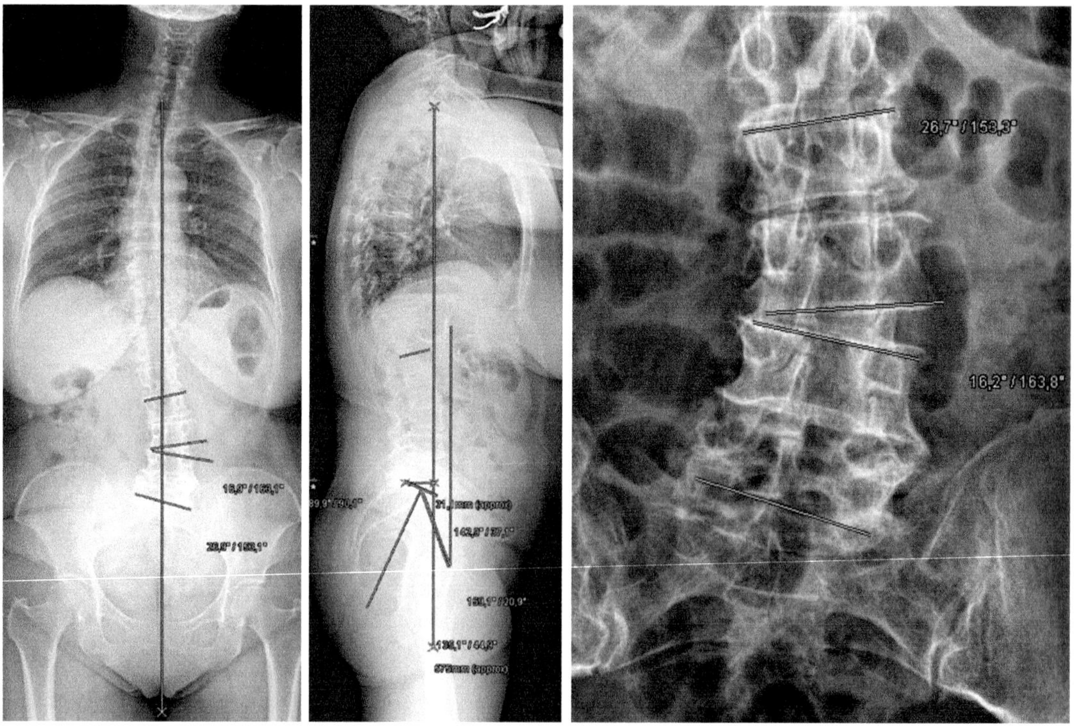

Fig. 13.1 Preoperative long-standing lateral and anteroposterior plus conventional x-rays. Preoperative coronal and sagittal x-ray with degenerative coronal malalignment. The coronal Cobb angle demonstrated a degenerative lumbar scoliosis of 27° with a corresponding apical and segmental Cobb angle of 17° (L3/L4). Sagittal balance analysis revealed an aligned profile identified as a LL of 37°, a PI of 45° with a corresponding PT of 20° and a SVA of <30 mm

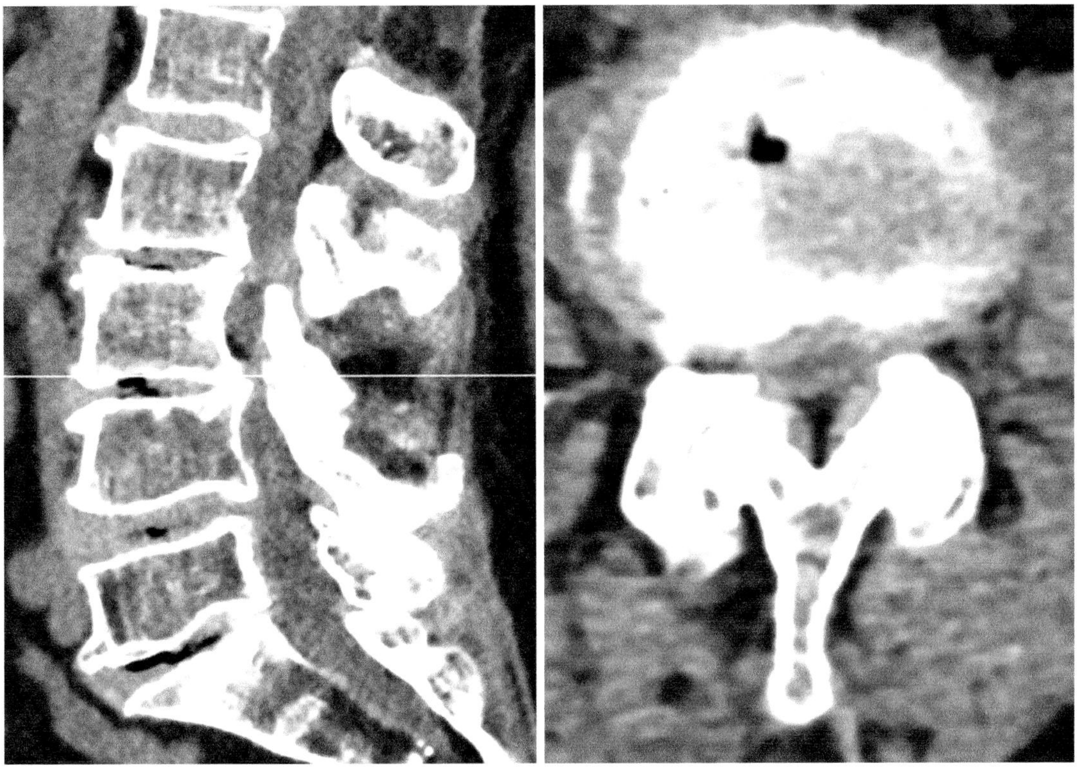

Fig. 13.2 Preoperative CT. A collapsed right-sided neuroforamen was seen at L3/L4 with a central and right-sided lateral recess stenosis aggravating the L3 and L4 radicular pain of the patient. The apex of the scoliotic curve was located at the segment L3/L4 with the end vertebrae L2 and L5 cranially and caudally

instrumentation L2–L5 with TLIF cage implantation at L2/L3, L3/L4 and L4/5 was performed. Smith-Peterson osteotomies were additionally carried out at L3/L4 and L4/L5 with derotation manoeuvres to realign the coronal profile (Fig. 13.4). Surgery was uneventful and the patient was discharged after 7 days.

During the postoperative inpatient stay, no additional brace was used and the patient was sent to physiotherapy daily. NRS improved to 5 after surgery and to 3 and 1 after 3 and 12 months, respectively. The walking distance improved to approximately 3000 metres and 6000 metres after 3 and 12 months. Routine postoperative radiological follow-up did not reveal any signs of implant-related complications, adjacent segment disease or proximal junctional kyphosis (Fig. 13.4). The LL improved to approximately 45° and the coronal Cobb angle to 8°.

13.3 Discussion of the Case

DLS is predominantly affecting the aging population and results in asymmetric degeneration succeeding in rotatory subluxation of functional spinal units of the lumbar spine [1]. Asymmetric degenerative lumbar changes caused by intervertebral disc and facet joint degeneration leads to a coronal plane deformity with lateral slippage. These degenerative changes often occur as a focal deformity including one motion segment at the mid portion of the lumbar spine (L3/L4 and L4/L5) with progressive degenerative changes adjacently. At first, the patients experience low back pain. Due to the coronal deformity, the convex curve opens the contralateral neural foramen and causes radiculopathy at the concave exiting nerve root [11]. In some cases, however, the degenerative changes affect multiple motion

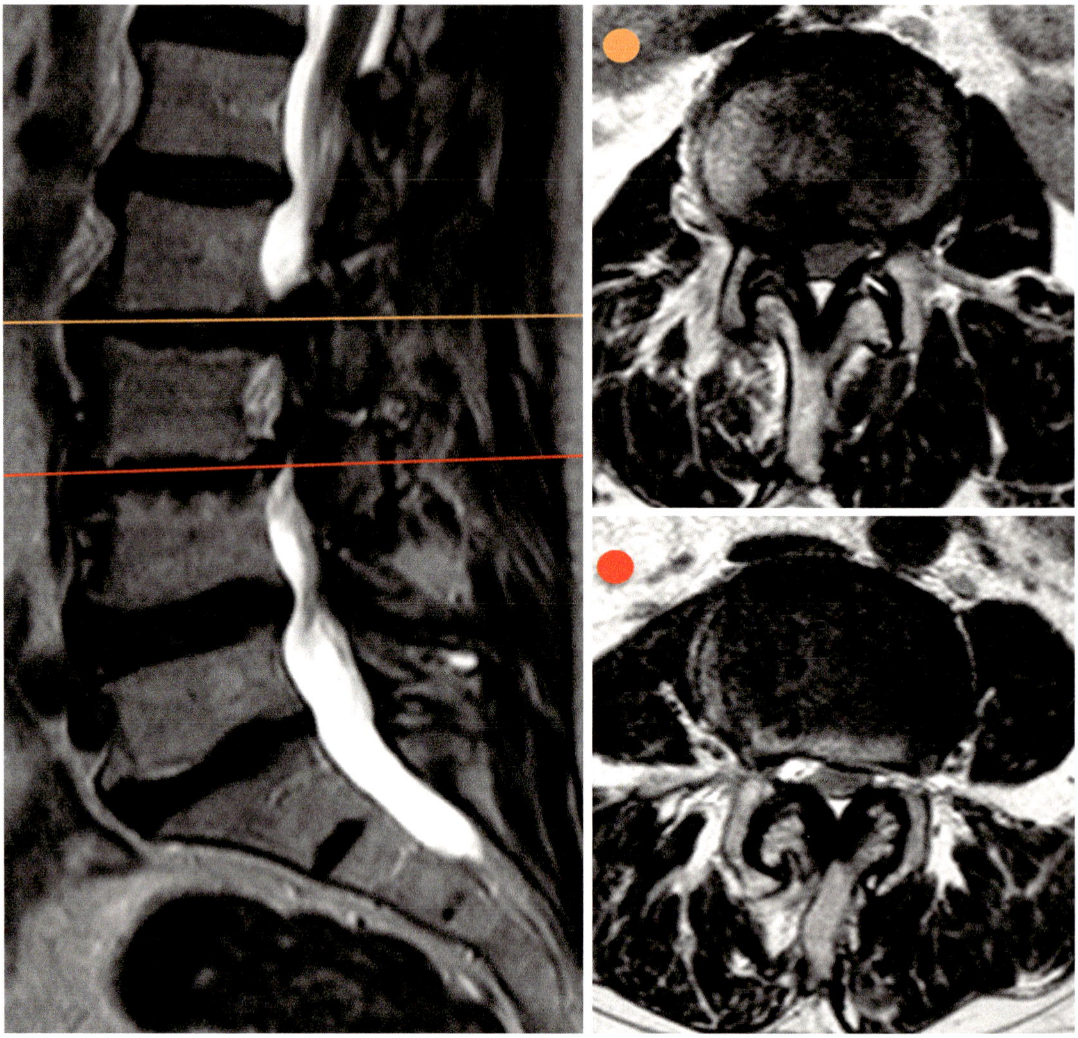

Fig. 13.3 Preoperative MRI. MRI confirmed a central and lateral canal stenosis at the levels L2/3 and L3/4, respectively. Additionally, the facet joints at these levels demonstrated effusion and pronounced hypertrophy

segments, so that extended lumbar curves with both sagittal and coronal deformities are present. DLS leads than to a significant reduction of quality of life with a high "burden of disease" level. Nevertheless, the first treatment steps for symptomatic adult degenerative lumbar scoliosis are non-operative involving pain medication, injection therapies and physical therapy. In case of refractory symptoms, a bundle of different surgical options is available. The surgical options largely depend on the clinical presentation of DLS, so that simple and potentially minimally invasive decompression procedures may be feasible in patients with predominantly claudicative symptoms.

In patients with multisegmental sagittally and/or coronally decompensated curves, the procedures might be expanded to long instrumented fusions including correction manoeuvres in both planes [2, 4, 23, 24]. Osteotomies, anterolateral approaches or combined procedures allow the surgeon to increase the degree of correction, however, the complication rate is simultaneously rising with this complex surgical armamentarium. The overall complication rate of DLS patients treated surgically has been

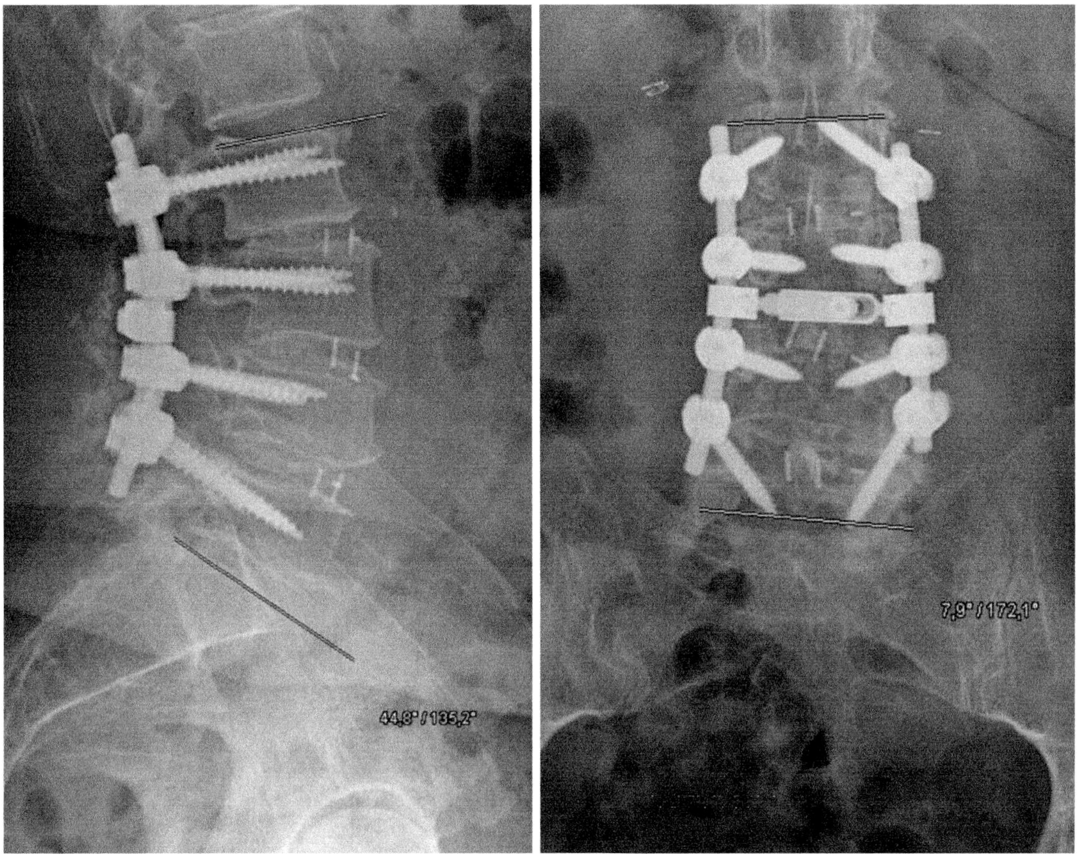

Fig. 13.4 Postoperative lateral and anteroposterior x-ray. Postoperative sagittal and coronal scans showed an improvement of LL to 45° and the coronal alignment improved to a Cobb angle of 8°. No signs of implant-related complications, adjacent segment disease or proximal junctional kyphosis were observed on follow-up, but there was some retrolisthesis at L2/L3

estimated at approximately 40%, and more than half of these patients required revision surgery for both mechanical as well as neurological complications [4]. In patients requiring osteotomies these rates are even higher. The number of instrumented vertebrae, extended fusions to the sacrum, osteotomies and a preoperative pelvic tilt over 26° have been determined as risk factors [4]. Due to the associated complication rate, however, short fusion techniques may be favoured over long constructs, especially in older patients with cardiovascular comorbidities, obesity or osteoporosis [9, 14]. All this complicates the treatment of DLS patients and questions whether surgical therapy should be performed at all and, if so, what surgical option should be used to improve the coronal and sagittal profile. To help choosing the appropriate surgical strategy, a bundle of classification systems is available. Berjano and Lamartina published a classification system based on the distribution of the symptomatic segments and the spinal alignment [2]. The authors describe the apical area of the patients' degenerative scoliotic curve as the apex of the main curve, a vertebra or a disc level (in the case presented L3). The end area is defined as the non-apical area adjacent to the end vertebra of the main lumbar degenerative curve. As a result, four types can be distinguished and the invasiveness of the surgical procedure increases from type 1 to type 4.

Other classification systems differentiate the etiological characteristics of the spinal deformity or morphological aspects based on the surgical outcome. The background of Aebi's classification system describes the cause of the deformity and Schwab's classification deals with the severity of the curve. The information to identify candidates for selective fusion based on the distribution of the symptomatic segments and the spinal alignment is still lacking [2, 13, 18, 19, 21].

13.3.1 Accordance with Literature Guidelines

The management of DLS patients remains an individual patient to patient decision. New surgically based classification systems have been published to aid in selecting the extent of the required procedure.

Level of Evidence: B to C
The level of evidence available is poor to moderate.

13.4 Conclusion and Take Home Message

The decision-making progress in the management of DLS patients is based on several factors including the clinical presentation, the age of the patient, the associated comorbidities and the spinopelvic sagittal and coronal alignment. Current classification systems may help surgeons to determine the invasiveness of the procedure based on the distribution of the symptomatic segments and the spinal alignment. Nevertheless, in view of the overall high complication and reoperation rates of adult deformity surgery, the invasiveness of the surgical procedure (simple decompression, instrumented fusion or osteotomies) should be determined critically. Overall, however, outcome is surprisingly good and patient satisfaction high, if patients are selected carefully.

Pearls

- Evaluate associated comorbidities to anticipate a potentially high complication rate especially in older patients
- Identify the affected and symptomatic segment(s)
- Reserve surgery after failed conservative treatment
- Always take the spinopelvic alignment into account
- Use classification systems to identify the cause and the severity of the deformity and use them to determine the invasiveness of the surgical procedure.
- Prefer simple decompression procedures to (multisegmental) instrumented fusion in case of predominant neurogenic claudication
- Long-term outcome seems to favour surgery over non-operative care

Editorial Comment

Lumbar degenerative scoliosis is a topic which is dominated by firm beliefs and strong opinions of experts, but almost no sound evidence at all. Therefore the decision making puts one everytime "between a rock and hard place". This chapter illustrates very well all the difficulties in that respect and the solution for this case worked well, for the time being one may add. Everything surrounding this difficult field is further elaborated in chapters 54–58 and 78 of the advanced modules. For the time being the message is, that whatever you do has disadvantages, like the high likelyhood of early adjacent segment degeneration and reoperation with this solution.

References

1. Aebi M. The adult scoliosis. Eur Spine J. 2005;14(10):925–48. https://doi.org/10.1007/s00586-005-1053-9.
2. Berjano P, Lamartina C. Classification of degenerative segment disease in adults with deformity of the lumbar or thoracolumbar spine. Eur Spine J. 2014; 23(9):1815–24. https://doi.org/10.1007/s00586-014-3219-9.
3. Carter OD, Haynes SG. Prevalence rates for scoliosis in US adults: results from the first national health and nutrition examination survey. Int J Epidemiol. 1987;16(4):537–44.
4. Charosky S, Guigui P, Blamoutier A, Roussouly P, Chopin D. Complications and risk factors of primary adult scoliosis surgery: a multicenter study of 306 patients. Spine (Phila Pa 1976). 2012;37(8):693–700. https://doi.org/10.1097/BRS.0b013e31822ff5c1.
5. Chin KR, Furey C, Bohlman HH. Risk of progression in de novo low-magnitude degenerative lumbar curves: natural history and literature review. Am J Orthop (Belle Mead NJ). 2009;38(8):404–9.
6. Faraj SS, Holewijn RM, van Hooff ML, de Kleuver M, Pellisé F, Haanstra TM. De novo degenerative lumbar scoliosis: a systematic review of prognostic factors for curve progression. Eur Spine J. 2016;25(8): 2347–58. https://doi.org/10.1007/s00586-016-4619-9.
7. Kebaish KM, Neubauer PR, Voros GD, Khoshnevisan MA, Skolasky RL. Scoliosis in adults aged forty years and older: prevalence and relationship to age, race, and gender. Spine (Phila Pa 1976). 2011;36(9):731–6. https://doi.org/10.1097/BRS.0b013e3181e9f120.
8. Kobayashi T, Atsuta Y, Takemitsu M, Matsuno T, Takeda N. A prospective study of de novo scoliosis in a community based cohort. Spine (Phila Pa 1976). 2006;31(2):178–82.
9. Lee C-H, Chung CK, Sohn MJ, Kim CH. Short limited fusion versus long fusion with deformity correction for spinal stenosis with balanced de novo degenerative lumbar scoliosis. Spine (Phila Pa 1976). 2017;42(19):E1126–32. https://doi.org/10.1097/BRS.0000000000002306.
10. Le Huec JC, Leijssen P, Duarte M, Aunoble S. Thoracolumbar imbalance analysis for osteotomy planification using a new method: FBI technique. Eur Spine J. 2011;20(Suppl 5):669–80. https://doi.org/10.1007/s00586-011-1935-y.
11. Liu H, Ishihara H, Kanamori M, Kawaguchi Y, Ohmori K, Kimura T. Characteristics of nerve root compression caused by degenerative lumbar spinal stenosis with scoliosis. Spine J. 2003;3(6):524–9.
12. Liu W, Chen XS, Jia LS, Song DW. The clinical features and surgical treatment of degenerative lumbar scoliosis: a review of 112 patients. Orthop Surg. 2009;1(3):176–83. https://doi.org/10.1111/j.1757-7861.2009.00030.x.
13. Lowe T, Berven SH, Schwab FJ, Bridwell KH. The SRS classification for adult spinal deformity: building on the King/Moe and Lenke classification systems. Spine (Phila Pa 1976). 2006;31(19 Suppl):S119–25. https://doi.org/10.1097/01.brs.0000232709.48446.be.
14. Phan K, Xu J, Maharaj MM, Li J, Kim JS, Di Capua J, et al. Outcomes of short fusion versus long fusion for adult degenerative scoliosis: a systematic review and meta-analysis. Orthop Surg. 2017;9(4):342–9. https://doi.org/10.1111/os.12357.
15. Pritchett JW, Bortel DT. Degenerative symptomatic lumbar scoliosis. Spine (Phila Pa 1976). 1993;18(6):700–3.
16. Robin GC, Span Y, Steinberg R, Makin M, Menczel J. Scoliosis in the elderly: a follow-up study. Spine (Phila Pa 1976). 1982;7(4):355–9.
17. Roussouly P, Gollogly S, Berthonnaud E, Dimnet J. Classification of the normal variation in the sagittal alignment of the human lumbar spine and pelvis in the standing position. Spine (Phila Pa 1976). 2005;30(3):346–53.
18. Schwab F, el-Fegoun AB, Gamez L, Goodman H, Farcy JP. A lumbar classification of scoliosis in the adult patient: preliminary approach. Spine (Phila Pa 1976). 2005;30(14):1670–3.
19. Schwab F, Lafage V, Farcy JP, Bridwell K, Glassman S, Ondra S, et al. Surgical rates and operative outcome analysis in thoracolumbar and lumbar major adult scoliosis: application of the new adult deformity classification. Spine (Phila Pa 1976). 2007;32(24): 2723–30. https://doi.org/10.1097/BRS.0b013e31815a58f2.
20. Schwab F, Patel A, Ungar B, Farcy JP, Lafage V. Adult spinal deformity-postoperative standing imbalance: how much can you tolerate? An overview of key parameters in assessing alignment and planning corrective surgery. Spine (Phila Pa 1976). 2010;35(25):2224–31. https://doi.org/10.1097/BRS.0b013e3181ee6bd4.
21. Schwab F, Ungar B, Blondel B, Buchowski J, Coe J, Deinlein D, et al. Scoliosis research society-schwab adult spinal deformity classification: a validation study. Spine (Phila Pa 1976). 2012;37(12):1077–82. https://doi.org/10.1097/BRS.0b013e31823e15e2.
22. Schwab FJ, Smith VA, Biserni M, Gamez L, Farcy JP, Pagala M. Adult scoliosis: a quantitative radiographic and clinical analysis. Spine (Phila Pa 1976). 2002;27(4):387–92.
23. Smith JS, Lafage V, Shaffrey CI, Schwab F, Lafage R, Hostin R, et al. Outcomes of operative and nonoperative treatment for adult spinal deformity:

a prospective, multicenter, propensity-matched cohort assessment with minimum 2-year follow-up. Neurosurgery. 2016;78(6):851–61. https://doi.org/10.1227/NEU.0000000000001116.

24. Transfeldt EE, Topp R, Mehbod AA, Winter RB. Surgical outcomes of decompression, decompression with limited fusion, and decompression with full curve fusion for degenerative scoliosis with radiculopathy. Spine (Phila Pa 1976). 2010;35(20):1872–5. https://doi.org/10.1097/BRS.0b013e3181ce63a2.
25. Tribus CB. Degenerative lumbar scoliosis: evaluation and management. J Am Acad Orthop Surg. 2003;11(3):174–83.
26. Watanuki A, Yamada H, Tsutsui S, En-yo Y, Yoshida M, Yoshimura N. Radiographic features and risk of curve progression of de-novo degenerative lumbar scoliosis in the elderly: a 15-year follow-up study in a community-based cohort. J Orthop Sci. 2012;17(5):526–31. https://doi.org/10.1007/s00776-012-0253-5.
27. Xu L, Sun X, Huang S, Zhu Z, Qiao J, Zhu F, et al. Degenerative lumbar scoliosis in chinese han population: prevalence and relationship to age, gender, bone mineral density, and body mass index. Eur Spine J. 2013;22(6):1326–31. https://doi.org/10.1007/s00586-013-2678-8.

14 Thoracolumbar Instrumentation and Fusion for Degenerative Disc Disease

Sven Kevin Tschoeke

14.1 Introduction

With the increase of an aging population worldwide, patient's expectations and demands for an improved independent lifestyle have led to innovative strategies in the treatment of degenerative disc disease. Aside from all conservative modalities, new surgical techniques attempt to enable a rapid recovery by reducing iatrogenic injury and complications with shorter operative times. Over the past two decades, the debate over which approach may achieve the highest fusion rates has been opened to a more global view on its efficacy of restoring the overall coronal and sagittal balance of the spine. Thus, the analyses of respective spinopelvic interrelations using modern full body radiographic imaging in an upright standing position have received closer attention and have since been fully included in our therapeutic management and strategical planning. Furthermore, the increasing number of failed primary surgeries and/or adjacent segment degeneration with secondary kyphotic deformity constitute a distinct entity of challenges with rather individual and case-dependent solutions. Today's advances in spinal instrumentation allow almost any operation to be performed in a minimally-invasive fashion. Regardless of selecting either the retroperitoneal corridor (ALIF, OLIF, LLIF) or traversing the spinal canal with or without osteotomy of the facet joints for segmental mobilsation (PLIF, TLIF, minimally-invasive-surgery (MIS)-TLIF), none of today's standard techniques have proven to be superior to another. Although each approach has its own risks and benefits, fusion rates or clinical outcomes appear to be similar [1]. However, there is fundamental consensus, that interbody fusion itself is preferable to posterolateral "on-lay" fusion techniques with less postoperative complications and lower rates of pseudarthrosis [2–4]. In conclusion, the surgeon must always consider all technical options to tailor the treatment to the patient's individual, but none the less realistic expectations.

This chapter aims to outline the individual strategical considerations when treating degenerative conditions of the thoracolumbar spine and highlight the importance of the overall clinical evaluation and imaging analyses. The following two cases shall demonstrate these objectives with regard to their individual surgical management, including different techniques targeted at treating the ostensible and causally determined clinical finding.

S. K. Tschoeke (✉)
Department of Spine Surgery, Klinikum Dortmund gGmbH, Dortmund, Germany
e-mail: kevin.tschoeke@klinikumdo.de

B. Meyer, M. Rauschmann (eds.), *Spine Surgery*, https://doi.org/10.1007/978-3-319-98875-7_14

14.2 Case Description

14.2.1 Case 1

49 yo female complaining of progressive low back pain and left-sided radiculopathy. Previous periradicular and facet joint injections failed to permanently improve her overall mobility. Low back pain and left-sided leg pain were distributed equally with the patient-reported VAS being 7/10 regardless of posture and exposure to every day activities. With a past history of idiopathic thoracolumbar scoliosis, her main complaints were rather focussed on the lumbar spine region. After months of unsuccessful conservative treatment, including a multimodal pain management (MPM), she was finally admitted to our department and scheduled for minimally-invasive decompression and fusion surgery.

14.2.2 Case 2

76 yo male with a history of previous decompression and fusion surgery at the L4/5 level in 2003 (Fig. 14.1a). After a decade of asymptomatic recovery, he returned to seek orthopaedic treatment for progressive back pain. The posterior screw-and-rod system was removed and the decompression and fusion extended to the adjacent L3/4 level in PLIF-technique in 2014 (Fig. 14.1b). With the development of progressive lumbar scoliotic deformity and sagittal imbalance, fusion was extended to the lower adjacent level 1 year later, thus resulting in a spondylodesis from L3 to S1, respectively (Figs. 14.1c and 14.2a). However, sagittal imbalance advanced to further immobilizing low back pain. In addition, the patient then developed a pathological fracture of the sacrum with further detrioration of his sagittal imbalance (Fig. 14.2b). After an initial uneventful conservative recovery, the patient fell a few months later and suffered an instable fracture of the L1 vertebra and was referred to our department for further treatment (Fig. 14.3). Consequently, the instrumentation was extended cranially to Th10, including a conventional open TLIF at the adjacent level L2/3 with multiple Ponte osteotomies to combine fracture stabilization and deformity correction. Ten months postoperatively, the patient developed newly increasing back pain in the mid and lower thoracic region. Follow-up EOS imaging demonstrated a gradual loss of correction with increasing sagittal imbalance (Fig. 14.4). Ultimately, the patient's pain level reached an immobilizing intensity, consequently leading to a CT of the thoracolumbar spine with subsequent confirmation of screw loosening from Th10 to Th12 (Fig. 14.5). Finally, the patient was scheduled for his fourth revision surgery.

14.3 Discussion of the Cases

14.3.1 Indication

14.3.1.1 Case 1

The indication for decompression and fusion surgery was based on the progression of immobilizing symptoms in line with a monthlong history of unsuccessfull interventional and conservative treatments. Although the majority of cases with mild radiculopathy in the absence of neurological impairment may very well be treated conservatively [5, 6], the patient's history including MPM was characteristic to revise the treatment strategy and not resume a conservative path. With the spine balanced in both the coronal and sagittal plane, the predominant symptoms were related soley to the lower lumbar spine spine region and associated with unilateral leg pain corresponding to an L4 and L5 radiculopathy, respectively. Moreover, the positive response to previous periradicular and facet joint injections at the L4/5 level confirmed the diagnostic findings (Figs. 14.6, 14.7, and 14.8) with regard to reducing symptoms temporarily, but not permanently. Thus, surgical treatment may involve decompression alone or in combination with a fusion procedure. To date, the necessity to add a fusion procedure in symptomatic cases with radiating leg pain and low back pain with or without spondylolisthesis, remains a matter of debate [7]. Although the definition of

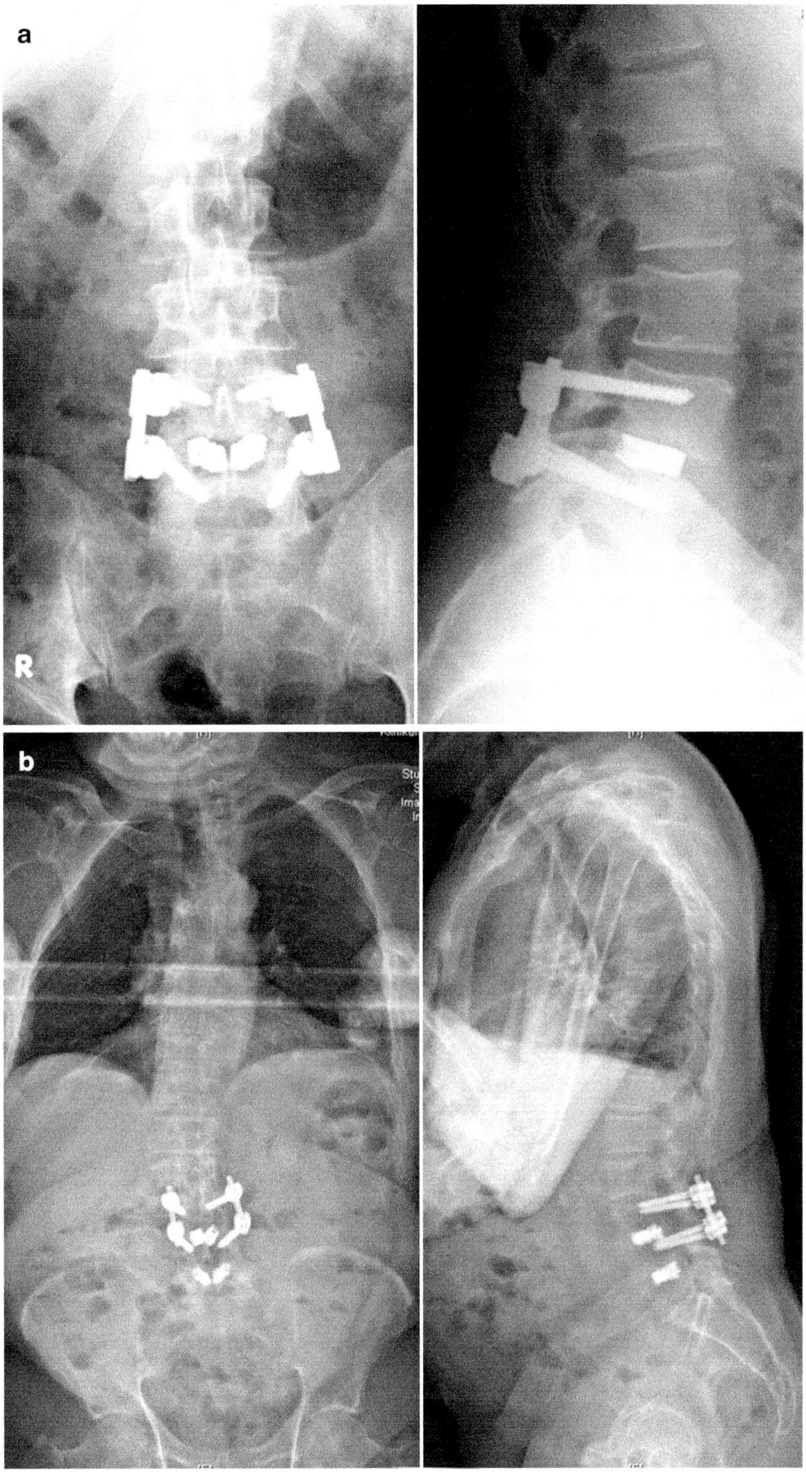

Fig. 14.1 Past history documentation of a 76yo male throughout a 13-year follow-up: (**a**) a.p. and lateral standing X-ray in 2003, (**b**) 2014 and (**c**) 2016

Fig. 14.1 (continued)

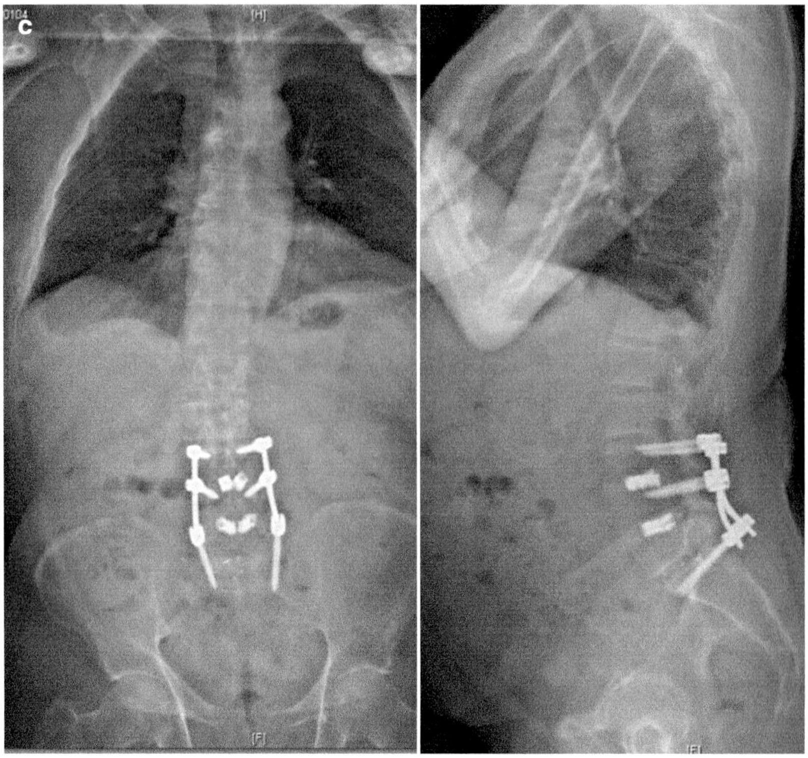

Fig. 14.2 Upright standing lateral total spine X-ray in (**a**) 2016 and (**b**) at 6 months follow-up after conservative treatment of a sacral fracture

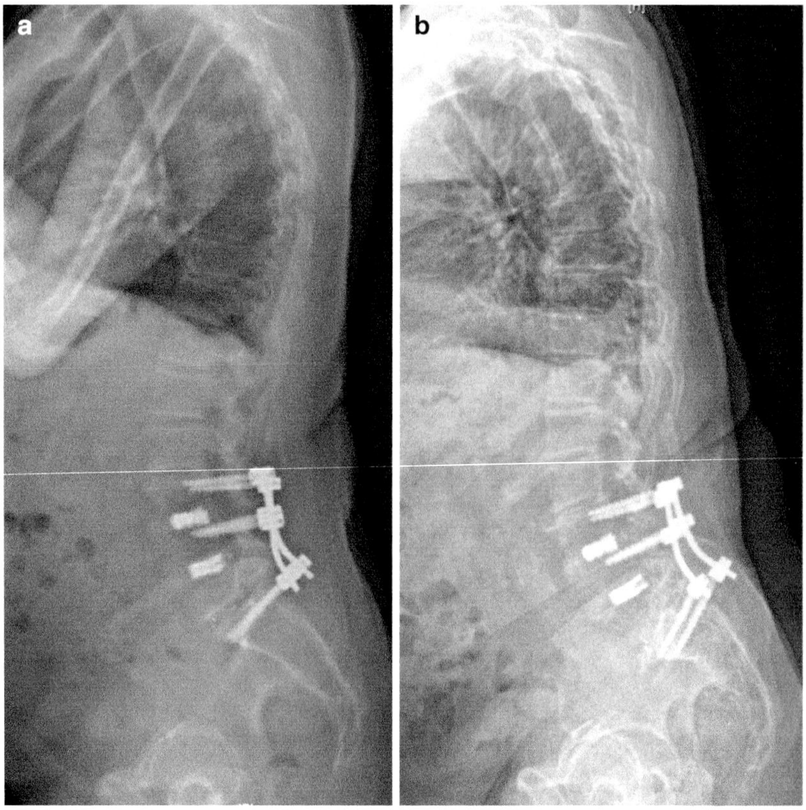

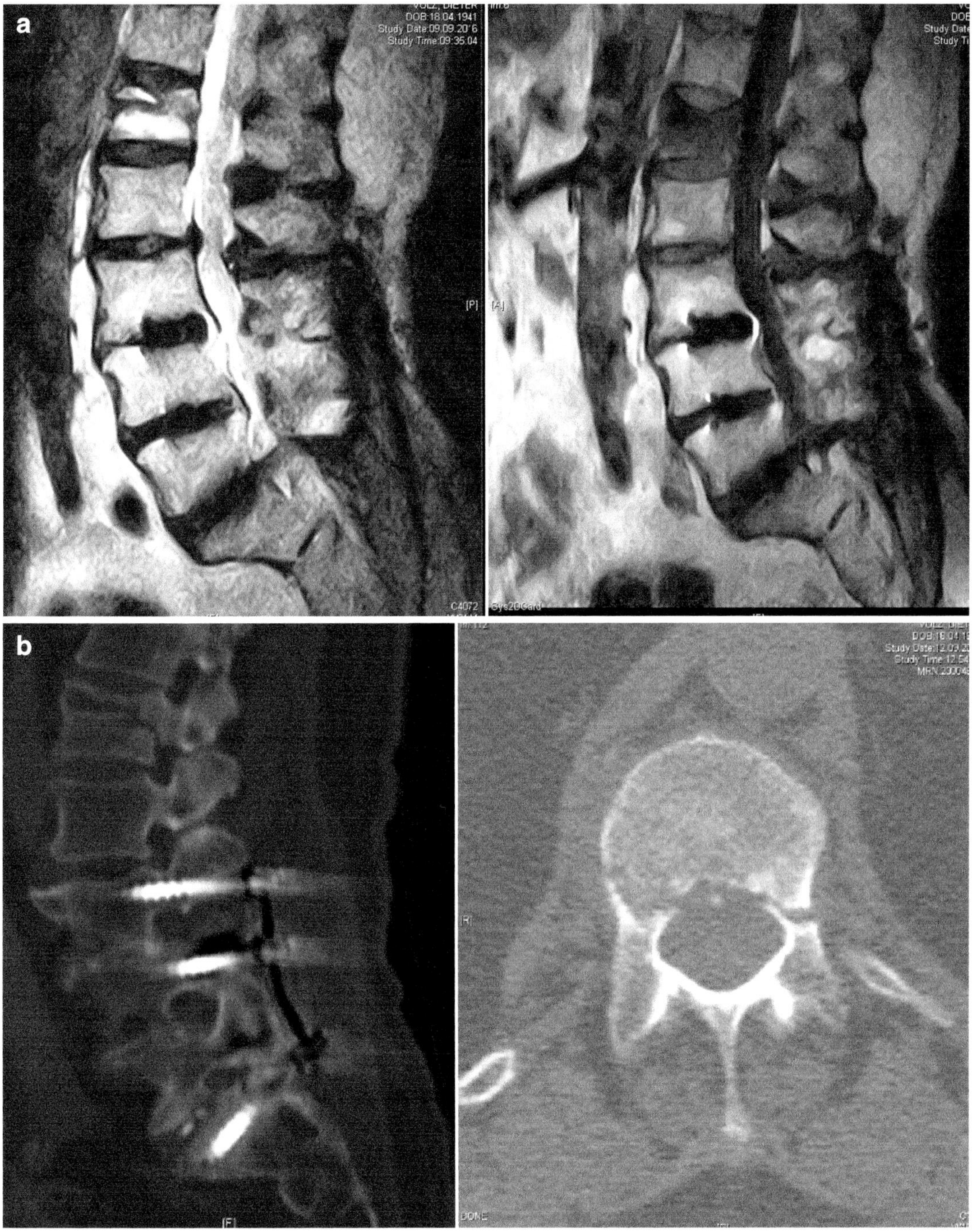

Fig. 14.3 (**a**) MRI showing the fracture at L1 in the T2-weighted (left) and T1-weighted (right) sequence with disc degeneration at the L2/3 level. (**b**) CT showing the instable L1 fracture involving both pedicles

instability is inconsistent [8], there are certain imaging characteristics that have been reported to predict a negative outcome when applying decompression alone in corresponding cases. These include a reduced disc space height of <6 mm, hypermobility at the spondylolisthetic level (<1.25 mm) and a high pelvic incidence with anterior sagittal imbalance [9–11]. In our Case 1 described here, these diagnostic parameters were complemented by the temporary pos-

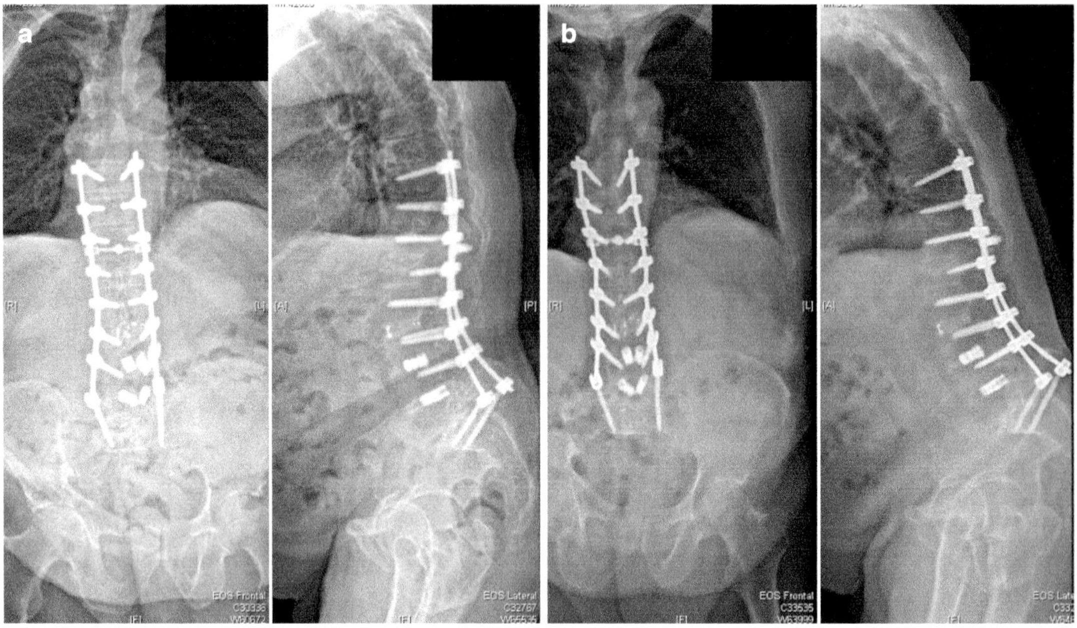

Fig. 14.4 (**a**) Postoperative result after extending the posterior screw-and-rod instrumentation to Th10 with fracture-level screws at L1 and an additional TLIF at L2/3, (**b**) 6 month postoperative follow-up demonstrating a progressive sagittal imbalance

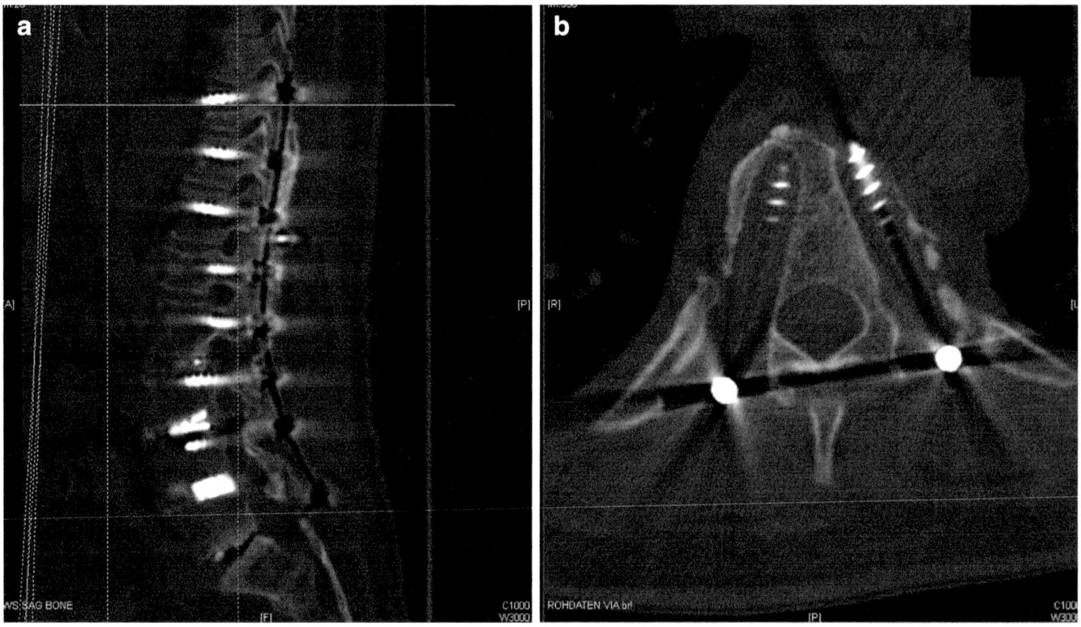

Fig. 14.5 Conventional CT at 1 year post-OP follow-up: (**a**) sagittal plane demonstrating screw loosening at Th10, 11 and 12 with a consolidated L1 vertebra, (**b**) axial plane at the Th10 level showing the large bony defect and screw migration

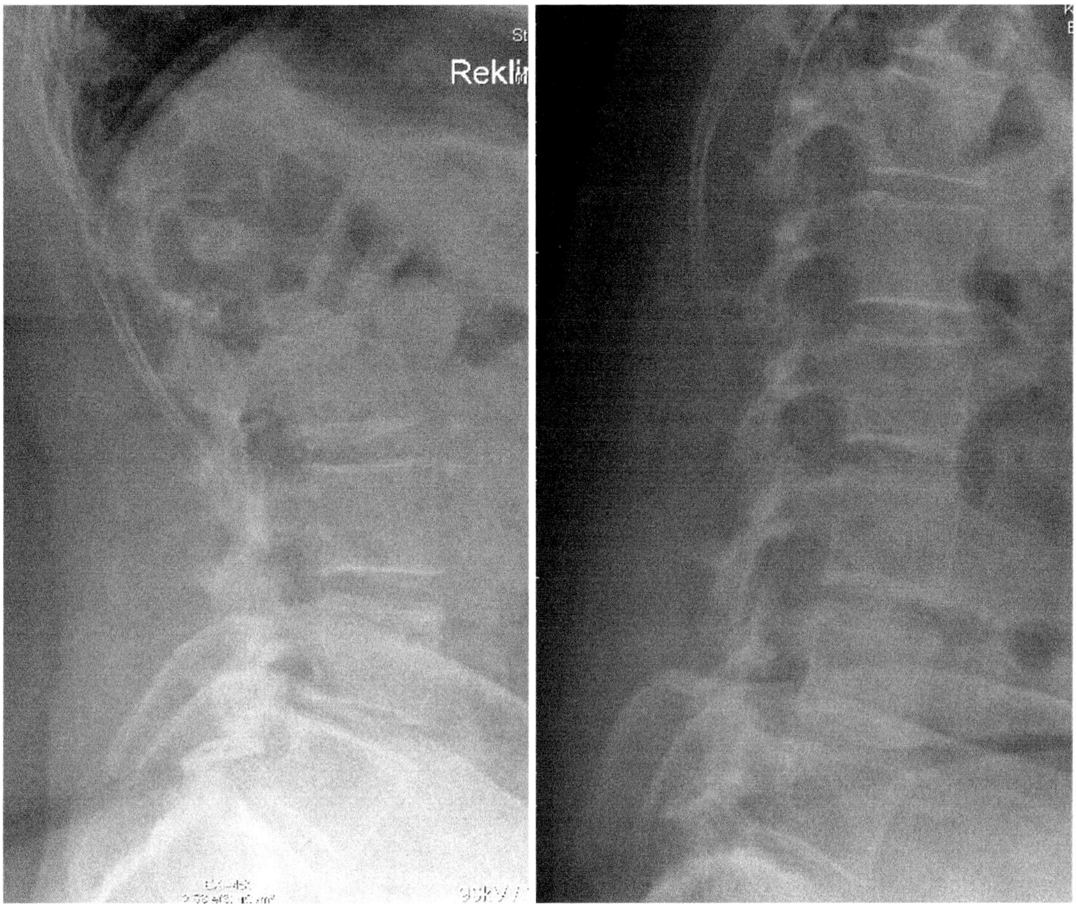

Fig. 14.6 Functional lateral X-rays showing a discrete instability with antelisthesis in anteflexion at the L4/5 level

itive response to both a periradicular injection and injections of the facet joints at the L4/5 level.

14.3.1.2 Case 2

Despite the previous surgery attempting to not only stabilize the L1 fracture, but also implement the correction of deformity, sagittal imbalance progressed to an immobilizing level of pain. Moreover, the patient complained of feeling restraint to actively convert any compensatory retroflexion of the pelvis or his thoracolumbar spine for the purpose of rebalancing a tolerable standing or walking posture. In addition to the significant screw loosening evident at the Th10, Th11 and Th12 level, the indication for revision surgery was given to reestablish a functional sagittal profile.

14.3.2 Choice of Approach

14.3.2.1 Case 1

Since the initial description of the PLIF technique by Briggs and Milligan in 1944, different methods of spinal segmental fusions have evolved, incorporating a variety of innovative implants with the option of autologous and synthetic bone grafting, and the use of pedicle screw fixation for posterior instrumentation [3]. In a

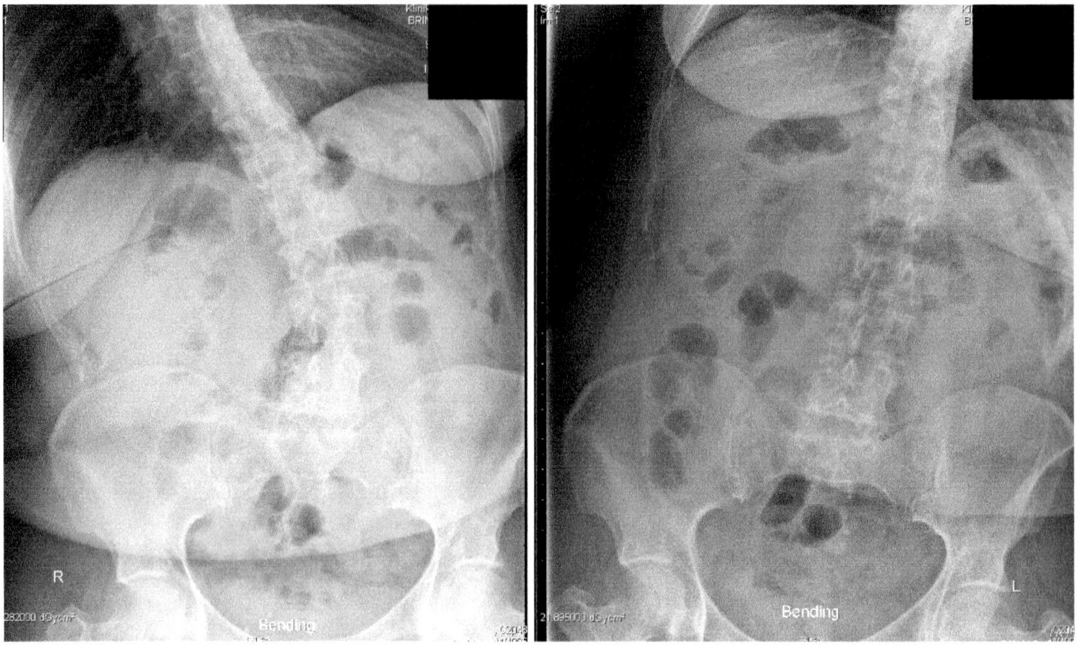

Fig. 14.7 Bending X-rays demonstrating translational instability at the L4/5 level

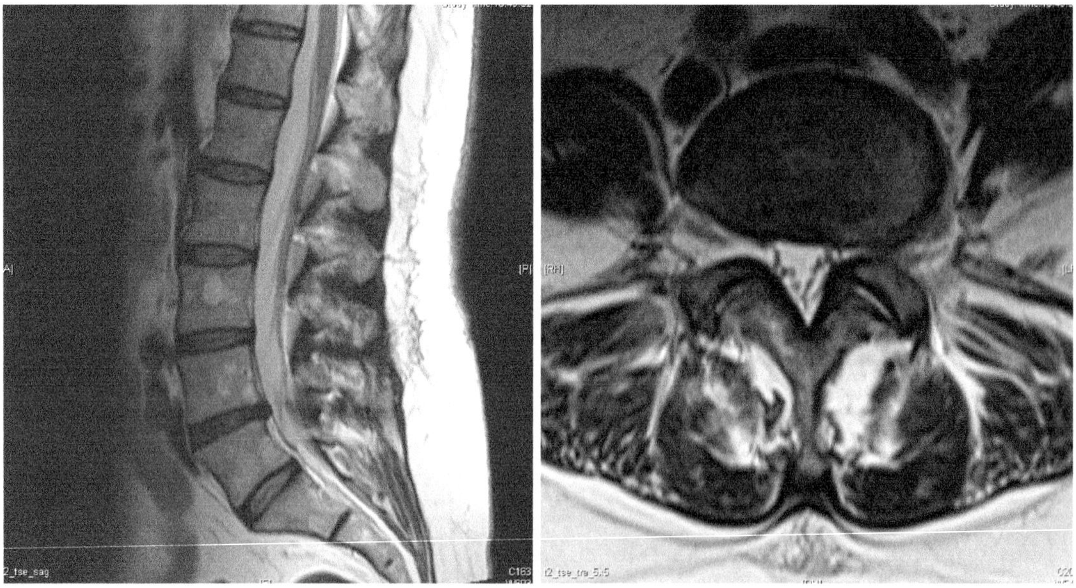

Fig. 14.8 MRI (T2-weighted images) of the lumbar spine demonstrating the degenerative disc in L4/5 with leftsided neuroforaminal stenosis

recent meta-analysis by Teng and colleagues, however, none of today's standard techniques (ALIF, OLIF/LLIF, TLIF and PLIF) stand out with significantly superior outcomes in either a direct of indirect comparison to another [1]. In a systematical search of the literature and subsequent inclusion of 30 studies, all approaches had similar fusion rates with complications such as incidental dural tears, motor or sensory deficits and visceral or vascular injuries being approach-related, but at a comparable rate throughout the included studies. Therefore, one must be careful in advancing a "one-fits-all" solution, since every approach has its own risks and benefits. Moreover, the socio-economical aspects of perioperative and postoperative care should also be taken into account, where a specific approach may be less effective in terms of implant costs, readmission rates, socio-professional reintegration and overall long-term patient-reported outcomes (PRO) [12]. The decision on which approach may be most appropriate to address all symptomatic and potentially modifiable factors is thus tailored to the individual case. In our Case 1, we therefore chose a minimally-invasive posterior procedure. To address the symptomatic left-sided radiculopathy and foraminal stenosis, the traversing L4 nerve root and spinal canal were accessed via a mini-open exposure in a modified Wiltse technique from the left. The two contralateral pedicle screws were placed percutaneously and the ipsilateral screws via the mini-open exposure in similar fashion. After performing a left-sided laminotomy and facetectomie for direct neural decompression, the disc space was thoroughly debrided and a titanium-coated PEEK cage including bone graft inserted in an oblique bridging fashion. After insertion of both rods, readjustment of lordosis was achieved via bilateral compression to complete the MIS-TLIF procedure. By utilizing the resected facet joint and bone from the laminotomy by punching only (no burr), this technique provided sufficient autologous bone graft without the additional need to harvest autologous bone from the iliac crest or resort any further bone substitution (Fig. 14.9).

In this particular case, a variety of alternative approaches would have been acceptable to achieve fusion at the L4/5 level. However, anterior approaches including the ALIF, LLIF and OLIF technique all require an additional form of autologous bone harvesting. In the majority of cases, harvesting of autologous bone is limited to the iliac crest, yet bearing an additional risk of postoperative immobilizing pain. Although there is an ongoing debate on whether the incidence of pain is strictly related to the harvesting site [13], its efficacy regarding fusion rates appears to be comparable to local bone harvested through the common posterior approaches to the lumbar spine, regardless of the choice of incision [14].

Yet, there are some advantages of anterior approaches that should be considered. While ALIF has proven to achieve a superior radiological outcome with improved restoration of postoperative disc height and segmental lordosis, OLIF and LLIF procedures have rendered the preservation of the anterior and posterior annular/ligamentous structures, equally permitting the insertion of wide cages resting bilaterally on the dense apophyseal ring and augmentation of disc height with indirect decompression of neural elements [1, 15].

However, ALIF, OLIF or LLIF at the L4/5 level with instability is not reasonable as a standalone procedure. Thus, complementing the respective treatment of the disc space with a posterior instrumentation (e.g. pedicle screw-and-rod system) is mandatory and requires a repositioning of the patient as an additional step in the operation.

Considering similar fusion rates amongst all four common approaches to the lumbar spine, each specific aspect and approach-related risk and benefit must be carefully weighed out with regard to the individual therapeutic goal.

14.3.2.2 Case 2

A characteristic challenge to any revision case is that there is no gold standard or generally accepted treatment guideline. In the particular setting of Case 2, the patient presented with all lumbar levels fused in addition to an angular kyphosis of the sacrum. Thus, all common approaches for lumbar fusion were exhausted. Furthermore, the cranial pedicle screws at Th10, 11 and 12 were severely loosened bilaterally due to the patient's repetitive attempt to actively convert to a rebalanced upright standing posture. As a result, our strategical considerations regarding the posterior instrumentation included two options: (1) Remove all loosened screws and extend the instrumentation cranially or (2) reduce

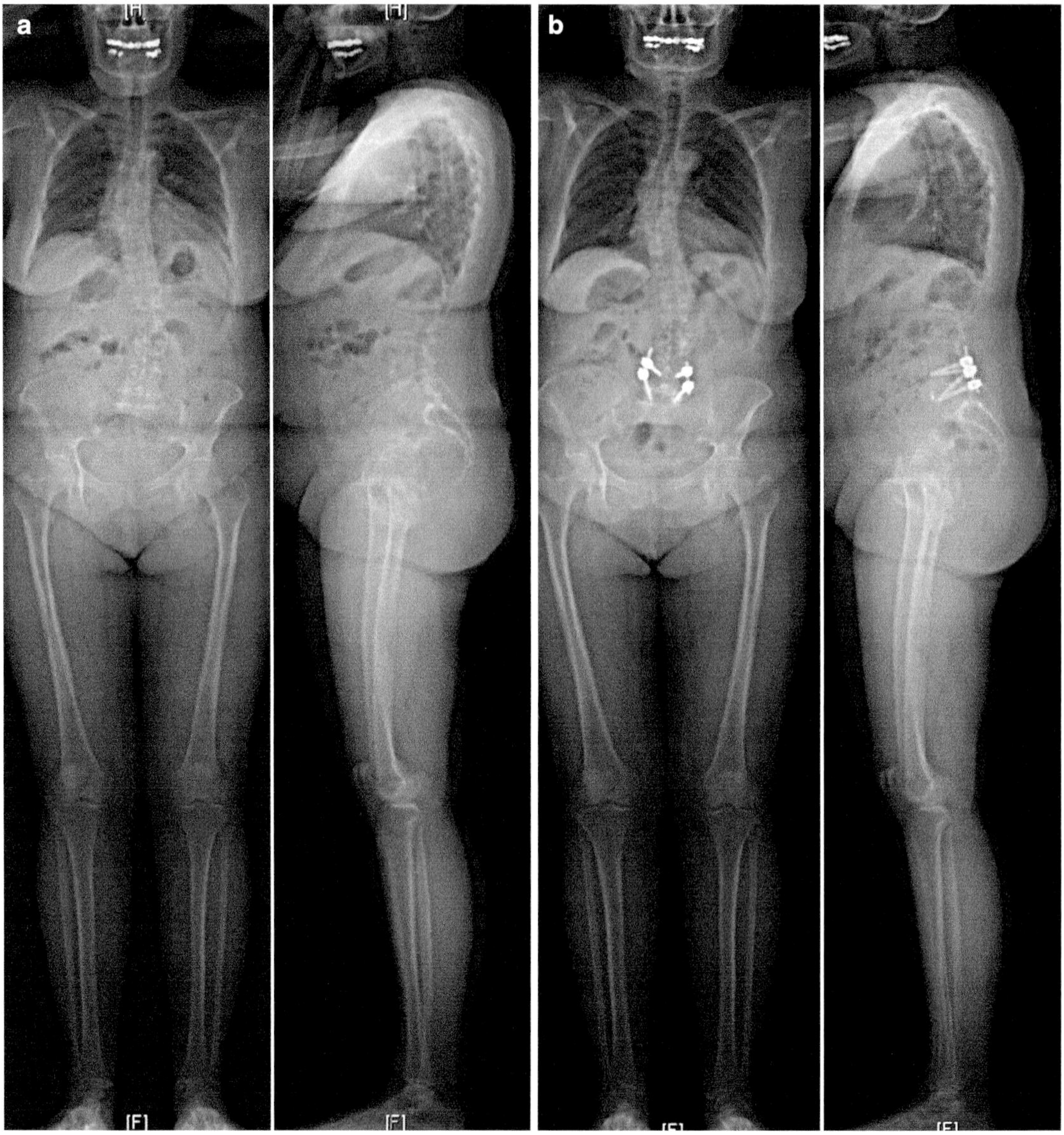

Fig. 14.9 EOS total spine imaging. (**a**) pre-operative upright standing ap and lateral, (**b**) 1 year post-operative follow-up upright standing ap and lateral

the instrumentation to the last cranially adjacent and intact motion segment.

In the event of any implant loosening or pseudarthrosis, insufficient bony fusion or hypermobility of the involved motion segment must be assumed. In cases where segmental fusion is mandatory to achieve sufficient stability and maintain the overall balance along with a functionally appropriate spinal alignment, the particular region must be addressed accordingly. However, in Case 2, the posterior instrumentation was initially extended to Th10 for stabilzation of an instable L1 fracture with regard to the existing lumbar fusion. In consideration of the meanwhile consolidated L1 fracture, intact thoracic and thoracolumbar discs and the patient's thoracolumbar discomfort, we interpreted his sense to be an indication of intact compensatory mechanisms

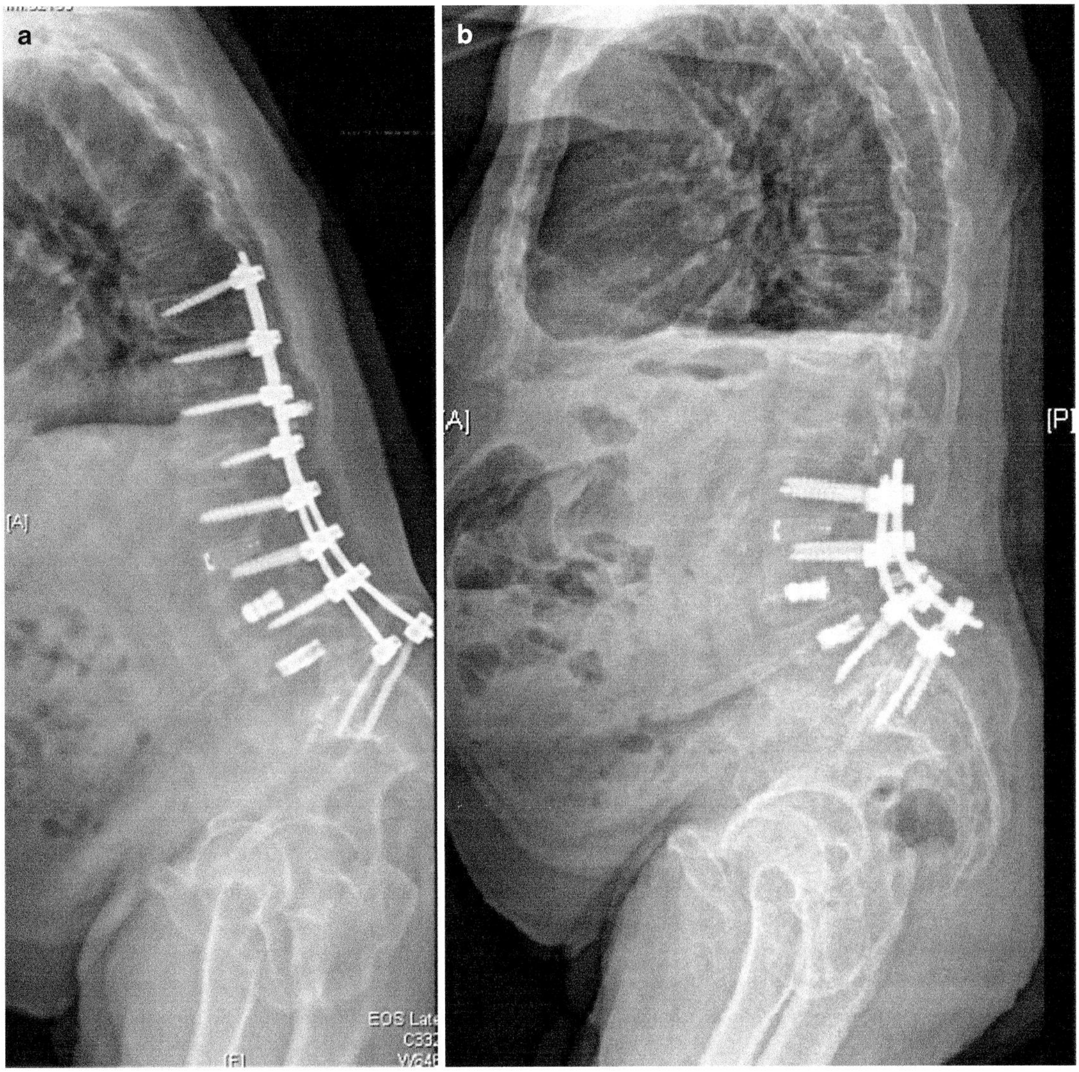

Fig. 14.10 (**a**) pre-operative lateral X-ray with sagittal imbalance, (**b**) 3-month postoperative follow-up after partial implant removal and PSO at L4

within the lower thoracic spine region. Hence, our approach was to follow the conviction, that implant removal may reestablish segmental motion in analogous manner to previous reports on thoracolumbar burst fractures [16–18].

In addition, the decreased lumbar lordosis demanded further attention to adequately rebalance the global sagittal profile. For this reason, we chose to include a pedicle subtraction osteotomy (PSO) at L4 to equally preserve the existing instrumentation and stability from L2 to S1 (Fig. 14.10).

In patients with fixed coronal or sagittal plane deformities of the lumbar and thoracolumbar spine, a single level PSO may generate a lumbar lordosis from 20 to 40 degrees with an approximate change in the sagittal vertical axis of up to 12 cm [19–21]. Although other techniques such as multiple segment Ponte osteotomies or a vertebral column resection (VCR) may similarly address hypolordotic or kyphotic deformities with subsequent sagittal imbalance, our Case 2 presented fused lumbar segments with the patient's demand to remobilize the structural dynamics of the thoracic and thoracolumbar region. Thus, our stretegy was to limit any manipulation to the already existing length of lumbar fusion by equally avoiding further immobilization of the cranially adjacent spine.

14.3.3 Accordance with the Literature Guidelines

Despite todays technical advances and improved surgical techniques, we must always acknowledge the fact that balance is a dynamic property which involves more than the bony alignment evaluated in diagnostic imaging. This suggests a more complex evaluation of the (aging) patient's abilities and requirements by equally considering the full portfolio of techniques with respect to the related risks and limitations. To date, there are no specific guidelines in the literature. Particularly revision cases demand an individual approach, preferebly managed in an interdisciplinary setting to allow for a patient-tailored and comprehensive evaluation.

14.4 Conclusions and Take Home Message

Both cases presented here display unexceptional encounters to the majority of spine surgeons. Careful evaluation and treatment of the major and foremost causally determined pathology is key to an overall good clinical outcome. In cases where the spine is well balanced, instrumentation and fusion should be limited to the pathological finding and equally preserve all dynamically intact structures involved to maintain the respective coronal and sagittal balance. In contrast, it may be very similar to liberate these structures and reactivate individual compensatory mechanisms in an otherwise fixed imbalanced posture. Despite aiming at correcting deformity by all means to restore a functional coronal and sagittal balance, soft tissue preparation should always be performed with reasonable care in either a minimally-invasive or conventional open fashion.

Pearls

- In the balanced spine, segmental pathologies may be addressed by "short segment" procedures.
- Selective periradicular or facet joint injections can aid the decision making between lumbar fusion versus non-fusion strategies.
- The choice of surgical approach and technique must give consideration to the therapeutic aim by equally including the patient's individual risks and conditions.
- Revision cases with signs of segmental hypermobility must be critically evaluated with regard to its relation of cause and effect. In justified case constellations, the revision strategy should preserve or reintegrate intact compensatory mechanisms supporting the overall sagittal balance of the spine.

Editorial Comment

This chapter illustrates in a nutshell that despite the fact, that a huge variety of techniques and instrumentations are available today, outcomes are often disappointing, especially with poorly localized low back pain. While the first patient went well, the second had many revisions and was never really satisfied. Why that is so, remains elusiveand explanations for it pure assumptions. By the way, the screw loosening illustrated here is according to our opinion not only caused by inadequate balance, but certainly also by an underlying low grade infection.

References

1. Teng I, Han J, Phan K, et al. A meta-analysis comparing alif, plif, tlif and llif. J Clin Neurosci. 2017;44:11–7.

2. Mobbs RJ, Sivabalan P, Li J. Minimally invasive surgery compared to open spinal fusion for the treatment of degenerative lumbar spine pathologies. J Clin Neurosci. 2012;19:829–35.
3. Mobbs RJ, Phan K, Malham G, et al. Lumbar interbody fusion: techniques, indications and comparison of interbody fusion options including plif, tlif, mi-tlif, olif/atp, llif and alif. J Spine Surg. 2015;1:2–18.
4. Eck JC, Hodges S, Humphreys SC. Minimally invasive lumbar spinal fusion. J Am Acad Orthop Surg. 2007;15:321–9.
5. Benditz A, Madl M, Loher M, et al. Prospective medium-term results of multimodal pain management in patients with lumbar radiculopathy. Sci Rep. 2016;6:28187.
6. Brunner M, Schwarz T, Zeman F, et al. Efficiency and predictive parameters of outcome of a multimodal pain management concept with spinal injections in patients with low back pain: a retrospective study of 445 patients. Arch Orthop Trauma Surg. 2018;138:901–9.
7. Liang HF, Liu SH, Chen ZX, et al. Decompression plus fusion versus decompression alone for degenerative lumbar spondylolisthesis: a systematic review and meta-analysis. Eur Spine J. 2017;26:3084–95.
8. Forsth P, Michaelsson K, Sanden B. Fusion surgery for lumbar spinal stenosis. N Engl J Med. 2016;375:599–600.
9. Barrey C, Jund J, Noseda O, et al. Sagittal balance of the pelvis-spine complex and lumbar degenerative diseases. A comparative study about 85 cases. Eur Spine J. 2007;16:1459–67.
10. Blumenthal C, Curran J, Benzel EC, et al. Radiographic predictors of delayed instability following decompression without fusion for degenerative grade I lumbar spondylolisthesis. J Neurosurg Spine. 2013;18:340–6.
11. Bourghli A, Aunoble S, Reebye O, et al. Correlation of clinical outcome and spinopelvic sagittal alignment after surgical treatment of low-grade isthmic spondylolisthesis. Eur Spine J. 2011;20(Suppl 5):663–8.
12. Qureshi R, Puvanesarajah V, Jain A, et al. A comparison of anterior and posterior lumbar interbody fusions: complications, readmissions, discharge dispositions, and costs. Spine (Phila Pa 1976). 2017;42:1865–70.
13. Sheha ED, Meredith DS, Shifflett GD, et al. Postoperative pain following posterior iliac crest bone graft harvesting in spine surgery: a prospective, randomized trial. Spine J. 2018;18(6):986–92.
14. France JC, Schuster JM, Moran K, et al. Iliac crest bone graft in lumbar fusion: the effectiveness and safety compared with local bone graft, and graft site morbidity comparing a single-incision midline approach with a two-incision traditional approach. Global Spine J. 2015;5:195–206.
15. Salzmann SN, Shue J, Hughes AP. Lateral lumbar interbody fusion-outcomes and complications. Curr Rev Musculoskelet Med. 2017;10:539–46.
16. Alanay A, Vyas R, Shamie AN, et al. Safety and efficacy of implant removal for patients with recurrent back pain after a failed degenerative lumbar spine surgery. J Spinal Disord Tech. 2007;20:271–7.
17. Jeon CH, Lee HD, Lee YS, et al. Is it beneficial to remove the pedicle screw instrument after successful posterior fusion of thoracolumbar burst fractures? Spine (Phila Pa 1976). 2015;40:E627–33.
18. Stavridis SI, Bucking P, Schaeren S, et al. Implant removal after posterior stabilization of the thoraco-lumbar spine. Arch Orthop Trauma Surg. 2010;130:119–23.
19. Bridwell KH. Decision making regarding smith-petersen vs. Pedicle subtraction osteotomy vs. Vertebral column resection for spinal deformity. Spine (Phila Pa 1976). 2006;31:S171–8.
20. Choi HY, Hyun SJ, Kim KJ, et al. Surgical and radiographic outcomes after pedicle subtraction osteotomy according to surgeon's experience. Spine (Phila Pa 1976). 2017;42:E795–801.
21. Kim YJ, Bridwell KH, Lenke LG, et al. Results of lumbar pedicle subtraction osteotomies for fixed sagittal imbalance: a minimum 5-year follow-up study. Spine (Phila Pa 1976). 2007;32:2189–97.

Lumbar Non-Fusion Techniques 15

Michael Stoffel

15.1 Introduction

Degeneration of the functional spinal unit (FSU) can lead to various pathologies like disc herniation, spinal stenosis, segmental instability, or intradiscal pain, respectively. This can result in back pain and – in case of nerve root irritation – sciatica.

Since pain educed by a degenerated joint is linked to its mobility, suppression of the latter should induce pain relief. Hence, spinal fusion became the golden standard treatment for disc arthrosis, degenerative segmental instability, and spondylolisthesis, respectively.

Nowadays, various fusion techniques exist with acceptable results. However, disadvantages arise from the high surgical effort associated with these techniques – where incidence and severity of complications rise with increased surgical complexity -, the risk of pseudarthrosis, and the increased incidence of adjacent level degeneration, resulting from the transfer of mechanical stress to adjacent segments [1, 2].

Since fusion rate and clinically successful pain relieve are not strictly interrelated in patients after spondylodesis, the complete immobilization of the FSU might not be an absolute prerequisite for pain relief in these patients.

These considerations led to the development of non-fusion techniques (AKA: dynamic techniques) in spine surgery with the following goals:

- relief pain caused by the degenerated FSU,
- maintenance or regain of stability,
- maintenance of mobility and function of the spine,
- reduction of stress transfer to adjacent FSUs as a longterm goal.

Non-fusion techniques can be divided into (a) joint replacement techniques (AKA: arthroplasty, prosthetics), where the nucleus pulposus (nucleus replacement), the whole disc (total disc replacement = TDR), or the facet joints (facet replacement), respectively, are removed and replaced, or (b) dynamic stabilization techniques, where posteriorly placed implants limit the range of motion in a FSU thereby leading to a redistribution of mechanical stress between the disc, the facet joint, and the implant (load sharing). In this group, pedicle-screw based dynamic systems (PDS) and interspinous process devices (IPD) exist.

Aim of the presented cases is to point out,

- in which clinical scenario the most popular non-fusion techniques (IPD, TDR, pedicle-screw based systems) might be used,

M. Stoffel (✉)
Department of Neurosurgery, Helios Klinikum Krefeld, Krefeld, Germany
e-mail: Michael.stoffel@helios-gesundheit.de

B. Meyer, M. Rauschmann (eds.), *Spine Surgery*, https://doi.org/10.1007/978-3-319-98875-7_15

- which pros and cons exist for their use in comparison to traditional fusion techniques,
- which level of evidence exists for clinical decision-making.

15.2 Case Description

15.2.1 Case 1

A 79 y/o male patient presents to our outpatient clinic with a 1 year history of progressive bilateral neurogenic claudication with a maximal walking distance of 200 meters, paravertebral and radiating pain (VAS 8) with right-sided predominance. The physical examination reveals no neurological deficit. His complaints are not responsive to pain killers or physiotherapy. He is a hobby volcanologist and significantly impaired in his activities of daily life. Due to a coronary heart disease and status post coronary stent (drug-eluting) implantation 1.5 years ago, he is on clopidogrel 75 mg (Fig. 15.1).

He is sent to his cardiologist for check-up prior to surgery, who agrees to the transient removal of clopidogrel perioperatively.

Monosegmental decompression via a right-sided approach (interlaminar fenestration) and bilateral decompression in undercutting technique is proposed as first tier therapeutic option. Implantation of a interspinous process device (IPD) is mentioned as alternative. Clopidogrel was paused 7 days prior to surgery, surgery was uneventful, and the patient left the hospital on post-op day 5. Clopidogrel was restarted on post-op day 7. Three months later he presented again in our outpatient clinic on a routine basis with completely resolved claudication.

15.2.2 Case 2

A 42 y/o male patient suffered from low back pain for app. 7 years with increasing severity exacerbating during sitting and trunk rotation with intermittent pseudoradicular bilateral sciatica. Visual Analogue Scale (VAS) back 6–7 and leg 4, Oswestry Disability Index (ODI) 37. Conservative treatment via the local pain clinics and inpatient rehabilitation remained without lasting benefit. Axial spondyloarthritis was ruled out by a rheumatologist. The patient's quality of life was significantly impaired and he was on sick leave (Fig. 15.2).

Diagnostic bilateral facet joint infiltrations L4/5 and sacroiliac joint infiltrations didn't lead to pain relief. Accordingly, the following therapeutic options were mentioned: total disc replacement (TDR), fusion, spinal cord stimulation, and continuation of conservative measures. TDR was recommended, the patient consented to the procedure, was operated via a left retroperitoneal approach, and a prosthesis was implanted.

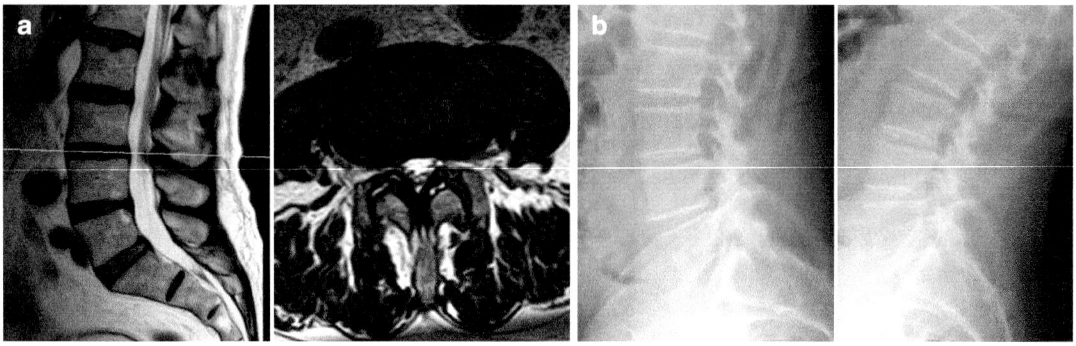

Fig. 15.1 (**a**) T2-weighted lumbar MRI exhibits bilateral facet joint hypertrophy causing narrowing of the recesses with right-sited predominance. In addition, a small facet joint cyst is detected on the right side. (**b**) Lumbar flexion-extension films rule out significant segmental hypermobility

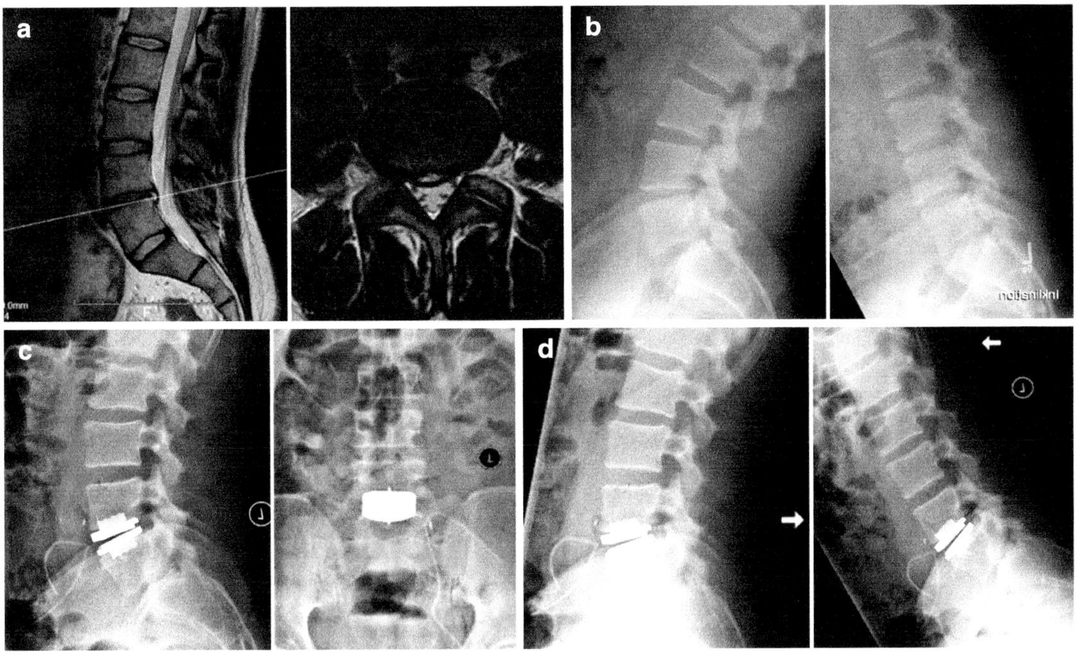

Fig. 15.2 (**a**) T2-weighted lumbar MRI exhibits a monosegmental degenerated disc L4/5 with reduced disc height, hypointense signal, a dorsal high intensity zone in the vicinity of the dorsal annulus and a disc protrusion. (**b**) Lumbar flexion/extension radiographs rule out segmental hypermobility. (**c** + **d**) a.p. and lateral radiographs and flexion-extension films on post-op day 2 confirm the adequate position of the implant and the mobility of the segment

Surgery was uneventful and the patient was discharged on post-op day 4. Post-operative physiotherapy was recommended. He came for routine follow-up 3 months post-op in our outpatient clinic. He was completely weaned from the pain killers, VAS back 2, VAS leg 0, ODI 18, and has resumed his work.

15.2.3 Case 3

A 48 y/o female presented to our outpatient clinic with a 9months' history of left-sided sciatica predominantly in the L5-dermatome (VAS 7), a L5-dysesthesia, and back pain of similar intensity. Two years ago, she had surgery for disc herniation in L4/5 und L5/S1 on the right side due to a foot drop. After surgery, she had good symptom relief for app. 15 months. The patient was on opioids and non-steroidals for at least 3 months. On physical examination, she was significantly obese (BMI 30), had diabetes, L5-hypesthesia, and a slight weakness of the left knee extension. The mobility of the lumbar spine was significantly reduced and she reported exacerbation of the back pain on spinal process pressure in the lower lumbar region (Fig. 15.3).

Bilateral medial nerve blocks for L4/5 und L5/S1 led to app. 80% reduction of back pain for 24 h. Surgery was offered including dynamic stabilization of L4/5 and L5/S1, decompression of the spinal recess and the foramina in both segments on the left side. Spondylodesis was mentioned as alternative.

Postoperatively, the sciatica disappeared completed, local back pain along the wound remained, and the patient was discharged on post-op day 8. Inpatient rehab was organized. Three months later, the patient exhibited no motor deficit anymore, denied sciatica or dysesthesia and a reported a VAS (back) 2 without pain medication.

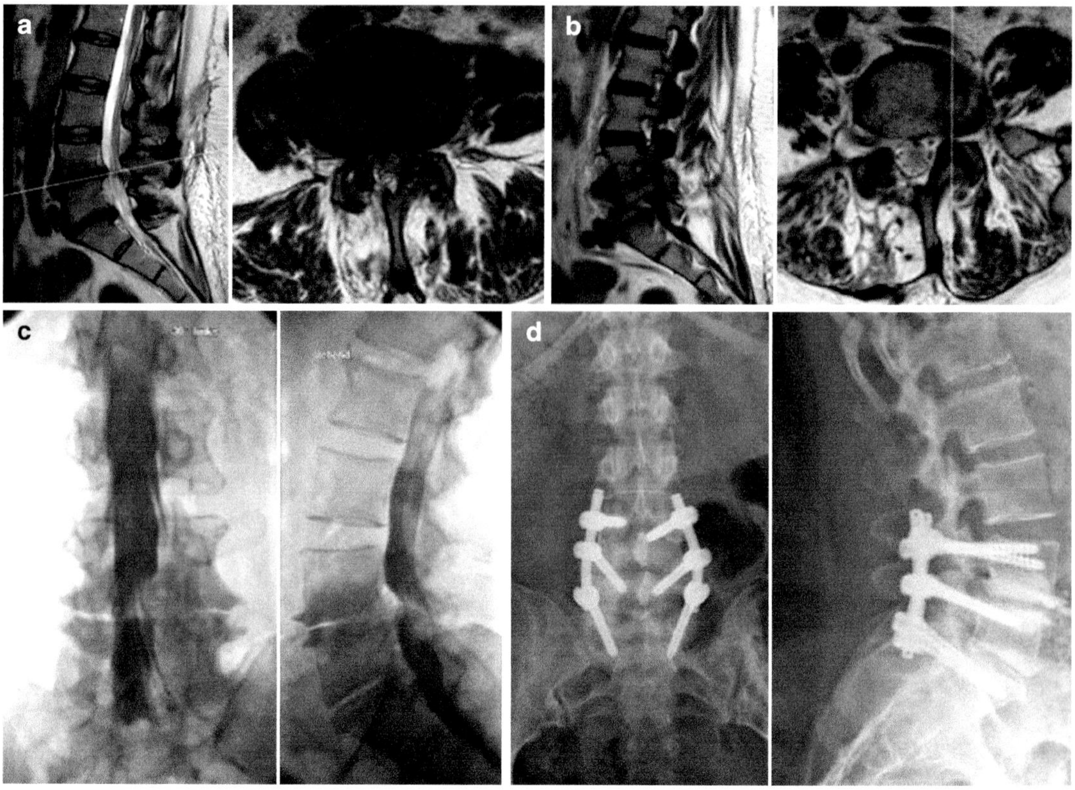

Fig. 15.3 (**a**, **b**) T2-weighted lumbar MRIs reveal disc degeneration and protrusion in L4/5 and L5/S1, status post interlaminar fenestrations in L4/5 and L5/S1, facet joint hypertrophy leading to recess stenosis in both segments and left-sided foraminal stenosis. The exact dimension of space occupation in the spinal canal is not unequivocally assessable due to scare tissue. (**c**) Myelography shows significant left-sided space occupation at L4/5 compressing the L4 und L5 root, disc space narrowing in L4/5 and L5/S1, and osteochondrosis. (**d**) Lumbar radiographs reveal proper implant placement L4, L5, and S1

15.3 Discussion of the Cases

15.3.1 Case 1

A. Why were things done this way

Spinal decompression via a microsurgical approach sparing the midline structures is currently the standard surgical option in patients with neurogenic claudication significantly impaired by their symptoms. Surgery is simple and the clinical benefit foreseeable and durable. Segment instability was ruled out. Platelet aggregation inhibition could be stopped prior to surgery. Therefore, no potentially increased risk of bleeding had to be expected. IPD-implantation appears a valid alternative in this case, however, much less durable and associated with a much higher reoperation rate.

B. Were they in accordance with the literature guidelines

According to the observational cohort of the SPORT-trial, patients with symptomatic spinal stenosis have a significantly better outcome compared to conservatively treated patients. The benefits of surgery are stable up to 8 years after surgery [3]. Concerning the technical realization of the decompression, laminotomy (uni- or bilateral) sparing the midline structures seems to be the current standard in Europe. Facet sparing laminectomy is still an alternative. A Cochrane Review summarizes 4 high-quality and 6 low-quality RCTs that compare laminotomy with laminectomy. Thereby, laminotomy and conventional laminectomy show similar effects on functional disability and leg pain. However, perceived recovery at final follow-up was better after bilateral laminotomy. Furthermore, the risk of iatrogenic instability and the severity of postoperative low back pain was less after uni- or bilateral laminotomy [4].

The effectiveness of IPDs in patients with neurogenic claudication was proven in a meta-analysis of two RCTs and eight prospective cohorts. All studies showed improvement in validated outcome scores after 6 weeks and 1 year. Pooled data based on the Zurich Claudication Questionnaire of the RCTs were more in favor of IPD compared to conservative treatment [5]. Compared to surgical decompression, IPDs showed no significant differences for low back pain, leg pain, ODI, and Roland Disability Questionnaire (RDQ) 12–24 months after the procedure, but a significantly higher risk of reoperation (odds ratio 3.34) [6]. This was confirmed in a recent RCT [7].

In patients dependent on platelet aggregation inhibitors, open surgery might be more prone to clinically significant rebleeding – a situation that might represent a niche for the use of percutaneous IPD placement.

As yet, the use of IPDs in the treatment of neurogenic claudication is not covered in a guideline.

C. How strong is the level of evidence available to date

Surgical decompression and the implantation of interspinous process devices improve clinical outcome in neurogenic claudication compared to nonoperative treatment (Level-I Evidence). The direct comparison of both procedures shows - at least in short-term – similar results in relieving symptoms of claudication, however, IPD proved to be much less durable than surgical decompression (Level-I Evidence).

15.3.2 Case 2

A. Why were things done this way

The patient suffered mainly from severe chronic low back pain with significant impact on his activities of daily life including work, refractory to conservative treatment. The MRI exhibited monosegmental degenerative disc disease (DDD) in L4/5. A significant contribution of the facet joints L4/5 and the sacroiliac joints to the generation of pain was ruled out by diagnostic infiltrations. Accordingly, the degenerated disc itself was the supposed pain generator and TDR or fusion would have been the first tier therapeutic options. TDR was our recommendation due to the potential advantages over fusion, i.e. maintenance of mobility and function of the spine and reduction of stress transfer to adjacent FSUs as mentioned above.

B. Were they in accordance with the literature guidelines

Due to results of the Norwegian Spine Study Group, patients with a history of low back pain for at least 1 year, an ODI of at least 30, and degenerative changes in one or two lower lumbar spine levels exhibit significantly better ODI-reduction after TDR than after rehabilitation [8]. Above that, low back pain, patients' satisfaction, SF-36 physical component, self efficacy for pain, and Prolo scale showed significant differences in favour of surgery in this study. Adjacent level disease was observed at similar frequencies at the 2-year follow-up in the surgical and the rehab group [9].

Six randomized controlled trials (RCTs) comparing TDR with spinal fusion for chronic back pain were summarized in a Cochrane Review [10]. Thereby, patients who underwent TDR had slightly better outcomes in terms of back pain and function 24 months after surgery than those who had fusion surgery, although the differences did not appear clinically significant.

Finally, there is growing evidence that the clinical outcome after lumbar TDR is durable over up to 10 years [11, 12].

C. How strong is the level of evidence available to date

The levels of evidence supporting TDR-surgery in this case are as follows:

- TDR superior to conservative treatment (Level-I Evidence)
- TDR at least not inferior to fusion surgery (Level-I Evidence)
- durable clinical outcome after TDR up to 10 years (Level-III Evidence)

As yet, no clear cut guideline for the indication of TDR is existing.

15.3.3 Case 3

A. Why were things done this way

The patient suffered from back pain and radiculopathy. Reason for the radiculopathy was compression of the nerve roots L4 and L5 on the left side, main reason for the back pain was disc degeneration in L4/5 and L5/S1 leading to disc height reduction and facet joint irritation in both segments, responsive to facet joint infiltration. Accordingly, a procedure including nerve root decompression and bisegmental stabilization seems the obvious causal therapy and only the method of stabilization seems questionable. In our experience, mono- or bisegmental dynamic stabilization in the degenerated spine achieves similar results to spondylodesis, however, with less surgical effort. Therefore, dynamic stabilization is our first choice when stabilization is indicated in degenerative disease other than spondylolysis or high-grade spondylolisthesis.

B. Were they in accordance with the literature guidelines

Reoperation for recurrent disc herniation leading to conservatively refractory pain is well established and – as known from a subgroup analysis of the SPORT-trial – patients will likely improve significantly following surgery, but possibly not as much as with primary discectomy [13]. The use of medial nerve blocks for short-term relief of facet-mediated chronic low back pain is suggested in the "Guideline update for the performance of fusion procedures for degenerative disease of the lumbar spine" [14]. Unfortunately, outcome prediction for subsequent lumbar fusion is not possible from the current literature [14]. The same guidelines consider lumbar fusion an option when disc herniation is associated with evidence of instability, chronic low-back pain, and/or severe degenerative changes [15]. The replacement of spondylodesis by a dynamic pedicle-screw based system seems a valid option in the degenerative spine. Thereby, the surgical step that provides the basis for solid fusion – e.g. discectomy and intervertebral cage implantation – can be spared, rendering the surgical procedure less invasive. Thereby, one of the potential advantages is that less complex procedures are also less prone to complications, a fact that could be proven in a RCT comparing different techniques for spondylodesis [2]. Various dynamic pedicle-screw based systems are on the market with different biomechanical ideas behind them. As yet, the most frequently studied systems are the Dynesis (Fa. Zimmer) and the Cosmic (Fa. Ulrich) system. Both systems have been investigated in numerous cohort studies and their efficacy to reduce preoperative back pain resulting from degenerative disease could be proven – at least on a short term basis (e.g. [16, 17]). However, no high-quality data comparing spondylodesis with dynamic stabilization are available. The data of an RCT on that topic are still pending.

C. How strong is the level of evidence available to date

The levels of evidence for reoperation for recurrent disc herniation is derived from subgroup analysis of an RCT and an observational cohort (Level-II Evidence). The decision for dynamic pedicle-screw based stabilization is based on cohort studies (Level-III Evidence).

15.4 Conclusions and Take Home Message

Interspinous process devices exhibit similar short-term relief of symptoms from neurogenic claudication than open decompression, but with a much higher reoperation rate. Accordingly, their use is reserved for niche indications – at maximum.

Patients with significant chronic low back pain refractory to conservative treatment, who reveal radiological signs of mono- or bisegmental disc degeneration, are potential candidates for lumbar TDR. Segment hypermobility and predominant facet joint syndrome should be ruled out.

Dynamic pedicle-screw based stabilization might be an alternative for spondylodesis in mono- or bisegmental degenerative disease, although sound data comparing these methods are not available so far.

Pearls

- IPDs don't seem to provide durable results and serve – at maximum – for niche indications
- Lumbar TDR is a valid option in selected cases of DDD – probably even with satisfying long-term results
- solid scientific results supporting the use of dynamic pedicle-screw based systems, although widely used and promising, are still pending

Editorial Comment

We strongly recommend to read this excellent chapter on a topic, that has produced considerable controversy in the last 20 years. A "hype" has been provoked initially for these new technologies leading to a massive overuse in unproven indications, which has then triggered an overreaction against them. So on most of them the majority of the spine community has closed the book already. This chapter now provides a very thorough and sober evaluation of the existing high-level evidence in this field. Overall it shows for IPDs (that is the stand-alone variant replacing decompression) and lumbar TDR to have a place in highly selected patients. However, acceptance within the community is questionable these days and the industry is probably not interested in the production of devices, which do not sell in high numbers. As it evolves, and evidenced by the preliminary data of a RCT comparing fusion with dynamic stabilization (unpublished data) pedicle-screw-based systems may have a place in low grade degenerative instabilities of the lumbar spine.

References

IPD

1. Ghiselli G, Wang JC, Bhatia NN, et al. Adjacent segment degeneration in the lumbar spine. J Bone Joint Surg Am. 2004 Jul;86-A(7):1497–503.
2. Fritzell P, Hägg O, Nordwall A, Swedish Lumbar Spine Study Group. Complications in lumbar fusion surgery for chronic low back pain: comparison of three surgical techniques used in a prospective randomized study. A report from the Swedish lumbar spine study group. Eur Spine J. 2003;12(2):178–89.
3. Lurie JD, Tosteson TD, Tosteson A, Abdu WA, Zhao W, Morgan TS, Weinstein JN. Long-term outcomes of lumbar spinal stenosis: eight-year results of the spine patient outcomes research trial (SPORT). Spine (Phila Pa 1976). 2015;40(2):63–76.
4. Overdevest GM, Jacobs W, Vleggeert-Lankamp C, Thomé C, Gunzburg R, Peul W. Effectiveness of posterior decompression techniques compared with conventional laminectomy for lumbar stenosis. Cochrane Database Syst Rev. 2015;(3).
5. Moojen WA, Arts MP, Bartels RH, Jacobs WC, Peul WC. Effectiveness of interspinous implant surgery in patients with intermittent neurogenic claudication: a systematic review and meta-analysis. Eur Spine J. 2011;20(10):1596–606.
6. Wu AM, Zhou Y, Li QL, Wu XL, Jin YL, Luo P, Chi YL, Wang XY. Interspinous spacer versus traditional decompressive surgery for lumbar spinal stenosis: a systematic review and meta-analysis. PLoS One. 2014;9(5):e97142.
7. Meyer B, Baranto A, Schils F, Collignon F, Zoega B, Tan L, LeHuec JC; NICE Trial Study Group. Percutaneous Interspinous Spacer vs Decompression in Patients with Neurogenic Claudication: An Alternative in Selected Patients?. Neurosurgery. 2017.

TDR

8. Hellum C, Johnsen LG, Storheim K, Nygaard OP, Brox JI, Rossvoll I, et al. Surgery with disc prosthesis versus rehabilitation in patients with low back pain and degenerative disc: two year follow-up of randomised study. BMJ. 2011;342:d2786.

9. Hellum C, Berg L, Gjertsen Ø, Johnsen LG, Neckelmann G, Storheim K, et al. Adjacent level degeneration and facet arthropathy after disc prosthesis surgery or rehabilitation in patients with chronic low back pain and degenerative disc: second report of a randomized study. Spine (Phila Pa 1976). 2012;37(25):2063–73.
10. Jacobs W, Van der Gaag NA, Tuschel A, de Kleuver M, Peul W, Verbout AJ, Oner FC. Total disc replacement for chronic back pain in the presence of disc degeneration. Cochrane Database Syst Rev. 2012.
11. Siepe CJ, Heider F, Wiechert K, Hitzl W, Ishak B, Mayer MH. Mid- to long-term results of total lumbar disc replacement: a prospective analysis with 5- to 10-year follow-up. Spine J. 2014;14(8):1417–31.
12. Plais N, Thevenot X, Cogniet A, Rigal J, Le Huec JC. Maverick total disc arthroplasty performs well at 10 years follow-up: a prospective study with HRQL and balance analysis. Eur Spine J. 2017.

Pedicle-screw based systems

13. Abdu RW, Abdu WA, Pearson AM, Zhao W, Lurie JD, Weinstein JN. Reoperation for recurrent intervertebral disc herniation in the spine patient outcomes research trial: analysis of rate, risk factors, and outcome. Spine (Phila Pa 1976). 2017;42(14):1106–14.
14. Watters WC 3rd, Resnick DK, Eck JC, Ghogawala Z, Mummaneni PV, Dailey AT, Choudhri TF, Sharan A, Groff MW, Wang JC, Dhall SS, Kaiser MG. Guideline update for the performance of fusion procedures for degenerative disease of the lumbar spine. Part 13: injection therapies, low-back pain, and lumbar fusion. J Neurosurg Spine. 2014;21(1):79–90.
15. Wang JC, Dailey AT, Mummaneni PV, Ghogawala Z, Resnick DK, Watters WC 3rd, Groff MW, Choudhri TF, Eck JC, Sharan A, Dhall SS, Kaiser MG. Guideline update for the performance of fusion procedures for degenerative disease of the lumbar spine. Part 8: lumbar fusion for disc herniation and radiculopathy. J Neurosurg Spine. 2014;21(1):48–53.
16. Stoll TM, Dubois G, Schwarzenbach O. The dynamic neutralization system for the spine: a multi-center study of a novel non-fusion system. Eur Spine J. 2002;11(Suppl 2):S170–8. Epub 2002 Sep 10
17. Maleci A, Sambale RD, Schiavone M, Lamp F, Özer F, von Strempel A. Nonfusion stabilization of the degenerative lumbar spine. J Neurosurg Spine. 2011;15(2):151–8. https://doi.org/10.3171/2011.3.SPINE0969. Epub 2011 May 13.

Management of Failed Back Surgery Syndrome

16

Ehab Shiban and Bernhard Meyer

16.1 Introduction

Failed back surgery syndrome (FBSS) has been initially defined as the end-stage following one or several operative procedures on the spine in order to relieve axial and/or radicular pain without positive effect. However, in many of these patients there might still be a spinal pathology causing their symptoms. The most common causes include residual/recurrent disc herniation, spinal stenosis, infection or mechanical instability following decompression. Therefore, another and much more suitable definition of FBSS was provided by the international association for the study of pain. Thereby FBSS is present when patients are suffering from spinal pain of unknown origin either persisting despite surgical intervention or appearing after surgical intervention for spinal pain originally in the same topographical location.

Because there is no clear and overall accepted definition of FBSS there is no valid data on incidence or prevalence. 20% to 40% of patients following spinal procedures are estimated to have FBSS. Treatment of FBSS depends on the underling condition. For patients with a clear patholtogy revision surgery can be recommended. Otherwise a multidisciplinary biopsychosocial rehabilitation or neuromodulation may be recommended. However, presence or absence of a spinal pathology on spinal imaging does not necessarily correspond with clinical findings [1]. Therefore treatment allocation of FBSS patients remains a challenging task is some cases.

This chapter will illustrate the different casus of FBSS and discuss the various treatment modalities with emphasis to their efficacy and level of evidence. At the end of this chapter the readers should be able correctly manage patients with FBSS.

The aim of the presented case is to illustrate a management algorithm and treatment allocation for patients with FBSS.

16.2 Case Description

A 62 year-old man presented with left sided S1 sciatica for the last 8 weeks. 6 Months prior the patient underwent a left sided microdiskectomy L5/S1 due to a soft herniated disc (Fig. 16.1). Thereafter he was pain free for 4 months. He had no clinically significant medical history and the physical examination revealed that he was unable to walk on his toes and that the ankle jerk reflex was diminished. Also he had severe pain with the straight-leg-raising maneuver to 40°. He was on

E. Shiban (✉) · B. Meyer
Department of Neurosurgery, Klinikum rechts der Isar, Technische Universität München, Munich, Germany
e-mail: Ehab.shiban@tum.de

B. Meyer, M. Rauschmann (eds.), *Spine Surgery*, https://doi.org/10.1007/978-3-319-98875-7_16

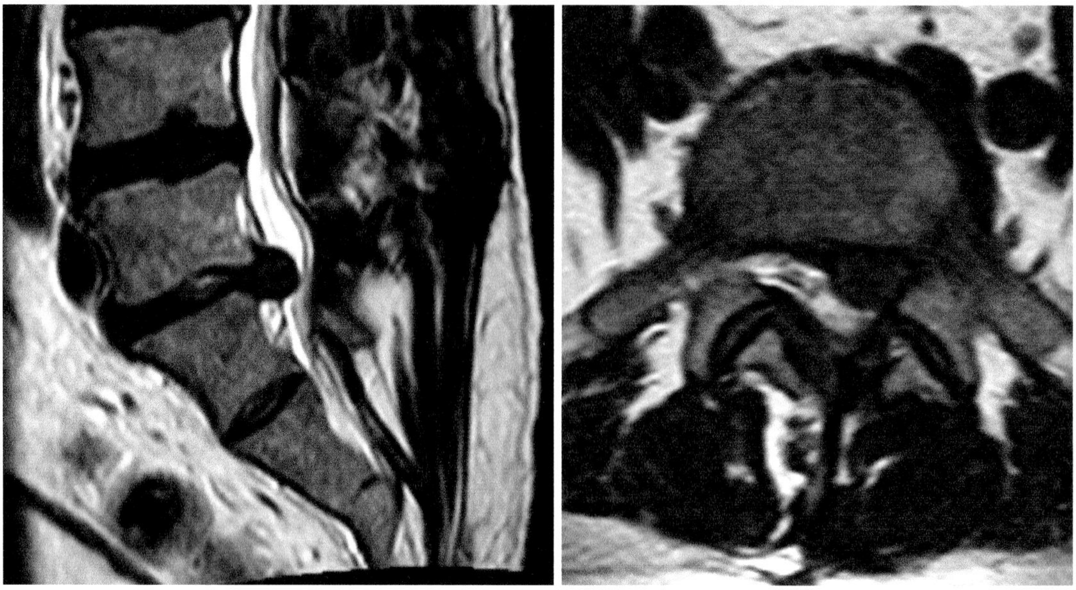

Fig. 16.1 MRI of the lumbar spine showing a clear right sided herniated disc at L5/S1

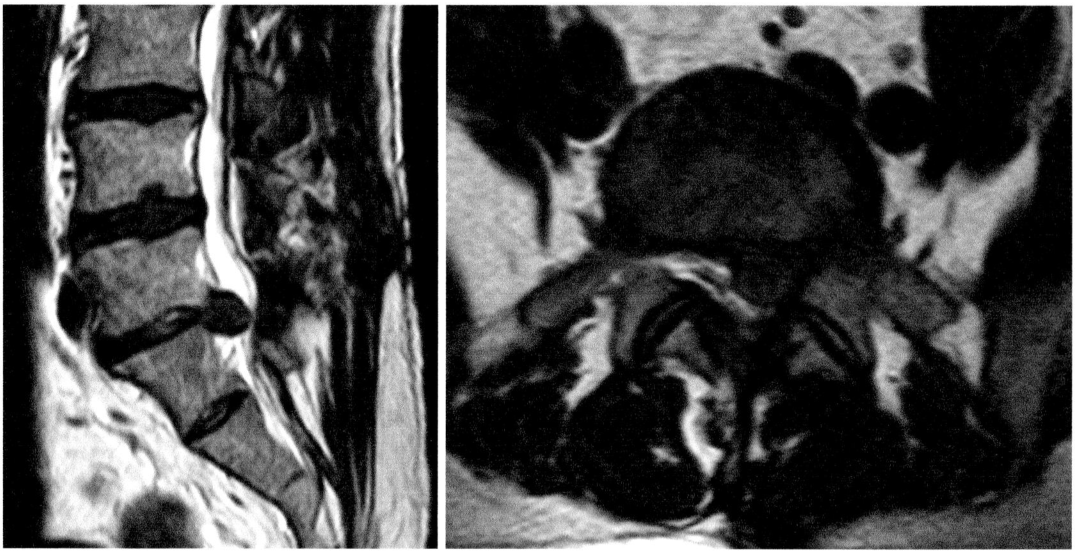

Fig. 16.2 MRI of the lumbar spine showing a clear right sided re-herniated disc at L5/S1

ibuprofen 800 mg twice daily without significant pain relief. Magnetic resonance imaging (MRI) showed a left sided recurrent herniated disc at L5/S1 (Fig. 16.2). The patient underwent elective re-microdiskectomy at L5/S1 and was pain free thereafter. At 12 months follow up the patient was still pain free.

16.3 Discussion of the Case

In this case we chose to perform surgery because the patient had a "true" recurrent herniated disc and did not achieve significant pain relief for 8 weeks following conservative treatment. It is generally accepted to treat recurrent disc herniation microsurgically following failed conservative treatment or in the presence of neurological deficits.

The assessment of patients with FBSS begins with a thorough history and physical examination. Thereby beside location of the pain the temporal relationship between pain and primary surgery has to be assessed. In cases in which the radicular pain persists in the immediate postoperative period is indicative of inadequate surgical treatment. A new onset of radicular pain immediately following surgery may be indicative of a misplaced pedicle screw, whereas a new onset of radicular pain one to 3 days following surgery in indicative of a postoperative hematoma or infection. Longstanding pain following surgery is however more difficult to asses, especially in multisegmental pathologies.

16.3.1 Imaging

The most simple and readably available imaging modality are X-rays. Thereby, spinal deformities, changes in lordosis and sagittal balance can be assessed. However, this not adequate fro assessment of spinal stenosis, nerve root compression or disc changes. The gold standard is gadolinium-enhanced MRI. The use on contrast enhancement allows to differentiae between postoperative fibrosis and disc herniation in most cases. However, the presence or absence of a recurrent herniated disc on postoperative imaging is sometime difficult to define, as most patients will have changes on spinal MRI that do not cause any symptoms [1]. In a multicenter randomized trial comparing surgery to prolonged conservative treatment for sciatica in patients with lumbar disk herniation, 33% of patients with favorable outcome and 35% of patients with unfavorable outcome had a recurrent disc herniation at one-year follow-up on magnetic resonance imaging [1]. Therefore, in unclear cases a diagnostic nerve block with only local anesthesia may be helpful in clarifying whether the changes on the MRI are symptomatic [4].

16.3.2 Management

For patients with FBSS and clear pathology of the index level with a corresponding clinical symptom then revision surgery in indicated. In the case of postoperative spinal infection, cerebrospinal fluid fistula or a clear recurrent disk herniation then revision surgery should be done (Fig. 16.3). For patients with low back pain without radicular pain, spinal claudication or with multisegmental degeneration conservative treatment with or without infiltration therapy should be initially performed. If there is no sufficient pain reduction then a trial of spinal cord stimulation can be recommended (Fig. 16.3).

Conservative treatment may include multiple modalities such as physical therapy, psychotherapy (stress reduction and cognitive behavioral therapy) [3] as well as facet joint infiltration or acupuncture [2]. All of these conservative measures should be done in addition to an optimized medical treatment plan.

If these conservative measure fail then a spinal cord stimulation (SCS) trial is warranted. SCS is an accepted treatment option for chronic pain. However, conventional SCS was preserved for FBSS patients with predominantly chronic neuropathic leg pain. In recent years the emergence of the high frequency stimulation method made low back pain a potential treatment target. A randomized multicenter RCT involving 198 participants illustrated the superiority of high-frequency SCS compared to conventional spinal cord stimulation for the treatment of back pain and leg pain [5].

16.3.3 Re-herniation: Surgical Approach

In those cases with a clear reherniation surgery has been shown to lead to favorable results. The choice between re-discectomy and re-discectomy with fusion for re-herniated disc is still a matter of some debate [6]. A survey among spine surgeons in the united stats identifying surgical treatment for re-herniation found that a surgeon practicing for 15–20 years was less likely to performed

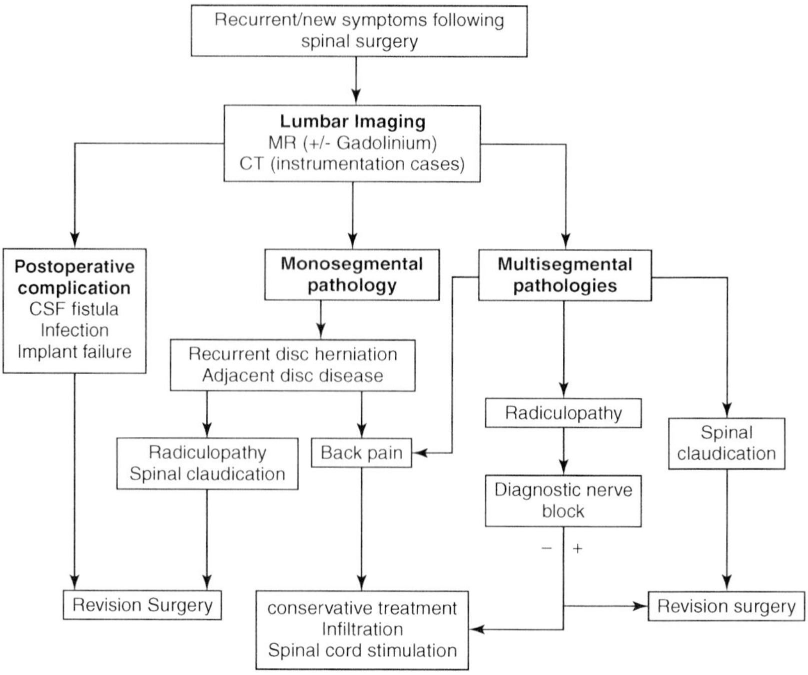

Fig. 16.3 Treatment algorithm for patients with failed back surgery syndrome

fusion for a re-herniated disc and surgeons performing more than 200 cases per year were more likely to perform fusion [8]. A recent meta-analysis of 37 studies with 1483 patients demonstrated that although greater improvement in back pain was achieved in patients undergoing re-discectomy and fusion compared to re-discectomy alone, the rate of satisfactory outcome was similar in both groups. Moreover, patients undergoing re-discectomy alone had a lower rate of surgery related complications [9]. In a small single center study 45 patients with first-time re-herniated disc were randomized for re-discectomy alone, re-discectomy with transforaminal lumbar interbody fusion or re-discectomy with posterolateral fusion. The three groups showed no significant differences with regard to the mean functional outcome, recovery rate or satisfactory rate [7].

16.3.4 Literature Guidelines

To date there are no guidelines or significant comparative studies to help surgeons in determining which approach would be most appropriate to treat re-herniated disc. The American Association of Neurologic Surgeons (AANS) 2014 guidelines report low-level evidence to support fusion for re-herniated disc. Therefore it is recommended to perform only re-discectomy for patients with re-herniation and radiculopathy without out [10].

16.4 How Strong Is the Level of Evidence Available to Date

16.4.1 Imaging

There is Level Ib evidence from multicenter RCT that there is a lack of distinguishability between radiographic evidence of herniation and symptomatic herniation [1].

16.4.2 Treatment

There is Level 2b evidence from a small single center RCT showing to difference between re-discectomy and re-discectomy and fusion for re-herniated disc [7]. There is Level Ib evidence from an industry sponsored multicenter spinal cord stimulation RCT showing favorable outcome of both leg and back pain in patients with FBSS using high-frequency stimulation compared to conventional stimulation [5].

16.5 Conclusions and Take Home Message

- In many of the patients with an alleged FBSS there might be a spinal pathology causing their symptoms. The most common causes include residual/recurrent disc herniation, spinal stenosis, infection or mechanical instability following decompression
- FBSS is best defined as a suffering from spinal pain of unknown origin either persisting despite surgical intervention or appearing after surgical intervention for spinal pain originally in the same topographical location
- In the case of postoperative spinal infection, cerebrospinal fluid fistula or a clear recurrent disk herniation then revision surgery should be done
- For patients with low back pain without radicular pain, spinal claudication or with multi-segmental degeneration conservative treatment is recommended
- New SCS stimulation techniques (High-frequency Stimulation) may be a promising alternative for patients with FBSS with predominantly low back pain

Pearls

- In many of the patients with an alleged FBSS there might be a spinal pathology causing their symptoms. The most common causes include residual/recurrent disc herniation, spinal stenosis, infection or mechanical instability following decompression
- FBSS is best defined as a suffering from spinal pain of unknown origin either persisting despite surgical intervention or appearing after surgical intervention for spinal pain originally in the same topographical location
- In the case of postoperative spinal infection, cerebrospinal fluid fistula or a clear recurrent disk herniation then revision surgery should be done
- For patients with low back pain without radicular pain, spinal claudication or with multisegmental degeneration conservative treatment is recommended
- New SCS stimulation techniques (High-frequency Stimulation) may be a promising alternative for patients with FBSS with predominantly low back pain

References

1. Barzouhi A, Vleggeert-Lankamp CL, Lycklama à Nijeholt GJ, Van der Kallen BF, van den Hout WB, Jacobs WC, Koes BW, Peul WC, Leiden-The Hague Spine Intervention Prognostic Study Group. Magnetic resonance imaging in follow-up assessment of sciatica. N Engl J Med. 2013;368(11):999–1007. Evidence Level Ib.
2. Cho Y-H, Kim CK, Heo KH, et al. Acupuncture for acute postoperative pain after back surgery: a systematic review and meta-analysis of randomized controlled trials. Pain Pract. 2015;15(3):279–91. Evidence Level Ia.
3. Cramer H, Haller H, Lauche R, Dobos G. Mindfulness-based stress reduction for low back pain. A systematic review. BMC Complement Altern Med. 2012;12(1):162. Evidence Level Ic.
4. Datta S, Manchikanti L, Falco FJ, Calodney AK, Atluri S, Benyamin RM, Buenaventura RM, Cohen SP. Diagnostic utility of selective nerve root blocks in the diagnosis of lumbosacral radicular pain: systematic review and update of current evidence. Pain Physician. 2013;16(2 Suppl):SE97–124. Evidence Level Ic.
5. Kapural L, Yu C, Doust MW, Gliner BE, Vallejo R, Sitzman BT, Amirdelfan K, Morgan DM, Brown LL, Yearwood TL, Bundschu R, Burton AW, Yang T, Benyamin R, Burgher AH. Novel 10-kHz High-frequency Therapy (HF10 Therapy) Is Superior to Traditional Low-frequency Spinal Cord Stimulation for the Treatment of Chronic Back and Leg Pain: The SENZA-RCT Randomized Controlled Trial. Anesthesiology. 2015;123(4):851–60. evidence based madecine 2B.
6. Drazin D, Ugiliweneza B, Al-Khouja L, Yang D, Johnson P, Kim T, Boakye M. Treatment of Recurrent Disc Herniation: A Systematic Review. Cureus. 2016;8(5):e622. Evidence Level Ic.
7. El Shazly AA, El Wardany MA, Morsi AM. Recurrent lumbar disc herniation: A prospective comparative

study of three surgical management procedures. Asian J Neurosurg. 2013;8(3):139–46. Evidence Level 2b.
8. Mroz TE, Lubelski D, Williams SK, O'Rourke C, Obuchowski NA, Wang JC, Steinmetz MP, Melillo AJ, Benzel EC, Modic MT, Quencer RM. Differences in the surgical treatment of recurrent lumbar disc herniation among spine surgeons in the United States. Spine J. 2014;14:2334–43. Evidence Level 2b.
9. Dower A, Chatterji R, Swart A, Winder MJ. Surgical management of recurrent lumbar disc herniation and the role of fusion. J Clin Neurosci. 2016;23:44–50. evidence based madecine 3A.
10. Wang JC, Dailey AT, Mummaneni PV, Ghogawala Z, Resnick DK, Watters WC 3rd, Groff MW, Choudhri TF, Eck JC, Sharan A, Dhall SS, Kaiser MG. Guideline update for the performance of fusion procedures for degenerative disease of the lumbar spine. Part 8: lumbar fusion for disc herniation and radiculopathy. J Neurosurg Spine. 2014;21:48–53. Evidence Level 5.

17 Surgical Treatment Options at the Sacroiliac Joint

Simon Bayerl, Dimitri Tkatschenko, Julius Dengler, and Peter Vajkoczy

17.1 Introduction

This case will address the possible treatment options of sacroiliac joint pain (SIP) including conservative treatment with intraarticular injections and radiofrequency denervation as well as operative fusion. SIP is a frequent cause for low back pain (LBP) with association of poor quality of life. Inflammation, pregnancy, trauma and especially previous spine surgeries are important triggers for SIP. Therefore Spine surgeons are frequently confronted with patients suffering from SIP. Making the diagnosis of SIJ dysfunction in the physical examination is difficult. It includes provocative maneuvers as FABER, distraction test, Oestgaard test, Gaenslen test and thigh thrust test. Even the diagnostic sensitivity of x-Ray, CT scans and MRI for SIP is low, but radiological diagnostics are essential to rule out other sources of LBP. Conservative treatment of LBP includes physical therapy, manual therapy and NSAID administration. Injections with steroids and local anesthetics or cryo and radiofrequency neurotomy may support the conservative treatment. However, in some cases the treatment of SIP is very difficult and even interventional approaches lead to a temporary pain relief only. In these cases fusion surgery of the SIJ can be offered. This case report describes a patient, who underwent all types of SIP treatment with physiotherapy, pain medication, intraarticular injections and radiofrequency neurotomy and finally minimally invasive fusion of the SIJ.

17.2 Case Description

A 78 y/o male patient presented himself to the outpatient department with chronic LBP localized in in the lower lumbar spine and the right gluteal region. Two years ago, a dorsal instrumentation with a dynamic pedicle screw-based system and additional microsurgical decompression for a L4/5 spinal canal stenosis was performed in an external hospital 2 years ago. The patient had experienced a pain relief for several months. In the further course a differently localized pain syndrome occurred, distinct from the initial pain. He reported on severe LBP (NRS 8/10) for several months with irradiation to the gluteal region and dorsal thigh on the right side. The neurological examination revealed mild dorsal flexor paresis, which had not changed for years. The Lasègue's sign was negative. The Oestgaard test was positive for the right SIJ. A CT myelogram showed no sign of spinal or foraminal stenosis with proper implant placement (Fig. 17.1a–c). Physiotherapy and pain medication resulted in insufficient pain relief.

S. Bayerl · D. Tkatschenko · J. Dengler · P. Vajkoczy (✉)
Department of Neurosurgery,
Charitè – Universitätsmedizin Berlin, Berlin,
Germany
e-mail: peter.vajkoczy@charite.de

B. Meyer, M. Rauschmann (eds.), *Spine Surgery*, https://doi.org/10.1007/978-3-319-98875-7_17

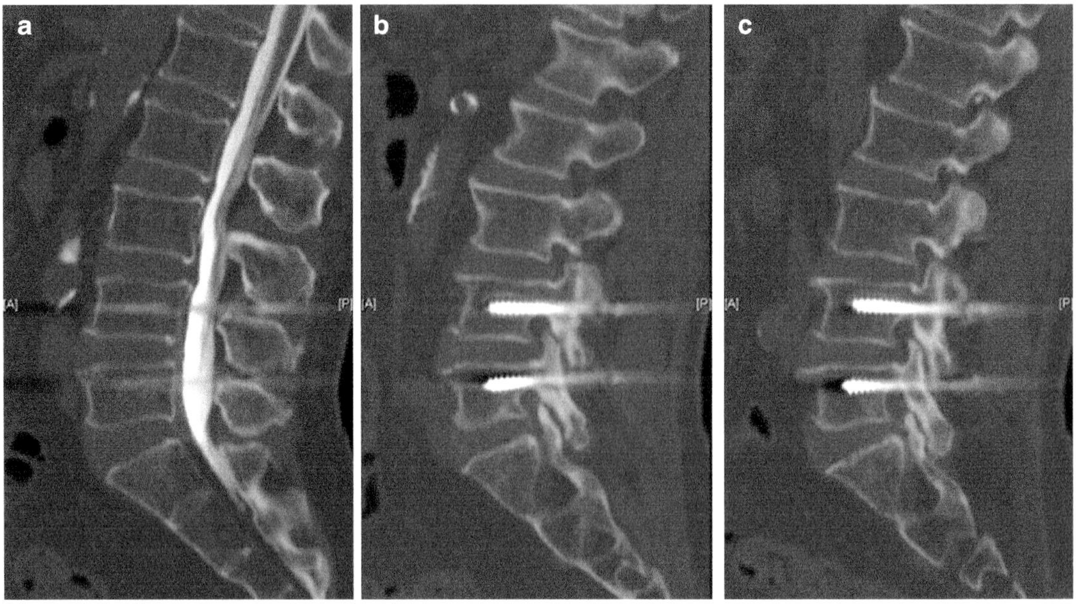

Fig. 17.1 CT myelogram. The CT myelogram (Sagittal view) shows proper implant placement with no signs of foraminal or spinal stenosis. (**a**) sagittal midline view, (**b**) sagittal right lateral view, (**c**) sagittal left lateral view. Confirmation of lack of spinal canal stenosis, radicular compression, or implant failure

The patient received infiltrations of the lumbosacral facet joints and the SIJ to detect the pain trigger. Repeated SIJ infiltrations under fluoroscopy resulted in a pain relief of 75% for several days, but he experienced an early pain recurrence. A right SIJ radiofrequency neurotomy was performed (bipolar and monopolar single-strip; Simplicity III probe®).

After denervation, the patient was free of pain for several months, but again the pain increased to the initial level despite an optimized conservative treatment. An additional intraarticular injection with contrast enhancement under fluoroscopic control resulted in a temporary complete pain relief and verified the diagnosis of Sacroiliac Joint Syndrome. As no alternative therapy was accessible a minimally invasive fusion of the right SIJ was offered. The iFuse Implant System® was used and three triangular titanium implants were placed across the SIJ using a lateral transiliac approach under fluoroscopic guidance. Postoperative x-ray of the pelvis showed proper implant placement (Fig. 17.2). The patient left the hospital 3 days after surgery. Six weeks of partial stress of the operated SIJ were recommended. In the follow-up outpatient visits the patient reported to be most of the time free of LBP for more than 2 years after surgery.

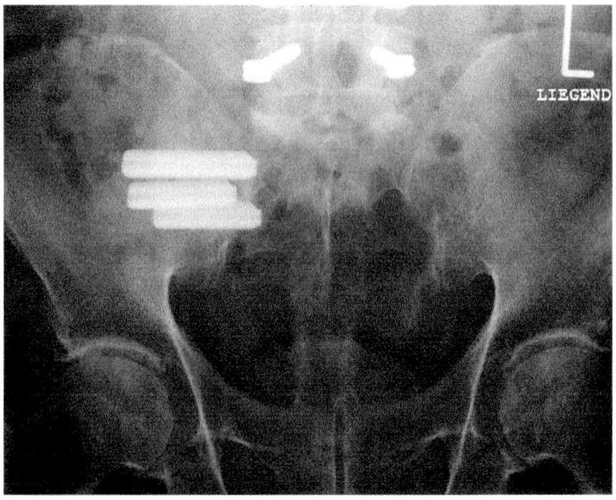

Fig. 17.2 SIJ fusion. Fluoroscopy (A/P) of triangular titanium implants for minimally-invasive SIJ fusion

17.3 Discussion of the Case

The patient suffered from chronic LBP after instrumentation and decompression at L4/L5. The examination with a pain syndrome localized in the lower lumbar spine and irradiation to the right gluteal region and thigh combined with a positive Oestgaard Test was suspicious for SIP. Repeated infiltrations with dramatic pain relief confirmed the diagnosis. Foraminal or spinal stenosis and implant failure or loosening were ruled out as the cause of LBP by CT myelogram. If a Sacroiliac Joint Syndrome is likely a stepwise escalating local therapy can be performed (Fig. 17.3).

The first line therapy for a SIP is a conservative treatment with physiotherapy and NSAIDs. If a satisfying pain relief cannot be achieved, staged infiltrations of the lumbar facet joints and the SIJ can be performed for diagnostic and therapeutic purpose. When the SIJ is detected as the main cause of LBP by provocative maneuvers and infiltrations, interventional neurotomy can be performed for a prolonged pain relief [1]. There are different denervation techniques for SIJ neurotomy, which can be used. Important is a complete denervation of all nerves arising from the dorsal foramina.

If radiofrequency therapy fails to enable a distinct long-term pain relief, a surgical fusion of the SIJ can be considered. However, it has to be stressed that the indication for surgical fusion of the SIJ must be regarded critically and, thus, should be limited to the few, selected cases that fail conservative therapy – in our experience these are less than 5% of all patients with chronic SIJ pain syndromes.

Before surgical fusion we recommend to perform an SIJ infiltration with contrast enhancement to prove the intraarticular injection of the local anesthetics and demonstrate its effect. Only if this injection leads to a drastic pain relief of at least 50% a SIJ fusion surgery should be performed.

There are many techniques to perform SIJ fusion. Already a century ago and lasting until today open surgeries were performed for SIJ fusion [2]. However, high implant failure rates and perioperative complications resulted in the development of minimal invasive techniques to perform SIJ fusion surgery. There are several techniques

Fig. 17.3 Management of SIP

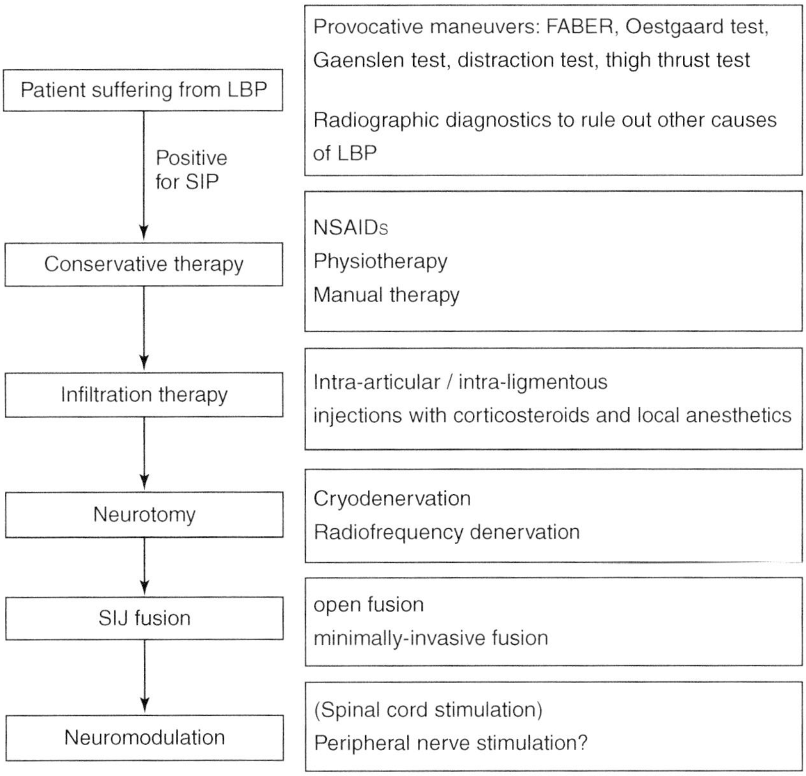

available. The most frequently used devices with the best clinical evidence are the distraction interference arthrodesis with neurovascular anticipation (DIANA®, SIGNUS Medizintechnik GmbH, Germany) and the triangular titanium implants (iFuse Implant System®, SI-Bone, Inc., San Jose, CA, USA). Results of an prospective observational study with inclusion of 171 patients with a 2 year follow-up could illustrate that the implantation of the DIANA®-device resulted in an improvement in pain and disability scores as well as in Quality of Life scores in [3]. However, there are no RCTs available. The highest amount of studies are available for the iFuse implant System®. Multicentre randomized controlled trials from a US and a European study group illustrated the effectiveness in minimally invasive SIJ fusion with this device concerning pain function and quality of life [4, 5]. The main complications of the surgical procedure are implant-related impingements on the S1 root, fractures, implant loosenings and hematomas. However, only in 2–3% of patients a revision surgery is required.

Another possible therapy for treatment of SIP is a neuromodulation approach. There is no evidence that Spinal Cord Stimulation is a good approach to address pain in the gluteal region. However, in a small case series peripheral nerve stimulation was shown be a promising therapy for SIP [6].

17.4 Conclusions and Take Home Message

Patients suffering from LBP due to SIJ dysfunction are frequently seen after fusion or decompression surgery of the lumbar spine. They report LBP and pain in the gluteal region and possibly pseudoradicular pain radiating into the lower extremities. Some patients report only temporary relief from conservative therapy, LA and steroid injections. To preserve the effect of injections a cryo or radiofrequency neurotomy of the dorsal rami innervating the SIJ is frequently used. Surgical options such as minimally-invasive SIJ fusion can be performed, if conservative treatment fails and the diagnosis of an SIP is confirmed clinically and via intraarticular infiltration. Peripheral Nerve Stimulation could become future therapy option, if randomized controlled trials confirm its effectivity.

Pearls and Pitfalls

- Conservative treatment for LBP from SIJ dysfunction is the gold standard
- Provocative maneuvers and LA injections to reveal the source of LBP are mandatory
- When discussing SIJ fusion intraarticular (not intraligamentous) injection for diagnostic reasons
- Surgical treatment only if all above measures fail and test results are unambigous
- Minimally-invasive SIJ fusion surgery is technically well established
- Peripheral nerve stimulation may be an option in the future

Editorial Comment

While we will not discuss probable shortcomings of the RCTs for MIS SIJ fusion and instead assume integrity of data, we strongly feel that a word of caution is necessary here. The results for efficacy and safety have been produced in the highly controlled environment of a RCT, where foremost indication, but also technique etc. are closely monitored. We are convinced, that efficacy rates will drop and safety issues increase dramatically when this device is used in an uncontrolled fashion outside a trial. SIJ pain is a diffuse and ill-defined yet ubiquitous "syndrom" and the surgical MIS technique is rather undemanding, both of which will set a very low threshold to use this device. Apart from the immediate increase of direct complications, we fear that a significant number of late low-grade-infection related implant loosenings will occur in the longer run. We therefore would only accept the use of this device under controlled conditions with rigid and complete post-market surveillance measures, such as mandatory data input into monitored registries including pre-, peri and postoperative as well as longterm data.

References

1. Aydin SM, Gharibo CG, Mehnert M, Stitik TP. The role of radiofrequency ablation for sacroiliac joint pain: a meta-analysis. PM R. 2010;2:842–51. https://doi.org/10.1016/j.pmrj.2010.03.035.
2. Buchowski JM, Kebaish KM, Sinkov V, et al. Functional and radiographic outcome of sacroiliac arthrodesis for the disorders of the sacroiliac joint. Spine J. 2005;5:520–8. https://doi.org/10.1016/j.spinee.2005.02.022.
3. Fuchs V, Ruhl B. Distraction arthrodesis of the sacroiliac joint: 2-year results of a descriptive prospective multi-center cohort study in 171 patients. Eur Spine J. 2018;27(1):194–204.
4. Dengler JD, Kools D, Pflugmacher R, et al. 1-year results of a randomized controlled trial of conservative management vs. minimally invasive surgical treatment for sacroiliac joint pain. Pain Physician. 2017;20:537–50.
5. Polly DW, Swofford J, Whang PG, et al. Two-year outcomes from a randomized controlled trial of minimally invasive sacroiliac joint fusion vs. Non-surgical management for sacroiliac joint dysfunction. Int J Spine Surg. 2016;10:28. https://doi.org/10.14444/3028.
6. Guentchev M, Preuss C, Rink R, et al. Long-term reduction of sacroiliac joint pain with peripheral nerve stimulation. Oper Neurosurg. 2017;13:634–8. https://doi.org/10.1093/ons/opx017.

18 Navigation of the Cervical, Thoracic and Lumbar Spine

Hanno S. Meyer and Yu-Mi Ryang

18.1 Introduction

Computer-assisted navigation (CAN) is a widely employed tool in spinal instrumentation surgery. It permits high-quality image guided placement of pedicle screws based on registration of preoperative or intraoperative spinal imaging data (e.g., preoperative or intraoperative CT images, intraoperative 3D fluoroscopy). The surgeon is thus provided with visual feedback showing the current planned screw placement trajectory superimposed on the imaging data of the patient. This is supposed to improve the safety and accuracy of pedicle screw placement and thus reduce complications potentially associated with screw misplacement, such as instability, neurological injury or revision surgery [1, 2].

CAN is applicable to the entire spine, i.e. for instrumentation of the cervical, thoracic and lumbosacral spine including the pelvis. The following case will demonstrate the use of CAN for spinal instrumentation.

The case will detail specific advantages and disadvantages of spinal navigation techniques with regard to:

- safety and accuracy
- image quality
- radiation exposure
- learning curve
- location (thoracolumbar versus cervical)

18.2 Case Description

A 64-year-old male patient suffered from thoracic back pain after he fell while sailing his boat. His neurological examination was normal. A CT scan showed a vertebral compression fracture of Th 6 and signs of osteoporosis (Fig. 18.1). The MRI scan was consistent with a recent injury (Fig. 18.2). There was no neural compression.

The patient had a history of cigarette smoking (50 pack years) and was otherwise healthy.

Analgesics did not provide sufficient pain relief. Instead, after a few weeks, the pain was increasing. The relative indication for surgery was discussed with the patient in detail. Taking medical history and age into account, it was eventually decided to proceed with minimally-invasive percutaneous posterior instrumentation. As in any spinal instrumentation performed in our department, CAN was used for pedicle screw placement (Figs. 18.3, 18.4, and 18.5).

As a first step, the navigation reference array was tightly attached to a spinous process via a small incision of skin and fascia (Fig. 18.3). Then, a 3D-scan was acquired (Fig. 18.4). During scanning,

H. S. Meyer · Y.-M. Ryang (✉)
Department of Neurosurgery, Klinikum rechts der Isar, Technische Universität München, Munich, Germany
e-mail: yu.ryang@tum.de

B. Meyer, M. Rauschmann (eds.), *Spine Surgery*, https://doi.org/10.1007/978-3-319-98875-7_18

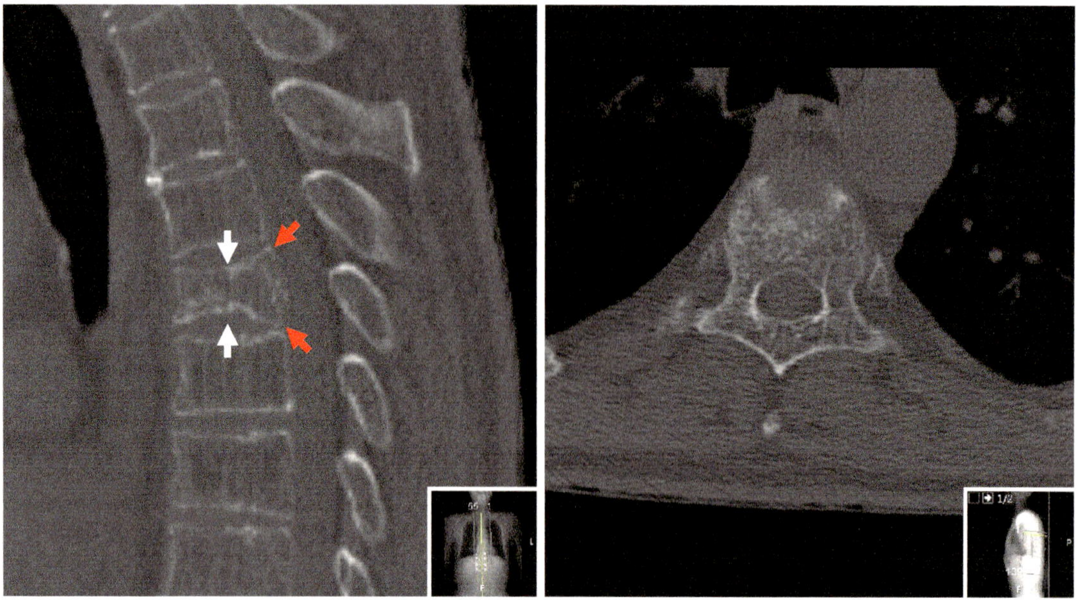

Fig. 18.1 CT Sagittal (left) and axial (right) slices of a CT scan showing a compression fracture of the vertebral body of Th 6. Both endplates are affected (white arrows), and there is height loss suggesting involvement of the posterior wall as well (red arrows). There is decreased cortical thickness as well as loss of trabecular bone structure, consistent with osteoporosis. The pedicles are intact, and there is no bony narrowing of the spinal canal

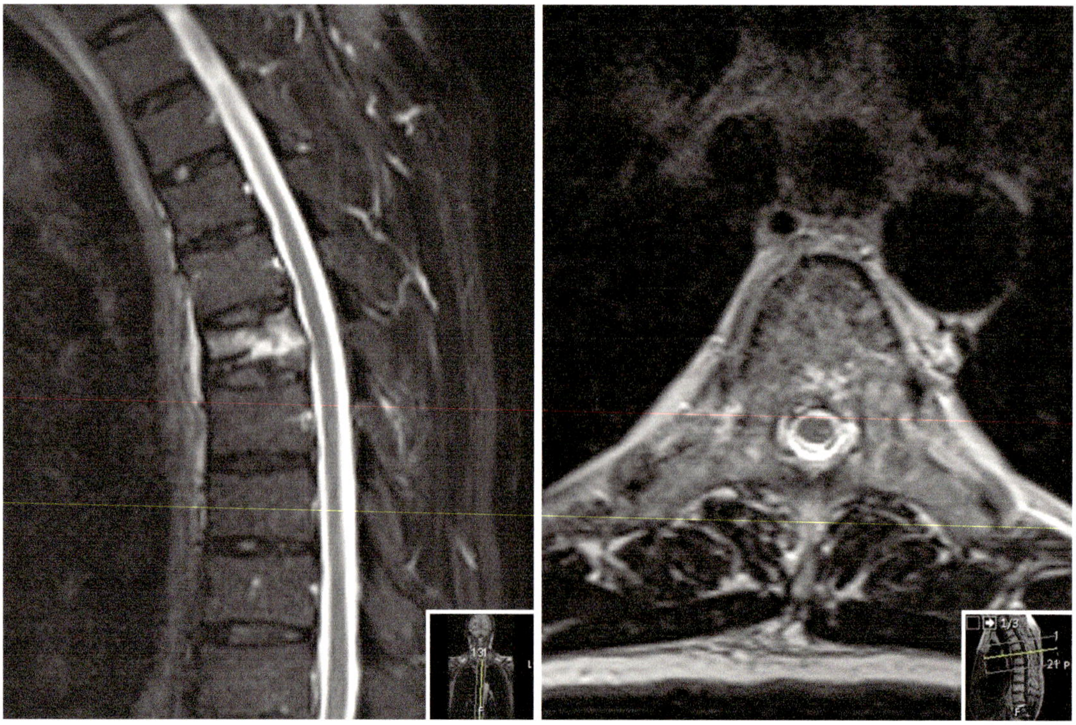

Fig. 18.2 MRI Sagittal (left) and axial (right) MRI slices. A STIR (Short Tau Inversion Recovery) sequence was acquired, providing sensitivity to bone marrow edema. There is substantial edema in the vertebral body of Th 6, suggestive of a recent injury. There is no significant spinal canal stenosis associated with the fracture

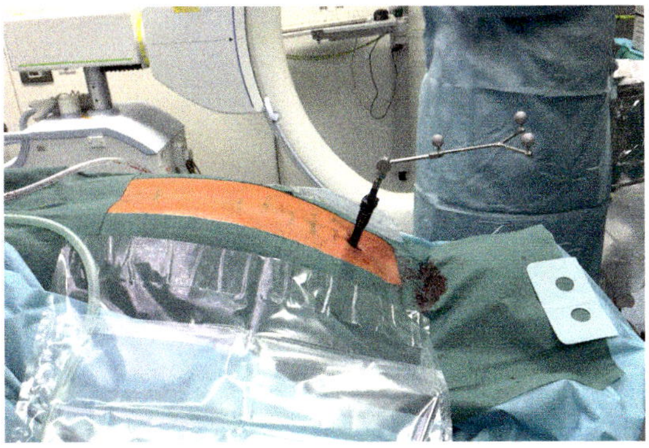

Fig. 18.3 Navigation reference array. This intraoperative picture shows the navigation reference array. Care must be taken to ensure tight attachment to the spine, which is usually achieved by clamping to a spinous process that is exposed via a small incision of the skin and fascia. The marker spheres can be detected by the navigation system's camera

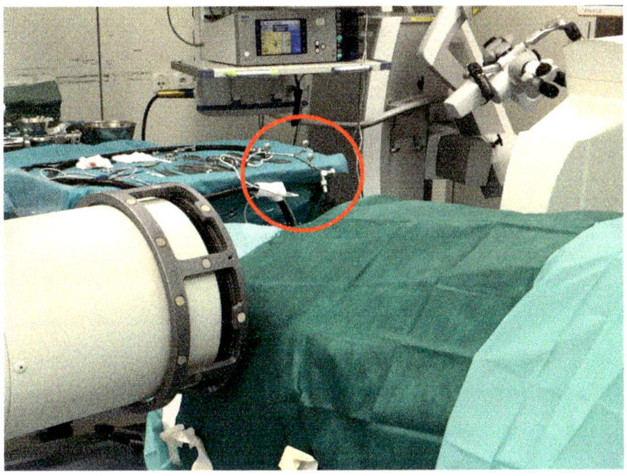

Fig. 18.4 Acquisition of 3D-fluoroscopy scan. The surgical field is covered to maintain sterility. The marker spheres (red circle) remain exposed to the field of view of the navigation system's camera, permitting 3D registration of the patient's anatomy with the acquired imaging data. Anesthesia should provide apnea during scanning to prevent movement artifacts

the OR staff could leave the operating room, eliminating radiation exposure. Anesthesia provided apnea to prevent movement artifacts after sufficient preoxigenation of the patient. Both the marker spheres of the reference array and the C-arm can be detected by the camera of the navigation system, permitting registration of the patient's anatomy with the acquired imaging data. The drill guide can be detected by the navigation system as well, enabling multiplanar visualization of the tip of the drill and

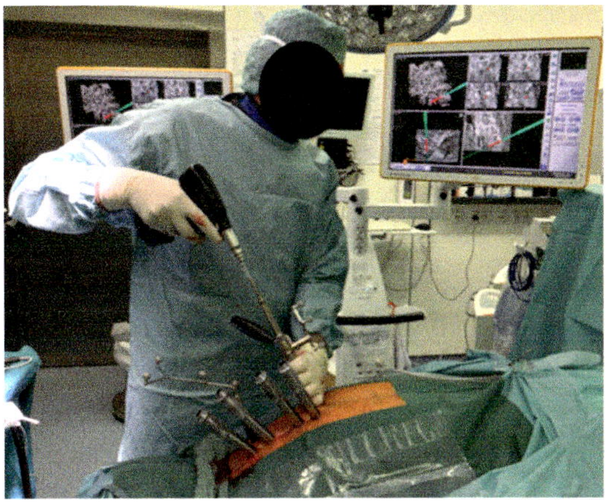

Fig. 18.5 Navigated pedicle screw placement. This intraoperative picture shows navigated placement of pedicle screws. Using a navigated drill guide with marker spheres that are detectable by the navigation system's camera, the tip of the drill as well as the current drilling trajectory can be superimposed on the 3D image set in three planes. This enables the surgeon to choose the ideal drilling trajectory based on visual feedback. After drilling, a k-wire is placed into the drill hole. The screw can then be placed via the k-wire along the navigated trajectory

the current drilling trajectory superimposed on the intraoperative 3D scan (Fig. 18.5). First, we confirmed that the registration succeeded by making sure that intraoperative landmarks (e.g., spinous processes) correspond to the respective structure in the image set. Then, pedicle screws could be placed without the need to expose anatomical landmarks, permitting a minimally invasive percutaneous approach while maintaining maximum accuracy. There was no need to perform imaging during screw placement, reducing the radiation exposure to surgeon and patient to a minimum as opposed to standard free-hand placement procedures using biplanar intraoperative fluoroscopy.

Pedicle screws were placed bilaterally in Th 4, 5, 7 and 8. A final control 3D-scan confirmed accurate placement of the screws. Prior to cement augmentation with PMMA. As a last step, rods were implanted using the caudal most existing skin incision.

There were no adverse events during or after surgery. The patient reported immediate pain relief. Standing radiography confirmed correct positioning of the implant (Fig. 18.6).

The patient was mobilized on the day of surgery and discharged home after 2 days. He was

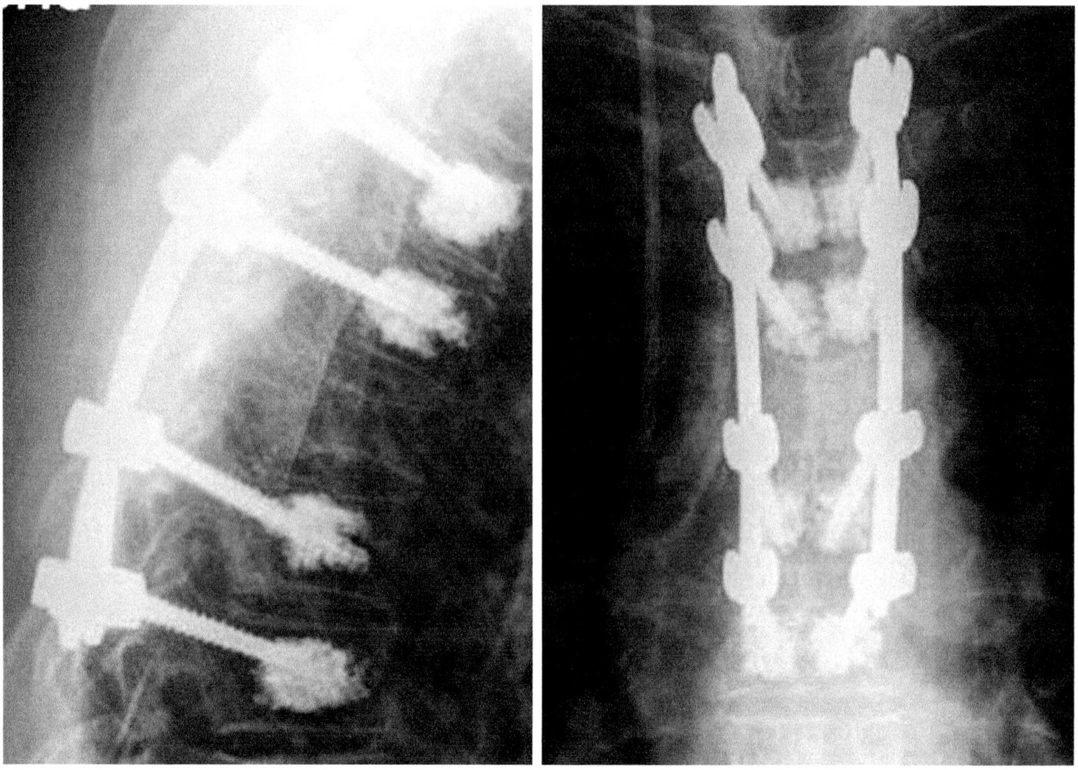

Fig. 18.6 Postoperative lateral (left) and a.p. (right) standing radiography confirm correct placement of the instrumentation system

referred to an endocrinologist to further investigate and treat the newly diagnosed osteoporosis.

18.3 Discussion of the Case

We present a standard case with instrumentation of the thoracic spine. We chose to use CAN for pedicle screw placement, as we do for any spinal instrumentation surgery involving pedicle screw placement in our department.

18.3.1 Navigation Techniques: Advantages and Disadvantages

18.3.1.1 Preop CT imaging for intraoperative Navigation

There are several CAN systems available, and there are also methodical differences. An important variable is the imaging modality. Imaging can be acquired preoperatively or intraoperatively. Excellent image quality is the biggest advantage of preoperative imaging (e.g., a CT scan.) A downside of preoperative imaging, however, is patient positioning for preoperative CT acquisition wich usually is supine in constrast to the prone position during surgery. This might be a source of possible imaging inaccuracy during surgery.

This technique works by point-by-point surface registration of the posterior vertebral lamina with a navigation probe (see Figs. 18.7, 18.8, and 18.9).

This way every vertebral level needs to be registered individually prior to instrumentation. This might take longer than using navigation systems working with intraoperative image acquisition techniques which usually have an automated registration.

Percutaneous minimally-invasive procedures can therefore not be performed since the posterior spinal elements need to be exposed with this technique. The superior image quality of this technique is of particular importance in the cervical spine where any PS inaccuracy can have devastating effects (vertebral artery injury if PS is placed too laterally or spinal cord injury in medial displacements). We therefore prefer CT-region matching with preoperative CT imaging for posterior instrumentations of the c-spine. Of importance is the high mobility of the c-spine in contrast to the thoracolumbar spine. We highly recommend to register every to be navigated vertebra individually prior to pedicle screw placement to enable for the highest possible accuracy.

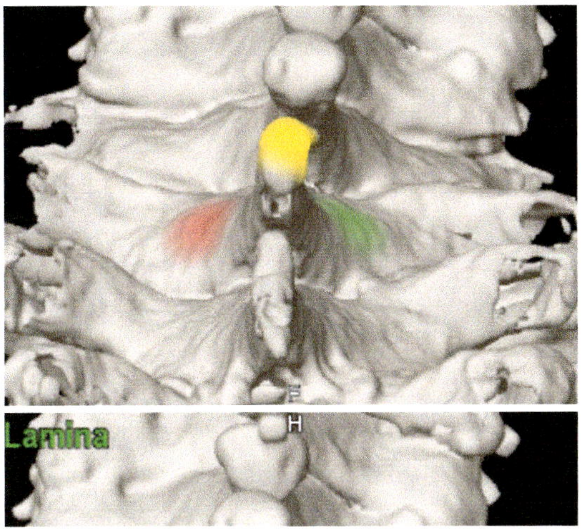

Fig. 18.7 Marked to be navigated posterior lamina of the cervical spine for CT-region matching navigation

Obviously, as in the present case, a percutaneous approach is not compatible with surface matching that requires exposure of at least the laminae of the vertebrae to be instrumented.

With the advent of intraoperative CT scanners this option might become obsolete one day, if these devices will hopefully become more affordable in the future.

18.3.1.2 Intraoperative 3D-fluoroscopy guided Navigation

Besides preop and intraop CT imaging most other navigation systems are based on intraoperative 3D-fluoroscopic image-guidance. Images are

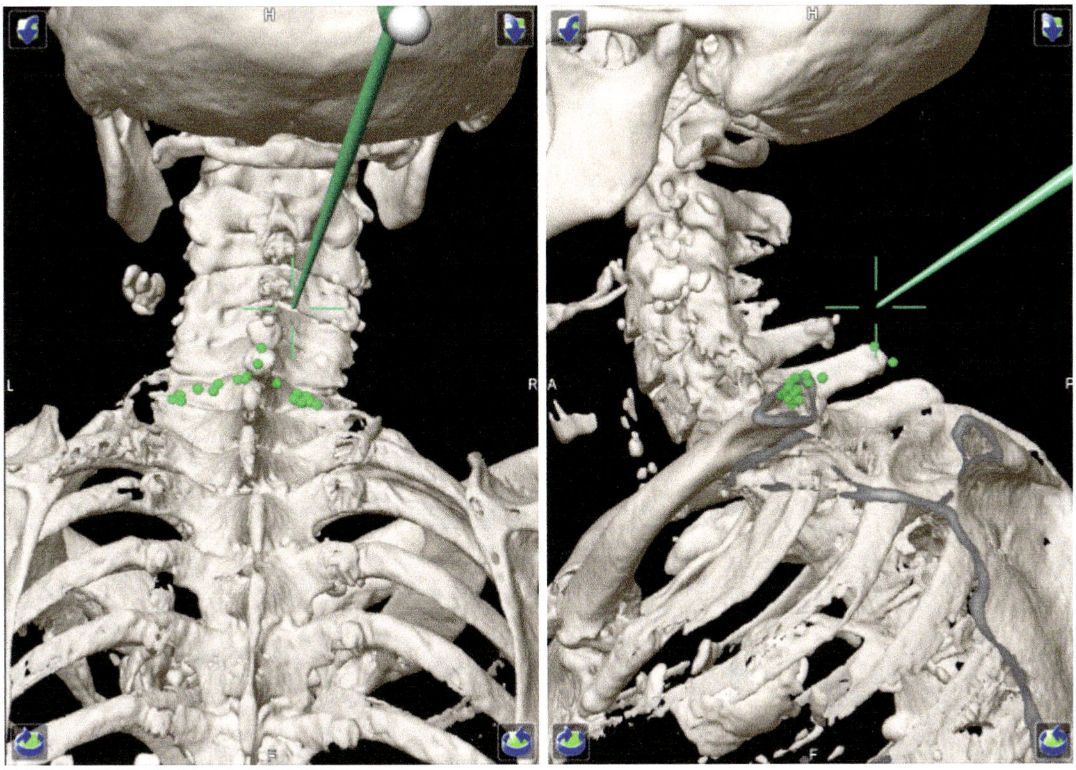

Fig. 18.8 Point-by-point registration of a posterior cervical spine lamina for CT-region matching registration

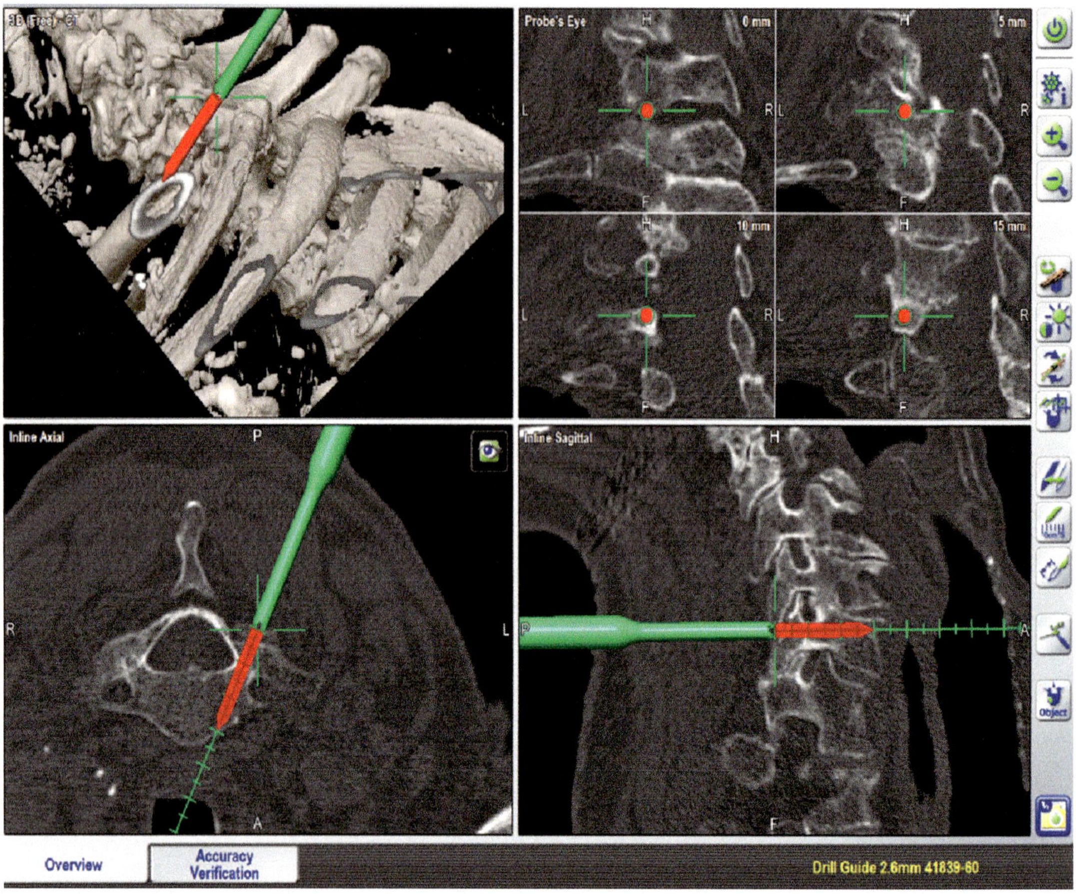

Fig. 18.9 Intraoperative CT-region matching based pedicle screw trajectory of the cervical spine

acquired intraoperatively after attachment of the reference array and registered automatically. This technique is therefore suitable for open as well as percutaneous minimally-invasive procedures. Depending on the system there are differences in image-quality and size of the field of view. In general image quality and gantry size are inferior to iCT, but these systems are less expensive.

For thoracolumbar instrumentations, we prefer intraoperative imaging for several reasons. The relatively low mobility of the thoracolumbar spine permits using one single scan for instrumentation of several segments. Available 3D-fluoroscopy imaging systems can acquire the entire lumbar spine and up to six or seven thoracic segments with one scan and modern systems with a larger field of view even enable navigation of the pelvis for S2-ala iliac screw placement. This makes intraoperative imaging the more efficient alternative when compared to surface matching in these cases. Moreover, the direct registration of the imaging data possibly provides higher accuracy than surface matching in the thoracolumbar spine, where post-scan-movements are less likely than in the cervical spine. This is consistent with the findings of a recent study comparing intraoperative with preoperative imaging – based navigation in scoliosis surgery [3].

Image quality which is up to date inferior to CT-imaging makes these systems less suitable for use in the cervical spine and the cervicothoracic region.

Patients with pathologically reduced bone mineral density or excessive obesity might also hamper image quality and reduce safety and accuracy.

18.3.1.3 Intraoperativ CT

Intraoperative CT definitely has advantages over other navigation systems. It produces the highest image quality, has the largest gantry and the largest field of view compared to other systems theoretically enabling navigation of the entire spine including the pelvis with one scan with a comparably low radiation dose. But of course, these systems come with a price and are the most expensive ones on the market today.

High investment costs are the downside of all intraoperative navigation systems available at the moment.

In general, CAN has many substantial advantages, accuracy being the obvious one. Based on more than 20 clinical trials that evaluated pedicle screw placement using CAN, there is no doubt that the procedure is safe and that it increases the accuracy of pedicle screw placement when compared to standard freehand (FH) pedicle screw instrumentation [1]. Whether this translates into a better clinical outcome for the patient has been analyzed by several meta-analyses. Most studies found only a trend towards improvement in clinically relevant outcome parameters, such as screw revision rates or neurological injury [1, 2, 4]. It has been argued that the difficulty in proving clinically relevant superiority of CAN over FH may be due to the known high success rates and safety profile of the latter method [1, 5]. Moreover, the variety of different CAN platforms adds heterogeneity to results in most studies [1]. Accordingly, using strict exclusion criteria, another meta-analysis found a significantly lower rate of screw-related complications in the CAN cohort as compared to the FH cohort [1, 6]. It can be assumed that future studies will add further evidence supporting the logical assumption that prevention of misplaced pedicle screws is beneficial to the patient.

Our case illustrates that CAN facilitates pedicle screw placement substantially. Mid-thoracic screws were placed through small skin / fascia incisions without the need to expose anatomical landmarks for orientation, as is usually required in FH instrumentation. One could argue that, given the technical effort associated with CAN, it should be limited to the most difficult cases only. However, in addition to providing facilitation and accuracy, there are two more facts supporting use of CAN whenever possible: First, CAN has been shown to eliminate radiation exposure to the OR staff and to significantly reduce the patient's effective dose of radiation exposure in a randomized prospective trial [7]. Thus, withholding it from patients and personnel is at least questionable. Finally, CAN is associated with a learning curve [8]. This needs to be overcome to fully benefit from its advantages, requiring its application on a regular basis.

Consequently, we argue that CAN should be implemented as standard procedure in the daily surgical routine of any spine surgery center [9].

As holds true for all navigation systems is the obligation of the surgeon to know the patient's anatomy and to check plausibility and accuracy of the navigation system repeatedly during surgery. All systems are prone to inaccuracy for example by unintended displacement or loosening of the reference array. Inaccuracy also increases with increasing distance of the reference array to the camera. The surgeon also needs to check the line of sight. Unnoticed blockage of the line of sight by an instrument, the surgeon or the instrumenting nurse during pedicle screw placement is also a possible source of inaccuracy.

Navigation therefore does not guarantee for accurate pedicle screw placement if these basic rules are not followed.

18.4 Conclusions and Take Home Message

CAN is a tool designed to assist in pedicle screw placement in spinal instrumentation surgery. It can facilitate the procedure, improve its accuracy, reduce the rate of revision surgeries by misplaced pedicle screws and possibly prevent associated complications. With CAN, radiation exposure is reduced for the patient and for the medical personnel. It is applicable to the cervical, thoracic and lumbar spine and to both open and minimally invasive approaches. However, there are technical nuances that are associated with advantages and disadvantages specific for the spinal region. Knowledge of the theory and technical application of CAN is crucial – inaccurate registration is useless, and the surgeon must be able to realize inaccurate navigation at any time during surgery. There is a learning curve for CAN, so it should be employed daily, on a regular basis. CAN should be used in spinal instrumentation surgery whenever possible.

- Computer-assisted navigation (CAN) is a useful tool in spinal instrumentation
- CAN increases pedicle screw placement accuracy, potentially leading to a better clinical outcome
- CAN significantly reduces the rate of revision surgeries due to PS screw misplacements
- CAN significantly reduces radiation exposure to medical staff and the patient
- CAN is useless when the registration fails, so knowledge of the theory and application of the technique is crucial
- CAN needs to be practiced, and there is a learning curve
- CAN should be standard in spinal instrumentation surgery
- CAN facilitates minimally-invasive spine procedures, esp. instrumentation
- CAN facilitates the increased use of percutaneous minimally-invasive procedures. Minimizing approach-related morbidity is crucial to reduce wound healing problems and infections in spinal tumor patients needing postoperative adjuvant radiation therapy
- CAN can help to better understand the complex anatomy of the spine

Pearls and Pitfalls

- Check plausibility and accuracy repeatedly
- Know the anatomy
- Do not entirely rely on the navigation
- Intraop imaging is still virtual reality
- Accuracy decreases with increasing distance of the reference array to the camera
- Unnoticed/unintended movement of the reference array during surgery can cause inaccurate pedicle screw placement
- Do not attach reference array on lamina of lytic or mobile spinous processes
- Avoid too tight attachment of the reference array, which might break the spinous process
- Ensure an unobstructed line of sight
- CT-region matching is not suitable for percutaneous procedures

Editorial Comment

Everything that needs to be known about spinal navigation today is described and discussed in this chapter by the senior author (YR), who has done extensive clinical research work in this field. Similar to chapter 7 the authors have chosen a non-degenerative case, which is not important in this instance, because technical principles are presented applicable to all pathologies. It is the editors' strong belief, that in the future navigation will be an integral part of all spinal surgeries/instrumentations. It is proven that it increases safety for the patient as well as the surgeon, by reducing misplacement rates and radiation exposure. It may be that these advantages are not "a big step", because adequate accuracy can also be achieved with a free-hand technique. However, one should remember, that progress in clinical science and ultimately patient care comes always in small steps. To translate the corresponding German phrase verbatim would be "the better is the enemy of the good". Neurosurgeons with a cranial focus are familiar with this development from an outsider technique to a standard of care over a time span of 20 plus years, because the beginnings of cranial navigation dates back to the late 80ies/early 90ies. The authors correctly convey very important principles for a successful implementation of spinal navigation. These include:

(a) Mandatory use in all (routine) cases for a successful integration into clinical routine to create confidence with the technique in the difficult cases, where it is actually needed and can be then applied without distracting from the actual surgery. Using it in the difficult case only is the most fatal mistake to be made.

(b) Resilience to the hardships of the learning curve needs to be anticipated and communicated to all team members to increase acceptance.

(c) The pitfalls of the technique need to be known and carefully avoided. As a rule of thumb, inaccuracies despite navigation are basically always related to the human factor and not the machine.

References

1. Overley SC, Cho SK, Mehta AI, Arnold PM. Navigation and robotics in spinal surgery: where are we now? Neurosurgery. 2017;80:S86–99.
2. Fichtner J, Hofmann N, Rienmüller A, Buchmann N, Gempt J, Kirschke JS, Ringel F, Meyer B, Ryang YM. Revision rate of misplaced pedicle screws of the thoracolumbar spine – Comparison of three-dimensional fluoroscopy navigation with freehand placement: a systematic analysis and review of the literature. World Neurosurg. 2018;109:e24–32.
3. Zhang W, Takigawa T, Wu YG, Sugimoto Y, Tanaka M, Ozaki T. Accuracy of pedicle screw insertion in posterior scoliosis surgery: a comparison between intraoperative navigation and preoperative navigation techniques. Eur Spine J. 2017;26:1756–64.
4. Verma R, Krishan S, Haendlmayer K, Mohsen A. Functional outcome of computer-assisted spinal pedicle screw placement: a systematic review and meta-analysis of 23 studies including 5,992 pedicle screws. Eur Spine J. 2010;19:370–5.
5. Kim YJ, Lenke LG, Bridwell KH, Cho YSS, Riew KD. Free hand pedicle screw placement in the thoracic spine: Is it safe? Spine (Phila Pa 1976). 2004;29:333–42.
6. Shin BJ, James AR, Njoku IU, Hartl R. Pedicle screw navigation: a systematic review and meta-analysis of perforation risk for computer-navigated versus freehand insertion. A review. J Neurosurg Spine. 2012;17:113–22.
7. Villard J, Ryang YM, Demetriades AK, Reinke A, Behr M, Preuss A, Meyer B, Ringel F. Radiation exposure to the surgeon and the patient during posterior lumbar spinal instrumentation: a prospective randomized comparison of navigated versus non-navigated freehand techniques. Spine (Phila Pa 1976). 2014;39:1004–9.
8. Ryang YM, Villard J, Obermuller T, Friedrich B, Wolf P, Gempt J, Ringel F, Meyer B. Learning curve of 3D fluoroscopy image-guided pedicle screw placement in the thoracolumbar spine. Spine J. 2015;15:467–76.
9. Meyer B, Ryang YM. Yes, We CAN! World Neurosurg. 2013;79:85–6.

Part III

Basic Module 3: Deformity

Natural Course and Classification of Idiopathic Scoliosis

19

Massimo Balsano and Stefano Negri

19.1 Introduction

Scoliosis is an elusive pathology in which a therapeutic decision must depend on an accurate prognostic stratification. It is defined as a three-dimensional deformity of the vertebral column which manifests itself in different forms, affecting the cervical, dorsal and lumbar regions. In more than 80% of scoliosis cases, a specific cause is actually not known (Idiopathic Scoliosis, IS).

Scoliosis Research Society (SRS) classified IS in two main categories about the age of onset:

- Early Onset Scoliosis (EOS) in children under 10 years old [1];
- Adolescent Idiopathic Scoliosis (AIS) in patients aged from 11 to 18.

AIS represents the 90% of idiopathic scoliosis. The estimated prevalence is 0.47–5.2%. Females are significantly more affected than males (1.5:1–3:1) [2].

19.2 Natural History

Learning about the natural history of idiopathic scoliosis is fundamental and the knowledge of it has an important role to prevent failures in the treatment.

The natural history of adolescent idiopathic scoliosis (AIS) may be divided into the short and long term.

A correct estimate of the risk of worsening is essential to identify patients worthy of treatment and at the same time to define patients who do not require it.

There are four major lines of long term studies which have investigated the natural history of AIS: the Swedish studies [3], the American with the Iowa cohort studies [4], the English [5] and the Italian [6] series. It is difficult to compare results of different studies; nevertheless, the main outcomes of these studies are summarized in Table 19.1.

Curve progression, back pain incidence, and psychosocial implications are the main topics analyzed to determine the real impact of scoliosis during life.

With skeletal maturity, curve progression slows substantially compared with the progression that is observed during the adolescent growth spurt.

In general, the increase in angular entity after skeletal maturity (coronal and axial rotation) causes a proportional increase of probability of progression and therefore decompensation of curves. Coronal Cobb >30°, progress at a rate of <1° per year [4, 5], where curves of major entity (>80–90°) have much slower progression's rate than smaller curves due to rigidity caused by degenerative changes.

M. Balsano (✉) · S. Negri
UOC Ortopedia e Traumatologia,
Regional Spinal Department, AOUI, Verona, Italy

B. Meyer, M. Rauschmann (eds.), *Spine Surgery*, https://doi.org/10.1007/978-3-319-98875-7_19

Table 19.1 The four mayor studies on the natural course of untreated AIS

Study	F-U (years)	N. Cases at F-U	Mean curve size (Cobb)	Progression after skeletal maturity	Mortality	Back Pain/Disability
Nilsonne et al. (1968) [3]	>45 (50–70)	52	No rx	48%	9.6%	19.2% (disabled to 75% or more)
Ascani et al. (1986) [6]	33 (15–47)	187	37% > 50°	All curves progressed after skeletal maturity (0.4°/yr). Thoracic curves between 50° and 59° progressed 0.56°/yr.	17% in severe curves	61% incidence of back pain. Psychological disturbances in 19%, (curves >40°)
Edgar et al. (1987) [5]	11 (0–27)	77	73°	>55° (>.0.5°/yr) Lumbar curves; increase in rotation > Cobb angle	–	Back pain in 79%
Weinstein et al. (2003) [4]	51 (44–61)	117	Thoracic 85°, thoracolumbar 90°, Lumbar 50°, double major 76°–79°	–	No increased mortality	61% of pts. had chronic pain, 22% Dyspnea

Thoracic curves have the highest tendency to progression. Thoracolumbar and lumbar curves have the highest propensity for developing lateral olisthesis during adulthood, and back pain may be more prominent and disabling.

The short term natural history of AIS indicates the behavior of the curves during growth and their tendency of evolution. This period is the most important for clinical and instrumental monitoring.

School screening programs have the risk of a high rate of false positives leading to unnecessary concerns for teenagers and their parents, as well as contributing to costly, unnecessary x-rays and specialist consultations [7].

On the other hand, there is evidence that school scoliosis patients detected by screening are less likely to need surgery than those patients who did not have screening [8].

The main indicator for short term progression of curves is the skeletal maturity at the time of evaluation. It can be assessed by the popular Risser test [9] and more recently by using elbow radiographs (AP and lateral projections) [10].

Mineral deposits in the iliac apophyses begin to appear at the anterolateral crest and progress medially towards the sacrum. Fusion of the calcified apophyses to the ilium then progresses in the opposite direction (medial-to-lateral).

According to the progression status of this process, which can be evaluated on standard radiograms, five progressive degrees (0–4) are described (Fig. 19.1).

At Risser 0–1 stages the incidence of progression is 25% for curves <20°, 70% for curves between 20° to 30° and 90% for curves >30°. At Risser 2–4 stages the incidence of evolution is 3% for curves <20°, 20% for curves between 20° to 30°, 30% for curves >30° and 50% for curves >45° [11].

Finally, we can summarize that age under 12, the absence of secondary sexual maturity signs, thoracic curves with severe vertebral rotation are the most negative prognostic factors for AIS progression.

19.3 Classification

The need to postulate shared classification' s principles has emerged to study and compare the clinical outcome of different types of curves.

Historically the fundamental curve patterns of AIS are:

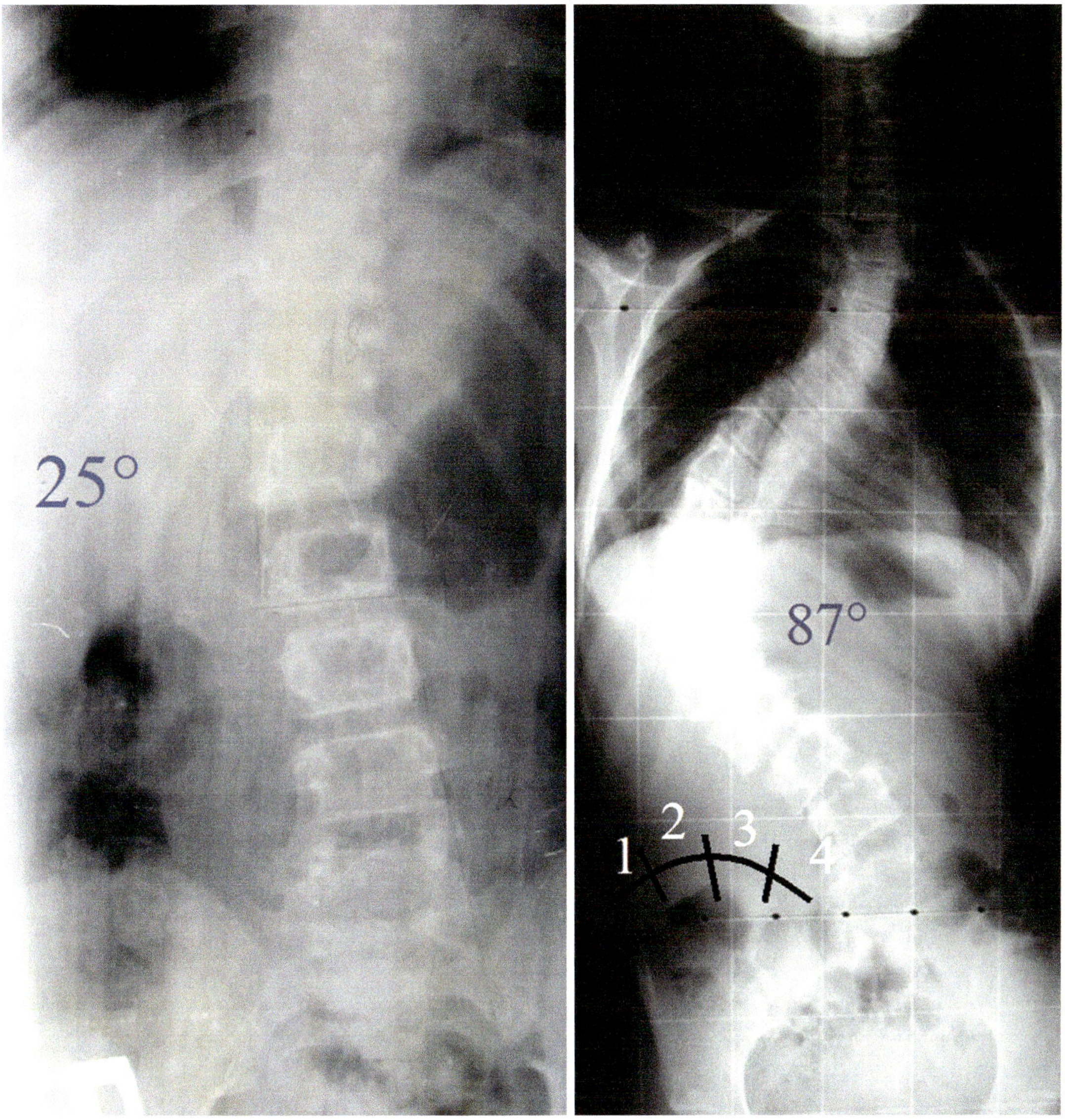

Fig. 19.1 Examples of Risser maturity test. Left: AIS with mild toraco-lumbar 25° Cobb (Risser 1) Right: Severe progression to 87° (Risser 3)

- Single major curve
  - Thoracic
  - Thoraco-lumbar
  - Lumbar
- Double major
  - Double thoracic
  - Double thoracic and lumbar
  - Double thoracic and thoraco-lumbar (Triple major).

The King-Moe classification [12] was the first to divide the different features of the curves in order to define the area of fusion. It derives from the experience of the surgical treatment of scoliosis with Harrington's instruments. These authors have the merit to be the first to describe important concepts, such as the stable vertebra, the structured and compensatory curve, but some controversies about sufficient interobserver and intarobserver reliability [13].

A total of 5 types are identified (Table 19.2, Figs. 19.2, 19.3, and 19.4).

Although this classification was widely used and has the merit of having guided the surgical treatment, there were many critical issues that emerged over the years.

First of all, the single thoraco-lumbar and lumbar major curves and the thoracic double majors were excluded. Second, the structuring criteria are not well explained, especially the relation to the reducibility of the curve at the side bending. Third, the sagittal curves profiles are not considered. Finally, the poor reliability of this classification combined with the advent of the segmental instrumentation and the obsolescence of Harrington's technique, the Lenke classification was introduced in 2001 [14]. This classification, which progressively becomes the most widely used and still considered the gold standard, is a two-dimensional radiographic assessment, coronal and sagittal, based on studies in postero-anterior (PA), latero-lateral (LL) and PA lateral bending, designed to determine the most appropriate fusion levels. It described six different types of curves (Table 19.3, Figs. 19.4 and 19.5).

Table 19.2 King-Moe classification [12]

I	Primary lumbar curve greater than the compensatory thoracic curve
II	Primary thoracic curve with compensatory lumbar curve
III	Short pure thoracic curve
IV	Long C-shaped thoracolumbar curve
V	Double thoracic curve with extension into cervical spine and compensatory lumbar curve

In this classification the lumbar spine modifier is very important because permits to identify the curves in A, B, C, based on the ratio between central sacral vertical line (CSVL) and the lumbar curve (Fig. 19.4).

The thoracic sagittal modifier permits according to thoracic kyphosis (T5-T12) to identify the profile as positive if >40° neutral in case of values included from 10° to 40° and negative if kyphosis <10° (Figs. 19.6 and 19.7).

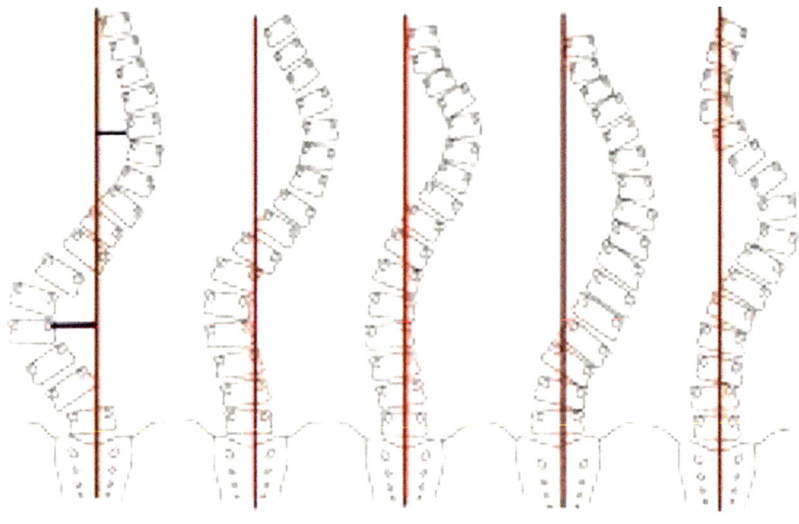

Fig. 19.2 Patterns of King-Moe classification

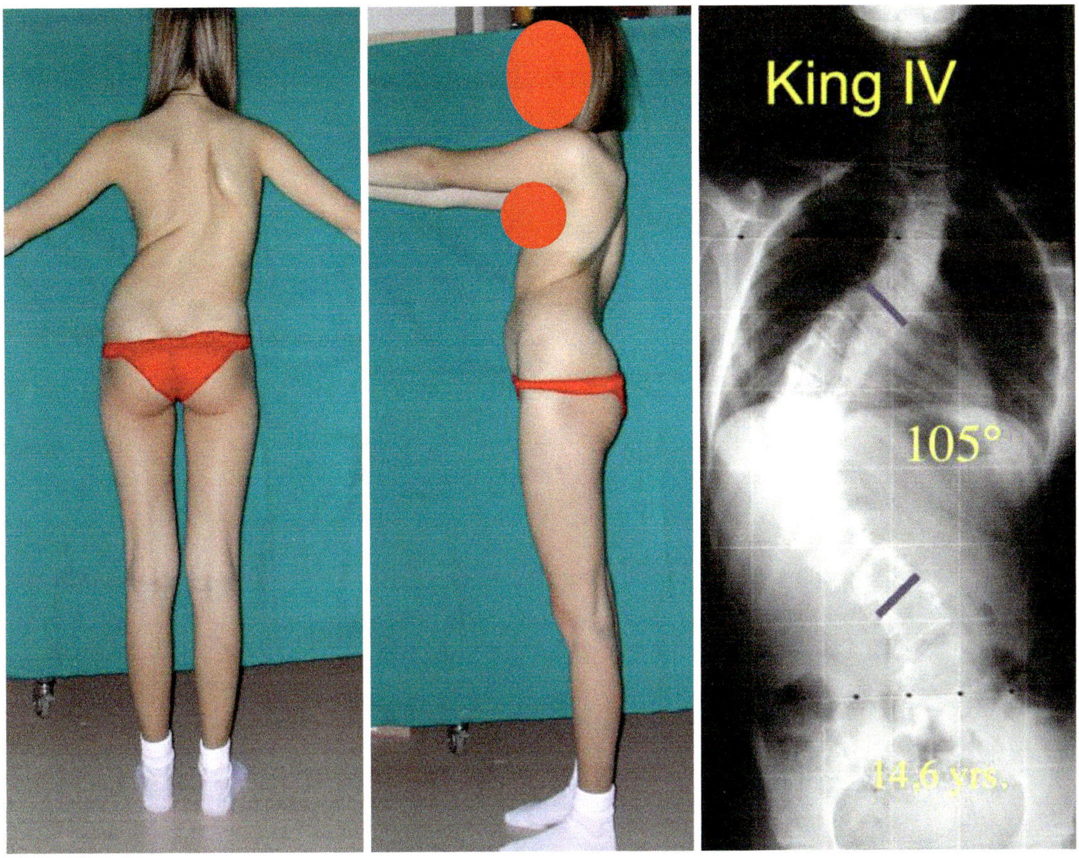

Fig. 19.3 Clinical and radiographic example of a King IV scoliotic curve in a 14 years old girl

Fig. 19.4 Clinical and radiographic example of a King II scoliotic curve in a 13 years old girl

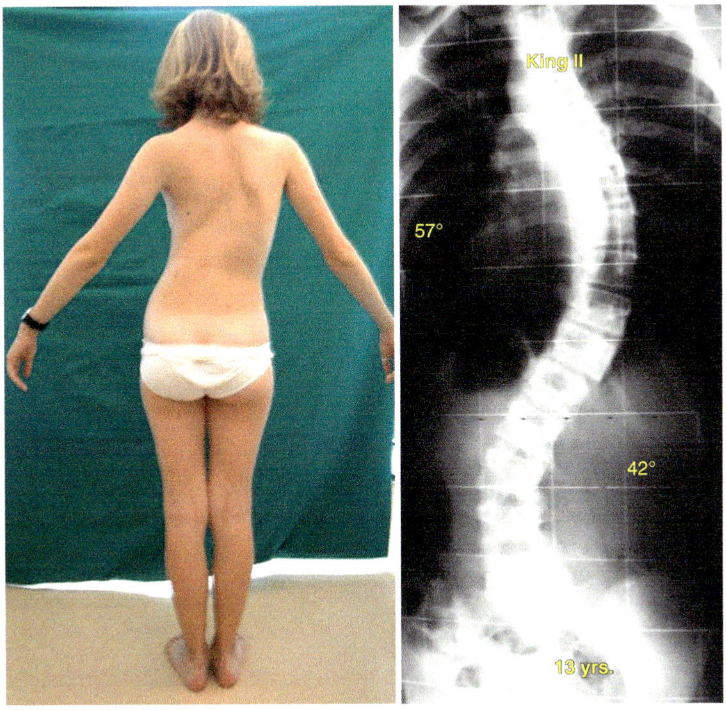

Table 19.3 Lenke classification

Type	Proximal Thoracic	Main Thoracic	Thoracolumbar/Lumbar	Curve Type
1	Non-structural	Structural (major[a])	Non-structural	Main thoracic (MT)
2	Structural	Structural (major[a])	Non-structural	Double thoracic (DT)
3	Non-structural	Structural (major[a])	Structural	Double major (DM)
4	Structural	Structural (major[a])	Structural (major[a])	Triple major (TM)[b]
5	Non-structural	Non-structural	Structural (major[a])	Thoracolumbar/lumbar (TL/L)
6	Non-structural	Structural	Structural (major[a])	Thoracolumbar/lumbar- main thoracic (TL/L – MT)
Minor curve structural criteria	Side bending cobb ≥25° T2-T5 kyphosis ≥ +20°	Side bending cobb ≥25° T10-L2 kyphosis ≥ +20°	Side bending cobb ≥25° T10-L2 kyphosis ≥ +20°	

[a]*Major* Largest Cobb measurement – always structural, *Minor* All other curves – may be structural or non-structural
[b]In type 4 curves (triple major), either the MT or the TL/L curve can be major, depending on the largest Cobb measurement. If the MT and TL/L are equal in magnitude, the MT will be considered the major curve

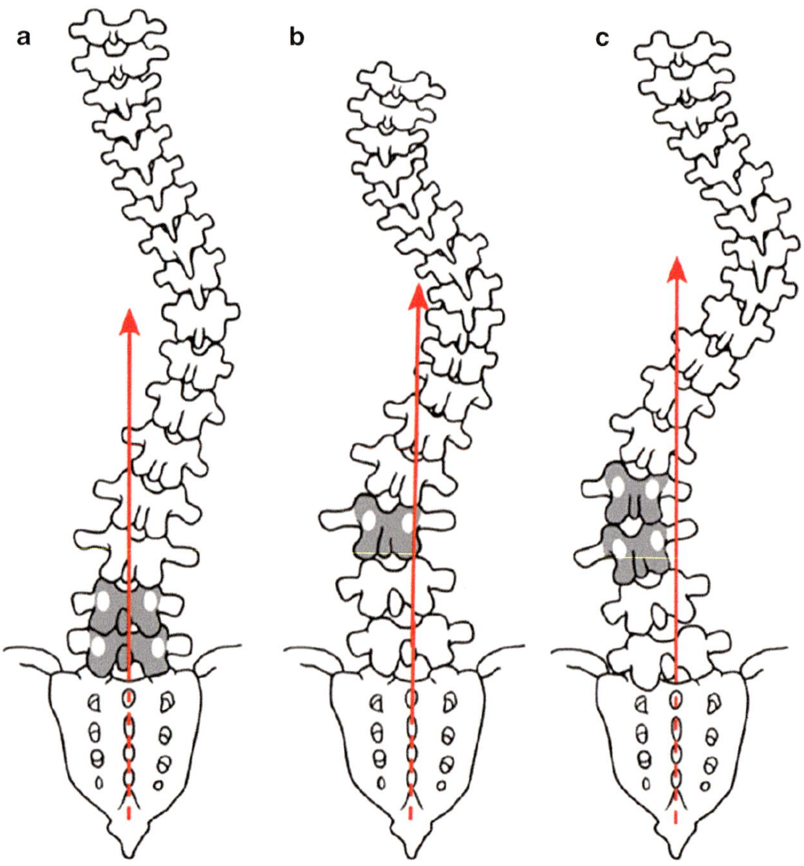

Fig. 19.5 Lumbar Modifier. (**a**) CSVL Between Pedicles (Apical Disc). (**b**) CSVL Touches Apical Pedicle (Apical Body). (**c**) The apical vertebral bodies are completely lateral to the CSVL (Apical Disc

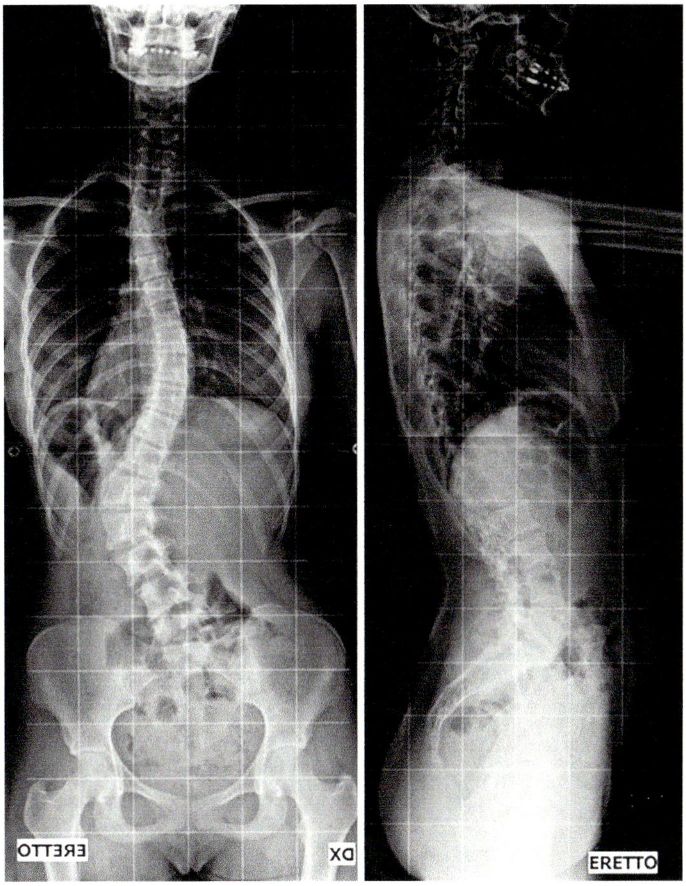

Fig. 19.6 Example of a Lenke VI curve in a 15 years old girl

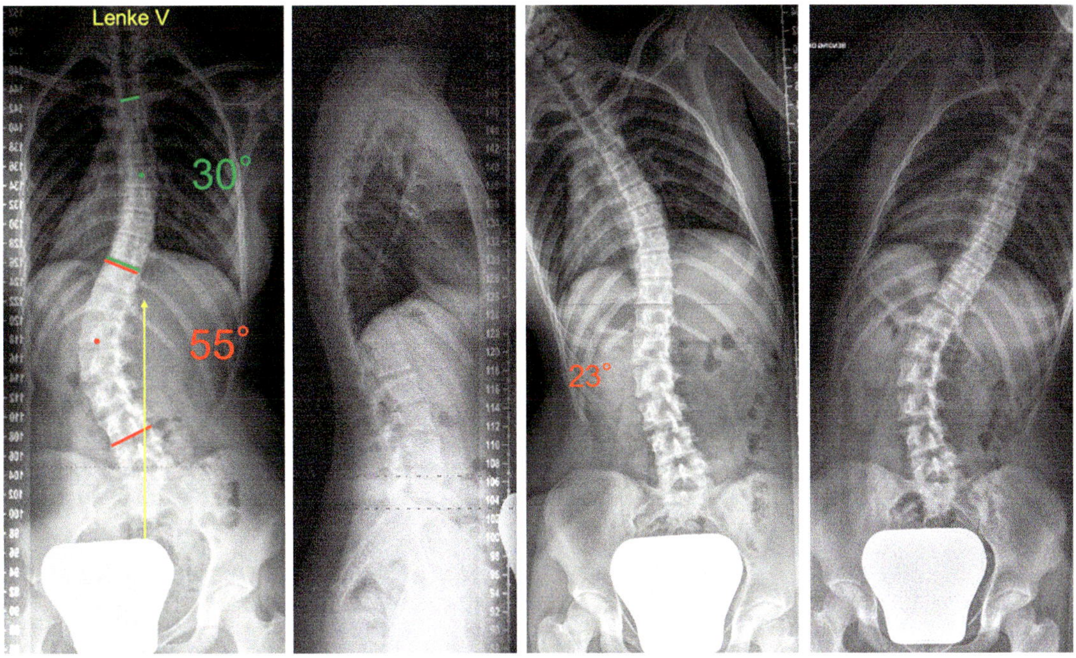

Fig. 19.7 Example of a Lenke V curve in a 13 years old girl, with high flexibility of both curves at the AP side bendings

19.4 Conclusions

The knowledge of the natural history of idiopathic scoliosis is fundamental, in order to understand the possible progression of the curves both at long and short term, and therefore helps to estimate with certain precision when to face the most suitable treatment, either conservative or surgical.

An incorrect attitude can lead to catastrophic progression of scoliosis, as, on the other hand, an incorrect diagnosis can lead to overtreatment.

Moreover, the classification of idiopathic scoliosis helps to understand the pathophysiological mechanisms that led to deformity and serves a great deal for the choice of the fusion area in surgical cases.

Pearls
- Adolescent Idiopathic Scoliosis evolution
- Natural History
- Classifications

Editorial Comment
Early scoliosis deformities and indication for further investigation can be done by clinical investigation. The so called "Adams bend forward-test" in combination with an scoliometer can help to determine, whether an x-ray has to be done or not. Angles above 7° should lead to a further radiological investigation.

References

1. Skaggs DL, Guillaume T, El-Hawary R, et al. Early onset scoliosis consensus statement, SRS Growing Spine Committee, 2015. Spine Deform. 2015;3:107. https://doi.org/10.1016/j.jspd.2015.01.002.
2. Konieczny MR, Senyurt H, Krauspe R. Epidemiology of adolescent idiopathic scoliosis. J Child Orthop. 2013;7:3–9. https://doi.org/10.1007/s11832-012-0457-4.
3. Nilsonne U, Lundgren K-D. Long-term prognosis in idiopathic scoliosis. Acta Orthop Scand. 1968;39:456–65.
4. Weinstein SL, Dolan LA, Spratt KF, et al. Health and function of patients with untreated idiopathic scoliosis. JAMA. 2003;289:559–67. https://doi.org/10.1001/jama.289.5.559.
5. Edgar MA. The natural history of unfused scoliosis. Orthopedics. 1987;10:931–9.
6. Ascani E, Bartolozzi P, Logroscino CA, et al. Natural history of untreated idiopathic scoliosis after skeletal maturity. Spine (Phila Pa 1976). 1986;11:784–9.
7. Yawn BP, Yawn RA. The estimated cost of school scoliosis screening. Spine (Phila Pa 1976). 2000;25:2387–91.
8. Labelle H, Stephens Richards B, De Kleuver M, Grivas TB, KDK L, Wong HK, Thometz J, Beausejour M, Turgeon I, Fong DY. SRS school screening task force report. In: Half-day courses. Non-operative spinal deformity treatment techniques, Sagittal plane deformity corrective techniques, Spinal deformity in Myelomeningocele, SRS abstract book. Lyon: Pre-Meeting Course; 2013. p. 52.
9. Risser JC. The iliac apophysis; an invaluable sign in the management of scoliosis. Clin Orthop. 1958;11:111–9.
10. Canavese F, Charles YP, Dimeglio A. Skeletal age assessment from elbow radiographs. Review of the literature. Chir Organi Mov. 2008;92:1–6. https://doi.org/10.1007/s12306-008-0032-9.
11. Lonstein JE, Carlson JM. The prediction of curve progression in untreated idiopathic scoliosis during growth. J Bone Joint Surg Am. 1984;66:1061–71.
12. King HA, Moe JH, Bradford DS, Winter RB. The selection of fusion levels in thoracic idiopathic scoliosis. J Bone Joint Surg Am. 1983;65:1302–13.
13. Cummings RJ, et al. Interobserver reliability and intraobserver reproducibility of the system of King et al for the classification of adolescent idiopathic scoliosis. J Bone Joint Surg Am. 1998;80-A:1107–11.
14. Lenke LG, Betz RR, Harms J, et al. Adolescent idiopathic scoliosis: a new classification to determine extent of spinal arthrodesis. J Bone Joint Surg Am. 2001;83-A:1169–81.

20 Diagnosis and Conservative Treatment of Adolescent Idiopathic Scoliosis: Case Presentation

Massimo Balsano and Stefano Negri

20.1 Patient History

12 years old female referred for scoliosis by a family pediatrician. She is 2 months postmenarchal and has no medical problems. She is engaged in typical activities for an adolescent female including volleyball and dance. Past medical history (PMH) and past surgical history (PSH) unremarkable.

She complaints of mild back pain localized at lumbar region, absent at rest and exacerbated by her sporting activities.

20.2 Examination

The patient is a healthy-appearing adolescent with near ideal body weight. The right shoulder is slightly higher with minimal waist line asymmetry. The right rib hump assessed with the Scoliometer® is 9° and in the lumbar left area is 10° (Fig. 20.1).

There is no clinical leg-length discrepancy. The skin has no abnormalities, and the neurological assessment is normal.

Radiographical AP Image (Fig. 20.2a): Idiopathic Scoliosis with right thoracic curve of 24°, apex in T8, and left lumbar curve of 25°, apex in L2, with axial rotation of lumbar and thoracic vertebral bodies, where in the lumbar curve the rotation is prevalent.

20.3 Diagnosis

Adolescent Idiopathic Scoliosis (AIS), Lenke 3, Lumbar modifier B, Risser 0.

20.4 Choice of Treatment

The mother is very careful about her daughter and seems compliant with medical indications.

Considering the morphological shapes of the curves, the clinical aspects, and the possible worsening of the scoliosis in a growing spine (70%) [1–3], we have treated the girl with a Cheneau brace (Fig. 20.3), wearing 22 h/day with exercises and physical therapy three times a week [4].

The choice of Cheneau brace for the patient has resulted from these considerations:

- It's a rigid brace, providing a 3D correction;
- The brace is opened anteriorly, providing a better compliance for the pulmonary function, chest and breasts;
- It's correction mechanism leads to the transfer of forces from the convex to the concave side of the curves, with a three-point acting system, with aimed overcorrection of the curves;
- It's well accepted by the patient and her family, with a high compliance.

M. Balsano (✉) · S. Negri
UOC Ortopedia e Traumatologia,
Regional Spinal Department, AOUI, Verona, Italy

B. Meyer, M. Rauschmann (eds.), *Spine Surgery*, https://doi.org/10.1007/978-3-319-98875-7_20

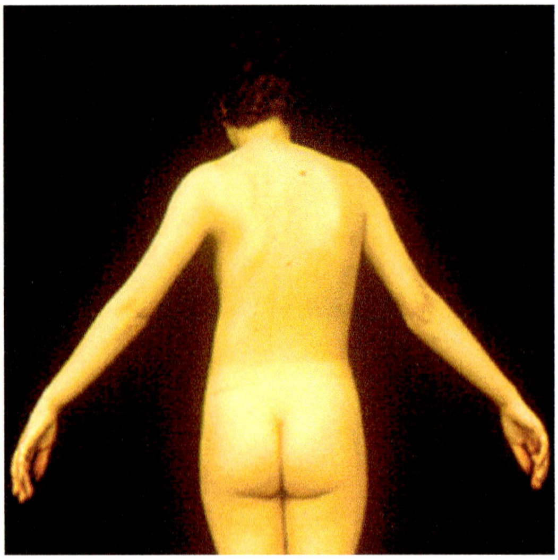

Fig. 20.1 Clinical image of the patient at the first observation. Note the shoulder and waists asymmetry

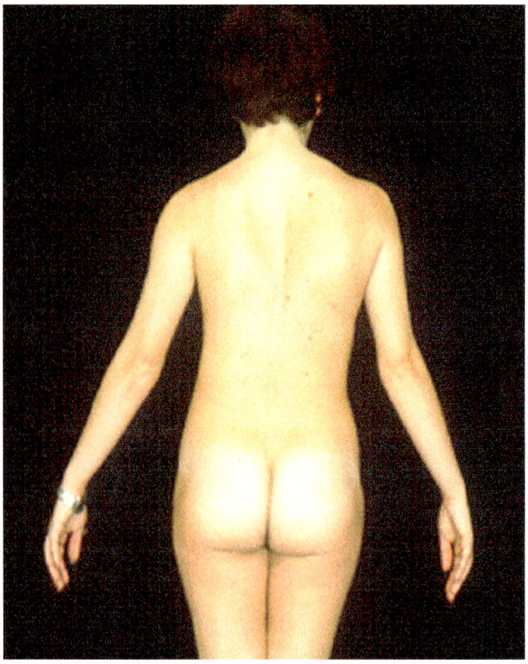

Fig. 20.3 Final clinical aspect: full recovery of the shoulders and waists asymmetry

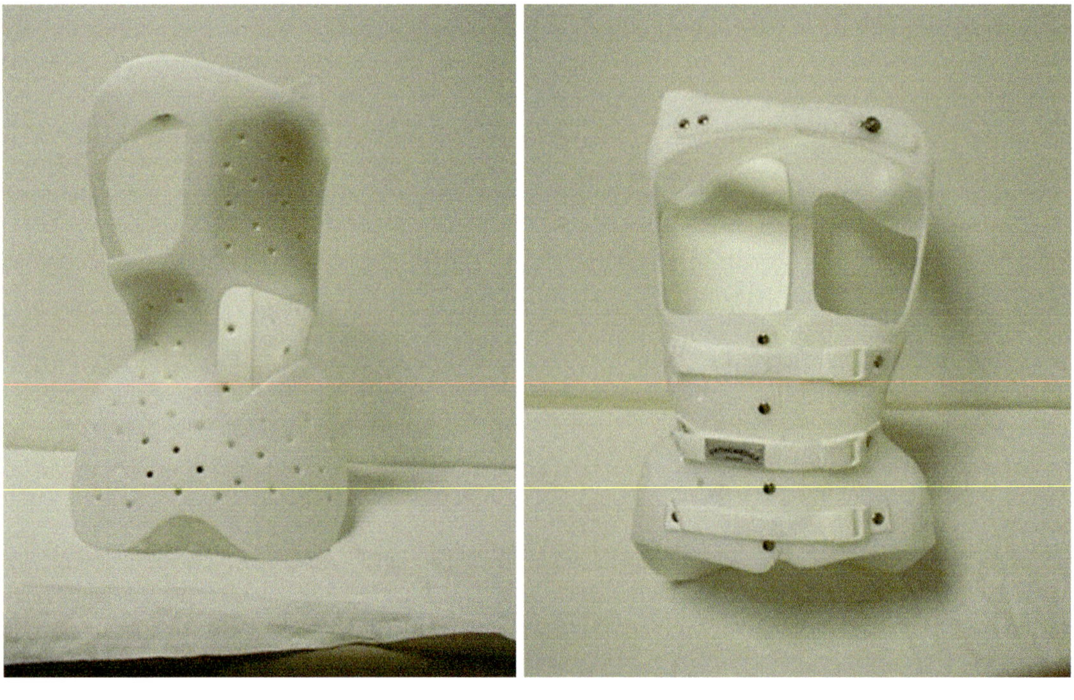

Fig. 20.2 Cheneau brace, posterior and anterior view

The purpose of brace treatment is always to arrest the possible evolution of the scoliosis and to avoid a surgical treatment with fusion.

The patient has followed our strict indications, with serial clinical controls every 3 months, and radiographic controls, wearing the brace at 3, 9 and 18 months from the beginning of treatment.

The final result, after 2 years of brace treatment, has showed a very good improving of clinical and radiographics aspects of the patient (Figs. 20.3 and 20.4).

20.5 Outcome

At 2-year follow-up, the patient was participating in all desired athletic activities without back pain or limitation. She was satisfied with her overall body alignment and shoulder balance. The thoracic scoliometer measurement was 2° and lumbar 3°.

20.6 Discussion

The aim of nonoperative treatment of AIS is to control the scoliosis either eliminating the need for surgery.

In this case the patient was successfully treated with the Cheneau brace, improving clinically, Functionally and radiographically.

The success of the result seems related to the starting point of the treatment, the choice of a 3D brace, and the perfect compliance of the patient and her family, that have strictly followed the medical prescriptions.

Pearls
- Adolescent Idiopathic Scoliosis
- Evolution
- Conservative treatment
- Brace treatment

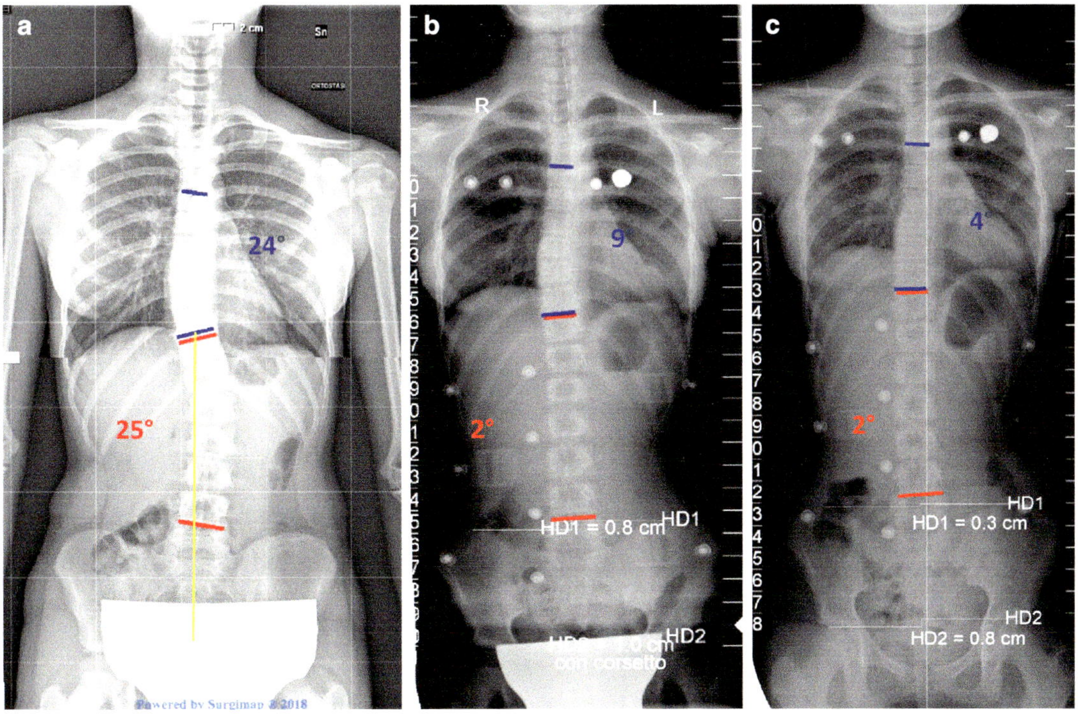

Fig. 20.4 (**a**) First X-Ray and observation: thoracic and lumbar curves (Lenke 3). (**b**) Second X-Ray after 3 months (in brace): hypercorrection of the lumbar curve. This indicated high flexible curve. (**c**) Third X-ray: 9 months later: optimal control of the curves and absence of worsening. (**d**) Fourth X-Ray: mild loss of correction. (**e**) Fifth X-ray: Final follow-up at 2 years

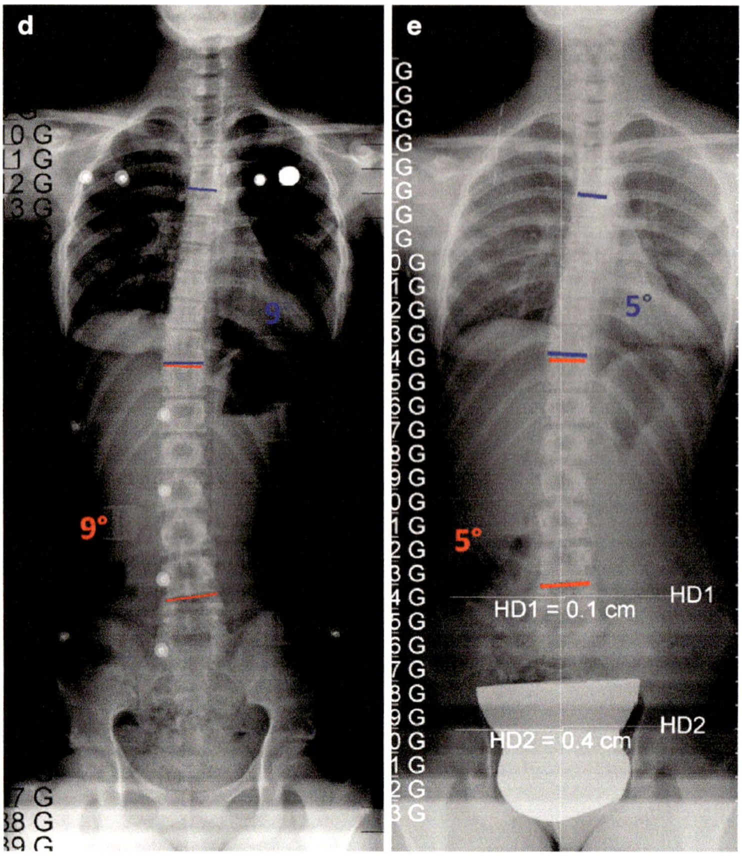

Fig. 20.4 (continued)

Editorial Comment

The right indication for a brace is mandatory on the maturity of the sceleton. The risser sign and the menarche in females as well as the votin break in males are important for decisionmaking for a brace. The result of treatment is always a progression stop. Almost always after treatment the scoliosis will have the same shape as at the beginning of the treatment.

References

1. James JIP. Idiopathic scoliosis: the prognosis, diagnosis, and operative indications related to curve patterns and the age at onset. J Bone Joint Surg Br. 1954;36B:35–49.
2. Aulisa AG, Guzzanti V, Marzetti E, et al. Correlation between compliance and brace treatment in juvenile and adolescent idiopathic scoliosis: SOSORT 2014 award winner. Scoliosis. 2014;9:6.
3. Weinstein SL, Pçonseti IV. Curve progression in idiopathic scoliosis. J Bone Joint Surg Am. 1983;65:447–55.
4. Weiss HR, Rigo M. The Cheneau concept of bracing. Actual standards. Stud Health Technol Inform. 2008;135:291–302.

Idiopathic Scoliosis: Operative Treatment

21

Ulf Liljenqvist

21.1 Introduction

This case will detail the aspects of posterior correction and selective fusion in an adolescent idiopathic thoracic scoliosis. It will highlight the rules of fusion lengths and the limits of selective fusion. The techniques of three-dimensional posterior correction are described.

21.2 Case Description

16 year old girl with a Lenke type 1 C modifier thoracic curve of 52° Cobbangle and a flexible lumbar curve of 40° that bends down to 12° on reverse bending films, thoracic kyphosis 37° (Fig. 21.1a–c). She has moderate pain on the concavity of the thoracic curve. Clinically, the left shoulder is down by 1,5 cm, rigth ribhump of 17°, left lumbar hump of 4° (Fig. 21.2a, b).

Operative treatment consisted of posterior segmental pedicle screw instrumentation in free-hand technique. Correction was done with reduction screws, segmental translation and derotation. Correction of the thoracic curve to 19° with spontaneous straigthening of the lumbar curve to 17° (Fig. 21.3a) On the left a 5.5 mm, slightly overbent Cobalt Chrome rod was placed to control thoracic kyphosis (Fig. 21.3b). For arthrodesis local bone plus calciumphosphate was used. Surgery under controlled hypotension with neuromonitoring.

One year postop. the patient is free from any pain and has resumed sport activities. Reduction of the rib hump to 9°, no lumbar hump (Fig. 21.4a, b). X-rays demonstrate slight increase of the lumbar curve with a fully balanced spine (Fig. 21.5a, b).

21.3 Discussion

In scoliotic curves exceeding 50° Cobbangle in adolescents surgical correction and instrumented fusion is recommended. In the majority of cases, posterior techniques are indicated including segmental pedicle screw instrumentation, segmental translational and derotation maneuvers and control of the sagittal plane [3, 4, 9]. Anterior correction is indicated in severely malrotated thoracolumbar curves and in some hypokyphotic thoracic curves with large ribhumps and larger secondary lumbar curves (Lenke type 1 C curves) [2, 6, 8].

The instrumented arthrodesis should include all structural curves, secondary flexible curves will straighten out spontaneously and do not

U. Liljenqvist (✉)
Department for Spine Surgery, St. Franziskus Hospital, Münster, Germany
e-mail: ulf.liljenqvist@sfh-muenster.de

B. Meyer, M. Rauschmann (eds.), *Spine Surgery*, https://doi.org/10.1007/978-3-319-98875-7_21

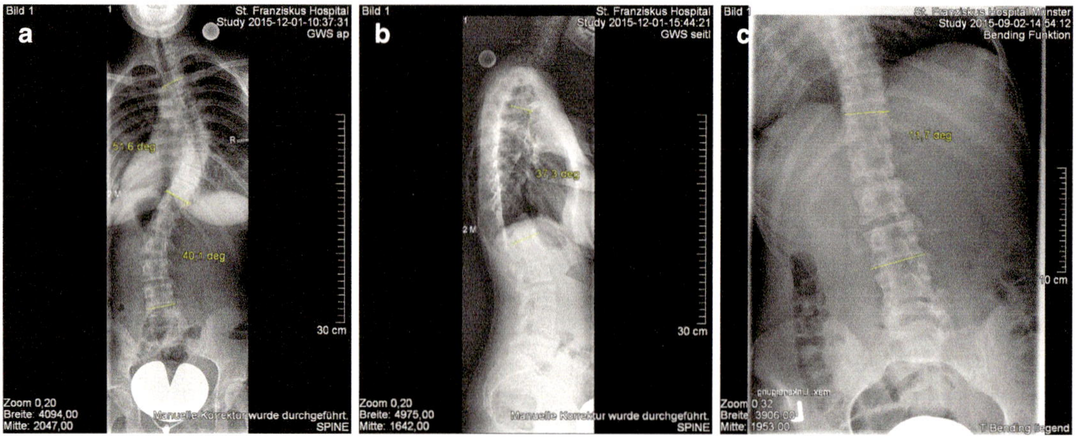

Fig. 21.1 (**a**–**c**) Preop. standing full spine X-ray ap and lateral (**a**, **b**) and reverse bending films (**c**)

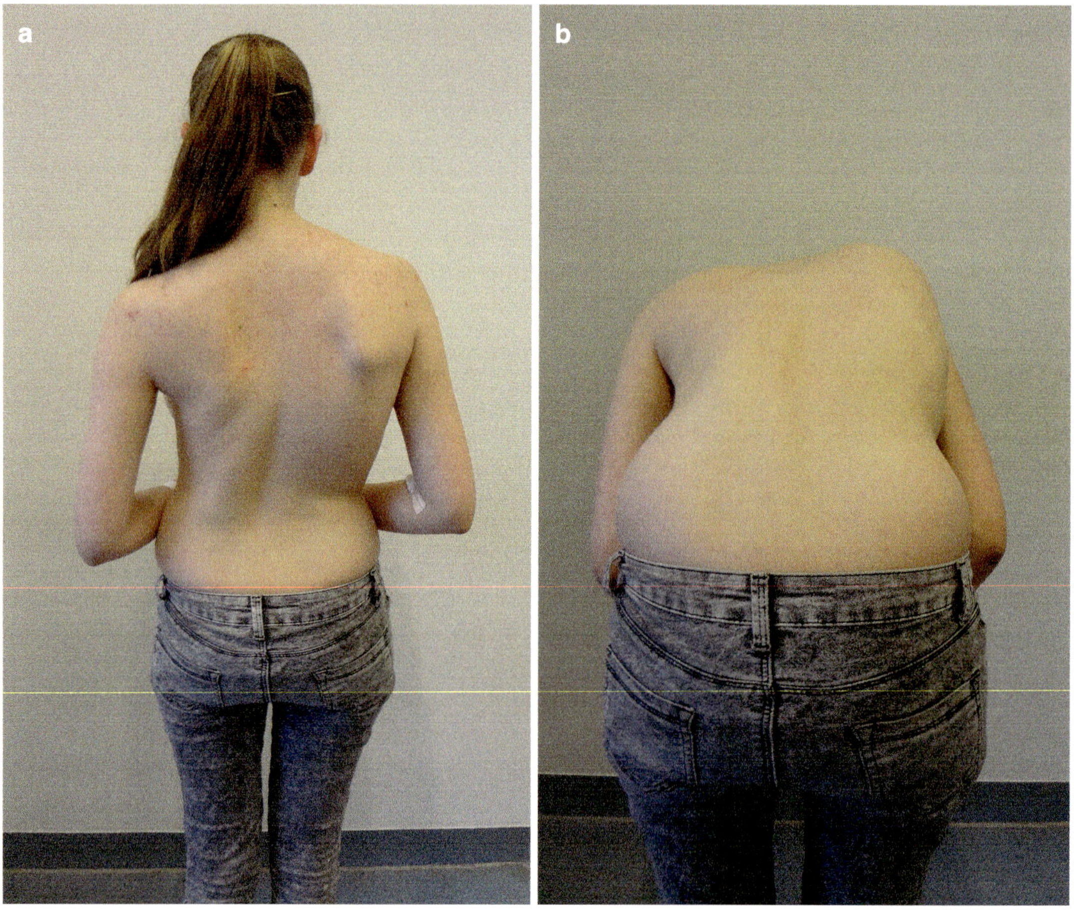

Fig. 21.2 (**a**, **b**) Preop. clinical pictures including forward bendning films (**b**)

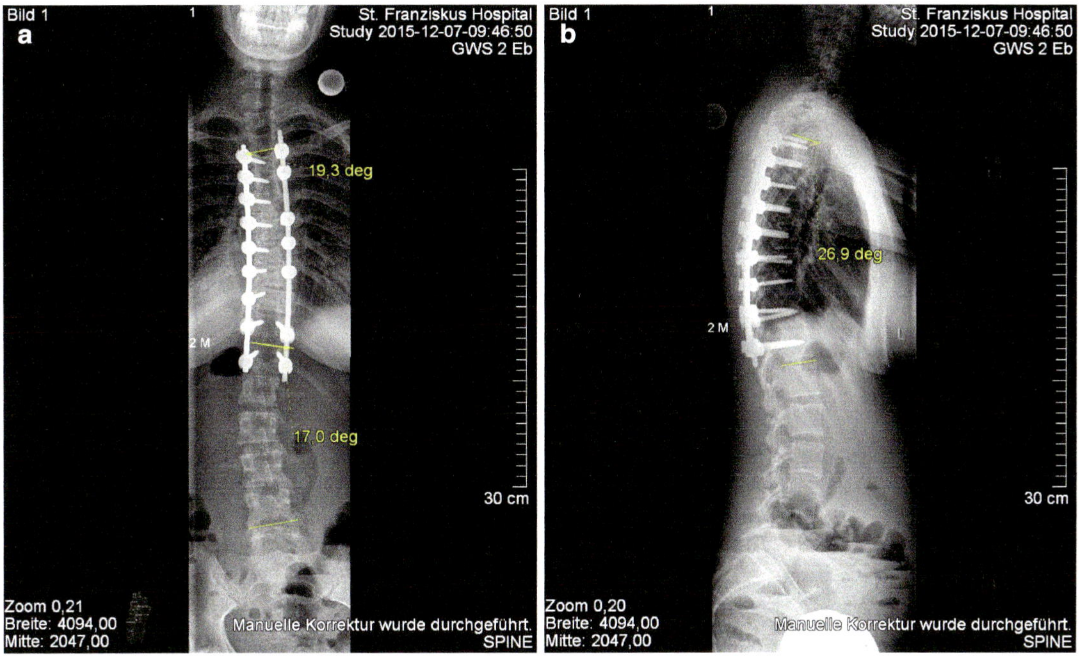

Fig. 21.3 (**a**, **b**) Postop. standing full spine X-ray ap and lateral

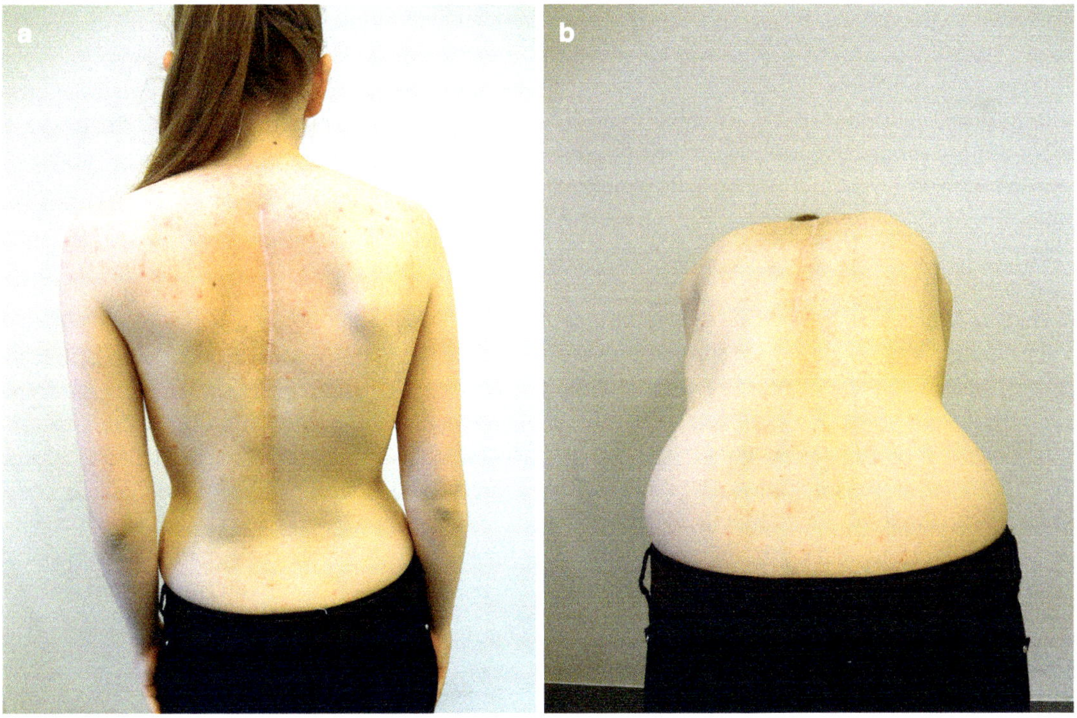

Fig. 21.4 (**a**, **b**) Clinical pictures 1 year postop

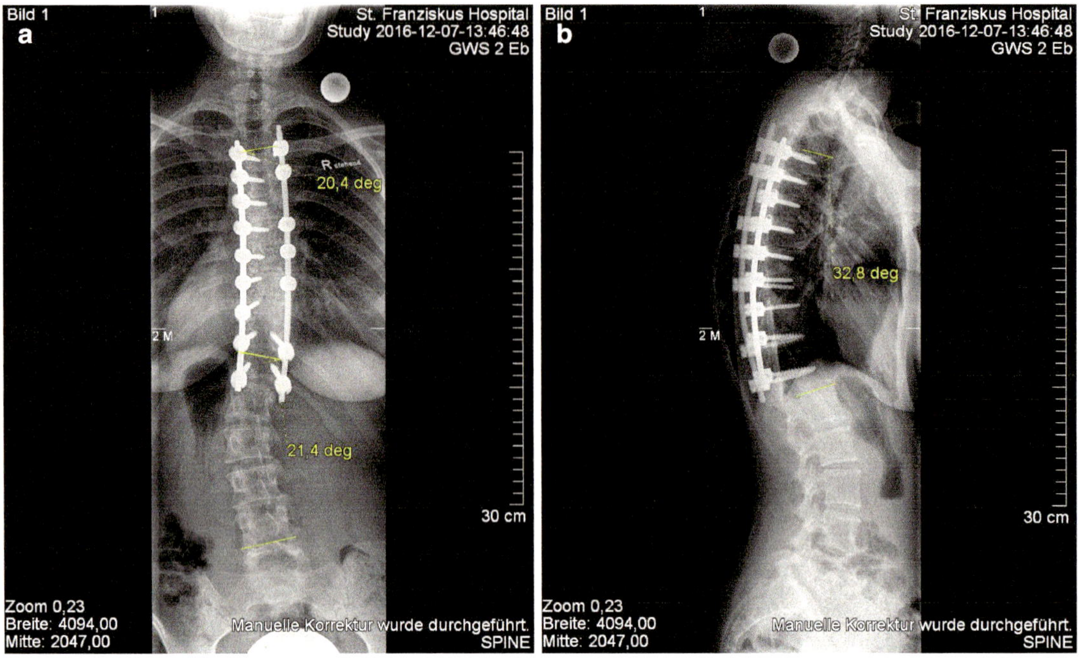

Fig. 21.5 (**a**, **b**) 1 year postop. standing full spine X-ray ap and lateral

need to be included into the fusion. A structural curve is characterized by a Cobbangle larger than 40–50°, a residual Cobbangle on the reverse bending films of >25° and a marked clinical malrotation (rib or lumbar hump). Accordingly, non-structural curves are flexible on the bending films and do have less marked malrotation. Severely hypo- or hyperkyphotic areas of the spine should be included into the fusion, as well [5, 7].

Upper instrumented vertebra is typically the upper endvertebra of the upper structural curve. The lowest instrumented vertebra (LIV) is normally the first vertebra of the lower structural curve that is touched by the central sacral vertical line. The LIV should be neutrally rotated and the disc below the LIV should be flexible, i.e. it should open up to both sides on both bending films [1].

21.4 Conclusions and Take Home Message

- selective thoracic fusion is feasible if the lumbar curve of is less than 50°, if it bends down to less than 25° on reverse bending films and if the lumbar hump is substantially smaller than the ribhump.
- the upper thoracic curve needs to be included (i.e. fusion cephalad to T2) if the rigth shoulder is down, if the upper thoracic curve is larger than 40°, if the residual upper thoracic curve on the reverse bending films is larger than 20° and if there is a substantial upper left ribhump
- segmental pedicle screws and a Cobalt Chrome rod on the concavity are golden standard
- anterior correction is indicated in severely malrotated thoracolumbar curves and in some hypokyphotic thoracic curves with large ribhumps

Pearls

- Selective fusion of the structural curve in multiple curve scoliosis
- Freehand segmental pedicle screw instrumentation as golden standard
- Anterior correction still indicated in rare cases of severly malrotated thoracolumbar curves and hypokyphotic thoracic curves

Editorial Comment

The indication for selective fusion in AIS is, reducing pain and the cosmetic aspect, but even more the reduction of degeneration in the lumbar spine. The selection of the lowest instrumented vetebra is very important to spare lumbar segments but do not create a "adding on phenomenon" in case of including not enough segments in the construct.

References

1. Bai J, Chen K, Wei Q, et al. Selecting the LSTV as the lower instrumented vertebra in the treatment of Lenke type 1A and 2A adolescent idiopathic scoliosis. Spine 2018;43:E390–8.
2. Bullmann V, Halm H, Niemeyer T, et al. Dual-rod correction and instrumentation of idiiopathic scoliosis with the Halm-Zielke instrumentation. Spine. 2003;15:1306–13.
3. Cao Y, Xiong W, Li F. Pedicle screw versus hybrid construct instrumentation in adolescent idiopathic scoliosis. meta-analysis of thoracic scoliosis. Spine. 2014;39:E800–10.
4. Lamerain M, Bachy M, Delpont M, et al. CoCr rods provie better frontal correction of adolescent idiopathic scoliosis treated by all-pedicle screw fixation. Eur Spine J. 2014;23:1190–6.
5. Lenke L, Betz R, Harms J, et al. Adolescent idiopathic scoliosis: a new classification to determine extent of spinal arthrodesis. J Bone Joint Surg Am. 2001;83:1169–81.
6. Liljenqvist U, Halm H, Bullmann V. Spontaneous lumbar curve correction in selective anterior instrumentation and fusion of idiopathic thoracic scoliosis of Lenke type C. Eur Spine J. 2013;22:S138–48.
7. Liljenqvist U, Lerner T, Bullmann V. Selective fusion of idiopathic scoliosis with respect tot he Lenke classification. Orthopade. 2009;38:189–92.
8. Schmidt C, Liljenqvist U, Lerner T, et al. Sagittal balance of thoracic lordoscoliosis: anterior dual rod instrumentation versus posterior pedicle screw fixation. Eur Spine J. 2011;20:1118–26.
9. Suk S, Kim J, Kim S, Lim D. Pedicle screw instrumentation in adolescent idiopathic scoliosis (AIS). Eur Spine J. 2012;21:13–22.

A Congenital Scoliosis Case Characterized with Contralateral Hemivertebrae

22

Alpaslan Senkoylu and R. Emre Acaroglu

22.1 Introduction

Congenital scoliosis is a complex spinal problem that may end up with a disaster if not treated properly. Pathology contains many challenges in every step starting by the patient's admission.

Aim of this case presentation is to discuss a complicated hemivertebra case with its diagnosis, natural history and treatment options.

22.2 Case Description

A 2-year old boy who complains of back deformity admitted to outpatient clinic. There was no other system abnormality in his history. However, elder brother was operated because of congenital scoliosis and hemivertebra excision was done 2 years ago. Physical examination revealed right sided loin and left sided rib humps (Fig. 22.1) and no neurology. P-A long cassette X-Ray demonstrated left T10 and right L2 hemivertebrae that were fully segmented according to CT scan (Fig. 22.2). Magnetic resonance imaging of whole spine showed no intraspinal anomaly (including syrinx, Chiari malformation, diastematomyelia) and spinal cord was ended at the level of L1.

Posterior hemivertebra excision, short segment pedicle segment fixation and fusion was done for the L2 hemivertebra at first session. Postoperative period was uneventful and same procedure was repeated for the T10 hemivertebra 3-month later (Fig. 22.3).

Surgical Technique Resection of hemivertebra is performed by a single stage posterior approach as mentioned, with fusion of the adjacent levels only by using pedicle screw fixation. The posterior elements of the spine and, in the thoracic spine, rib head of hemivertebra on convex side are exposed subperiosteally at the affected levels. One level above and one level below 4 mm diameter pedicle screws are inserted. Then, transverse process of hemivertebra at the convex side is excised (together with rib head at thoracic spine) and body of the hemivertebra is dissected retroperitoneally (or via extrapleural approach) with the finger or Harrington's elevator. This allows us better orientation and less blood loss. Lamina and pedicle of index level is removed with Kerrison rongeur or high-speed burr. Exciting nerve root should be protected at lumbar level, but it can be sacrificed at thoracic level. After control of epidural bleeding body of hemivertebra is resected with adjacent discs and cartilaginous end plates. Compression of the pedicle screws at the convex

A. Senkoylu
Gazi University, Ankara, Turkey

R. E. Acaroglu (✉)
Ankara Spine Center, Ankara, Turkey

B. Meyer, M. Rauschmann (eds.), *Spine Surgery*, https://doi.org/10.1007/978-3-319-98875-7_22

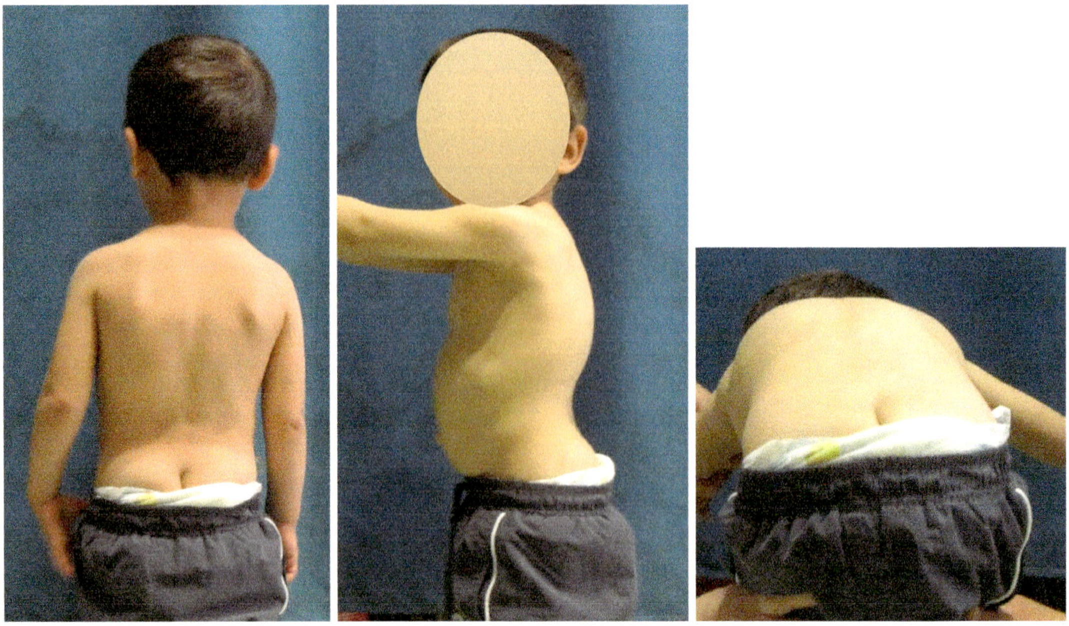

Fig. 22.1 Clinical pictures of 2-year-old boy. Forward bending test shows a right sided loin and left sided rib hump

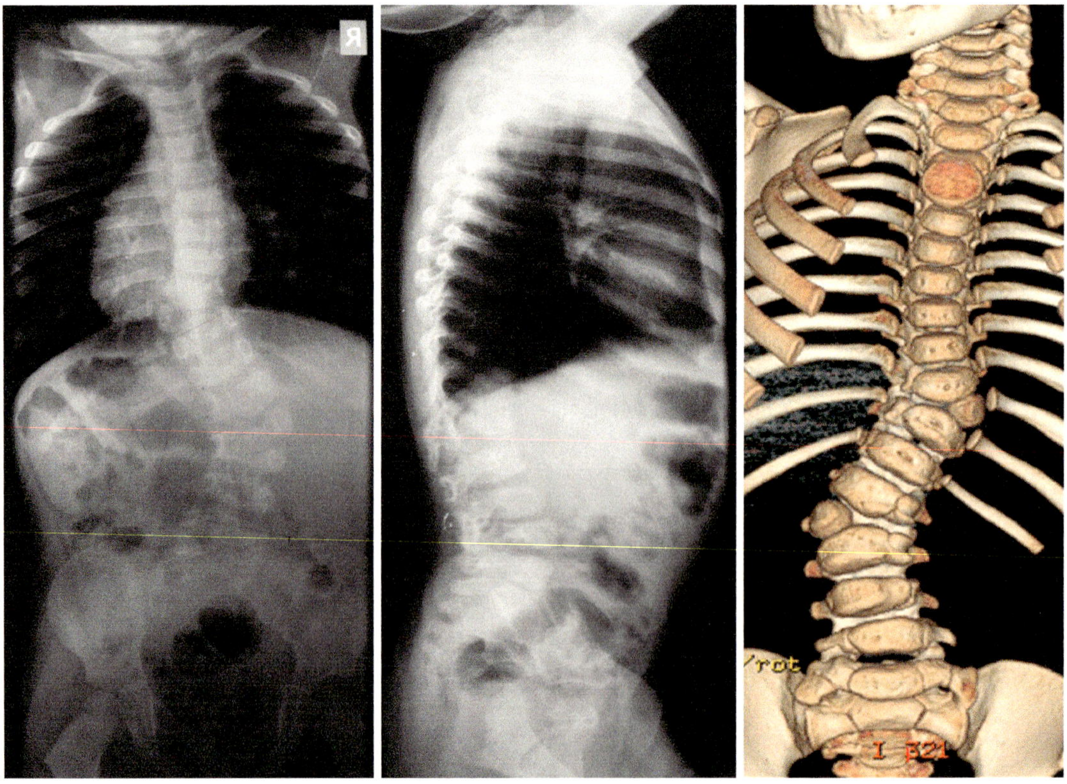

Fig. 22.2 P-A and Lateral long cassette X-ray and 3D reformatted CT scan (c) of the patient show contralateral hemivertebrae at T10 and L2 levels

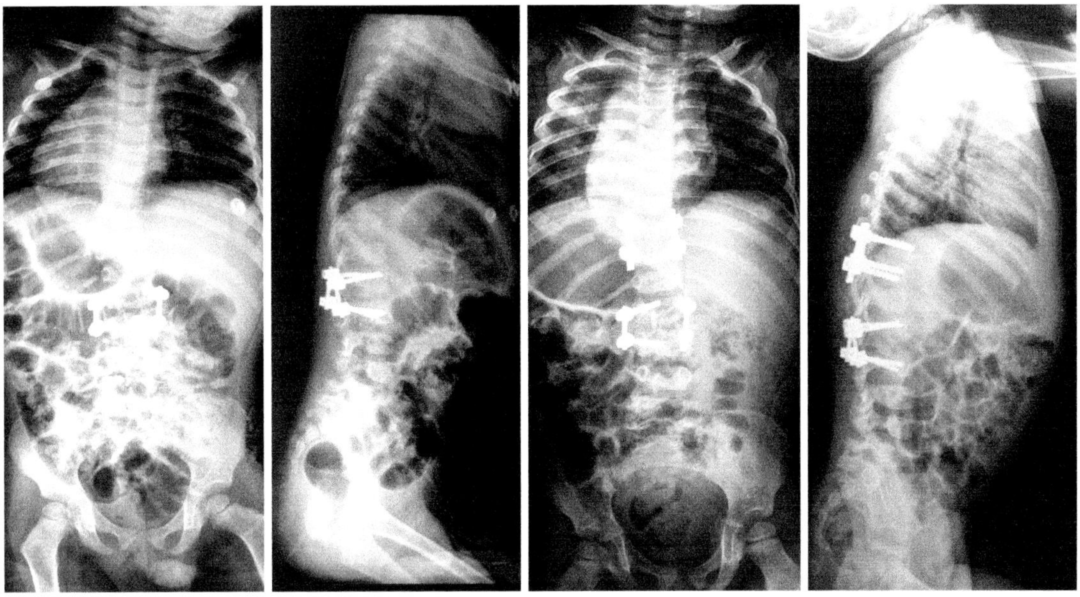

Fig. 22.3 Postoperative P-A and Lateral X-ray examinations of both sessions. There was an apparent shoulder imbalance in the control X-ray of first session which was corrected by the contralateral hemivertebra resection with second operation

side is done by the assistance of application three-point bending to the trunk of the patient. This prevents screw loosening due to direct excessive stress. Local bone is used for one level fusion (Fig. 22.3). Patients can be mobilized freely with a TLSO. TLSO can be weaning of 3 months, postoperatively.

There was no any postoperative complication. Patient has been following for 6 years and now he is 8-year-old with a balanced spine in all three planes (Fig. 22.4).

22.3 Discussion of the Case

Congenital scoliosis is the most frequent congenital deformity of the spinal column. It can be classified as defect of formation or defect of segmentation, yet most malformations have combined features of these deformities. Hemivertebra should be defined under the failure of formation group [1]. Natural history which is important for decision making differs according to anatomic location of hemivertebra. It has been well defined that locations at lumbar and thoracolumbar junction have bad prognosis and, presumably, progress. However, hemivertebra located in middle and upper thoracic spine is compensated well and may not need operation [2]. Morphology of the deformity also an important factor for prognosis. Worst scenario for the prognosis is fully segmented hemivertebra (two growth plates) and contralateral unsegmented bar. Estimated progression rate as fast as 10° a year according to Mc Master. Table 22.1 shows the hierarchic ranking from bad prognosis to good prognosis [2–4].

There is a consensus in the literature that hemivertebra should be treated as soon as possible after the diagnosis if it is located certain anatomic regions. Early treatment prevents extension and structural differentiation of deformity and also compensatory curves. Posterior resection, short level instrumentation and fusion is accepted a gold standard by the current literature [5, 6].

Preoperative whole spine MRI is crucial for the patients who planned the surgical intervention since the intraspinal anomalies are frequently possible

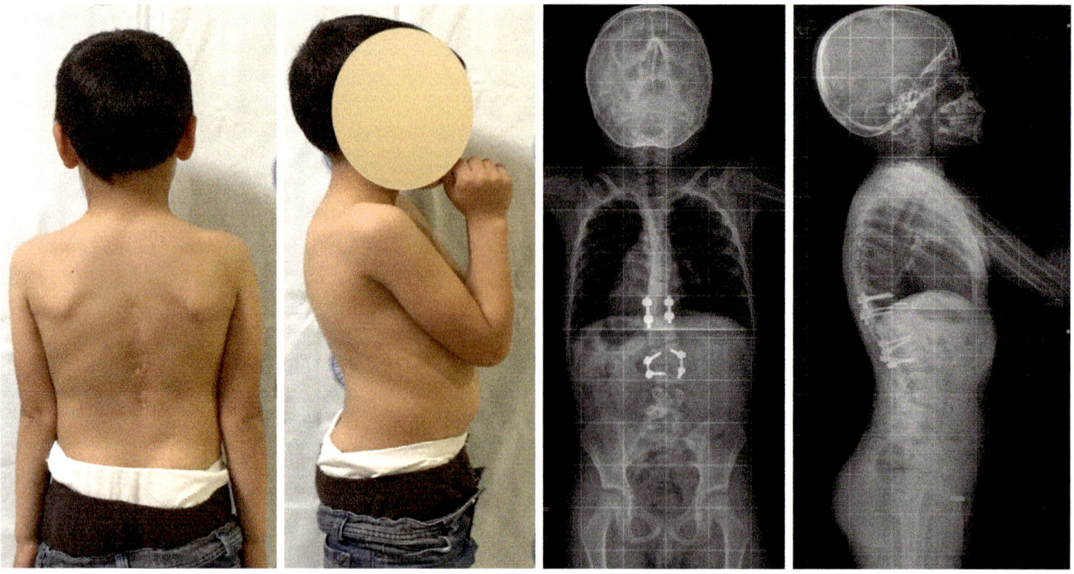

Fig. 22.4 Acceptable correction is maintaining after 6-year

Table 22.1 Grading of morphologies from the worst to bad prognosis

Fully segmented hemivertebra with a contralateral unsegmented bar
Unilateral unsegmented bar
Two consecutive fully segmented hemivertebrae
Fully segmented hemivertebra
Semisegmented hemivertebra
Wedge vertebra
Incarcerated hemivertebra
Block vertebra

Adapted from McMaster and Arlet et al. [2–4]

with congenital deformities [7]. We also performed whole spine MRI in order the check spinal cord anomalies. CT scan also was taken for detailed evaluation of pathoanatomy and found that there were only two contralateral hemivertebra without segmentation defect (Fig. 22.2). Hemivertebra excision was performed to L2 level. The first decision was a possible follow-up for the contralateral hemivertebra located at T10 level. However, clinical and x-ray examination revealed an uneven shoulder balance after the index operation (Fig. 22.3). T10 hemivertebra was also excised for preventing further coronal decompensation. Mid-term follow-up showed a balanced spine (Fig. 22.4).

22.4 Conclusions and Take-Home Message

In conclusion, congenital scoliosis is a complex spinal problem that needs detailed preoperative work out. Immediate surgical intervention should be done in special circumstances. Parents should be informed well for possible need of remedial interventions.

Pearls and Pitfalls

- Advanced imaging studies should be done for possible intraspinal anomaly and detailed anatomic interpretation
- Early surgical intervention should be done hemivertebrae located lumbar and thoracolumbar junction
- Surgeon's competency is crucial for this intervention
- Patient should be followed up closely until the end of adolescent period

References

1. Moe JH, Winter RB, Bradford DS, et al., editors. Scoliosis and other spinal deformities. Philadelphia: Saunders; 1978. p. 131–202. (Level of Evidence is 4).
2. McMaster MJ, Ohtsuka K. The natural history of congenital scoliosis. A study of two hundred and fifty-one patients. J Bone Joint Surg. 1982;64–A:1128–47. (Level of Evidence is 3).
3. McMaster MJ, David CV. Hemivertebra as a cause of scoliosis. J Bone J Surg-B. 1986;68(B):588–92. (Level of Evidence is 3).
4. Vincent A, Odent T, Aebi M. Congenital Scoliosis. Eur Spine J. 2003;12:456–63. (Level of Evidence is 4).
5. Ruf M, Jürgen H. Posterior Hemivertebra Resection With Transpedicular Instrumentation: Early Correction in Children Aged 1 to 6 Years. Spine. 2003;28(18):2132–8. (Level of Evidence is 3).
6. Chang DG, Kim JH, Ha KY, Lee JS, Jang JS, Suk SI. Posterior Hemivertebra Resection and Short Segment Fusion With Pedicle Screw Fixation for Congenital Scoliosis in Children Younger Than 10 Years. Spine. 2015;40(8):E484–91. (Level of Evidence is 3).
7. Batra S, Ahuja S. Congenital Soliosis: Management and Future Directions. Acta Orthop Belg. 2008;74:147–60. (Level of Evidence is 4).

23 Delayed Neurological Deficit and Surgical Site Infection After Pedicle Subtraction Osteotomy in a Revision Case

Susana Núñez-Pereira and Ferran Pellisé

23.1 Introduction

This case highlights 2 feared complications of adult deformity surgery: the development of a new neurological deficit and deep surgical site infection. The neurological deficit in this patient had a delayed onset. This is an atypical occurrence, and its management differs from that of deficits detected on intraoperative neuromonitoring. As to the surgical site infection, the patient was at high risk for this complication. Following appropriate treatment, she had an infection relapse 13 months later, which required a partial 2-stage implant exchange.

23.2 Case Description

23.2.1 Background

Patient: a 71-year-old woman

Comorbidities: hypertension, type II diabetes, allergy to non-steroidal anti-inflammatory drugs

She had undergone 4 previous lumbar surgeries:

Instrumented L4/5 fusion in 2000
Instrumentation lengthening and L3/4 fusion in 2006
L3 pedicle subtraction osteotomy (PSO) in 2010
Revision surgery to treat cerebrospinal fluid leakage in 2010

During the last revision surgery, samples sent to the microbiology laboratory yielded coagulase-negative staphylococci (CoNS). The patient completed an 8-week course of antibiotics and wound healing was uneventful. At follow-up visits, she reported persistent imbalance and instability (Fig. 23.1), but no low back pain. CT scans showed solid fusion. Because of the persistent symptoms, she was scheduled for an L4 PSO in 2012. Preoperative neurological examination using the ASIA score indicated an intact neurological status with no sensory or motor deficits. At the preoperative evaluation, the ODI and SRS-$22_{subtotal}$ scores were 64.4 and 2.06, respectively.

23.2.2 Surgical Procedure

The patient underwent implant removal, instrumentation from T12 to ilium, L5/S1 transforaminal lumbar interbody fusion (TLIF), and L4 PSO. Antibiotic prophylaxis with cotrimoxazole

S. Núñez-Pereira
Spine Unit, Hospital Universitario Donostia, Donostia/San Sebastián, Spain

F. Pellisé (✉)
Department of Orthopaedic Surgery, Spine Unit, University Hospital Vall d'Hebron, Barcelona, Spain
e-mail: 24361fpu@comb.cat

B. Meyer, M. Rauschmann (eds.), *Spine Surgery*, https://doi.org/10.1007/978-3-319-98875-7_23

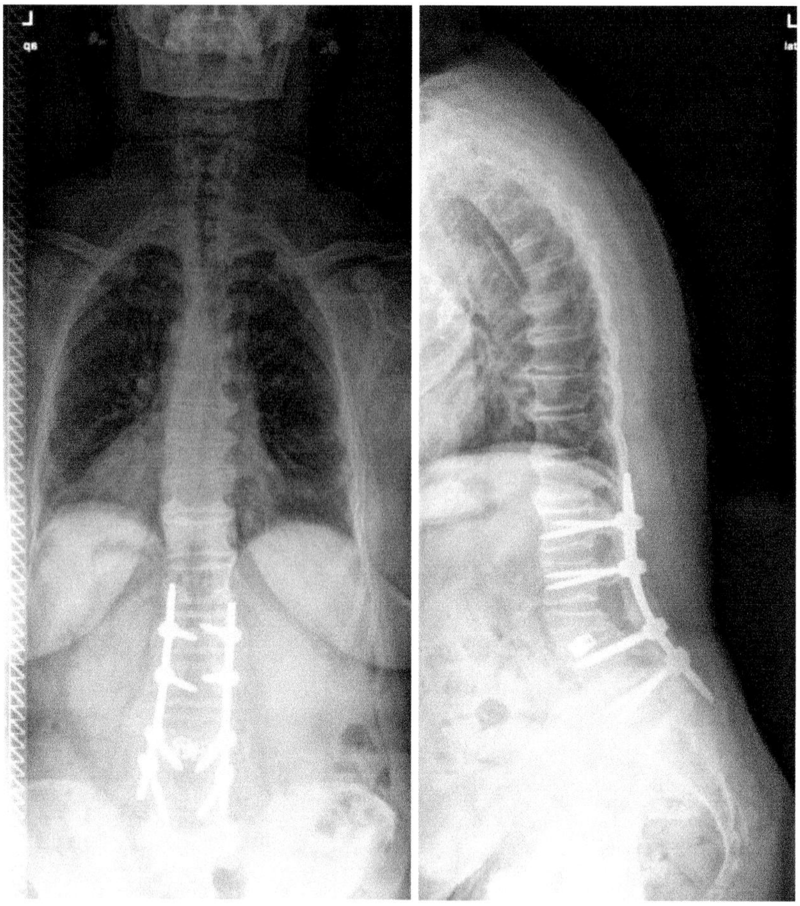

Fig. 23.1 Preoperative radiographs

was administered, as it provided the best coverage for the CoNS causing the previous infection. Surgery lasted 585 min and the estimated blood loss was 2300 mL. Intraoperative neuromonitoring, including motor evoked potentials (MEP) somatosensory evoked potentials (SSEP), and electromyography, was uneventful throughout the procedure. Wound closure included application of topical vancomycin. The patient was extubated in the evening and showed full motor scores in both lower extremities.

23.2.3 Neurological Complication

Three days after surgery, new weakness developed in the bilateral hip flexors and knee extensors (right 1–2/5, left 2–3/5) and the patient was unable to stand. On CT examination, the implants were properly positioned and there was some postoperative hematoma, but no clear signs of dural sac compression (Fig. 23.2). Due to the acute neurological changes and her inability to maintain an upright position, a revision was planned to examine all the affected nerve roots. MRI was not available at such short notice, and it was decided not to delay surgery until MRI could be performed. It is unlikely that the MRI findings would have changed the decision to carry out revision surgery in the situation of acute neurological impairment.

Revision surgery was performed the following day. Cotrimoxazole was used for antibiotic prophylaxis. The L2 to L5 nerve roots were bilaterally exposed and further decompressed along the foramina. The intraoperative findings were quite unremarkable, and the operating surgeon did not detect any stenotic areas. After

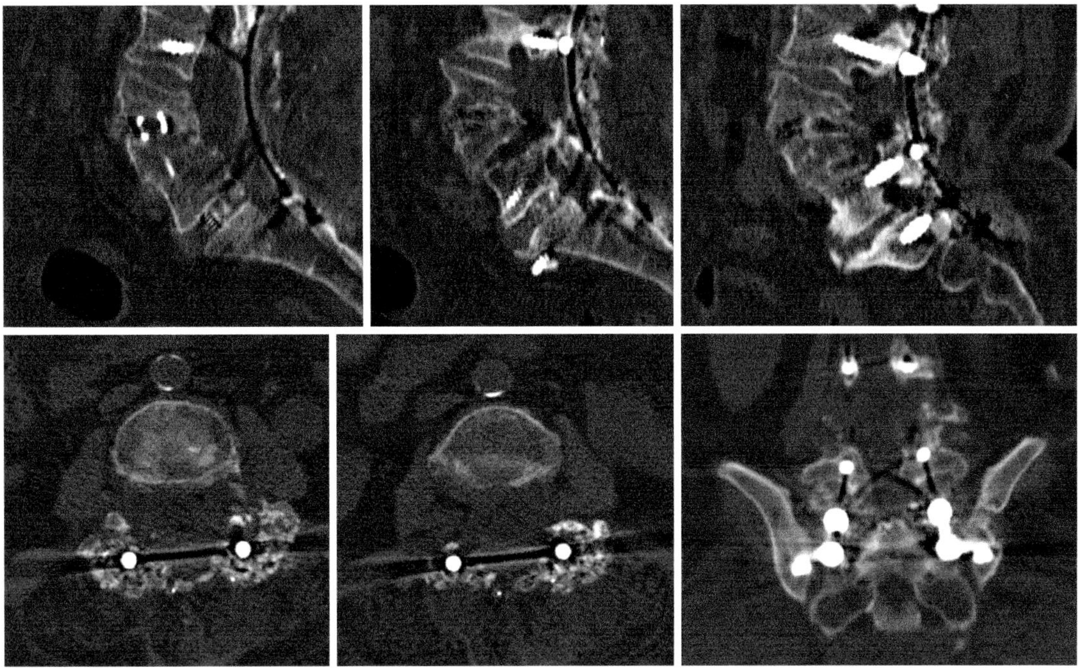

Fig. 23.2 Postoperative CT images

surgery, the motor deficit improved, and 3 days after revision, weakness was 4/5 in both extremities. The motor deficits had fully recovered by 2 years after surgery. The postoperative MRI examination ruled out ischemia and showed no remaining compression (Fig. 23.3).

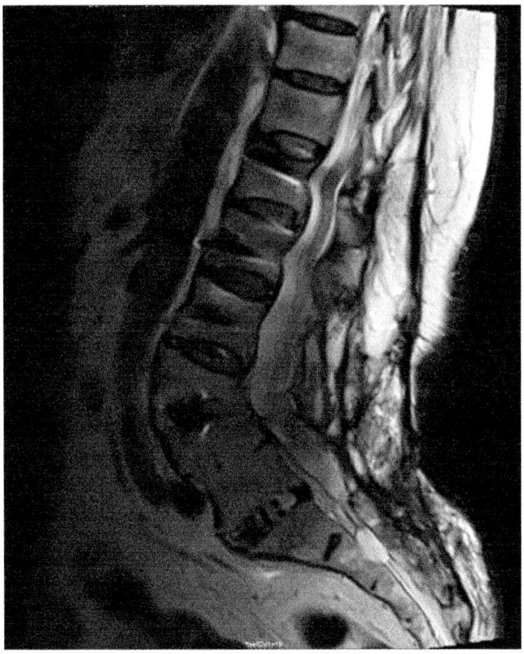

Fig. 23.3 Postoperative MRI showing no signs of ischemia or compression

23.2.4 Infectious Complication

Initial wound healing was good, but on day 14 after revision surgery, the wound showed a purulent secretion with no signs of sepsis. Two days later, surgical debridement and wound lavage were carried out. The implants were left in place. Culture of intraoperative samples yielded *Escherichia coli* resistant to ampicillin and gentamicin. Tailored antibiotic therapy was started. After completing a 2-week course of intravenous antibiotics, the wound had healed successfully and the patient was discharged with an additional 3-month oral antibiotic regimen. Further wound healing was uneventful and follow-up visits showed no other complications. One year after surgery, the patient consulted because of a fistula with secretions on the left side of the wound. CT examination showed solid fusion of the construct. The patient was scheduled for a new surgical debridement and 2-stage implant exchange. The implants on the left side, connected with the fistula, were removed (Fig. 23.4). *E.coli* grew in all samples, and showed the same resistance pattern as the strain from the previous infection. Three weeks after partial removal of the instrumentation and antibiotic treatment, reinstrumentation was performed (Fig. 23.5). The patient received oral ciprofloxacin for 6 months following the debridement procedures. Wound healing was uneventful in both staged surgeries.

23.2.5 Final Follow-Up

Two years after the last revision procedure, the patient has full strength and is able to stand and walk without aids. She still has some dysesthesia in both feet, which makes her feel insecure. The dysesthesia is likely related with her diabetic polyneuropathy. The spine is well balanced, with a GAP score of 2, and the x-rays show good correction and solid fusion (Figs. 23.6 and 23.7). However, the patient's perception of her current status is unfavorable. At 5 years following the

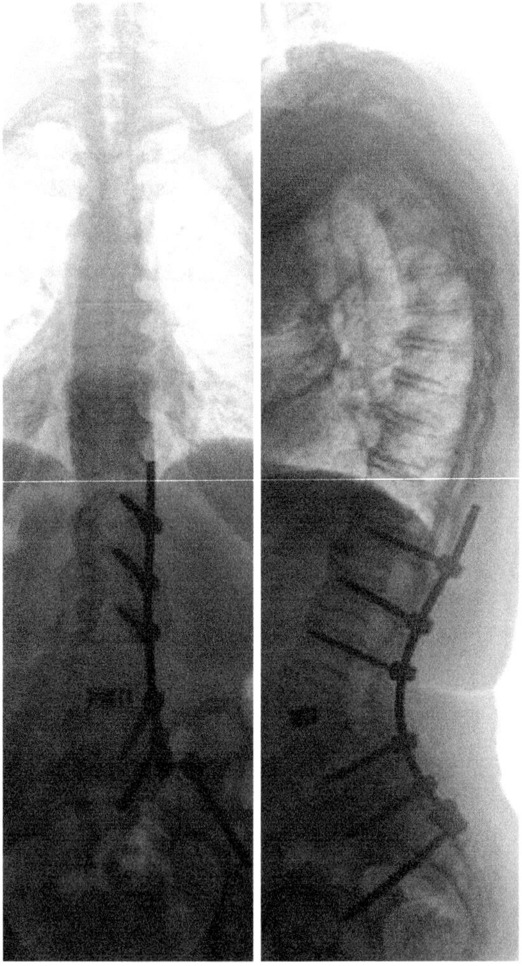

Fig. 23.4 Partial implant removal

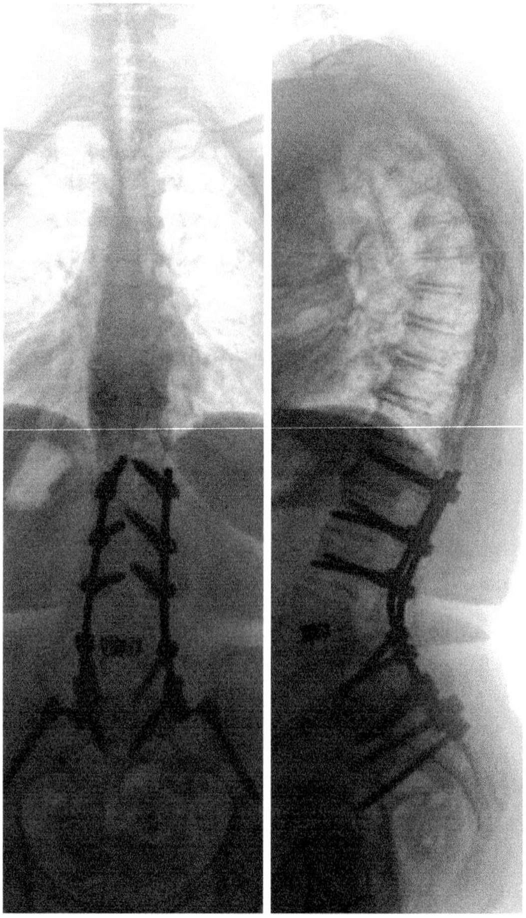

Fig. 23.5 Radiographs following reinstrumentation

original procedure, the ODI and SRS-22$_{subtotal}$ scores were 52.5 (−11.9) and 3.83 (+1.77).

23.3 Discussion

The case presented describes a relatively high-risk patient with diabetes and 4 previous surgeries, who experienced 2 major complications of spinal deformity surgery, both requiring revision surgery. Complex surgeries, as quantified by the Adult Deformity Surgery Complexity Index (ADSCI) are clearly related with a higher risk of developing major complications [1]. Acknowledging this risk is paramount to plan proper perioperative and postoperative care, and to provide adequate counseling for the patient.

As is true for any complex reconstruction procedure of the adult spine, PSO surgery is associated with a degree of neurological risk [2]. A reasonable explanation for the neurological deficit occurring 3 days after the procedure could not be found. Intraoperative neuromonitoring had been uneventful and the patient's neurological examination immediately after surgery was normal. The literature contains few reported cases of delayed postoperative neurological deficit. The largest series includes 92 cases and is the result of a survey carried out in deformity surgeons by the SRS [3]. The cause of the deficit was unknown in 42% of patients, and was attributable to ischemic injury in 38%, cord edema in 4%, and cord compression caused by the instrumentation or a hematoma in 16%. Among the total, 68%

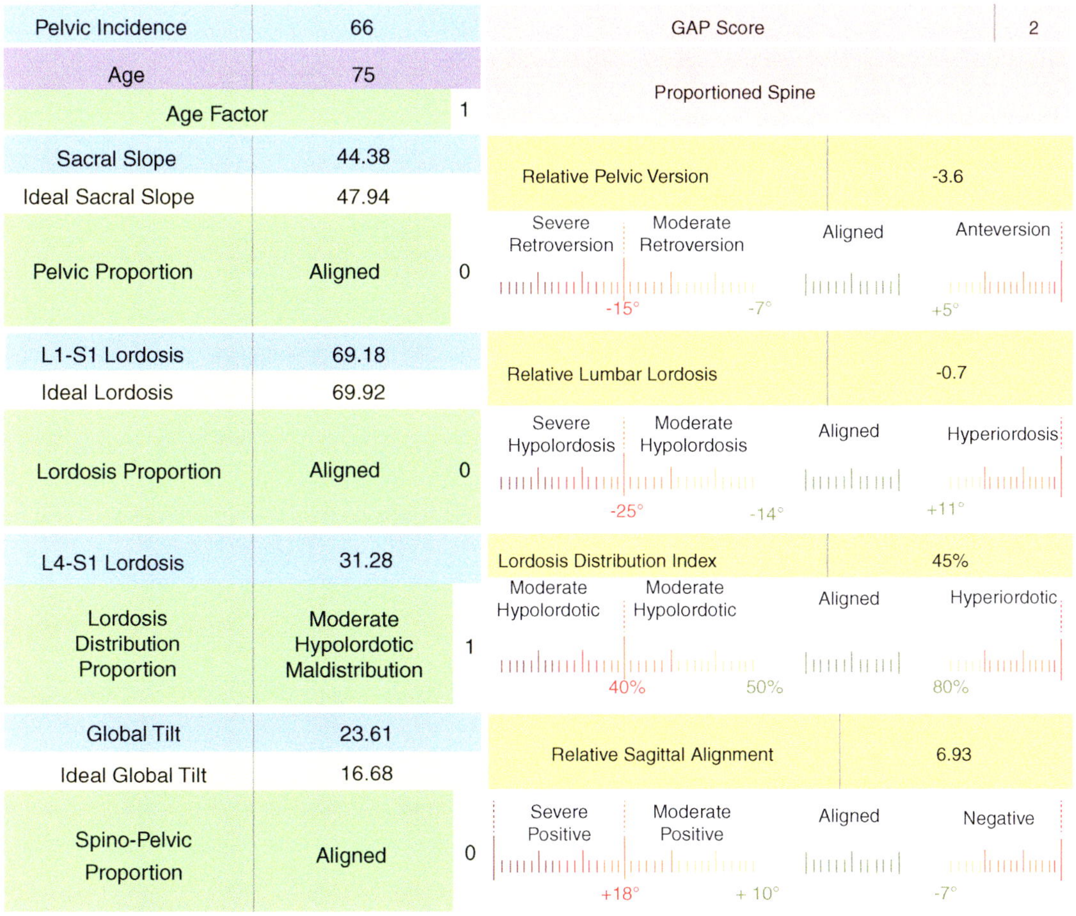

Fig. 23.6 Final alignment according to the GAP Score

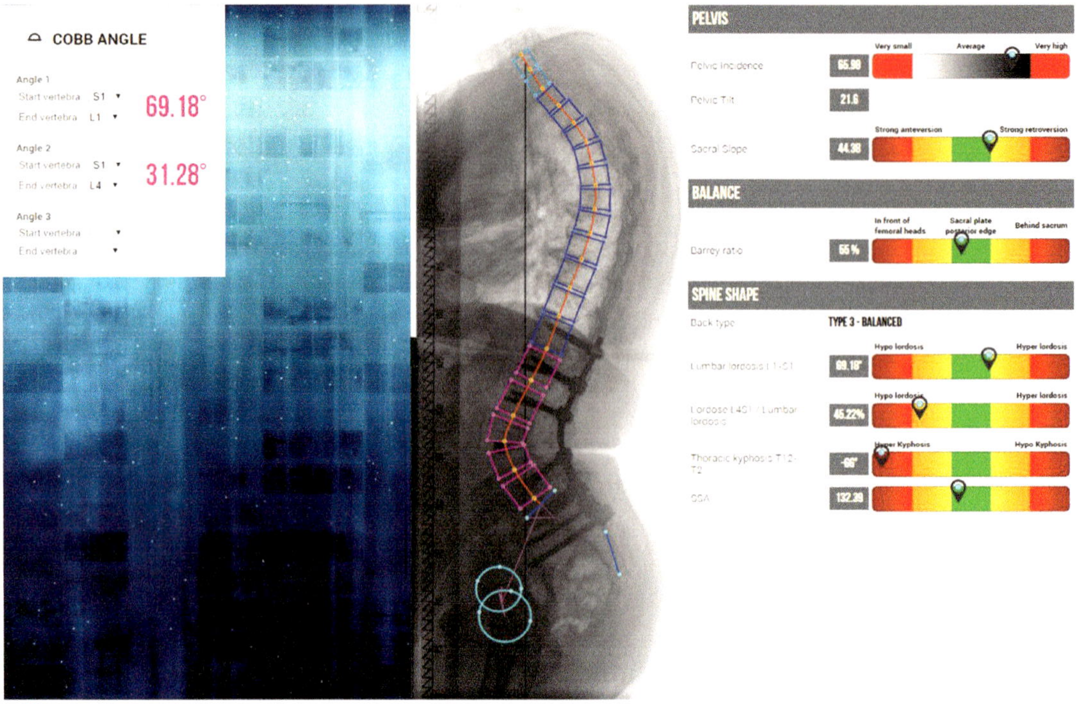

Fig. 23.6 (continued)

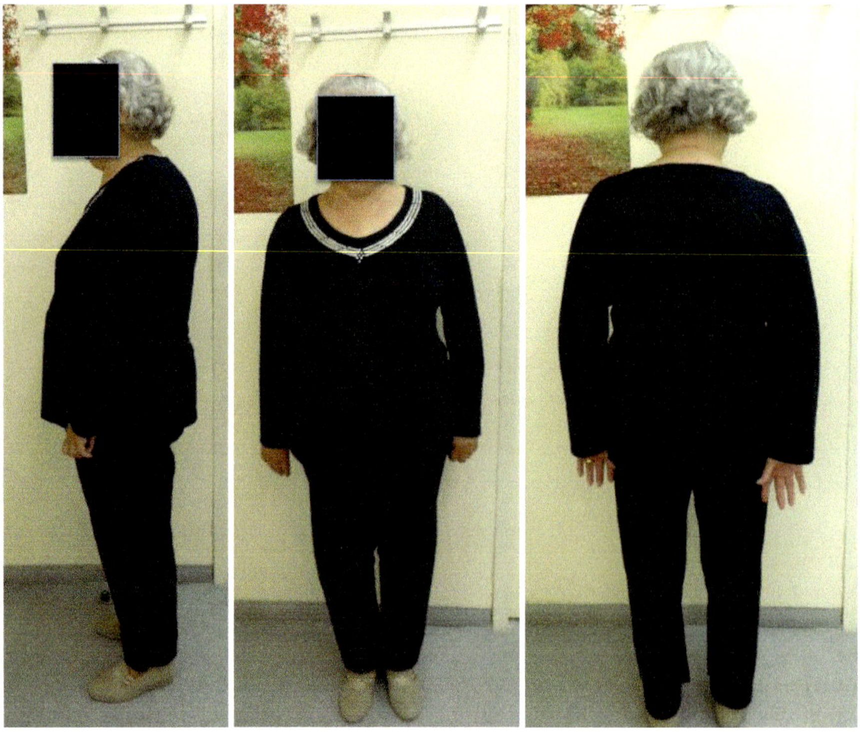

Fig. 23.7 Clinical photographs at final follow-up

underwent revision surgery. The prognosis for recovery was found to be better in patients with cord compression than in those with an ischemic cause (86% vs 51%, $p = 0.048$).

The patient reported here had no signs of compression due to the instrumentation. Some hematoma was seen on CT, but there were no clear signs of dural sac compression. In a previously operated patient, such as the one described, the scarred dural sac may not tolerate compression resulting from osteotomy shortening, and buckling can occur. In a review of 12 PSOs with postoperative neurological deficits [4], some degree of dorsal impingement or subluxation was thought to be the cause in 7 patients, and dural buckling in the remaining 5 patients. Only 3 of the 12 patients had permanent impairment.

Decision-making in this setting is especially challenging as there is pressure "to do something", but there are no clear guidelines or rules to rely on. Due to the considerable disability implied by this type of complication, revision surgery was carried out the following day to investigate residual dural compression or buckling. The intraoperative findings were rather unremarkable, and therefore, all the nerve roots were further decompressed. Dexamethasone was administered for 24 h. Shortly after revision, the neurological symptoms improved, which suggested that further decompression had provided some relief to the neural structures. We cannot know whether the patient might have improved without revision surgery. However, the evidence that compression-related neurological deficits have a better prognosis for recovery supports the idea that the area should be inspected to ensure that all neural structures are free.

Regarding the surgical site infection, the patient had several factors placing her at a high risk for this complication: 4 previous surgeries, a previous infection at the same site, diabetes mellitus, and a long, complex procedure. Dexamethasone administration for 24 h after revision surgery is an additional risk factor for infection. Prophylactic measures included tailored antibiotic prophylaxis and further standard of care measures, such us preoperative skin lavage with chlorhexidine. At the time of revision surgery, an indwelling catheter remained in place from the first procedure. This is a plausible port of entry for gram-negative bacteria (GNB) [5], and the most likely source of infection in our patient. To provide broader coverage against GNB, a combination of gentamycin with standard prophylaxis is an option. However, the strains causing our patient's infection were gentamycin resistant; hence, it is likely that the addition of gentamycin to the prophylactic regimen would not have changed the final outcome in this particular case.

Infection relapse has been described in around one quarter of patients with spinal surgical site infections [6]. The risk factors for treatment failure are uncertain. Some authors have suggested that long-term antibiotic suppression therapy may be helpful to avoid relapses [7], but the available evidence does not suffice to support this measure in all patients. Furthermore, there are no available guidelines on the ideal duration of antibiotic treatment in this clinical situation. In general, antibiotics are given for 3 months, as was done in the present case. Implant removal is usually the best treatment option for infection relapses several months later, as it is the only way to remove the biofilm of microorganisms adhering to the implants. Regarding reinstrumentation, a higher loss of correction rate has been described in adolescent idiopathic scoliosis patients undergoing implant removal without reinstrumentation for late infection [8], but there are no data regarding this issue in adult spinal deformity. Nonetheless, higher rates of implant failure and rod breakage are associated with 3-column osteotomies [9]; hence, it seems reasonable to enhance support with reinstrumentation to avoid further failures. As the infection was confined to only one side, half the implants could remain in situ, providing some stability at the beginning. Regarding the antibiotic treatment to use, there are no standards for cases of relapse. After consultation with the hospital Infectious Diseases Department, directed antibiotic treatment was given for 6 months, and there were no further relapses after 5 years of follow-up.

Pearls

- Delayed onset neurological deficits after PSO might be related to compression and dural buckling or ischemia
- Revision surgery is justified to ensure nerve root decompression and optimise final neurological outcome
- Implant exchange should be considered in cases with recurrent SSI not solved with debridement, antibiotics and implant retention

Editorial Comment

Surgical site infection is a increasing problem in complex spine surgery. The philosophy of early agressive debridement is always recommended. No "wait and see strategy" should be performed. Vacuum assisted closiure, would be an alternative of tretament with promising results concerning woundhealing.

References

1. Pellisé F, Vila-Casademunt A, Núñez-Pereira S, Domingo-Sàbat M, Bagó J, Vidal X, et al. The adult deformity surgery complexity index (ADSCI): a valid tool to quantify the complexity of posterior adult spinal deformity surgery and predict postoperative complications. Spine J. 2018;18(2):216–25.
2. Kelly MP, Lenke LG, Shaffrey CI, Ames CP, Carreon LY, Lafage V, et al. Evaluation of complications and neurological deficits with three-column spine reconstructions for complex spinal deformity: a retrospective scoli-risk-1 study. Neurosurg Focus. 2014;36(5):E17.
3. Auerbach JD, Kean K, Milby AH, Paonessa KJ, Dormans JP, Newton PO, et al. Delayed postoperative neurologic deficits in spinal deformity surgery. Spine (Phila Pa 1976). 2016;41(3):E131–8.
4. Buchowski JM, Bridwell KH, Lenke LG, Kuhns CA, Lehman RA, Kim YJ, et al. Neurologic complications of lumbar pedicle subtraction osteotomy: a 10-year assessment. Spine (Phila Pa 1976). 2007;32(20):2245–52.
5. Núñez-Pereira S, Pellisé F, Rodríguez-Pardo D, Pigrau C, Sánchez JM, Bagó J, et al. Individualized antibiotic prophylaxis reduces surgical site infections by gram-negative bacteria in instrumented spinal surgery. Eur Spine J. 2011;20(Suppl 3):397–402.
6. Maruo K, Berven SH. Outcome and treatment of postoperative spine surgical site infections: predictors of treatment success and failure. J Orthop Sci. 2014;19(3):398–404.
7. Kowalski TJ, Berbari EF, Huddleston PM, Steckelberg JM, Mandrekar JN, Osmon DR. The management and outcome of spinal implant infections: contemporary retrospective cohort study. Clin Infect Dis. 2007;44(7):913–20.
8. Muschik M, Lück W, Schlenzka D. Implant removal for late-developing infection after instrumented posterior spinal fusion for scoliosis: Reinstrumentation reduces loss of correction. A retrospective analysis of 45 cases. Eur Spine J. 2004;13(7):645–51.
9. Smith JS, Shaffrey CI, Klineberg E, Lafage V, Schwab F, Lafage R, et al. Complication rates associated with 3-column osteotomy in 82 adult spinal deformity patients: retrospective review of a prospectively collected multicenter consecutive series with 2-year follow-up. J Neurosurg Spine. 2017;27(4):444–57.

Operative Treatment of High-Grade Spondylolisthesis

24

Dezsö Jeszenszky and Markus Loibl

24.1 Introduction

This chapter will outline the special clinical and radiological characteristics of spondylolisthesis. The pathogenesis, classification, and indication for surgery will be discussed, together with the surgical strategies and techniques used in its treatment. The aim of the presented case is to highlight the surgical options for addressing high-grade spondylolisthesis in the authors' experience, and to examine the existing evidence with respect to:

- choice of approach
- extent of instrumentation
- extent of reduction
- interbody fusion

At the end of the chapter, the reader should be aware of the potential pitfalls and be able to formulate a conclusive approach when planning and performing surgery for the treatment of high-grade spondylolisthesis.

D. Jeszenszky (✉) · M. Loibl
Department of Spine Surgery, Schulthess Klinik, Zürich, Switzerland
e-mail: dezsoej.jeszenszky@kws.ch; markus.loibl@kws.ch

24.2 Pathogenesis, Classification and Diagnosis of Spondylolisthesis

Spondylolisthesis is a condition in which one vertebra translates anteriorly in relation to the adjacent caudal vertebra. Typically, the clinical manifestation of spondylolisthesis is back pain due to segmental degeneration and instability, and radicular pain due to neural compression. Gravity and longitudinal muscle contraction around the lordotic lumbar spine apply forces to the lower lumbar vertebrae pushing them anteriorly and inferiorly. These forces are counteracted by the facet joints, posterior arches, pedicles, and discs. In spondylolisthesis, one or more of these structures fails, which results in the lower lumbar vertebrae translating and rotating forwards relative to the sacrum or caudal vertebra [1].

Historically, two classification systems have been important in describing the variability of presentation of spondylolisthesis. The **Wiltse classification** divides spondylolisthesis into five categories: dysplastic, isthmic, degenerative, traumatic, and pathologic (Table 24.1) [2]. Dysplastic spondylolisthesis is most often observed at the L5-S1 level, typically with deficient development of the bony hook (inferior facet of L5) and the catch (superior facet of S1). Isthmic spondylolisthesis is characterized by a defect of the pars interarticularis between the joints. Secondary changes of the shape of the L5

B. Meyer, M. Rauschmann (eds.), *Spine Surgery*, https://doi.org/10.1007/978-3-319-98875-7_24

Table 24.1 Wiltse classification of spondylolisthesis

I. Dysplastic		Congenital
II. Isthmic		Defect in the pars interarticularis
	IIA	Spondylolytic – stress fracture of pars region
	IIB	Pars elongation
	IIC	Acute pars traumatic fracture
III. Degenerative		Due to a long standing intersegmental instability
IV. Post-traumatic		Acute fracture of the posterior elements beside the pars region
V. Pathologic		Destruction of the posterior elements from generalized or localized bone pathology

Table 24.2 Marchetti and Bartolozzi classification of spondylolisthesis

1982	1994
Developmental	
Due to lysis	High dysplastic
Due to elongation	With lysis
Traumatic	With elongation
Acute fracture	Low dysplastic
Stress fracture	With lysis
	With elongation
Acquired	
Iatrogenic	Traumatic
Pathologic	Acute fracture
Degenerative	Stress fracture
	Post-surgery
	Direct surgery
	Indirect surgery
	Pathologic
	Local pathology
	Systemic pathology
	Degenerative
	Primary
	Secondary

vertebra or sacral dome can be present as stress-related changes. In degenerative spondylolisthesis, in contrast, the most commonly affected level is L4-5, and the bony hook and pars interarticularis are intact. For this reason, anterior translation of more than 1 cm is rarely observed. However, it is commonly associated with spinal stenosis.

Marchetti and Bartolozzi further classified spondylolisthesis into developmental and acquired, based on the presumed etiology (Table 24.2) [3]. With the refinement of their classification in 1994 they combined the dysplastic and isthmic groups, and then divided them on the basis of their behavior. The high versus low dysplasia categories are useful for predicting progression (Figs. 24.1 and 24.2).

The **Meyerding scale** provides a common metric for quantifying the extent of anterior translation, where the inferior vertebral body is divided into four equal sections to allow five possible grades (I to V). The anterior translation is graded on the basis of the percentage of the inferior vertebral body that is uncovered as a result of the anterior translation [4]. More than 50% uncovered S1 endplate equals a grade III. In a grade V spondylolisthesis (spondyloptosis), the L5 vertebral body completely translates anteriorly and falls off the sacrum. Grades III, IV and V slips are considered as high-grade spondylolisthesis. Spondyloptosis occurs in a distinct minority of patients with spondylolisthesis, representing just 1% of all cases. Even experienced spine surgeons encounter a limited number of these patients.

The diagnosis of spondylolisthesis is based on radiologic evaluation of the lumbar spine with anteroposterior and lateral radiographs, as well as dynamic radiographs in flexion and extension. Computed tomography [5] can be helpful to assess the bony lumbosacral junction and other lesions of the posterior elements. Magnetic resonance imaging (MRI) is highly sensitive in the detection of degenerative changes such as disc degeneration or stenosis at the level of the spondylolisthesis.

24.3 Conservative Treatment and Indications for Surgery in High-Grade Spondylolisthesis

The presented classifications help the surgeon to decide which patients are most likely to benefit from surgery. It is reasonable to attempt

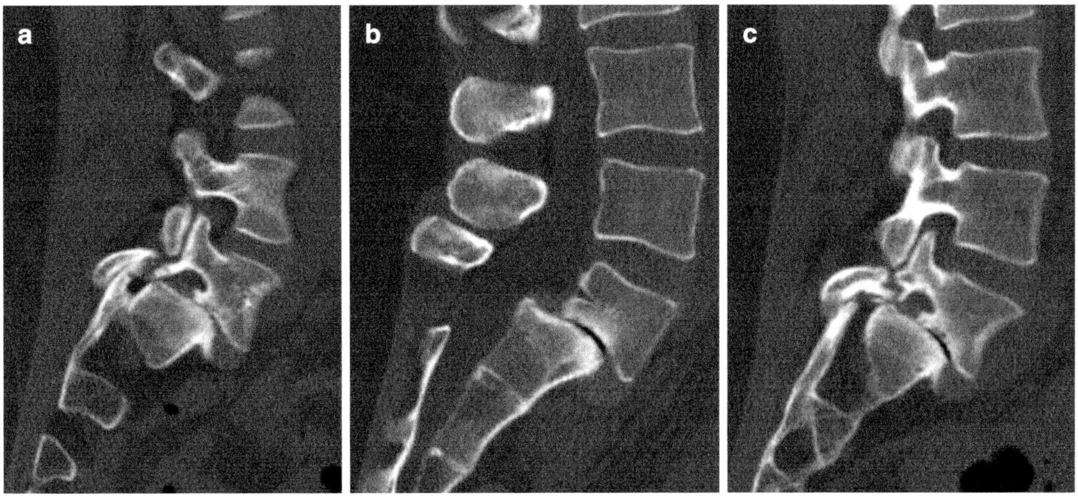

Fig. 24.1 Sagittal CT reconstructions of the lumbar spine on the right (**a**), midline (**b**) and left (**c**) of a patient with low dysplastic spondylolisthesis. Note maintained shape of sacrum and low slip angle. Patient aged 40 years

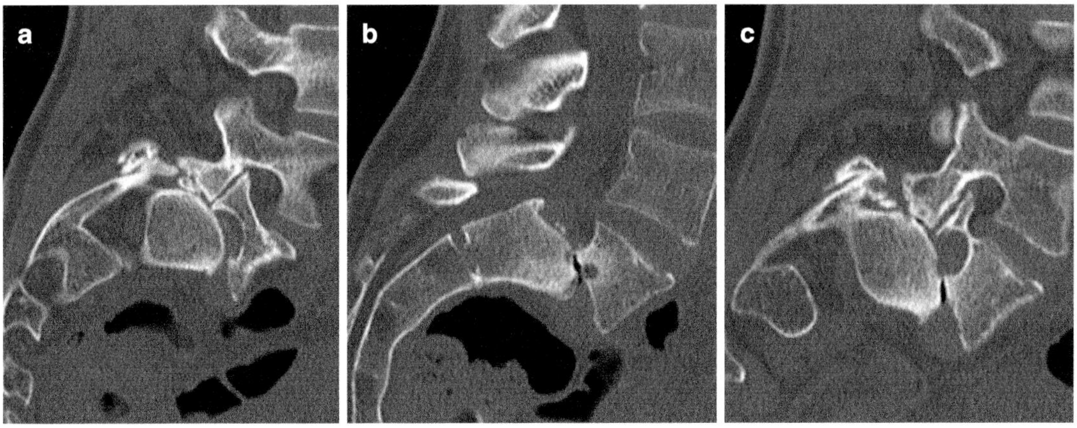

Fig. 24.2 Sagittal CT reconstructions of the lumbar spine on the right (**a**), midline (**b**) and left (**c**) of a patient with high dysplastic spondylolisthesis. Note rounding of sacrum despite degenerative changes of the disc and higher slip angle. Patient aged 28 years

conservative management in asymptomatic adolescents and adults with low and high dysplastic spondylolisthesis [4]. Conservative management typically comprises a course of physical therapy, focusing on core muscle strengthening, and adjuvant medical treatment, consisting of anti-inflammatory drugs and muscle relaxants. Epidural injections (anaesthetic and steroids), as well as injections into and around the pars articularis may alleviate the pain [6].

Radiographic progression during conservative management is rare (about 3%); however, especially before the adolescent growth spurt, children should be followed regularly to exclude slip progression [7].

Surgery can be considered in adolescents with high dysplastic spondylolisthesis and in symptomatic patients with low dysplastic spondylolisthesis. Surgery is usually required for patients with high-grade spondylolisthesis and continued low back pain and/or radicular pain despite conservative treatment, or in the case of neurologic deficit or postural or gait changes. Moreover, surgical treatment is recommended for asymptomatic children with anterior translation of more than 50% and for asymptomatic mature adolescents with anterior translation of more than 75%, or in general if progression is noted [4].

24.4 Case Description High-Grade Spondylolisthesis

A 20 year-old female patient was referred due to increasing back pain over several years. She reported low back pain after 15 min of standing or walking. Leg pain was denied. Non-steroidal anti-inflammatory drugs and physical therapy were initially helpful but no longer provided relief from the pain. After radiologic evaluation of the lumbar spine, anteroposterior and lateral radiographs revealed a Grade V lumbosacral spondylolisthesis with spina bifida occulta (Fig. 24.3). CT and MRI scans demonstrate typical characteristics of spondyloptosis (Figs. 24.4 and 24.5).

The patient was operated in our institution via a posterior approach with the aim of anatomic reduction and instrumented fusion from L5 to S1. Intraoperatively, the neural elements were decompressed widely. The L4 vertebra was incorporated temporarily for improved construct strength during reduction (Fig. 24.6).

The surgery went well under continuous neurophysiologic monitoring, including somatosensory and transcranial electrical stimulation, and electromyography. Plain anteroposterior and lateral lum-

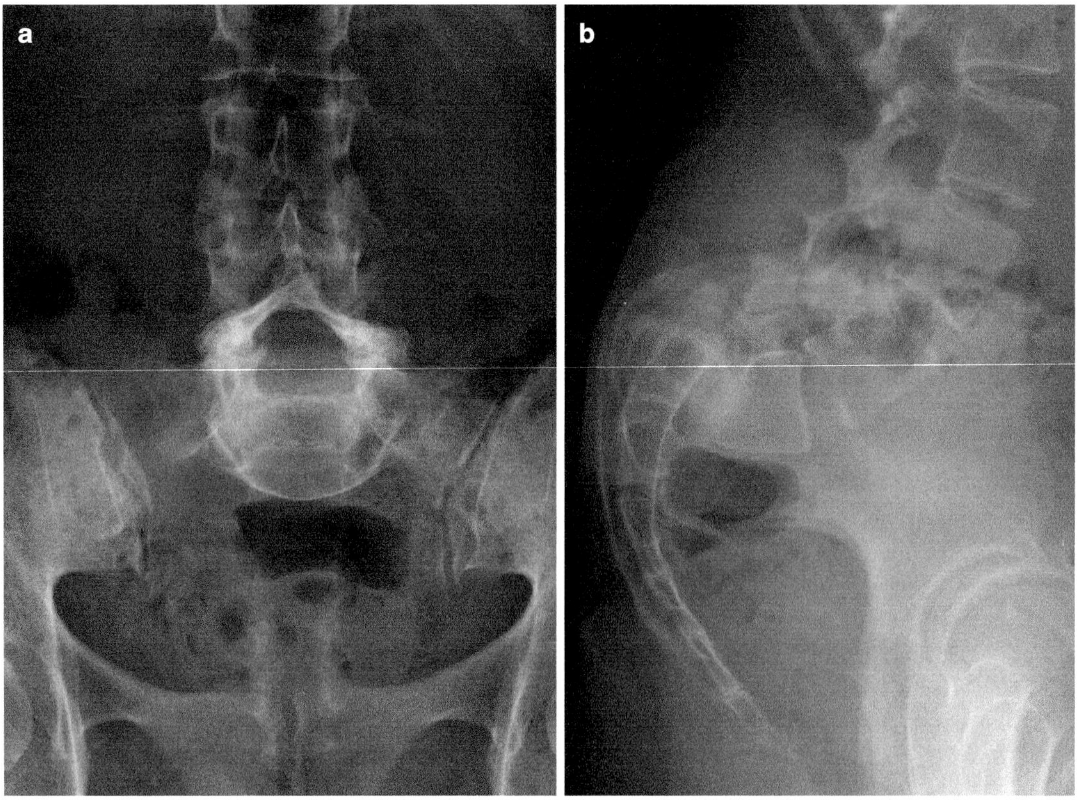

Fig. 24.3 Radiographs of the lumbar spine on outpatient visit. The radiographs demonstrate a Grade V lumbosacral spondylolisthesis with extreme lumbosacral kyphosis and spina bifida occulta. Anteroposterior (**a**) and lateral (**b**) radiographs

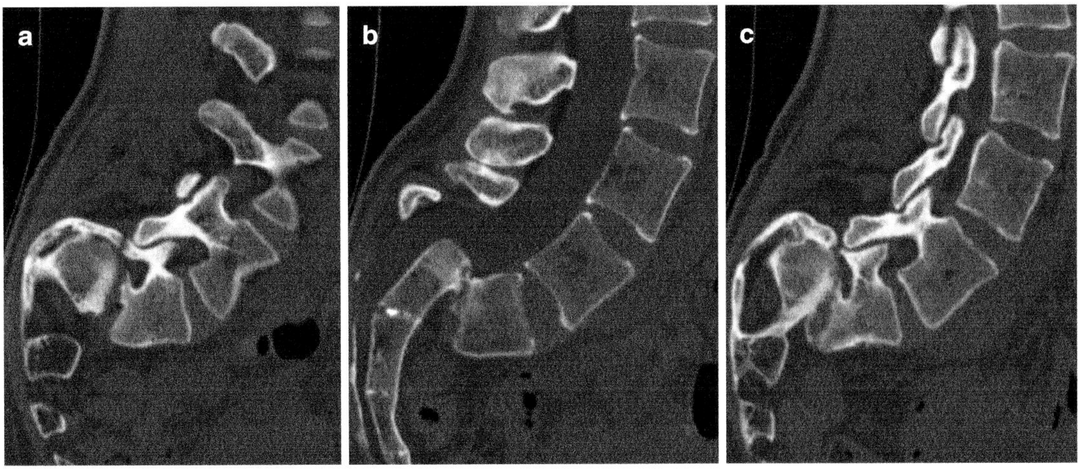

Fig. 24.4 Preoperative CT scan. The CT scan demonstrates dysplasia of the posterior elements of L5, including a bilateral pars interarticularis defect and trapezoidal shape of the L5 vertebral body. Sagittal CT reconstructions on the right (**a**), midline (**b**) and left (**c**)

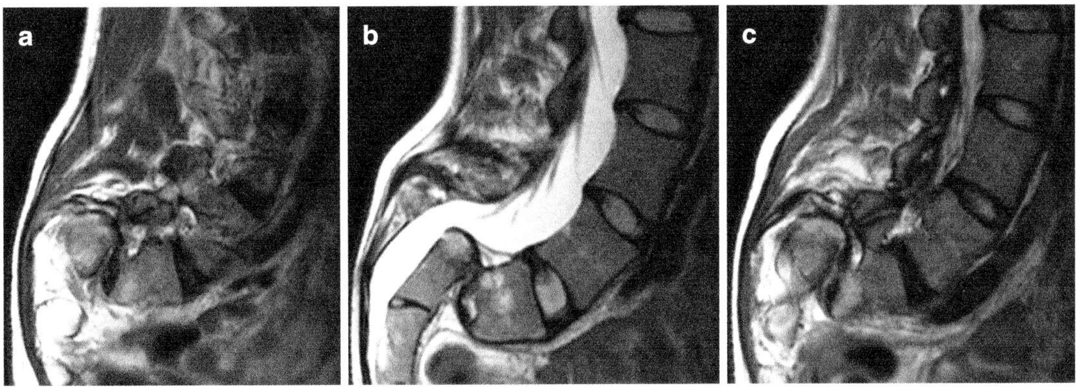

Fig. 24.5 Preoperative MRI scan. The MRI scan confirms severe bilateral narrowing of the L5 and S1 neural foramina. Sagittal MRI reconstructions on the right (**a**), midline (**b**) and left (**c**)

bar radiographs obtained postoperatively revealed successful slip reduction and partial kyphosis correction (Figs. 24.7 and 24.8). Sagittal CT reconstructions demonstrated solid lumbosacral fusion at 5 years' follow-up (Fig. 24.9).

24.5 Discussion of the Case

24.5.1 Indication

The presented patient suffered from back pain only, with no leg pain or neurologic deficit. The clinical indications for surgical treatment of high-grade spondylolisthesis include low back pain and/or radicular pain resistant to conservative treatment, progression of the lumbosacral deformity, and the presence of neurologic deficit [8]. In this case of spondyloptosis, with back pain after 15 min of standing, the threshold for surgical treatment was very low, despite neurologic complication rates associated with slip reduction of up to 45% [9]. The primary goal of surgery is to relieve the pain and the neurologic symptoms (if present).

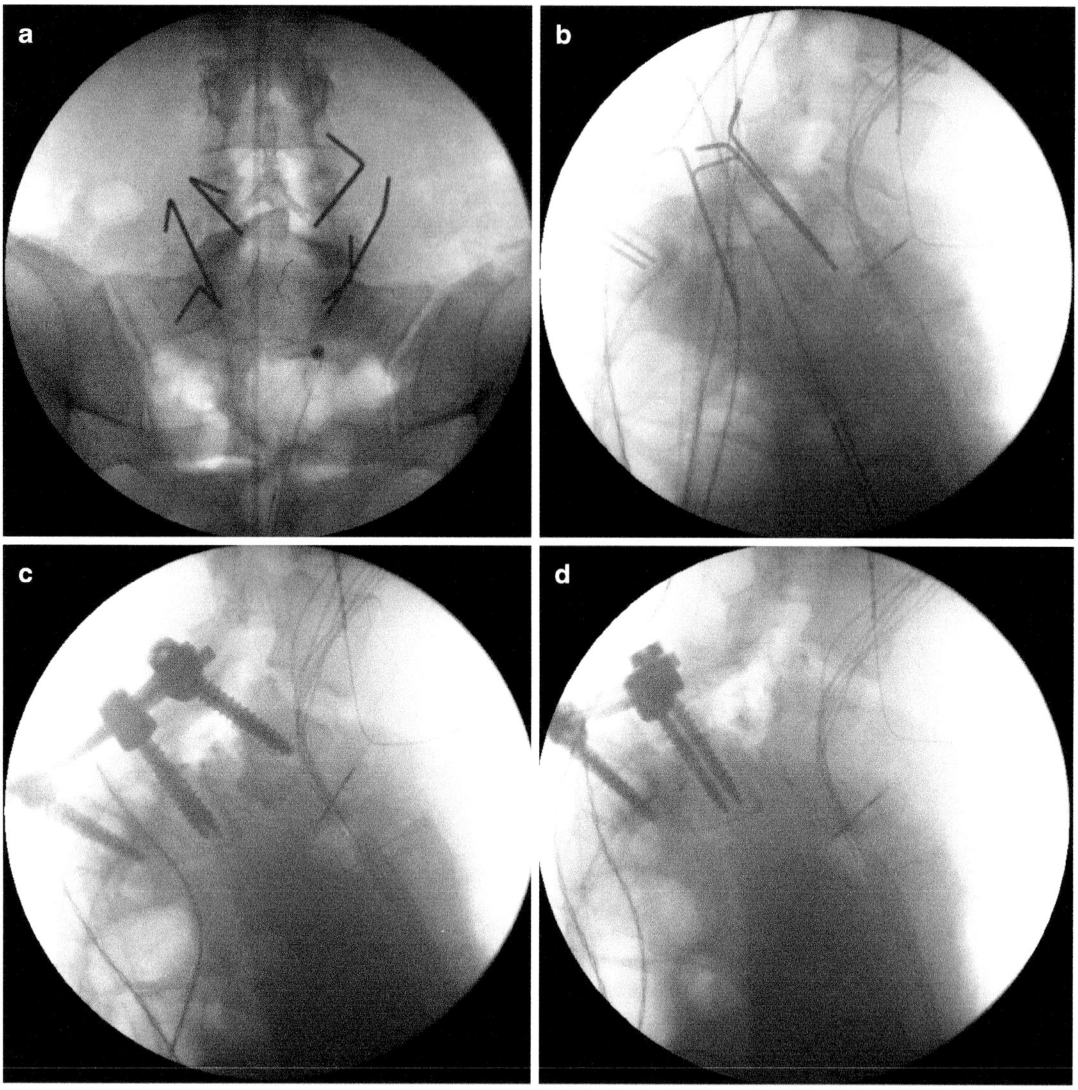

Fig. 24.6 Intraoperative Fluoroscopy. Intraoperatively the L4 vertebra was incorporated temporarily for improved construct strength during reduction. Anteroposterior (**a**) and lateral (**b**) fluoroscopy after K-wire placement, and lateral fluoroscopy after pedicle screw fixation and reduction with incorporation of L4 (**c**) and segment liberation L4/5 (**d**)

24.5.2 Choice of Approach

There are several anterior and posterior (or combined) surgical treatment strategies (dorsal, dorsoventral, dorsal-ventro-dorsal) [8, 10] that aim to provide stable instrumentation, restoration of sagittal balance, reduction of the spondylolisthesis, and solid lumbosacral fusion [8]. In our experience, anterior release and reduction can be achieved from posterior in a safe manner with direct vision and control of the neural structures at risk. The reduction is maintained by dorsal instrumentation with the use of pedicle screws inserted in L5 and S1. After reduction, ventral support is required to allow dorsal compression forces. The authors prefer titanium cages, or bone-on-bone anterior support and fusion, for definitive support of the anterior column. While some colleagues advocate posterior instrumentation combined with ventral support

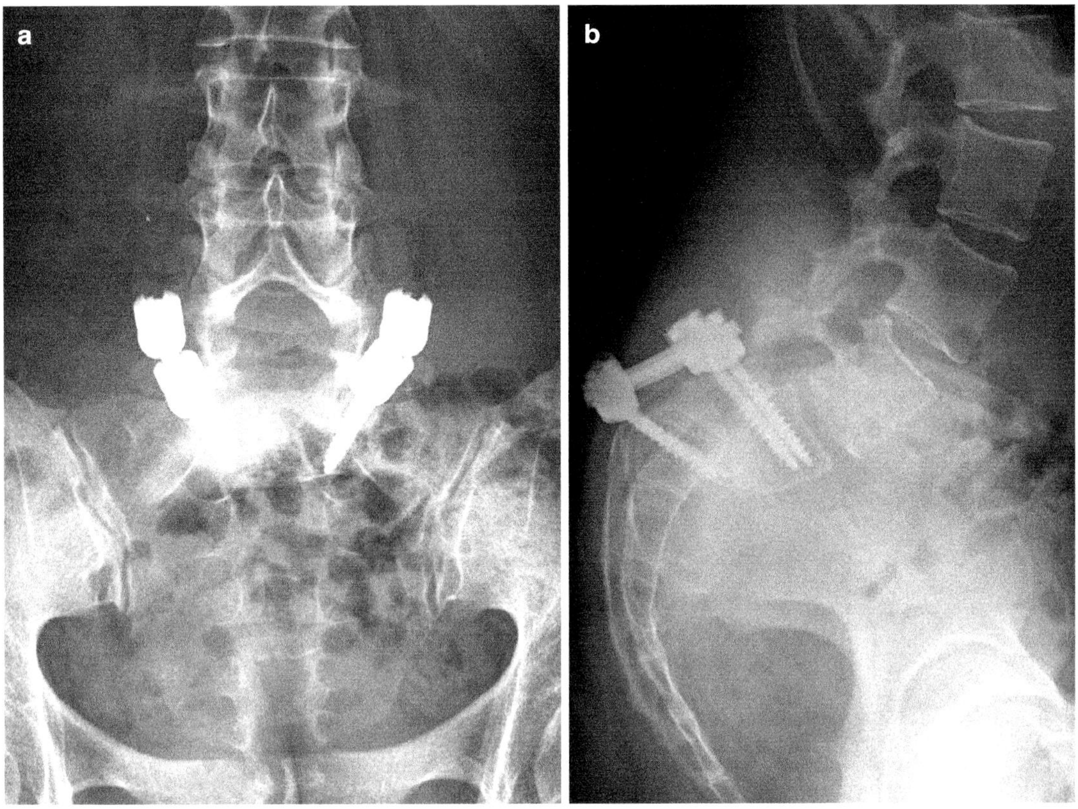

Fig. 24.7 Postoperative radiographs of the lumbar spine. The radiographs demonstrate pedicle screw fixation L5 and S1 with slip reduction and partial kyphosis correction. Anteroposterior (**a**) and lateral radiograph (**b**)

in the form of anterior lumbar interbody fusion (ALIF), the majority of experienced spine surgeons will use a posterior approach for instrumentation, release, reduction, and interbody fusion, since the plane of the former L5-S1 intervertebral disc space in high-grade spondylolisthesis is difficult to access from anterior due to segmental kyphosis. Moreover anterior approach-related complications can be avoided by posterior treatment strategies [8, 9, 11, 12]. Anterior fusion may, however, be useful for revision cases or pseudarthrosis [5]. Based on the existing evidence, lumbosacral interbody fusion is left to the individual surgeon's preference with posterior or transforaminal access (PLIF or TLIF) [13] or transsacral strut grafting and screw fixation [10].

24.5.3 Extent of Instrumentation

Instrumentation from L4 to S1 is a debatable issue as it sacrifices the L4/5 disc. To date, there are no guidelines on how to improve construct strength during reduction and in the postoperative phase. The authors and other colleagues believe that temporary incorporation of L4 has advantages for the reduction manoeuvre [8, 11], since screw purchase in severely dysplastic L5 pedicles can be weak and unreliable. Moreover, the shear stress on L5 screws is considerable during reduction, risking a loss of reduction or implant loosening. For this reason, several authors even propose a permanent supplementary L4 anchorage to reduce stress on the individual pedicle screw and to enable the instrumentation

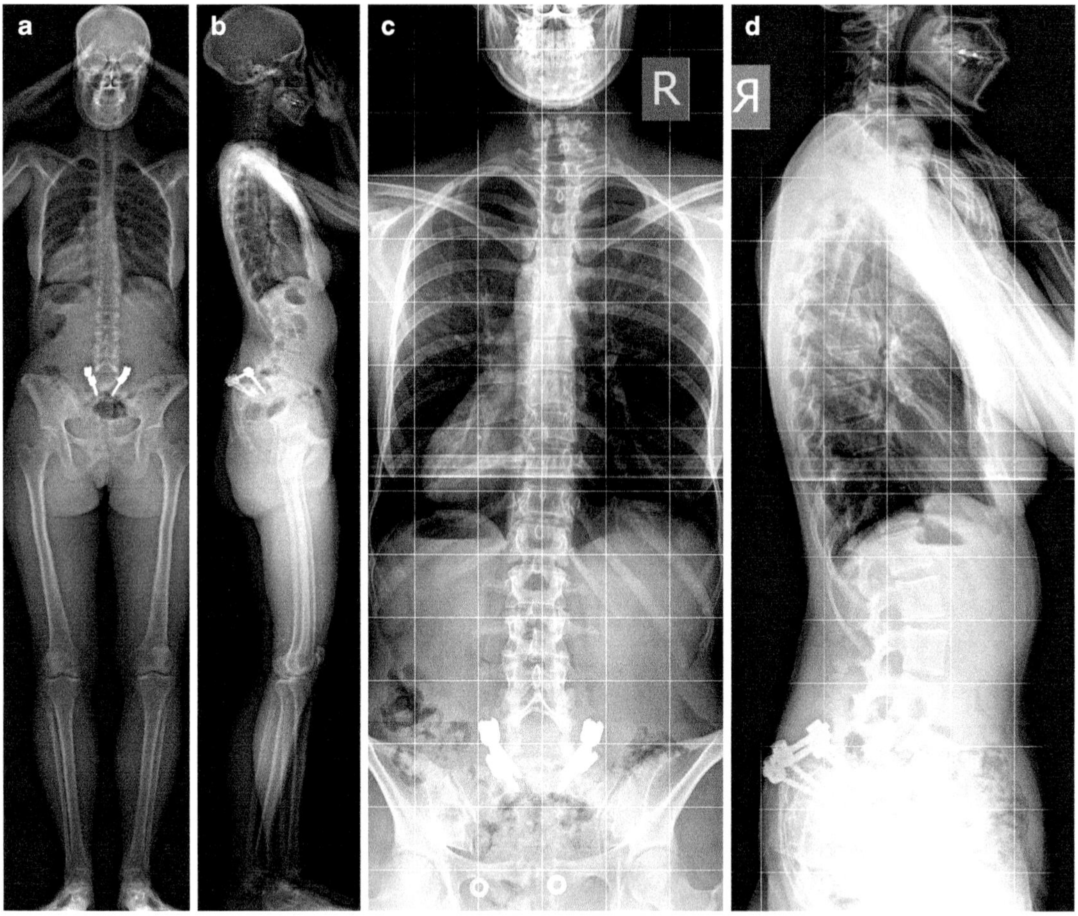

Fig. 24.8 Postoperative radiographs of the whole body and spine after 5 years. The radiographs demonstrate persistent improved sagittal alignment without adjacent segment pathology. Anteroposterior (**a**, **c**) and lateral radiograph (**b**, **d**) of the whole body (**a**, **b**) and spine (**c**, **d**)

to end on a more horizontal vertebra [12, 14]. Segment liberation L4/5 can be considered after reduction, as in the presented case.

24.5.4 Extent of Reduction

The correction of the underlying lumbosacral deformity has been attracting increasing attention in the literature [13]. In high-grade spondylolisthesis, there is conflicting evidence regarding the relative merits of in situ fusion versus instrumented fusion with reduction and restoration of spino-pelvic balance. Although some authors consider the results of in situ fusion to be satisfactory, most spine surgeons maintain that it is associated with an unacceptable rate of pseudarthrosis, slip progression, and other shortcomings, especially when treating older adolescents and adults.

It is generally accepted that the goal of reduction is to improve the sagittal alignment and not necessarily to correct the anterior translation completely. However, to date, there is no consensus on the necessity to reduce the lumbosacral deformity and to perform a neural decompression.

Hresko et al. reported two distinct groups of patients with either "balanced" or "unbalanced" pelvis in high-grade spondylolisthesis [15]. Patients with an "unbalanced" pelvis include those who stand with a retroverted pelvis and a vertical

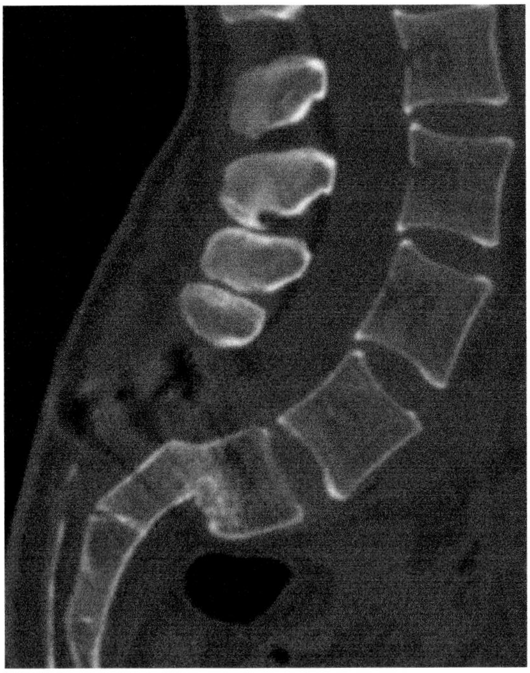

Fig. 24.9 Sagittal midline CT reconstruction. Postoperative CT scan on outpatient visit after 5 years. The CT scan demonstrates complete slip reduction and solid lumbosacral fusion with notable discrepancy of the L5 and S1 area

sacrum, characterized by a high pelvic tilt (PT) and a low sacral slope. Martiniani et al. supported the hypothesis that complete reduction of the L5/S1 slippage with restoration of segmental lordosis and correction of the sacral position (reduction of the PT towards normal values) should be carried out in patients with an "unbalanced" pelvis [13]. Based on the authors´ experience and that of other colleagues, anatomic reduction of the local lumbosacral translation and correction of the overall sagittal profile should be aimed for in all patients to reduce shear forces at the lumbosacral junction to a physiological level [8].

The reduction of a severe L5 slip is usually associated with elongation of the lumbosacral junction and the corresponding neural structures, which can lead to neurological complications in up to 45% of patients [9]. The risk of neurologic injury is directly related to the extent of reduction sought. For this reason, shortening of the lumbosacral junction by sacral dome resection has been proposed as a key component to reduce neurological complications such as L5 radiculopathy [14]. A few spine surgeons have extended the concept of spine shortening to the resection of a significant part of the — or even the entire — fifth vertebra (so-called Gaines procedure) to facilitate reduction and reduce stretch radiculopathy [16, 17]. Despite this, transient L5 radiculopathy after reduction is frequent. Schär et al. demonstrated that with the use of intraoperative neuromonitoring (IONM) the risk of irreversible L5 radiculopathy is minimal [9]. In the case of IONM signal changes that recover intraoperatively, full clinical recovery can be expected within 3 months.

In cases such as the one presented here, both the literature and our own experience advocate complete reduction of the L5/S1 anterior translation with correction of segmental kyphosis with the shortest fusion possible under continuous IONM to prevent neurological complications.

24.5.5 Interbody Fusion

After reduction of high-grade spondylolisthesis, reconstruction of the ventral column and lumbosacral interbody fusion in combination with posterolateral fusion are essential to ensure long-term lumbosacral junction stability. Adequate bony surfaces between the bodies of L5 and S1 are required for anterior column fusion. Ventral support allows for a strong dorsal compression force to reduce shear forces, and to avoid narrowing of the neuroforamen. The authors prefer titanium cages in combination with autologous bone graft, with faster healing of cancellous chips compared with corticocancellous bone blocks. Ventral support and interbody fusion can be accomplished by anterior or posterior approaches.

In the presented case, due to the discrepancy of the L5 and S1 vertebral body (Fig. 24.9), lumbar interbody fusion was performed without a cage.

24.5.6 Accordance with the Literature Guidelines

Based on current evidence, guidelines for the treatment of high-grade spondyolisthesis cannot be derived from the literature. The indication for treatment reported here was in accordance with current consensus. The choice of surgical approach — reduction of the slippage and restoration of segmental lordosis — was challenging, but concordant with current expert opinion.

Level of Evidence: C

The evidence base for the management of high-grade spondylolisthesis is poor, with the available literature comprising at best retrospective cohort studies.

24.6 Conclusions and Take Home Message

The surgical treatment of high-grade spondylolisthesis remains controversial. The present discussion concentrates on two points: is reduction of spondylolisthesis indicated and how should it be accomplished? From a biomechanical point of view, the objective of surgical treatment is to reduce shear forces at the lumbosacral junction by reduction of the spondylolisthesis, correction of the sagittal deformity, dorsal tension-band forces, and secure ventral support.

Pearls

- the main indications for surgery are low back pain and radicular pain resistant to conservative treatment, progression of the lumbosacral deformity, and neurologic deficit
- the role of deformity correction and restoration of spino-pelvic balance requires further clarification
- instrumentation, release, reduction and interbody fusion can be achieved from posterior in a safe manner with direct vision and control of the neural structures at risk
- with the use IONM, complete reduction of the L5/S1 slip can be performed with minimal risk of irreversible L5 radiculopathy

Editorial Comment

Reposition and defining the number of segments is an difficult decision. Lamartinas definition of the unstable zone can help to make a decision if only one or two vertebras should be included in the instrumentation to reduce the risk of adjacent segment failure.

References

1. Edwards C, Weidenbaum M. Spondylolisthesis: introduction. The textbook of spinal surgery. Philadelphia: Lippincott-Raven; 2011. p. 553–5.
2. Wiltse LL, Newman PH, Macnab I. Classification of spondylolisis and spondylolisthesis. Clin Orthop Relat Res. 1976;117:23–9.
3. Marchetti PC, Bartolozzi P. Classification of spondylolisthesis as a guideline for treatment. The textbook of spinal surgery. Philadelphia: Lippincott-Raven; 1997. p. 1211–54.
4. Rahman RK, Perra J, Weidenbaum M. Wiltse and Marchetti/Bartolozzi classification of spondylolisthesis – guidelines for treatment. The textbook of spinal surgery. Philadelphia: Lippincott-Raven; 2011. p. 556–62.
5. Molinari RW, Bridwell KH, Lenke LG, Ungacta FF, Riew KD. Complications in the surgical treatment of pediatric high-grade, isthmic dysplastic spondylolisthesis. A comparison of three surgical approaches. Spine. 1999;24:1701–11.
6. Sencan S, Ozcan-Eksi EE, Cil H, et al. The effect of transforaminal epidural steroid injections in patients with spondylolisthesis. J Back Musculoskelet Rehabil. 2017;30:841–6.
7. Danielson BI, Frennered AK, Irstam LK. Radiologic progression of isthmic lumbar spondylolisthesis in young patients. Spine. 1991;16:422–5.
8. Ruf M, Koch H, Melcher RP, Harms J. Anatomic reduction and monosegmental fusion in high-grade developmental spondylolisthesis. Spine. 2006;31:269–74.
9. Schar RT, Sutter M, Mannion AF, et al. Outcome of L5 radiculopathy after reduction and instrumented transforaminal lumbar interbody fusion of high-grade L5-S1 isthmic spondylolisthesis and the role of intraoperative neurophysiological monitoring. Eur spine J. 2017;26:679–90.
10. Lakshmanan P, Ahuja S, Lewis M, Howes J, Davies PR. Transsacral screw fixation for high-grade spondylolisthesis. Spine J. 2009;9:1024–9.
11. Shufflebarger HL, Geck MJ. High-grade isthmic dysplastic spondylolisthesis: monosegmental surgical treatment. Spine. 2005;30:S42–8.

12. Lengert R, Charles YP, Walter A, Schuller S, Godet J, Steib JP. Posterior surgery in high-grade spondylolisthesis. Orthop Traumatol Surg Res: OTSR. 2014;100:481–4.
13. Martiniani M, Lamartina C, Specchia N. "In situ" fusion or reduction in high-grade high dysplastic developmental spondylolisthesis (HDSS). Eur Spine J. 2012;21(Suppl 1):S134–40.
14. Min K, Liebscher T, Rothenfluh D. Sacral dome resection and single-stage posterior reduction in the treatment of high-grade high dysplastic spondylolisthesis in adolescents and young adults. Eur Spine J. 2012;21(Suppl 6):S785–91.
15. Hresko MT, Labelle H, Roussouly P, Berthonnaud E. Classification of high-grade spondylolistheses based on pelvic version and spine balance: possible rationale for reduction. Spine. 2007;32:2208–13.
16. Obeid I, Laouissat F, Bourghli A, Boissiere L, Vital JM. One-stage posterior spinal shortening by L5 partial spondylectomy for spondyloptosis or L5-S1 high-grade spondylolisthesis management. Eur Spine J. 2016;25:664–70.
17. Gaines RW, Nichols WK. Treatment of spondyloptosis by two stage L5 vertebrectomy and reduction of L4 onto S1. Spine. 1985;10:680–6.

25 Parameters of Spino-Pelvic Balance, Etiology and Pathogenesis of Disturbed Spino-Pelvic Balance

Aurélie Toquart and Cédric Y. Barrey

These cases will focus on the way to analyze and understand disturbed spino-pelvic balance in adults for clinical practice.

After describing the main parameters for sagittal balance assessment, we will describe in details 3 clinical situations: balanced, compensated and imbalanced.

25.1 Context

First, it is important to define the normal spino-pelvic balance and describe the most relevant parameters.

The spinopelvic balance implies an economic posture of the spine above the pelvis and the lower limbs in order to place the axis of gravity into a physiological position with minimum musculature action. It takes into consideration the relationship between pelvic morphology and pelvic position and the curvatures of the spine above [1–6].

The pelvic incidence (PI), which reflects the shape of the pelvis (morphological parameter), represents a fundamental parameter. PI is defined as the angle from a line perpendicular to the mid-point of the sacral endplate and a line connecting this point to the center of the femoral heads. It's an individual parameter, not affected by the posture or the pelvis position and considered as quasi-invariable for a subject after the end of growth.

Geometrically, PI is equal to the algebraic sum of the sacral slope (SS) and the pelvic tilt (PT), two posture-dependent measurements (positional parameters), used to describe pelvic orientation: PI = SS + PT.

Clinical significance for spino-pelvic parameters are summarized in Table 25.1.

To describe the shape of the spine, it is commonly used the regional angles as thoracic kyphosis (TK) and lumbar lordosis (LL). They represent positional parameters, therefore affected by the position of the subject and also by the degenerative changes of the spine.

A significant correlation between the PI and the LL has already been demonstrated (correlation around 0.6–0.7) [1]. Some formulae exist in the literature, for instance:

PT theoric = 0.37 × PI − 7 [2]
LL L1-S1 theoric = 0.54 PI + 32.56 [3]

The limitation of such formulas is that the relation between LL and PI is not strictly linear and using just one formula has limitations, especially for the extreme values. The relation between the two parameters varies according to

A. Toquart · C. Y. Barrey (✉)
Department of Spine and Spinal Cord Surgery, University Hospital Pierre Wertheimer (GHE), Claude Bernard University of Lyon 1, Hospices Civils de Lyon, Lyon, France
e-mail: cedric.barrey@chu-lyon.fr

B. Meyer, M. Rauschmann (eds.), *Spine Surgery*, https://doi.org/10.1007/978-3-319-98875-7_25

Table 25.1 Clinical insights for spinopelvic parameters [6]

Nature of the parameter	Anatomical structure involved	Parameter	Clinical insight
Anatomical	Pelvis	PI	Pelvis shape
Positional	Pelvis	PT	Position of the pelvis related to the femoral heads
Positional	Pelvis	SS	Inclination of the pelvis
Positional	Spine	LL	Curve in extension above the sacral plate to maintain the balance
Positional	Spine	TK	Provide resistance and rigidity to the spine
Positional	Spine and pelvis	C7 ratio	Position of C7 vertebra above the pelvis (reflects the relative position of the whole spine above the pelvis)
Positional	Spine, pelvis and lower limbs	TPA	Position of the whole pelvic-spine complex above the lower limbs

PI pelvic incidence, *PT* pelvic tilt, *SS* sacral slope, *LL* lumbar lordosis, *TK* thoracic kyphosis, *TPA* T1-pelvis angle

the value of PI. Utilization of PI classes (six classes of PI, each 10°, from class I to class VI), previously published [5] gives full account of the variation of the relation between PI and LL. In fact, LL is equal to PI + 13/18 for low PI values (class I and II), equal to PI + 6/9 for medium values (class III and IV) and LL is quasi-equal to PI for high PI values (class V and VI), Table 25.2.

In one of our series [4], we divided the normal population into 6 groups (6 classes) of patients, according to their PI, every 10°, and the theoretical PT, SS and LL depending on their PI. We use

Table 25.2 Theoretical values for PI and PT using the distribution into 6 PI classes from I to VI [6]

PI class	PI (°)	PT_{th} (°)	LL_{th} (°)
I	<38	4	PI + 18
II	38–47	8	PI + 13
III	48–57	12	PI + 9
IV	58–67	16	PI + 6
V	68–77	20	PI + 2
VI	>78	24	PI-5

it daily, to calculate the lack of lumbar lordosis for example.

The nature of the formula used to determine the theoretical value of lumbar lordosis has a clear impact on the result, especially for the extreme values. As example, with 30° PI, theoretical LL should be 40°, 43° and 48° according to Schwab, LeHuec and Barrey-Roussouly calculation method. With 80° PI, theoretical LL should be 90°, 68° and 75° according to Schwab, LeHuec and Barrey-Roussouly calculation method. Table 25.3.

Not only the global magnitude of the lumbar lordosis is important to consider but also the distribution of the lordosis along the lumbar spine. It is important to keep in mind that 2/3 of the lordosis is given by the L4-S1 segment only and that 40% is provided by L5S1.

In parallel to regional analysis, global alignment has to be evaluated. To assess the global sagittal balance, the SVA is commonly used (sagittal vertical axis), which is the horizontal distance between the postero superior S1 corner and the vertical line passing through the C7 center. It should be less than 50 mm. If it's superior, there is an anterior sagittal imbalance (positioning of C7 plumb line forward).

Instead of measuring a linear distance, we recommend to use angular and/or ratio parameters to characterize the positioning of C7 in relation to the sacrum. Angular parameter is represented by the spino-sacral angle (SSA), initially described by P. Roussouly, and the C7 ratio, initially reported by C. Barrey, corresponds to the SVA/sacro-femoral distance ratio (SVA/SFD). These two parameters have already been reported and validated [5].

Table 25.3 Impact on the method used to calculate the theoretical lordosis

Pelvic Incidence	LLth Schwab	LLth Le Huec	LLth Barrey–Roussouly
Formula	**PI + 9°**	**PI/2 + 28**	**PI Class**
30°	40° Not enough	43°	48°
40°	50°	48°	53°
50°	60°	53°	59°
60°	70°	58°	66°
70°	80° Too much	63°	72°
80°	90°	68°	75°

The SSA (spino sacral angle) was defined as the angle between the sacral plate and the line connecting the centroid of C7 vertebral body and the midpoint of the sacral plate. In the normal population the mean value of this angle is 135 ± 8°.

SFD is the horizontal distance between the vertical bicoxo-femoral axis and the vertical line passing through the posterior corner of the sacrum. In the normal population the mean value of the C7 ratio (=SVA/SFD) is – 0.9 ± 1(−1.9; 0.1).

In clinical practice, regarding the global balance, three situations can be described:

1. Balanced with no compensation (normal spinopelvic balance)
2. compensated sagittal balance (2A: completely compensated and 2B: partially compensated
3. Imbalanced (globally imbalanced with the insufficiency of the compensatory mechanisms)

In this chapter, we intend to describe one case of each situation.

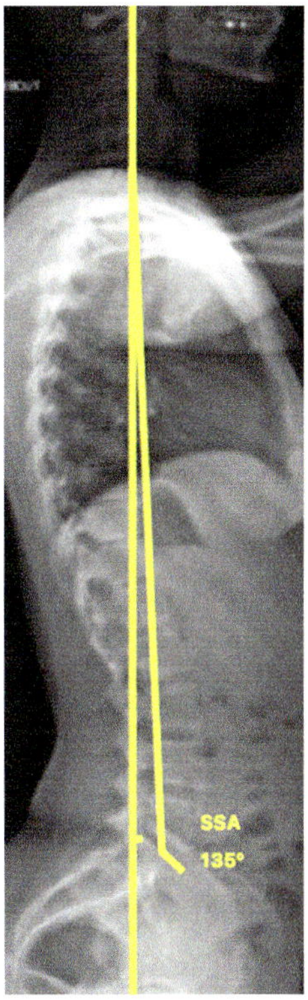

Fig. 25.1 Assessment of global alignment with measurement of SVA and SSA

25.2 Cases Description

25.2.1 Case 1

Balanced with normal spinopelvic alignment.

This case is a 26 years old asymptomatic woman.

First, concerning the global balance, we can observe that SVA is less than 50 mm (−2 mm), SSA is exactly 135° and C7 ratio measured to −2/12 = −0.17 (normal), Fig. 25.1.

Secondly, concerning the pelvic incidence, this was calculated to 37° (low PI), so she belongs to the first PI group (class I), Fig. 25.2.

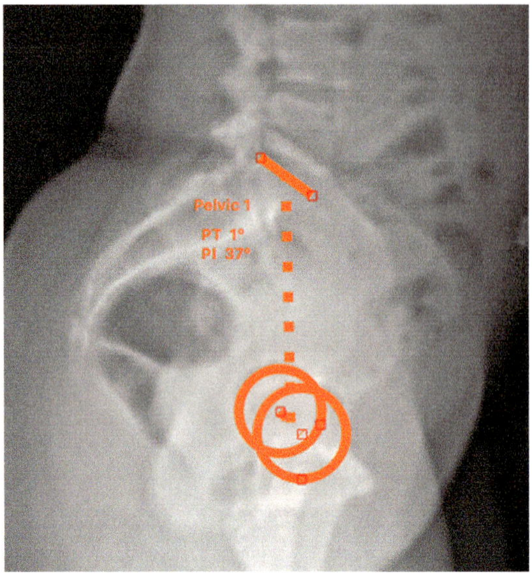

Fig. 25.2 Measurement of pelvic parameters: PI, PT and SS

Seeing the value of PI, theoretical PT should be 4°. Finally, the measured PT is 1°. These two values are very close and PT can therefore be considered as normal. SS is measured to 36° for a theoretical value of 33°.

Concerning now the spinal parameters, LL is 58° for a theoretical of 55° (PI + 18 = 37 + 18 = 55°), Fig. 25.3.

Regarding the distribution of lordosis along the lumbar spine, we noted that the L4-S1 lordosis (40°) represents 2/3 of L1-S1 lordosis (58°).

Finally, seeing all the parameters calculated, this woman can consequently be considered as well-balanced with no sagittal alignment disorder.

25.2.2 Case 2

The compensated sagittal balance, which represents a compromise situation characterized by the preservation of the global balance but at the price of compensation mechanisms (thoracic hypokyphosis, extension of thoraco-lumbar junc-

Fig. 25.3 Measurement of spinal curves: lumbar lordosis and thoracic kyphosis

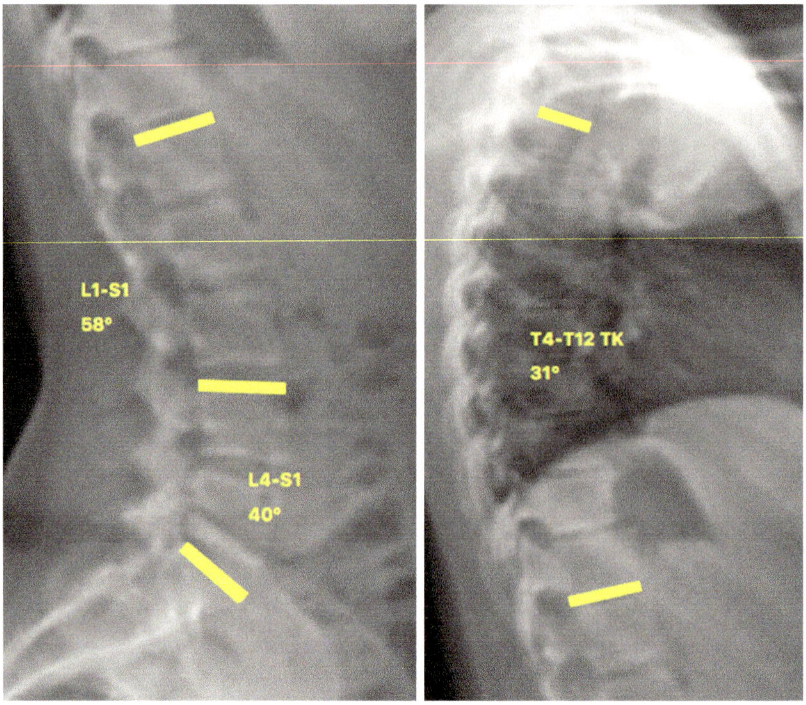

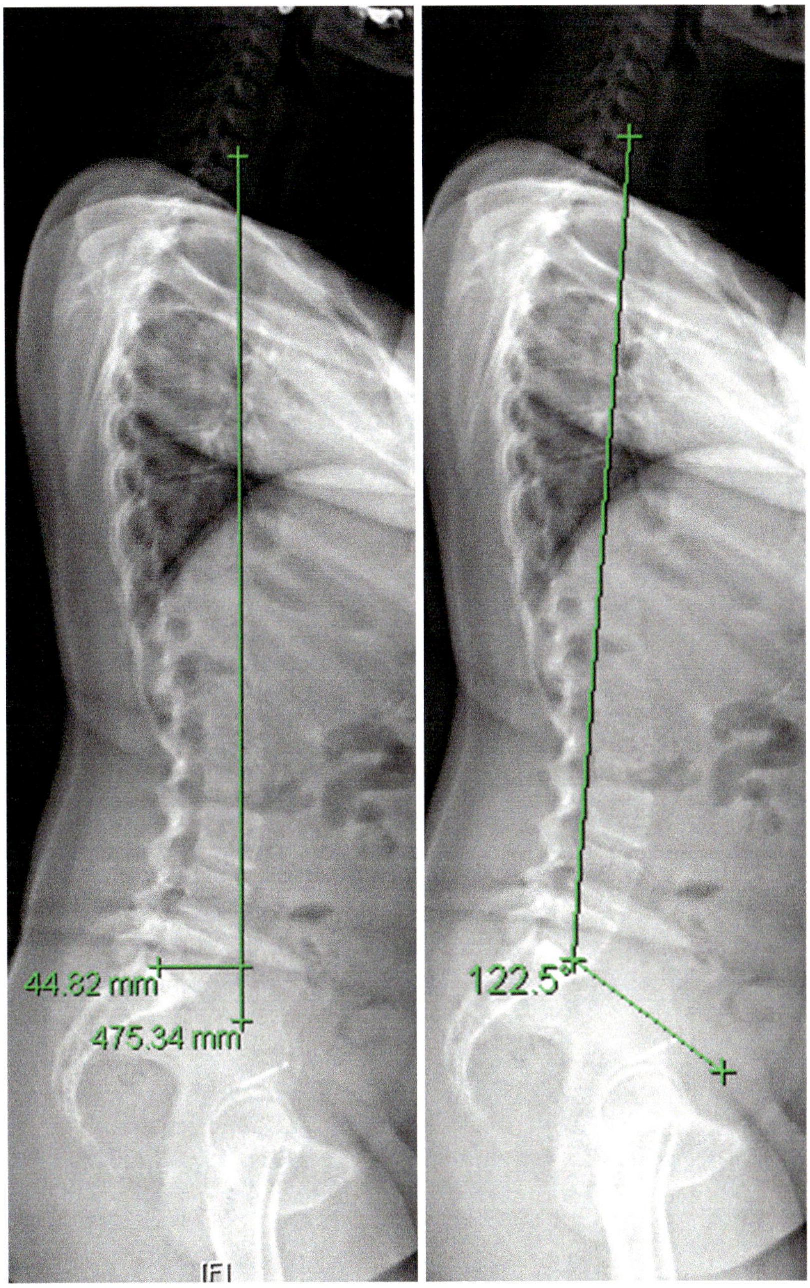

Fig. 25.4 Assessment of global alignment: SVA is measured to 44.8 mm and SSA to 122.5°

tion, pelvic retroversion and/or flexion of the knees).

This 40 years old woman presented with chronic low back pain for many years.

We can observe that the SVA is less than 50 mm (44.8 mm), the SSA close to 135° +/− 8 (122.5°) and C7 ratio to 0.88 (less than 1), Figs. 25.4 and 25.5.

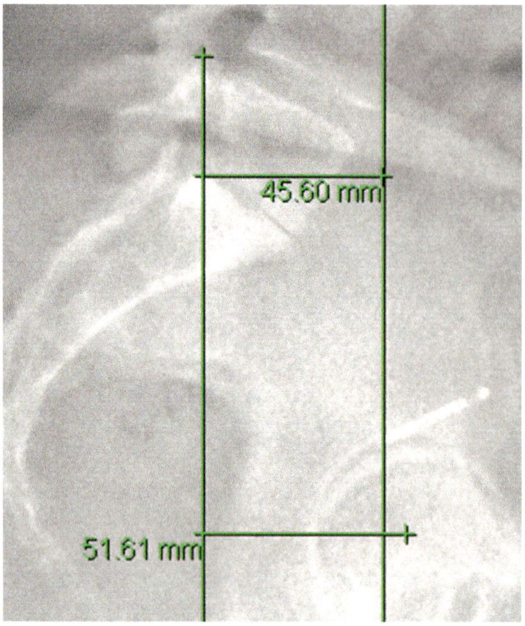

Fig. 25.5 Calculation of C7 ratio (=SVA/SFD = 45.6/51.6 = 0.88)

The global alignment is preserved however we noted that the PT, SS and LL were not into the normal ranges.

Indeed, the PI was measured to 64° (PI group number IV), Fig. 25.6. According to our table, the theoretical PT should be 16° with SS around 48°. In fact, PT was increased, measured to 28°, i.e. retroverted pelvis, and SS was decreased, measured to 36° only.

The L1-S1 Lordosis (LL) was measured to only 45°, for a theoretical value of 69° (LL theoretical = PI + 5 = 69°). We can therefore estimate that there is a lack of lordosis around 25°. The L4-S1 Lordosis was only 15°, i.e. representing 1/3 of the existing LL and only 1/5 of the theoretical lordosis, whereas it should represent approximately 2/3 of the LL. According to the expected theoretical values, L1-S1 Lordosis should be around 70° and so L4-S1 should be around 46° (2/3 of 70).

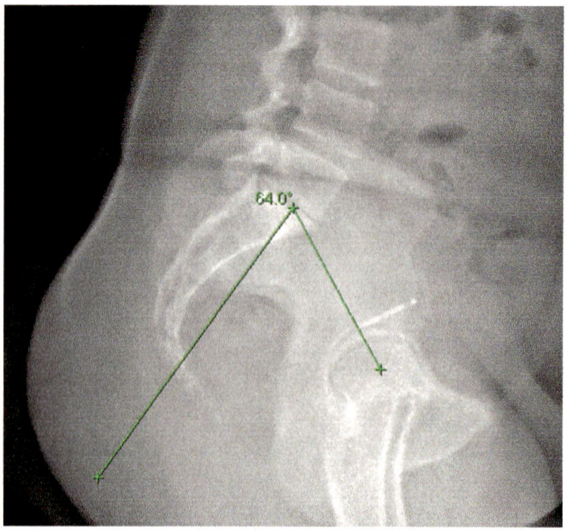

Fig. 25.6 Measurement of the pelvic parameters: PI, SS and PT

Reduction of thoracic kyphosis (hypokyphosis) is another compensatory mechanism permitting to limit the anterior translation of the axis of gravity, Fig. 25.7. It is typically observed in young patients with flexible and non-degenerative thoracic spine, like this case.

25.2.3 Case 3

Imbalanced. The compensatory mechanisms are not enough efficient to maintain the sagittal alignment.

The case is a male, 48 y-old, complaining of low back pain and walking disability. We observed significant increase of the SVA (measured to 131 mm for a normal of <50 mm), Fig. 25.8. C7 plumb-line is located in front of the femoral heads. The patient is in an anterior imbalanced situation.

We can also note that the values of SSA and C7 ratio are clearly abnormal (only 81° for SSA and 1.4 for C7 ratio, much more than 1), Fig. 25.9. The patient is globally imbalanced.

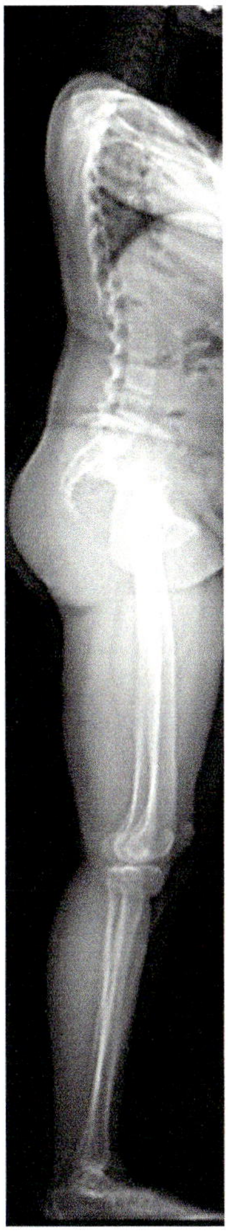

Fig. 25.7 Full body X-rays demonstrated the flat spine above the pelvis with reduction of both lumbar and thoracic curves

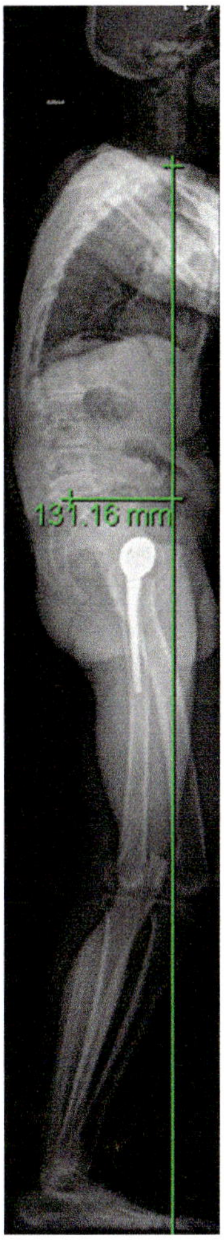

Fig. 25.8 Full body (EOS™ system) showing the spinal deformity with anterior sagittal imbalance. SVA is clearly augmented calculated to >130 mm

Concerning the pelvic parameters, we found first that PI was measured to 50° (PI group class III), Fig. 25.10. Taking into consideration this PI value, PT should be 12° and SS 38°. In fact, we calculated that SS was only 5° and that PT was strongly increased to 45°. The augmentation of PT corresponds to pelvis retroversion, i.e. hip extension. However, this pelvic retroversion is not enough to compensate the loss of lumbar lordosis and did not succeed to maintain the spinopelvic balance and the overall sagittal alignment.

Concerning now spinal parameters, the L1-S1 Lordosis is almost zero, measured to only 3° (for a theoretical LL = PI + 9, i.e. 59°), so there is a lack of 56°, Fig. 25.11. In fact, the loss of lordosis was due to severe and multilevel degenerative

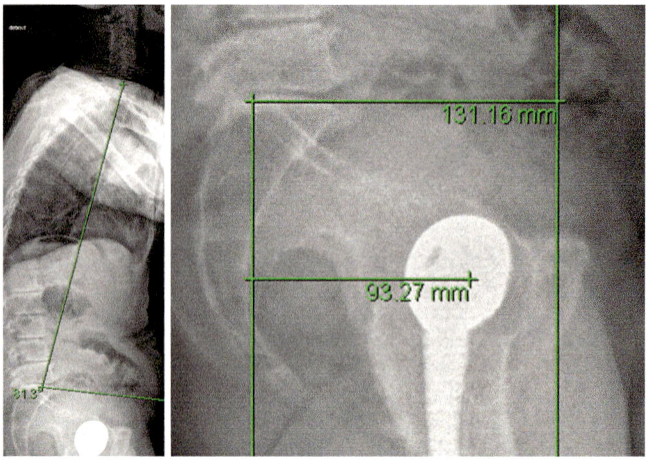

Fig. 25.9 Measurement of the SSA (81°) and calculation of the C7 ratio (131/93 = 1.4)

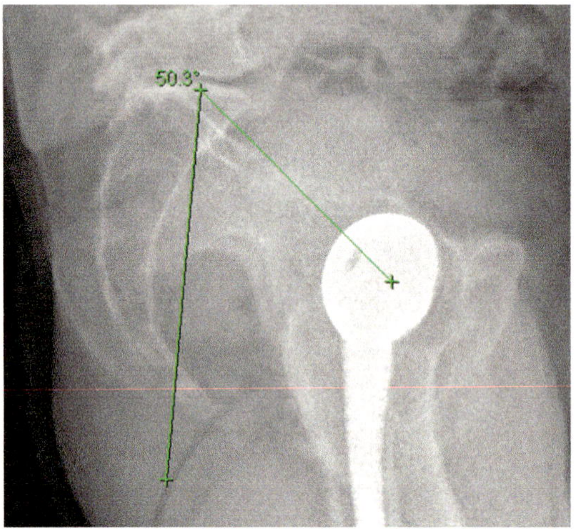

Fig. 25.10 Measurement of the pelvic parameters: PI, SS and PT

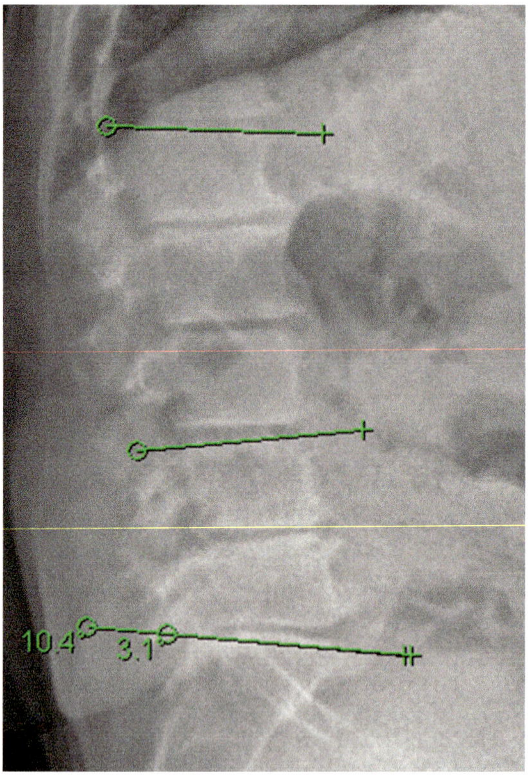

Fig. 25.11 Analysis of the lumbar curve with calculation of L1-S1 and L4-S1 lordosis

disc diseases and represents the cause of the sagittal imbalance. The L4-S1 Lordosis was only 10° and the TK 36°.

The surgery consisted of T10-pelvis instrumentation with PSO at L4. After surgery, we can observe a real improvement in his sagittal balance, Fig. 25.12. The SVA is now less than 40 mm (35.6), the SSA close to 135 +/− 8 (123°) and C7 ratio less than 1.

Also, the pelvic parameters are now close to the theoretical values (SS = 34° for theoretical SS of 40° and PT = 16° for theoretical PT of 12°, with an unchanged PI to 50°).

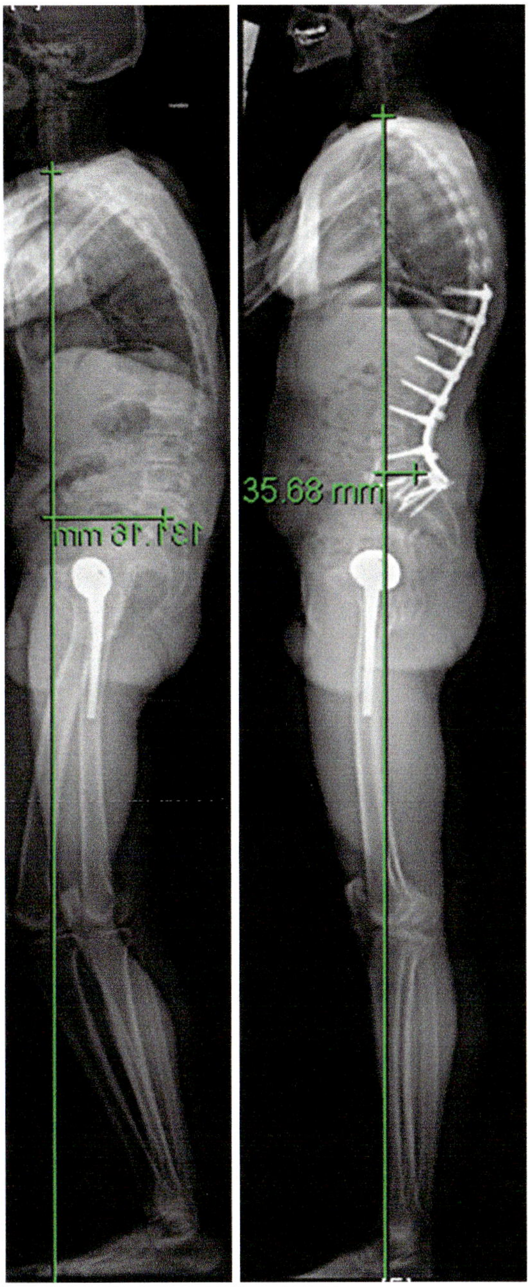

Fig. 25.12 After surgery, SSA was measured to 123°, SVA to 35.6 mm and C7 ratio to 0.77 (SVA/SFD = 35.6/46.3 = 0.77)

Regarding the distribution of the lumbar lordosis along the lumbar spine, L1-S1 Lordosis is exactly 60° (expected theoretical LL = 59°) and the L4-S1 at 46°, that is to say a little bit more than 2/3 of L1-S1 lordosis, Fig. 25.13.

The TK is 51°, it increased about 15°, without any surgical correction. It probably means that there was a moderate hypokyphosis to compensate the sagittal imbalance before the surgery. Restoration of the physiological LL permitted to eliminate the need for compensation mechanisms.

25.3 Discussion

Through this chapter and the 3 clinical cases presented, we have seen the importance of analyzing the spinopelvic balance before surgery in the context of spinal degenerative diseases.

Disturbed spinopelvic balance in adults is most of the time due to a lack of lumbar lordosis, or a thoracic kyphosis increasement [1–3]. The first etiology of these spinal curvatures changes is the aging of the spine, with arthritis and disc degeneration.

Sometimes, more rarely, it can be due to a non-degenerative spinal pathology, such as Scheuermann, or camptocormia, with a stiff global kyphosis. It can also be due to a post-traumatic kyphosis or post-operative hypolordotic instrumentation (iatrogenic flat back).

Spinal kyphotic deformity induces a forward translation of the center of mass of the trunk that can be countered by several compensating mechanisms [4]. If the whole spine is fixed, the compensating mechanisms are located at the level of the pelvis and lower limbs. The main compensating mechanism is the pelvic retroversion, which is demonstrated by increased PT. However, the spontaneous pelvic retroversion can be insufficient to maintain balance if the deformity is too great. The last mean is to flex the knees and extend the ankles. This is a compromise situation and if pelvis retroversion may result into a better sagittal balance situation, it generally induces walking disability and chronic fatigue [4].

If the spine is flexible, which is typically the case in young adult, it can be involved in the compensating mechanisms. The most typical example is the lumbar degenerative kyphosis where the thoracic spine is usually hypokyphotic, and the cervical spine hyperlordotic.

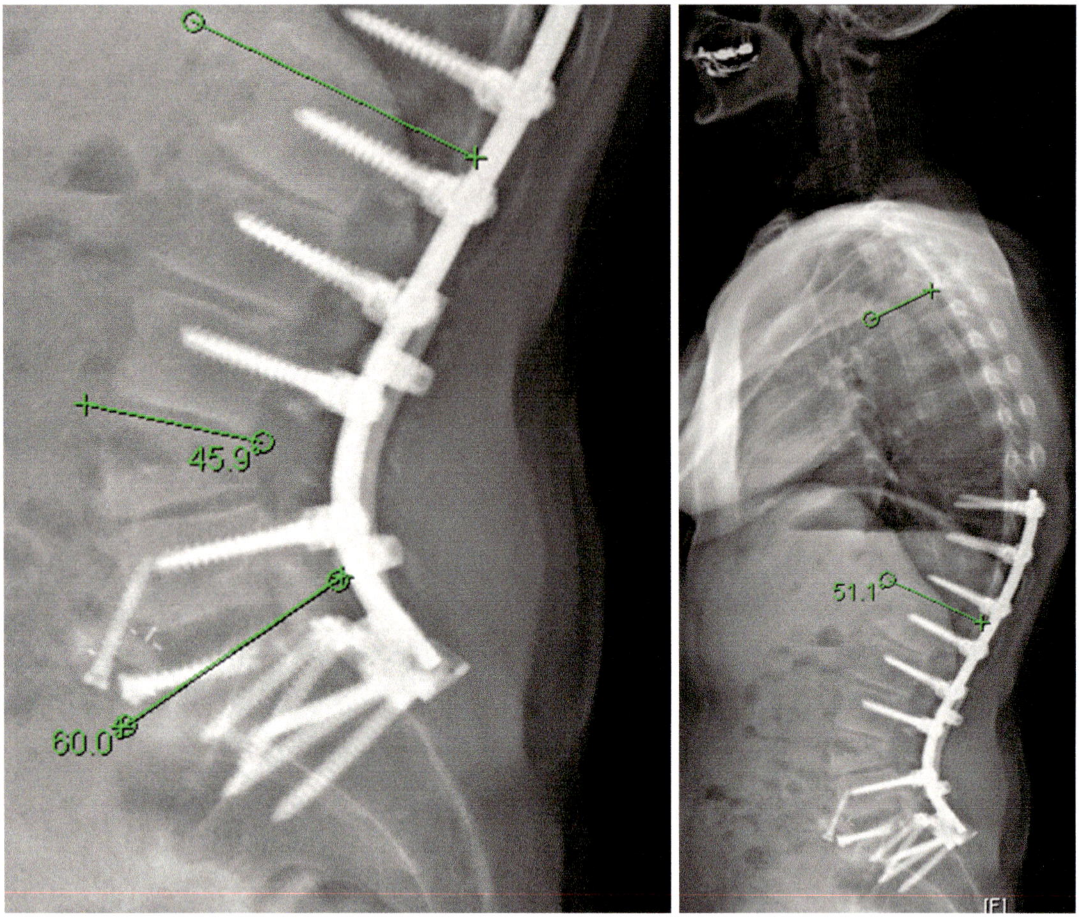

Fig. 25.13 Measurement of pelvic parameters post-operatively: PI = 50°, SS = 34° and PT = 16°

25.4 Conclusion and Take-Home Messages

To assess the spino pelvic balance into the context of adult spinal deformity before a surgery, we previously reported a 3-steps algorithm [4–6].

The first step is to measure the pelvic incidence in order to determine the expected theoretical values of the spino-pelvic positional parameters and in particular the value of the theoretical LL. Seeing the relation of PI and LL, using classes of PI is more relevant and more precise than using a unique formula.

The second step is to evaluate the global sagittal alignment by analyzing the positioning of C7 related to the pelvis. Concerning the most relevant parameters, we recommend to use SVA, SSA and C7 ratio.

Finally, the last step is to look for the compensatory mechanisms in spinal area (extension of the TL junction, reduction of the thoracic kyphosis); in the pelvic area (only 1 compensation mechanisms, i.e. pelvis retroversion); and in lower limbs area (knee flexion).

After a meticulous and systematic analyzing of sagittal alignment, next step is the planning of the corrective surgery and this is the subject of another chapter (Chap. 54).

Editorial Comment

The spino-pelvic parameters are very important tools for planning a surgery with a good outcome. The surgeon has also to take in mind, that compensation of adjacent regions (iliosacral joint; hip's and flexibility of thoracic segments) which are mandatory to produce good results without failures in the adjacent segments.

References

1. Vaz G, et al. Sagittal morphology and equilibrium of pelvis and spine. Eur Spine J. 2002;11(1):80–7.
2. Vialle R, et al. Radiographic analysis of the sagittal alignment and balance of the spine in asymptomatic subjects. J Bone Joint Surg Am Vol. 2005;87A(2):260–7.
3. Gille O. PhD thesis, Ecole Nationale Superieure des Arts et Metiers, Paris; 2006.
4. Barrey C, et al. Compensatory mechanisms contributing to keep the sagittal balance of the spine. Eur Spine J. 2013;22:S834–41.
5. Barrey C, et al. Sagittal balance of the pelvis-spine complex and lumbar degenerative diseases. A comparative study about 85 cases. Eur Spine J. 2007;16(9):1459–67.
6. Barrey C, et al. Current strategies for the restoration of the adequate lordosis during lumbar fusion. World J Orthop. 2015;6(1):117–26.

Diagnosis, Classification and General Treatment Options for Hyperkyphosis

26

Mohammad Arabmotlagh and Michael Rauschmann

The physiological sagittal shape of the spine consists of kyphosis of thoracic spine and lordosis of cervical and lumbar spine. Normal range of thoracic kyphosis and lumbar lordosis are 20–45° and 40–60°, respectively [1]. The sum of these curvatures aims to keep the spine in sagittal balance, a condition with lowest energy consumption during standing position. The sagittal balance is characterized by the plump line, which is drawn vertically from the center of the C7 vertebral body down to the sacrum. In normal condition, the plump line bisects the sacral endplate. A variety of conditions may lead to increasing segmental (angular) or regional (arcuar) kyphosis. Compensatory mechanisms exist to counteract the shift of the trunk to the forward as hyperlordosis of cervical and lumbar spine, reclination of pelvis and flexion of knees. Exhaustion of these compensatory mechanism result in the shift of the plump line anterior to the femoral head axis and sagittal imbalance of the spine. Table 26.1 illustrates etiologic conditions that result in kyphotic deformities.

M. Arabmotlagh (✉)
Spine Department, Academic University Hospital Sana Klinik Offenbach, Goethe University Frankfurt, Offenbach, Germany

M. Rauschmann
Department of Spine Surgery, Sana Klinikum Offenbach, Offenbach, Germany

26.1 Patient Evaluation

Patients should be examined in standing position with knees as straight as possible. Patients with imbalanced spine try to compensate with knee flexion and backward rotation of the pelvis. The grade of knee flexion should be taken into account, when analyzing spine parameters on lateral view x-ray. Hip flexion contraction may limit the compensatory mechanism of the pelvis. The effect of hip and knee on spine posture can be removed by sitting position. If an imbalanced spine improves in sitting position, the cause may lie in hip flexion contraction, which can be proved by Thomas maneuver. Examination in supine position may reveal the flexibility of the deformity, which can be illustrated with lateral view x-ray with a bolster underneath the apex of the deformity. Attention should be paid on myelopathy signs as gait pattern and pathologic reflexes.

26.2 Radiologic Evaluation

X-ray images in lateral and ap view of the whole spine from occiput to the end of sacrum with femoral heads should be performed. The sagittal balance is evaluated by the plump line, which is drawn vertically from the center of C7 vertebral body down. With a balanced spine, the plump line falls on the anterior edge of S1 endplate. The spine is significantly imbalanced if plump line falls

B. Meyer, M. Rauschmann (eds.), *Spine Surgery*, https://doi.org/10.1007/978-3-319-98875-7_26

Table 26.1 Pathologic conditions that result in kyphotic deformity of Spine

Degenerative process	Trauma	Inflammation	Growth	Neuromuscular
Loss of disc space height Osteoporosis	Posttraumatic Postoperative Tumor Osteoporosis	Infection Ankylosing spondylitis	Scheuermann Congenital Postural	M. Parkinson

anterior to the femoral head axis. On the frontal plane, the spine is balanced if the vertical line dropped from C7 spine process falls on the sacrum midline. For the evaluation of the spine flexibility, x-ray in lateral view is performed in supine position with a bolster underneath the apex of the deformity to prove any opening of the disc spaces.

Any neurologic abnormality, angular kyphosis or any other irregular deformity of the spine without obvious underlying cause, require MR-imaging of the whole spine. CT scanning is helpful in cases of complex deformities for structural illustration of the spine.

26.3 Treatment Options

Surgical treatment options for correction of spine deformities involve dorsal instrumentation combined with varying osteotomy techniques. The spectrum of osteotomies ranges from partial removing of interlaminar bone, which represents the least invasive technique, to resection of one or more vertebral bodies as the most invasive technique. With increasing degree of osteotomy, the potential for correction of the deformity as well as the risks of the operation increase. The type of osteotomy selected, depends on the degree of the deformity and on the flexibility of the spine. The first osteotomy of the spine was described by Smith-Petersen (SPO) to treat the hyperkyphosis of ankylosing spondylitis by opening up the anterior column through dissection of anterior disc space and anterior longitudinal ligament and simultaneous closing the posterior wedge after resection of posterior elements in lumbar spine [2]. With the classic SPO a maximum correction of 30° is possible. The center of rotation through this osteotomy is in the posterior anulus of the disc. Thus, the correction maneuver results in lengthening of the spine anteriorly. This may lead to the rupture of great vessels running anterior to the spine, a very serious complication that was reported in numerous studies [3]. Older patients were more frequent involved in this complication due to the atherosclerotic changes and consequently loss of the flexibility of vessels in elderly people. Wilson reported few years later a modification of SPO which was limited to only posterior osteotomy without anterior opening [4]. Aim of this technique was to avoid anterior lengthening of the spine and subsequent rupture risk of the anterior vessels. Today, a wedge osteotomy of posterior column without opening of anterior disc space is commonly referred to SPO. This technique requires some mobility of the disc space anteriorly. Without opening of the anterior column, a maximum correction of 10° in each segment is possible.

Ponte described 1984 multisegment closing wedge osteotomy of thoracic spine to treat scheuermann kyphosis by a Λ shape interlaminar osteotomy with resection of flavum ligament and osteoclasia of adjacent laminae as well as facet joints [5]. With Ponte-procedure the anterior column of spine is preserved and the correction is achieved by the forceful compression through segmental pedicle screws. The center of rotation is at the posterior disc anulus as with SPO. This results in slight opening of anterior disc space with a maximum of 10° correction of each segment (Figs. 26.1 and 26.2).

With pedicle-subtraction osteotomy (PSO) the correction is completely achieved by closing of the resected wedge without lengthening of the anterior column. Thomasen described this method to avoid anterior lengthening and to save the anterior vessels [6]. Technically, PSO is performed following instrumentation of the spine. After resection of the lamina and facet joint, the pedicles are removed completely, vertebral body is decancellated through the base of the pedicles and the lateral cortical wall of the vertebral body is removed in a posteriorly based wedge manner.

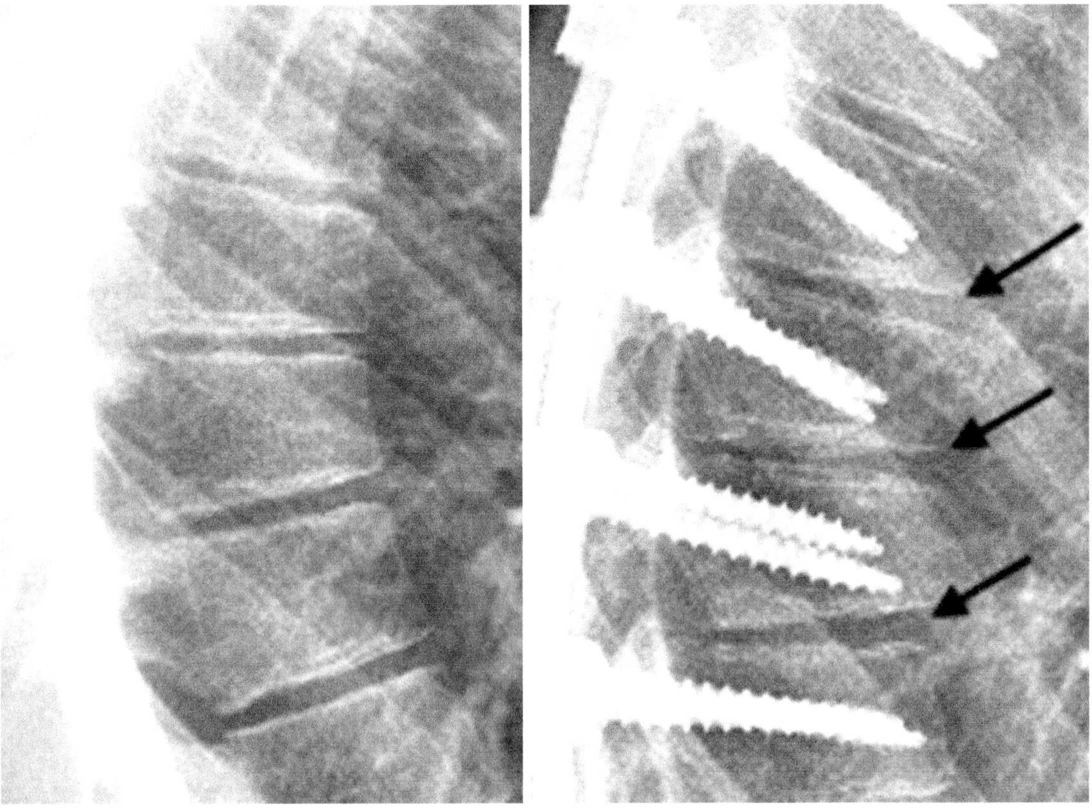

Figs. 26.1 and 26.2 Pre- and postoperative x-ray in lateral view of thoracic spine with scheuermann kyphosis. Correction was achieved with multiple Ponte osteotomies. Arrows indicate anterior opening of disc spaces

The anterior cortex and longitudinal ligament are preserved. The correction is achieved by closing the gap through compression of adjacent pedicle screws (Figs. 26.3 and 26.4). Attention should be paid to remove sufficient amount of the lamina to avoid compression to the neural structures by closing the wedge. Compared to SPO, PSO is associated with more blood loss during the vertebral resection. With PSO a correction up to 30° can be achieved in the osteotomized vertebral body. PSO is the procedure of choice in fixed kyphotic deformities of all etiologies. Despite the rule that the correction should be performed where the deformity is located, PSO is usually performed at L2 or L3, for example in case of fixed global imbalance of the spine or ankylosing spondylitis. These levels offer some advantages as this area distal to the conus is less risky with regard to neurologic complication by manipulation of dural sac. Further, the more distally the osteotomy the more correction can be achieved

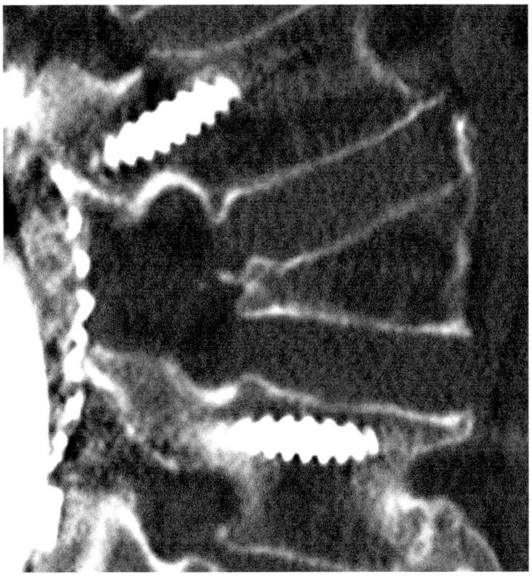

Fig. 26.3 Postoperative CT scan of pedicle subtraction osteotomy of L2. Shape of vertebral body after posterior based wedge resection

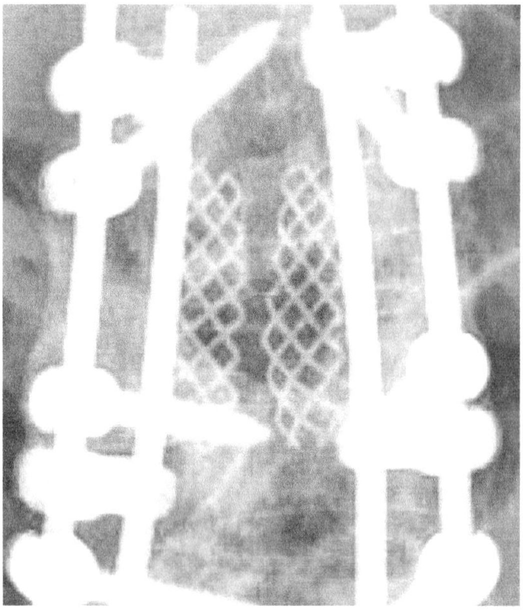

Fig. 26.4 Postoperative x-ray in ap view demonstrate the double rod technique and the use of a titanium mesh to bridge the posterior bone gap for deposition of bone graft to achieve more stable instrumentation and bony fusion of the osteotomy

due to the long lever arm. Recent studies support to perform PSO at more distal levels, even at L5, to achieve the main lordotic curve at lumbosacral junction [7]. However, if the deformity is in cervicothoracic spine, as with ankylosing spondylitis, PSO can be performed in the upper thoracic spine below C7 where vertebral arteries run outside the vertebra. Simultaneous deformity in frontal plane can be addressed by asymmetric wedge resection of the PSO. Long term complication of PSO is failure of instrumentation as break of rods. This may occur when posterior bony fusion does not take place due to the wide posterior osteotomy and open disc space anteriorly. This complication can be avoided either by bridging the posterior gap with bone graft or by selection of the vertebra for PSO where adjacent disc spaces are fused anteriorly. Some authors recommend dorsal instrumentation with double rod each side to achieve a more stable situation.

For correction of severe deformities in frontal and sagittal plane, vertebral column resection (VCR) is a powerful technique (Figs. 26.5, 26.6, and 26.7). With this technique, a complete cross-

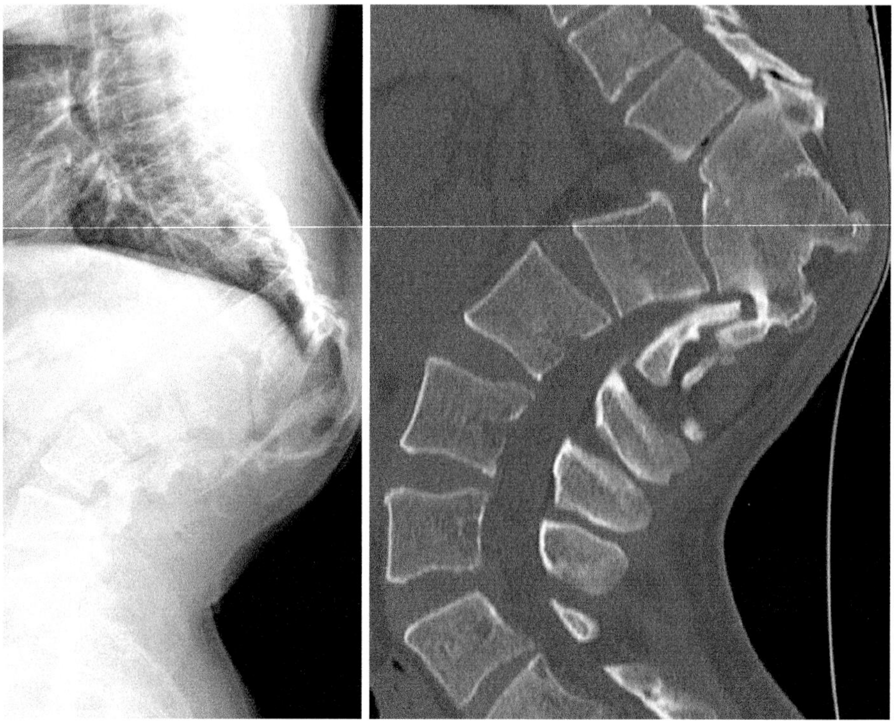

Figs. 26.5 and 26.6 Preoperative x-ray and CT scan of severe posttraumatic rigid kyphosis. Vertebral column resection was selected to correct the kyphosis

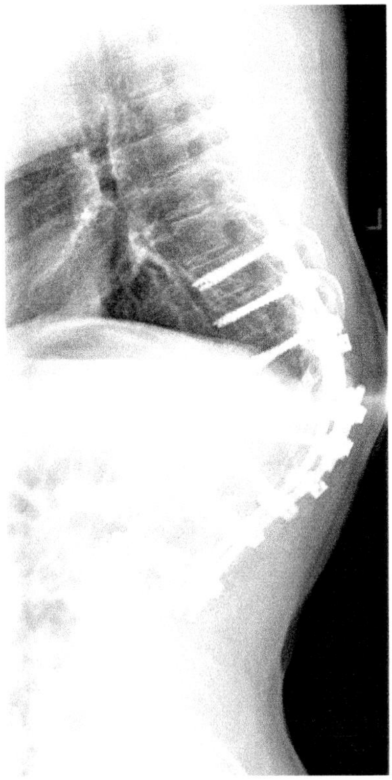

Fig. 26.7 Postoperative x-ray after vertebral column resection. A correction of 50% was achieved. Due to intraoperative loss of neural function that was detected by neuromonitoring, the correction was performed partially

sectional resection of bony and ligamentous tissue of spine is carried out, which enables multiplanar correction of the deformity. Preoperative planning of resection area is crucial for a sufficient correction of the deformity that ranges from one to more vertebral bodies. Appropriate indication for VCR are rigid angular kyphoscoliosis or congenital scoliosis due to hemivertebral formation. Sometimes implantation of a cage anteriorly is necessary to bridge the gap after vertebral resection. However, this technique is very challenging, requires experienced surgical team and is associated with high rate of neurological complication. Neurological complication results from either direct injury to neural structures or disturbances of blood supply. Neuromonitoring with SSEP and MEP is routinely recommended during surgery to control neural function.

26.4 Take Home Message

Several pathologic conditions may lead to a short or large curve hyperkyphosis of spine. The spine and the adjacent joints are able to compensate the hyperkyphosis to some extent. A symptomatic sagittal imbalance of spine emerges, when these compensatory mechanisms fail.

A thorough clinical and radiological evaluation is crucial to detect the location, the extent and the mobility of the deformity as well as the compensatory mechanisms of organism to counteract the deformity.

Several osteotomy techniques are available for correction of hyperkyphosis. They range from partial posterior osteotomy to complex multilevel vertebral body resection. With increasing degree of osteotomy, the potential for correction as well as the risks of operation increase.

Pearls

- Hip and knee joints compensate for spine deformities. They have to be considered and examined to evaluate the full extent of the spine balance
- Flexible and regional deformities can be addressed by one-column osteotomy technique as Ponte-osteotomy, whereas rigid deformities require three-column osteotomy techniques as PSO or VCR
- Wide decompression of spinal canal is needed for PSO and VCR to avoid stenosis after correction
- Use temporary rods for controlled and stepwise correction maneuver to avoid dislocation of screws

References

1. Bernhardt M, Bridwell K. Segmental analysis of the sagittal plane alignment of the normal thoracic and lumbar spine and thoracolumbar junction. Spine. 1989;14:717–21.
2. Smith-Petersen MN, Larson CB, Aufranc OE. Osteotomy of the spine for correction of flexion

deformity in rheumatoid arthritis. J Bone Joint Surg Am. 1945;27:1–11.
3. Fazl M, Bilbao JM, Hudson AR. Laceration of the aorta complicating spinal fracture in ankylosing spondylitis. Neurosurgery. 1981;8:732–4.
4. Wilson MJ, Turkel JK. Multiple spinal wedge osteotomy; its use in a case of Marie-Strumpell spondylitis. Am J Surg. 1949;77:777–82.
5. Ponte A, Vero B, Siccardi G. Surgical treatment of Scheuermann's hyperkyphosis. In: Winter RB, editor: Progressing Spinal Pathology: Kyphosis. Bologna; Aulo Gaggi. 1984. p. 75–81.
6. Thomasen E. Vertebral osteotomy for correction of kyphosis in ankylosing spondylitis. Clin Orthop Relat Res. 1985;(194):142–52.
7. Alzakri A, Boissiere L, Cawley DT, Bourgli A, Pointillart V, Gille O, Vital JM, Obeid I. L5 pedicle subtraction osteotomy: indication, surgical techniques and specifities. Eur Spine J. 2018;27: 644–51.

27 Scheuermann Kyphosis and Ankylosing Spondylitis

Mohammad Arabmotlagh
and Michael Rauschmann

27.1 Case 1: Scheuermann Kyphosis

27.1.1 Introduction

This case presents a young man with scheuermann's kyphosis. Clinical features, radiological evaluation, decision making of treatment options and surgical procedures are presented.

27.1.2 Case Description

Sixteen years old young man presenting with pronounced curvature of the spine, which has been noticed by his parents. He has no pain and is doing his sport's activity without any limitation. The pronounced curvature is felt as a disturbing "hump" that is embarrassing him.

The physical examination reveals no neurologic deficits. The Adams forward bending test shows an increased kyphotic curve of midthoracic region without any rotation of the spine. The increased kyphotic curve is not flexible and cannot be corrected with hyperextension of the spine. The secondary sexual characteristics are developed and the parents report that the puberty vocal change has been 2 years ago.

X-ray imaging of whole spine in ap and lateral view was performed in standing position (Fig. 27.1). The thoracic kyphosis is 81° (normal range 30–50°) according to Cobb method measured as the angle between inferior endplate of T12 and superior endplate of T3, so far visible. The apex of the kyphosis is at T9 level and the vertebral bodies in this region are anteriorly wedged (T7 – T11). Further, some irregularities of the endplates are present, as indicated by arrows (Fig. 27.1).

Based on clinical and radiological features, the diagnosis was made as scheuermann kyphosis. The young patient is skeletally mature and no more growth is expected. The patient was informed about the pathology and the relatively good prognosis as well as about the therapy options. Therapy options included (1) conservative treatment with physiotherapy to strengthen the trunk musculature and observation and (2) operative correction of the hyperkyphosis.

After thorough discussion with patient and his parents the decision was felt for operative treatment. To prepare the surgery, an additional x-ray in lateral view in supine position with a hypomochleon underneath the apex was made (Fig. 27.2). This position results in opening of the

M. Arabmotlagh (✉)
Spine Department, Academic University Hospital Sana Klinik Offenbach, Goethe University Frankfurt, Offenbach, Germany

M. Rauschmann
Department of Spine Surgery, Sana Klinikum Offenbach, Offenbach, Germany

B. Meyer, M. Rauschmann (eds.), *Spine Surgery*, https://doi.org/10.1007/978-3-319-98875-7_27

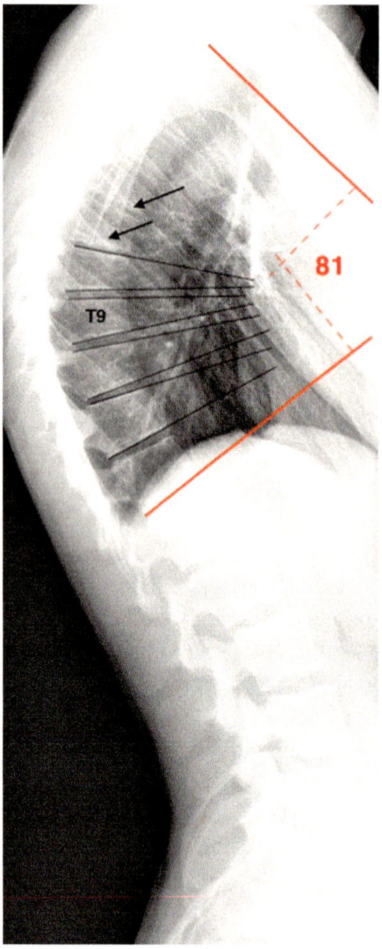

Fig. 27.1 Lateral view x-ray of spine shows thoracic kyphosis of 81°, apex of kyphosis at T9 and anteriorly wedged vertebral bodies T7 to T11. Arrows indicate irregularities of vertebral endplates

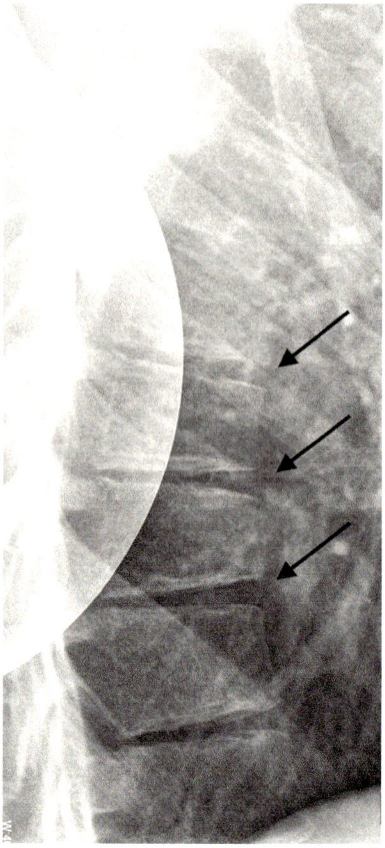

Fig. 27.2 X-ray of thoracic spine in supine position with a bolster underneath the apex of kyphosis shows opening of disc spaces (arrows)

disc space and indicates the mobility of the segments in this region of spine (arrows). Further, MR-imaging of whole spine was performed to rule out any neurological pathology as well as stenosis of the spinal canal (Fig. 27.3). To determine the extent of spinal fusion, the lateral view x-ray was evaluated. The proximal fusion level should include the kyphotic end vertebra, which is T3 in this case. The distal fusion level should include the sagittal stable vertebra. This is the most proximal vertebra that is touched by posterior sacral vertical line (Fig. 27.4), which is L2 in this case.

The operation was performed through posterior-only approach with multilevel Ponte osteotomies of apical kyphotic region and posterior instrumentation of T3 to L2 by segmental pedicle screws. The correction was achieved by cantilever forces with pre-molded bilateral rods and segmental compression. Attention was paid to correct not more than 50% of thoracic kyphosis. During the entire operation time neuromonitoring with SSEP and MEP control was performed. A peridural catheter was placed at the end of the operation for postoperative pain control.

The patient was mobilized immediately after the operation with physiotherapeutic support. Postoperative x-ray control was performed in lateral and ap view in standing position (Fig. 27.5). The hyperkyphosis was corrected to 53°. The patient was released from the hospital 7 days after surgery.

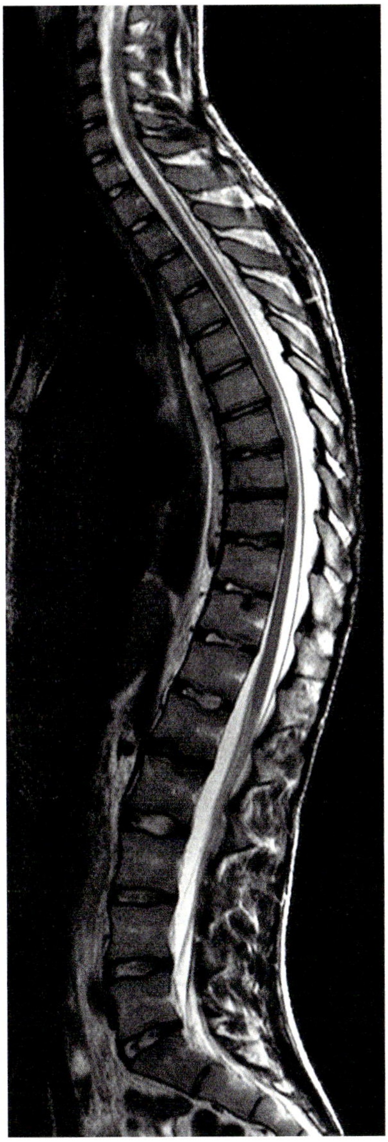

Fig. 27.3 MRI scan of whole spine illustrating the spinal canal which is recommended preoperatively to rule out any spinal canal pathology

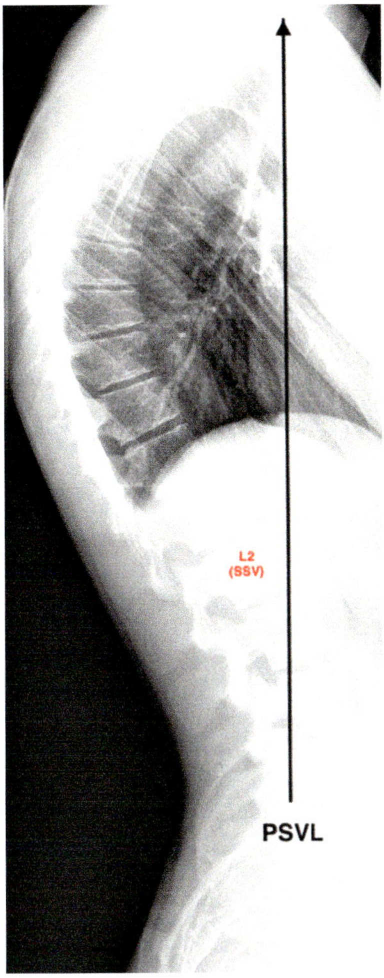

Fig. 27.4 Posterior sacral vertical line (PSVL) is drawn vertically from posterior edge of sacral endplate to identify the sagittal stable vertebra (SSV). SSV is the first vertebra from proximal that touches the PSVL. It is recommended to include SSV into instrumentation distally

27.1.3 Discussion

Indications for operative treatment of scheuermann's kyphosis are (1) progression of kyphosis despite conservative treatment, (2) painful thoracic kyphosis greater than 70–80° or thoracolumbar kyphosis greater than 40°, and (3) cosmetic issue that is not acceptable for the patient. Thoracolumbar kyphosis or angular kyphosis are more likely to be disabling and therefore are more considered for operative treatment. Conservative treatment include physiotherapy to strengthen the trunk muscles and temporary bracing to release the muscles which are overstressed by keeping the spine straight. If patients are skeletally immature bracing is considered to correct the deformity. In our case, the puberty vocal change occurred 2 years ago which indicates that puberty growth spurt is passed. X-ray of pelvic crest (Risser sign) or elbow may deliver more information about further growth potential.

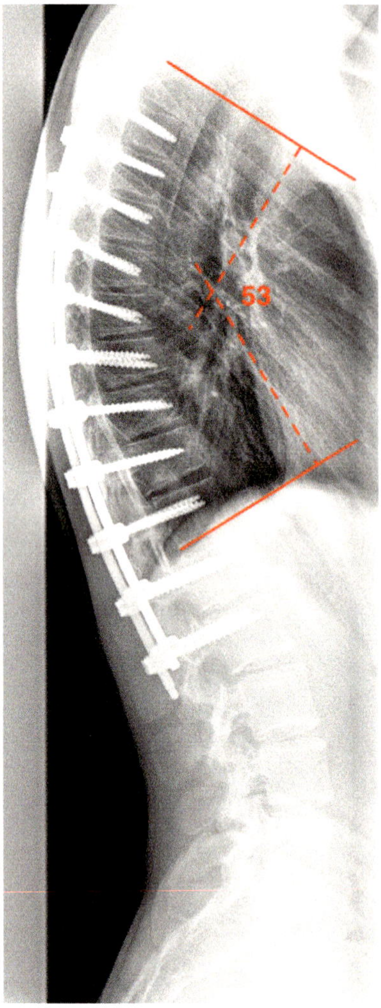

Fig. 27.5 Lateral view x-ray of spine after the operation shows correction of thoracic kyphosis to 53°

Mature skeletal system and absence of back pain do not necessitate conservative treatment options. In literature, the indication for operative treatment of scheuermann kyphosis is controversially discussed due to the natural history of the deformity. There are two studies reporting about natural history by long term follow up of patients with scheuermann kyphosis [1, 2]. Both have shown that patients with scheuermann kyphosis claim more frequently about back pain but the daily life was not significantly affected by the deformity. Limitation of cardiopulmonary function was only observed with severe thoracic kyphosis greater than 100°. These factors and risks of operation should be discussed with patient if operative treatment is considered.

One of the complications by the operative treatment is the junctional kyphosis adjacent to the instrumented spine. One study reported that proximal junctional kyphosis occurred more often than distal but distal junctional kyphosis was more often associated with symptoms and re-operation [3]. It was shown that proximal junctional kyphosis occurred when instrumentation of spine was short to proximal end vertebra of kyphosis and the deformity was overcorrected. To prevent proximal junctional kyphosis, it is recommended to correct less than 50% of the deformity. Other study reported about the occurrence of distal junctional kyphosis and suggested to extend the instrumentation to the sagittal stable vertebra [4]. The sagittal stable vertebra was defined as the first vertebra from proximal which touches the posterior sacral vertical line. According to these data, it is crucial to determine the extent of instrumentation preoperatively. The inclusion of the upper end vertebra of kyphosis proximally and the sagittal stable vertebra distally is recommended.

All studies reporting about results of operative treatment of scheuermann kyphosis have low level of evidence. All of them were retrospectively performed and the surgical techniques used were not uniform, including posterior only or combined anterior-posterior procedures with different implant materials as with hooks or with modern pedicle screw instrumentation. Long term results of operative correction are lacking. There is no data comparing the natural history of scheuermann kyphosis with the results of operative correction.

27.1.4 Conclusions and Take Home Message

The knowledge of natural history of scheuermann kyphosis is very important and should be considered in the process of decision making.

Operative treatment is considered when (1) progression of the deformity is observed, (2) pain is not controlled despite of conservative treatment, and (3) cosmetic issue is not acceptable for the patient.

According to data available, it is recommended to include the upper end vertebra of the kyphosis proximally and the sagittal stable vertebra distally in the instrumentation to avoid junctional kyphosis.

27.2 Case 2: Ankylosing Spondylitis

27.2.1 Introduction

This case presents a young woman 29 years old with ankylosing spondylitis. Clinical features, radiological evaluation, decision making of treatment options and surgical procedures are presented.

27.2.2 Case Description

Young woman claims about back pain in lumbar area since over one year. Pain disappears during rest and increases with ambulation. Sometimes back pain is over the entire spine. She claims also about difficulty to stand upright and to get horizontal gaze. She feels more convenient holding the buggy during walking. She has continuous pain medication with ibuprofen. There was trauma in the history.

The physical examination reveals forward shift of the trunk and bended knees to compensate the arcuar thoracic hyperkyphosis. Percussion over the upper part of lumbar spine is painful, range of motion of the spine is strongly limited and painful. There is little change in thoracic circumference after deep inspiration and expiration. Examination of hip joints shows full range of motion without any limitation. The truncal flexed deformity did not change as the patient was sitting or lying in supine position. Neurologic examination reveals no deficits.

X-ray imaging of whole spine in ap and lateral view was performed in standing position (Fig. 27.6). Lumbar spine is straight without any lordosis. The thoracic kyphosis is 80°. Pelvis is

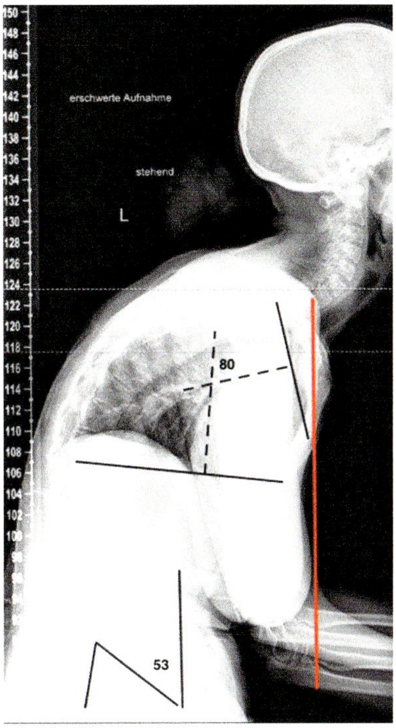

Fig. 27.6 Lateral view x-ray of whole spine in standing position prior to the operation. Plump line is red, pelvic tilt is 53° and thoracic kyphosis is 80°

rotated backward with almost vertical sacrum. Pelvic tilt amounts over 50° and sacral slope is almost horizontally. Plump line is far anterior to the femoral head axis. CT scan of the spine showed ossification of facet joints throughout the spine and of costotransversal joints (Fig. 27.7). Anterior longitudinal ligament was ossified only in the midthoracic spine (Fig. 27.8). A discontinuation of dorsal ossification was recognized at L2/3 level. At this level, the facet joints were not fused.

Based on clinical and radiological features, ankylosing spondylitis (AS) was supposed as the diagnosis. In contrast to typical AS patients, in our case pain increased during daily activity and disappeared with rest. Further, pain was not localized on the sacroiliac joint but on the upper part of the lumbar spine corresponding to the site, where the dorsal ossification was discontinued and facet joints were open. A x-ray guided infiltration of the facet joints with local anesthesia resulted in an almost complete pain relief for few hours.

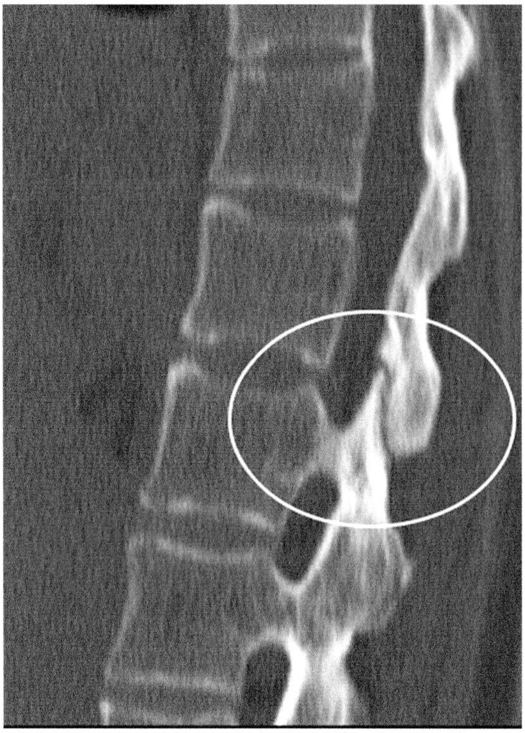

Fig. 27.7 CT scan of lumbar spine shows fusion of facet joints, open disc space and discontinuation of posterior ossification al level L2/3

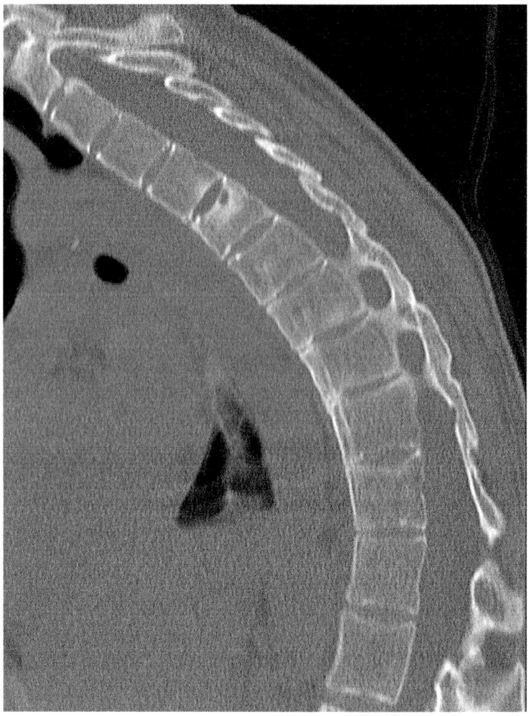

Fig. 27.8 CT scan of thoracic spine shows ossification also of disc space and of anterior longitudinal ligament

In this case, two problems were to be addressed: (1) painful mobility of level L2/3 and (2) the sagittal imbalance of the trunk. Thus, surgical treatment was recommended to achieve fusion of L2/3 and to correct the sagittal deformity by a modified wedge osteotomy (Smith-Petersen osteotomy).

The operation was performed through a posterior-only approach with a single level Smith-Petersen osteotomy at L2/3 and posterior segmental pedicle screw instrumentation 3 segments above and below the osteotomy. The correction was achieved by implantation of a cage in the anterior part of the L2/3 disc space and posterior compression of the pedicle screws.

The patient was mobilized immediately after the operation with physiotherapeutic support. She was very satisfied with her new posture. Postoperative x-ray control was performed in lateral and ap view in standing position (Fig. 27.9). The osteotomy led to 25° segmental angulation and the sagittal imbalance was markedly corrected.

27.2.3 Discussion

In the present case, a patient with ankylosing spondylitis (AS) was treated. The sagittal alignment was markedly imbalanced with anterior shift of the trunk and plump line anterior to the femoral head axis. The deformity consisted of fixed loss of lumbar lordosis and thoracic hyperkyphosis. Pelvic incidence was about 50°. Hip joints had neither flexion contraction nor any radiological degenerative changes. Special feature of the spine was ossification of dorsal elements with open disc space. The focus of back pain was found to be at L2/3. Thus, the main deformity was located in the thoracolumbar spine without involvement of hip joints and the source of pain was at level L2/3.

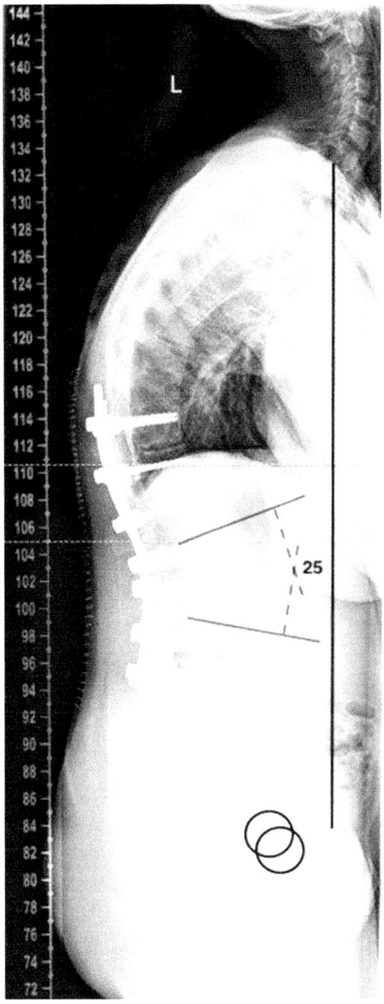

Fig. 27.9 Lateral view x-ray of whole spine in standing position after the operation. Posterior instrumentation from T12 to L5 and opening wedge osteotomy (Smith-Petersen) L2/3 with implantation of a cage anterior into the disc space. An angular lordosis of 25° was achieved at level L2/3. Plump line is markedly shifted back but still anterior to the femoral head axis

This constellation suggests that correction can be performed in the lumbar spine. An osteotomy in lumbar spine offers two advantages. The lower the osteotomy is performed in the spine, the more correction effect on flexion deformity can be achieved due to the long lever arm. Secondly, with respect to neurologic complications the osteotomy is performed distal to the conus in a safe area.

After determination of the level of osteotomy, the question arises how much correction is needed? There was high grade thoracic kyphosis and the pelvic incidence was about 50°. According to the study of Roussouly [5] pelvic incidence, which has a constant value after the end of the growth, correlates positively with lumbar lordosis. Consequently, a lumbar lordosis of about 50° is desired.

Options to correct the deformity were open wedge osteotomy (Smith-Petersen), multisegment closing wedge osteotomy (Ponte), and pedicle-subtraction osteotomy [6]. The multisegment Ponte osteotomy requires some flexibility of the spine and therefore this technique is not appropriate. Both other techniques, Smith-Petersen and pedicle-subtraction osteotomy, were able to address the deformity. Smith-Petersen osteotomy was also an option because disc space L2/3 is not completely fused. For 50° correction, osteotomy of 2 levels are necessary since a maximum correction of 30° is possible at a single level (see Chap. 26). In this case Smith-Petersen osteotomy was selected to avoid wedge resection of the vertebral body with excessive bleeding and due to the young age of the patient with healthy and flexible vessels. However, despite 2-level osteotomy, the osteotomy was performed at single level.

Postoperatively, patient was satisfied with her new posture. The postoperative x-ray in lateral view (Fig. 27.9) showed an angular correction of 25°. The plump line was markedly shifted back to the femoral head axis but was still significantly anterior to it. Thus, the correction was only partly achieved. For a complete correction, a 2-level osteotomy should have been carried out, as preoperative evaluation had suggested.

A large number of biomechanical and clinical studies are available with regard to sagittal balance of spine and corrective techniques of spine deformities. The level of evidence is, however, low due to the huge variability of patients that have been treated, the lack of controls, and retrospective methods used in all studies [7].

27.2.4 Conclusions and Take Home Message

The reconstructive surgery of ankylosing spondylitis deformity is very complex. The reduced bone quality and loss of spine flexibility expose these patients to high operation risks.

A thorough clinical and radiological evaluation is needed to determine the major component of the spine deformity, whether it is a thoracolumbar, thoracic or cervicothoracic deformity. Attention should be paid for flexion contracture of hip joints and may be treated with arthroplasty prior to correction of spine deformity.

Several surgical techniques are available to correct the deformity. Each of them has advantages and limitations that should be weighed out in the process of surgical decision making.

Pearls

- Surgical correction of scheuermann kyphosis with pedicle screw instrumentation and multilevel Ponte osteotomies can be performed with posterior only approach
- The whole deformity of scheuermann kyphosis is to be included in the instrumentation with the lowest vertebra touching the posterior sacral vertical line
- Avoid overcorrection to prevent proximal junctional kyphosis
- The correction of rigid deformity of the spine with ankylosing spondylitis requires three-column osteotomy techniques
- Poor bone quality in ankylosing spondylitis is the challenging point in the surgical treatment of this disease. Multiple level instrumentation, at least 3 levels above and below the osteotomy site, is suggested to avoid failure of instrumentation

Editorial Comment

The risk of neurological complications in the correction of kyphotic deformities is even higher then in scoliotic cases. Therefore neuromonitoring in corrections especially in the thoracic spine is strongly recommended.

Performing the correction, after the osteotomy is made, the procedure should be assisted by tilted the operating table instead inducing the force for correction just by compression on the pedicle screws.

References

1. Murray PM, Weinstein SL, Spratt KF. The natural history and long-term follow-up of scheuermann kyphosis. J Bone Joint Surg Am. 1993;75(2):236–48.
2. Ristolainen L, Kettunen JA, Heliövaara M, Kujala UM, Heinonen A, Schlenzka D. Untreated scheuermann's disease: a 37-year follow-up study. Eur Spine J. 2012;21:819–24.
3. Lonner BS, Newton P, Betz R, Scharf C, O'Brien M, Sponseller P, Lenke L, Crawford A, Lowe T, Letko L, Harms J, Shufflebarger H. Operative management of scheuermann's kyphosis in 78 patients. Spine. 2007;32(24):2644–52.
4. Cho KJ, Lenke LG, Bridwell KH, Kamiya M, Sides B. Selektion of the optimal distal fusion level in posterior instrumentation and fusion for thoracic hyperkyphosis. The sagital stable vertebra concept. Spine. 2009;34(8):765–70.
5. Roussouly P, Gollogly S, Berthonnaud E, Dimmet J. Classification of the normal variation in the sagittal alignment of the human lumbar spine and pelvis in the standing position. Spine. 2005;30(3):346–53.
6. Bridwell KH. Decision making regarding Smith-Petersen vs. pedicle substraction osteotomy vs. vertebral column resection for spinal deformity. Spine. 2006;31(19):S171–8.
7. Kim KT, Park KJ, Lee JH. Osteotomy of the spine to correct the spinal deformity. Asian Spine J. 2009;3(2):113–23.

Surgical Correction and Special Features in Traumatic and Congenital Kyphotic Deformities

28

Sleiman Haddad, Antonia Matamalas, and Ferran Pellisé

28.1 Introduction

The term kyphosis is derived from Greek and is used to describe a "hump". As the word implies, in spine, it is used for sagittal spinal curves with anterior concavity. The normal spine has two areas physiologically aligned in kyphosis: the thoracic spine and the sacrum. Pathological kyphosis can be found in any part of the spine and can be due to a variety of etiologies including congenital or developmental anomalies, trauma, infection, inflammatory diseases or degenerative disc disease among others. It therefore can affect any age group.

Congenital kyphosis is usually caused by anterior formation defect or segmentation failure. This form of anterior tethering in a growing spine can cause a progressive deformity. Severity of the resultant deformity varies according to type of defect, location and the number of affected vertebrae. Not only the deformity can cause a sagittal malalignment and imbalance, in severe cases it can result in neurological cord compression. Surgical treatment in congenital kyphosis is recommended for significant, progressive and unstable deformities to restore normal sagittal alignment, prevent sagittal imbalance and preserve neurological structures.

Most symptomatic posttraumatic kyphotic deformities occur at the thoracolumbar junction. They are mainly caused by a loss of the anterior vertebral column height or support. Indications for surgical treatment in these cases are correction of the deformity, neurological decompression and stabilization of the injury in acute cases. In installed deformities, the main objective of surgery would be to correct the resulting sagittal malalignment.

In this chapter, we will be presenting a clinical case of each etiology and discuss the rationale for treatment of kyphotic deformity in these scenarios. We will be reviewing the various surgical techniques available for each case, guide the reader through the decision making and discuss other relevant considerations.

28.2 Case Description

28.2.1 Congenital Kyphosis Case

An 18-month child was referred to our clinics with a progressive angular kyphosis in thoracolumbar area. Clinical exam revealed a partially flexible thoracolumbar hump with no associated neurological abnormalities. Full-body standing X-Rays showed a congenital spine dislocation with a segmental kyphosis measuring 52° between

S. Haddad · A. Matamalas · F. Pellisé (✉)
Department of Orthopaedic Surgery, Spine Unit, University Hospital Vall d'Hebron, Barcelona, Spain
e-mail: 24361fpu@comb.cat

B. Meyer, M. Rauschmann (eds.), *Spine Surgery*, https://doi.org/10.1007/978-3-319-98875-7_28

T10-L2 (Fig. 28.1). CT scan showed an hypoplasia of L1 vertebral body with dysplasia of posterior facets and T10-L2 kyphotic deformity of 38° (Fig. 28.2). Facet joints could be seen clearly dislocated bilaterally. A small rotational component was also present. MRI of the whole spine confirmed an angular kyphosis due to a formation defect of L1 vertebral body (type 1). There was no cord compression or myelopathy nor other associated intracanal abnormalities (Fig. 28.3). We recommended surgery in his case due to the severity of the deformity and the high risk of progression and neurological impairment. The patient was operated on at 20 months of age. Through a midline posterior approach, the spine was subperiosteally exposed and 3.5 mm (cervical) pedicle screws were bilaterally inserted from T11 to L3 while skipping L1. We then proceeded to perform

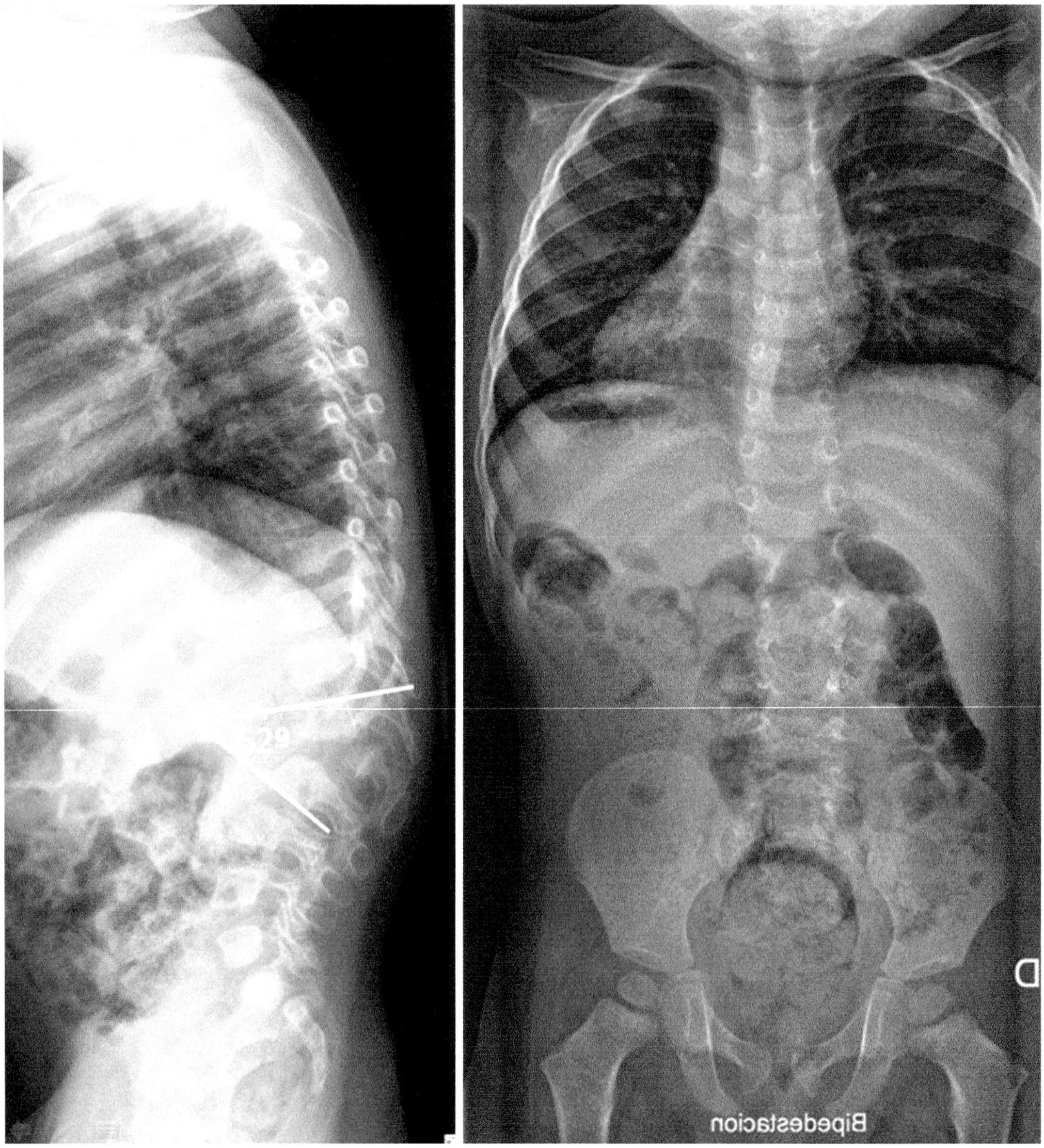

Fig. 28.1 AP and lateral X-rays of a 18 month old toddler with a congenital L1 kyphosis and dislocation. Regional kyphosis measured 52° and the T12-L1 facet joints were clearly dislocated

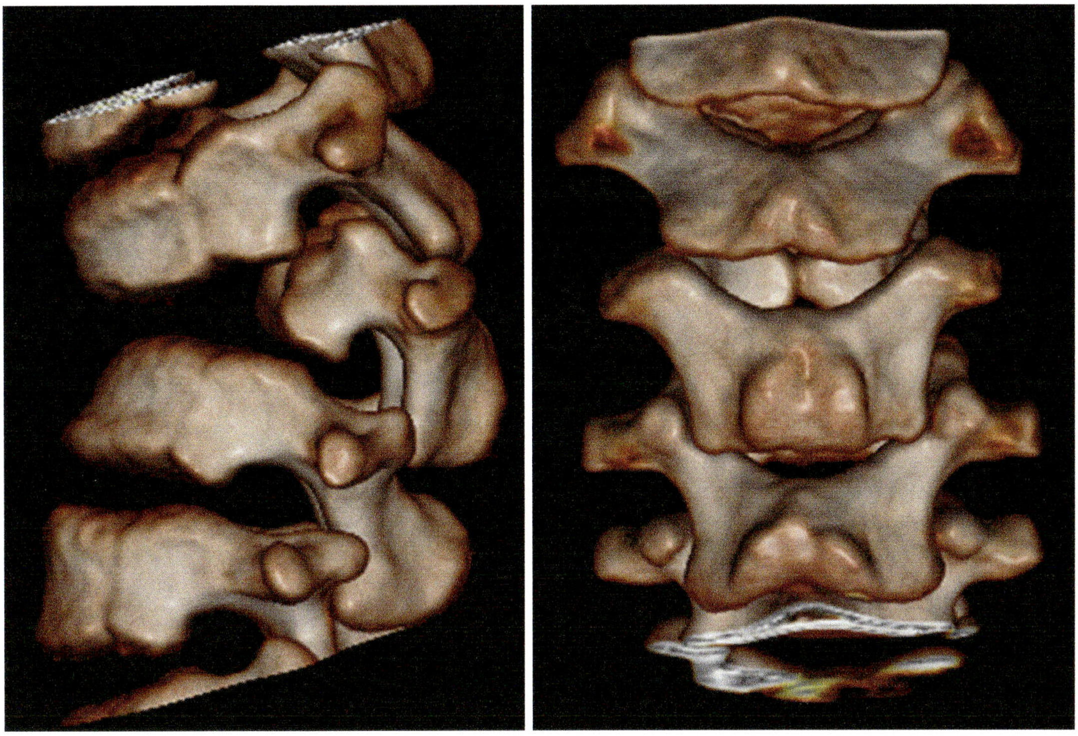

Fig. 28.2 3D reconstruction of the CT scan showing a relatively preserved posterior arch with dysplastic and naked facets and a regional kyphosis of 38°

a posterior vertebral column resection (PVCR) of the L1 including the discs above and below. Progressive stepwise correction of the deformity was performed under neuromonitoring, anterior column reconstruction was done with a mesh cage impacted with local bone graft. Final construct was done with physiologically aligned rods tightened under compression. A rigid thoracolumbar orthosis was prescribed after surgery until fusion was achieved. 2 years after surgery he had a very satisfactory course with complete fusion and no recurrence of the deformity (Fig. 28.4).

28.2.2 Postraumatic Deformity Case

A 61 year-old female was referred to our clinics for surgical assessment. She refers a fall from her own height 8 months prior to presentation when she was diagnosed with an L1 fracture. She was initially treated conservatively with an external rigid brace for 3 months. Unfortunately she progressively developed a disabling severe low back pain that did not respond to conservative treatment. On clinical examination she had a thoracolumbar kyphosis but seemed to conserve a fair sagittal balance. Her deformity was rigid and did not correct on forced extension nor when she laid down. Her neurological assessment was unremarkable.

Whole spine standing films showed a consolidated L1 fracture with a resultant regional kyphosis of 38° (Fig. 28.5). She however could maintain a sacral vertical axis (SVA) of 5.4 cm at the expenses of a hyperextension of the lower lumbar spine (L2-S1 Lordosis 71°, L4-S1 65°). The pelvis was retroverted (PT 20°, SS 31° for PI of 50°, GT 35°). Her GAP score was 9. In summary, the patient presented with a Type II sagittal imbalance due to a fracture in thoracolumbar area. The deformity was fixed and angular over the L1. Surgery was prescribed due to the severity of her symptoms and deformity. Taking into account the fixed and angular nature of the deformity, the thoracolumbar location and the shape of the deformed

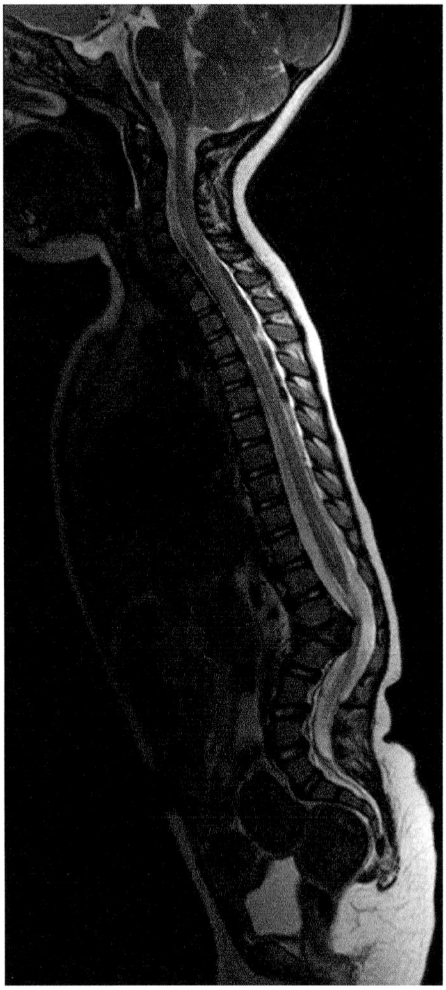

Fig. 28.3 Mid-sagittal cut of a of a T2 weighted whole spine MRI ruling out any neurological compression, myelopathy or intracanal malformation

vertebra with significant loss of anterior vertebral body height, we opted for a PVCR. For this purpose, we resected the wedged L1 vertebral body including the discs above and below to reconstruct segmental morphology, restore anterior column support and enhance fusion. We reconstructed the anterior column using a carbon-fiber cage with local bone graft. Posterior stabilization was achieved with cemented pedicle screws from T5 to L3. By extending to T5 we avoided ending the instrumentation at the thoracic natural apex, therefore, preventing possible Proximal Junctional Kyphosis (PJK). Intraoperative imaging confirmed the appropriate placement of the spinal anchors and adequate sagittal alignment reconstruction of the thoracolumbar junction. Prophylactic vertebroplasty was performed in the first vertebrae above and below the instrumentation to prevent further fractures at these levels. Local and homologous bone grafts were placed over the decorticated posterior elements to further enhance fusion. Intraoperative neuromonitoring was unaltered throughout surgery. The patient did not have any major intraoperative nor perioperative complications. Four years after surgery her pain and disability had improved significantly. She was well aligned, (SVA 2 cm, GT 16°, LL 51°, L4-S1 38°, SS 34°, PT 16°, GAP 1 for age) and the T12-L2 kyphosis measured 1° (Fig. 28.6).

28.3 Discussion of the Cases

The treatment of severe fixed angular kyphotic deformity presents a technical challenge to the spinal surgeon. It requires a proper understanding of the deformity and the resulting compensatory mechanisms as well as mastery of the osteotomy techniques.

Congenital kyphosis is due to defect of formation, of segmentation or both. Segmentation defects involve more than 2 vertebrae and usually result in a regular deformity. It is usually detected in the adolescent age group, has a small progression potential due to its late development and does not cause any direct threat to neurological elements. Defects of formation are more common and usually occur over a single level, although multiple level involvements have been well described. Progression is the rule in these cases and the risk of neurological compromise is of special concern. The congenital dislocated spine has been defined as the potentially most serious form of congenital kyphosis with an abrupt single-level sagittal displacement of the spinal canal [2]. The facet joints are often hypoplastic and/or dislocated. Progression to neurological injury is almost universal. Neurological impairments may rarely be noted at birth or may develop later in about 10–12% of cases of congenital kyphosis, mainly during adolescence [3]. In congenital dislocation, neurological injury occurs much earlier. Consequently, congeni-

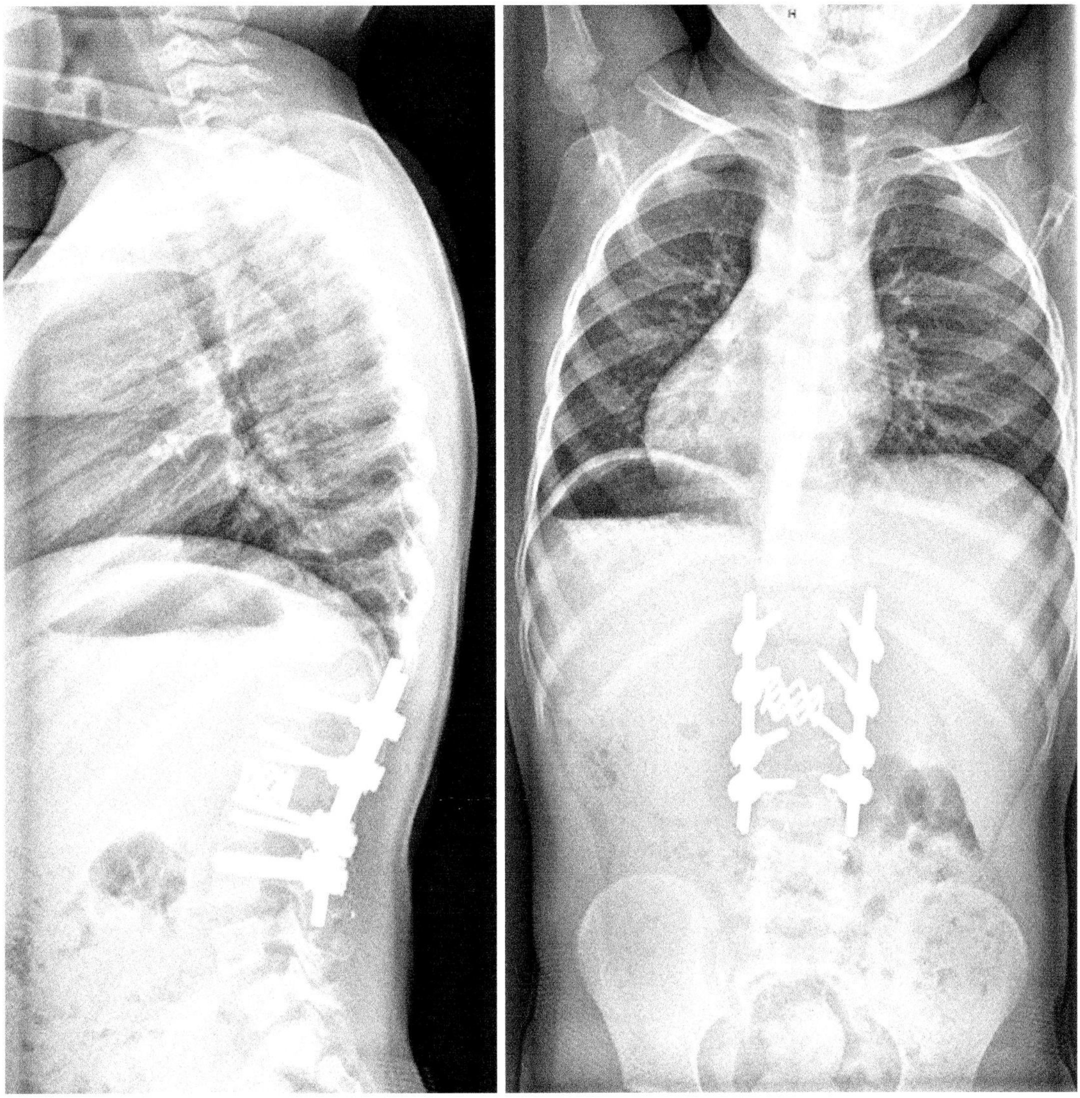

Fig. 28.4 2 year postoperative AP and lateral X-rays showing satisfactory reconstruction of the thoracolumbar junction

tal dislocation is a surgical urgency that requires early stabilization. There is no established age at which it can be approached, and therefore should be treated as early as possible.

Established posttraumatic kyphotic deformities on the other hand do not usually progress overtime. In addition, the neurological injury is sustained with the initial trauma and rarely – if any- develops overtime. A notable exception might be Kummell's pseudoarthrosis where a deficient anterior support can lead to deformity progression, fatigue of the posterior elements, local instability and in extreme cases, neurological compromise.

Surgical indications and goals of treatment vary between both groups. In congenital deformity, the indications are mainly deformity progression and neurological compromise. Therefore the objectives are to halt the progression, restore the physiological alignment and protect neurological structures. These objectives should be achieved with corrections over as few segments as possible to allow for growth. The correction should also be

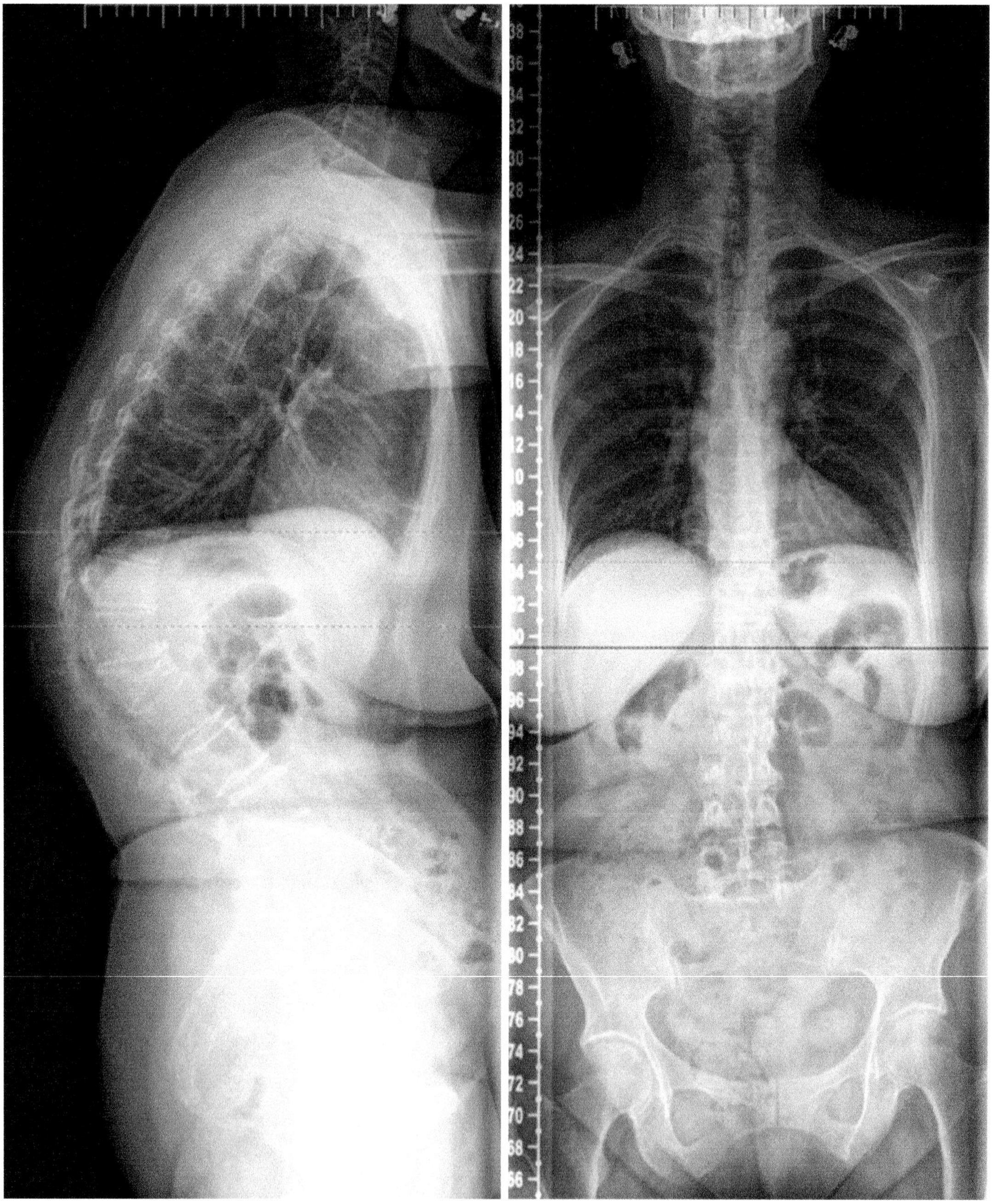

Fig. 28.5 AP and lateral standing whole spine xrays of a 61-year-old lady with sagittal malalignment due to an L1 osteoporotic fracture healed with residual regional kyphosis measuring 41°

maintained throughout growth and patients should graduate in an acceptable state. On the other hand, patients with traumatic kyphosis complain of gross deformity, or from pain and disability secondary to an altered sagittal alignment. Goals of treatment in this group include restoring a balanced and harmonious sagittal alignment by correcting the local kyphosis and eliminating the compensatory curves, achieving solid fusion.

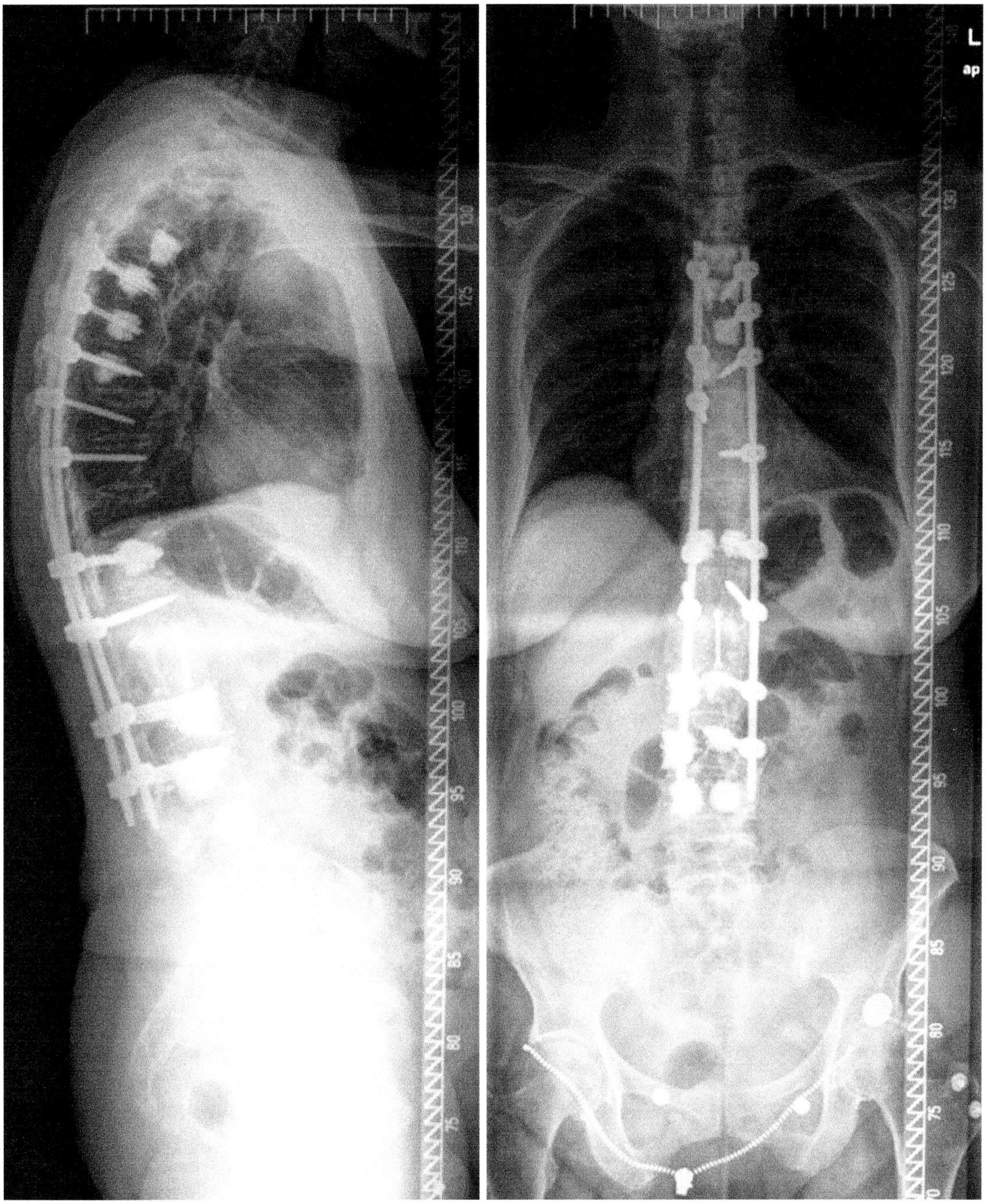

Fig. 28.6 4 years postoperative AP and lateral x-rays. The patient maintained a satisfactory sagittal alignment and had no subsequent junctional failure or new fracture

The initial workup always includes a whole spine standing X-rays to assess global spine sagittal alignment. The main driver is usually the congenital malformation or the traumatic injury. In both groups it is usually angular and can be stiff or fixed. Compensatory mechanisms, generally include recruitment of adjacent segments, mainly flattening the thoracic spine above the kyphosis and/or increasing the lumbar lordosis. When these are not enough, the pelvis is retroverted in an effort to bring the center of gravity backward towards the sacrum. If these mechanisms fail, the patient then recruits the knees. When all available compensatory mechanisms have been exhausted the patient develops a positive sagittal imbalance [4]. Measuring the SVA or the global tilt can help the surgeon assess the global alignment. Global tilt is independent of patient's position and does not need any calibration of the x-ray [5]. Flexibility can be assessed during clinical encounter or by using a flexion extension xray, or supine xrays over bolsters. Also, comparing standing xrays to supine scans (either MRI or CT) can be helpful. The deformity can be either: (1) totally flexible; (2) partially flexible or (3) fixed [6].

Additional workup includes a CT scan to assess bony anatomy and flexibility. It assists the surgeon in his decision-making and surgical planning. An MRI scan is also in order whenever a neurological injury is suspected or as part of initial workup in patients with congenital deformities. Clinical manifestations of intracanal abnormalities are frequently initially absent and up to 30% of patients with congenital vertebral anomalies have intraspinal malformations detectable by MRI. These include tethered cord, diastematomyelia, diplomyelia, and syringomyelia. Some of these might alter the surgical plan. Finally, an MRI scan also can detect occult concomitant vertebral malformation at other levels.

There is no role for bracing in congenital dislocation and traction has been associated with paraplegia. Segmentation defects can be treated differently depending on the magnitude of the deformity and whether or not correction is desired. In small deformities detected early, a short posterior fusion might suffice. Instrumentation can be avoided especially in younger patients. If the deformity is significant, the surgeon can opt for multiple anterior releases or vertebral column resection, depending on the magnitude of the deformity and the number of involved vertebrae. The use of posterior instrumentation and closing under compression is advised. However, if the patient is too small for instrumentation, a hyperextension cast could be used. Our case shows that instrumented fusion is possible at very early ages using small diameter screws. In defects of formation with kyphosis smaller than 50°, and if the deformity is detected very early, an isolated posterior fusion or tethering can suffice. These deformities are partially flexible and amenable to reduction under compression. Again, fusion can be instrumented or using local grafting techniques and extension bracing. In these cases, a second surgery might be needed to increase fusion rates. Avoiding instrumentation, Winter and Moe reported satisfactory outcomes in 12/17 patients (71%) younger than 5 years [7]. If the deformity is greater than 50° and the vertebral body is very hypoplasic, vertebral resection is recommended. This can be done through a staged anterior/posterior approach or through an all-posterior approach. Authors recommend PCVR as it allows for a better control of the deformity and neurological elements while decreasing surgical and anesthetic times as well as additional morbidities from two surgeries. The anterior column can be reconstructed using a structural graft such as a rib or a fibula, or using a mesh cage.

Whereas a flexible deformity distributed over various segments can be treated with posterior column osteotomies, the mainstay of treatment of severe and rigid angular kyphosis is surgical correction using three column osteotomies. This is specially true in posttraumatic deformities. Several three-column osteotomy techniques have been described, where a circumferential excision of one or more vertebral bodies is performed, through a combined anterior-posterior or a sole posterior approach. As evidence regarding the safety and feasibility of three column spinal osteotomies has increased and instrumentation has become more reliable and powerful (e.g., thoracic pedicle screws vs. hooks or hybrid constructs), more patients have been treated via a single posterior surgical approach aimed at one or more apical kyphotic vertebrae. Despite being circumferential posterior osteotomies, the primary difference of PVCR versus the pedicle subtraction osteotomy (PSO) is that with PVCR both the spinal cord and the impinging wedge fragment are identified under direct vision from the lateral side, thus allowing for confirmation of complete decompression. Therefore, PVCR can be safely performed at the level of the cord and more than one vertebrae can be excised. This provides the powerful translation and shortening necessary to correct great rigid deformities. Therefore, PVCR can offer better control of angular deformities than PSO [8]. The amount of correction achieved by PSO is limited to anatomical constrains. PSO in lumbar adult spine can achieve a 25–30° [6, 9]. The amount of correction obtained in the pediatric population is much less due to the smaller size of the vertebral body and smaller pedicular wedge. In the thoracic spine PSOs are less frequently indicated [6]. Moreover, authors do not recommend PSOs in the context of a traumatic wedged vertebra. First of all, the amount of correction is less, as the superior cut can only be parallel to the superior endplate and therefore following the wedged angle. In addition it is technically challenging to follow the superior endplate without breaching it or damaging it. Finally, a PSO in the context of a wedged vertebra results in a flattened and shortened vertebral body between two mobile discs, which increases significantly the pseudoarthrosis rate. Although shortening of the cord is considered safe, too much shortening may be dangerous. On the other hand, with PVCR the amount of correction is only limited by the spinal cord and PVCR restores the height of the anterior column.

Up to date, there is no enough literature comparing advantages of PVCR compared with staged anterior-posterior osteotomies (APVCR). Nevertheless, anterior transthoracic procedures have gradually fallen out of favor because of several factors, mainly due to the difficulties in approaching the concavity of the angular kyphosis in deformities greater than 60°. Correction by pure distraction of the anterior column can cause severe stretching of the spinal cord. Irrespective of whether they are staged or performed as a single procedure, combined anterior-posterior procedures are a major surgical undertaking and the associated medical and surgical morbidity can be considerable. Theoretically PVCR has a number of advantages over APVCR: reduction of operative time and blood loss, maintenance of spinal stability and neurological control throughout the whole procedure, more reliable reconstruction of spinal column, less postoperative morbidity and more effective corrections. However, more recent literature did not find any significant differences in blood loss or complication rate between both approaches [9]. Surgical time, surgery through a single approach and anesthestic time as well as full simultaneous control of the deformity and the spinal cord still favor PVCR.

Cancellous bone graft is traditionally used at the site of VCR, anterior column reconstruction may be done with strut grafts or cages. In patients with weak bone, we prefer to reconstruct the anterior column with carbon fiber cages that have big footprint. A larger footprint distributes the load more homogenously, recruits the lateral cortices of the adjacent vertebral bodies and decreases the loading pressure. This would ultimately decrease the rate of subsidence that might be encountered with mesh cages.

During the surgical correction of the deformity, rods are sequentially exchanged after the osteotomy or can be bent in situ. The surgeon should have excellent visual control of the cord during this stage and it is highly advisable to have spinal cord monitoring. These are essential to ensure the safety of the technique. The authors recommend for the routine use of IONM including assessment of both motor and sensory tracts, free-run electromyography and nerve root testing.

Somatosensory evoked potential (SEP) monitoring alone is known to reduce post-operative paraplegia by 50–60% but paraplegia can still occur without SEP warning, most of the times due to anterior spinal artery syndrome, which only affects the vascular territory of the anterolateral column of the spinal cord. Spinal cord perfusion may be compromised even at normal systemic blood pressure when intraoperative mechanical stress is applied to neural tissue. The introduction of motor evoked potentials (MEP) has allowed for monitoring the corticospinal tracts (CT) individually, with changes correlating highly with post-surgical neurological outcomes. Muscle motor evoked potentials triggered by transcranial electrical stimulation (Tc-MEP, mMEP) evaluate the function and the flux of motor outputs from motor cortex, CT, nerve roots, and peripheral nerves. Tc-MEPs have a reported sensitivity of 75–100% and specificity of 84–100% for the detection of iatrogenic motor deficits. Most of the permanent spinal cord injuries are thought to be associated with changes to the blood supply of the thoracic cord. Excessive traction or shortening of the cord during deformity reduction as well as mechanical impingement can also cause permanent damage if left unrevised. Except for vascular insult, MEPs can point out more precisely the moment that spinal cord is stressed in PVCR and thus allowing for correction to be reversed to the state immediately before any changes in potentials. Transient nerve root injury however remains the most common neurologic complication in PVCR. To avoid neurological complications, common strategies include maintaining blood supply to the spinal cord by preserving the neurovascular bundle on one side and also avoiding hypotensive anesthesia.

Wound infection and/or hematoma after these types of procedure are also a major concern and can affect between 5% and 10% of the cases. They may be prevented with meticulous technique and optimal nutritional status.

28.4 Conclusions and Take Home Message

Including Pearls and Pitfalls

Both of our cases were sharp, angular deformities in thoracolumbar area. In the congenital kyphosis, posterior vertebral column resection and replacement of the insufficiently formed vertebral body was considered the best option to correct the deformity, restore segmental anterior column support and achieve long-lasting circumferential fusion. In the posttraumatic deformity case, we chose PVCR over PSO for two main reasons. Firstly, the magnitude of the correction needed over a single segment could be better achieved with VCR. Secondly, authors prefer VCR to PSO when the vertebral body is significantly wedged and discs above and below are mobile. A PSO in these cases can easily violate the remaining endplates and leave a "floating" osteotomized vertebral body with a high risk of pseudoarthrosis and mechanical failure.

References

1. Pellise F, Vila-Casademunt A, European Spine Study G. Posterior thoracic osteotomies. Eur J Orthop Surg Traumatol: Orthop Traumatol. 2014;24(Suppl 1):S39–48.
2. Zeller RD, Ghanem I, Dubousset J. The congenital dislocated spine. Spine. 1996;21(10):1235–40.
3. Winter RB, Moe JH, Wang JF. Congenital kyphosis. Its natural history and treatment as observed in a study of one hundred and thirty patients. J Bone Joint Surg Am. 1973;55(2):223–56.
4. Barrey C, Roussouly P, Le Huec JC, D'Acunzi G, Perrin G. Compensatory mechanisms contributing to keep the sagittal balance of the spine. Eur Spine J. 2013;22(Suppl 6):S834–41.
5. Obeid I, Boissiere L, Yilgor C, Larrieu D, Pellise F, Alanay A, et al. Global tilt: a single parameter incorporating spinal and pelvic sagittal parameters and least affected by patient positioning. Eur Spine J. 2016;25(11):3644–9.
6. Bridwell KH. Decision making regarding Smith-Petersen vs. pedicle subtraction osteotomy vs. vertebral column resection for spinal deformity. Spine. 2006;31(19 Suppl):S171–8.
7. Winter RBMJ, Lonstein JE. A review of family histories in patients with congenital spinal deformities. Orthop Trans. 1983;7:32.
8. Papadopoulos EC, Boachie-Adjei O, Hess WF, Sanchez Perez-Grueso FJ, Pellise F, Gupta M, et al. Early outcomes and complications of posterior vertebral column resection. Spine J. 2015;15(5):983–91.
9. Saifi C, Laratta JL, Petridis P, Shillingford JN, Lehman RA, Lenke LG. Vertebral column resection for rigid spinal deformity. Glob Spine J. 2017;7(3):280–90.

Part IV

Basic Module 4: Spinal Fractures

Epidemiology & Classification 29

Matti Scholz and Frank Kandziora

29.1 Introduction

In Germany annually, about 500,000 people of all ages are injured. It is estimated that about around 10,000 people suffer from a relevant injury to the spine. Approximately 70% of these relevant spinal injuries are located in the thoracic and lumbar spine. As high biomechanical loads occur due to the transition from the rigid thorax to the flexible lumbar spine a high percentage of fractures are located in the thoracolumbar junction.

Most spinal fractures are compression fractures involving exclusively the anterior column. Due to severe flexion or extension moments, anterior and/or posterior lesions of the tension band are possible. Finally, the combination of translational, distraction and/or rotational forces might lead to complex fracture dislocations.

Injuries to the spine can be easily and reliably classified using the AOSpine Injury Classification System (Fig. 29.1) [1]. Furthermore, the AOSpine Severity Score (AOSIS) might support the treating physician whether to treat a spinal fracture operatively or conservatively [2, 3].

This chapter will outline the specifics of diagnosing a traumatic thoracolumbar fracture, appropriate fracture classification using the AOSpine Injury Classification System and choosing the appropriate treatment strategy by using the AOSpine Severity Score (AOSIS). At the end of this chapter the reader should be able to classify different spinal fractures according to the morphology, the neurological status and potentially existing treatment modifiers.

The presented case was selected to show different fracture morphologies in a polytraumatized patient. This case will detail the algorithm to analyze spinal fractures to select the proper classification and treatment for each fracture.

29.2 Case Description

A 45 years old female was injured during a suicidal jump from the third floor of a building, due to a medical induced psychosis. After initial treatment and stabilization on scene she was transferred to a nearby local hospital. After X-ray diagnosis and detection of multiple spinal fractures (Fig. 29.2), patient was transferred by helicopter to our hospital. Therefore she arrived approximately 2.5 h after the initial trauma at our Emergency Room.

M. Scholz (✉) · F. Kandziora
Zentrum für Wirbelsäulenchirurgie und Neurotraumatologie, Berufsgenossenschaftliche Unfallklinik Frankfurt am Main, Frankfurt am Main, Germany
e-mail: matti.scholz@bgu-frankfurt.de

B. Meyer, M. Rauschmann (eds.), *Spine Surgery*, https://doi.org/10.1007/978-3-319-98875-7_29

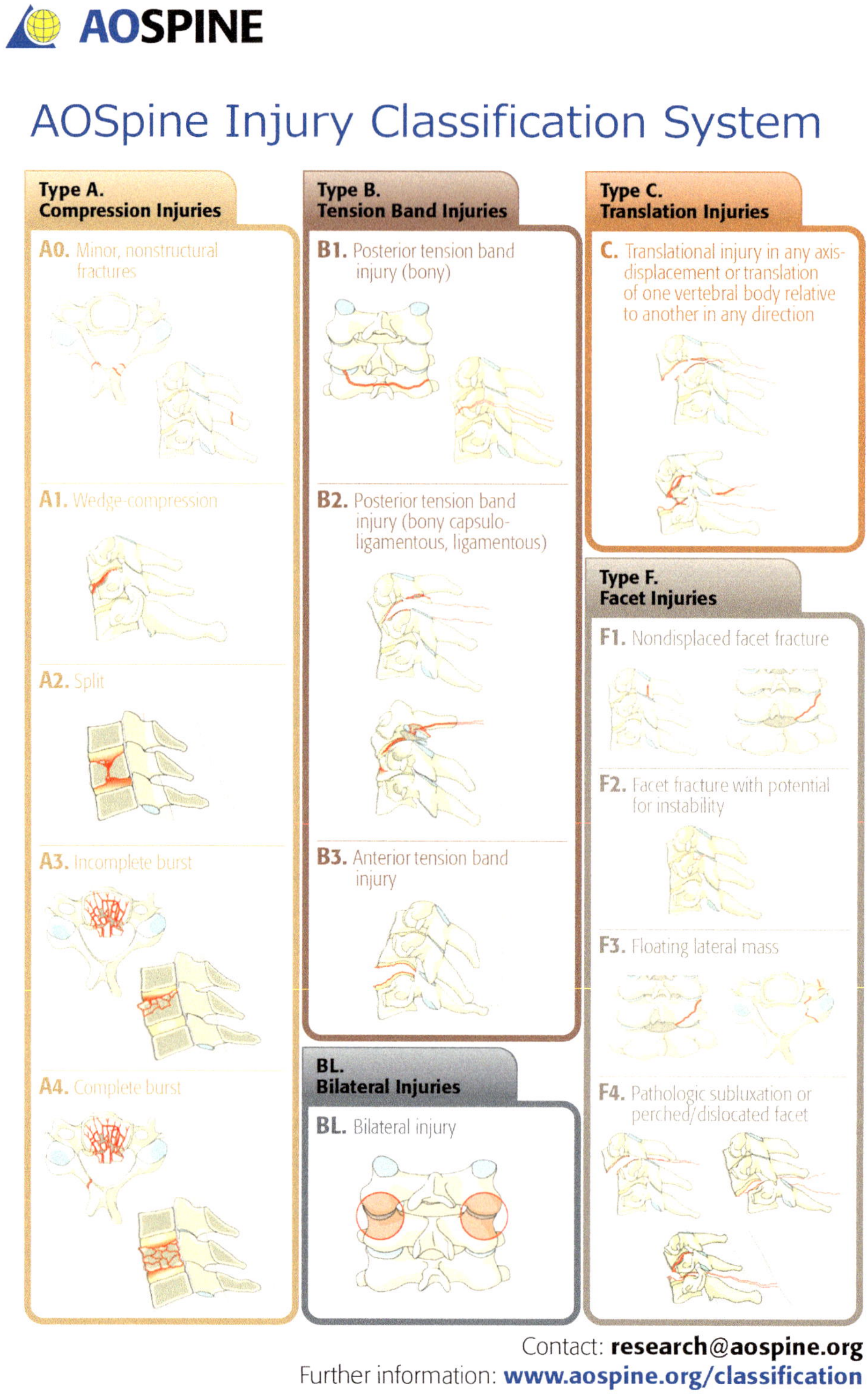

Fig. 29.1 Thoracolumbar AOSpine Injury Classification System and algorithm for morphologic classification

AOSPINE

AOSpine Injury Classification System

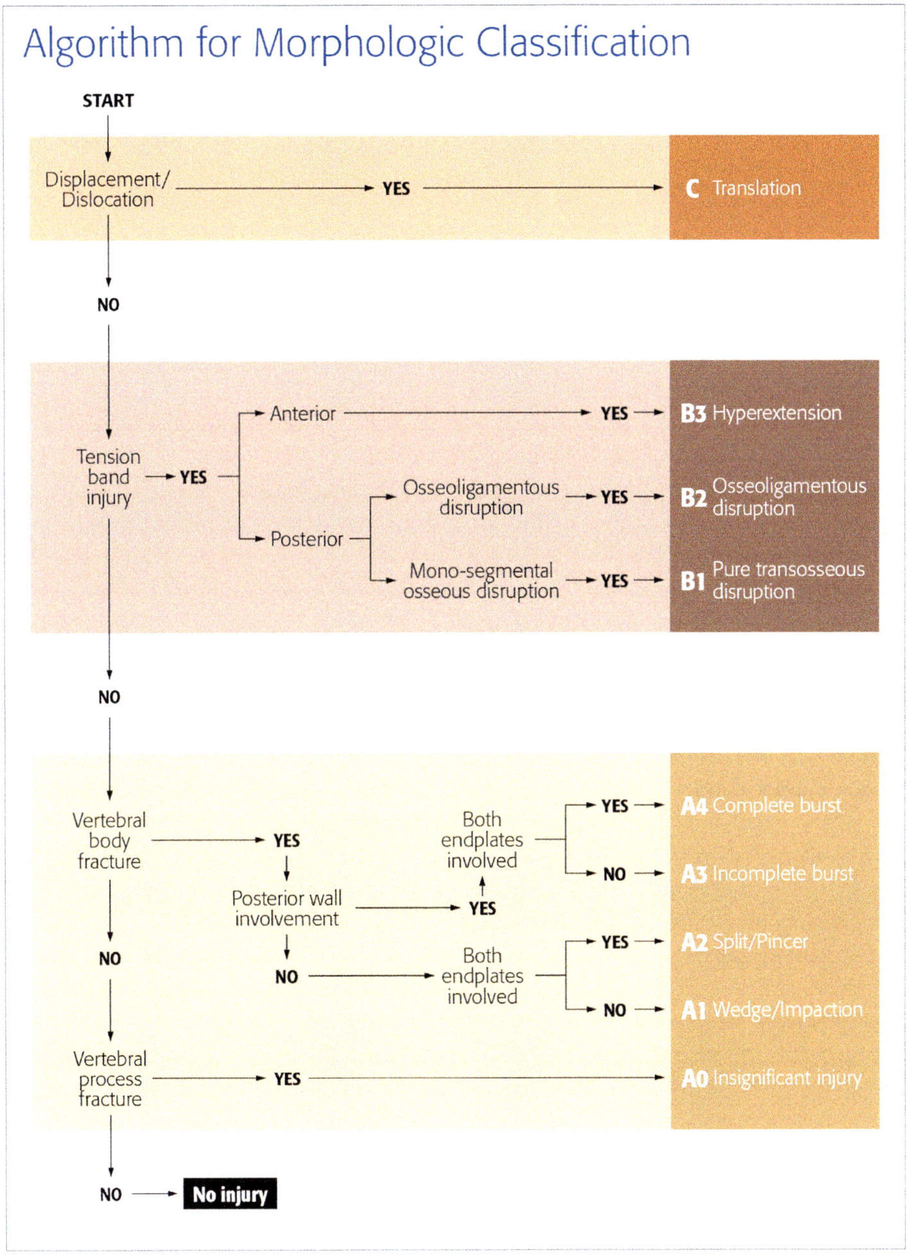

Fig. 29.1 (continued)

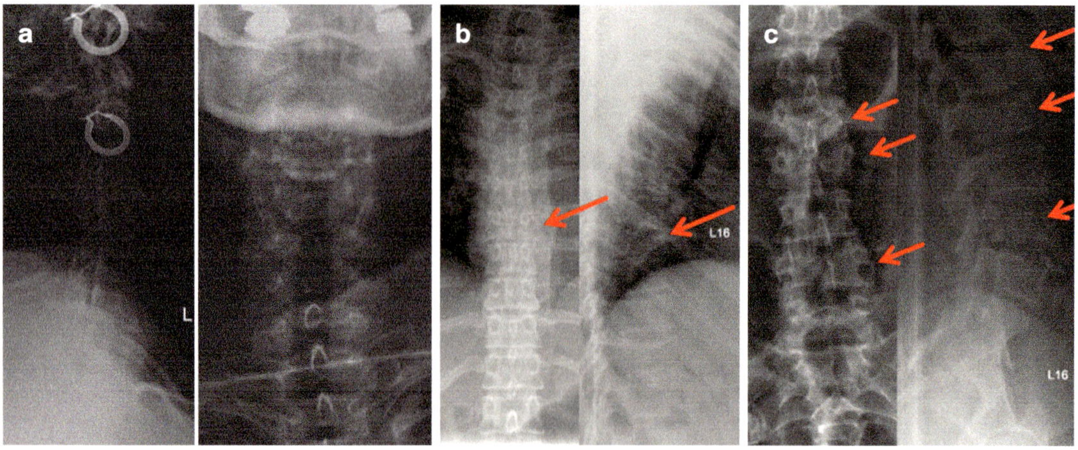

Fig. 29.2 Native X-rays immediately after trauma detecting multiple traumatic thoracolumbar fractures (**a**) cervical X-ray (**b**) thoracic x-ray and (**c**) lumbar x-ray in a-p. and lateral plane

Primary survey showed an awake patient with a GCS of 13 without an A, B or C problem due to the ATLS screening. Neurological examination showed a severe "D" problem with paraparesis of the lower legs (motor function grad II) with disturbed bilateral sensation. Sacral dermatoma including perianal area are spared and the patient showed an intact sphincter tonus. According to the ASIA Scale she was scored as ASIA C. Furthermore several bruises and cuts were detectable and patient complained about severe back pain and pain in her left wrist. The upper extremities showed no neurological abnormalities. Due to the severe pain patient was sedatetd and orally intubated after the primary survey to perform adequate diagnostics. Thereafter patient was diagnosed with the standard polytrauma protocol including a "head to feet" computed tomography including 2D reconstructions in coronal and sagittal plane (Fig. 29.3).

Each vertebra was screened according to the AOSpine algorithm for morphologic classification. No injury was showing a translational or distractional fracture pattern. A posterior tension band injury (B-type) was evident in the level L1/2 (Fig. 29.4) and L3/4 (Fig. 29.5). There were no signs of anterior tension band rupture (B3) or pure osseous disruption. Therefore both fractures are classified as B2 fractures.

Excluding the already diagnosed B2 fractures, remaining fractures were screened for posterior wall involvement. Posterior wall was involved at the level L1 (Fig. 29.6) and Th7 (Fig. 29.7). Th7 and L1 fracture showed additionally involvement of both endplates and were classified as A4 fracture.

The fracture at the level Th4 (Fig. 29.8) showed no posterior wall involvement but a coronal split involving both endplates. Hence this fracture was classified as A2 fracture. The remaining fracture at the level L5 (Fig. 29.9) showed no vertebral body involvement but a fracture of the right transverse process and the spinous process not affecting the vertebral stability. This fracture finally was classified as A0 fracture.

Finally the following diagnoses were documented. Spinal fractures are listed in order from most severe to last severe. Injuries of the same subtype are ordered from cranially to caudally [1, 4]:

- SCI sub L1 with paraparesis (motor function grade II) and sacral sparing (ASIA –C)
- L1/2 AOSpine B2, L1 A4 fracture
- L3/4 AOSpine B2, L4 A4 fracture
- Th7 AOSpine A4 fracture (complete burst fracture)
- L1 AOSpine A4 fracture with lamina split
- Th4 AOSpine A2 fracture (coronal split fracture)
- L5 AOSpine A0 fracture (right proc. transversus + proc. spinosus)
- Coccygeal fracture sub S4 (A1 according to the AOSpine sacral classification)
- left radius fracture (AO C3.3)
- bilateral lung contusion
- cuts at hands, knees and multiple bruises

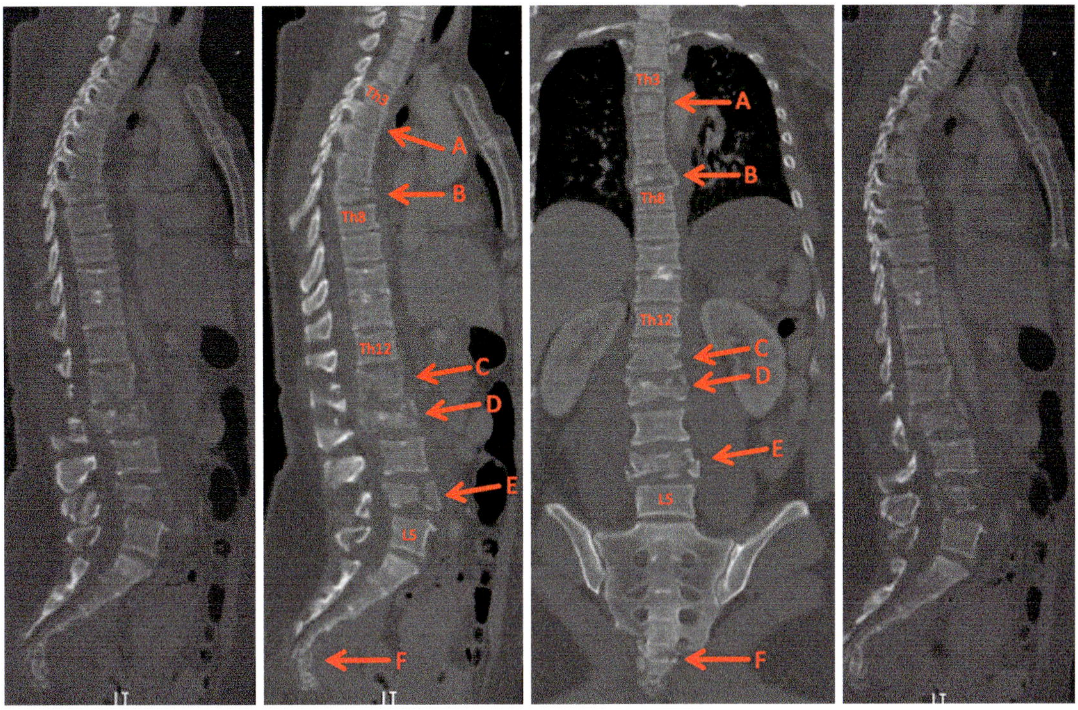

Fig. 29.3 Sagittal and coronal reconstructions of the thoracolumbar trauma-scan. The trauma scan showed several spinal fractures involving the vertebrae Th4, Th7, L1, L2, L4, L5 and the os coccyges

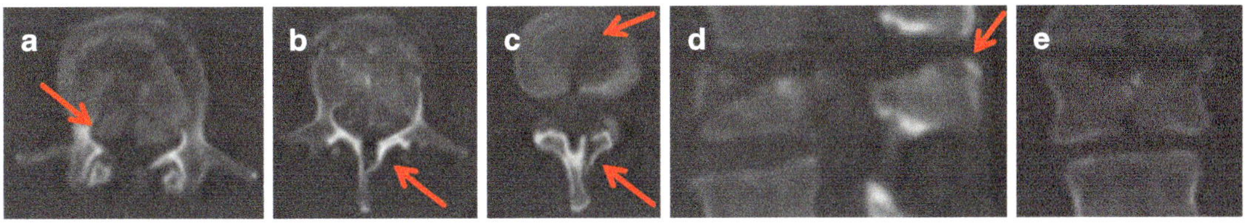

Fig. 29.4 CT findings at the level L2 with tension band injury L1/2, complete anterior burst fracture with severe spinal canal encroachment and left posterior lamina split

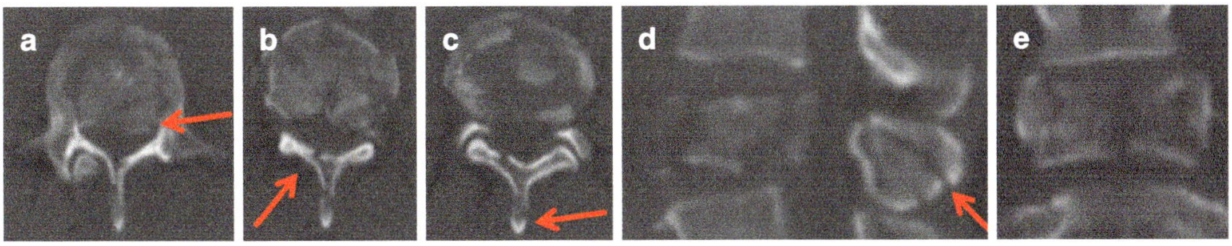

Fig. 29.5 CT findings at the level L4 with tension band injury L3/4, complete anterior burst fracture with 50% spinal canal encroachment and right posterior lamina split

To assess treatment indication, AOSIS was scored for the most severe fracture. B2 fractures are scored with 6 points and additional 4 points was given for the incomplete neurological deficit (ASIA C). Hence the patient was finally scored with 10 points for the L1/2 and L3/4 injury, constituting an indication for operative treatment according to AOSIS. The A4 fracture in Th7 was scored with 5 points indicating operative or conservative treatment. The A2 fracture in Th4 was scored with 2 points indicating conservative treatment.

Patient was treated primary by posterior stabilization Th11/12-L3-L5 and decompression (Fig. 29.10). Furthermore a posterior bisegmental fixation was performed, to stabilize the Th7 fracture. One week later the treatment was completed by anterior fusion including corporectomy L1 + 2 and L4 followed by left sided retroperitoneal vertebral body replacement using two expandable cages (Fig. 29.11).

Patient was treated 5 months in our paraplegic unit and improved with her neurological function. 9 months after the primary operation she is able to walk for about 20 min with a little support by a companion person. She is back home, has resolved her psychological disorders and is moved with her family to a new apartment on the ground floor.

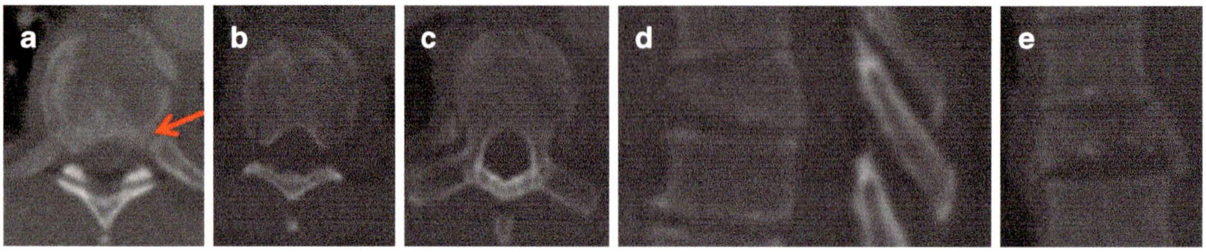

Fig. 29.6 CT findings at the level Th7 without C- and B-type lesion but posterior wall and both endplates involved

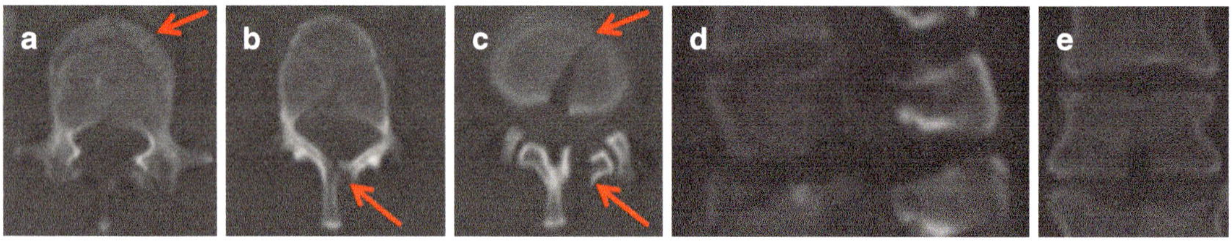

Fig. 29.7 CT findings at the level L1 without C- and B-type lesion but posterior wall and both endplates involved due to a sagittal split of the vertebra and the left side of the lamina

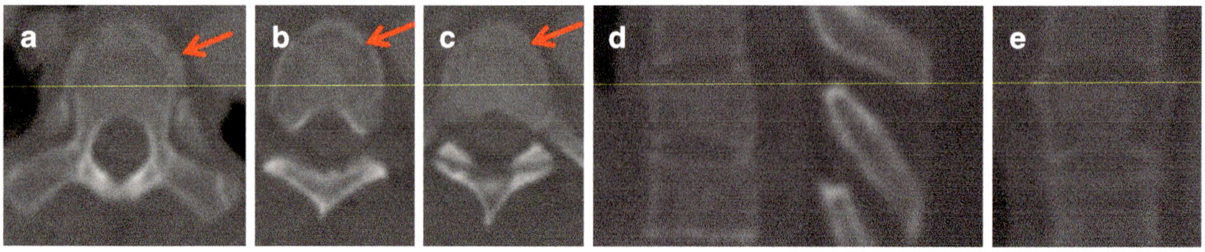

Fig. 29.8 CT findings at the level Th4 without C-, B-type lesion and without posterior wall involvement. Fracture is running in the coronal plan involving both endplates

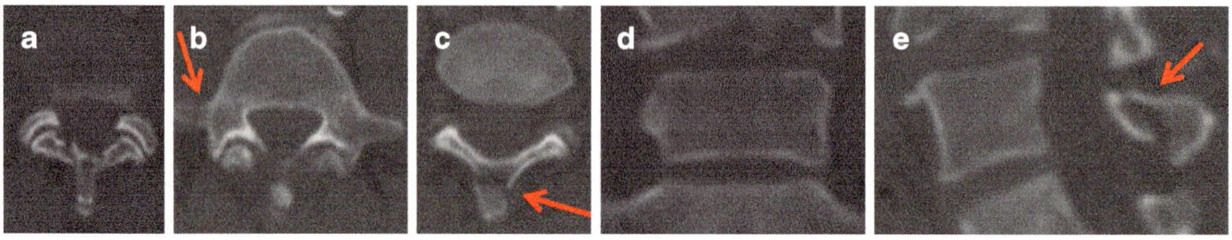

Fig. 29.9 CT findings at the level L5 without C- and B-type lesion and without lesion of the vertebral body. Red arrow demonstrating fracture of the right transverse process and spinous process

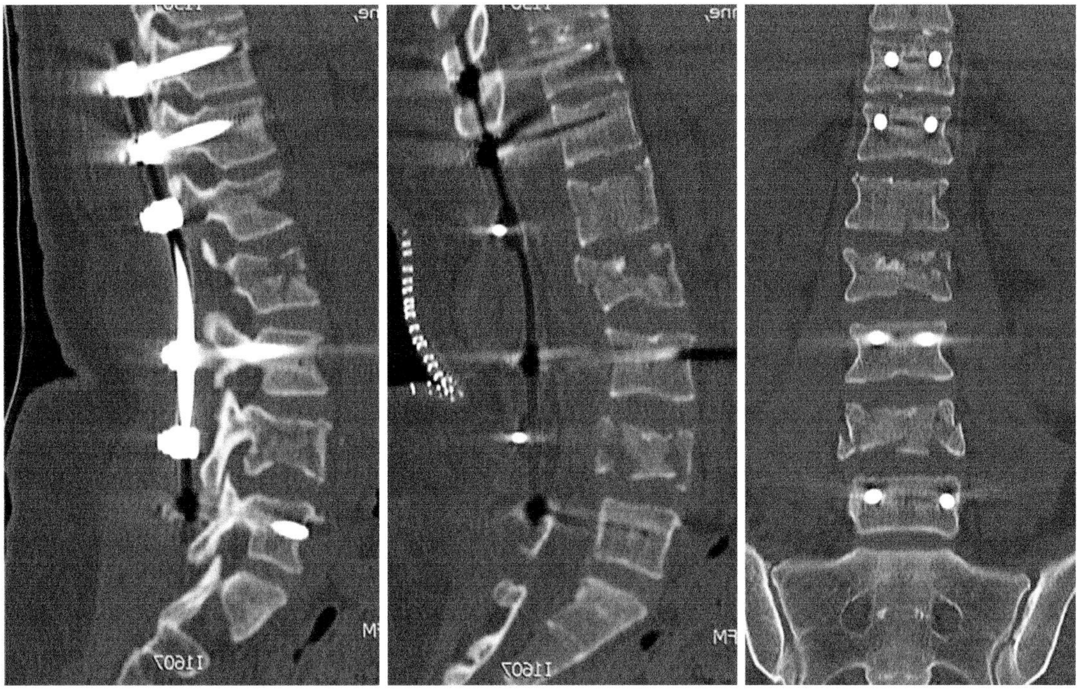

Fig. 29.10 CT scan after posterior decompression and stabilization Th11/12-L3-L5

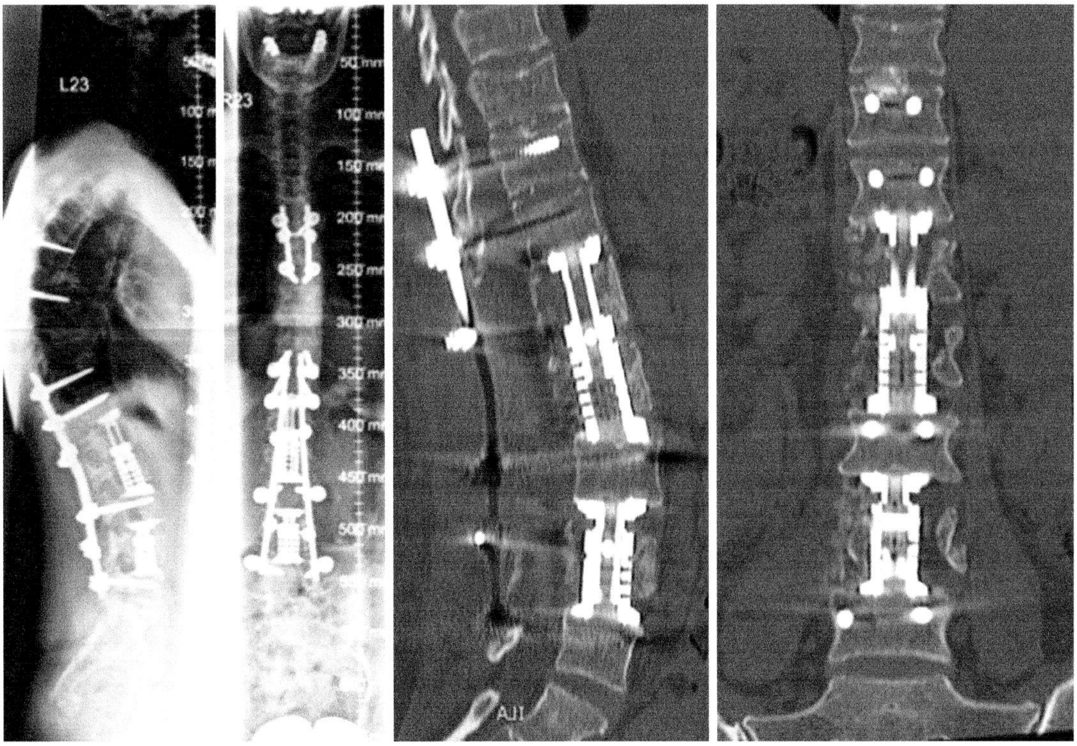

Fig. 29.11 Full spine standing X-ray 9 months after the primary injury revealing a coronal and sagittal balanced spine. CT scan is demonstrating advanced fusion with perfect implant positioning

29.3 Discussion of the Case

A challenging case with multiple fractures was presented. With the presented case several important steps from diagnosing until final treatment might be discussed.

29.3.1 Diagnosis

Plain X-ray images of the spine are an important screening tool to detect spinal injuries. However, in case of a polytrauma or if a spinal fracture is suspected after native radiological imaging, a computed tomography is the standard diagnostic tool. Accordingly to the given x-ray images of the presented case (Fig. 29.1) with inadequate information's regarding posterior wall, tension band or facet joint involvement; it is impossible to establish a definitive treatment strategy. Based on the computed tomography images spinal fractures might be classified accordingly to the AOSpine Injury Classification System with respect to: dislocation (C-type), insufficiency of the tension belt (B-type), anterior compression with or without posterior wall involvement (A-type). If a ligamentous injury (B-type) cannot be safely ruled out prior conservative treatment, or if there is a neurological deficit without correlation to the CT findings, an additional MRI diagnostics should be performed. The presented case demonstrated obvious a posterior tension band injury at two level in the lumbar spine. The traumatic bony stenosis of the spinal channel at L1/L2 explained the neurological deficit; hence a further MRI diagnosis was not necessary in the presented case.

29.3.2 AOSpine Injury Classification System

Similar to the Magerl classification, the severity of the injury increases in the same way as the degree of classification. The AOSpine Injury Classification System differentiates between three basic types of injury analogous to the Magerl classification. However, the classification is no longer based on the applied force vector, but on the degree of instability, regardless of whether this was caused by distraction or rotation injuries:

Main injury types:

Type A: Compression fractures

Typ B: Tension Band injury: failure of the posterior tension band (discoligamentous or osseous) or failure of the anterior ligamentous or osseous tension band (hyperextension injuries of the anterior column without signs of translational instability)

Typ C: Translational injuriy in any direction with posterior tension band failure and / or anterior column injury.

To obtain the correct classification radiological images should be screened according to the algorithm for morphologic classification (Fig. 29.1) from c-type to a-type. For further details please have a look into the original publication [1].

29.3.3 Indication for Operative or Conservative Treatment

The Thoracolumbar AOSpine Injury Score (TL AOSIS) was developed by the AOSpine Knowledge Forum Trauma and refined using a modified Delphi method and several online surveys conducted within a global professional body (AOSpine) [5]. The TL AOSIS should enable the link between classification and treatment recommendation. It should also allow further differentiation of the severity (0–12 points) of a thoracolumbar spinal injury. For this purpose, the individual classification proportions morphology, neurological damage and modifiers were assigned to scores reproduced in Table 29.1.

TL AOSIS suggests that patients with zero to three points (0–3) should be treated conservatively, more than five points (>5) surgically, and four to five (4–5) points either conservatively or surgically. This deliberately chosen "blurring" should take into account regionally different therapeutic concepts, available resources, experience of the treating physician and additional patient-specific aspects not considered in the

Table 29.1 AOSpine Score for thoracolumbar injuries (Thoraco-Lumbar **AOS**pine **I**njury-**S**core – **TL AOSIS**)

Classification	Points
Type A-injury	
A0	0
A1	1
A2	2
A3	3
A4	5
Type B injury	
B1	5
B2	6
B3	7
Type C – injury	
C	8
Neurological damage	
N0	0
N1	1
N2	2
N3	4
N4	4
Nx	3
Patient related modifiers	
M1	1
M2	0

classification, which may also play a decisive role in the choice of therapy [6].

29.4 Conclusions and Take Home Message

Fracture classification is important to evaluate stability. A correct classification using the AOSpine classification and the use of an appropriate scoring system (AOSIS) assists in the guidance of treatment.

Pearls

- Simple classification based on morphological criteria
- Good inter- and intraobserver reliability
- Classification includes patient neurological status and modifiers which may alter treatment decision
- TL AOSIS is helpful to determine treatment strategy

Editorial Comment

The editors strongly advocate the use of the AO Spine system to classify spinal injuries rationally and comparably. The consequences may vary regionally within Europe, which is acknowledged by us. This case description illustrates very well the highly structured and efficient work up and treatment of severe injuries as they are standardized in large trauma centers in German speaking countries. Despite the editors' personal preference for this approach, it needs to be stressed that no level 1 evidence exists for this type of management, which explains and also justifies the above mentioned regional differences.

References

1. Vaccaro AR, Oner C, Kepler CK, et al. AOSpine thoracolumbar spine injury classification system: fracture description, neurological status, and key modifiers. Spine. 2013;38:2028–37. https://doi.org/10.1097/BRS.0b013e3182a8a381.
2. Kepler CK, Vaccaro AR, Schroeder GD, et al. The thoracolumbar AOSpine injury score. Global Spine J. 2015;6:329–34. https://doi.org/10.1055/s-0035-1563610.
3. Vaccaro AR, Schroeder GD, Kepler CK, et al. The surgical algorithm for the AOSpine thoracolumbar spine injury classification system. Eur Spine J. 2015;25:1–8. https://doi.org/10.1007/s00586-015-3982-2.
4. Reinhold M, Audigé L, Schnake KJ, et al. AO spine injury classification system: a revision proposal for the thoracic and lumbar spine. In: European Spine Journal. Berlin Heidelberg: Springer; 2013. p. 2184–201.
5. Schroeder GD, Vaccaro AR, Kepler CK, et al. Establishing the injury severity of thoracolumbar trauma: confirmation of the hierarchical structure of the AOSpine thoracolumbar spine injury classification system. Spine. 2015;40:E498–503. https://doi.org/10.1097/BRS.0000000000000824.
6. Verheyden AP, Hölzl A, Ekkerlein H, et al. Recommendations for the treatment of thoracolumbar and lumbar spine injuries. Unfallchirurg. 2011;114:9–16. https://doi.org/10.1007/s00113-010-1934-1.

30 Pre-Hospital Management, Physical Examination & Polytrauma Management

Philipp Schleicher and Frank Kandziora

30.1 Introduction

This case will detail the following problems:

1. Pre-hospital management of spinal injuries
2. How to immobilize the spinal injured patient
3. Prioritization of treatment in multiple injured patients.

30.2 Case Description

On a weekday afternoon, a 50 year-old male was found lying beside a motorcycle in a small city nearby. Upon the time of paramedics' arrival, his eyes were open spontaneously, there was no verbal response at all, but he showed extension movements on painful stimuli (Decerebrate response, GCS = 4 + 1 + 2 = 7). Frothy secret was coming out of his mouth. The breathing sounds were attenuated bilaterally. Due to an obvious airway problem, a likely breathing disorder and an obviously impaired consciousness, the paramedic team placed two large-bore iv-lines and performed endotracheal intubation whilst manual c-spine immobilization.

He was ventilated with 100% oxygen. Using a log roll maneuver, he was put on a vacuum mattress and a hard cervical collar was mounted under continuous manual c-spine stabilization.

Emergency department (ED) delivery was about 1 h and 15 min after the accident.

At the time of ED delivery, his vital signs were: heart rate 140/min, blood pressure 99/75 mmHg, oxygen saturation 95%, respiratory rate 12/min (mandatory CPPV ventilation), body temperature 35.7 °C.

According to ATLS standard, a chest and pelvis X-ray were performed. This revealed a bilateral hematothorax, which was decompressed by chest tubes immediately. Right after placing the chest tubes, 300 ml blood was drained. Further drainage was not observed and cardio-respiratory parameters improved.

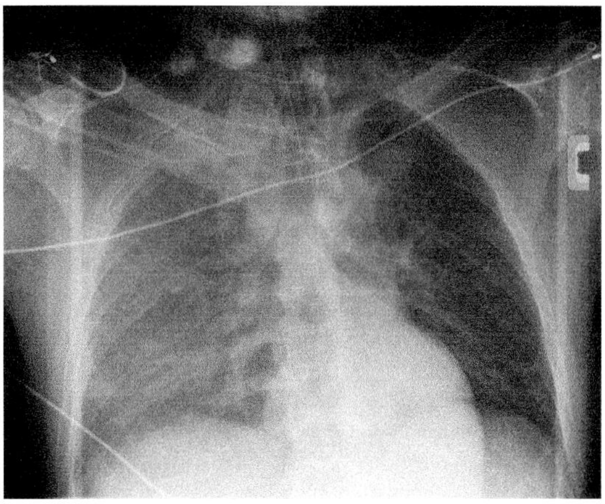

P. Schleicher (✉) · F. Kandziora
Zentrum für Wirbelsäulenchirurgie und Neurotraumatologie, Berufsgenossenschaftliche Unfallklinik Frankfurt am Main, Frankfurt am Main, Germany
e-mail: philipp.schleicher@bgu-frankfurt.de

B. Meyer, M. Rauschmann (eds.), *Spine Surgery*, https://doi.org/10.1007/978-3-319-98875-7_30

Due to the major trauma mechanism, a CT trauma scan was done.

The CT-scan showed an obvious unstable Jefferson burst fracture of the atlas with fragmentation of both lateral masses (Gehweiler IIIB/IV) and a flexion-distraction injury T5-T6 with burst fracture of both vertebrae (AO Spine B2,NX).

A fracture of the sternal manubrium at the same level of the thoracic spine fracture indicated a severe instability, sometimes referred to as "floating thorax". Despite the complete burst morphology of T5 and T6, the spinal canal was not compromised. By the time of CT diagnostics, the thoracic spine injury appeared to have the highest treatment priority (Fig. 30.1).

Beside the hematothorax, there was no further thoracic or abdominal injury. There were no imaging signs of traumatic brain injury (TBI) or cerebral hypoxemia. The Jefferson type atlas injury was likely to cause a vertebral artery injury, so a CT angiogram was made subsequently, showing no injury of neither of the two vertebral arteries.

Another finding was a decent widening of the C4–5 disc space adjacent to the spontaneously fused cervical spine segments C5–7, which raised suspicion of a hyperextension injury (Fig. 30.2).

At this timepoint, there was no recent information about the motor function of the extremities. An injury to the spinal cord was likely due to the thoracic spine fracture morphology.

To gain more information on spinal cord compression/injury and on the assumed hyperextension injury at C4–5, an MRI of the cervical and thoracic spine was added immediately.

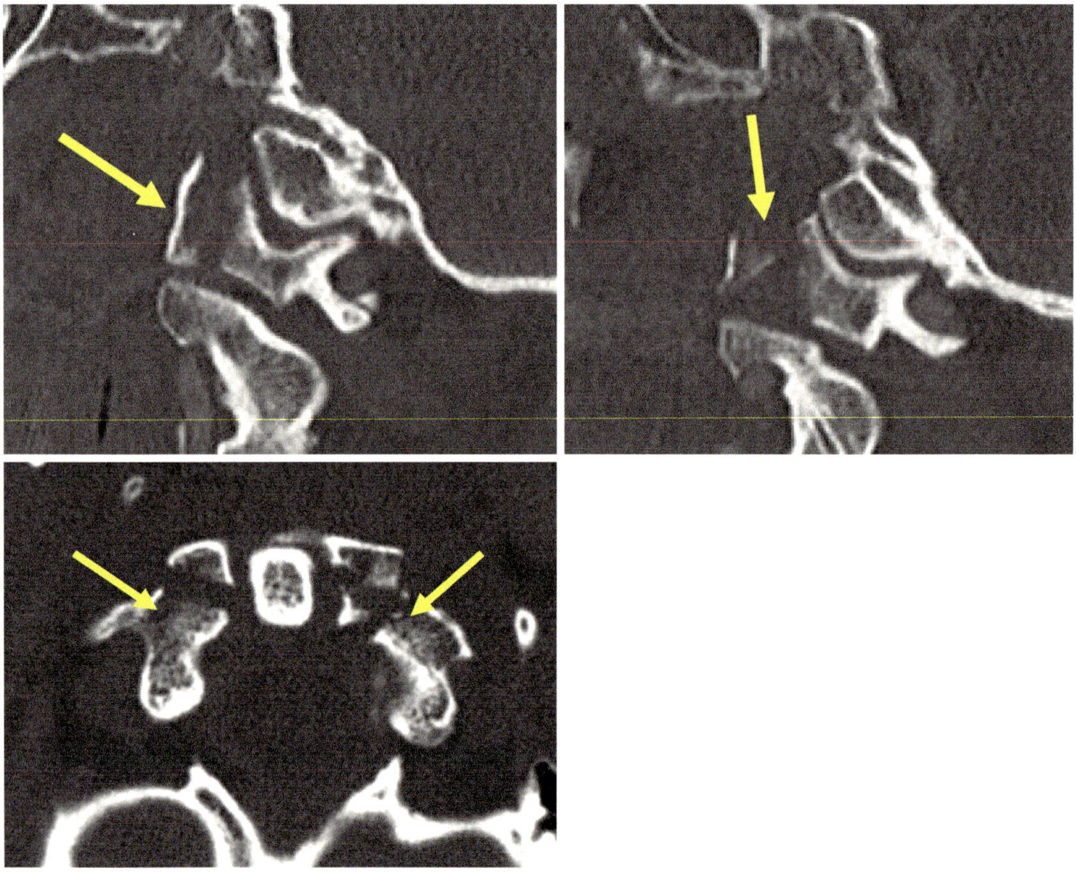

Fig. 30.1 Jefferson type atlas fracture with fragmentation of both lateral masses. It was classified as Gehweiler IIIB / IV; Dickman IIA

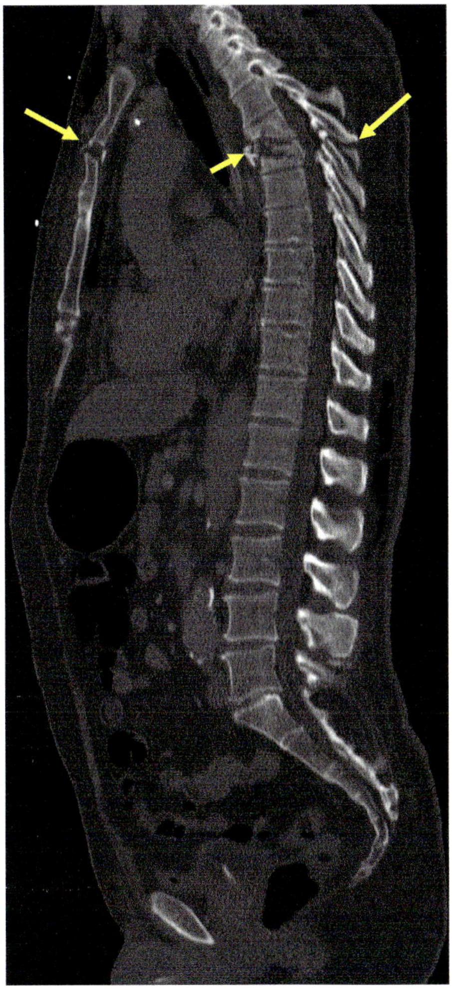

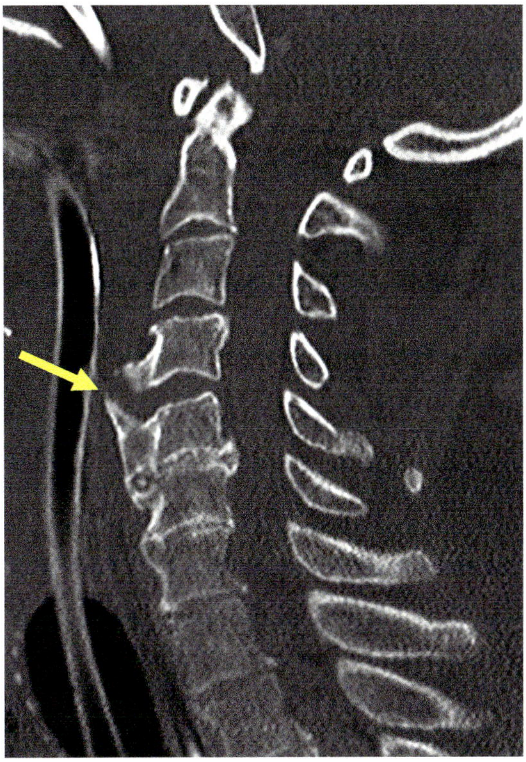

Fig. 30.2 Sagittal CT-scan of the cervical spine. The subtle widening of the disc space compared to the adjacent segments and the spontaneous fusion below this raised suspicion for a disco-ligamentous injury of this segment. MRI was added

The MRI showed no definite signs of spinal cord injury at neither level, but some retropulsed posterior wall fragments in contact with the anterior cord at the T5–6 level. The C4–5 disc was ruptured with some prevertebral hematoma and a hyperintense disc signal on T2-imaging, confirming a hyperextension injury adjacent to a bisegmental spontaneous fusion of C5–7 (AO Spine B3,M3,NX) (Fig. 30.3).

Despite a small effusion in the anterior atlanto-dental joint, there were no further signs of cranio-cervical instability, such as a lesion to the transverse atlantal ligament, to the tectorial membrane or widening of the occipito-atlantal joint space.

After having completed diagnostics with CT traumascan, CT angiogram and MRI about 90 min after ED delivery, the injurity severity score (ISS) could be calculated and added up to an ISS of 29.

The final diagnoses were:

1. Severe blunt chest injury with
   (a) multiple bilateral rib fractures
   (b) bilateral hematothorax
   (c) bilateral pulmonary contusion
   (d) sternal fracture
2. Jefferson Fracture of the Atlas, Type Gehweiler IIIB/Dickman IIA
3. Hyperextension injury C4–5, Type AOSpine B3, NX
4. Flexion-Distraction injury T5–6, Type AOSpine B2, NX

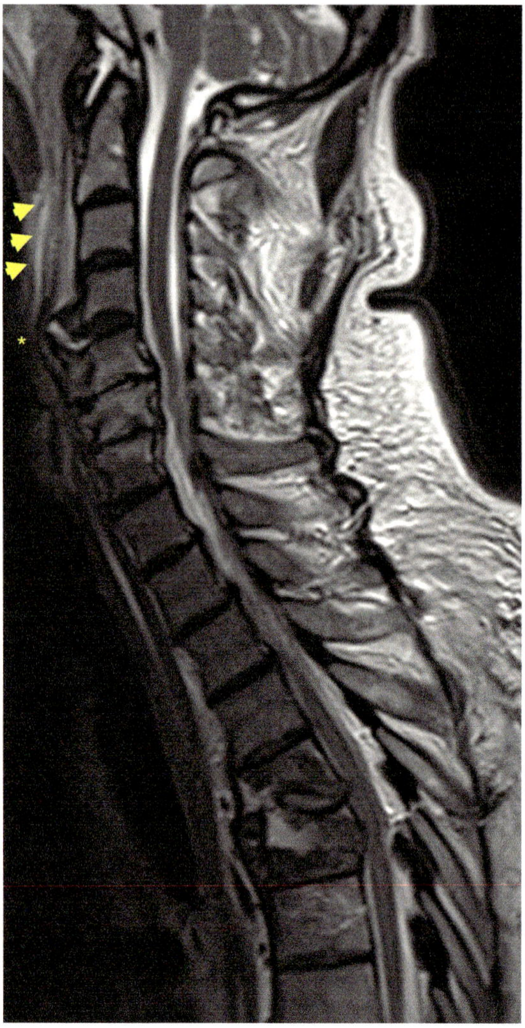

Fig. 30.3 T2-weighted sagittal MRI of the cervical and thoracic spine. The disc space C4–5 showed a hyperintense signal (asterisk) and a prevertebral fluid effusion was visible (arrowheads), both indicating a transdiscal injury in this segment. The spinal cord appears intact at all three injury sites, but at T6, moderate anterior as well as posterior compression might be present

30.3 Treatment

Initial treatment of the immediately life-threatening hematothorax was finished about 10 min after ED delivery, then the next step was surgical stabilization and decompression of the most unstable and most dangerous spinal injuries as an urgent day-1-surgery.

So, **anterior cervical discectomy and interbody fusion (ACDF) at the C4–5 level** was performed first and then the patient was turned to perform **posterior thoracic decompression and fusion T3–4 to T7–8**. OR time was 70 min for ACDF and 2 h and 5 min for the posterior procedure. Blood loss was 50 cc and 700 cc, respectively. There were no complications during the two procedures. Intraoperatively, the unstable rupture of the C4–5 disc could be confirmed. Day-1 surgical procedures were finished about 6.5 h after ED delivery and approximately 8 h after trauma. The patient was kept ventilated and sedated for another 3 days, until respiratory circulatory and inflammatory parameters had improved slightly (Figs. 30.4 and 30.5).

The final surgical step – **temporary posterior occipitocervical (C0-C3) stabilization** for treatment of the Jefferson type atlas fracture was performed on the fourth day after trauma. In this procedure, OR time was 2 h and 10 min, blood loss was about 200 cc (Fig. 30.6).

After this last procedure, there were no further unstable lesions, which facilitated **rotorest kinetic therapy**.

Due to his severe thoracic trauma, respiratory weaning was prolonged significantly. Extubation was achieved 14 days after trauma and he could be transferred to regular ward on the 16th day after admission. Neurologic examination after extubation showed full motor and sensory function of all extremities.

He was able to walk without any aids and could be discharged to outpatient treatment approximately 4 weeks after trauma.

30.4 Discussion of the Case

This case demonstrates very well many aspects of trauma treatment in the prehospital and early clinical period.

In the prehospital trauma setting, it is important to "read" the trauma scene and to get a feeling of the involved energy acting on the patient's body. In this case, the emergency team had to assume a high speed bicycle accident, which has a high probability for any kind

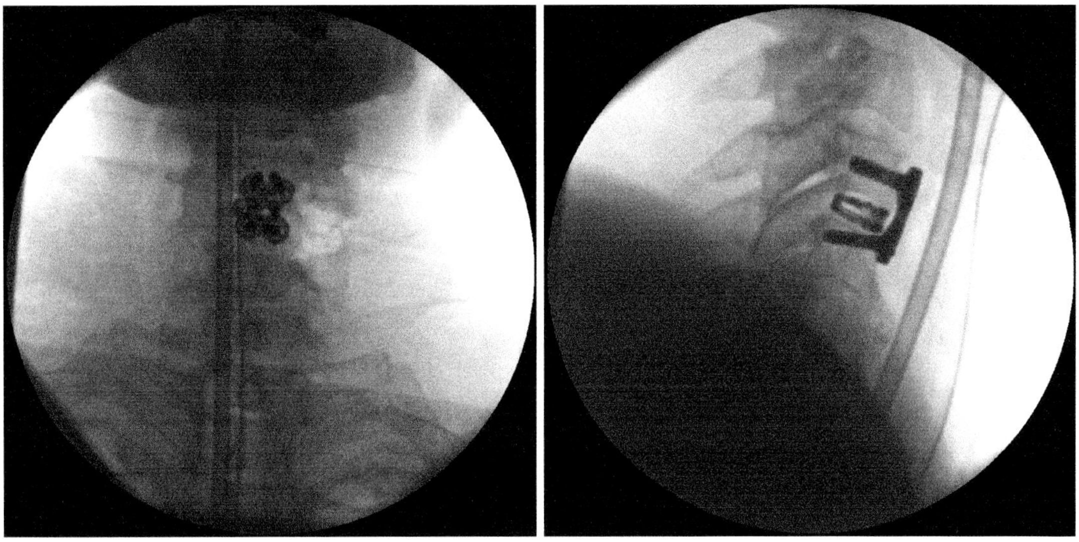

Fig. 30.4 Intraoperative fluoro view after decompression and plate stabilization of C4–5

Fig. 30.5 Postoperative x-ray after thoracic stabilization T3–4 to T7–8 and decompression T5–6

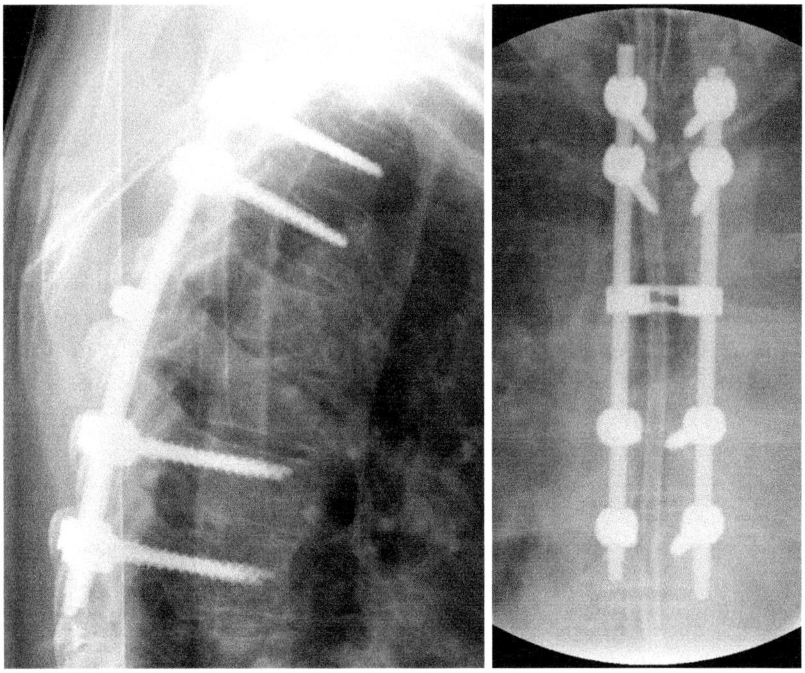

of severe injury, especially spinal injuries. Patients with multiple injuries (ISS >16) have a probability of 30–36% for a severe spinal injury [1, 2].

The first step in this case is to ensure a proper airway without putting any further movement to the cervical spine. Manual immobilization is the safest way to protect the c-spine while airway

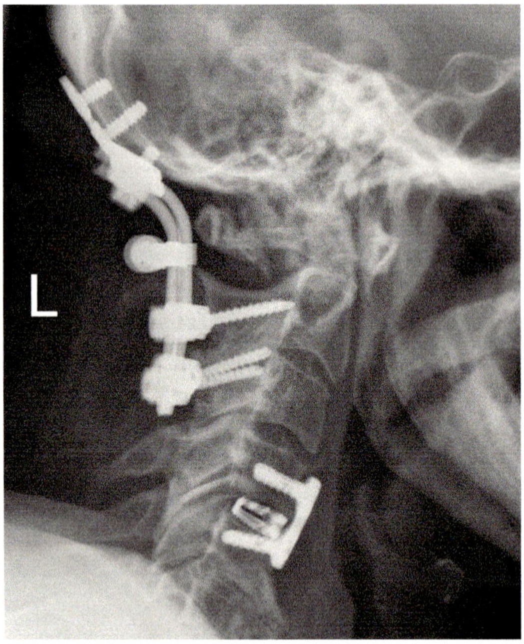

Fig. 30.6 Postoperative x-ray after final occipito-cervical stabilization

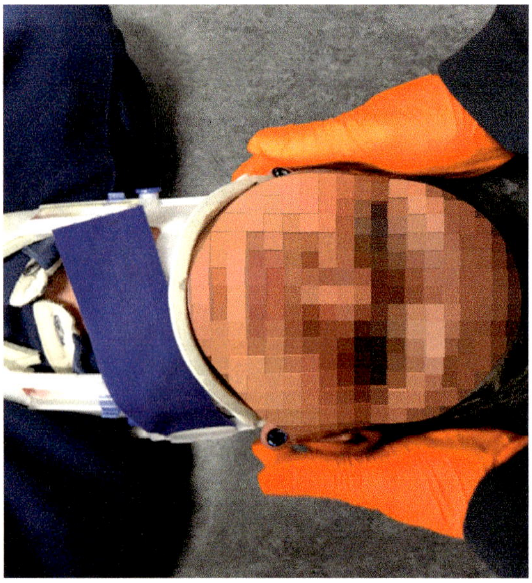

Fig. 30.7 Manual inline stabilization of the head and cervical spine after mounting a hard cervical collar. Cervical collars alone do not provide sufficient stability and should always be combined with other measures

management. A cervical collar alone is not able to sufficiently protect the cervical spine against dangerous movements (Fig. 30.7) [3, 4].

After completion of the primary survey, transport priority has to be set. In critically injured patients, with severe, life-threatening injuries, a whole body immobilization might be skipped to accelerate transfer to definitive surgical care. In our case, these instability criteria were met (impaired consciousness, attenuated breathing sounds), so the indication for a whole body immobilization could be discussed.

For any other patients with trauma mechanisms susceptible to spinal injuries, whole spine immobilization is recommended. For immobilization of the whole spine, there are basically two methods established: after having stabilized the cervical spine with a hard cervical collar, the patient is either placed and strapped onto a spine board or molded into a vacuum mattress [5]. The authors prefer the vacuum mattress, because this method can better adopt to specific needs in the individual patient, such as severe hyperkyphosis in Bechterev's disease or lifting the upper body in traumatic brain injury.

When placing the patient onto a flat surface one must also consider the relationship between the occiput and the thorax: adult patients, especially with thoracic hyperkyphosis might need a pillow beneath the head to prevent hyperextension of the cervical spine, whereas children have an occiput greater than the thorax, so the thorax should be put on some blankets or pillows to prevent hyperflexion of the spine (Fig. 30.8).

Since hard collars alone will not sufficiently stabilize the c-spine during transport, it is mandatory to fix the head additionally: either with so called head blocks or by molding the vacuum mattress tightly around the head [6]. The head fixation to be placed AFTER strapping the rest of the patient's body to the spine board/vacuum mattress, otherwise inadvertent displacement of the body against the fixed head might lead to fatal damage of the cervical spine (Fig. 30.9).

During transportation in a critically injured patient, oxygenation and blood pressure

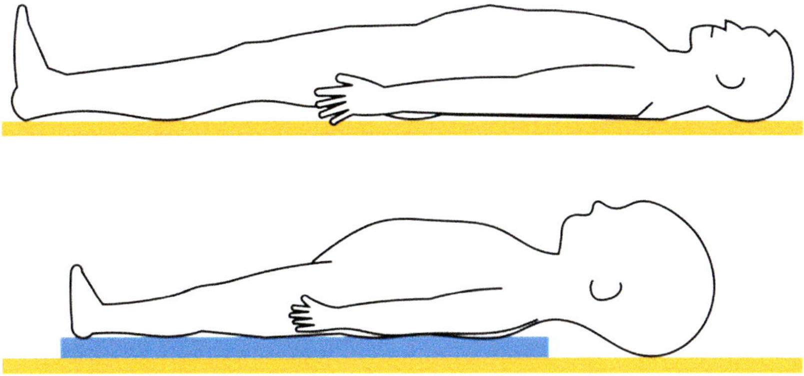

Fig. 30.8 Note the different relationship between the occiput and the rest of the body in children and adults. For a proper spinal immobilization in children, putting the body on some extra blankets is recommended

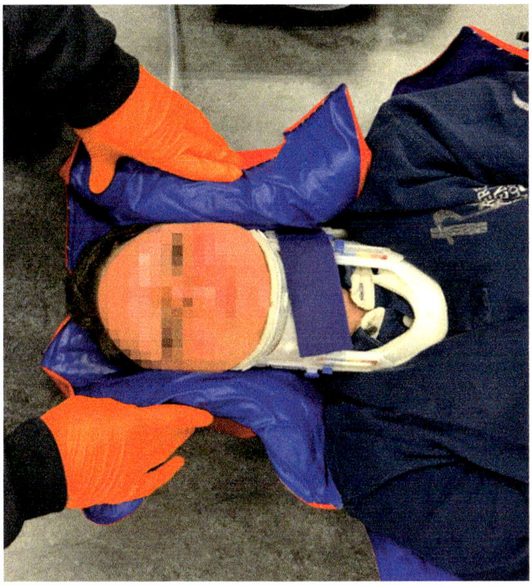

Fig. 30.9 For transportation, additional head fixation is mandatory. It can be easily solved by molding the vacuum matress around the head

management are the major issues, especially in spinal trauma. The spinal cord is very sensitive to hypoxia, so oxygen saturation should be kept over 95% and the mean arterial blood pressure should be kept above 85–90 mmHg [7].

In our case, early *inhospital* treatment followed strictly the ATLS-protocol, with initially solving the breathing disorder (Type "B" problem) by decompression of the thorax. After exclusion of any further thoracic, abdominal and pelvic lesions, which might have led to a circulatory disorder (Type "C" problem), the spinal injuries with potential spinal cord injury (Type "D" problem) had the highest priority [8].

A high dose steroid regime to protect the spinal cord was abandoned due to the concomitant pulmonary injuries and an unclear neurological status. The neuroprotective effect of high-dose steroids is questioned, while pulmonary and gastro-intestinal complications have been reported. So recent guidelines recommend this as an *optional* treatment regimen only in an isolated spinal cord injury, not in the multiple trauma setting [4].

Early surgical decompression and stabilization of spinal injuries within <72 h has shown to improve patient outcome in terms of hospital stay, ICU-stay, ventilator hours and sepsis rate. Especially thoracic spine fractures in combination with a severe thoracic injury will benefit from early surgical treatment [1].

The effect of early decompression on neurologic outcome is still under discussion, but data supporting a positive effect are increasing [9].

In this special case, it was necessary to prioritize three different spinal injuries (upper cervical, lower cervical and thoracic spine), which is not uncommon in polytrauma patients [10].

Our decision to start with the lower c-spine lesion was driven by several factors:

1. The anterior procedure could be performed without turning the patient, so further manipulation of the whole spine was minimized,

whereas treatment of the thoracic spine first would have necessitated a prone position with a high risk of cervical dislocation.
2. An impending C4–5 spinal cord injury will impair the patients functional ability much more than a possible T5–6 lesion.
3. The anterior procedure is usually a quick procedure with little blood loss, so the risk of general decompensation before fixing the other injuries is minimized.

The decision to fix the upper c-spine lesion as the last step was driven by the fact, that Jefferson/ Gehweiler III Type lesions are usually quite benign in terms of acute neurologic damage. The instability symptoms associated with these injuries usually develop at a later timepoint, due to chronic instability and joint incongruence. Additionally, the procedure is sometimes technically demanding and might be associated with a significant amount of blood loss, so it is recommended to be performed at a later timepoint, when the most critical period is over.

Usually, in typical Gehweiler Type III fractures, a C1–2 stabilization or even a C1-ring osteosynthesis is sufficient and will save as much motion as possible for the patient's head movement. In this case, the lateral masses of C1 were involved into the fracture (Gehweiler Type IV component), which put some doubts on screw purchase in the C1- lateral masses. Although significantly reducing the patient's flexion-extension ability, temporary occipito-cervical stabilization was favored therefore. Implant removal after bony consolidation of the fracture is planned.

The ACDF procedure in lower cervical spine fractures is an established method with a low approach-related morbidity, good decompression options and high stabilization performance with modern angle stable implants. Especially in the hyperextension (Type B3) injuries, restoration of the anterior tension band is the most important step from a biomechanical point of view – and this is best achieved by placing a plate in front of the spine.

Posterior long-segment stabilization with pedicle screws and decompression via laminectomy is also an established method for treatment of unstable thoracic burst fractures. An additive anterior column support could be discussed, but in the thoracic spine the lesion is usually subjected to bending moments rather than axial compression like in the thoraco-lumbar junction [11]. Furthermore, the anterior surgical approach in T5–T6 is challenging, while adding more fixation points in the rigid thoracic spine will not cause a significant loss of motion.

30.5 Conclusions and Take Home Message

The incidence of spinal injuries in multiple injured patients is high, so a spinal injury should be assumed in every major trauma until the opposite is proven.

Prehospital treatment basically consists in the sensible application of spinal immobilization and providing a sufficient perfusion to the potentially injured spinal cord.

During inhospital polytrauma management, spinal injury treatment has a lower priority than Airway management ("A"), breathing disorders ("B") or circulatory disorders ("C"), but even then, fixing spinal injuries will support the treatment of these injuries also.

This justifies surgical treatment of unstable spinal fractures as emergency procedures, so called "day-1-surgeries".

When priorizing different spinal injuries, one must balance the ongoing risk for further spinal cord injury against the "second hit" effect of the surgical trauma.

Pearls
- Every major trauma MUST rise suspicion for a spinal injury
- If a spinal injury is suspected, spinal immobilization is mandatory until the spine is cleared definitely
- Whole body spinal immobilization can only be skipped in critical, life-threatening injuries, which require immediate surgical intervention

- In the multiple trauma setting, the most important and most difficult issues are
  - to keep the overview,
  - to prioritize properly
  - to stay sensitive to subtle details, which may have fatal consequences and
  - to react flexible on unexpected findings

Pitfalls
- To overlook subtle signs for significant injury. Being distracted by the most severe injury or skipping important diagnostic measures in order to save time might drive you into catastrophy
- To rely on solitary cervical collar for spinal stabilization
- To fix a hyperkyphotic patient onto a flat spineboard might worsen or even create a spinal injury.

Editorial Comment

This chapter illustrates and underscores the most important principle for pre-hospital and early in-house care following trauma with suspected injury to the spine: Know your predefined, structured modus operandi and never deviate from it!

References

1. Bliemel C, Lefering R, Buecking B, Frink M, Struewer J, Krueger A, et al. Early or delayed stabilization in severely injured patients with spinal fractures? Current surgical objectivity according to the trauma registry of DGU: treatment of spine injuries in polytrauma patients. J Trauma Acute Care Surg. 2014;76(2):366–73.
2. Eggers C, Stahlenbrecher A. Verletzungen der BWS und LWS. Unfallchirurg. 1998;101(10):779–90.
3. Kwan I, Bunn F, Roberts IG. Spinal immobilisation for trauma patients. Cochrane Lib. 2001;(2):CD002803.
4. Ahn H, Singh J, Nathens A, MacDonald RD, Travers A, Tallon J, et al. Pre-hospital care management of a potential spinal cord injured patient: a systematic review of the literature and evidence-based guidelines. J Neurotrauma. 2011;28(8):1341–61.
5. Mahshidfar B, Mofidi M, Yari AR, Mehrsorosh S. Long backboard versus vacuum mattress splint to immobilize whole spine in trauma victims in the field: a randomized clinical trial. Prehosp Disaster Med. 2013;28(5):462–5.
6. Báez AA, Schiebel N. Is routine spinal immobilization an effective intervention for trauma patients? Ann Emerg Med. 2006;47(1):110–2.
7. Bernhard M, Gries A, Kremer P, Böttiger BW. Spinal cord injury (SCI)—prehospital management. Resuscitation. 2005;66(2):127–39.
8. Lendemans S, Ruchholtz S. S3-Leitlinie Polytrauma/Schwerverletzten-Behandlung. Unfallchirurg. 2012;115(1):14–21.
9. Fehlings MG, Vaccaro A, Wilson JR, Singh A, Cadotte DW, Harrop JS, et al. Early versus delayed decompression for traumatic cervical spinal cord injury: results of the surgical timing in acute spinal cord injury study (STASCIS). PLoS One. 2012;7(2):e32037.
10. Henderson RL, Reid DC, Saboe LA. Multiple noncontiguous spine fractures. Spine. 1991;16(2):128–31.
11. Briggs AM, Van Dieën JH, Wrigley TV, Greig AM, Phillips B, Lo SK, Bennell KL. Thoracic kyphosis affects spinal loads and trunk muscle force. Phys Ther. 2007;87(5):595–607.

Spinal Cord Injury

31

Sandro M. Krieg

31.1 Introduction

Traumatic spinal cord injury (SCI) usually results in impairment of sensory, motor, or autonomic functions. Incidence and main origin of SCI can be country-specific and varies to some extend (Figs. 31.1 and 31.2) [16].

The prevalence of SCI was reported to be globally between 236 and 1009 per million which yet remains quite difficult to obtain [16].

The acute and chronic management of SCI patients needs considerable interdisciplinary resources. Besides the psychological and physical burden of these patients, the economic burden of SCI is high, considering an estimated lifetime cost of $3.03 million per patient [16]. These cost culminate due to the acute care, long-term physiotherapy but also due to the high rate of acute and long-term complications, such as pressure ulcers, bladder dysfunction and infection, bowel dysfunction, wound infections, instrumentation failure, respiratory problems, and chronic pain. Physicians being involved in the treatment of SCI, knowledge of current and emerging therapeutic approaches is crucial to provide optimal treatment and long-term outcomes for these complex patient cohorts.

This chapter will therefore outline the specifics of traumatic SCI, its typical clinical course, mandatory preoperative imaging, surgical approaches and medical management. Moreover, the rationale and evidence for the steps is discussed. At the end of this chapter the reader should be aware of the problems and pitfalls we face when treating SCI patients. The aim of the presented case is therefore to emphasize these various aspects in the diagnosis and treatment of this disease. Such specifics are:

- Acute phase treatment
- Surgical indication
- Medical management
- Avoidance of typical complications

31.2 Case Description

A 51 y/o female patient returned home drunken with bruises at the head and arm and went to bed. The next morning she did not wake up properly and her husband called the paramedics. Upon arrival in the emergency department neurological examination showed some upper extremity movement but paraplegia from C7 downwards with absent anal sphincter tone and no bladder control; reflexes and sensitivity absent. Thus, SCI was graded according to the American Spinal

S. M. Krieg (✉)
Department of Neurosurgery, Klinikum rechts der Isar, Technische Universität München, Munich, Germany
e-mail: Sandro.Krieg@tum.de

B. Meyer, M. Rauschmann (eds.), *Spine Surgery*, https://doi.org/10.1007/978-3-319-98875-7_31

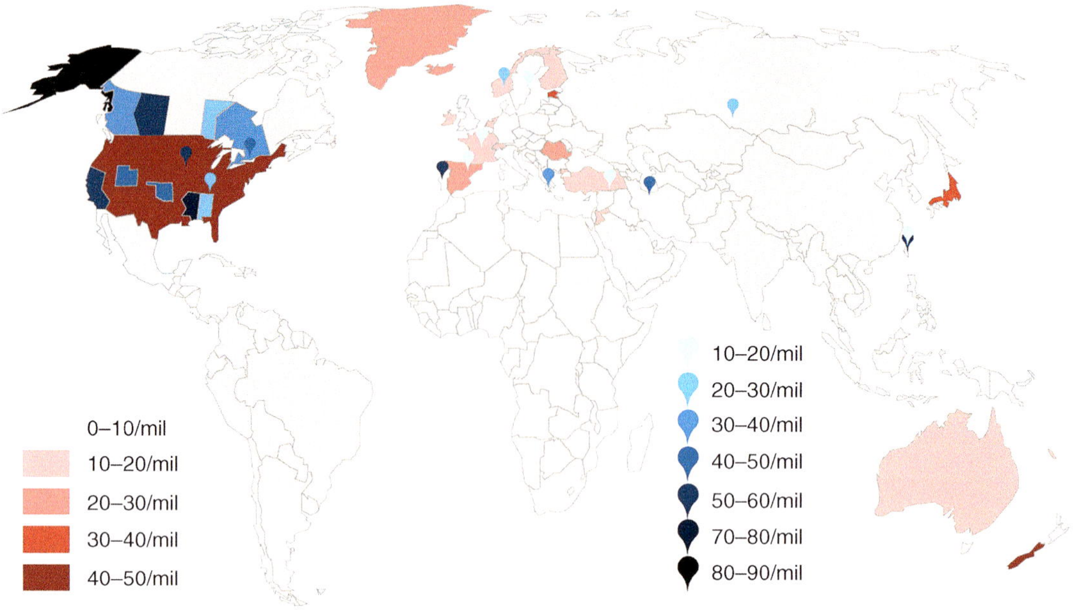

Fig. 31.1 Incidence map worldwide. (Figure 2 from Singh et al. 2014: Relative annual incidences of SCI worldwide [16])

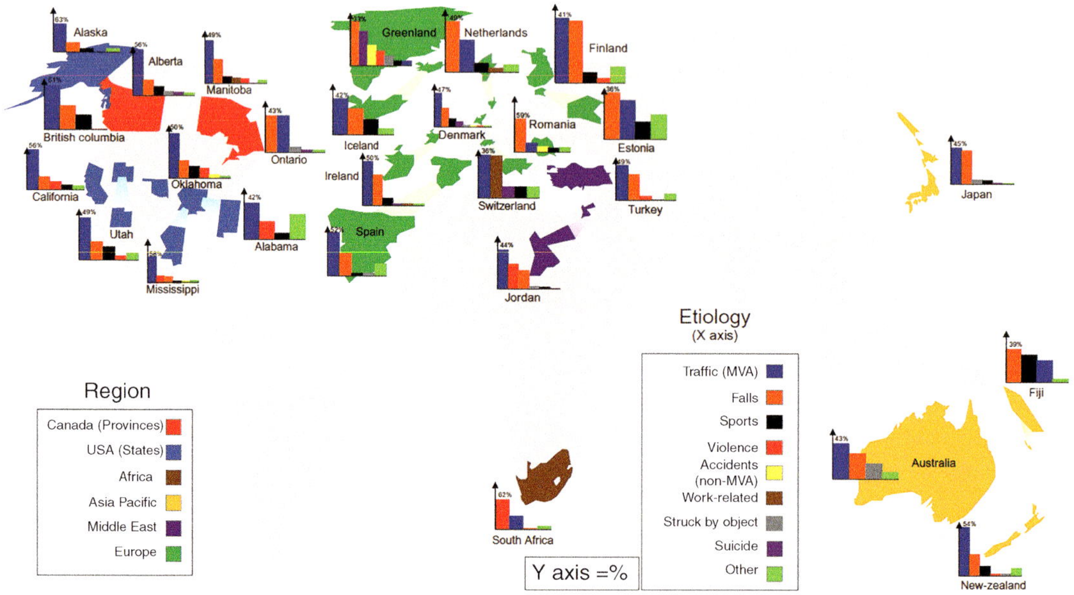

Fig. 31.2 Causes of SCI worldwide. (Figure 6 from Singh et al. 2014: Causes of SCI severely vary worldwide from motor vehicle accident (MVA) to falls, sports, violence, non-MVA accidents, work-related, or suicide [16])

Injury Association (ASIA) Impairment Scale (AIS) to ASIA grade A. CT scan showed bilateral facet joint luxation at C6/7 with translation; otherwise no further injuries (Fig. 31.3). An MRI scan was performed in order to rule out further discoligamentous injury in other levels (Fig. 31.4).

The patient was immediately taken to the OR and dorsoventral instrumentation was performed at C6/7 including repositioning, anterior decompression, anterior cage and plating plus dorsal lateral mass screws in C6/7 (Fig. 31.5).

The patient was postoperatively taken to the ICU where she stayed for 4 days. She did not develop respiratory problems and was discharged to rehabilitation at the seventh postoperative day. Neurological examination at discharge was improved to ASI C from C7 downward, no bladder or anal sphincter control).

31.3 Discussion of the Case

31.3.1 Initial Management

While the initial trauma causes the initial irreversible injury, the remaining spinal cord tissue requires optimal care in order to minimize secondary injury mechanisms. Thus, these patients should be directly transferred to tertiary care centers being able to take care of the spinal injury, further traumatic injuries, such as hip fractures, vascular injuries or traumatic brain injury, but also the further management of spinal shock and in-hospital complications.

First Responders need to quickly and properly assess and manage trauma patients on scene. After advanced trauma life support (ATLS) protocols' primary points like airway, breathing, and circulation, a full assessment of injuries including neurological functions is crucial. Worth noting, periods of hypotension <90 mmHg correlate withworse neurological outcome in SCI [11, 19]. Respiratory problems especially occur in patients with high cervical (C0–5) SCI thus requiring immediate ventilation. Up to 50% of patients with even incomplete SCI require tracheostomy during the in-hospital stay; a number which is even higher for high cervical SCI [20].

In the emergency room it can be difficult to stabilize critical patients whilst evaluating multiple systems for further injury. Especially in polytraumatized SCI patients neurogenic (requires vasopressors) and hypovolemic (requires crystalloid fluid or blood products) shock can be present. Early whole body CT scan can provide a quick assessment of all critical injuries. To get a quick and good clinical picture

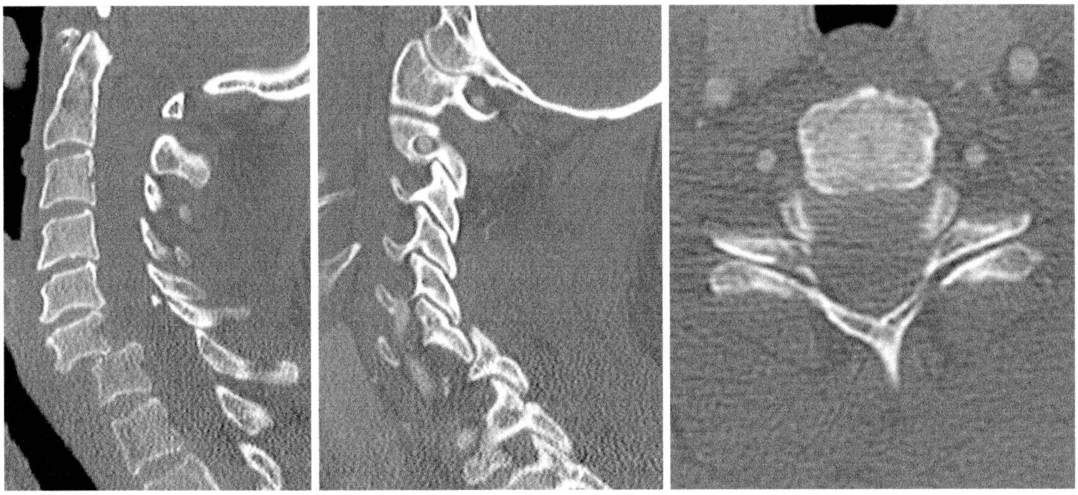

Fig. 31.3 CT scan in the emergency room. The CT scan shows a bilateral facet joint luxation at C6/7 with translation in the sagittal midline (**a**), sagittal facet joint plane (**b**), and axial slice (**c**)

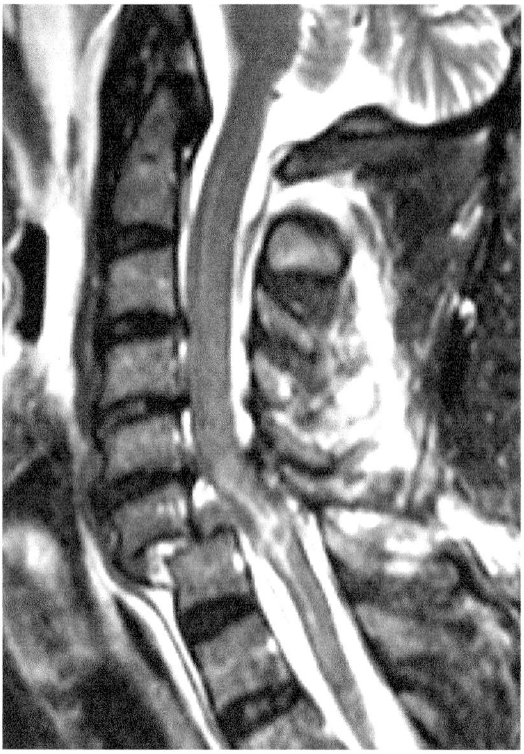

Fig. 31.4 Preoperative MRI. This sagital preoperative MRI scan shows a monoesegmental injury including severe myelomalacia with no further discoligamentous injury in other levels

of the patient in this situation, the trauma team should include a spine surgeon for early evaluation of neurological function. Yet, the neurological examination is mostly reduced to achieve a quick general picture of motor, sensory, and autonomous functions without delaying other procedures including CT scan. However, it should include all relevant factors allowing ASI grading once the patient is stabilized [14]. In this situation please differentiate between neurogenic shock (life-threatening loss of sympathetic tone causing declined peripheral resistance) and spinal shock (flaccid paralysis from the injured level downwards), which is usually related to ASI A or B SCI [5]. A rectal examination provides information of the autonomous system and the sacral roots and evaluates tone, sensation and contraction.

In the case presented at the beginning of this chapter, initial management when the patient didn't wake up properly; most likely due to neurogenic shock and hypotension. An early trauma CT scan showed no concomitant fractures, which needed to be ruled out considering the unknown injury mechanism and potentially undetected high blood loss.

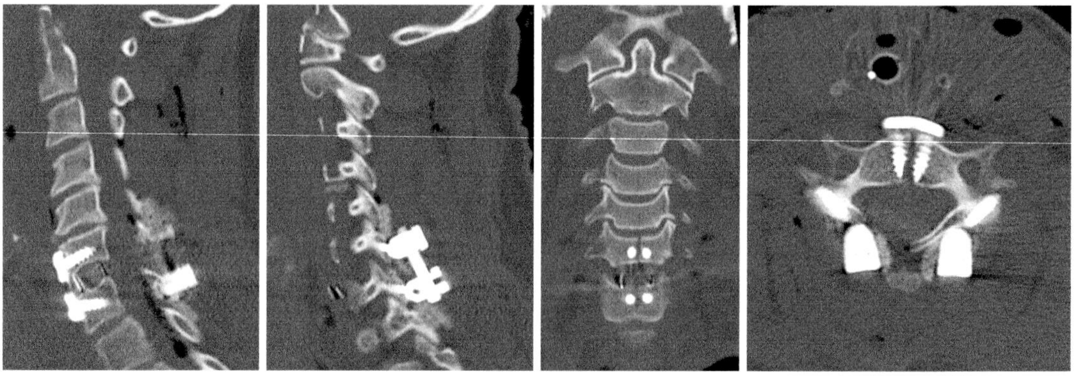

Fig. 31.5 Postoperative CT scan. The CT scan shows the dorsoventral instrumentation and realignment via anterior cage and plating plus dorsal lateral mass screws in C6/7 in the sagittal midline (**a**), sagittal facet joint (**b**), coronal (**c**), and axial plane (**d**)

31.3.2 Indication for Surgery

As outlined above, there are many factors affecting the initial concept of timing and order of polytraumatized patients with SCI. Both, the Thoracolumbar Injury Classification and Severity Score (TLICS) and the Subaxial Cervical Spine Injury Classification and Severity Score (SLIC) are broadly used for such decision-making guidance [6, 18]. For both, the integrity of the posterior ligamentous or discoligamentous complex, injury morphology, and the neurological status are the major factors (please see Chaps. 30 and 34 for details). Concerning our patient, the SLIC score was 9 and therefore indicating surgery. However, in terms of present SCI, the score is very easy to interpret: any SCI plus spinal canal involvement means surgical treatment.

31.3.3 Timing of Surgery

There is still some debate concerning the timing of surgery. Length of overall hospital and ICU stay and medical complications are lower with early surgery (defined as within the first 24 h after injury), especially in polytraumatized patients [4]. Concerning neurological outcome after SCI, early vs. delayed decompression trials showed inconsistent results. However, today, most studies and authors will agree that early decompression shows superior neurological outcome with an average AIS improvement of 2 within the first 6 months [9, 13]. Yet, proper resuscitation of patients prior to surgery is required [7, 10, 20]. We also need to be aware that the currently published evidence on surgical decompression within the first 24 h does not mean any cut-off time point for our daily practice rather than a statistical flaw. It is the result from grouping patients <24 h and >24 h for statistical analysis in order to obtain proper group sizes and not based on pathophysiology. In the contrary: when considering the pathophysiology of SCI, any spinal cord compression not only means direct disruption of fibers, it also means pressure onto the spinal cord tissue resulting in reduced perfusion and oxygen supply causing further cell death namely the so-called secondary injury [20]. Currently further evidence in the frame of randomized controlled trials is lacking but the gut feeling, clinical experience, and pathophysiology tell us that decompression needs to be done as early as safely possible. Since the patient in our illustrative case was then fully stable in terms of respiration and circulation, immediate instrumentation and fusion was performed resulting in early recovery of two ASI grades within 7 days.

31.3.4 Required Imaging

SCI is a clinical diagnosis. However, we rely on imaging in order to localize the injury correctly and to reveal accompanying vascular injuries as well as non-symptomatic other spinal injuries. For SCI CT is the imaging of choice due to its quick and broad availability, its accuracy in detection and the ability to easily examine also ventilated patients. Depending on the mechanism of injury, CT angiography is recommended in most cases due to traumatic dissection of the carotid, vertebral or even aortic artery [3]. The use of MRI in the acute trauma patient is limited to awake patients with severe pain or to awake or ventilated patients with a neurological deficit, which cannot be properly explained by the CT scan. Moreover, guidelines recommend MRI in the first 48 h after trauma in elderly patients to exclude potential cervical injury [19]. In terms of estimating prognosis of spinal cord injury, however, there has been an increase in articles demonstrating that MRI is able to quantify the spinal cord integrity by diffusion tensor imaging and functional MRI [17]. Coming back to our SCI patient, clinical symptoms and CT imaging showed consistent results. Yet, due to the suspected further discoligamentous injury to other parts of the cervical spine, an immediate MRI scan was performed to properly guide the surgical approach. Very early decompression was still possible and further intraspinal hematoma could be ruled out that way. After surgery, early recovery of the lower extremity pareses indicated potential spinal cord recovery.

31.3.5 Surgery

Besides decompression of the spinal cord in case of spinal cord compression on the imaging, the optimal method of spinal stabilization depends on the morphology of ligamentous and bony injury including injury mechanism and neurological status. In general, incomplete SCI is usually treated more aggressively than complete SCI by most surgeons since it shows that the primary injury did not destroy the whole spinal cord function initially thus further (so-called secondary) injury can occur and needs to be avoided. Spinal shock may make this differentiation more difficult in clinical reality. The particular approaches are described in Chaps. 33, 34, 35, 36, 37, 38, 39, 40, and 41.

31.3.6 Postoperative Management of SCI

Along with the objective for surgical decompression, the primary therapeutic goal of SCI management is the reduction of the secondary injury. This secondary injury includes mechanisms starting instantaneously but lasting for several weeks, such as breakdown of the blood–brain barrier, inflammatory cytokines, sodium- and calcium-mediated cell injury, glutamate-related excitotoxicity, vasospasm, ischemia and apoptosis [14]. On a macroscopic level, this secondary injury can be worsened due to spinal instability, systemic hypoxia, systemic hypotension, or low supply of glucose. Due to these secondary mechanisms, the initial primary injury expands as secondary injury in size, which causes worse neurological outcome.

Consequently, besides the management of concomitant injuries, monitoring and optimizing respiratory, cardiac, and circulatory parameters is crucial in order to reduce mortality and improve neurological and medical outcome [15]. Thus, a mean arterial pressure (MAP) >85 mmHg for 7 days after injury is recommended [15]. Along with those measures further neuroprotective strategies have been investigated extensively in the past:

Systemic or local hypothermia is used by many centers since ages. Clinical evidence is however sparse and only demonstrated in animal studies and one retrospective case–control study with a trend towards better functional recovery after hypothermia (43% vs. 21%) [14]. One prospective nonrandomized study is still ongoing (NCT01739010).

Methylprednisolone inhibits inflammation and membrane lipid peroxidation and is therefore seen as a treatment option for SCI. While current AANS/CNS guidelines do not recommend its use, the latest Cochrane review recommended Methylprednisolone as a treatment option [2, 19]. It includes 8 randomized controlled trials with very different results ending in showing no neurological benefit. A short application 8 h after SCI for 24 h showed significant motor improvement. Yet, wound infection and gastrointestinal bleeding doubled while it lead to lower mortality. Therefore while the Cochrane review's concludes with the effectiveness of Methylprednisolone, the AANS/CNS guidelines do not recommend it also emphasizing the lacking FDA approval for this indication. Additional data from the STASCIS trial shows us, nonetheless, reduced complications by 44% in SCI patients receiving Methylprednisolone [9]. In contrast to the general idea of the abovementioned measures, including surgical decompression, to reduce secondary injury, regenerative approaches aim on inducing spinal repair mechanisms. They are mostly experimental and outlined in several high quality articles [1, 14].

The SCI patient outlined at the beginning of this chapter was monitored on the ICU where she never showed any impairment of respiration or circulation due to the injury below C4. She was then transferred to an intermediate care unit of our department until discharge due to the higher staff requirements to care SCI patients. A permanent catheter was kept until she was transfered to the rehabilitation unit.

31.3.7 Bowel and Bladder Function

As part of SCI bowel and bladder function can be impaired in a transient or permanent manner. This can cause serious sequelae, such as urinary tract infection or even renal damage. One year after SCI, 33% of patients were admitted to a hospital because of bladder issues [20]. Thus, today, instead of using the Valsalva maneuver intermittent self-catheterization is recommended. In terms of bowel function 3 different patterns of bowel dysfunction were defined [12]:

- Pattern A (SCI above T-7): no control of abdominal muscles; spinal sacral reflexes present
- Pattern B (SCI below T-7): with control of abdominal muscles; sacral reflexes present
- Pattern C (SCI below T-7): with control of abdominal muscles; no sacral reflexes

Chronic treatment is done via timed eating and rectal stimulation if required. Prokinetic medication can be used. For patients suffering recurrent problems with bowel function, colostomy is an option.

31.3.8 Accordance with the Literature Guidelines

As discussed above, there are several guidelines available, which are in part contradictory [8, 19, 20]. Though, for most steps of treatment including indication of surgery there is a consensus of the majority of peers. This is also true for the treatment algorithm through which our illustrative patient went.

In some cases crucial steps of treatment will still depend on the decision of the individual surgeon (Table 31.1).

Table 31.1 Evidence of guideline

Topic	Level of AANS/CNS recommendation	Guideline/recommendation
Hypotension	Level III	Correction of hypotension to systolic blood pressure >90 mmHg as soon as possible
	Level III	Maintenance of mean arterial blood pressure between 85 and 90 mmHg for 7 days
Hypoxia	None	Hypoxia (PaO_2 <60 mmHg or O_2 saturation <90%) should be avoided [3]
ICU monitoring	Level III	SCI patients should be managed in an ICU setting with cardiac, hemodynamic, and respiratory monitoring to detect cardiovascular dysfunction and respiratory insufficiency
Immobilization	Level II	Patients with SCI or suspected SCI (except in penetrating injury) should be immobilized
	Level III	Spinal immobilization should be performed with rigid cervical collar and supportive blocks on a backboard with straps
Specialized centers	Level III	SCI patients should be transferred expediently to specialized centers of SCI care
Examination	Level II	The ASIA ISNCSCI examination should be performed and documented
Imaging	Level I	No cervical imaging is required in awake trauma patients that have no neck pain/tenderness, normal neurological examination, normal range of motion, and no distracting injuries
	Level I	CT is recommended in favor of cervical X-rays
	Level I	CT angiography is recommended in patients who meet the modified Denver screening criteria [4]
Neuroprotection	Level I	Methylprednisolone is not recommended[a]
Spinal cord decompression	None	Surgical decompression prior to 24 h after SCI can be performed safely and is associated with improved neurological outcome [5**]
	Level III	Early closed reduction of fracture/dislocation in awake patients without a rostral injury is recommended, and pre-reduction MRI does not appear to influence outcome

This table (Table 1 from Martin et al. [14]) shows the current best practice guidelines and their level of evidence as a small collection of relevant data from the 2013 AANS/CNS guidelines [14, 19]

Current best practices for the diagnosis and management of SCI. Listed are several key recommendations, many of which are from the 2013 updated guidelines from the Joint Section on Disorders of the Spine and Peripheral Nerves of the American Association of Neurological Surgeons and the Congress of Neurological Surgeons [2**]

[a]Martin et al. do not agree with this guideline

Level of Evidence: A
The level of evidence available to date is considerably good for most aspects of treatment.

31.4 Conclusions and Take Home Message

Today we have considerably fair scientific evidence for the best practice in the acute management of SCI. While some issues under debate might be solved by larger and clear randomized controlled trials, we will also see some new treatments which will be established in the next one or two decades; like pharmaceuticals disrupting mechanisms underlying secondary injury, cellular therapies, hypothermia, and biomaterials.

Pearls
- SCI is mostly traumatic
- it requires immediate decompression in the majority of cases; the evidence on optimal timing ist yet sparse
- level of evidence on perioperative management is still inconclusive in many cases

Editorial Comment
This is a very good chapter and highly recommended reading, because it discusses excellently an important topic with still according to us unnecessary controversy and great regional variations. When and how a patient with an SCI is treated depends within Europe alone very much on where he resides, but not on what an appropriate and sober interpretation of the evidence in the literature would actually dictate. Apart from mere fatalistic and sometimes uninformed attitudes, there are very often organizational obstacles that cause deviations from the best of care for these patients. We are convinced, that surgical decompression and stabilization should be performed as an absolute emergency (if no other life threatening (!) injuries prohibit it) irrespective of ASIA grade, i.e. complete versus incomplete. It is counterproductive to lead sophisticated scientific discussions, because there will never be data from several RCTs to definitely prove that early intervention is beneficial. We think, if there is only a slight doubt that delay in treatment may harm the patient and on the other hand early surgery poses not more risks, then there is no argument at all to postpone or delay treatment. In an industrialized and whealthy environment like Europe, organizational issues should never be an argument to do so. This chapter also illustrates that fatalism if confronted with complete injuries is no longer appropriate, because patients with complete cervical SCI -opposed to thoracic ones- may recover in a relevant number of times. The discussion about this should clearly be in the center of attention and not the useless one on how (front, back, both, which sequence...) to operate bilateral locked facets. According to us that decision should also be left to the individual surgeon's discretion. There are many ways to skin the proverbial cat.

References

1. Ahuja CS, Nori S, Tetreault L, Wilson J, Kwon B, Harrop J, et al. Traumatic spinal cord injury-repair and regeneration. Neurosurgery. 2017;80(3S):S9–S22. https://doi.org/10.1093/neuros/nyw080.
2. Bracken MB. Steroids for acute spinal cord injury. Cochrane Database Syst Rev. 2012;1:CD001046. https://doi.org/10.1002/14651858.CD001046.pub2.
3. Bromberg WJ, Collier BC, Diebel LN, Dwyer KM, Holevar MR, Jacobs DG, et al. Blunt cerebrovascular injury practice management guidelines: the Eastern Association for the Surgery of Trauma. J Trauma. 2010;68(2):471–7. https://doi.org/10.1097/TA.0b013e3181cb43da.
4. Carreon LY, Dimar JR. Early versus late stabilization of spine injuries: a systematic review. Spine (Phila Pa 1976). 2011;36(11):E727–33. https://doi.org/10.1097/BRS.0b013e3181fab02f.

5. Ditunno JF, Little JW, Tessler A, Burns AS. Spinal shock revisited: a four-phase model. Spinal Cord. 2004;42(7):383–95. https://doi.org/10.1038/sj.sc.3101603.
6. Dvorak MF, Fisher CG, Fehlings MG, Rampersaud YR, Oner FC, Aarabi B, et al. The surgical approach to subaxial cervical spine injuries: an evidence-based algorithm based on the SLIC classification system. Spine (Phila Pa 1976). 2007;32(23):2620–9. https://doi.org/10.1097/BRS.0b013e318158ce16.
7. El Tecle NE, Dahdaleh NS, Hitchon PW. Timing of surgery in spinal cord injury. Spine (Phila Pa 1976). 2016;41(16):E995–E1004. https://doi.org/10.1097/BRS.0000000000001517.
8. Fehlings MG, Tetreault LA, Wilson JR, Kwon BK, Burns AS, Martin AR, et al. A clinical practice guideline for the management of acute spinal cord injury: introduction, rationale, and scope. Global Spine J. 2017;7(3 Suppl):84S–94S. https://doi.org/10.1177/2192568217703387.
9. Fehlings MG, Vaccaro A, Wilson JR, Singh A, Cadotte D, Harrop JS, Aarabi B, Shaffrey C, Dvorak M, Fisher C, Arnold P, Massicotte EM, Lewis S, Rampersaud R. Early versus delayed decompression for traumatic cervical spinal cord injury: results of the Surgical Timing in Acute Spinal Cord Injury Study (STASCIS). PLoS One. 2012;7(2):e32037. https://doi.org/10.1371/journal.pone.0032037.
10. Furlan JC, Noonan V, Cadotte DW, Fehlings MG. Timing of decompressive surgery of spinal cord after traumatic spinal cord injury: an evidence-based examination of pre-clinical and clinical studies. J Neurotrauma. 2011;28(8):1371–99. https://doi.org/10.1089/neu.2009.1147.
11. Hadley MN, Walters BC. Introduction to the guidelines for the management of acute cervical spine and spinal cord Injuries. Neurosurgery. 2013;72(Suppl 2):5–16. https://doi.org/10.1227/NEU.0b013e3182773549.
12. Hughes M. Bowel management in spinal cord injury patients. Clin Colon Rectal Surg. 2014;27(3):113–5. https://doi.org/10.1055/s-0034-1383904.
13. Lenehan B, Fisher CG, Vaccaro A, Fehlings M, Aarabi B, Dvorak MF. The urgency of surgical decompression in acute central cord injuries with spondylosis and without instability. Spine (Phila Pa 1976). 2010;35(21 Suppl):S180–6. https://doi.org/10.1097/BRS.0b013e3181f32a44.
14. Martin AR, Aleksanderek I, Fehlings MG. Diagnosis and acute management of spinal cord injury: current best practices and emerging therapies. [journal article]. Curr Trauma Rep. 2015;1(3):169–81. https://doi.org/10.1007/s40719-015-0020-0.
15. Ryken TC, Hurlbert RJ, Hadley MN, Aarabi B, Dhall SS, Gelb DE, et al. The acute cardiopulmonary management of patients with cervical spinal cord injuries. Neurosurgery. 2013;72(Suppl 2):84–92. https://doi.org/10.1227/NEU.0b013e318276ee16.
16. Singh A, Tetreault L, Kalsi-Ryan S, Nouri A, Fehlings MG. Global prevalence and incidence of traumatic spinal cord injury. Clin Epidemiol. 2014;6:309–31. https://doi.org/10.2147/CLEP.S68889.
17. Stroman PW, Wheeler-Kingshott C, Bacon M, Schwab JM, Bosma R, Brooks J, et al. The current state-of-the-art of spinal cord imaging: methods. NeuroImage. 2014;84:1070–81. https://doi.org/10.1016/j.neuroimage.2013.04.124.
18. Vaccaro AR, Lehman RA Jr, Hurlbert RJ, Anderson PA, Harris M, Hedlund R, et al. A new classification of thoracolumbar injuries: the importance of injury morphology, the integrity of the posterior ligamentous complex, and neurologic status. Spine (Phila Pa 1976). 2005;30(20):2325–33.
19. Walters BC, Hadley MN, Hurlbert RJ, Aarabi B, Dhall SS, Gelb DE, et al. Guidelines for the management of acute cervical spine and spinal cord injuries: 2013 update. Neurosurgery. 2013;60(Suppl 1):82–91. https://doi.org/10.1227/01.neu.0000430319.32247.7f.
20. Yue JK, Winkler EA, Rick JW, Deng H, Partow CP, Upadhyayula PS, et al. Update on critical care for acute spinal cord injury in the setting of polytrauma. Neurosurg Focus. 2017;43(5):E19. https://doi.org/10.3171/2017.7.FOCUS17396.

32 Upper Cervical Spine Trauma

Yu-Mi Ryang

32.1 Introduction

32.1.1 Objective 1: OC Luxation (Difficulties in Assessment and Treatment, Prognosis)

Atlantooccipital dislocation (AOD) or occipitoatlantal dislocation (OAD) is a rare but serious injury of the upper c-spine caused by a traumatic ligamentous disruption of the craniocervical junction. This injury usually occurs after high-energy/-velocity accidents and is associated with a high morbidity and a mortality rate of 20–30% amongst all traumatic c-spine injuries. It can be easily overlooked but needs to be considered especially after high-impact trauma and in field resuscitation. Once deemed fatal (in earlier days only 1/3 of patients reached the hospital alive), better emergency management and the widespread availability of CTs led to better on site survival and more frequent recognition and more timely diagnosis of this injury improving mortality rates and neurological outcome. This has in consequence led to an increasing incidence of this injury [1].

This chapter will show a case of AOD with a typical trauma mechanism and typical clinical signs and symptoms. Aim of this case is to raise the sensitivity for this rare traumatic injury. Recognition of AOD requires experience and the awareness of the existence of this often times overlooked serious injury.

This case will detail the following problems such as:

– recognition of this rare and potentially fatal injury
– choice of imaging
– management of this injury

At the end of this chapter the reader should be aware of the problems and pitfalls in recognition and treatment of AOD.

These injuries are classified according to **Harris** into three types:

Type I: Anterior dislocation of the occiput
Type II: Posterior dislocation of the occiput
Type III: Axial dislocation of the occiput

32.1.1.1 Case Description

A 53 y/o male construction worker fell headway from a scaffold of 3 m height. He was awake initially with no neurological deficit and referred to a tertiary peripheral hospital. There he soon developed respiratory insufficiency and a bilateral N. VI palsy. He was intubated on site and transferred to the ER of a level I trauma center.

On presentation in the ER the patient was intubated, sedated and ventilated. Pupils were

Y.-M. Ryang (✉)
Department of Neurosurgery, Klinikum rechts der Isar, Technische Universität München, Munich, Germany
e-mail: yu.ryang@tum.de

B. Meyer, M. Rauschmann (eds.), *Spine Surgery*, https://doi.org/10.1007/978-3-319-98875-7_32

miotic and reactive to light. The cranial CT showed no signs of trauma, except for a traumatic subarachnoid hemorrhage in the craniocervical junction (Fig. 32.1). Sagittal reconstructions of the CT-angiogram revealed extension of the tSAH around the spinal cord of the entire c-spine (Fig. 32.2). Trauma mechanism and neurological deterioration of the patient with respiratory insufficiency and bilateral N. VI palsy raised the suspicion of an injury of the occipitocervical junction. On closer inspection of the CT-scan revealed the AOD (Fig. 32.3). MRI was performed immediately confirming AOD (Fig. 32.4).

The patient received surgery with posterior occipitocervical fixation from the occiput with an occiput plate to C2–3 with C2 isthmic and C3 lateral mass screws the same day (postop CT-scan Fig. 32.5).

After surgery the patient was weaned from the ventilator and could be extubated within the next days. He had no new neurological deficit. The N. VI palsy was remitting over the next few weeks. Two weeks after admission the patient experienced a sudden onset of severe dyspnea and cardiac arrest needing CPR and emergency intubation. Pulmonary CT showed a fulminant pulmonary embolism leading to the subsequent death of the patient (Fig. 32.6).

32.1.1.2 Discussion of the Case

Clinical and Radiological Assessment

The greatest difficulty in AOD is the timely recognition and treatment of this traumatic c-spine injury. This is necessary, because it is a purely ligamentous lesion with subtotal or total rupture of the occipitocervical ligaments which is highly unstable and therefore life-threatening. Clinical assessment of these patients usually is difficult or impossible since the majority lose consciousness, are cardiopulmonary unstable and need intubation at the trauma site. In field resuscitation or a comatous patient are therefore highly suggestive for AOD, especially after high impact trauma and a patient of younger age. Visible signs of hyperflexion or -extension injuries such as lacerations of the back of the head or forehead are more signs suggesting AOD.

When suspecting AOD it is imperative to avoid any unnecessary movement of the patient, especially any extension manoeuvre that can cause neurological deterioration in up to 10%. We recommend performing early CT and MRI of the cranium and the c-spine with CTA and / or MRA especially of the carotid arteries to rule out dissections.

Indication

Since AOD must be considered a highly unstable ligamentous injury, early fixation is necessary.

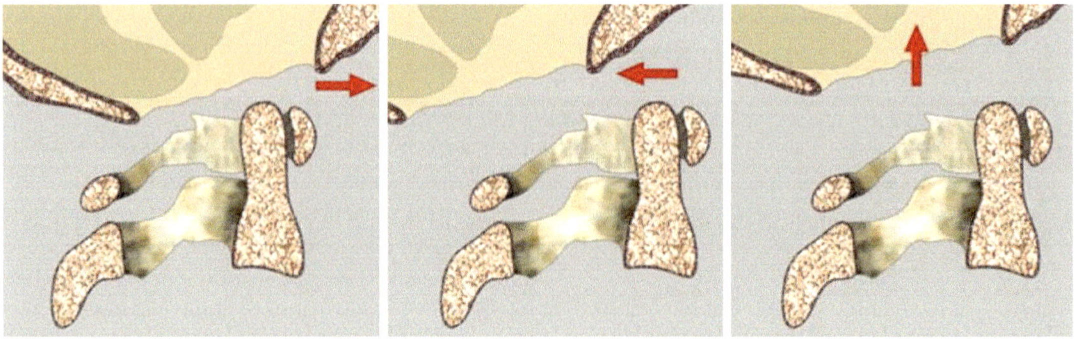

Fig. 32.1 Harris classification [2]

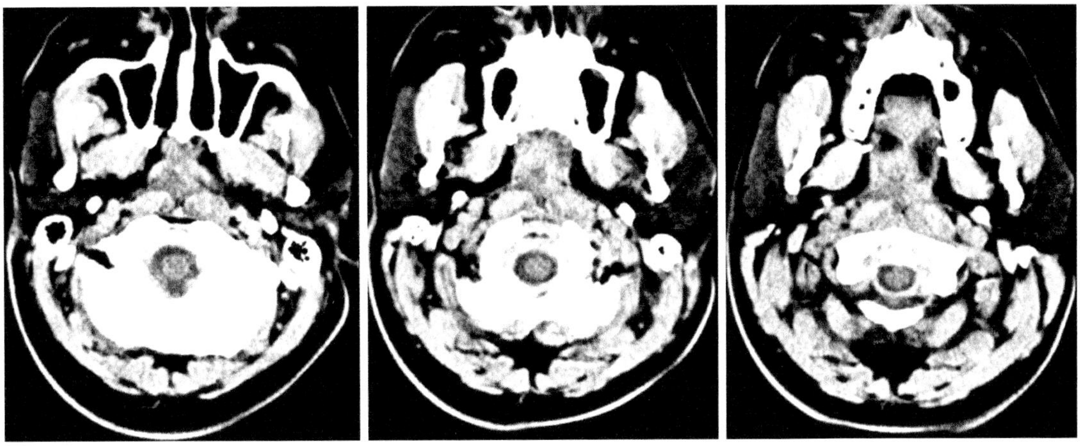

Fig. 32.2 Cranial CT scan showing traumatic subarachnoid hemorrhage in the craniocervical junction as an indirect sign of AOD

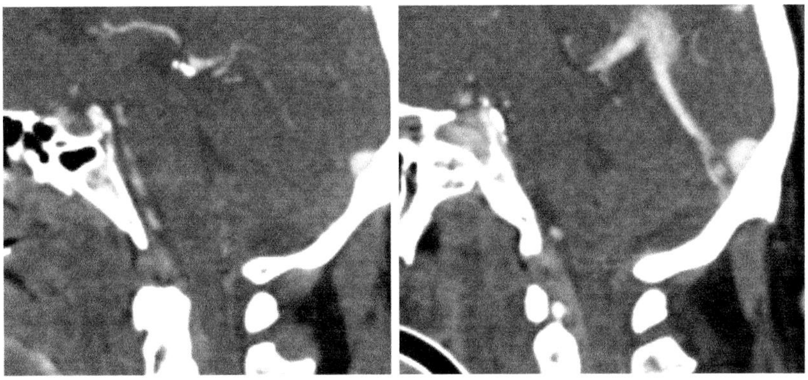

Fig. 32.3 CTA showing traumatic subarachnoid hemorrhage in the craniocervical junction and the c-spine

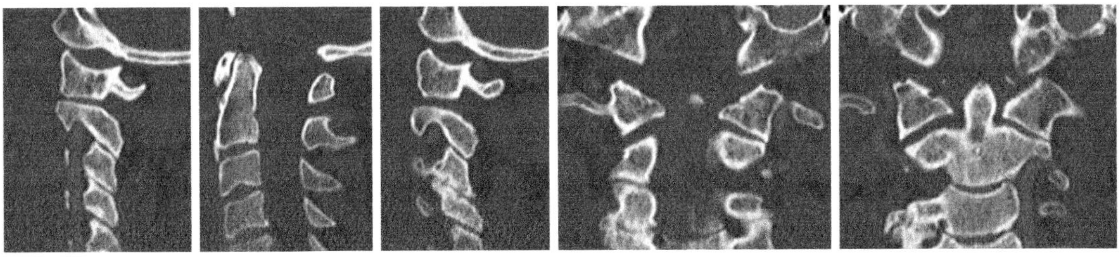

Fig. 32.4 Sagittal and coronal CT scans of the c-spine showing an abnormal distance between the occipital condyles and C1

Choice of Treatment

These injuries need to be fixed immediately. Treatment with internal fixation and fusion is recommended.

Accordance with the Literature Guidelines

Our treatment is accordance with the treatment guidelines of the Joint Section on Disorders of the Spine and Peripheral Nerves of the American

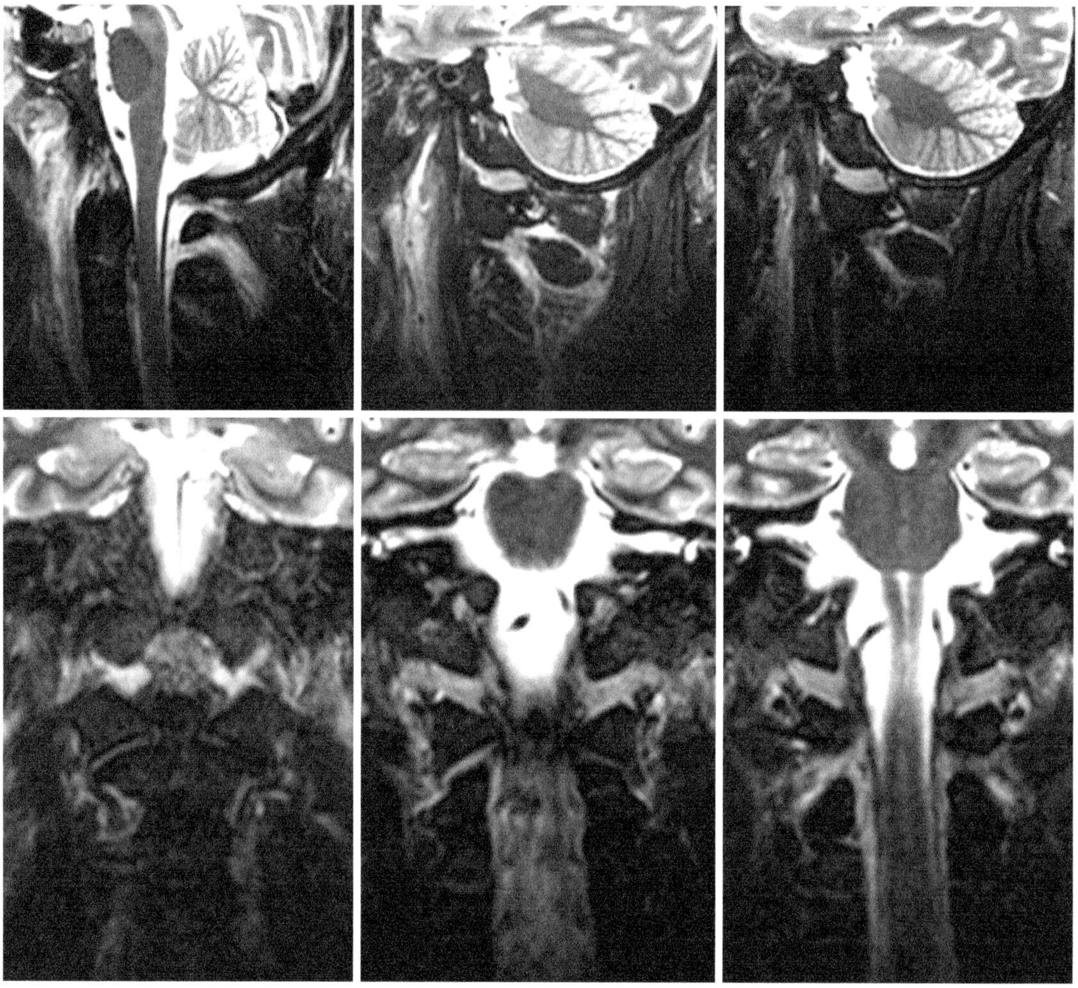

Fig. 32.5 Craniocervical sagittal and coronal STIR-weighted MRI showing hyperintensities between clivus and the apex of the dens and in the gaping occipitocervical joint space

Association of Neurological Surgeons and the Congress of Neurological Surgeons.

How Strong is the Level of Evidence Available to Date

Current recommendations in adults are based on level III evidence with regard to diagnostics and treatment.

For pediatric patients there is a level I recommendation for CT imaging to determine the condyle-C1-interval.

32.1.2 Objective 2: C2 Fracture (Treatment Options Surgical/ Problems with Halo)

C2 injuries comprise of fractures of the odontoid, traumatic spondylolisthesis and atypical axis fractures.

In this chapter we will discuss a case of a traumatic odontoid fracture (tOF) since these are the most frequent injuries of the c-spine (10–15%). The frequency of tOFs increases with age.

Pearls and Pitfalls

- Early and timely recognition and surgery are crucial for this potentially fatal injury.
- Look out for indirect signs of AOD such as:
  - Trauma mechanism (hyperextension/flexion injury)
  - High energy trauma
  - Patient age (ligamentous injuries predominant in younger patients)
  - tSAH in the craniocervical junction on CT as an indirect sign of ligamentous disruption of the craniocervical junction
  - In field resuscitation as an indirect sign of a high-energy trauma and traumatic lesion of the craniocervical junction with affection of the brainstem.
- Not only look for osseous lesions, but also look for ligamentous lesions, which are hard to detect on CT or x-ray.
- Always check alignment, i.e. check for pathological condyle-C1-interval (CCI), atlanto-dental interval (ADI)
- Traction is not recommended in AOD. Be careful with cervical orthosis or any other cervical immobilization device. They might exert traction leading to neurological deterioration with a potentially fatal outcome.

They are classified into three types according to **Anderson and D'Alonzo** [3]:

Type I: Fracture through the tip; unstable
Type II: Fracture through the base of neck; usually unstable
Type IIA: Comminuted type II fracture; usually unstable
Type III: Fracture through body of C2; usually stable

or according to **Grauer** (Fig. 32.7):
Type I: Fracture through odontoid tip
Type IIA: Transverse fracture line through base of neck, non-displaced
Type IIB: Anterior-superior to posterior-inferior fracture line or displaced type II fracture
Type IIC: Anterior-inferior to posterior-superior fracture line or comminuted type II fracture
Type III: Fracture including at least one of the superior articular C2 facets

Type I fractures with avulsion of the alar ligaments are very rare. Type II fractures are the most frequent tOF.

In younger patients the trauma mechanism usually is a high impact/velocity trauma after a fall from great height or after a motor vehicle accident. In contrast the trauma mechanism in elderly patients usually is a low energy trauma, such as a simple fall in a domestic environment.

Therefore the fatality at the time of accident in younger patients is reported to range between 25% and 40%, whereas there is basically no reported mortality in elderly patients. Eighty percent of patients with type II fractures are neurologically intact, 10% have a minor and 10% a significant neurological deficit. The main complaint usually is neck pain.

This case will detail the following problems concerning the treatment modality (conservative vs. surgical management) with regard to:

- age and bone quality
- fracture type and anatomical conditions
- surgical technique
- factors affecting outcome and morbidity and mortality

At the end of this chapter the reader should be aware of the problems and pitfalls in the treatment of tOF, especially with regard to age (young vs old patient).

32.1.2.1 Case Description

A 45-year old male patient fell from a ladder from approximately 4 m height. He was unconscious shortly and complained of severe neck pain on regaining consciousness. He was brought

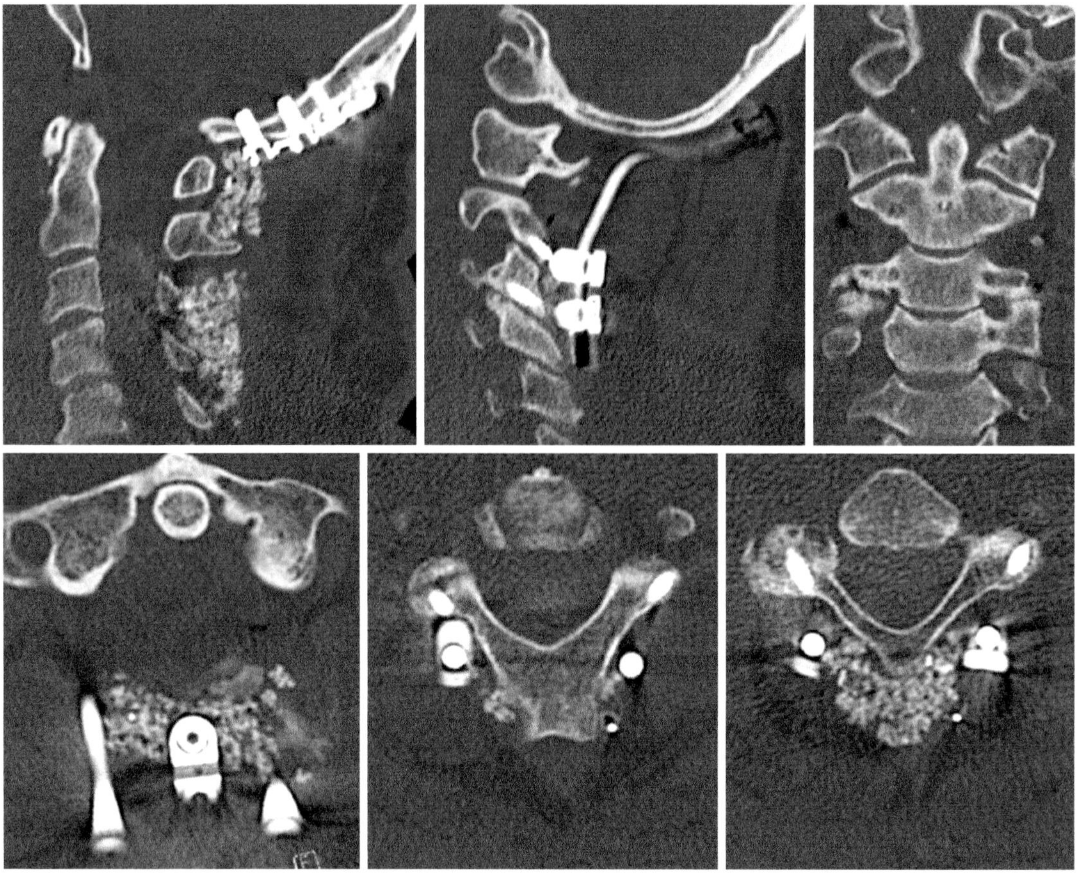

Fig. 32.6 Postoperative sagittal, coronal and axial CT-scans after posterior occipitocervical fixation

to the ER awake and without neurological deficit. A CT scan of the cervical spine showed a non-dislocated traumatic odontoid fracture type IIB (Fig. 32.7). An MRI confirmed the acute type IIB tOF (STIR weighted MRI) and ruled out any further discoligamentous injuries (Fig. 32.8).

The patient was immobilized in a hard collar and received surgery with an anterior odontoid screw fixation in Böhler technique using biplanar c-arm fluoroscopy within 7 days after trauma (Figs. 32.9 and 32.10). Surgery was uneventful. The hard collar was removed and the patient was mobilized the next day. The postoperative CT scan showed correct fracture alignment and a correct position of the anterior odontoid lag screw (Fig. 32.11). The patient was discharged on the second postoperative day with improved neck pain (VAS 3/10) and without neurological deficit.

32.1.2.2 Discussion of the Case

Indication

Type II fractures are the most common tOF. Since these fractures are usually unstable they need to be immobilized. There is still an ongoing debate concerning the treatment modality especially in elderly patients, which is being investigated in an ongoing prospective European multicentre trial (INNOVATE Trial). Treatment options vary from conservative treatment with a hard collar or halo vest to surgical treatment via anterior approaches such as anterior transarticular C1/2 fixation, an

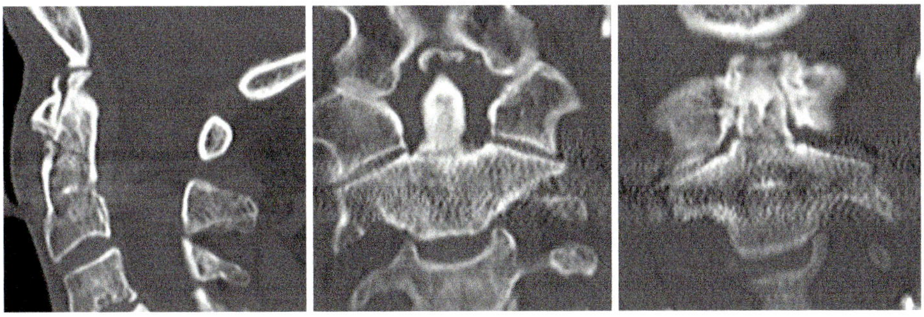

Fig. 32.7 Sagittal and coronal CT scan showing non-dislocated traumatic odontoid fracture type IIB

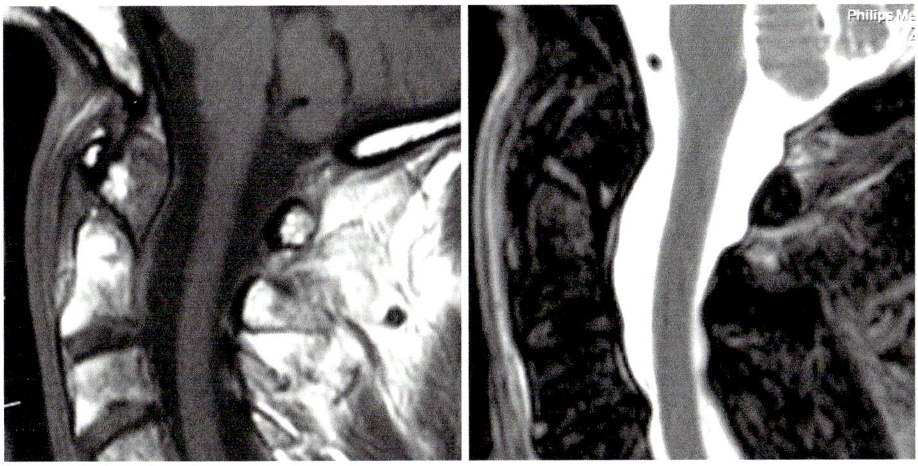

Fig. 32.8 Sagittal MRI (T1 and T2-STIR weighted images) showing a traumatic odontoid fracture type IIB

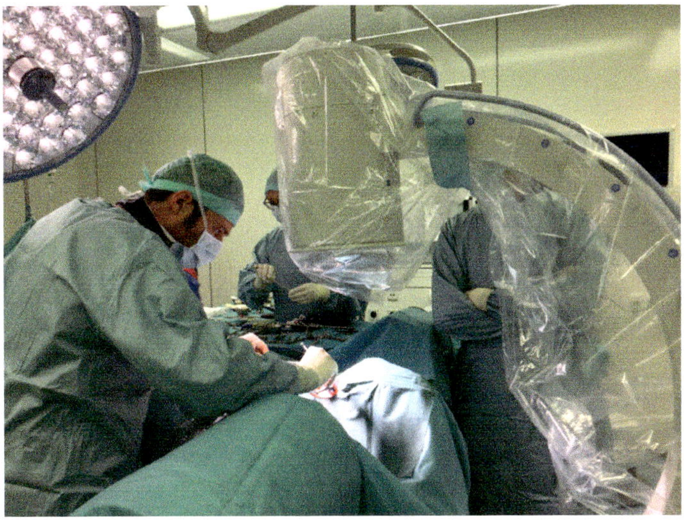

Fig. 32.9 Intraoperative set up with biplanar fluoroscopy using two c-arms placed a.p. and laterally around the patient

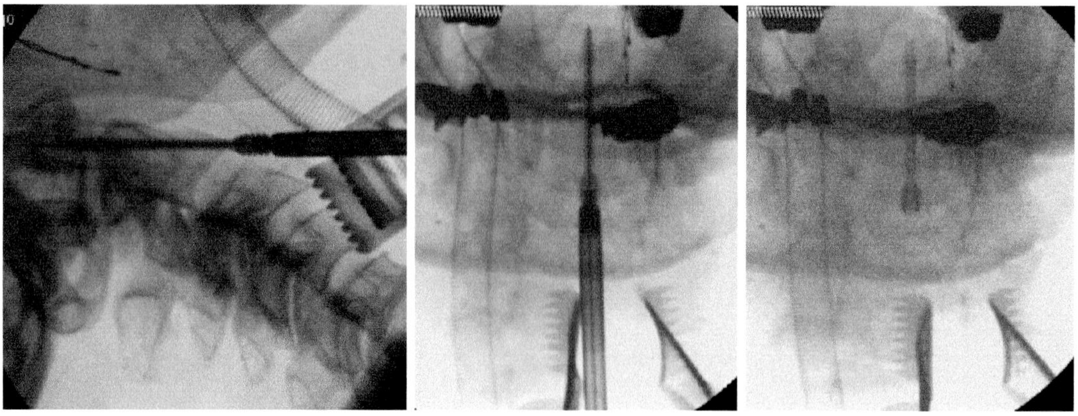

Fig. 32.10 Intraoperative lateral and a.p. fluoroscopic images of inserted k-wire and anterior odontoid lag screw

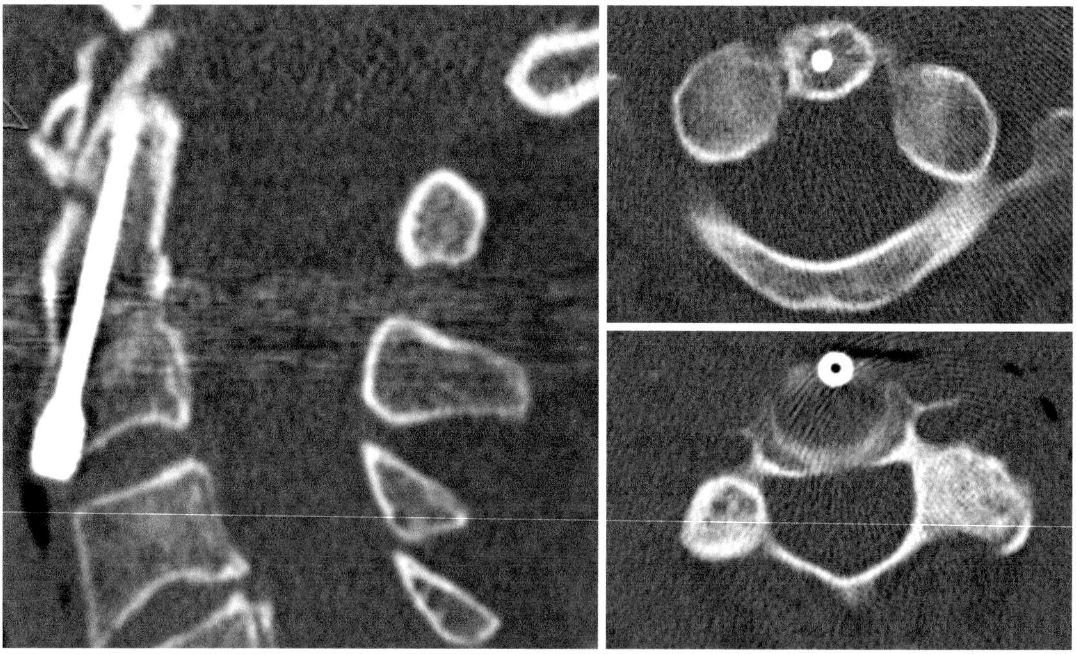

Fig. 32.11 Postoperative CT after anterior odontoid screw fixation

anterior odontoid screw fixation or a combination of both techniques with one or two odontoid screws to posterior fixations such as posterior transarticular C1-C2 fixation in Magerl technique [11] (Fig. 32.12a) or posterior C1 lateral mass-C2 isthmic or pedicle screw fixation in Harms-Goel technique with a polyaxial screw rod system [9, 10] (Fig. 32.12b).

Choice of Treatment

There is no class I evidence on how to treat tOF. Class II evidence recommends surgery for type II tOF in elderly patients ≥50 years of age. A prospective multicenter trial was able to significantly improve functional outcome, increase fusion rate and reduce mortality in surgically treated elderly patients. Also the nonunion rate

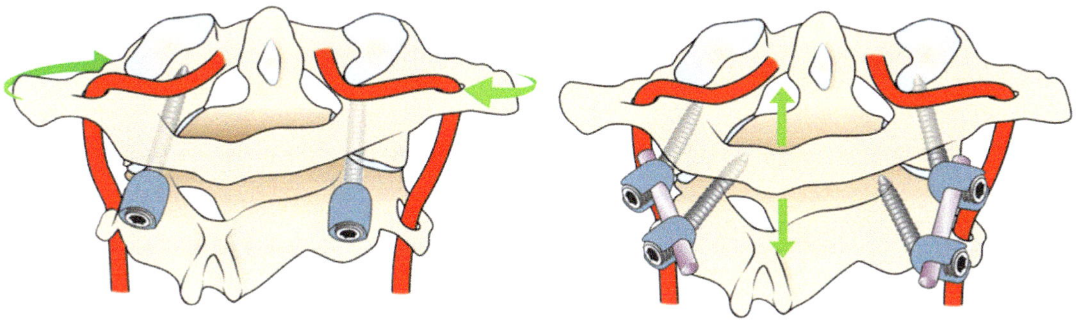

Fig. 32.12 Posterior transarticular C1-C2 fixation technique after Magerl (**a**, left); posterior C1-C2 fixation technique after Harms-Goel (**b**, right). (Courtesy of AOSpine) (Source: AO Surgery Reference, www.aosurgery.org) (© Copyright by AO Foundation, Switzerland)

is reported to be 21-times higher in patients ≥50 years of age compared to younger patients if treated conservatively [5, 6]. Therefore for these patients surgery is recommended with a strong recommendation for posterior fixation [7]. Class III evidence indicates that factors such as patient age, fracture type/displacement, secondary loss of reduction and delayed treatment are associated with nonunion [5]. Immobilization in a halo vest can be administered in non-displaced type II fractures. However, it is associated with a high mortality rate of up to 40% in elderly patients [8]. Surgery should be considered in displaced fractures of ≥5 mm, comminuted fractures or inability to achieve or maintain fracture alignment with external immobilization [5]. Fusion rates are reported to be >90% for anterior and posterior surgical fixations alike. However, there are some contraindications concerning some surgical techniques. Whereas the Harms-Goel technique is universally applicable for any kind of tOF in any patient even in displaced fractures, which can be openly reduced during surgery, the Magerl technique is unsuitable in displaced fractures or patients with a kyphotic thoracic spine since the entry point for the drill is approximately at the level of Th1. Also the rate of vertebral artery injuries is reported to be higher than with the Harms-Goel technique.

Anterior odontoid screw fixation (AOSF) is a relatively easy and minimally-invasive technique. However, it is not suitable in patients with barrel chest, thoracic kyphosis or patients with a very short neck, in osteoporosis or reduced bone mineral density and in type IIC fractures. If these factors are not taken into account prior to surgery, the failure rate can be as high as 36% (loss of correction, non-union, delayed fusion, pseudarthrosis) and is associated with an increased risk of postoperative dysphagia and pneumonia in elderly patients. Therefore we recommend using this technique only in patients <50 years of age with good bone quality and non-displaced type IIA and IIB fractures.

Why Were Things Done this Way

This patient had a non-displaced type IIB fracture and his age was below 50 years of age. Therefore we decided to treat him surgically with an anterior odontoid screw fixation (AOSF).

Our **treatment recommendation** for tOF is:

Type I:	External immobilization
Type II:	Younger patient with type IIA or non-displaced type IIB:
	Anterior odontoid screw fixation
	Older patient or type IIC:
	Posterior atlantoaxial fixation
Type III:	Stable: External immobilization
	Unstable: Atlantoaxial fixation

Accordance with the Literature Guidelines

Our treatment is accordance with the treatment guidelines of the Joint Section on Disorders of the Spine and Peripheral Nerves of the American Association of Neurological Surgeons and the Congress of Neurological Surgeons.

How Strong is the Level of Evidence Available to Date

Current recommendations are based on level II and III evidence.

32.2 Conclusions and Take Home Message

Surgery should be considered in unstable type II and III odontoid fractures. AOSF should be restricted to younger patients with normal bone mineral density and non-displaced type IIA + B fractures. There is growing evidence that elderly patients benefit from surgery compared to conservative treatment with a strong recommendation for posterior C1-C2 fixation.

Pearls and Pitfalls

- Type II odontoid fractures are the most common c-spine fractures
- Elderly patients seem to benefit from surgery compared to conservative management with regard to functional outcome, quality of life, mortality and fusion rate
- There is a strong recommendation for posterior C1-C2 fixation in elderly patients
- The Harms-Goel technique is universally applicable in any odontoid fracture type
- The Magerl technique is unsuitable in displaced fractures and certain anatomical conditions (thoracic kyphosis, high riding vertebral artery)
- AOSF should preferably applied in younger patients with non-displaced fractures (type IIA and IIB) and good bone quality
- AOSF is contraindicated in osteoporosis and comminuted fractures or fracture lines ascending from anterior-inferior to posterior-superior
- Osteoporosis is the most important risk factor for tOF in the elderly [12]
- tOF in the elderly are associated with higher failure and higher morbidity and mortality rates irrespective of the treatment modality

32.2.1 Objective 3: Isolated C1 Ring Fracture

Atlas fractures account for approx. 3–13% of c-spine fractures. About 56% are isolated C1 ring fractures, 44% are combined C1-C2 fractures. Typical Jefferson fractures with combined fractures of the anterior and posterior C1 ring are found in one third of patients.

Approx. 9% have additional other c-spine fractures and 21% have associated head injuries.

The typical trauma mechanism is axial loading by jumping headfirst into shallow water or falls directly on the cranial vertex. Patients are usually neurologically intact.

C1 ring fractures are classified after **Gehweiler et al.** [13] (Fig. 32.13):

- **Type 1**: Isolated anterior ring fracture
- **Type 2**: Isolated posterior ring fracture
- **Type 3**: Combined anterior and posterior ring fracture "Jefferson fracture"
  3a: Intact transverse atlantal ligament (TAL) (stable)
  3b: Disrupted TAL (unstable)
- **Type 4**: Isolated lateral mass fracture (rare)
- **Type 5**: Isolated transverse process fracture (very rare)

The most relevant fractures are the combined anterior and posterior C1 ring fractures type 3b better known as Jefferson fractures. It is crucial to assess the integrity of the transverse atlantal ligament (TAL) because its integrity determines whether a type 3 fracture is stable (type 3a, TAL intact) or unstable (type 3b, TAL disrupted).

Type 3b fractures are further classified after **Dickmann et al.** [14] (Fig. 32.14):

- **Type IA:** Interligamentous central TAL lesion
- **Type IB:** Interligamentous TAL lesion near the lateral mass
- **Type IIA:** Isolated osseous TAL avulsion
- **Type IIB:** Osseous TAL avulsion with lateral mass fracture (Gehweiler type 4)

Treatment of isolated C1-ring fractures therefore mainly depends on the integrity of the transverse atlantal ligament (TAL). A non-displaced

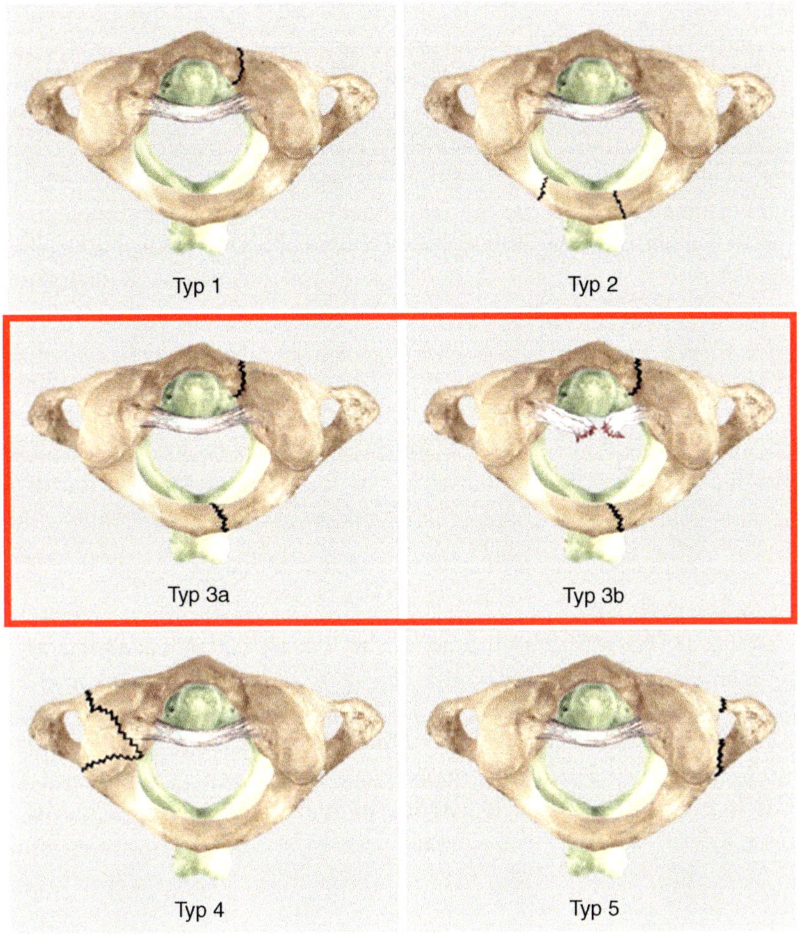

Fig. 32.13 Gehweiler classification of atlas fractures. Gehweiler type 3a = stable Jefferson fracture; Gehweiler type 3b = unstable Jefferson fracture (from [17])

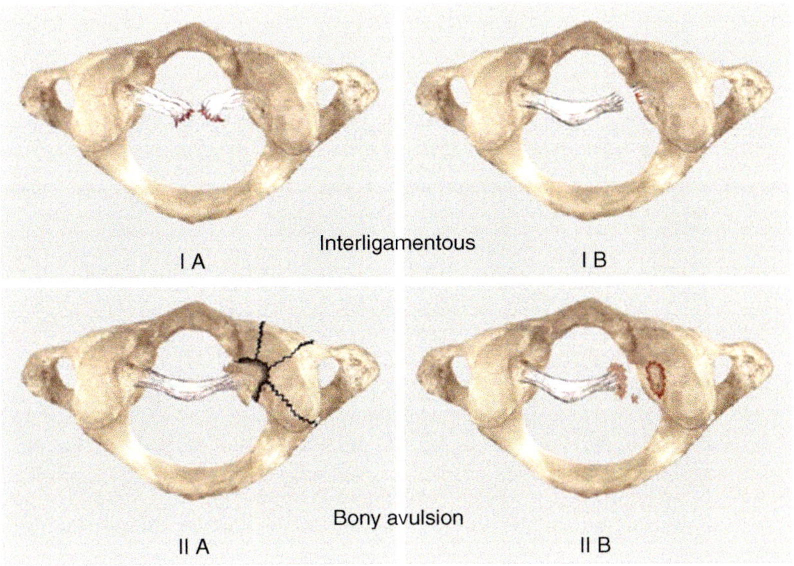

Fig. 32.14 Dickmann classification of transverse atlantal ligament (TAL) lesions (from [17])

atlas fracture with an intact TAL might be treated by immobilization alone, while all other atlas fractures should be treated surgically. C1-ring osteosynthesis should be considered in dislocated atlas fractures with intact or non-displaced osseous avulsion of the TAL. In displaced and/or intraligamentous TAL rupture an atlantoaxial fusion should be performed (see flowchart Fig. 32.19).

In combined C1-C2 fractures the C2 fracture type dictates the treatment modality (s. C2 fractures).

The purpose of this case is to delineate the importance and difficulties to adequately diagnose and treat C1 fractures with regard to:

- adequate diagnostic imaging
- correct classification
- treatment options
- the importance of the integrity of the transverse atlantal ligament (TAL)

Adequate diagnostic clinical and imaging work-up is essential to assess potentially unstable C1 fractures which are solely determined by the integrity of the transverse atlantal ligament (TAL). TAL integrity is also the main factor in decision-making as to which treatment modality should be applied.

At the end of this chapter the reader should be aware of the problems and pitfalls in the correct classification and treatment of isolated C1 fractures.

32.2.1.1 Case Description

A 25 y/o female fell on her head while tussling with her 5 y/o son. She presented to her GP for neck pain (VAS 7/10) who prescribed oral pain medication. Due to persisting neck pain despite oral analgesics she admitted herself to the ER 1 week after trauma. Because of her young age it was decided to perform plain as well as flexion/extension radiographs instead of a CT scan to minimize radiation exposure. Radiographs revealed an atlantoaxial instability with an increased atlanto-dental interval (ADI) of >3 mm (Fig. 32.15). On presentation she fortunately was neurologically intact and provided with a cervical orthosis. To properly assess the extent of osseous and ligamentous injury to the atlantoaxial complex a CT scan and MRI with STIR-weighted images were necessary which confirmed a right-sided Jefferson burst fracture (anterior and posterior ring) with osseous avulsion of the transverse atlantal ligament (TAL) (Gehweiler type 3b/Dickmann type IIB) and slight displacement of the odontoid peg (Figs. 32.16 and 32.17). A posterior C1-ring osteosynthesis was performed. Surgery was uneventful and the patient could be discharged from hospital without a cervical orthosis with improved neck pain (VAS 3/10) on the second postoperative day. Postoperative a.p. and lateral radiographs showed correct alignment of the atlantoaxial complex and correct positioning of the osteosynthesis material (Figs. 32.18 and 32.19).

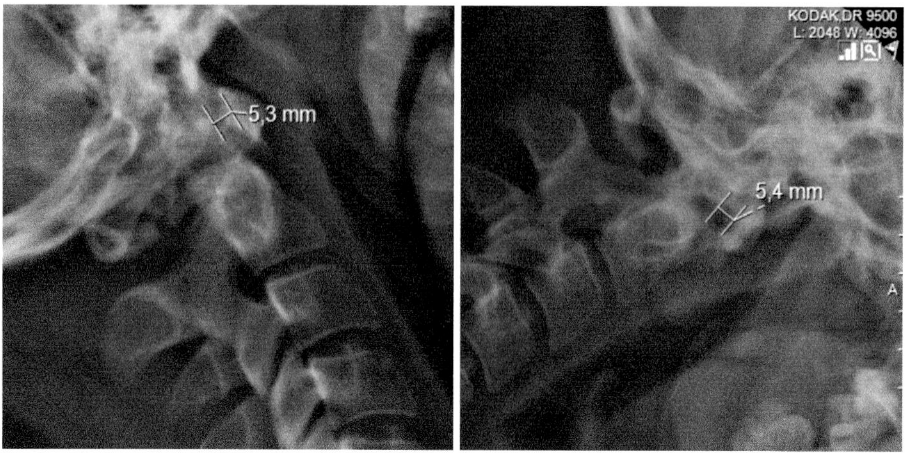

Fig. 32.15 Pathological atlanto-dental interval (ADI >3 mm) on flexion/extension radiographs

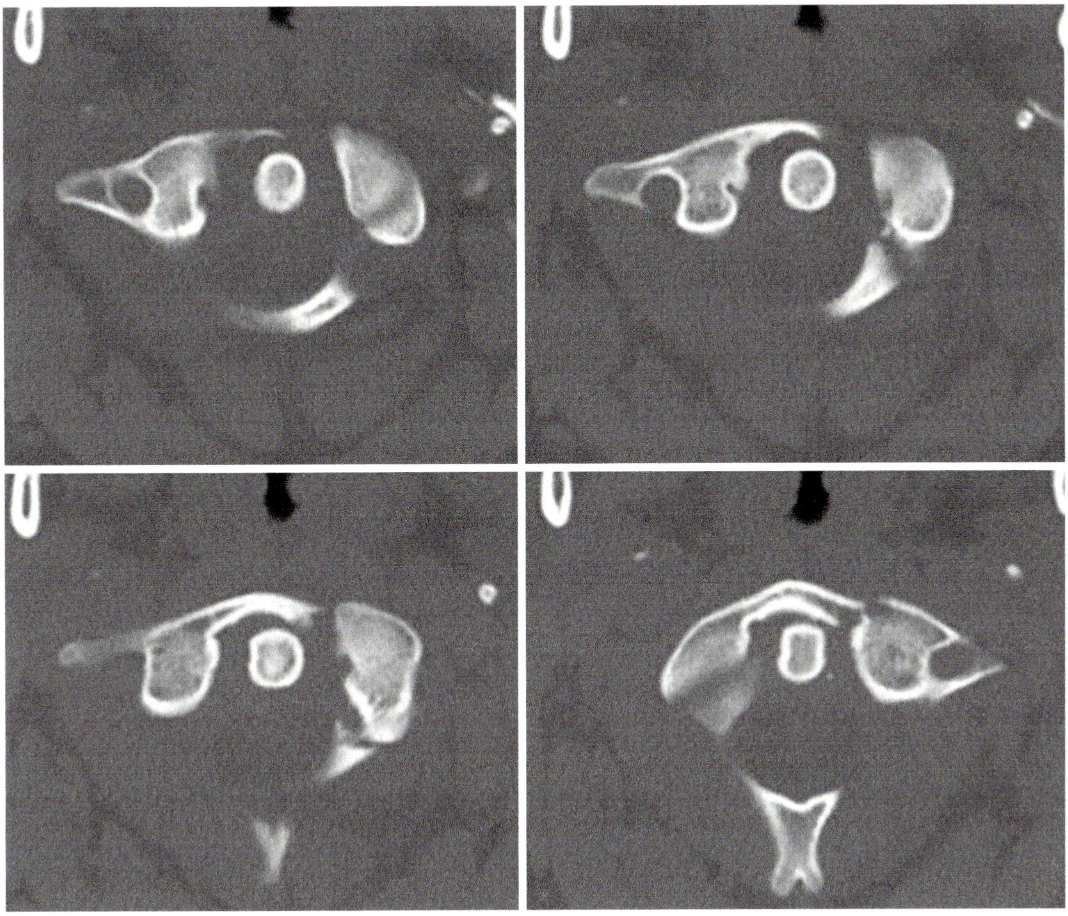

Fig. 32.16 Axial CT-scan of a right-sided Jefferson fracture (combined anterior and posterior C1-ring fracture) Gehweiler type 3b/Dickmann type IIB

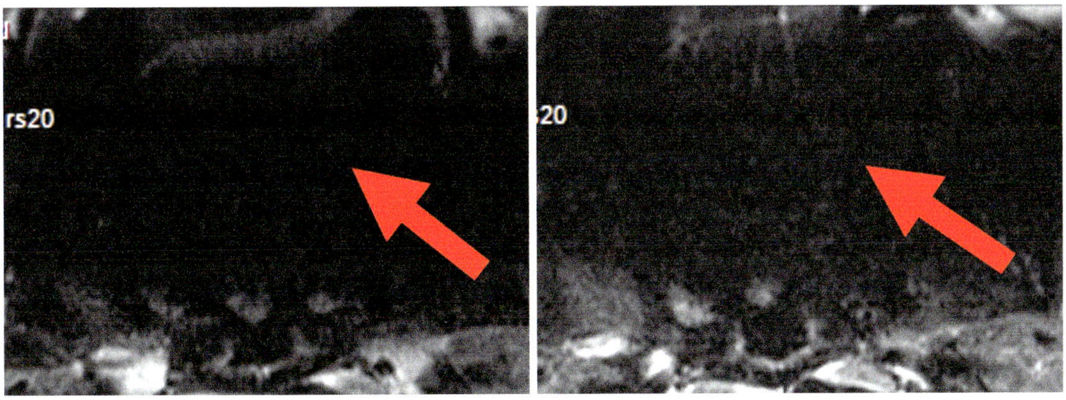

Fig. 32.17 Gehweiler type 3b/Dickmann type IIB fracture with osseous avulsion of the transverse atlantal ligament (TAL)

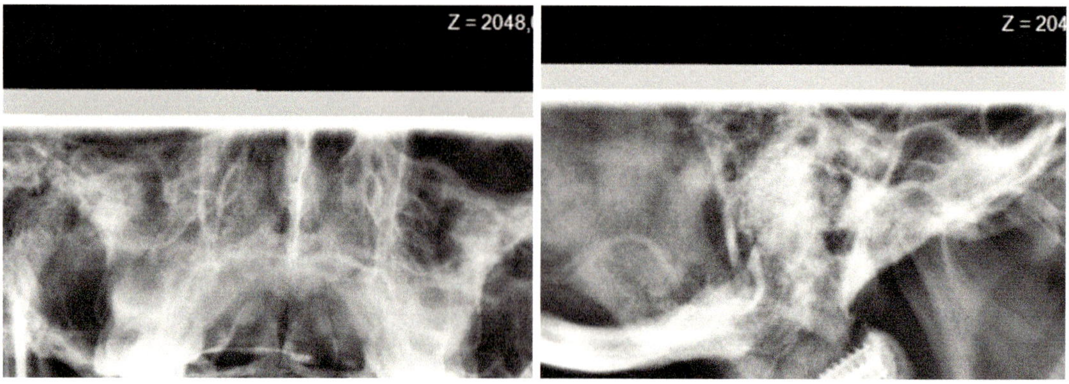

Fig. 32.18 Postoperative a.p. and lateral radiographs after C1-ring osteosynthesis with C1 lateral mass screws and a connecting rod

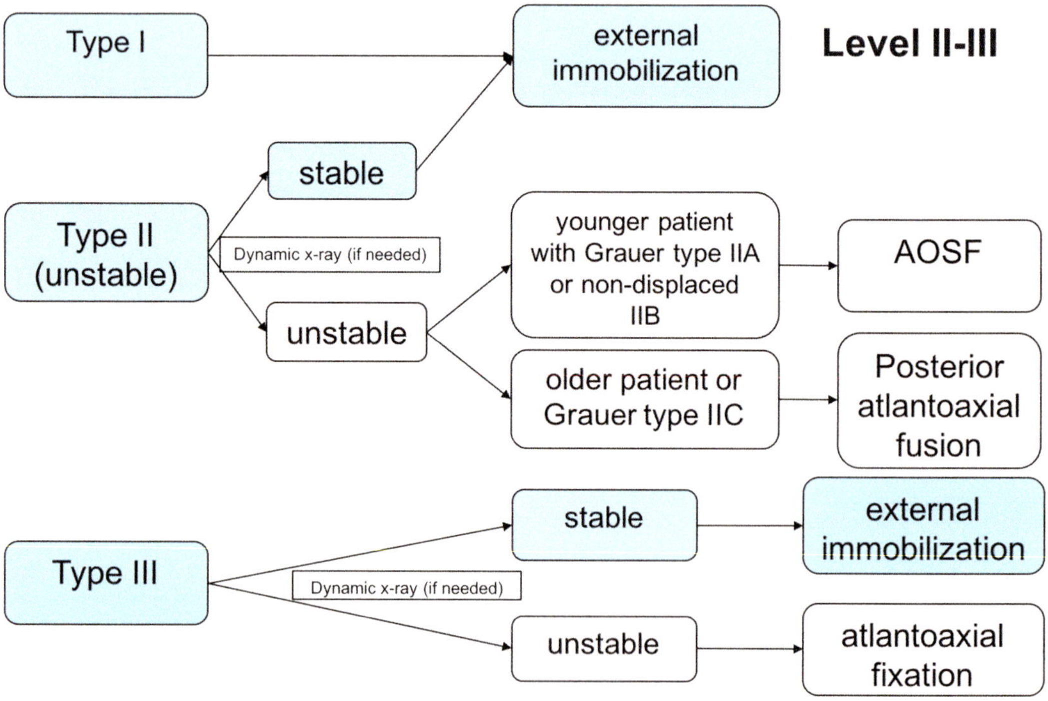

Fig. 32.19 Flowchart on the recommended treatment of atlas fractures

32.2.1.2 Discussion of the Case

Why Were Things Done this Way

This patient had a C1-ring fracture Gehweiler type 3b, Dickmann type IIB equalling an unstable fracture with an osseous TAL avulsion. Therefore she was treated with a C1-ring osteosynthesis.

Were they in Accordance with the Literature Guidelines

Our treatment is accordance with the treatment guidelines of the Joint Section on Disorders of the Spine and Peripheral Nerves of the American Association of Neurological Surgeons and the Congress of Neurological Surgeons.

How Strong is the Level of Evidence Available to Date

Up to date only level III evidence is available [15, 16].

32.3 Conclusions and Take Home Message

Assessment of the integrity of the transverse atlantal ligament (TAL) is crucial in the decision making for treatment of isolated C1-ring fractures. MRI imaging with STIR-sequences is essential to properly assess TAL and other ligamentous injuries. Flexion/extension radiographs might be helpful to confirm instability in cases with indistinct MRI findings.

Pearls and Pitfalls

- Integrity assessment of the TAL is crucial for treatment decision
- MRI and if needed flexion/extension radiographs should be performed to assess TAL integrity and other discoligamentous injuries
- An atlanto-dental interval (ADI) of >3 mm is an indirect sign of atlantoaxial instability
- C1 fractures Gehweiler type 3a with an intact TAL can usually be treated with external immobilization
- C1 fractures Gehweiler type 3b with a disrupted TAL can be treated with a halo orthosis. However, the reported morbidity and mortality especially in the elderly is considerably high, therefore surgical fixation might be the superior treatment option

Editorial Comment

This is highly recommended reading regarding modern concepts of upper cervical spine trauma. Especially the motion-preserving osteosynthesis of unstable isolated C1-ring fractures and the fact that a posterior Harms/Goel construct is the surgical treatment of choice for odontoid fractures in the elderly.

References

Level of Evidence II (Diagnosis)/III (Treatment)

1. Theodore N, Aarabi B, Dhall SS, et al. The diagnosis and management of traumatic atlanto-occipital dislocation injuries. Neurosurgery. 2013;72(Suppl 2):114–26.
2. Kandziora F, Schnake K, Hoffmann R. Injuries to the upper cervical spine. Part 1: Ligamentous injuries. Unfallchirurg. 2010;113:931–43.
3. Anderson LD, D'Alonzo RT. Fractures of the odontoid process of the axis. J Bone Joint Surg Am. 1974;56:1663–74.
4. Grauer JN, Shafi B, Hilibrand AS, et al. Proposal of a modified, treatment-oriented classification of odontoid fractures. Spine J. 2005;5(2):123–9.
5. Ryken TC, Hadley MN, Aarabi B, et al. Management of acute combination fractures of the atlas and axis in adults. Neurosurgery. 2013;72(Suppl 2):151–8.
6. Vaccaro AR, Kepler CK, Kopjar B, et al. Functional and quality-of-life outcomes in geriatric patients with type-II dens fracture. J Bone Joint Surg Am. 2013;95(8):729–35.
7. Harrop JS, Hart R, Anderson PA. Optimal treatment for odontoid fractures in the elderly. Spine (Phila Pa 1976). 2010;35(21 Suppl):S219–27.
8. Majercik S, Tashjian RZ, Biffl WL, et al. Halo vest immobilization in the elderly: a death sentence? J Trauma. 2005;59(2):350–6; discussion 356–8.
9. Harms J, Melcher RP. Posterior C1-C2 fusion with polyaxial screw and rod fixation. Spine (Phila Pa 1976). 2001;26:2467–71.
10. Goel A, Laheri V. Plate and screw fixation for atlanto-axial subluxation. Acta Neurochir. 1994;129:47–53.
11. Magerl F. Spondylodesis of the upper cervical spine. Acta Chir Austriaca. 1982;43(Suppl):69.
12. Käsmacher J, Schweizer C, Valentinitsch A, et al. Osteoporosis is the most important risk factor in traumatic odontoid fractures in the elderly. J Bone Miner Res. 2017;32(7):1582–8.

Level of Evidence III

13. Gehweiler JA, Osborne RH, Becker RF. The radiology of vertebral trauma. Philadelphia: Saunders; 1983.
14. Dickmann CA, Greene KA, Sonntag VK. Injuries involving the transverse atlantal ligament: classification and treatment guidelines based upon experience with 39 injuries. Neurosurgery. 1996;38:44–50.
15. Hadley MN, Walter PC, Grabb PA, et al. Isolated fractures of the atlas in adults. In: guidelines for the management of acute cervical spine and spinal cord injuries. Neurosurgery. 2002;50(3 suppl):S120–4.
16. Ryken TC, Aarabi B, Dhall SS, et al. Management of isolated fractures of the atlas in adults. Neurosurgery. 2013;72(Suppl 2):127–31.
17. Kandziora F, Schnake K, Hoffmann R. Injuries to the upper cervical spine. Part 2: Osseous injuries. Unfallchirurg. 2010;113:1023–41.

Subaxial Cervical Trauma

33

Rodolfo Maduri and John M. Duff

In this chapter, we discuss two specific entities. The first is a fracture dislocation in the subaxial cervical spine, and the second is a burst fracture also of the subaxial spine. We will describe each case, its management and the rationale behind it.

33.1 Case 1: Cervical Spine Fracture Dislocation Injury

33.1.1 Introduction

Acute fracture-dislocations of the cervical spine are rare, accounting for the 9% of the overall injury of the cervico-thoracic spine. Cervico-thoracic fracture dislocation is defined as fracture of the neural arch or vertebral body with true facet subluxation, mono – or bilateral [1]. This invariably involves high energy trauma and patients often present with multisystem injuries. The purpose of this case presentation is to outline the diagnostics of cervical spine fracture dislocation, its management in the emergency department, and its surgical management. Specifically, we look at radiological investigation, particularly the role of MR imaging. We also look at the use of closed reduction techniques including traction, and finally surgical treatment.

33.1.2 Case Description

A 57 year old patient presented to a local hospital by ambulance with neck pain following a bicycle accident. He had a transient loss of consciousness and complained of severe neck pain. He was evaluated clinically with a normal examination. Cervical spine Xrays were interpreted as normal. The patient was sent home with simple analgesics.

The patient came back to the same hospital 4 days later with persistent severe neck pain and new onset pain and weakness of the right arm. The diagnostic CT scan of the whole spine showed a C7-T1 fracture dislocation and bilateral perched facets with fracture of the posterior arch of C7 (Fig. 33.1 Panel a). A semi-rigid collar was placed and he was transferred to our institution. His neurological examination on arrival revealed a mild right triceps weakness and his right triceps reflex was diminished. The remainder of his neurological examination was entirely normal. Specifically, there were no signs of spinal cord injury (ASIA E).

The cervical MRI confirmed the presence of a traumatic disc herniation with disc materiel behind the body of C7, without direct spinal cord compression.

R. Maduri · J. M. Duff (✉)
Department of Clinical Neurosciences, University Hospital of Lausanne, CHUV, Lausanne, Switzerland

B. Meyer, M. Rauschmann (eds.), *Spine Surgery*, https://doi.org/10.1007/978-3-319-98875-7_33

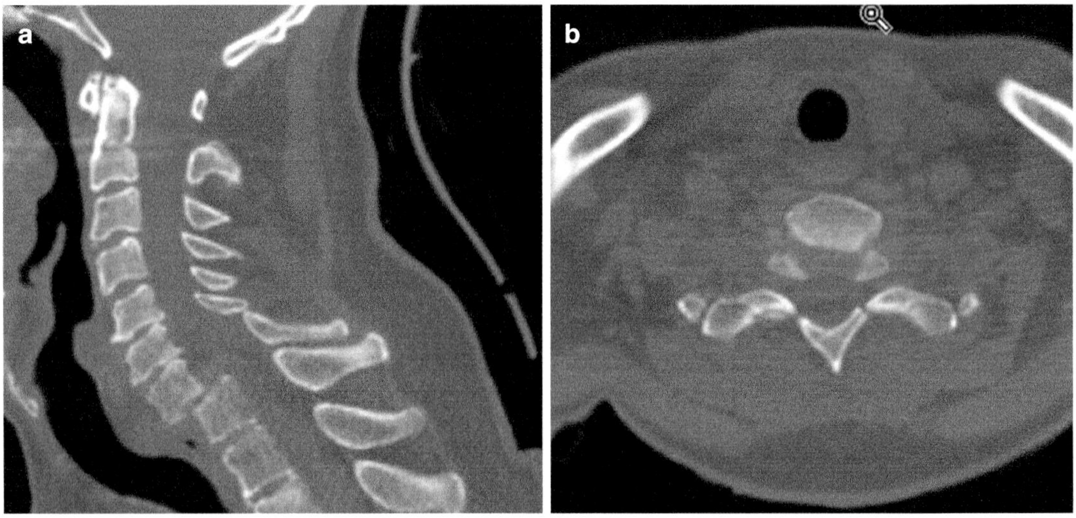

Fig. 33.1 Panel (**a**) Sagittal CT scan of the cervical spine showing a traumatic spondylolisthesis of C7 on T1 with bilateral perched facets Panel (**b**) axial cervical CT scan showing fracture of the posterior arch of C7

Due to the highly unstable injury, surgical open reduction and fixation was chosen as an immediate treatment. It was felt that traction using a Gardiner-Wells tongs to attempt a closed reduction in an awake patient was not advisable due to the presence of a large traumatic disc herniation in the spinal canal, which can cause additional neurological injury.

Using spinal cord monitoring, the patient was placed supine on a radiolucent Jackson table. The head was positioned carefully in a horseshoe headholder under electrophysiologically monitoring and 3 kg of in line traction. The cervical spine alignment was checked using 2D lateral fluoroscopy. There was no change compared with preoperative imaging.

A standard C7-D1 anterior discectomy (ACD) was performed, assisted by gentle distraction with Caspar pins between the vertebral bodies. No cage was placed into the disc space. The skin was closed with staples, and the patient was turned over into the prone position. The C6-T1 posterior elements were exposed through a midline skin incision. Bilateral upper T1 facetectomies were done using a high speed drill, which allowed reduction between C7 and T1. Following open reduction, the facet joints were curetted out and local bone was packed into the joints, followed by pedicle screws placement at C7 and at T1 using 2D fluoroscopic guidance. The posterior wound was closed, and the patient was again turned into the supine position. The anterior cervical incision was reopened, an interbody cage was placed into the C7-T1 disc space, and an anterior plate was placed from C7 to T1.

The postoperative period was uneventful with a partially recovered C8 deficit. The postoperative imaging (Fig. 33.2 Panel a, b and c) showed a satisfactory fracture reduction, and implant placement.

33.1.3 Discussion of the Case

According to the revised AO Spine classification [6], this is a type C injury, with a B component and an F4 component (pathologic perched/dislocated facet).

In case of acute cervicothoracic dislocation with bilateral perched facets in a stable patient, as described in the present case, treatment objectives are to decompress neural elements, restore spinal alignment and to achieve immediate spine stabilization and ultimately bone fusion.

Spine realignment may be accomplished either through a closed reduction with cervical traction or through an open posterior reduction. Traction and attempted closed reduction could be an initial treatment option here were it not for the traumatic disc herniation. This should

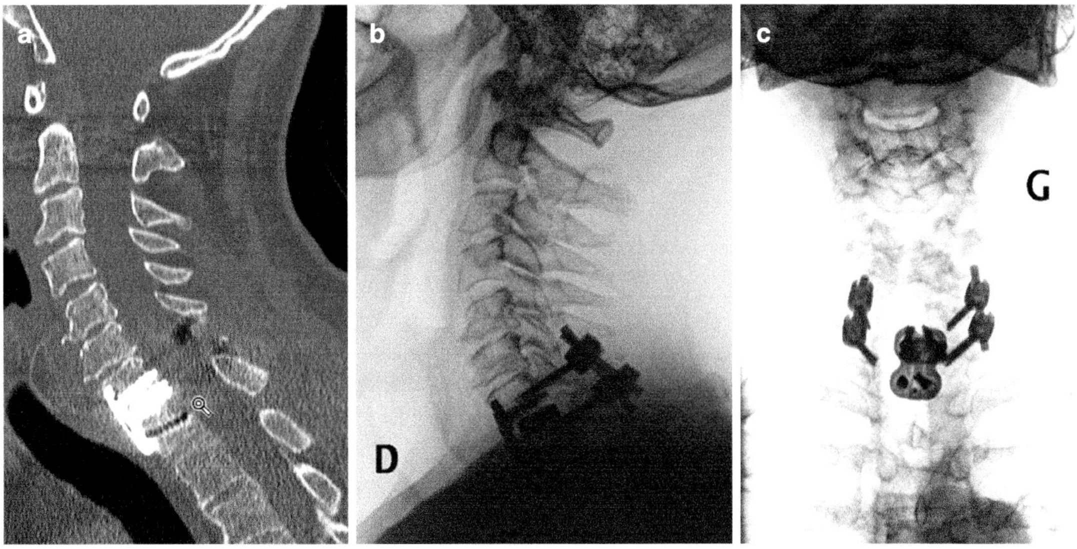

Fig. 33.2 Panel (**a**) postoperative sagittal CT scan of the cervical spine showing restoration of sagittal alignment. Panel (**b**) and (**c**) postoperative cervical standing X-rays

be done only in a cooperative patient and not in a patient with an associated head injury or in an intoxicated state. This can be done using 2D flurorscopic guidance if the fracture subluxation can be properly visualized. The technique is using a halo ring (Gardner Wells tongue) with pins fixed at 2–3 cm anterior to the external acoustic meatus to achieve flexion. The amount of weight required for reduction ranges from 5–10 lbs per level to as much 80% of the patient's body weight.

Open reduction is an alternative for direct spine realignment or after failed closed reduction.

The maintenance of spine realignment and fusion may be achieved through a rigid external immobilization, anterior arthrodesis with plate fixation and/or posterior arthrodesis.

Healing with halo vest immobilization is more probable if there are fracture fragments over the articular facets in case of a bi-pedicular fracture which could make realignment easier than, for example, locked facets [3]. Close radiological follow up is needed to rule out fracture dislocation [4].

In our case, due to the ongoing nerve root compression, open reduction through an anterior and posterior approach was chosen to realize also a direct foraminal decompression at C7-D1 level and to achieve fusion through pedicular screw.

The treatment strategy was in accord to the actual literature evidence Level III.

33.1.4 Conclusions and Take Home Message

- Fracture dislocation of the cervical spine spine are unstable fractures requiring spinal reduction and fusion.
- Closed reduction may be attempted using traction in an awake and alert patient where there is no traumatic disc herniation. If this fails, or if there is a traumatic disc herniation confirmed on MRI, we would advocate open decompression and reduction, as performed in this case.
- Cervical CT scan and MRI are both important in the diagnostic workup

33.2 Case 2: Subaxial Cervical Burst Fracture

33.2.1 Introduction

Burst fractures of the cervical spine are due to vertical compression load to failure in the subaxial cervical spine. These fractures are associated in 26% of cases with spinal cord injury and require early surgical treatment to decompress the spinal cord and restore spinal alignment [5].

Here we present a case of subaxial burst fracture. We discuss the diagnosis, the treatment strategy including surgical decompression, reduction, and segmental reconstruction with fixation.

33.2.2 Case Description

A 30 year old lumberjack was struck on the head by a falling tree branch. He was immediately unresponsive at the scene. Emergency services placed the patient on a backboard with a cervical collar, following which he was transferred to our institution for further management.

On arrival, he had a Glasgow Coma Score of 10, and he was intubated due to an agitated state. He was hemodynamically stable. A rapid neurological evaluation prior to intubation confirmed a generalized weakness of his 4 extremities (probable ASIA C) [8].

The head CT scan showed a right temporoparietal fracture with a small right acute subdural hematoma. An intracranial pressure (ICP) monitor was placed.

The CT scan of the spine showed a C4 "split burst" fracture with kyphosis (Fig. 33.3 Panel a).

Using the AO classification [6, 9] this fracture is classified as type A4 + B3 + F2.

After placement of the ICP monitor, surgery was performed for the cervical fracture.

The first stage was an anterior approach. The patient was placed in supine position the head slightly extended in a neutral position. A right transverse incision was performed at the level of the C3-C4 disc space. After standard exposure, using the microscope, C3-C4 and C4-C5 discectomies were performed. A corpectomy of C4 was performed and all fragments were removed as far as the posterior longitudinal ligament. An expandable PEEK cage was then placed in the corpectomy defect and its position was verified with fluoroscopy, followed by anterior plate fixation.

In the postoperative period, repeat neurological examination confirmed a post-traumatic cervical myelopathy with an ASIA D grade.

The cervical MRI realized after the anterior surgery showed spinal cord T2 hyperintensity at the level of injury (C4) confirming the posterior ligamentous complex (PLC) injury.

A second stage surgery with posterior fixation was carried out several days later. The patient was placed in a prone position with the head fixed in a three-point Mayfield headholder. A midline incision was carried out to expose the posterior elements from C3 and C5. Under 3D fluoroscopic navigation, pedicle screws were placed at C3 and C5 with rod placement. The facet joints at C3/4 and C4/5 were drilled and curetted, and

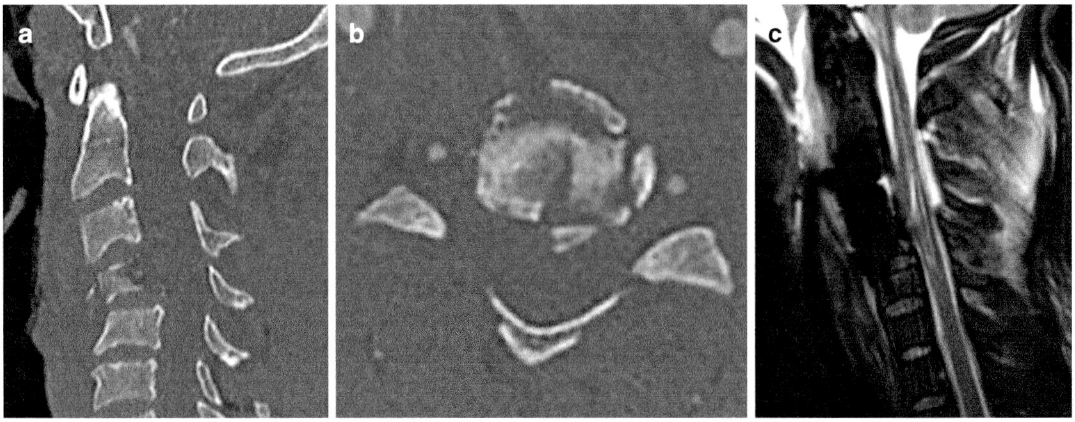

Fig. 33.3 Panel (**a**) and (**b**) Sagittal and Axial CT scan of the cervical spine showing a "split burst" fracture of C4 associated with cyphosis of the subaxial spine. Panel (**c**) shows the postoperative MRI after C4 corpectomy and anterior fixation shows the disruption of the posterior ligamentous complex (PLC)

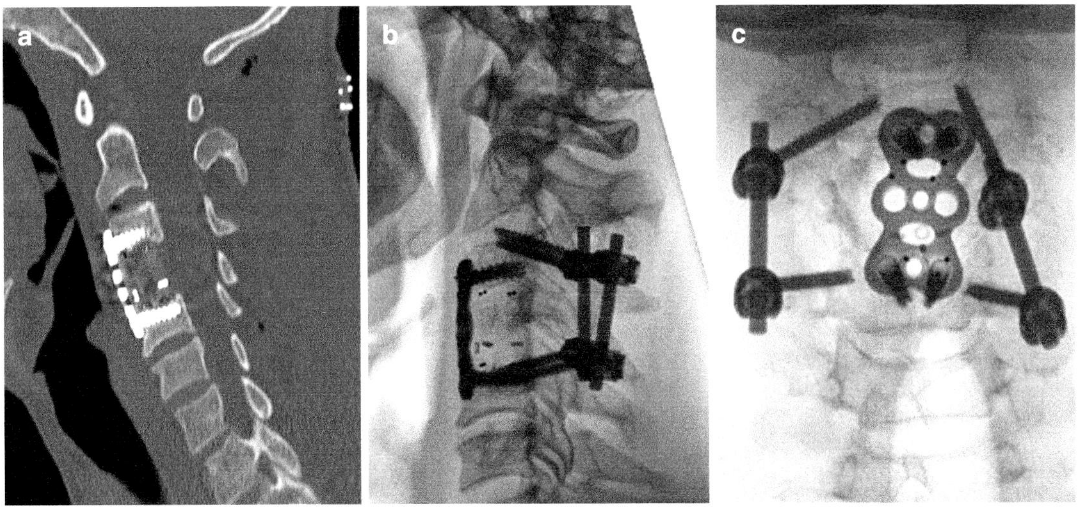

Fig. 33.4 Panel (**a**) postoperative sagittal CT scan of the cervical spine showing restoration of the anterior column support with cage and plate placement. Panels (**b**) and (**c**) postoperative lateral and anteroposterior cervical standing X-rays

local bone was placed into these joints to facilitate bone fusion.

Postoperative imaging (Fig. 33.4 Panel a, b and c) showed a satisfactory decompression and fracture reduction.

33.2.3 Discussion

Subaxial flexion-compression fractures are often unstable injuries, particularly with disruption of PLC [9]. Such injuries require surgical stabilization. This case is an example of axial loading sufficient for vertebral body failure and disruption of the posterior ligamentous complex by hyperflexion. As is often the case, there is an associated spinal cord injury. Spinal cord injury in the absence of significant translation tells us that there has been signification deformation of the spinal column at the moment of impact, returning to a more normal position by elastic recoil. This indicates associated soft tissue, and more specifically, ligamentous injury. Corpectomy and cage placement restores anterior column support, and the posterior fixation restores the posterior tension band.

As this is a compressive injury, it is reasonable to consider traction, either preoperatively to help stabilize the fracture segment, or intraoperatively to help restore alignment. The presence of a skull fracture with the possibility of a craniotomy precluded the use of traction in this case.

Early surgical intervention was chosen in this case because of severe instability and an existing spinal cord injury. However, precise timing of surgery is controversial [7].

Closed reduction is indicated in awake patients with no traumatic disk herniation documented with cervical MRI.

Spinal ralignment and stabilization may be achieved through anterior, posterior or anterior and posterior approaches. Anterior approaches are indicated when adequate reduction is achieved through simple traction, no disk herniation is documented on preoperative MRI and the patient is neurologically intact. Posterio fixation alone is indicated in case of subaxial flexion-compression injuries with disrupted PLC and preserved spinal alignment.

Toh et al. [5] compared anterior versus posterior stabilization for burst and teardrop fractures and found that anterior decompression and fusion restored spinal canal diameter by 60%, as compared with only 6% with posterior stabilization. If the spine can be realigned easily with traction, then a posterior stabilization alone may be performed in neurologically intact patients.

Cervical pedicle screw fixation has been shown to be biomechanically a very robust construct comparable to lateral mass screw constructs [2].

The treatment strategy is based on level III evidence.

33.2.4 Conclusions and Take Home Message

- Subaxial cervical burst fracture are usually treated surgically. Additional PLC, disruption requires additional posterior fixation. MRI is essential to define the operative strategy.
- Early (<24 h) decompression with vertebral reconstruction through an anterior approach may improve neurological outcome.
- When indicated, posterior fixation with pedicle screw fixation provides enhanced stability over lateral mass screw fixation, but is technically more demanding and is not always necessary.

Editorial Comment

This chapter illustrates managment aspects for 2 more common type of subaxial fractures. We think the surgeries performed represent state of the art and it should be a given in the year 2019 that these injuries are clear indication for surgery. According to us it is also a given that in fractures with an SCI as in case 2 surgery should be performed as an emergency no matter what time of the day or night. The question how to manage an injury like the one in the first case is very old and not very productive. It should be left at the treating surgeon's decision, if he wants to use traction first, or go for open reduction, or start front or back etc. On a personal note, I never use preoperative traction and a direct anterior approach and reposition after discectomy is always feasible and my preference. A posterior construct can then be done in the same or a second stage.

References

1. Amin A, Saifuddin A. Fractures and dislocations of the cervicothoracic junction. J Spinal Disord Tech. 2005;18:499–505.
2. Duff J, Hussain MM, Klocke N, Harris JA, Yandamuri SS, Bobinski L, et al. Does pedicle screw fixation of the subaxial cervical spine provide adequate stabilization in a multilevel vertebral body fracture model? An in vitro biomechanical study. Clin Biomech (Bristol, Avon). 2018;53:72–8.
3. Ramieri A, Domenicucci M, Cellocco P, Lenzi J, Dugoni DE, Costanzo G. Traumatic spondylolisthesis and spondyloptosis of the subaxial cervical spine without neurological deficits: closed re-alignment, surgical options and literature review. Eur Spine J. 2014;23(Suppl 6):658–63.
4. Sonntag VK. Management of bilateral locked facets of the cervical spine. Neurosurgery. 1981;8:150–2.
5. Toh E, Nomura T, Watanabe M, Mochida J. Surgical treatment for injuries of the middle and lower cervical spine. Int Orthop. 2006;30:54–8.
6. Vaccaro AR, Koerner JD, Radcliff KE, Oner FC, Reinhold M, Schnake KJ, et al. AOSpine subaxial cervical spine injury classification system. Eur Spine J. 2016;25:2173–84.
7. Fehlings MG, Tetreault LA, Wilson JR, Kwon BK, Burns AS, Martin AR, Hawryluk G, Harrop JS. A clinical practice guideline for the management of acute spinal cord injury: introduction, rationale, and scope. Global Spine J. 2017;7(3 Suppl):84S–94S. https://doi.org/10.1177/2192568217703387. Epub 2017 Sep 5.
8. Ditunno JF, Young W, Donovan WH, Creasey G. The international standards booklet for neurological and functional classification of spinal cord injury. American Spinal Injury Association. Paraplegia. 1994;32(2):70–80. (ISSN: 0031-1758).
9. Vaccaro AR, Koerner JD, Radcliff KE, et al. AOSpine subaxial cervical spine injury classification system. Eur Spine J. 2016;25(7):2173–84. https://doi.org/10.1007/s00586-015-3831-3. [published Online First: Epub Date].

34 Management Criteria for Thoracic, Thoracolumbar and Lumbar Fractures

Esat Kiter and Nusret Ok

34.1 Introduction

Classification of the vertebral fractures to encourage an optimal treatment protocol has long been in the interest of spine surgeons. In the past, although many morphology-based or mechanistic classification systems have been proposed, none of them has lasting influence on daily practice. In the last two decades, the spine community focused on developing a classification system incorporating morphology, mechanism, and clinical factors relevant for surgical decision. However, even in the current classification systems, treatment protocols always have a gray zone which allows the surgeon to make his own decision.

In this chapter, we underline the role of very basic factors in the evaluation of the patients which may affect the surgeon's decision, including.

- importance of reading radiological images,
- physical examination and history which give you very important clues about the posterior ligamentous complex (PLC).

E. Kiter (✉) · N. Ok
Pamukkale University, Department of Orthopedics, Denizli, Turkey

34.2 Case Description

A 37-year-old male patient was admitted to the emergency department due to traffic accident. During the car crash, he was seated on the front passenger seat with a fasten belt. His major complaint was back pain on the posterior thoracic area. His neurological examination findings were normal. There were no any additional (i.e., cranial, skeletal, or intraabdominal) traumatic morbidity and he was free from skin abrasion on the anterior thorax. Plain X-rays showed a T12 fracture (Fig. 34.1). A computed tomography (CT) scan was ordered (Fig. 34.2) by the emergency department and the patient, was, then referred to a spine surgeon.

His treatment was planned in a conservative manner, and the Jewett brace was applied. On the second day of hospital stay, the patient was ambulated with brace. Ambulation was well-tolerated by the patient with acceptable pain. However, X-rays within the Jewett brace in the standing position (Fig. 34.3) showed increased kyphosis at the fracture site due to the instability.

Although neurological condition was stable during the ambulation, an operative intervention was indicated. Posterior *in situ* fixation was performed with a less invasive trans-muscular approach (Fig. 34.4). The patient was followed for 7 years postoperatively without any complication.

B. Meyer, M. Rauschmann (eds.), *Spine Surgery*, https://doi.org/10.1007/978-3-319-98875-7_34

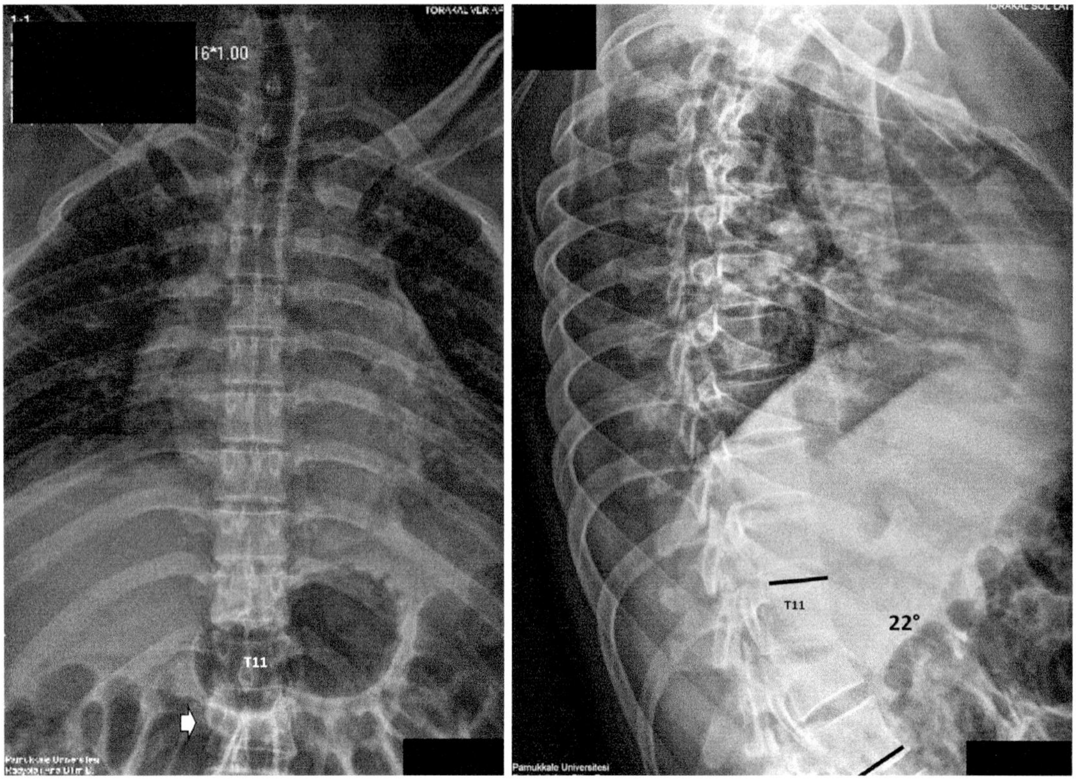

Fig. 34.1 Plain X-rays at the initial admission. Anteroposterior (AP) and lateral X-ray of the patient. Superior end plate collapse of T12 is apparent. Local kyphotic angle is 22° in the lying measurements. Interspinous distance is markedly increased between T11 and T12 (which is not noticed by the surgeon)

34.3 Discussion of the Case

34.3.1 Indication

This case is typical flexion distraction injury of the spine. According to the AOSpine Thoracolumbar Injury Classification System (AO-TLICS), this is type B2 injury with osteoligamentous failure [7] and is credited with 6-point [2].

According to the AO-TLICS classification, surgical treatment is recommended for patients with more than five points, and conservative treatment is recommended for those with three points and below. The treatment method depends on the decision of the surgeon in the injury scores between these values [8].

The PLC consisting of supraspinous ligament, interspinous ligament, ligamentum flavum, and the facet joint capsules. This complex is responsible for the tension band effect in the posterior spinal column and has significant contributions on spinal stability [6]. However, morphological and mechanical descriptions emphasizing the bone morphology of the fractured spinal cord have been remained on the agenda for many years. Radiological imaging of the PLC has become recommended with the magnetic resonance imaging (MRI) technology which was developed in the early 1980s. However, this evaluation method is expensive and may not be available in all healthcare centers. One of the criticized features of the TLICS classification, which was defined in 2005 and used commonly for a while, has brought MRI into the forefront.

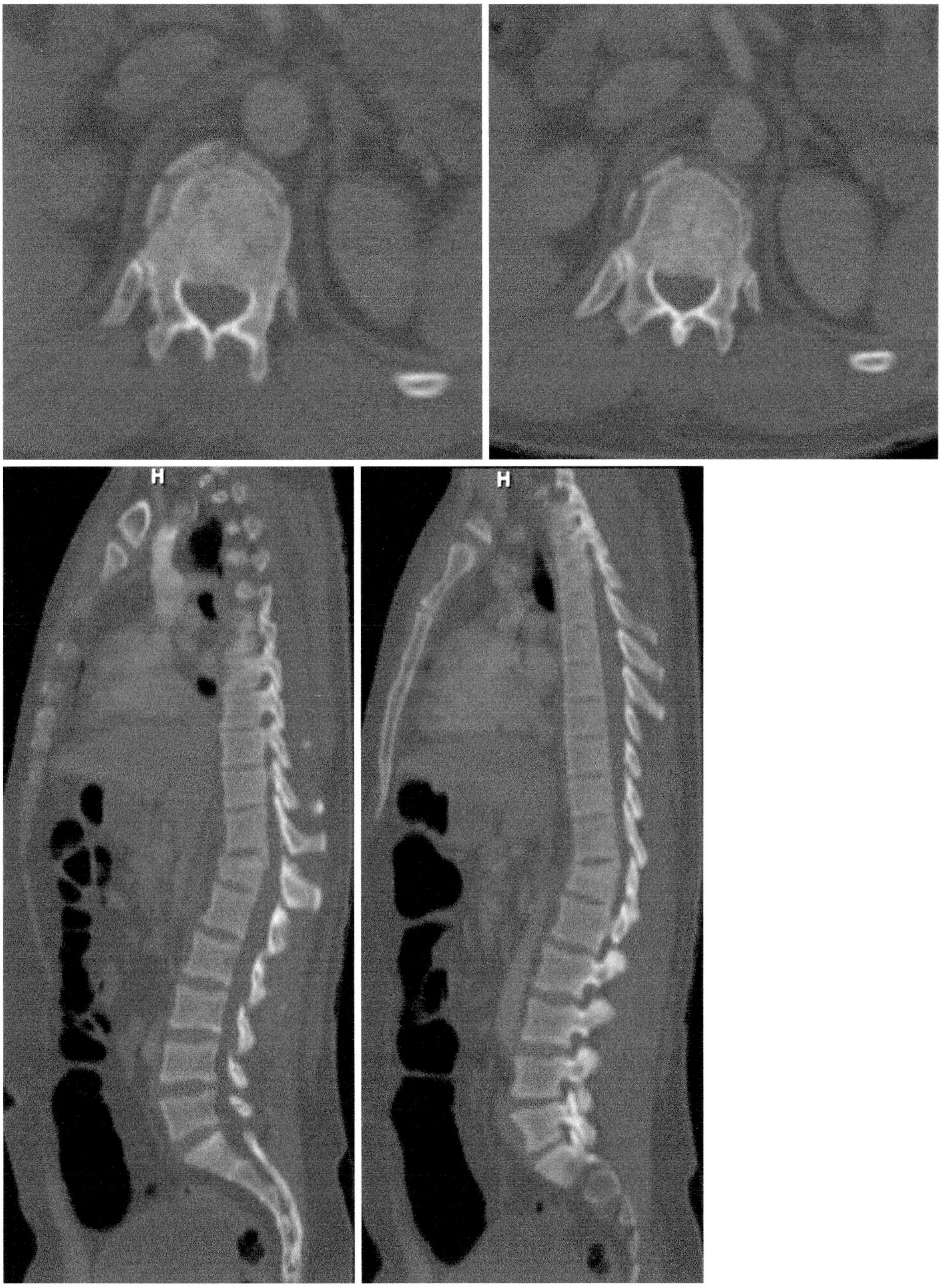

Fig. 34.2 CT scan. CT scan showing a vertebral body fracture with superior end plate plus posterior wall involvement. There are no bony fractures at the posterior elements of the spine

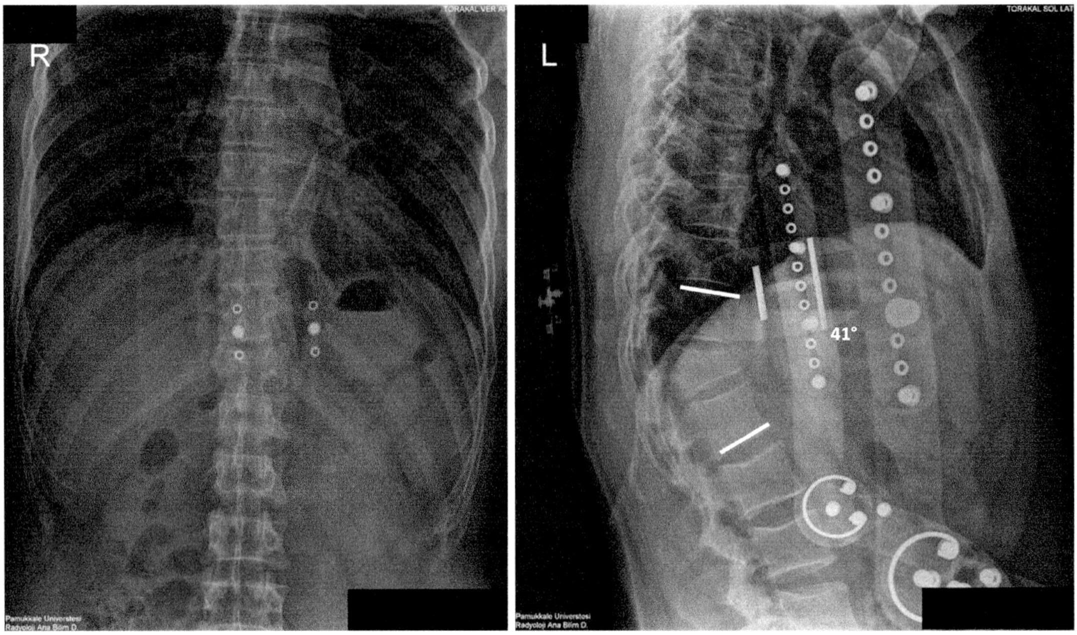

Fig. 34.3 Standing X-rays after ambulation. On the lateral view, increasing of the kyphosis (41°) is noticeable. The gap between T11 and T12 spinous process is still present

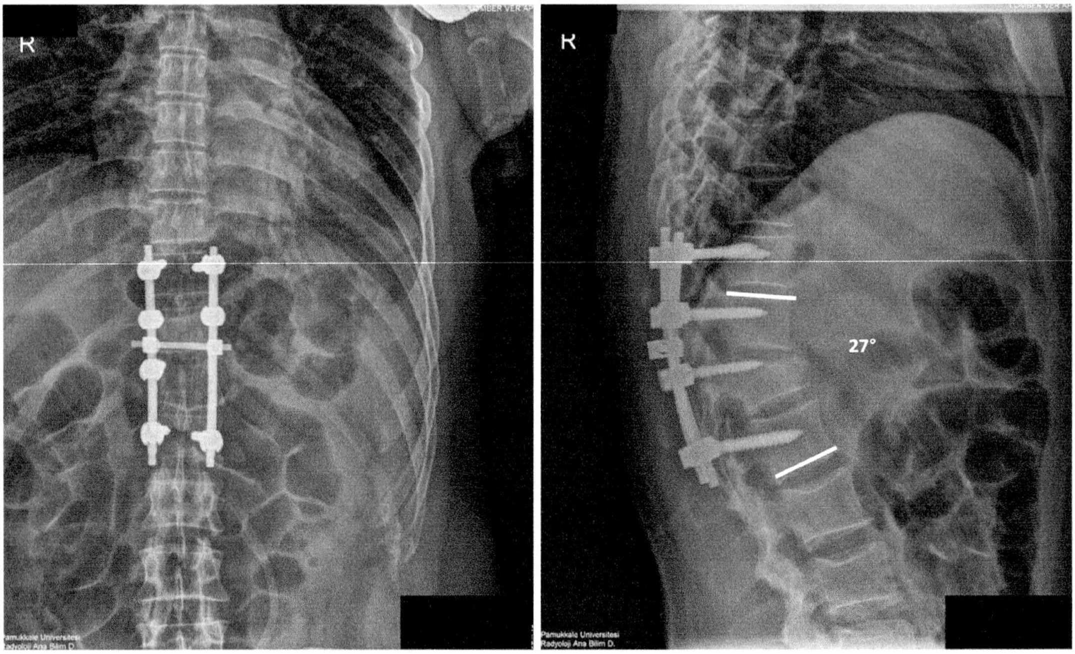

Fig. 34.4 Postoperative x-rays of the patient. In situ (correction achieved with prone position) fixation with trans-paravertebral approach (less invasive). One-side intermediate screw was placed

34.3.2 What Was Wrong?

What was wrong in this case was that PLC injury was not noticed at the first examination. Accordingly, it was considered as AO-TLICS classification type A3 (3 points) injury, and conservative treatment was planned. The main reason of this was that the increase in interspinous distance was not considered in direct graphs, and no interspinous palpation and physical examination were performed. The surgeon made the first diagnosis by basically evaluating the CT images. These tomographic images are not-standing (supine) obtained graphs, and they give limited information about the injury mechanism, if there is no fracture in the posterior elements.

The diagnosis of PLC injury cases, in particular, can be made with simpler methods and, therefore, not performing MRI should not be considered as a fault in this case.

34.3.3 Surgical Technique

Basically, posterior tension band repair is sufficient for these types of cases. These types of cases are treated with percutaneous pedicle fixation in present practise. However, percutaneous fixation system was not available 7 years ago in local conditions. Less invasive transparavertebral muscle approach was popular in that period [4], and the patient was treated as fusionless with the less invasive method.

This treatment has advantages, compared to the conventional open screw application [5]. The distal level was kept short and was ended in construct L1, since the intermediate screw was applied [1, 3].

34.4 Conclusions and Take Home Message

In conclusion, PLC injury rules out all type A fractures and almost all of the conservative treatment options. Therefore, it should be evaluated carefully. In addition, MRI is useful in the evaluation of this kind of injuries, but is not a gold standard. Obeying the fundamental hierarchy in the evaluation of the patient (i.e., good anamnesis and physical examination) should be a surgical discipline which should be kept in mind. However, this case reminds us that it is possible to make the right diagnosis even with the simplest imaging method without the need for complex imaging methods.

Pearls

- Obeying the fundamental hierarchy in the evaluation of the patient should be kept in the mind
- It is possible to make right diagnosis even with the simplest method, if you know where you should check
- PLC injury excludes almost all of the conservative treatment options

Editorial Comment

There is considerable variety on how (agressively) unstable thoracolumbar fractures are treated throughout Europe with surgery. The level of evidence for or against it is too low for firm conclusions, which is the reason why we observe this. In a situation like this it is essential to reliably classify the injury in a reproducible manner, to have an estimate if conservative treatment, that is bracing is a reasonable option.

References

1. Anekstein Y, Brosh T, Mirovsky Y. Intermediate screws in short segment pedicular fixation for thoracic and lumbar fractures: a biomechanical study. J Spinal Disord Tech. 2007;20(1):72–7. https://doi.org/10.1097/01.bsd.0000211240.98963.f6.
2. Kepler CK, Vaccaro AR, Schroeder GD, Koerner JD, Vialle LR, Aarabi B, et al. The Thoracolum bar AO spine injury score. Global Spine J. 2016;6(4):329–34. https://doi.org/10.1055/s-0035-1563610.
3. Mahar A, Kim C, Wedemeyer M, Mitsunaga L, Odell T, Johnson B, et al. Short-segment fixation of lumbar burst fractures using pedicle fixation at the level of the fracture. Spine (Phila Pa 1976). 2007;32(14):1503–7. https://doi.org/10.1097/BRS.0b013e318067dd24.

4. Pang W, Zhang GL, Tian W, Sun D, Li N, Yuan Q, Zhang B, et al. Surgical treatment of thoracolumbar fracture through an approach via the paravertebral muscle. Orthop Surg. 2009;1(3):184–8. https://doi.org/10.1111/j.1757-7861.2009.00032.x.
5. Sun XY, Zhang XN, Hai Y. Percutaneous versus traditional and paraspinal posterior open approaches for treatment of thoracolumbar fractures without neurologic deficit: a meta-analysis. Eur Spine J. 2017;26(5):1418–31. https://doi.org/10.1007/s00586-016-4818-4.
6. Vaccaro AR, Rihn JA, Saravanja D, Anderson DG, Hilibrand AS, Albert TJ, et al. Injury of the posterior ligamentous complex of the thoracolumbar spine: a prospective evaluation of the diagnostic accuracy of magnetic resonance imaging. Spine (Phila Pa 1976). 2009;34(23):E841–7. https://doi.org/10.1097/BRS.0b013e3181bd11be.
7. Vaccaro AR, Oner C, Kepler CK, Dvorak M, Schnake K, Bellabarba C, et al. AOSpine spinal cord injury & trauma knowledge forum. AOSpine thoracolumbar spine injury classification system: fracture description, neurological status, and key modifiers. Spine (Phila Pa 1976). 2013;38(23):2028–37. https://doi.org/10.1097/BRS.0b013e3182a8a381.
8. Vaccaro AR, Schroeder GD, Kepler CK, Cumhur Oner F, Vialle LR, Kandziora F, et al. The surgical algorithm for the AOSpine thoracolumbar spine injury classification system. Eur Spine J. 2016;25(4):1087–94. https://doi.org/10.1007/s00586-015-3982-2.

35 Posterior Surgical Management of Thoracic and Lumbar Fractures

Yann Philippe Charles

35.1 Introduction

Unstable thoracolumbar fractures and trauma leading to severe kyphosis are usually treated surgically. There is no clear consensus whether open or percutaneous instrumentation should be preferred, and the necessity of grafting remains debated [1]. Currently, there is an increasing trend towards Minimally Invasive Surgery (MIS), since percutaneous instrumentation decreases the risk for bleeding and infection during the perioperative period, and it shortens the length of hospitalization [2]. Clinical trials comparing open and percutaneous techniques indicate that MIS leads to lower pain and disability scores at short-term, whereas clinical results are similar after 6 months [3, 4]. There is only little evidence on long-term outcomes after posterior percutaneous instrumentation. However, clinical results and sagittal alignment are maintained effectively with MIS if the right surgical strategy has been chosen according to the fracture type, the patient's age and general health status [5, 6].

This case description will outline the management of an incomplete burst fracture at the thoracolumbar junction without neurological impairment. The rationale for a posterior surgical treatment is discussed. The aim of the presented case is to emphasize specific aspects that should help the reader in clinical and technical decision making with an MIS approach. The discussion will focus on the following technical aspects:

- The different possibilities posterior closed fracture reduction techniques,
- The indication and limits for an additional anterior column support by vertebral body expansion and cement augmentation,
- The indication and specific need for an anterior column reconstruction and grafting with MIS,
- The use of percutaneous instrumentation as a temporary internal fixator.

35.2 Case Description

A 52-year old female patient was admitted at our emergency department after a motor vehicle accident with an estimated speed of 120 km/h. She was conscious and well oriented. Her blood pressure was 140/90 mmHg and her pulse rate 84/min. Clinical examination evidenced a hematoma at the right hypochondrium. Pulmonary auscultation remained normal and an abdominal tenderness was noted when palpating the right upper quadrant and epigastric region. She further reported back pain around the thoracolumbar junction. Her neurological status and examination

Y. P. Charles (✉)
Service de Chirurgie du Rachis, Hôpitaux Universitaires de Strasbourg, Strasbourg, France
e-mail: yann.philippe.charles@chru-strasbourg.fr

B. Meyer, M. Rauschmann (eds.), *Spine Surgery*, https://doi.org/10.1007/978-3-319-98875-7_35

of the limbs were normal. Routine chest and pelvic x-rays were performed in the emergency room and evidenced fractures of the 9th and 10th right ribs, while a pelvic ring fracture was ruled out. Because of the high velocity trauma, a total body CT scan was performed with injection of contrast media. A small subcapsular liver hematoma was evidenced without active bleeding. CT imaging of the spine showed an incomplete burst fracture of T12 (Fig. 35.1), classified as A3 type according to the new AO classification [7].

An abdominal echography was performed after 2 days, showing that there was no progression of the liver hematoma prior spinal operation. Positioning the patient prone on a Jackson table with the thoracolumbar junction in slight lordosis allowed almost complete reduction of the fracture. She was then operated using a percutaneous approach that consisted of a balloon kyphoplasty at T12 in order to complete the reduction. Because of the posterior wall involvement, the vertebral body expansion was then followed by a percutaneous instrumentation in order to stabilize the segment T11-L1 (Fig. 35.2).

The patient ambulated without a brace from day one after surgery with the aid of a physical therapist. She gained full autonomy until day 5 and was discharged at home with paracetamol and tramadol as pain medication. The first out clinic follow-up visit was scheduled 6 weeks postoperatively. The patient was pain free and did not require analgesics. Physical therapy was started aiming for strengthening of the paravertebral musculature. The patient was able to return to work as a schoolteacher after 2 months.

A routine follow-up visit was scheduled at 6-month follow-up. As the patient was very sportive, she asked if an implant removal might be considered prior starting horse riding competition again. A CT scan showed a complete bony consolidation of the T12 vertebral body (Fig. 35.3), and percutaneous removal of the instrumentation was performed after 9 months.

The postoperative follow-up was uneventful and the patient returned to sports activities. An MRI of the thoracolumbar spine was performed for research purposes at 2-year follow-up (Fig. 35.4). The sagittal T2 sequence showed that the T11-T12 disc remained well hydrated despite the compression fracture and the underlying cement augmentation in the T12 vertebral body. Furthermore, the aspect of the paravertebral musculature at the fracture and instrumented levels remained normal on axial views and low fat infiltration was evidenced. Although not routinely used in clinical practice, this MRI showed the

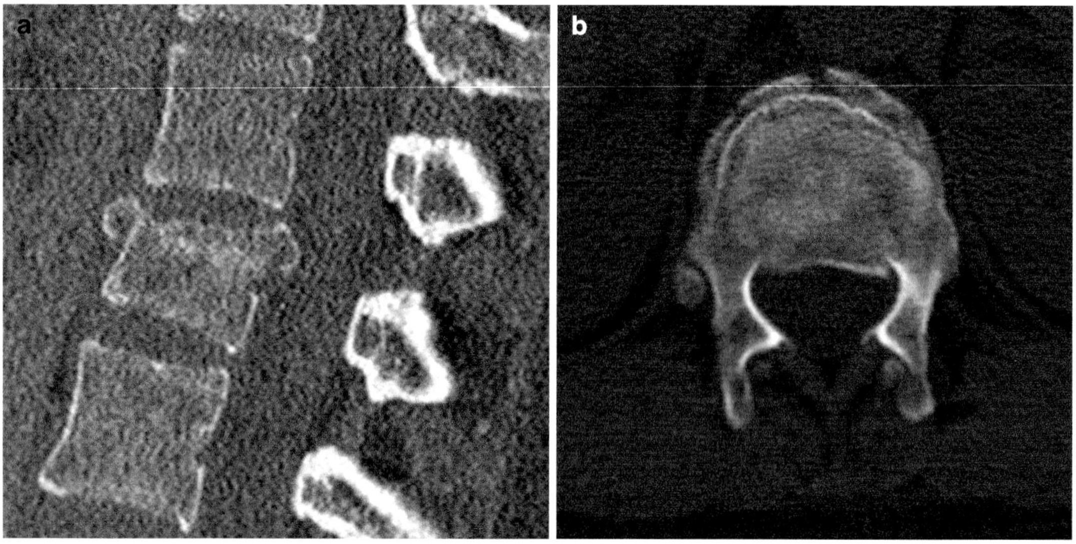

Fig. 35.1 CT scan performed at emergency admission showing an incomplete burst fracture on sagittal (**a**) and axial (**b**) reconstructions

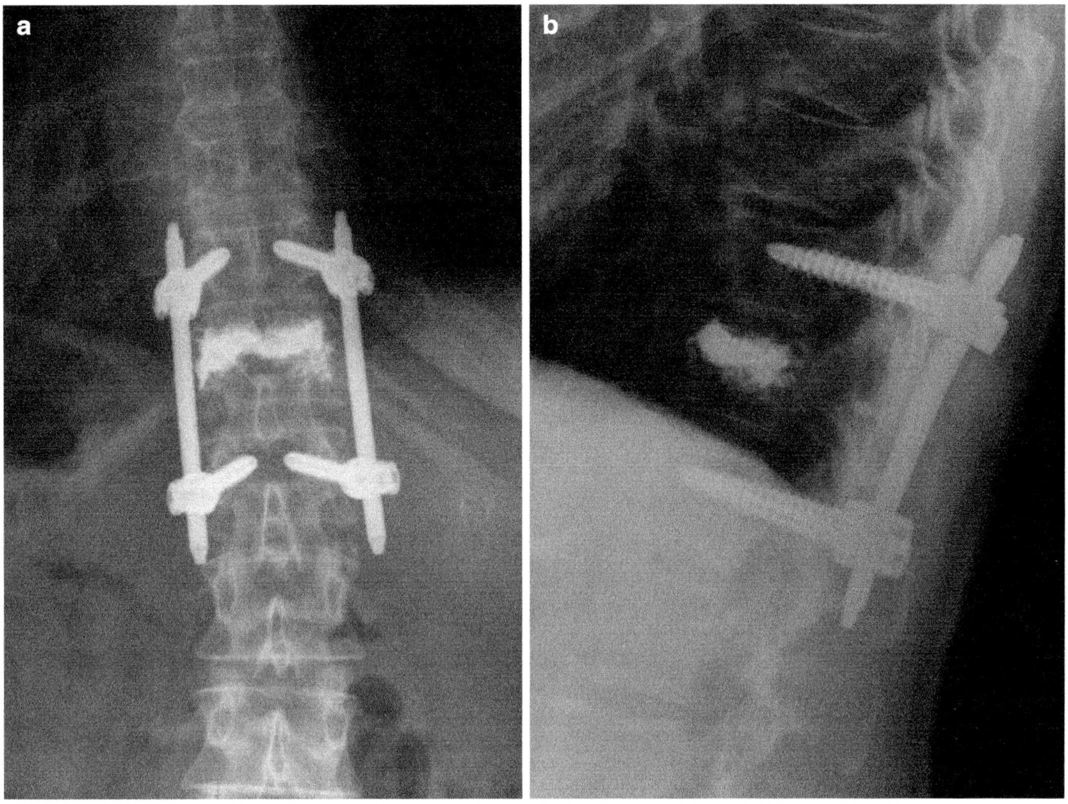

Fig. 35.2 Postoperative anterior-posterior (**a**) and lateral (**b**) radiographs showing percutaneous instrumentation between T11-L1 and kyphoplasty at T12

advantage of muscle preservation through an MIS procedure.

35.3 Discussion of the Case

35.3.1 Indication

This case illustrated a common incomplete burst fracture of the thoracolumbar junction. As there was no neurologic impairment and a minor posterior wall displacement, conservative treatment might have been discussed using a Böhler type brace for 3 months [1]. This treatment leads to consolidation, but a recurrent vertebral body collapse with loss of correction at the fractured level might be observed. In the case of A3 fractures at T12 or in the lumbar spine, short percutaneous pedicle screw instrumentation represents an adequate alternative, which stabilizes the fractured segment and allows the patient to stand up postoperatively without the need for an additional brace. Longer instrumentation might be recommended in the thoracic spine by covering the kyphotic apex by instrumenting 2 levels above and below the fractured level. In cases of severe posttraumatic kyphosis at the thoracolumbar junction, multi-level instrumentation might also be considered if more reduction is needed through the instrumentation itself.

35.3.2 Reduction Techniques

MIS uses principles derived from classic fracture treatment principles, and similarities exist between open and percutaneous techniques. Prone positioning of the patient with a slight lordosis at the thoracolumbar junction reduces kyphosis at the fracture level. This closed

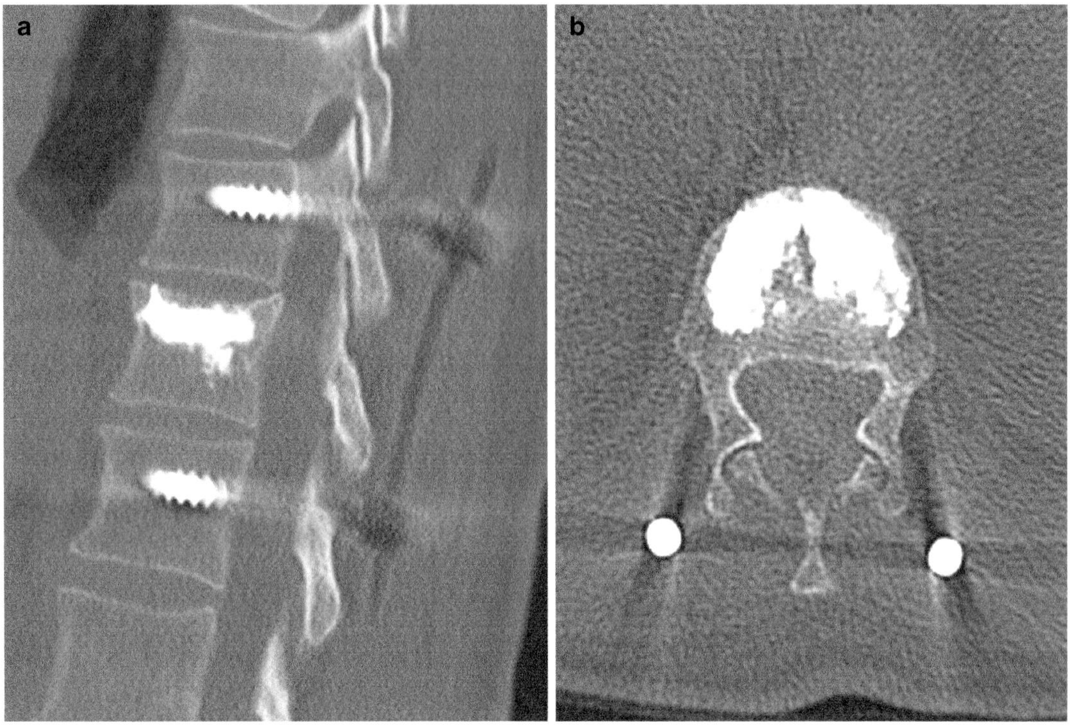

Fig. 35.3 CT scan performed at 6 months postoperatively showing an anatomic consolidation of T12 on sagittal (**a**) and axial (**b**) reconstructions

reduction can be enhanced by leg and halo traction depending on fracture instability. The AO-principle is commonly used is used in burst fractures. A parallel distraction is realized first on Schanz screws in open surgery or monoaxial screws when using an MIS technique. This maneuver creates ligamentotaxis and is followed by an angulation of the monoaxial system in order to restore lordosis in a second step [8]. As an alternative, MIS persuader systems or percutaneous monoaxial long arm screws are efficient for fracture reduction [6]. Pre-bent lordotic rods are progressively inserted into monoaxial screws above and below the fracture, which stretches the spine and creates lordosis with ligamentotaxis at the fracture (Fig. 35.5). Add-on techniques, such as in situ contouring corrects kyphosis by bilateral lordotic rod bending inside the patient, which lengthens the anterior column. The cranial endplate and posterior wall fragments are reduced by ligamentotaxis. The use of pure titanium or cobalt-chromium rods with an appropriate elastic modulus is mandatory for this technique [9]. Alternatively, monoaxial screws at the fracture level may enhance reduction by lifting the endplate directly [3].

35.3.3 Anterior Column Support

If the fracture type represents a pure bony lesion like a Chance fracture, classified as B1 type according to the new AO classification [7], a single posterior percutaneous osteosynthesis is sufficient. An additional vertebral body expansion might be considered in order to maintain reduction at long-term if a vertebral body collapse was present in the fracture type. Kyphoplasty represent one option to consolidate incomplete burst fractures (A3) in combination with posterior instrumentation. Cement injection into the fractured cranial vertebral body would allow an immediate stabilization of the achieved reduction and prevent from recurrence

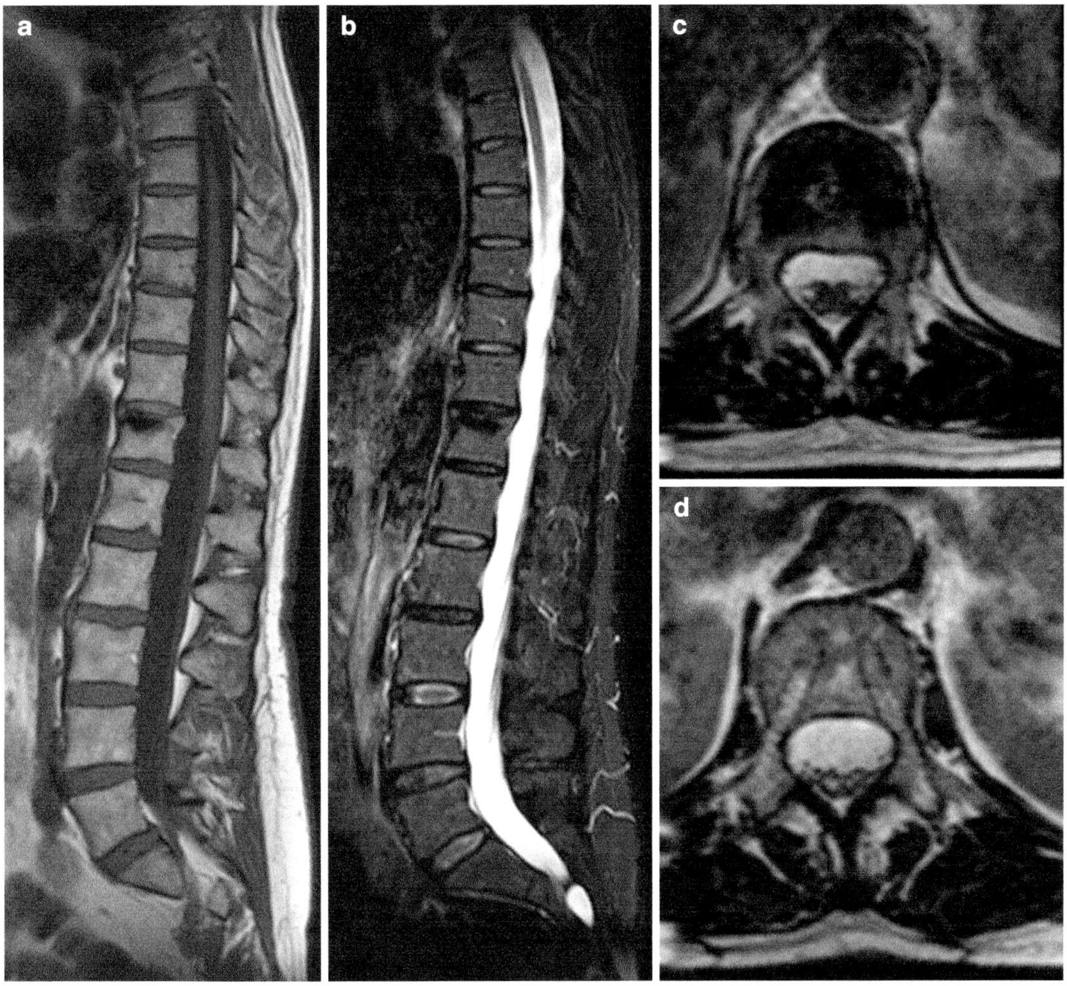

Fig. 35.4 MRI of the thoracolumbar spine performed after implant removal at 2-year follow-up, showing a well-hydrated T11-T12 disc on sagittal T1 (**a**) and T2 (**b**) sequences, and a preserved paravertebral musculature with minor dystrophy at the fracture level (**c**) and instrumented level L1 (**d**)

of kyphosis when the patient stands up postoperatively [5, 10]. In the present case, kyphoplasty was used prior to instrumentation since fracture reduction was mainly obtained by prone positioning of the patient. If this first step of closed reduction had remained insufficient on lateral fluoroscopy, it might have been recommended to complete the reduction by percutaneous instrumentation first. This sequence enhances the ligamentotaxis effect at the anterior column, thus creating an "eggshell" which is then completed by a kyphoplasty.

Anterior fusion might be considered in major anterior column defects. A select mono-segmental fusion is indicated in incomplete burst fractures (A3) if reduction occurred mainly in the cranial adjacent disc rather than in the fractured vertebra. Single level anterior fusion might also be indicated in hyperextension one-level disco-ligamentous injuries (B3). A complete anterior column reconstruction might be preferable in pincer type fractures with disc incarceration in the vertebral body (A2), complete burst fractures (A4) or flexion-distraction fractures with an anterior burst component (B2) [6]. Select anterior fusion with MIS is essential when treating unstable thoracolumbar fractures associated with ligamentous injuries, since percutaneous

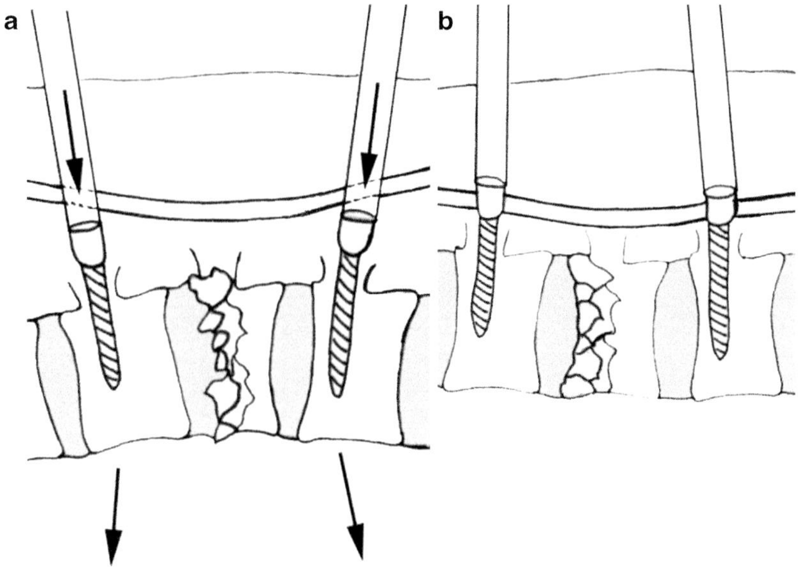

Fig. 35.5 Percutaneous fracture reduction using monoaxial long arm screws and pre-bent lordotic rods which are progressively pushed into the screw heads (**a**). This maneuver creates an elongation of the fractured spinal segment with ligamentotaxis and lordosis once the 90-degree connection between rods and screws is achieved (**b**)

instrumentation does not enable bone grafting like open posterior fusion [3, 4].

35.3.4 Temporary Internal Fixation

Percutaneous instrumentation can be used as temporary internal fixator, which is removed through small skin incisions after consolidation. This allows treating thoracolumbar fractures without damaging paravertebral muscles as posterior dissection is avoided [11]. When using a combined approach of posterior osteosynthesis and select anterior column fusion, removal of the instrumentation is beneficial in younger patients if motion of non-fused lumbar segments can be restored [6]. The combination of kyphoplasty and percutaneous osteosynthesis with subsequent removal of instrumentation allows a management without fusion of incomplete burst fracture. It might be legitimist, when questioning cement injection in younger patients. However, this practice led to adequate clinical and radiologic outcomes without long-term adverse events [5, 10]. Furthermore, this strategy seems justified in A3 fractures as the cranial intervertebral disc is usually contained during the compression mechanism of the injury [12]. It remains unclear, whether cement injection under the cranial endplate inhibits nutrition of the disc by diffusion. The follow-up MRI of this case has shown that the nucleus remained well hydrated. This finding underlined that an incomplete burst fracture does not necessarily lead to cranial disc degeneration if the segment is temporarily maintained by percutaneous instrumentation.

35.4 Conclusions and Take Home Message

Incomplete thoracolumbar fractures without neurologic impairment can be treated efficiently with an MIS procedure. Fracture reduction and stabilization is achieved by percutaneous instrumentation in combination with kyphoplasty within the first days after trauma. This approach has the advantage of preserving the paravertebral musculature. Clinical outcome and sagittal alignment are usually satisfactory on short- and long-term. In younger and physically active patients, instrumentation removal might be discussed if range of motion of non-fused segments can be expected in the lumbar spine or at the thoracolumbar junction.

Pearls

- Preoperative analysis of CT images should rule out facet joint and discoligamentous injuries if percutaneous instrumentation without fusion is indicated.
- Proper prone positioning and reduction using monoaxial screws represent efficient techniques for fracture reduction.
- Expansion and cement augmentation of the fractured vertebral body allow an immediate anterior column strengthening, which lowers the risk for recurrent kyphosis in the early postoperative period.

Editorial Comment

This article illustrates nicely the concept of "internal bracing" as an alternative to external bracing of an incomplete burst fracture. The only thing I would have made differently is to use no cement and short index screws instead.

References

1. Scheer JK, Bakhsheshian J, Fakurnejad S, Oh T, Dahdaleh NS, Smith ZA. Evidence-based medicine of traumatic thoracolumbar burst fractures: a systematic review of operative management across 20 years. Global Spine J. 2015;5(1):73–82.
2. Court C, Vincent C. Percutaneous fixation of thoracolumbar fractures: current concepts. Orthop Traumatol Surg Res. 2012;98:900–9.
3. Lee JK, Jang JW, Kim TW, Kim TS, Kim SH, Moon SJ. Percutaneous short-segment pedicle screw placement without fusion in the treatment of thoracolumbar burst fractures: is it effective? Comparative study with open short-segment pedicle screw fixation with posterolateral fusion. Acta Neurochir. 2013;155(12):2305–12.
4. Vanek P, Bradac O, Konopkova R, Lacy P, Lacman J, Benes V. Treatment of thoracolumbar trauma by short-segment percutaneous transpedicular screw instrumentation: prospective comparative study with a minimum 2-year follow-up. J Neurosurg Spine. 2014;20(2):150–6.
5. Zairi F, Aboukais R, Marinho P, Allaoui M, Assaker R. Minimally invasive percutaneous stabilization plus balloon kyphoplasty for the treatment of type A thoraco lumbar spine fractures: minimum 4 year's follow-up. J Neurosurg Sci. 2014;58(3):169–75.
6. Charles YP, Walter A, Schuller S, Steib JP. Temporary percutaneous instrumentation and selective anterior fusion for thoracolumbar fractures. Spine (Phila Pa 1976). 2017;42(9):E523–31.
7. Vaccaro AR, Oner C, Kepler CK, Dvorak M, Schnake K, Bellabarba C, Reinhold M, Aarabi B, Kandziora F, Chapman J, Shanmuganathan R, Fehlings M, Vialle L, AOSpine Spinal Cord Injury & Trauma Knowledge Forum. AOSpine thoracolumbar spine injury classification system: fracture description, neurological status, and key modifiers. Spine (Phila Pa 1976). 2013;38(23):2028–37.
8. Weiß T, Hauck S, Bühren V, Gonschorek O. Repositioning options with percutaneous dorsal stabilization. For burst fractures of the thoracolumbar junction. Unfallchirurg. 2014;117(5):428–36.
9. Charles YP, Walter A, Schuller S, Aldakheel D, Steib JP. Thoracolumbar fracture reduction by percutaneous in situ contouring. Eur Spine J. 2012;21(11):2214–21.
10. Fuentes S, Blondel B, Metellus P, Gaudart J, Adetchessi T, Dufour H. Percutaneous kyphoplasty and pedicle screw fixation for the management of thoraco-lumbar burst fractures. Eur Spine J. 2010;19(8):1281–7.
11. Ntilikina Y, Bahlau D, Garnon J, Schuller S, Walter A, Schaeffer M, Steib JP, Charles YP. Open versus percutaneous instrumentation in thoracolumbar fractures: magnetic resonance imaging comparison of paravertebral muscles after implant removal. J Neurosurg Spine. 2017;27(2):235–41.
12. Loriaut P, Mercy G, Moreau PE, Sariali E, Boyer P, Dallaudière B, Pascal-Moussellard H. Initial disc structural preservation in type A1 and A3 thoracolumbar fractures. Orthop Traumatol Surg Res. 2015;101(7):833–7.

36 Anterior Surgical Management of Thoracic and Lumbar Fractures

Jens Castein and Frank Kandziora

36.1 Introduction

The posterior stabilisation is the Gold Standard in the operative treatment of spinal fractures. We want to focus on the question which cases might benefit from an additional anterior stabilisation.

A common situation in the clinical practice is, that after a posterior stabilisation the question of an additional anterior operation arises.

Although the scientific evidence for the need of an additional anterior stabilisation is low, we think that in many cases the result of the therapy can be improved with an additional anterior operation.

The following example shows a typical case, in which we would recommend an additional anterior decompression und stabilisation.

Even though in the everyday clinical practice the cases might be not so straightforward, we think that for the demonstration of the principles this case is a prime example.

J. Castein (✉) · F. Kandziora
Zentrum für Wirbelsäulenchirurgie und Neurotraumatologie, Berufsgenossenschaftliche Unfallklinik Frankfurt am Main, Frankfurt am Main, Germany
e-mail: jens.castein@bgu-frankfurt.de

36.2 Case Description

A 33 year old man lost control over his car because of unknown reasons. After the initial treatment at the accident site he was transferred with a helicopter to our emergency room. The patient arrived 3 h after the accident.

The clinical examination showed evidence for a spinal cord injury with a paraplegia below T 6 and a residual sensibility corresponding to an ASIA B type lesion.

The X-rays and CT-scan showed fractures of the rips 4–7 on the left side and a bilateral lung contusion.

The reason for the paraplegia was a luxation fracture T 6/7 (AOS C) with a incomplete cranial burst-split of the T 8 (AOS A4).

According to the new AOS-Classification it was a T 6/7 C, T 6/A4, T 7/A 3, T 8/A4, M0, N3 injury (Figs. 36.1 and 36.2).

As an emergency operation we performed an instrumentation T 4,5 on T 8,9,10 with an realignment of the spine and a wide decompression of the spinal canal T 6,7.

As a second step we did an additional anterior thoracoscopic assisted corpectomy T 6,7 and partially T 8 (endplate) with anterior clearance of the spinal canal because there was still a fragment left behind T 5 and the patient showed no neurological improvement after the posterior decompression (Fig. 36.3).

B. Meyer, M. Rauschmann (eds.), *Spine Surgery*, https://doi.org/10.1007/978-3-319-98875-7_36

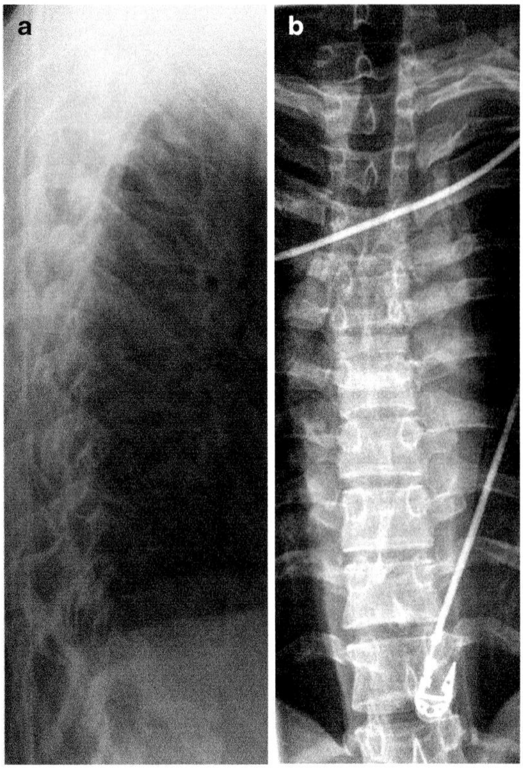

Fig. 36.1 The x-rays from the emergency room in lateral (**a**) and in a.p.-view (**b**) show the fractures of the vertebral bodies T 6,7 and 8 and the anterior displacement of T 6 representing a C-type injury of T 6/7

In the further clinical course we transferred the patient to our paraplegic unit for further rehabilitation.

During his stay in the hospital, which lasted 7 months, the patient learned to walk again.

He is now able to walk for short distances without any help. Unfortunately his is still suffering of an atactic gait and a neurogenic bladder (Figs. 36.4 and 36.5).

36.3 Discussion of the Case

In the upper thoracic spine (T 1–5) we would recommend as an anterior approach a costotransversectomy.

For the vertebral bodies T 5/6 to T 11 a transthoracic approach is used. Most surgeons recommend a left sided approach for the lower thoracic spine because on the right side the liver is difficult to mobilize. For the mid to upper thoracic spine T 5–8 a right-sided approach is preferred.

If it is done in a thoracoscopic or a classic open approach should be chosen by the surgeon depending on his experience and the existing equipment. In our clinic we often use a mini-open approach in combination with thoracoscopy. Especially in cases where the vertebral body has to be replaced, a purely endoscopic operation is not possible because for bringing in the implant an incision of a certain size is unavoidable.

For the vertebral bodies L 2, 3 und 4 we use an XLIF - eXtreme Lateral Interbody Fusion – approach. With this lateral retroperitoneal approach the vertebral bodies can be accessed with a small incision and no large vessels have to be mobilized, which makes it a pretty safe approach.

The vertebral body of L1 can typically be accessed with both approaches. We mostly use the XLIF-approach. Although for the surgeon it is sometimes a bit challenging to mobilize the rib cage, the mayor benefits of the retroperitoneal approach would be that the function of the lung is not compromised and the postoperative pain is much less with no need for a thoracic drainage.

For the replacement of L 5 a classic pararectal retroperitoneal ALIF approach is necessary. Of course L 2–4 can also be reached with an ALIF approach. But in our experience the XLIF approach is causing less bowl irritation and the risk of injuring large vessels is considerably less.

When it is planned from the beginning of the therapy that the patient receives a combined posterior-anterior approach and he suffers of osteoporosis it is advisable to do a posterior cement augmentation of the adjacent vertebral bodies. The anterior implant can rest on the cement filling which will reduce the risk for implant subsidance.

In thoracolumbar fractures we mostly do single level fusions with a resection of the disc and the crushed bony fragments in A3 fractures with at least 2/3 vertebral body height left. There must be a large enough part of bone, where the implant

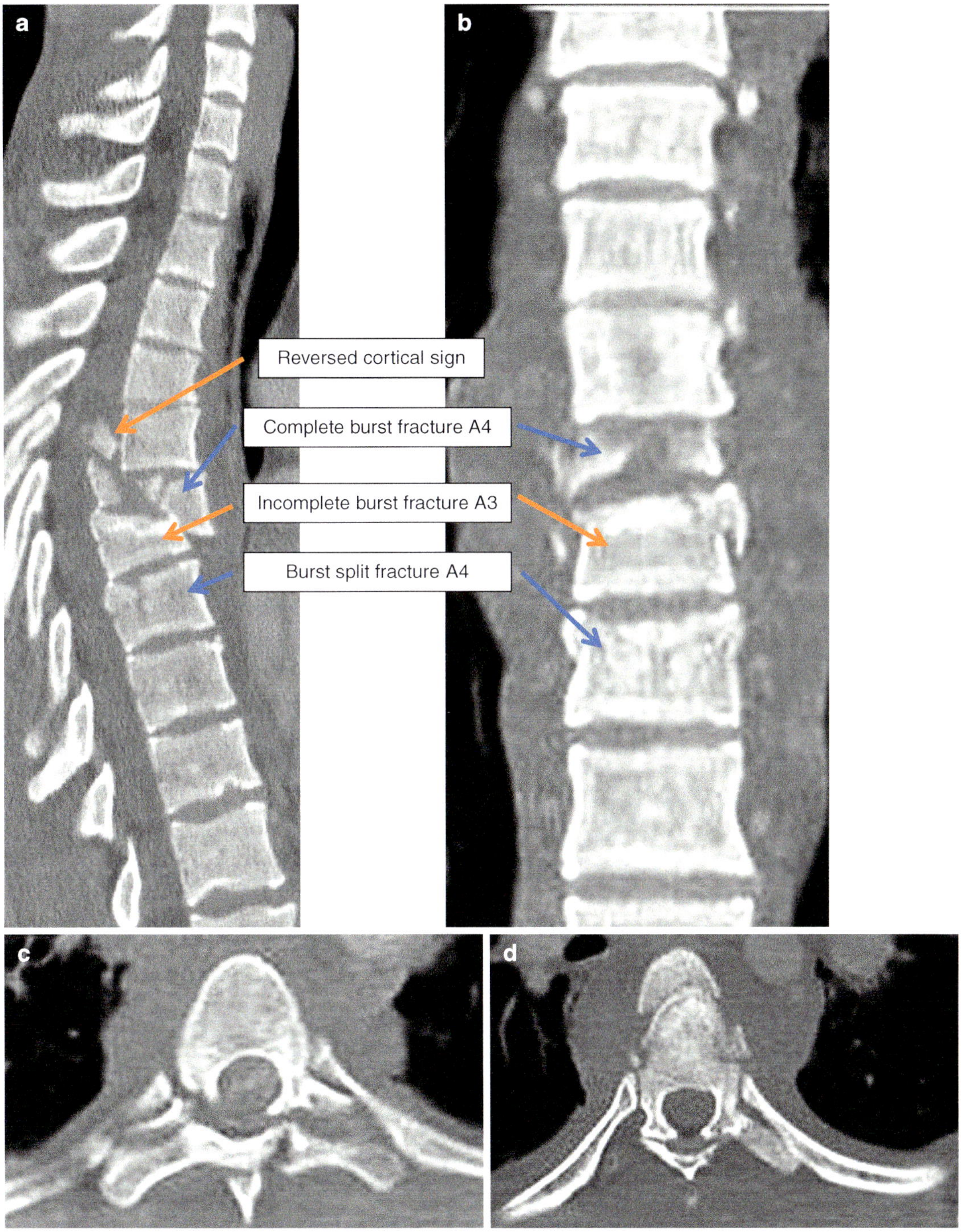

Fig. 36.2 In the CT-Scan further details of the fractures can be seen. Panels (**a**), (**b**), (**c**) and (**d**) show the complete extent of injury in sagittal, coronal and axial cuts

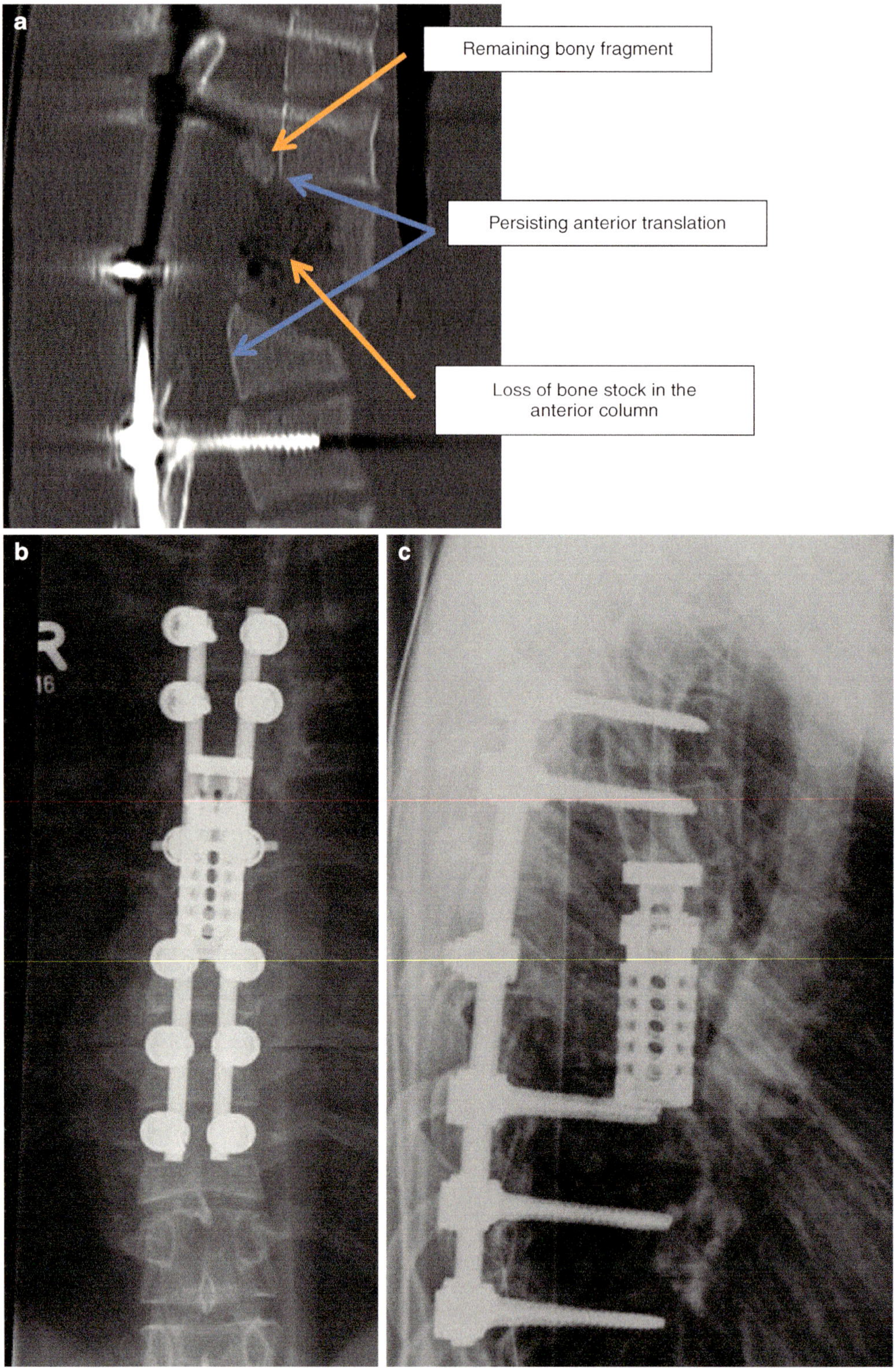

Fig. 36.3 The postoperative CT (**a**) showed a remaining bony fragment which still compromises the dural sac, a significant loss of bone stock in the anterior spinal column and a persisting anterior translation. The postoperative x-rays (**b+c**) showed an excellent positioning of the implants with a good correction of the kyphosis but with a mild residual scoliosis

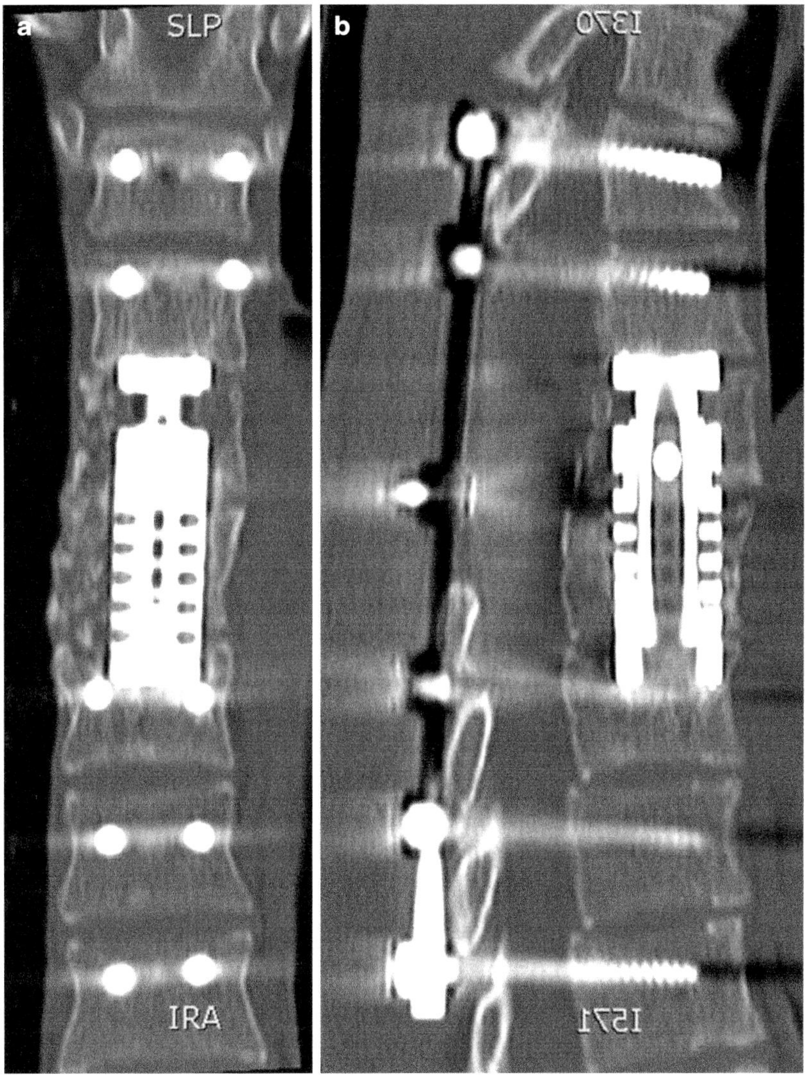

Fig. 36.4 Six months after the trauma the CT-scan showed a good bony integration of the implants with no sign of implant loosening Panels (**a**), (**b**), (**c**) and (**d**) show the complete extent of injury in sagittal, coronal and axial cuts

can be anchored. Depending on the case we use a combination of autologous bone graft and a ventral plate or cage with a screwed design. There is no evidence in the literature for the supremacy of a specific technique.

If the thoracolumbar fracture is a complete burst fracture or an incomplete burst with an impression of the vertebral body of more than 2/3 we would recommend a vertebral body replacement. In these cases we are using expandable titanium cages. Widely used autologous bone grafts as a stand-alone technique are associated with donor site pain, risk of non-union and increased correction loss [1].

Concerning the implants there seems to be a trend that expandable and non-expandable titanium cages have the same fusion rate but expandable cages enable more intraoperative correction [2].

If the fracture is in the lower lumbar or the mid or upper thoracic spine we restrict the indication for an anterior approach.

In incomplete burst fractures of the lower lumbar spine with an impression of the vertebral body not more than 2/3 of the vertebra und a more or less preserved lordosis a loss of correction is unlikely because most of the load in the lumbar spine is carried by the posterior column.

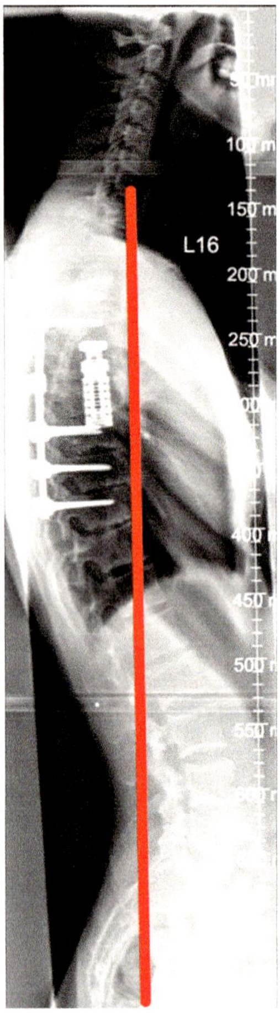

Fig. 36.5 The whole spine x-ray after 6 months in standing position showed a physiological sagittal balance

In our clinic fractures in the upper und mid thoracic spine are operated from posterior including 2 levels above and below the broken vertebra. We think that in these regions it is precarious to do just 1 level above and below because the vertebral bodies are rather small and only small screws can be used. Additional reasons for this concept are that loosing motion segments in these regions is not as critical as in the thoracolumbar or lumbar spine and a loss of correction in these regions is better tolerated by the patients according to Glassman et al. [3]. So in these regions even complete burst fractures are treated only by a posterior approach when the kyphosis is moderate. It is not possible to define a cut off for "moderate kyphosis" but often a whole-spine x-ray helps to see how the patient is affected by the kyphosis and how much he has to compensate.

In former days a long segment posterior stabilization was the common surgical procedure for stabilizing spinal fractures.

The more modern concept is a short segment fixation for saving as much motion segments as possible especially in the thoracolumbar und lumbar spine.

Although posterior stabilization as a stand-alone procedure is a sufficient therapy for many spinal fractures, it has some disadvantages as a stand-alone solution. The most frequent problem is a progressive loss of the initial correction. There seems to be a relation between the destruction of the anterior column and the correction loss after a posterior stand-alone stabilization. Knop et al. for example found a clear correlation between the preoperative wedge angle of the vertebral body and the postoperative loss of reduction [4].

We think that loss of reduction and persisting kyphosis is one of the biggest problems in the treatment of thoracolumbar fractures.

Among others Glassman [3] showed in 2005 that a positive sagittal balance – which means kyphosis – is linear associated with a deterioration in health status measures including the SF-12 an ODI-Scores. Because of the linear association, a cut off angle in terms of a critical degree can't be determined. The deterioration depended on the region of the kyphosis with the thoracolumbar as a critical region only excelled by the lumbar region.

Kyphosis might also accelerate degeneration in the adjacent spinal levels. In an in-vivo animal model (sheep) Oda [5] showed that a fusion L3–5 in kyphosis versus an in-situ fusion lead to significant degenerative changes of the cephalad facet joints.

On the other hand the patients with an additional anterior operation have more blood loss, a longer duration of the operation and the hospital stay and a possible higher rate of complications [6].

So what could help in decision making by taking into consideration that clear evidence for a better *clinical outcome* with an anterior-posterior procedure is still lacking [6]?

A system which can be helpful is the Cormack Load Sharing Classification [7].

Table 36.1 The Cormack load sharing classification system

Amount of comminution	Points	Amount of correction of kyphotic deformity	Points
<30%	1	3° or less	1
30–60%	2	3° to 9°	2
>60%	3	10° or more	3
Displacement of fracture segments			
0–1 mm	1		
At least 2 mm but <u>less</u> than 50% of the cross sectional area of the vertebral body	2		
More than 2 mm but <u>more</u> than 50% of the cross sectional area of the vertebral body	3		

Cormack et al. analysed a series a patients who received short segment instrumentation because of a vertebral fracture. A point system was developed that grades: The amount of damaged vertebral body, the spread of the fragments in the fracture site and the amount of corrected traumatic kyphosis. Table 36.1 shows how the point system works.

Every patient in this series, who had broken screws, had 7 points or more.

The author himself mentions that the classification system has some weaknesses. There were only a small number of patients examined (28 patients) and the system does not contain any assessment of the posterior ligaments. However it remains helpful in evaluating the stability of the anterior column.

Very important for considering an anterior operation is if there are still bony fragments displaced into the spinal canal and causing neural compression. This was the case in our patient. After the initial posterior operation a CT was done, which still showed a fragment compromising the dural sac. Additionally the patient didn't improve in his neurologic function. So these facts encouraged us to indicate an additional anterior operation.

An anterior approach always has the benefit to resect fragments anterior to the dural sac in a save way especially in the thoracic spine where the dural sac should not be mobilized.

Another problem which is recognized since years but still not solved is the role of the intervertebral disc. With increased force on the vertebral body there is an increased force on the intervertebral disc and like any other cartilage tissue the disc has very limited potential for regeneration. An injured disc will not heal and might cause chronic pain. So this might be an argument for additional anterior surgery for the price of sacrificing motion segments.

The crucial point is that although there are some classifications for qualifying the injury of the disc for example from Sander et al. there is no guideline for implementing this into clinical decision making [8].

Also important are the comorbidities of the patient. Especially if the patient has a serious lung disease it might be better to do a longer posterior instrumentation than a short combined anterior-posterior instrumentation. On the other hand residual pulmonary problems due to a persistent hamatothorax might trigger an anterior stabilisation during an pulmonary operation.

In our example case we did an additional anterior operation for 4 reasons:

1. There was a severe destruction of the vertebral bodies (Cormack Classification >7 points)
2. After the initial posterior operation the spinal canal was still compromised and the patient had a persisting neurologic deficit
3. Because of the young age of the patient we wanted to restore a physiological sagittal balance
4. To increase the stability because there was still some anterior translation after the initial posterior operation

36.4 Conclusions and Take Home Message

Clear guidelines for an additional anterior approach can't be derived from the literature.

Evidence Level: C

Although evidence is lacking everyone who is involved in the treatment of spinal fractures should have a clear concept of how to treat these patients.

A summary our concept reduced to a take home message will be described in the following.

According to the recommendations of the Spine Section of the German Orthopaedic and Trauma Society (DGOU/Verheyden et al.) we regularly recommend an additional anterior approach in cases where:

- The vertebral body is more than one third of its height impressed
- There are still bony fragments displaced in the spinal canal and lead to a compression of spinal cord or nerve roots
- The initial kyphotic angle is more than 15–20° or the scoliosis is more than 10°
- The disc is caved in the vertebral body or displaced into the spinal canal

Why?

A widely destruction of the vertebral body predicts postoperative reduction loss after posterior only stabilisation and the more the initial kyphotic angle the more severe the injury is and the more likely a reduction loss will occur [4]. We think that especially in the long term a severe kyphosis at the thoracolumbar junction will matter. At the latest when degeneration of the lumbar spine hinders the compensatory hyperlordosis.

Furthermore a severe damage of the disc will not heal and might cause on going pain.

If there are still bony fragments anterior of the dural sac it might be safer especially in thoracic spine to take them out from an anterior approach.

On the other hand we don't recommend an additional anterior approach in every case.

In A3-type lesions (AOSpine Classification) with only minimal involvement/displacement of the posterior wall, a kyphosis <15° and a good bone quality an additional anterior approach is not necessary.

Also most transosseous B- or C-type lesions (AOSpine-Classification) with only a small bony defect and maybe in a patient with ankylosing spondylitis show good results with long posterior stabilisation only.

And of course severe comorbidities especially of the lung make a long posterior instrumentation more favorable.

In the upper and lower thoracic spine we often restrict the therapy to posterior stabilization two levels above and below even in complete burst fractures considering the kyphosis and degree of destruction of the vertebral body. In these regions sacrificing motion segments is not as critical as in the thoracolumbar or lumbar spine and because of the small vertebral bodies a longer stabilization is needed anyway.

Pearls

- In spite of lacking evidence we recommend an additional anterior approach when the anterior column has a large bony defect (e.g. the vertebral body height is diminished more the 30% or both endplates are broken), which is the case in most A3 type-lesions and all A4-type lesions especially when a short segment stabilisation is planned (According to the recommendations of the Spine Section of the German Orthopaedic and Trauma Society [DGOU/Verheyden et al.]).
- For A3-type lesions an anterior monosegmental fusion is recommend. A4-type lesions should get a vertebral body replacement.

Pitfalls

- In patients with a severe lung illness or a history of complex abdominal operations the need for an additional anterior approach should be questioned critically. These patients might profit from a longer posterior instrumentation without an anterior approach.

Editorial Comment

The authors show according to us a clear-cut case in which an anterior reconstruction should be performed. Despite the fact that there is no high level evidence, the authors provide a very sound line of arguments on when or when not anterior reconstruction is to be considered.

References

1. Smits AJ, Polack M, Deunk J, et al. Combined anteroposterior fixation using a titanium cage versus solely posterior fixation for traumatic thoracolumbar fractures: a systematic review and meta-analysis. J Craniovertebr Junction Spine. 2017;8(3):168–78.
2. Eleraky MA, Duong HT, Esp E, Kim KD. Expandable versus nonexpandable cages for thoracolumbar burst fracture. World Neurosurg. 2011;75(1):149–54.
3. Glassman SD, Bridwell K, Dimar JR, Horton W, Berven S, Schwab F. The impact of positive sagittal balance in adult spinal deformity. Spine (Phila Pa 1976). 2005;30(18):2024–9.
4. Knop C, Blauth M, Bastian L, Lange U, Kesting J, Tscherne H. Frakturen der thorakolumbalen Wirbelsäule. Unfallchirurg. 1997;100:630–9.
5. Oda I, Cunningham BW, Buckley RA. More does spinal Kyphotic deformity influence the biomechanical characteristics of the adjacent motion segments? An in vivo animal model. Spine. 1999;24(20):2139.
6. PP Oprel P, Tuinebreijer WE, Patka P, den Hartog D. Combined anterior-posterior surgery versus posterior surgery for thoracolumbar burst fractures: a systematic review of the literature. Open Orthop J. 2010;4:93–100.
7. McCormack T, Karaikovic E, Gaines RW. The load sharing classification of spine fractures. Spine (Phila Pa 1976). 1994;19(15):1741–4.
8. Sander AL, Laurer H, Lehnert T, El Saman A, Eichler K, Vogl TJ, Marzi I. A clinically useful classification of traumatic intervertebral disk lesions. AJR Am J Roentgenol. 2013;200(3):618–23. https://doi.org/10.2214/AJR.12.8748.

37 Sacral Fractures

Ulas Yildiz and Frank Kandziora

37.1 Introduction

Sacral fractures have historically been an overlooked entity due to their heterogeneous nature. Furthermore they are complex in nature and pose diagnostic challenges and technical difficulties for treatment. They can be differentiated into traumatic (70%) and atraumatic (approx. 30%) etiology. Since the world's older population continues to grow at an unprecedented rate, in nearby future the ratio will change in favor of atraumatic fractures (e.g. sacral insufficiency fractures). The traumatic sacral fracture is the result of a severe high-energy trauma and typically part of a pelvic ring injury. Such high forces lead to damage and disruption of the soft tissue surrounding the pelvis. In contrast the atraumatic fracture occurs in the form of an osteoporotic or insufficiency fracture without a history of trauma. Therefore multiple injuries are rare in these patients. These characteristics make it necessary to differentiate in planning the operative care. Numerous classification systems and the lack of valid therapeutic algorithm lead to a case by case decisions in treatment, depending on the local organizational structures (orthopedics, neurosurgeons or/and trauma surgeons).

This article compares two different fracture entities which were operated in basically the same manner. Both injuries deal with a lumbopelvic instability. Besides the differences between osteoporotic and traumatic fractures and the pitfalls in operative care, the aim of this article is to assess the characteristics and choice of treatment due to the complexity of sacral fractures.

37.2 Case Description

37.2.1 Case I: Trauma

A 22 year old female sustained multiple injuries in a road traffic accident. She was travelling by car and suffered a head-on collision with another vehicle at a speed of approximately 50 kilometers per hour.

After being admitted to our hospital, the patient reported of a lower back pain and presented with a deformity of the right hand. During further clinical and neurological examination she showed a light sensorimotor deficit of the right L5 nerve root. Tibialis somatosensory evoked potentials in the additional neurophysiological evaluation were within normal measures suggesting a nerve root contusion (Fig. 37.1).

The initial imaging revealed a fracture of the os hamatum and a fracture-luxation of the os triquetrum combined with a carpal luxation of the right hand.

U. Yildiz (✉) · F. Kandziora
Zentrum für Wirbelsäulenchirurgie und Neurotraumatologie, Berufsgenossenschaftliche Unfallklinik Frankfurt am Main, Frankfurt, Germany
e-mail: Ulas.yildiz@bgu-frankfurt.de

B. Meyer, M. Rauschmann (eds.), *Spine Surgery*, https://doi.org/10.1007/978-3-319-98875-7_37

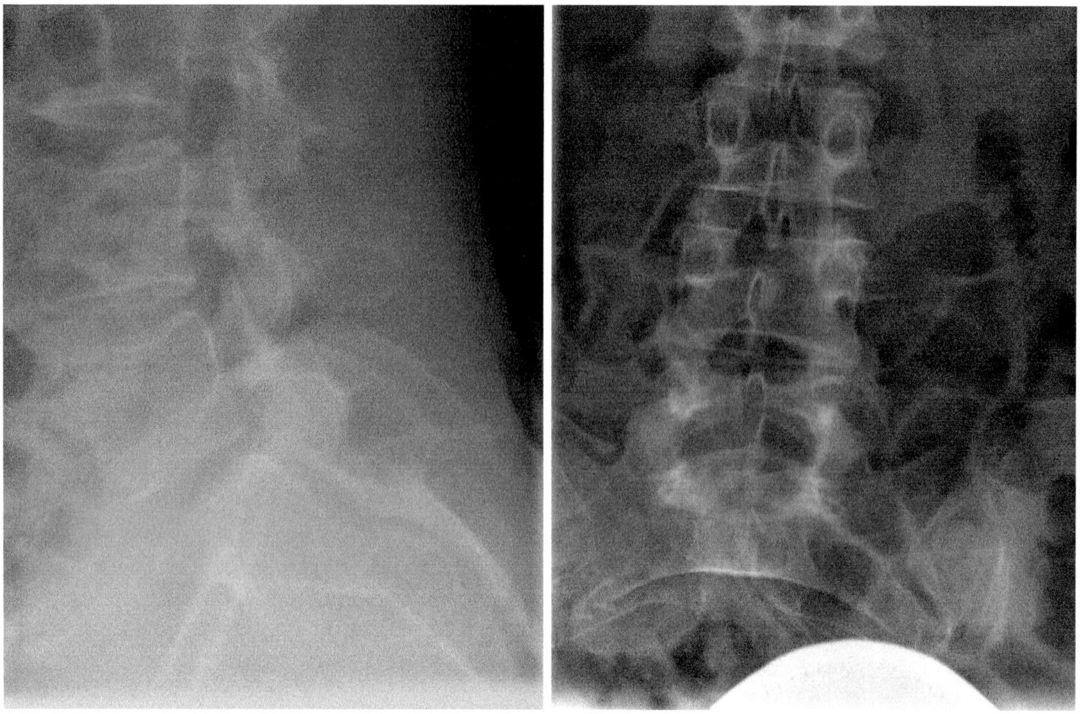

Fig. 37.1 The X-ray indicates a fracture of the right Massa lateralis with a cortical disruption

First plain X-rays of the sacral bone indicated a fracture of the right Massa lateralis. Supplementary Ct-scan showed a complex bilateral H-type fracture of the sacrum with major dislocation of the right base and the right sacral wing below (Figs. 37.2 and 37.3). The fracture lines involved all three zones described in Denis Classification [1], affecting the central canal but sparing the neural structures within. The translational flexion injury in the central mass of the sacrum could be further subclassified into type II, according to sagittal plane alignement by Roy-Camille [2]. No radiographic entrapment of the L5 nerve root could be detected.

Surgical approach was done by a midline incision from the L3 to the S4 segment, followed by dissecting the paraspinal musculature subperiosteally off the posterior elements of L4 through S4 and lateral dissection to the posterior superior iliac spines bilaterally. Screws were placed through both L4 and L5 pedicles under fluoroscopic guidance. After exposing the PSIS (posterior superior iliac spina) a small recess was created with a bone chisel 1 cm caudally and medially of the PSIS to prepare the entry point of the iliac fixation. This was done to prevent prominence of the screw head which can cause a serious discomfort for the patient. To create the tract of both ilium screws, a probe was used, following the trajectory from the PSIS to the AIIS (anterior inferior iliac spina). After probing and ensuring that there were no cortical breeches or penetrations, the screw length was determined and set under fluoroscopy, aiming towards the AIIS. The rods were inserted, reduced und connected to the screw heads. In order to increase the rigidity of the rod-screw construction and to minimize axial rotation, regarding the highly unstable H-type fracture of the sacrum, a transverse connector was attached. Decompression of the nerve root L5 was not carried out, since the neurophysiological test was without pathological finding.

No complications or adverse events occurred during postoperative course. The patient was mobilized as tolerated. Follow-up consisted of upright radiographs after mobilization, along with pelvic inlet and outlet imaging. To detect bone formation and consolidation, a Ct-Scan was performed in an outpatient setting 3 months after surgery. Fortunately her motor and sensory functions recovered.

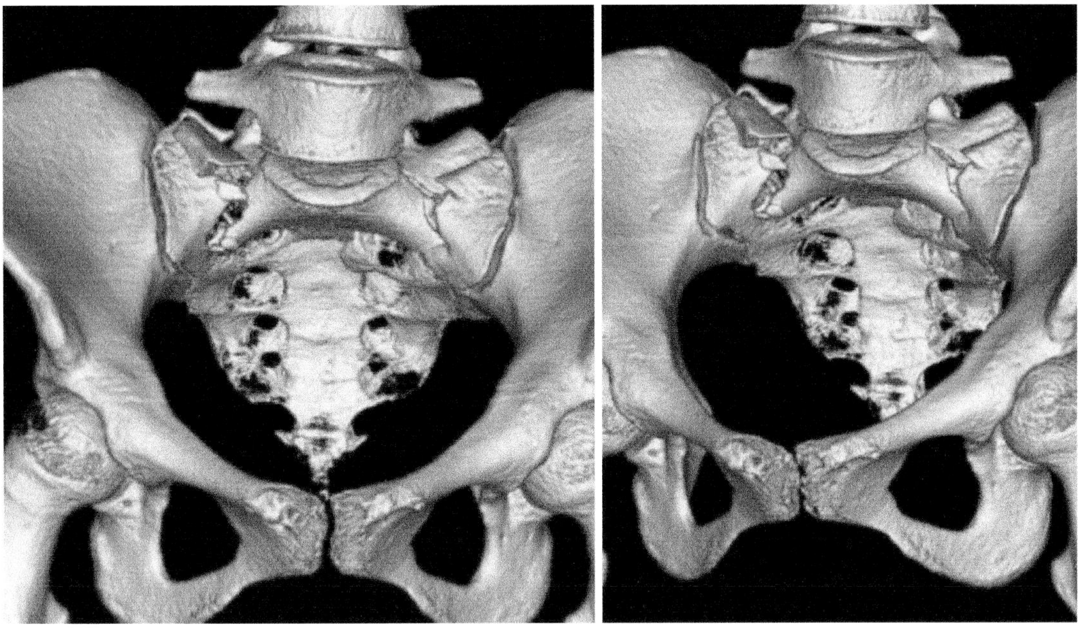

Fig. 37.2 Additional digital reconstruction of the initial Ct-scan could verify fractures on both Massa lateralis, the right base with a fragment more dislocated

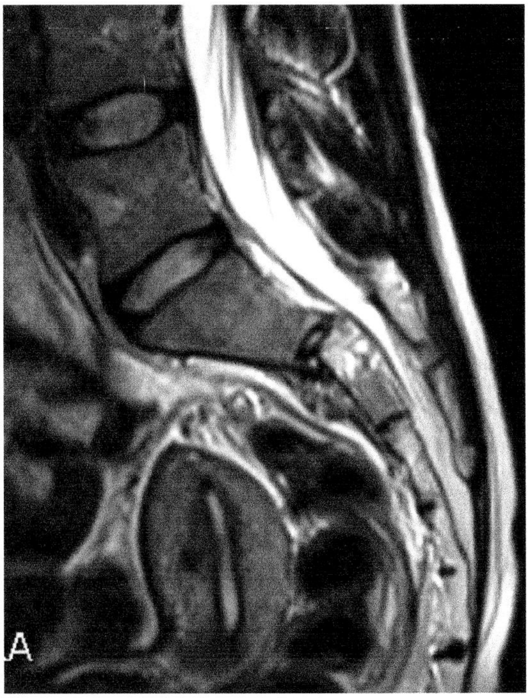

Fig. 37.3 MRI-scan showing flexion injury with translational displacement inbetween S1 and S2 according to type II in Roy-Camille Classification with a presacral hematoma

After osseous consolidation of the sacral fracture an implant removal was scheduled 4 months after surgery to liberate the lumbar segments (Figs. 37.4, 37.5 and 37.6).

37.2.2 Case II: Osteoporosis

An 81 year-old patient suffered a fall during epileptic convulsion. During initial treatment and diagnostic workup in an external clinic, he complained of lower immobilizing back pain.

After assessing a hyperextension fracture-dislocation of the segment L5/S1 type B3 according to AO Spine Classification, the patient was relocated to our department for further operative care. Dual-energy X-ray absorptiometry revealed an osteoporotic bone mineral density. Since the S1 endplate was disrupted, the conjunction between the lumbar spine and the pelvic ring was separated along with the soft tissue (Fig. 37.7).

Then a spondylodesis between L5 and S1 and a fixation of the lumbosacral spine to the pelvic ring was aimed by utilizing an instrumentation from L4 to S1 with S2 alar iliac screw fixation.

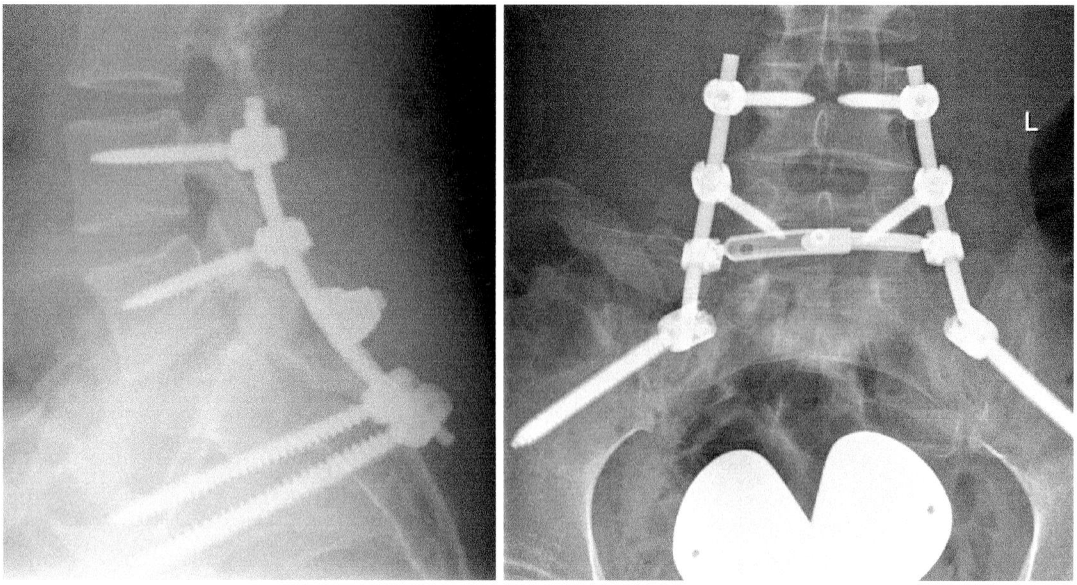

Fig. 37.4 Postoperative X-rays

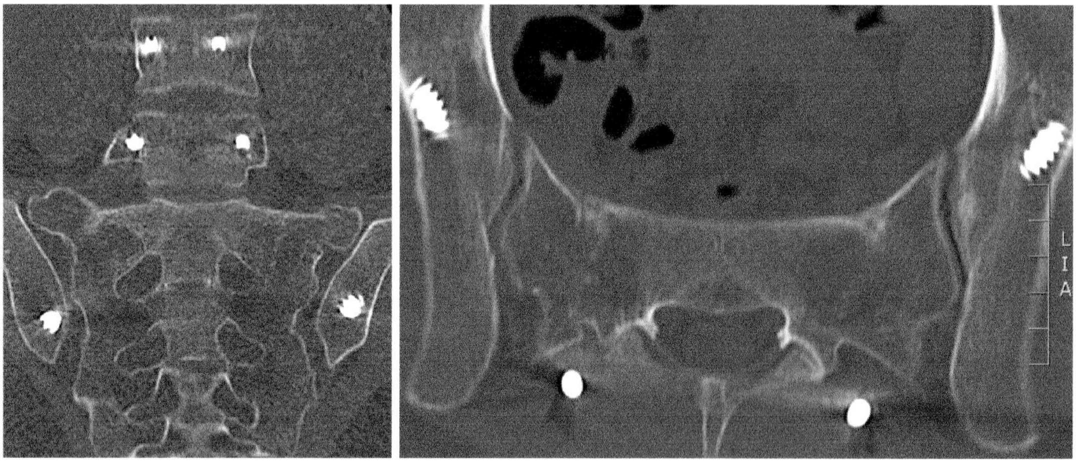

Fig. 37.5 3-months postoperative CT imaging

Surgical procedure was performed in the same manner as in the case before except for the iliac fixation. The technique of S2 alar iliac screw fixation was chosen because of lower screw prominence and enhanced biomechanical strength compared to the iliac screws. Demineralized bone matrix was added around the fully resected facet joints L5/S1.

S2 alar iliac screws bridge the sacroiliac joint directly and alter the sacroiliac joint surface. Hence it is predominantly useful in patients where already degenerative SI-joint problems exist preoperatively, while it should be avoided in young patients with healthy SI-joints especially if an implant removal is expected (Fig. 37.8).

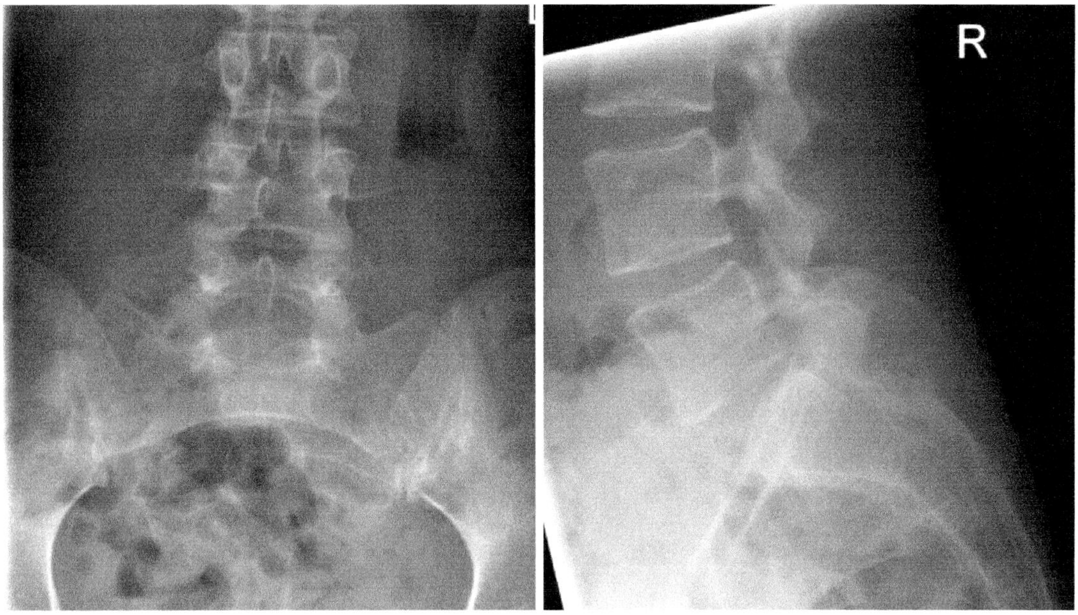

Fig. 37.6 After implant removal

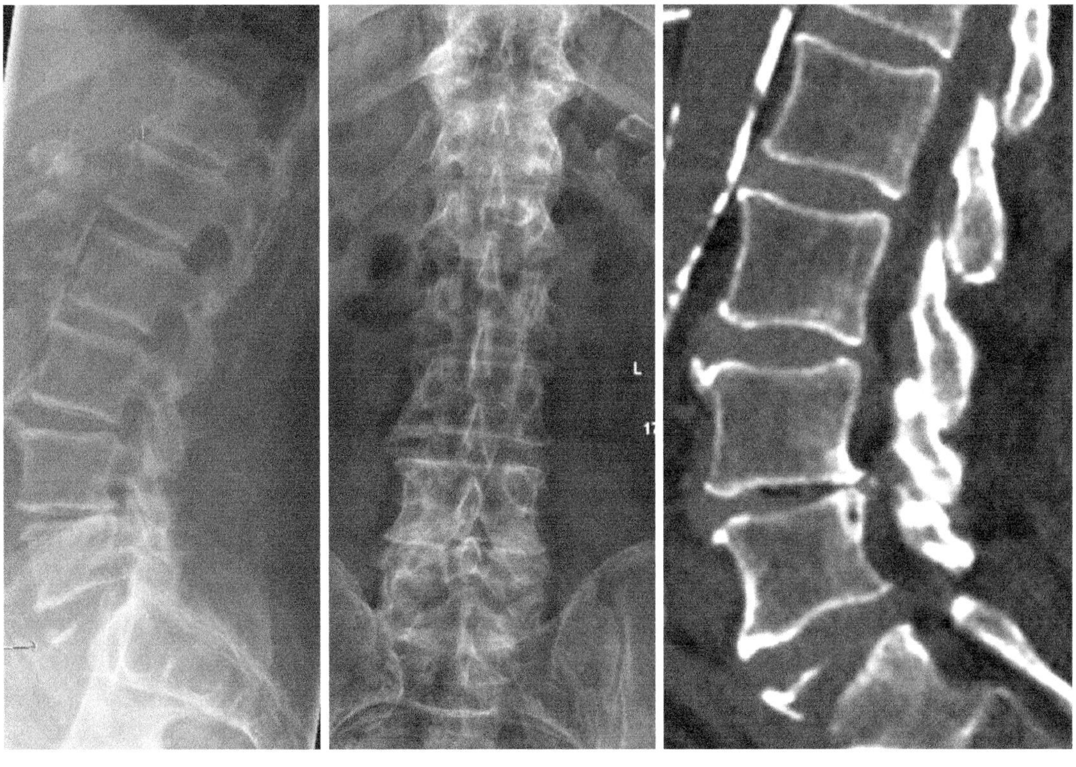

Fig. 37.7 Hyperextensionfracture, note that the endplate S1 is torn out with a bigger gap in the L5-S1 segment

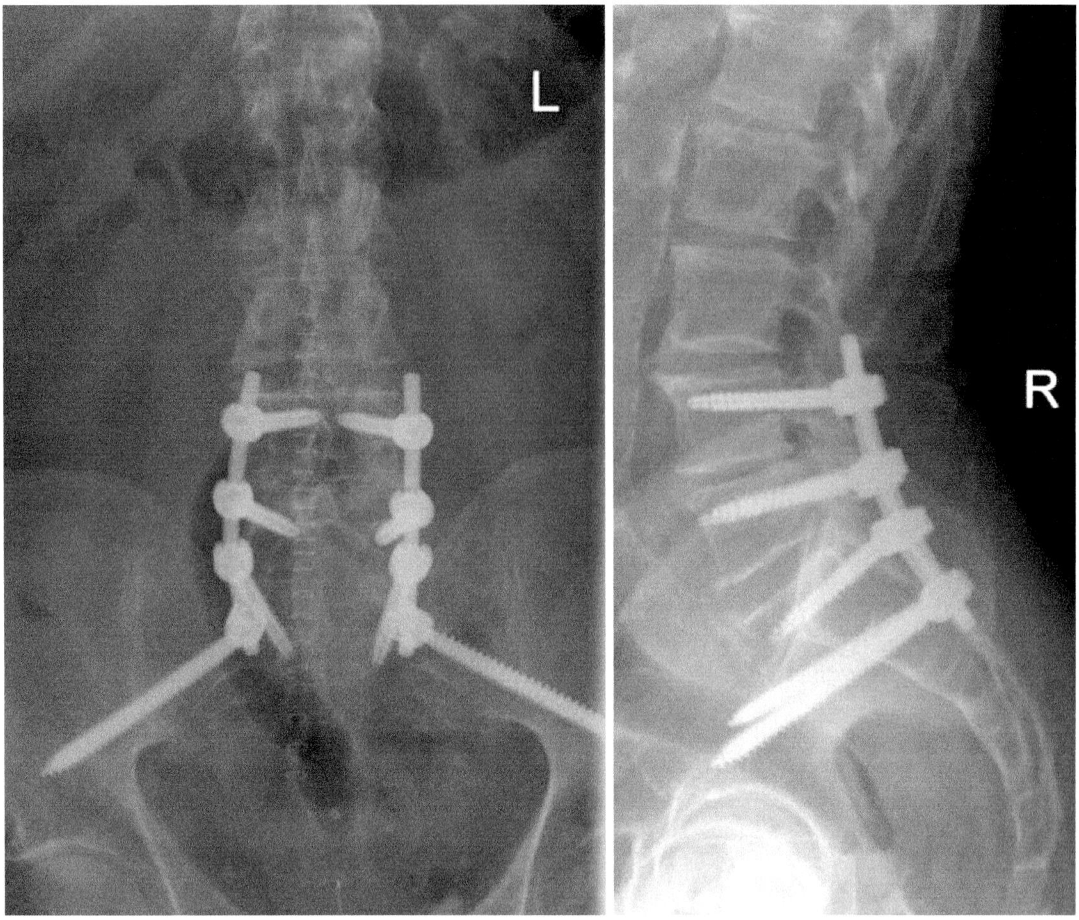

Fig. 37.8 Postoperative X-rays

A second surgical intervention was performed for additional anterior load-bearing support as well as to restore sagittal balance and spinal contour. Preoperative imaging of the pelvic blood vessels revealed an adequately wide corridor within the bifurcation of the iliac veins. Through a midline incision between the umbilicus and the symphysis the posterior abdominal wall was reached by bluntly freeing the parietal peritoneum. A lordotic ALIF cage was inserted into the resected disc L5/S1 to bridge the gap. Four integrated divergent locking screws were inserted to add a significant mechanical stability.

Initial postoperative care consisted of early mobilization to prevent ileus and atelectasis. Early oral feeding led to regular bowel movements and normal stool frequency. Opioid-based analgesia could be reduced by the time the patient was discharged, while the patient was able to mobilize himself independently (Figs. 37.9 and 37.10).

37.3 Discussion of the Cases

Numerous classification systems for sacral fractures evolved over the past years due to the diversity of this injury. The most commonly used is the Denis or Roy-Camille Classification [1, 2] referring to the location of the fracture or its grade of dislocation. Denis et al. divided the sacrum into 3 zones in relation to the sacral foramina with the highest frequency of neurological impairment for zone III injuries, medial

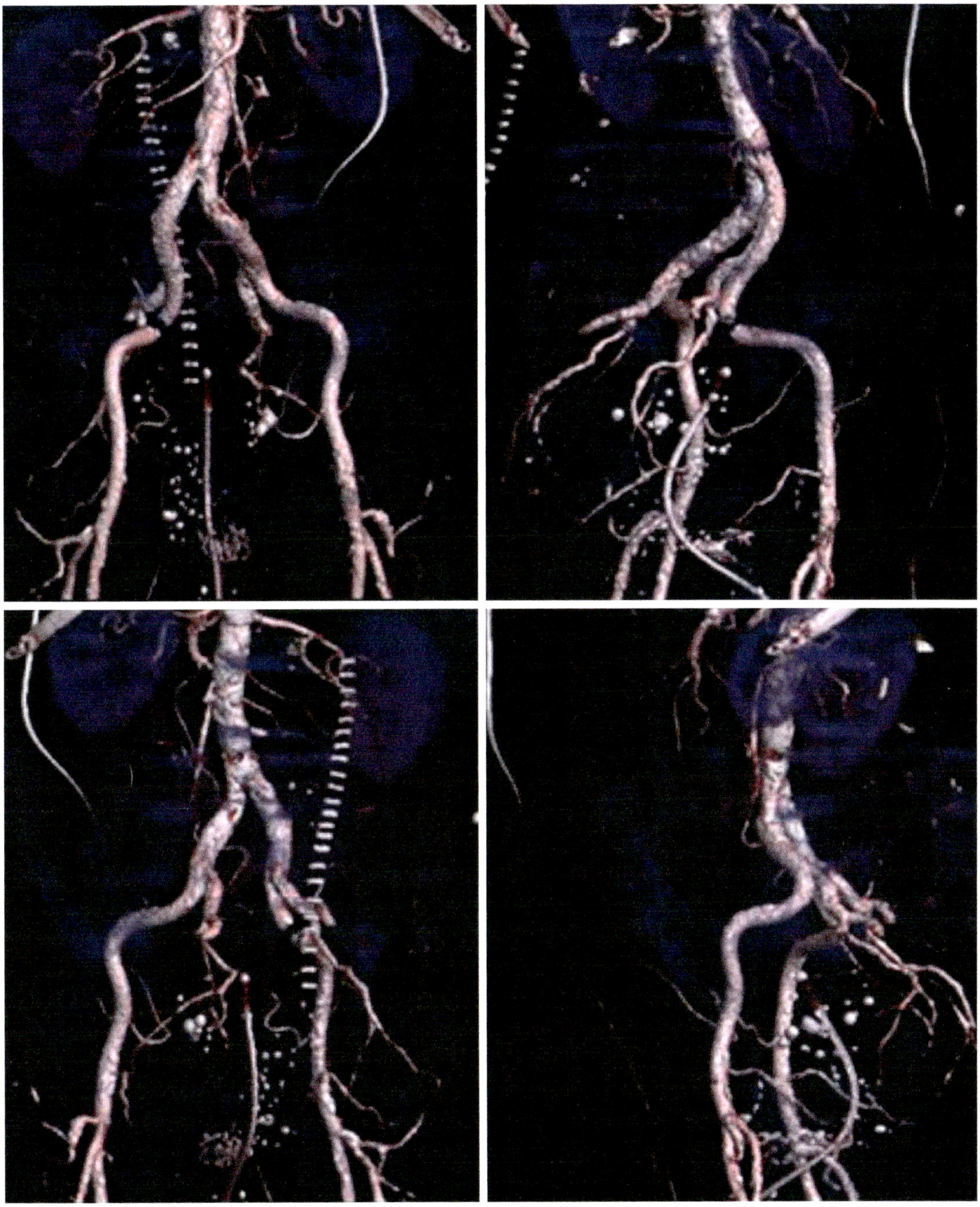

Fig. 37.9 3D imaging of the blood vessels to clarify the corridor of the iliac veins

to the sacral foramina. Vertical fractures in zone III rarely present neurologic deficits, the main cause are transverse fractures type II or III in Roy-Camille Classification which are associated with cauda equine syndrome or lumbosacral plexus dysfunction [3, 4]. Injuries along the sacral foramina usually lead to radiculopathies.

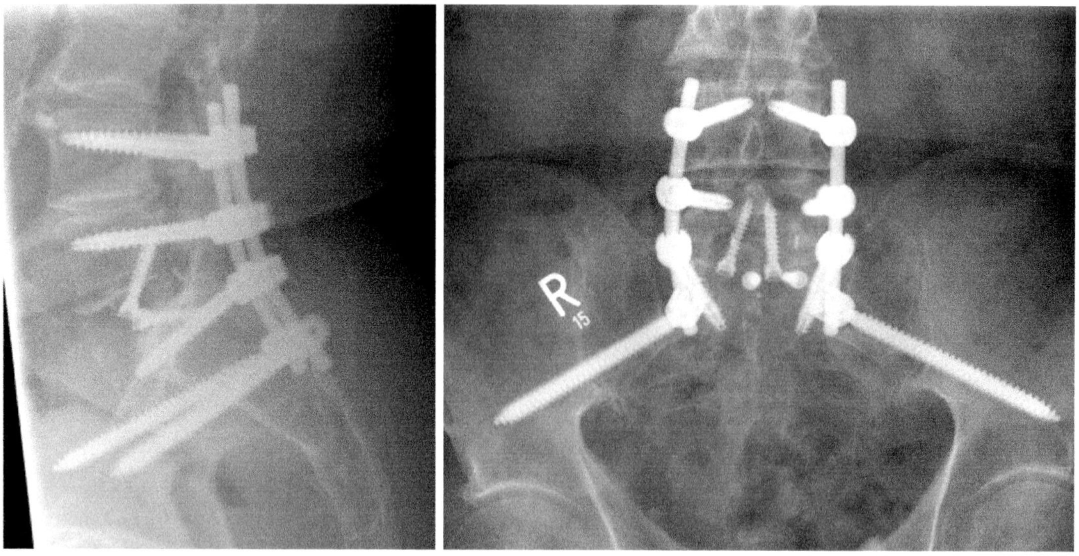

Fig. 37.10 Postoperative X-rays with an interbody gaft

In order to take account for the characteristics and their complications, a universally accepted sacral fracture classification was established by the AOSpine [5]. It is a 3 stage classification which distinguishes the grade of instability. Type A does not affect the spinopelvic stability whereas type B fractures occur unilaterally with a posterior pelvic instability and type C bilaterally with a concomitant spinopelvic dissociation. This system aims to achieve international acceptance and describes injuries based on fracture morphology, neurologic status and case specific modifiers. Secondary to its use for trauma cases, disregarding the specifics of osteoporotic or metabolically impaired bone, it has so far not reached wide distribution.

In terms of fragile bone Rommens et al. introduced the classification of fragility fractures of the pelvic ring [6]. Compared to pelvic ring lesions of younger adults, the osteoporotic bone fails to bear the daily load, ranging from low-energy to physiological load. Many fracture patterns show a certain dynamic process. Linstrom et al. have found that walking causes alternate weight bearing with stress to both sacral ala [7]. This may induce a uni- or bilateral fracture within the reduced bone stock. After losing the lateral support the forces transmitted downward from the spine to the sacrum produce high impact at the central portion of the sacrum. That in turn causes an anteriorinferior vector in the upper part of the sacrum which may lead into a transverse fracture.

From this point of view the comprehensive classification of Rommens et al. may be just a snapshot of pelvic ring lesions but reflects the clinical and morphological characteristics in a better way. This detailed system allows to understand and predict the stability and prognosis of the lesion. Despite a well-understandable structure, however, this classification system has so far found little use due to its complexity.

The trauma case needs to be classified as type C3 referring to AOSpine with a displaced H-type fracture. Due to its transverse fracture displacement it has a higher likelihood of neurological impairment. As one would expect, in a higher dislocated case, this should have led to a cauda equine syndrome or lumbosacral plexus dysfunction. But neither occurred, because of the limited dislocation and the widely intact spinal canal. Instead she only presented with a sensorimotor radiculopathy of the right L5 nerve root. The greater dislocation of a bone fragment from the right-sided base of the sacrum with a presumably compromised iliolumbar ligament resulting in an indirect "stretch" of the L5 radix may be an explanation for the neurologic symptom. Because of preoperative intact neurophysiological testing and its peripheral affection as well as the missing direct nerve root compression, direct surgical decompression was not carried out. We expected to achieve sufficient decompression by indirect reduction with concomitant ligamentotaxis. An open reduction was performed to evaluate and address the fracture dislocation. The transverse displacement involves a spinopelvic instability and demands a rigid spino-pelvic stabilization. In vertically unstable sacral fractures a spinopelvic stabilization counteracts the shear forces and is thereby mandatory to exclude the fractured sacrum from weight bearing. A transverse connector was attached to prevent axial rotation. This allowed early weight-bearing and facilitated nursing care. Alternative options for internal fixation, including percutaneous iliosacral screws, transiliac bars, sacral rods or isolated posterior plates do not provide adequate fixation for early mobilization in our hands.

Even though the osteoporosis case suffered a low energy trauma, the FFP Classification cannot be applied due to the missing corresponding subdivision. This fracture type should rather be classified as B3-type in AOSpine Classification comparable to a U-shaped lesion. Due to reduced bone stock, a spinopelvic fixation technique was performed to achieve a reliable implant anchoring, secure stability and prevent pseudarthrosis. Since exclusively the endplate of S1 was torn out, pedicle screws were applied from L4 to S1. S2 Alar-Iliac screws were chosen because of their lower prominence, increased ability to directly connect to proximal fixation, less extensive dissection of soft tissue and their greater likelihood of enhanced biomechanical strength compared to the iliac screw technique. Under the assumption of an extensive disruption of the ligaments and soft tissue, an ALIF-Cage was inserted into the segment L5/S1 in order to secure the anterior support and induce a bone fusion.

37.3.1 Comparing Both Cases

The young trauma patient had a fixation following the principles of a temporary stabilization. After consolidation and bone formation, the implants were removed to liberate all affected joints. The osteoporosis case on the other hand received a permanent fusion of the L5-S1 segment. Since elderly patients commonly have calcified und rigid adjacent ligaments and soft tissue, in case of a trauma they usually suffer from a wide lesion of both, soft tissue and fragile bone structure. Considering this, a sufficient support of anterior and dorsal structures was needed to allow early mobilization.

37.4 Conclusion and Take Home Message

High speed trauma must be followed by high-resolution diagnostic workup, specifically a multislice polytrauma Ct-Scan. If there is an accompanying neurological deficit, an MRI scan should be performed promptly in order to rule out intraspinal hematoma or affection of neuronal structures. The current therapeutic methods are based on the stability criteria of the pelvic ring. During the initial hours following trauma the primary focus remains on optimizing patient survival by limiting ongoing hemorrhage into the retroperitoneal perisacral region. External pelvic clamp or external fixateur is recommended during emergency care. In case of a compensated state, however, internal fixation offers better nursing care and mobilization. Furthermore, this allows to bridge the weight-bearing from the lower lumbar spine bypassing the injured sacrum directly to the ileum.

In elderly patients there is usually a lack of trauma history and plain radiographs of the pelvic ring are performed standardly to exclude fractures. In prospective studies, up to 60–80%, and in retrospective studies around 50% of osteoporotic sacral fractures remained undetected in conventional X-rays [8, 9]. If affected patients complain of persistent pain Ct, MRI or scintigraphy are indispensable to verify a fracture. Conservative treatment is generally promising in atraumatic sacral fractures or after low-energy trauma provided that the patient has no neurological deficits and can be mobilized. Unstable fractures should be closely examined, otherwise they can lead to further complications due to neglected treatment. In terms of a necessary surgical intervention, a definitive solution with adequate stabilization should be sought out in the interest of the patient. Sacral fractures require long-segment fixation, especially in osteoporotic bone, with an additional Iliac or S2 Alar-Iliac screw in order to resist flexion moments. Specifically at L5-S1, pseudarthrosis is very common with lumbosacral fusions. With the objective to minimize the risk of pseudarthrosis an interbody graft should be utilized.

Pearls
- Maintain a high index of suspicion for fracture in metabolically impaired bone
- MRI Scan is the gold standard in management of suspected osteoporotic sacral fracture

References

1. Denis F, Davis S, Comfort T. Sacral fractures: an important problem. Retrospective analysis of 236 cases. Clin Orthop Relat Res. 1988;227:67–81.
2. Roy-Camille R, Saillant G, Gagna G, Mazel C. Transverse fracture of the upper sacrum. Suicidal jumper's fracture. Spine. 1985;10(9):838–45.
3. Bellabarba C, Stewart JD, Ricci WM, et al. Midline sagittal sacral fractures in anterior—posterior compression pelvic ring injuries. J Orthop Trauma. 2003;17(1):32–7.
4. Rodrigues-Pinto R, Kurd MF, Schroeder GD, et al. Sacral fractures and associated injuries. Global Spine J. 2017;7(7):609–16.
5. Bellabarba C, Schroeder GD, Kepler CK, et al. The AOSpine sacral fracture classification. Global Spine J. 2016;6(1_suppl):s-0036-1582696-s-0036.
6. Rommens PM, Hofmann A. Comprehensive classification of fragility fractures of the pelvic ring: recommendations for surgical treatment. Injury. 2013;44(12):1733–44.
7. Linstrom NJ, Heiserman JE, Kortman KE, et al. Anatomical and biomechanical analyses of the unique and consistent locations of sacral insufficiency fractures. Spine. 2009;34(4):309.
8. Gotis-Graham I, McGuigan L, Diamond T, et al. Sacral insufficiency fractures in the elderly. Bone Joint J. 1994;76(6):882–6.
9. Ries T. Detection of osteoporotic sacral fractures with radionuclides. Radiology. 1983;146(3):783–5.

Spine Injuries in the Elderly

38

Maria Wostrack and Bernhard Meyer

38.1 Introduction

In the elderly the risk of traumatic fractures is rising due to an increased risk of falls caused by cerebrovascular and cardiac diseases. Another problem is the altered bone metabolism leading to increased bone fragility and fracture tendency. Thus even minor trauma such as domestic falls often leads to significant spine injuries.

Both most common fracture types in the elderly are osteoporotic vertebral body compression fracture in the thoracolumbar spine and Anderson and D'Alonzo type II odontoid fracture in the upper cervical spine [3].

Due to operative difficulties caused by the loss of the bone mineral density on one hand, and perioperative complications caused by medical comorbidities on the other, the decision in favor of surgical procedure is usually restrained. In contrast to the clearly evident benefits of surgical treatment of a for instance hip fracture, definitive guidelines for treatment of spine fractures in the elderly are missing.

The chapter will elucidate the existing dilemma between surgical therapy for osteoporotic fractures in elderly patients harboring high perioperative morbidity, versus conservative treatment potentially leading to an insufficient healing and neurological impairment. The rationale for both, conservative options and surgical approaches is discussed in this chapter based on the two most common types of geriatric spine fractures.

38.2 Case 1

38.2.1 Case Description

A 95 y/o female patient with a history of apoplexy and dementia stumbled and fell down on the back of her head. The externally performed CT scan and the MRI showed an Anderson and D'Alonzo type 2 odontoid process fracture (Figs. 38.1 and 38.2). After diagnostics and fixation in a Miami-J collar, the patient was transferred to our clinic. The patient suffered from strong neck pain. The neurological examination showed no deficits.

The patient underwent C1-C2 posterior by C1-C2 arthrodesis using the Goel and Harms technique (fixation of the C1 lateral masses and C2 isthmus using polyaxial screws) (Fig. 38.3).

No new deficits occurred after surgery. A perioperatively-acquired pneumonia was successfully treated by systemic application of a calculated antibioticum for 1 week. The patient was

M. Wostrack (✉) · B. Meyer
Department of Neurosurgery, Klinikum rechts der Isar, Technische Universität München, Munich, Germany
e-mail: maria.wostrack@tum.de

B. Meyer, M. Rauschmann (eds.), *Spine Surgery*, https://doi.org/10.1007/978-3-319-98875-7_38

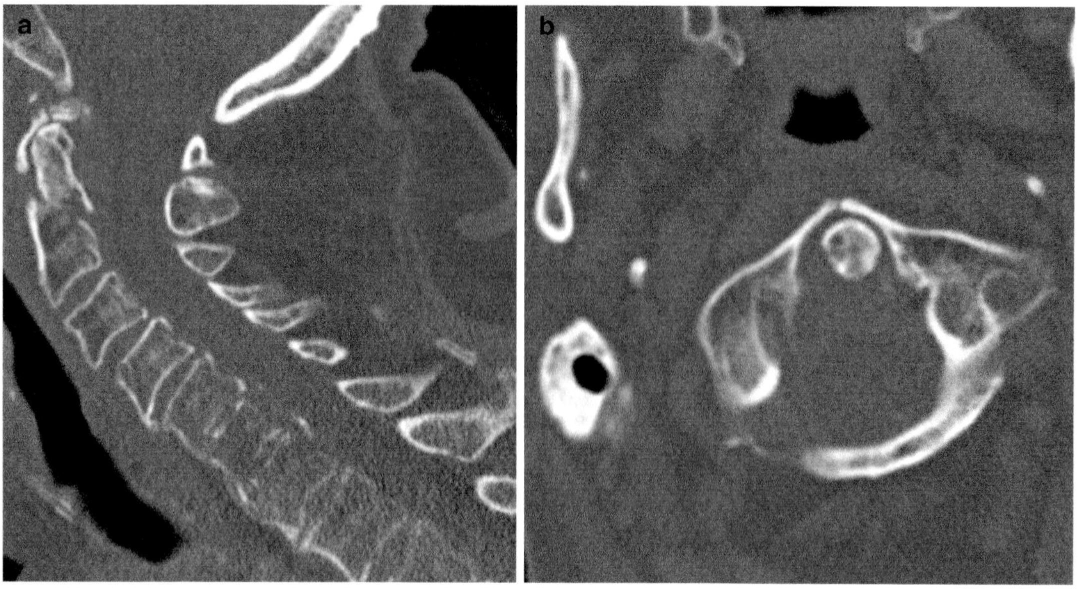

Fig. 38.1 Initial CT Scan. Sagittal (**a**) and axial (**b**) CT scan rendering type II odontoid fracture

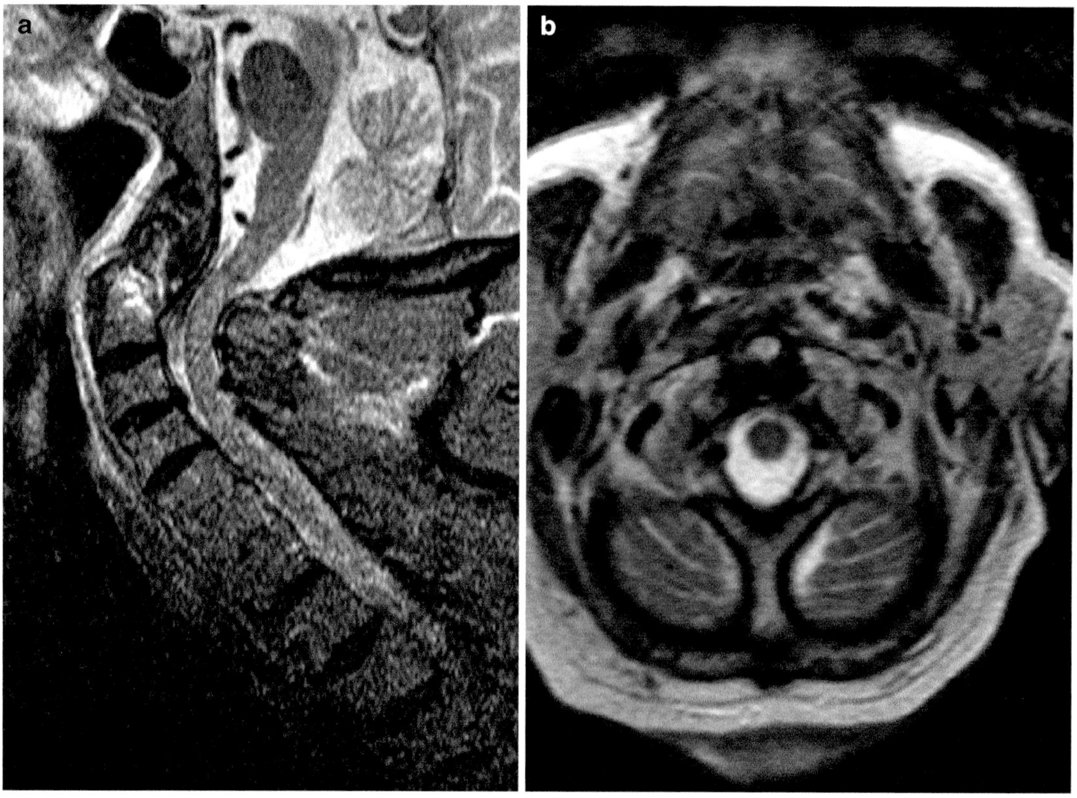

Fig. 38.2 Preoperative MRI. Sagittal STIR MRI (**a**) showing pathological signal enhancement along the C1/C2 complex; the sagittal and additionally axial images (**b**) are indicative for the disruption of the transverse ligament of the atlas

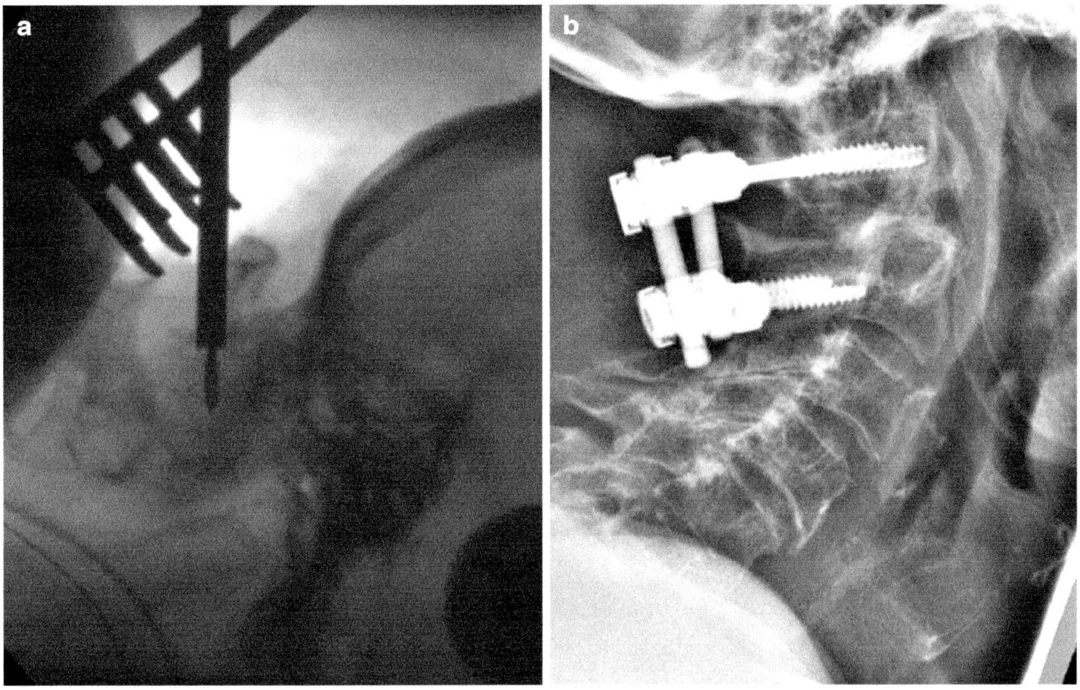

Fig. 38.3 Posterior screw-rod C1-C2 fixation. (**a**) Posterior C1-2 fixation is performed with lateral mass screws placed in C1 (**a**) and isthmic screws in C2. Drilling is guided by anatomic landmarks and lateral fluoroscopy. (**b**) X-ray check showing appropriate results after surgery

discharged back to her nursing home in a clinically and neurologically stable state 2 weeks after the surgery.

38.3 Case 2

38.3.1 Case Description

A 77 y/o female patient with a known history of osteoporosis presented to our outpatient department with progressive lumbar pain. The patient had fallen about 2 months ago. Additionally the patient reported to suffer from chronically back pain and claudication symptoms since about 9 months. Her complaints were progressive despite conservative treatment with high-dose morphine-derived analgetics. CT and MR-imaging revealed a consolidated osteoporotic compression fracture of the L1 with a consecutive kyphotic deformity (Fig. 38.4). Based on the imaging findings and the clinic described above, the patient was then offered surgical therapy.

The patient underwent a two-stage surgery: percutaneous dorsal correction sponylodesis with augmented pedicle screw fixation Th10-11-12 and L2-3-4 and pedicle subtraction osteotomy at the level of L1 in the first step, followed by a vertebral body replacement of the L1 2 days later (Fig. 38.5).

No postoperative neurological deficits or medical complications were observed. The patient was transferred to a rehabilitation clinic 10 days after the second surgery. At discharge, the patient presented with residual wound pain, she was able to walk short distances without assistance.

38.4 Case Discussion

38.4.1 Indication

38.4.1.1 Odontoid Fractures

Independent of the applied treatment these injuries are associated with high morbidity and mortality. The fracture-associated mortality is

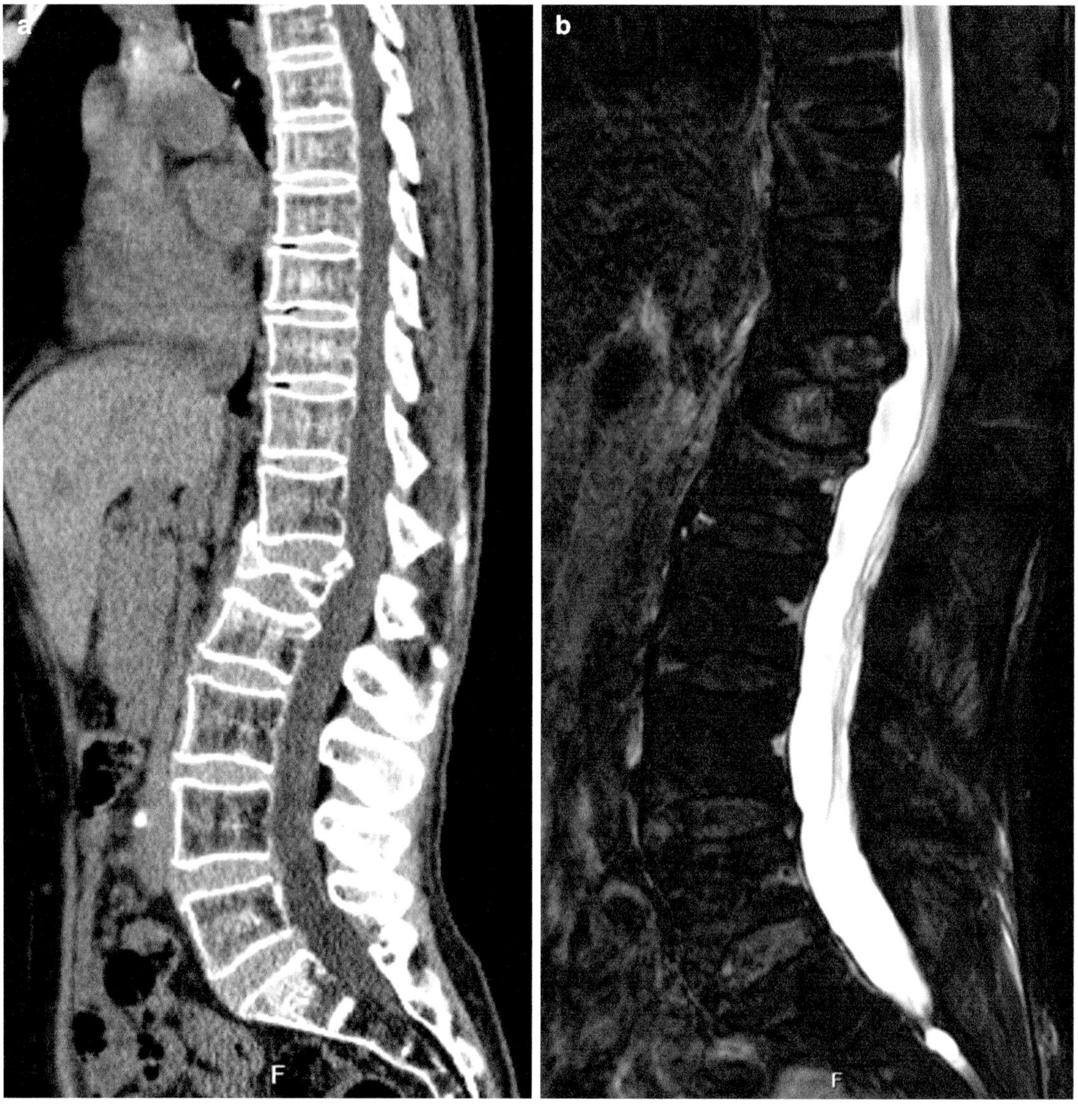

Fig. 38.4 Initial diagnostic. Sagittal CT in (**a**) and T2 STIR MR-imaging (**b**) revealed a consolidated osteoporotic compression fracture of the L1 with a consecutive kyphotic deformity

increased especially in the first 12 weeks after the injury, at 1 year the mortality rate is still at 37.5% [34].

Osteoporotic changes, a poor blood supply of the fracture gap, and degeneration-associated impaired biomechanics lead to a disrupted healing of the fracture resulting in an increased rate of pseudoarthrosis of up to 85% [8]. Especially patients with dislocated odontoid fractures seem to be predisposed to a nonunion and an increased risk of mortality [12].

The optimal management for type II fractures remains controversial. No Level A evidence-based guidelines are available so far.

Overall, four different options for the treatment of type II odontoid fractures have been described: the conservative regimes include rigid and non-rigid immobilization, and the two surgical approaches are anterior screw fixation of the odontoid and posterior fusion of the C1/2 complex.

According to larger retrospective series and metaanalyses, mortality rates with conservative

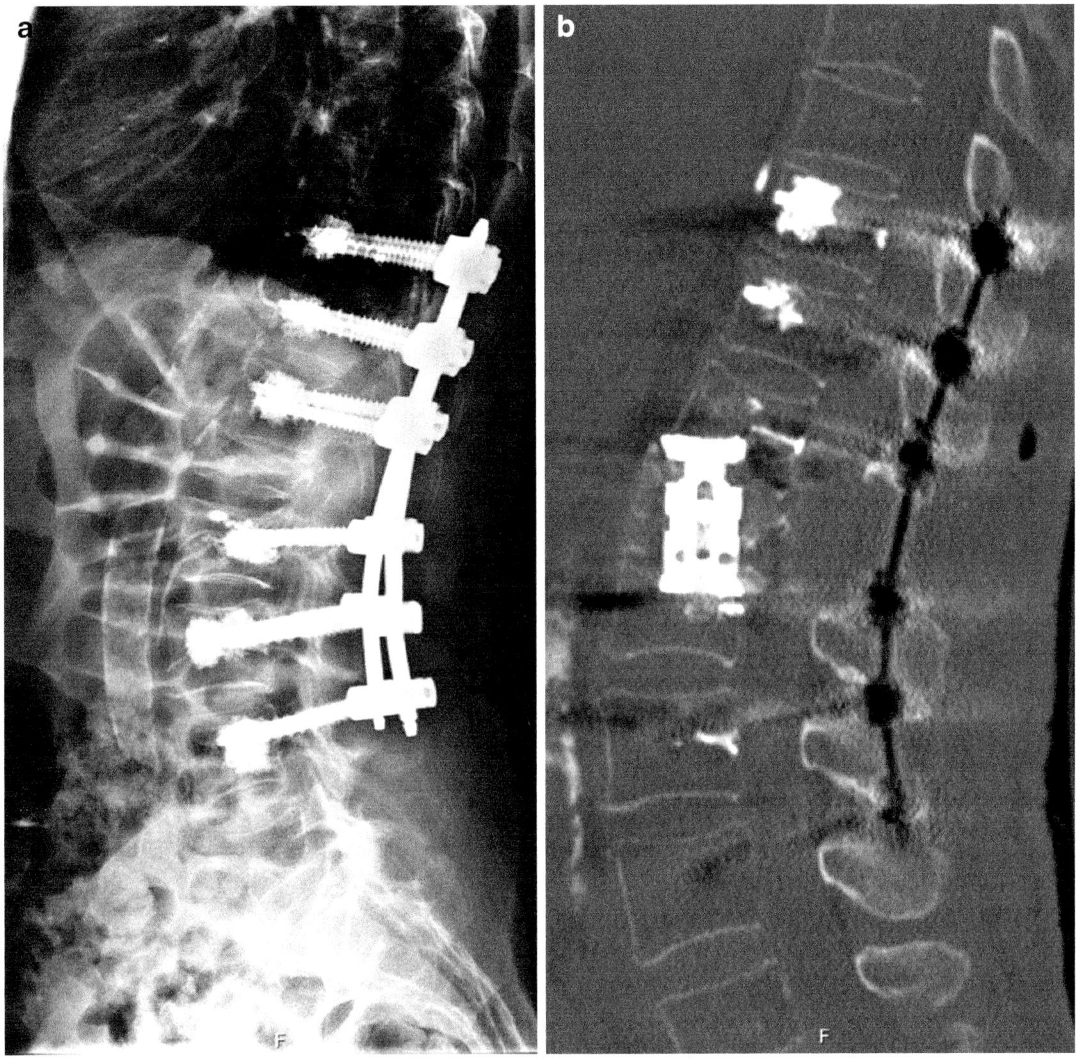

Fig. 38.5 (**a**) Postoperative Image. **a** Sagittal control X-Ray after cement augmented pedicle screw fixation Th 10-11-12 and L 2-3-4 and correction of kyphotic deformity; (**b**) Sagittal CT scan shows the final result after anterior spinal fusion performed in a second step

treatment by an immobilization in collars or halo-thoracic bracing vary between 33% and 45% [25]. Conversely the perioperative mortality rates are reported to be significantly lower ranging between 6% and 41% [8, 9, 13, 29, 35]. Chapman et al. could demonstrate in their large retrospective multicenter study a significant 30-day survival advantage (7% vs 22%) and a trend toward improved longer-term survival (38% vs 51%) for operatively treated over non-operatively treated patients [5]. The fusion rates by non-operative techniques are reported to reach 70%, however precisely in the elderly the risk of osseous non-union is highly increased with conservative immobilization, as found by a case-control study based on Class II data [19]: The odds ratio of this study indicated that the risk of failure for halo immobilization was 21 times higher in patients aged 50 years or more. Regarding the fusion rates, surgical treatment may provide significantly more beneficial results, than conservative options, leading in up to 100% to osseous union [8, 35]. Stable non-union – or fibrous union – could be an adequate aim in the treatment of odontoid fractures, if the patient is asymptomatic and the dynamic X-rays show no instability at the site of the fracture [18, 25]. The main concern in these cases is the risk of a delayed myelopathy in patients with established osseus non-union of the odontoid [7]. Indeed, it is unclear over what period of time the myelopathy would develop: in most cases it takes several years for the relevant clinic to appear. This theoretically would make this problem negligible in the elderly population. However, the majority of elder patients with non-union after conservative treatment still require delayed surgery within 90 months after trauma because of their clinically relevant symptoms [31].

This data together suggests a trend toward more favorable outcomes of surgically treated patients.

38.4.1.2 Vertebral Body Compression Fracture

Osteoporotic compression fractures, mostly A-fractures according to the AO classification, are very frequent in the elderly affecting 117 in 100,000 people. The thoracolumbar junction is the most commonly involved site. Typical signs are acute back pain, motor and vegetative deficits, claudicatio spinalis, imobilization, and substantial decrease in quality of life. Conservative treatment includes analgesia, bed rest, and a concomitant medical treatment of osteoporosis. Although most fractures heal well with nonoperative procedures, up to 30% of fractures can develop painful nonunion, progressive kyphosis, and neurological deficit. For patients who develop severe pain not responding to nonoperative measures and painful nonunion, percutaneous cement augmentation procedures including vertebroplasty or kyphoplasty have been suggested in acute stages. However, in case of healed (old) osteoporotic fractures with established kyphotic deformity and sagittal imbalance, as well as relevant symptoms such as disabling pain or neurological deficits, more extensive intervention including dorsal pedicle screw-rod fixation and decompression by one- or multilevel laminectomy may be considered [17]. If indicated, the surgery should proceed as a minimally invasive percutaneous approach to minimize the blood loss, duration of the procedure, and perioperative complications in elderly patients. In cases with additional relevant deformity and/or burst fracture, a corporectomy of the fractured vertebral body should be performed for the ventral decompression. Spinal instrumentation and fusion may be combined with an osteotomy in order to achieve a correction of the segmental kyphosis. There is no clear evidence of the advantages and disadvantages of these complex interventions in the elderly. The indication is given rather as an ultima ratio in case of progressive deformity and symptoms despite intensive conservative therapy. Only few case series and expert opinions reporting on this subject are available [2, 11, 23, 27]. Fortunately, complex instrumented procedures are only needed in about 5% of all symptomatic osteoporotic compression fractures [30].

38.4.2 Surgical Approach

38.4.2.1 Odontoid Fractures

Amongst different surgical techniques, posterior fixation of the C1/2 complex using C1 lateral mass and C2 istmus screws by Goel/Harms is the most effective option for treatment of odontoid fractures with fusion rates approaching 100% [10, 20].

A higher failure rate with the direct anterior screw fixation technique has been claimed in the elderly population, mainly due to the advanced osteoporosis leading to increased rates of screw-loosening and non-union [1]. Additional arguments against this technique are a higher risk for postoperative pneumonia and dysphagia after surgery, insufficient healing and reposition in cases with transverse atlantal ligament injuries or fracture dislocation. These facts together allow to provide strong recommendations against anterior fixation in the elderly [14].

38.4.2.2 Vertebral Body Compression Fracture

Osteosynthesis in patients with consolidated compression fractures can result in high complications rates due to the osteoporosis, comorbidities and commonly increased risks of mechanical failures of implants and rates of pseudarthrosis in the elderly. Pedicle screw loosening and adjacent-level vertebral body fracture are common sequela among patients with osteoporosis. In order to decrease these operative risks, it is necessary to keep the surgery as less invasive as possible. Performing a percutaneous osteosynthesis can be a reasonable option, which would minimize surgical time, blood loss, muscle trauma, and infection risks leading to shorter in-hospital stay and rehabilitation [27, 28]. Additionally, the use of fenestrated pedicle screws with PMMA cement augmentation allows to increase the pull-out strength of the screws to more than double of the non-augmented fixation and to prevent the above-mentioned osteoporosis – associated risks [6].

In cases with considerable thoracic kyphosis, correction of the deformity may become necessary. Different surgical techniques have been discussed for the correction of the osteoporotic spine including anterior spinal fusion, posterior fusion alone, PSO, and combined anterior and posterior surgery [26, 28, 32]. Still, there is no consensus and no evidence regarding which is the most appropriate approach. The indication should be put in place very carefully and tailored individually depending on patients comorbidities, severity of symptoms, and extent of osteoporotic changes.

Even if the surgery was performed perfectly, one should be aware of the not uncommon late complications, such as loosening of pedicle screws or subsequent vertebral compression fractures within adjacent segments.

38.4.3 Conservative Treatment

38.4.3.1 Odontoid Fractures

In patients who are not suitable for surgery, non-operative fixation should be considered as an alternative treatment option. The described conservative therapy includes non-rigid external immobilization using a hard cervical collar and/or the rigid external fixation by halo vest.

The halo vest associated morbidity, particularly in the elderly, has been increasingly highlighted by several authors with mortaity of 40% and morbidity of more than 50% [15, 25]. Based on a series of 50 patients, Tashjian et al. have found that the mortality and morbidity rates in patients with halo vest were 42% and 66% while that in the patients treated by surgery or collars were 20% and 36%, respectively [33]. Another study by Majercik et al. found that old patients with halo vest had a significantly higher mortality than old patients treated with surgery or collar (6 and 12%) and a 20 times higher mortality than young patients (40% vs 2%) [21]. This makes the use of halo today nearly obsolete.

The non-rigid external immobilisation using a hard cervical collar is an in exceptional cases acceptable form of treatment for type II odontoid fractures for old patients with inappropriately high surgical risks. The osseous fusion rates are described to reach up to 70%, the rates of stable fibrous union are approximately 90% [24]. However, not to forget is that the conservative management with cervical collars also bears addtional specific complications, such as decubital ulcers, which may occur in up to 10% of cases [18].

38.4.3.2 Vertebral Body Compression Fracture

Most pain-related symptoms from vertebral compression fractures in acute stages are resolved with conservative management comprising of analgesic medication, physical therapy and short bed rest [22]. In case of a fracture healed in a deformity without signs of instability or neurological deficits, conservative therapy can be attempted. The role of bracing in treatment of osteoporotic compression fractures is not quite clear. There is some concern regarding the placement of increased stress on the posterior elements of the spine when extension bracing is used. Furthermore, bracing bears additional risks, particularly in the elderly population, such as decubitus ulcers with subsequent soft-tissue infections, diminished pulmonary capacity and weakening of the axial musculature [4].

Level of Evidence
Odontoid Fractures: C

The level of evidence available to date is relatively low. Due to the lack of class I studies, no definitive conclusions can be drawn regarding the optimal treatment of type II odontoid fractures or consolidated thoracolumbar compression fractures in the elderly. There are no comparative studies prospectively comparing surgical options. An international cooperative registry study (INNOVATE) is underway to prospectively assess fracture healing and clinical outcome after surgical versus conservative treatment of odontoid fractures in the elderly patient, with a specific emphasis on the very old patient [16].

Instrumentation for Vertebral Body Compression Fracture: D

The evidence is extremely low. No prospective studies and only a few small retrospective series have evaluated benefits and harms of complex reconstruction surgeries for osteoporotic compression fractures. Therefore, the indication for these approaches should be very strict and reserved for selected patients with progressive deformities and disabiling symptoms.

38.5 Conclusions and Take Home Message

Regardless of the applied treatment, osteoporotic fractures in the elderly bear per se a high risk of poor outcome and death due to increased rates of preexisting comorbidities and immobilization-associated impact. The primary goal of the fracture treatment in the elderly is to achieve the fastest possible restoration to the degree of the pre-traumatic mobilization.

The most common two types of spinal fractures in the elderly are the type II odontoid fracture in the cervical spine, and the vertebral body compression fracture in the thoracolumbar spine.

The surgery of the type II odontoid fracture is advocated in the majority of cases because of the increased risk for the development of an unstable pseudarthrosis, morbidity and and mortality in case of an insufficient treatment. The dorsal fixation of the C1/C2 complex provides the most appropriate surgical approach in terms of fusion and comparably low perioperative risks for failure or complications.

Osteoporotic compression fractures in the thoracolumbar spine may be treated conservatively with pain medication and moderate immobilization if the pain level is low, neurological deficits are absent, and the patient appears to benefit from conservative measures. Spinal deformities in patients with osteoporosis are complex to treat because of their disabling and progressive nature. For fractures with severe collapse that leads to neurological deficit and increasing deformity, instrumented stabilization and decompression can be considered. Using minimally invasive approach including percutaneous fixation with cement-augmented screws may provide acceptable results.

Pearls

- The earliest possible mobilization is the main goal of the therapy
- Keep in mind the increased risk of non-fusion and high fracture associated mortality rates especially with conservative treatment regimes
- Odontoid fracures: dorsal fixation of the C1/C2 complex provides the most appropriate surgical approach in terms of fusion and perioperative risks
- Dorsal intrumentation for osteoporotic compression fractures is reserved for selected patients with progressive symptomatic deformities, disabiling symptoms and neurological deficits

Editorial Comment

Surgical treatment of the 2 most common fractures in the elderly is outlined in this chapter. There is basically no reasonable evidence for the management described in case 2, so indication should be restricted to the ones outlined below. My personal opinion for odontoid insufficiency fractures in the elderly is that a posterior C1-2 construct is the treatment of choice. If conservative treatment is considered, a soft collar is sufficient to have the fracture heal in a rigid pseudarthrosis. A Halo is obsolete and has higher risks than surgery.

References

1. Andersson S, Rodrigues M, Olerud C. Odontoid fractures: high complication rate associated with anterior screw fixation in the elderly. Eur Spine J. 2000;9:56–9.
2. Behrbalk E, Uri O, Folman Y, Rickert M, Kaiser R, Boszczyk BM. Staged correction of severe thoracic kyphosis in patients with multilevel osteoporotic vertebral compression fractures. Global Spine J. 2016;6:710–20.
3. Blauth M, Lange UF, Knop C, Bastian L. Spinal fractures in the elderly and their treatment. Orthopade. 2000;29:302–17.
4. Chang V, Holly LT. Bracing for thoracolumbar fractures. Neurosurg Focus. 2014;37:E3.
5. Chapman J, Smith JS, Kopjar B, Vaccaro AR, Arnold P, Shaffrey CI, Fehlings MG. The AOSpine North America Geriatric Odontoid Fracture Mortality Study: a retrospective review of mortality outcomes for operative versus nonoperative treatment of 322 patients with long-term follow-up. Spine (Phila Pa 1976). 2013;38:1098–104.
6. Choma TJ, Pfeiffer FM, Swope RW, Hirner JP. Pedicle screw design and cement augmentation in osteoporotic vertebrae: effects of fenestrations and cement viscosity on fixation and extraction. Spine (Phila Pa 1976). 2012;37:E1628–32.
7. Crockard HA, Heilman AE, Stevens JM. Progressive myelopathy secondary to odontoid fractures: clinical, radiological, and surgical features. J Neurosurg. 1993;78:579–86.
8. Deng H, Yue JK, Upadhyayula PS, Burke JF, Suen CG, Chan AK, Winkler EA, Dhall SS. Odontoid fractures in the octogenarian: a systematic review and meta-analysis. J Neurosurg Sci. 2016;60:543–55.
9. Dhall SS, Yue JK, Winkler EA, Mummaneni PV, Manley GT, Tarapore PE. Morbidity and mortality associated with surgery of traumatic C2 fractures in octogenarians. Neurosurgery. 2017;80:854–62.
10. Dickman CA, Sonntag VK. Posterior C1-C2 transarticular screw fixation for atlantoaxial arthrodesis. Neurosurgery. 1998;43:275–80; discussion 280–271.
11. Elder BD, Lo SF, Holmes C, Goodwin CR, Kosztowski TA, Lina IA, Locke JE, Witham TF. The biomechanics of pedicle screw augmentation with cement. Spine J. 2015;15:1432–45.
12. Evaniew N, Yarascavitch B, Madden K, Ghert M, Drew B, Bhandari M, Kwok D. Atlantoaxial instability in acute odontoid fractures is associated with nonunion and mortality. Spine J. 2015;15:910–7.
13. Graffeo CS, Perry A, Puffer RC, Carlstrom LP, Chang W, Mallory GW, Clarke MJ. Deadly falls: operative versus nonoperative management of Type II odontoid process fracture in octogenarians. J Neurosurg Spine. 2017;26:4–9.
14. Harrop JS, Hart R, Anderson PA. Optimal treatment for odontoid fractures in the elderly. Spine (Phila Pa 1976). 2010;35:S219–27.
15. Horn EM, Theodore N, Feiz-Erfan I, Lekovic GP, Dickman CA, Sonntag VK. Complications of halo fixation in the elderly. J Neurosurg Spine. 2006;5:46–9.
16. Huybregts JG, Jacobs WC, Peul WC, Vleggeert-Lankamp CL. Rationale and design of the INNOVATE trial: an international cooperative study on surgical versus conservative treatment for odontoid fractures in the elderly. BMC Musculoskelet Disord. 2014;15:7.
17. Kashii M, Yamazaki R, Yamashita T, Okuda S, Fujimori T, Nagamoto Y, Tamura Y, Oda T, Ohwada T, Yoshikawa H, Iwasaki M. Surgical treatment for osteoporotic vertebral collapse with neurological deficits: retrospective comparative study of three procedures--anterior surgery versus posterior spinal shorting osteotomy versus posterior spinal fusion using vertebroplasty. Eur Spine J. 2013;22:1633–42.
18. Koech F, Ackland HM, Varma DK, Williamson OD, Malham GM. Nonoperative management of type II odontoid fractures in the elderly. Spine (Phila Pa 1976). 2008;33:2881–6.
19. Lennarson PJ, Mostafavi H, Traynelis VC, Walters BC. Management of type II dens fractures: a case-control study. Spine (Phila Pa 1976). 2000;25:1234–7.
20. Maiman DJ, Larson SJ. Management of odontoid fractures. Neurosurgery. 1982;11:471–6.
21. Majercik S, Tashjian RZ, Biffl WL, Harrington DT, Cioffi WG. Halo vest immobilization in the elderly: a death sentence? J Trauma. 2005;59:350–6; discussion 356–358.
22. McConnell CT Jr, Wippold FJ 2nd, Ray CE Jr, Weissman BN, Angevine PD, Fries IB, Holly LT, Kapoor BS, Lorenz JM, Luchs JS, O'Toole JE, Patel ND, Roth CJ, Rubin DA. ACR appropriateness criteria management of vertebral compression fractures. J Am Coll Radiol. 2014;11:757–63.
23. Mesfin A, Komanski CB, Khanna AJ. Failure of cement-augmented pedicle screws in the osteoporotic spine: a case report. Geriatr Orthop Surg Rehabil. 2013;4:84–8.
24. Muller EJ, Schwinnen I, Fischer K, Wick M, Muhr G. Non-rigid immobilisation of odontoid fractures. Eur Spine J. 2003;12:522–5.
25. Muller EJ, Wick M, Russe O, Muhr G. Management of odontoid fractures in the elderly. Eur Spine J. 1999;8:360–5.
26. Okuda S, Oda T, Yamasaki R, Haku T, Maeno T, Iwasaki M. Surgical outcomes of osteoporotic vertebral collapse: a retrospective study of anterior spinal fusion and pedicle subtraction osteotomy. Global Spine J. 2012;2:221–6.
27. Pesenti S, Blondel B, Peltier E, Adetchessi T, Dufour H, Fuentes S. Percutaneous cement-augmented screws fixation in the fractures of the aging spine: is it the solution? Biomed Res Int. 2014;2014:610675.
28. Ponnusamy KE, Iyer S, Gupta G, Khanna AJ. Instrumentation of the osteoporotic spine: biomechanical and clinical considerations. Spine J. 2011;11:54–63.
29. Ryang YM, Torok E, Janssen I, Reinke A, Buchmann N, Gempt J, Ringel F, Meyer B. Early morbidity and mortality in 50 very elderly patients after posterior atlantoaxial fusion for traumatic odontoid fractures. World Neurosurg. 2016;87:381–91.

30. Shen M, Kim Y. Osteoporotic vertebral compression fractures: a review of current surgical management techniques. Am J Orthop. 2007;36:241–8.
31. Smith JS, Kepler CK, Kopjar B, Harrop JS, Arnold P, Chapman JR, Fehlings MG, Vaccaro AR, Shaffrey CI. Effect of type II odontoid fracture nonunion on outcome among elderly patients treated without surgery: based on the AOSpine North America geriatric odontoid fracture study. Spine (Phila Pa 1976). 2013;38:2240–6.
32. Suk SI, Kim JH, Lee SM, Chung ER, Lee JH. Anterior-posterior surgery versus posterior closing wedge osteotomy in posttraumatic kyphosis with neurologic compromised osteoporotic fracture. Spine (Phila Pa 1976). 2003;28:2170–5.
33. Tashjian RZ, Majercik S, Biffl WL, Palumbo MA, Cioffi WG. Halo-vest immobilization increases early morbidity and mortality in elderly odontoid fractures. J Trauma. 2006;60:199–203.
34. Venkatesan M, Northover JR, Wild JB, Johnson N, Lee K, Uzoigwe CE, Braybrooke JR. Survival analysis of elderly patients with a fracture of the odontoid peg. Bone Joint J. 2014;96-B:88–93.
35. Yang Z, Yuan ZZ, Ma JX, Ma XL. Conservative versus surgical treatment for type II odontoid fractures in the elderly: grading the evidence through a meta-analysis. Orthop Traumatol Surg Res. 2015;101:839–44.

39 Spinal Trauma in Patients with Ankylosing Spinal Conditions

Dominique A. Rothenfluh and David Kieser

39.1 Introduction

Ankylosing spinal conditions are a constellation of mixed conditions causing fusion of the spine. The most well recognized condition is ankylosing spondylitis (AS), which is a systemic chronic autoimmune spondyloarthropathy typically affecting younger males in the third decade of life and causing progressive spinal fusion in a caudal to cranial direction commencing at the sacro-iliac joints. It is believed to affect 0.2% of the Caucasian population (lower in other populations) and 90% of patients are HLA-B27 positive. Most have the classic radiographic appearance of squaring of the vertebra with "shiny corners" at the attachments of the annulus fibrosis (Romanus lesions), marginal syndesmophytes, osteopenia and ultimately a bamboo spine. Other spondyloarthropathies causing ankylosis of the spine include psoriatic arthritis, enteropathic arthritis and chronic reactive arthritis. However, multi-level spinal ankylosis is rare in these conditions and in those with an ankylosed spine their presentation, workup and treatment is similar to AS.

When injured, the spine can fracture anywhere but most often fractures in the mid-cervical and cervicothoracic junction (80%) and less at the thoracolumbar junction. Most commonly, these fractures are extension type unstable fractures involving all three columns typically through the intervertebral disc. The stiff fractured spine acts as long bone fractures and therefore secondary dislocation and deterioration of neurologic status is common. A peculiarity of these fractures is the high epidural haemorrhage rate [6], which increases the risk of neurological injury and mortality. However, due to the progressive compressive effect of the haemorrhage, neurological symptoms often present late and therefore clinicians should be aware of this progressive phenomenon.

In ankylosed spine, particularly in AS, stress shielding in the fused spine and increased bony resorption leads to osteoporosis contributing to a higher fracture risk. Many fractures therefore occur as a result of a low energy trauma mechanism and about 50% are missed on standard plain x-ray films [3]. It is important to note that up to a third of ankylosing patients with a spinal injury will have an unrecognized non-contiguous injury level and nearly 80% of these will result in a neurological injury if not treated early, therefore a whole spine CT or MRI scan is necessary [2].

D. A. Rothenfluh (✉)
Oxford University Hospitals NHS Foundation Trust, Nuffield Orthopaedic Centre, Oxford, UK

D. Kieser
University of Otago, Department of Orthopaedic Surgery and Musculoskeletal Medicine, Christchurch School of Medicine, Christchurch, New Zealand

B. Meyer, M. Rauschmann (eds.), *Spine Surgery*, https://doi.org/10.1007/978-3-319-98875-7_39

The present case should illustrate that innocuous injuries can result in unstable spinal fractures and that they are hard to identify clinically and on standard radiographs.

39.2 Case Description

A 69 year old female with a known history of AS presented to the emergency department after a fall from standing height at home landing onto her left shoulder sustaining a proximal humerus fracture. She had mild bruising around her eyes and along the bridge of her nose in the distribution of her glasses' frame. She did not complain of any neurological concerns but did complain of mild neck pain. She was discharged in a shoulder immobilizer for the management for her proximal humerus fracture but returned 4 days later due to continued neck pain. Her cervical spine x-ray showed prevertebral soft tissue swelling at the C5/6 level, but no fracture line could be identified (Fig. 39.1).

Cross-sectional CT scan imaging revealed the chalk-stick fracture affecting all three columns (Fig. 39.2).

She therefore underwent C4–7 anterior stabilization with a compression plate. She made an unremarkable recovery with serial radiographs illustrating fracture union (Fig. 39.3). She has subsequently been discharged.

39.3 Discussion of the Case

39.3.1 Diagnosis

This case illustrates the challenges in diagnosing unstable three-column spinal injuries in patients with ankylosing spinal conditions. The patient sustained a fairly innocuous fall, all be it sufficient enough to cause an undisplaced proximal humerus fracture. However, this minor trauma was sufficient to cause a potentially unstable chalk-stick fracture in her ankylosed spine. The distracting injury sustained to her proximal

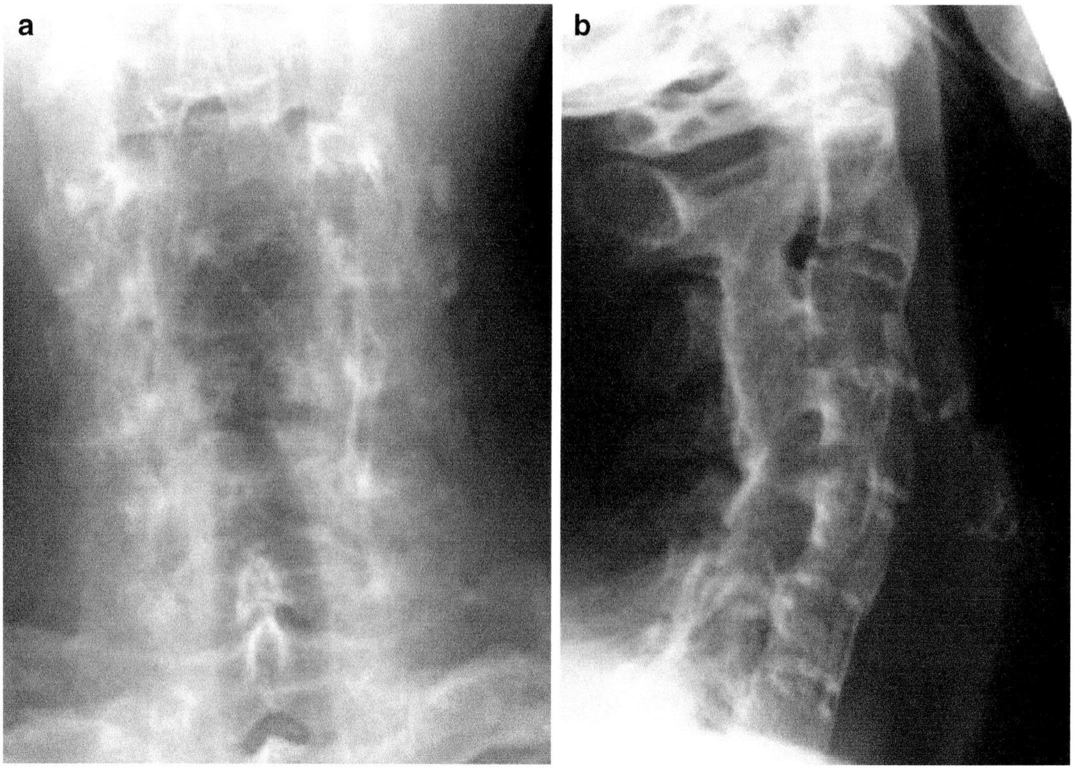

Fig. 39.1 AP and lateral erect cervical x-rays demonstrate prevertebral soft tissue swelling but fail to identify the fracture

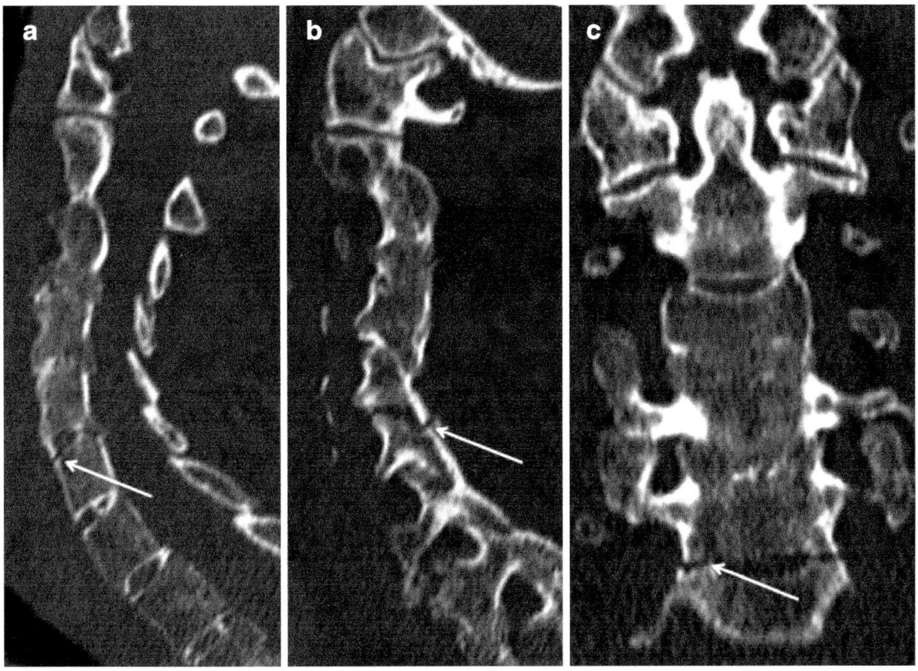

Fig. 39.2 Midline (**a**) and para-central (**b**) sagittal, as well as a coronal (**c**) CT scan. The arrows point to the 3-column chalk-stick fracture

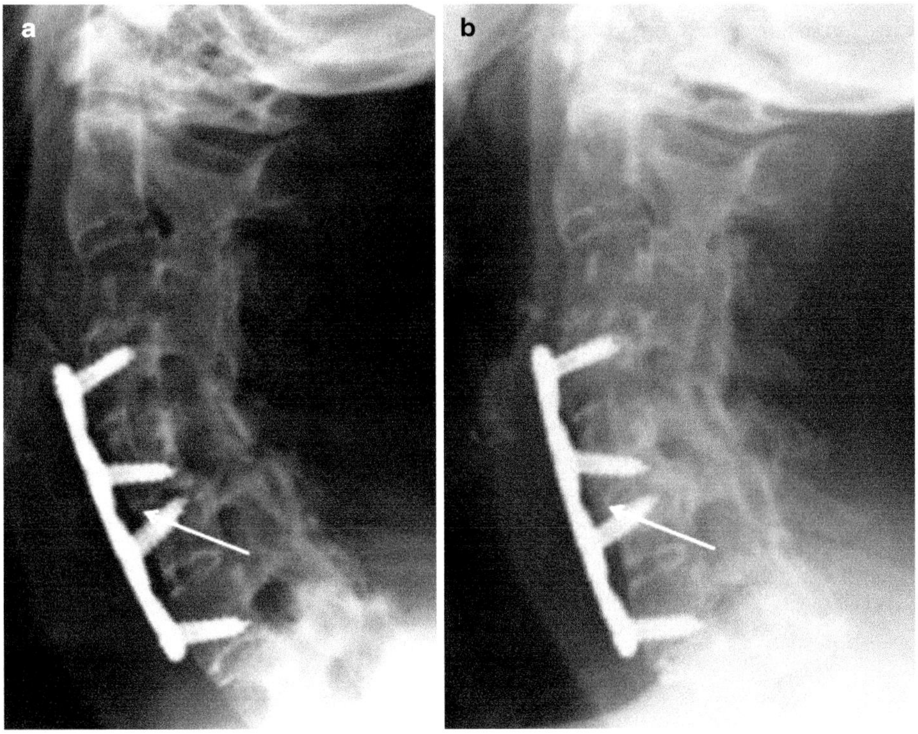

Fig. 39.3 Immediate post-operative (**a**) and 6-month post-operative (**b**) lateral erect x-rays. The arrow illustrates the fracture line

humerus limited her initial recognition of neck pain. However, in retrospect the clinicians should have recognized the injury pattern to her periorbital region suggesting forehead impact and an extension injury to her neck. A recognition of the importance of increased vigilance in patients with AS may have ensured the patient obtained appropriate spinal imaging at first. In addition, the radiographs attained on her re-presentation are challenging to interpret. It was only with heightened awareness of the subtleties of fractures in AS that the pre-vertebral soft tissue swelling was identified and cross-sectional imaging attained.

The present case illustrates a rather common scenario in fractures in the ankylosed spine, whereby either a low energy trauma does not prompt imaging or it is missed on conventional radiographs. An up to 50% rate of failing to identify fractures in these patients using standard radiographs has been reported and therefore cross-sectional imaging should take precedence and is mandatory to exclude or confirm a diagnosis [3]. It is of note, however, that CT and MRI are complementary and neither can detect 100% of fractures. Particularly in injuries of the posterior column, MRI is useful as they may be missed with a CT [5].

39.3.2 Choice of Approach and Fixation

The principles of surgical stabilization of ankylosing spinal conditions are similar to those of long bone fractures. Because of the long lever arms and high local force at the fracture site, fixation with long constructs and multiple fixation points are required. This is particularly important in those with associated osteopenia which is a frequent finding in ankylosed spines, particularly AS. The intervertebral discs (IVD) of the ankylosed segments do not need to be spared as their function has been eliminated by the fusion. However, the surgeon needs to be mindful of the challenges of fixation due to osteoporosis and deformity.

Given the potentially unstable injury of fractures in ankylosed spines with a risk of neurologic injury upon secondary dislocation, operative intervention was chosen to ensure optimal stability and healing of the fracture. She did not have an epidural haematoma which influenced the decision on an anterior versus posterior approach. Instead, an anterior approach was selected because her extension-type injury was felt to have resulted in anterior tension failure and an anterior approach would allow to ensure accurate reduction and compression of the fracture.

While there remains a paucity of literature on the specific management of spinal trauma in ankylosing spinal conditions especially with regard to the surgical approach, posterior approaches seem to be the more commonly chosen surgical technique for stabilization of subaxial fractures of the cervical spine [4]. The advantages of a posterior approach seem to be the possibility of easily extending the fixation to decrease the lever arm on the fractured segment and access to perform a multilevel decompression in the presence of a neurologic deficit or epidural hematoma. It may also be easier to access the spine from posterior in the presence of a significant kyphotic deformity of the cervical spine. However, the posterior approach may be more invasive than an anterior approach. The failure rate of anterior fixation has been reported to be up to 50% in one study [1]. If inadequate fixation is found in the anterior approach particularly due to reduced bone density, an additional posterior fixation is required. While anterior-posterior approaches are the most invasive, they are indicated especially in cases of coincident deformity correction during fracture fixation. In the present case, anterior fixation was adequate and resulted in healing of the fracture.

39.4 Conclusions and Take Home Message

Fractures of the subaxial cervical spine in ankylosing spine conditions are frequently missed due to the low energy trauma mechanism, distracting injuries and the fact that 50% of fractures are not visible on standard radiographs. A high level of suspicion is thus required and cross-sectional imaging such as CT or MRI of the whole spine mandatory. Close attention to the patients' neurological status needs to be maintained due to the high rate of epidural hemorrhage. These fractures are typically unstable and delayed diagnosis and conservative treatment may result into loss of alignment, secondary dislocation and a neurological deficit. While the majority of fractures are treated surgically using a posterior approach, an anterior approach can result into healing of the fracture if adequate fixation is achieved. Due to reduced bone density and the long bone nature of the fracture, long fixations should be chosen.

Pearls

- 50% of fractures of the subaxial cervical spine in ankylosing spine conditions are missed on standard radiographs
- Cross-sectional imaging is mandatory with a high-level of suspicion even after low energy traumas such as simple falls
- Attention needs to be maintained to the neurological status due to the high rate of epidural hematomas
- The majority of fractures are treated surgically using a posterior approach, an anterior approach can result into healing of the fracture if adequate fixation is achieved

Editorial Comment

In addition to all the caveats regarding injuries in this patient group, I would like to add that per SOP in my unit a patient with an AS condition even after minor trauma is assumed to have a spinal fracture until proven otherwise. To rule out a fracture a CT and MRI of the complete spine is mandatory. Every fracture in these patients is to be regarded as highly unstable, because it is essentially a long-bone fracture and surgery is basically the treatment of choice in all cases.

References

1. Einsiedel T, Schmelz A, Arand M, Wilke HJ, Gebhard F, Hartwig E, Kramer M, Neugebauer R, Kinzl L, Schultheiss M. Injuries of the cervical spine in patients with ankylosing spondylitis: experience at two trauma centers. J Neurosurg Spine. 2006;5(1):33–45.
2. Finkelstein JA, Chapman JR, Mirza S. Occult vertebral fractures in ankylosing spondylitis. Spinal Cord. 1999;37(6):444–7.
3. Koivikko MP, Koskinen SK. MRI of cervical spine injuries complicating ankylosing spondylitis. Skelet Radiol. 2008;37(9):813–9.
4. Westerveld LA, Verlaan JJ, Oner FC. Spinal fractures in patients with ankylosing spinal disorders: a systematic review of the literature on treatment, neurological status and complications. Eur Spine J. 2009;18(2):145–56.
5. Whang PG, Goldberg G, Lawrence JP, Hong J, Harrop JS, Anderson DG, Albert TJ, Vaccaro AR. The management of spinal injuries in patients with ankylosing spondylitis or diffuse idiopathic skeletal hyperostosis: a comparison of treatment methods and clinical outcomes. J Spinal Disord Tech. 2009;22(2):77–85.
6. Wu CT, Lee ST. Spinal epidural hematoma and ankylosing spondylitis: case report and review of the literature. J Trauma. 1998;44(3):558–61.

Part V

Basic Module 5: Tumors of Spine and Inflammatory Diseases

40 Vertebral Osteomyelitis: Etiology, Pathogenesis, Routes of Spread Symptoms and Diagnosis

Christoph Fleege and Michael Rauschmann

40.1 Introduction

With 2–7% of all osteomyelitis, spondylodiscitis is rare, but is the third most common form of osteomyelitis after the femur and tibia [1]. The disease occurs more frequently in the sixth decade of life. Basically, a distinction is made between unspecific, also pyogenic and specific infections. While unspecific spondylodiscitis is a problem of developed industrialized countries, tuberculous spondylodiscitis, the most important specific form, is more prevalent in developing and emerging countries. However, due to increasing globalization, these statements are no longer completely true. Both nonspecific and specific spondylodiscitis have seen an increase in the number of diagnoses over the last few decades. The causes of these changes are not only the demographic development but also the medical advances in diagnostics. While incidence in the past has been reported as 1:250.000, studies and registry data currently show an increase of up to 5:100.000 with an increase in old age [2–4]. Despite improved diagnostics, the average time between the onset of first symptoms and diagnosis is between 2 and 6 months [5]. The delay of initial treatment by more than 60 days leads to a poorer clinical course [6].

The pediatric spondylodiscitis is also a rare entity with an incidence of 1:250.000, often as an unspecific kind caused by Kingella kingae and Staphylococcus aureus and a high rate of specific infections mainly in Africa and South Asia [7].

Since the main problem consists of securing the diagnosis and the specific detection of the germs in clinical routine, this chapter will mainly describe the etiology, pathologenesis and diagnosis.

The case presented shows a typical course of disease and a standardized diagnostic algorithm.

40.2 Case Description

A 56-year-old patient, with lumbar back pain, radiating into the right hip was presented. Five month back, he was suffering from a pharyngeal mucous membrane inflammation (aphthae) which was treated with local cortisone application.

Furthermore the following secondary diagnoses were observed: obesity BMI 40.2, NIDDM, nicotine abuse, chronic obstructive pulmonary disease and osteoarthritis of the right hip. At the time of admission he had the following blood investigations: Leucocytes 13/nl, CRP 13.7 mg/dl (norm <0.5) (Figs. 40.1 and 40.2).

C. Fleege (✉)
Spine Department, Orthopaedic University Hospital Friedrichsheim, Frankfurt, Germany
e-mail: c.fleege@friedrichsheim.de

M. Rauschmann
Department of Spine Surgery, Sana Klinikum Offenbach, Offenbach, Germany

B. Meyer, M. Rauschmann (eds.), *Spine Surgery*, https://doi.org/10.1007/978-3-319-98875-7_40

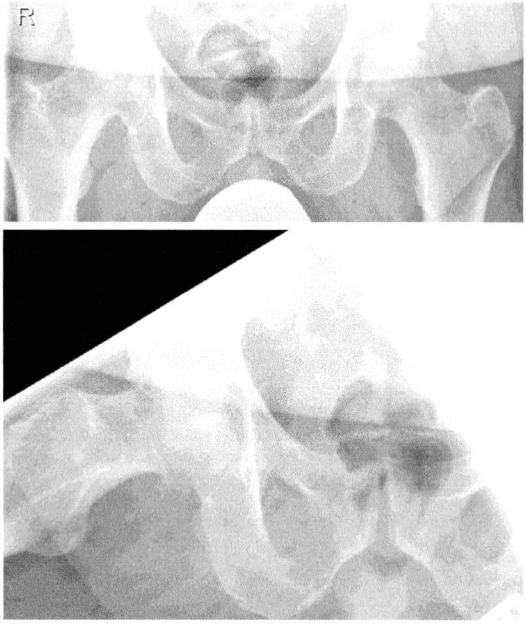

Fig. 40.1 x-ray pelvic ap and Lauenstein view right at the first time of admission

The MRI scans (T1 and T2-weightening) didn't show any signs of inflammation at the whole spine, but a central spinal stenosis. Due to a severe Osteoarthritis of the right hip and the clinical limitations of movement of the hip joint, the indication for a total hip replacement was performed. Due to the increased infectious parameters, normalization should be awaited.

4 month later, the patient was seen by the department of infectious diseases with joint and back pain, weight loss and reduced general condition. Until this time, no antibiotic therapy was performed.

Radiological diagnostics algorithm was performed (Figs. 40.3, 40.4, 40.5 and 40.6):

In conclusion the x-ray, mri and ct-scan showed clear signs of a unspecific spondylodiscitis L2/3 with a small inflammatory reaction for the psoas muscle on the right side. Blood investigations: Leucocytes 12.5/nl, CRP 14.1 mg/dl (norm <0.5). Subfebrile temperatures to moderate fever of 38.4 °C.

Further investigations were implemented. Therefore, blood cultures were taken on three different times. After three sterile results, an x-ray guided fine-needle biopsy was performed (Fig. 40.7).

The result of the sampling from the disc compartments were also sterile. The histological result showed floride and older inflammatory reactions with no evidence of specific infection.

Initiation of an empirical antibiotic therapy with Fosfomycin 2g 1-0-1 and Imipenem 0.5g 1-1-1 intravenous, after 10 days oralization to Levofloxacin 500 mg 1-0-1 and Clindamycin 300 mg 1-1-1-1 for the following 6 weeks (Figs. 40.8 and 40.9).

Six month after diagnosis a normalization of the laboratory parameters of infection and a significant reduction of lumbar back pain (VAS 2), without any medication was investigated. Only an inguinal pain on the right side was seen. Therefore the patient could return to work 9 month after starting of symptoms. Due to the low pain, currently a hip replacement isn't planned.

The illustrated case shows a structured algorithm of the diagnosis with a nonspecific anamnesis and nonspecific symptoms, the performance of a radiological diagnosis and measures to lead a germ detection by blood culture and biopsy.

40.3 Case Discussion

40.3.1 Etiology

Spondylodiscitis is caused by bacteria as the cause of specific, pyogenic infection and by mycobacteria, brucelles, and fungi as the cause of specific infections, and in very rare cases by parasites.

References show a certain constancy in the description of the pathogens, however, variations in selected patient groups with specific risk factors can be observed. The most common pathogen of pyogenic spondylodiscitis is Staphylococcus aureus with 20–80% of cases, followed by Gram-negative bacteria (leader E. coli) with 4–30% and streptococci/enterococci with 5–30% (leader Streptococcus epidermidis) [8–10].

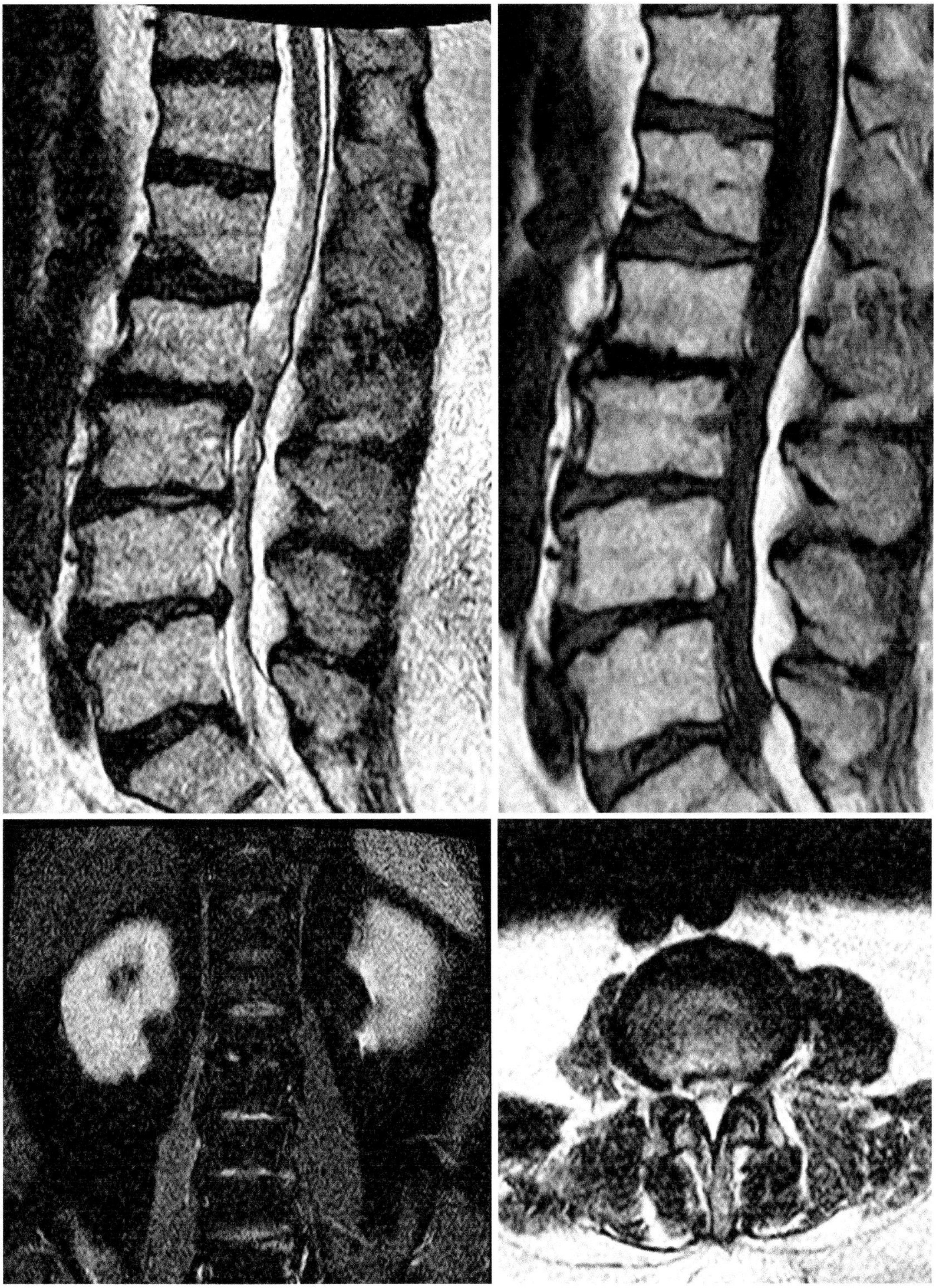

Fig. 40.2 Magnetic resonance imaging lumbar spine at the same time

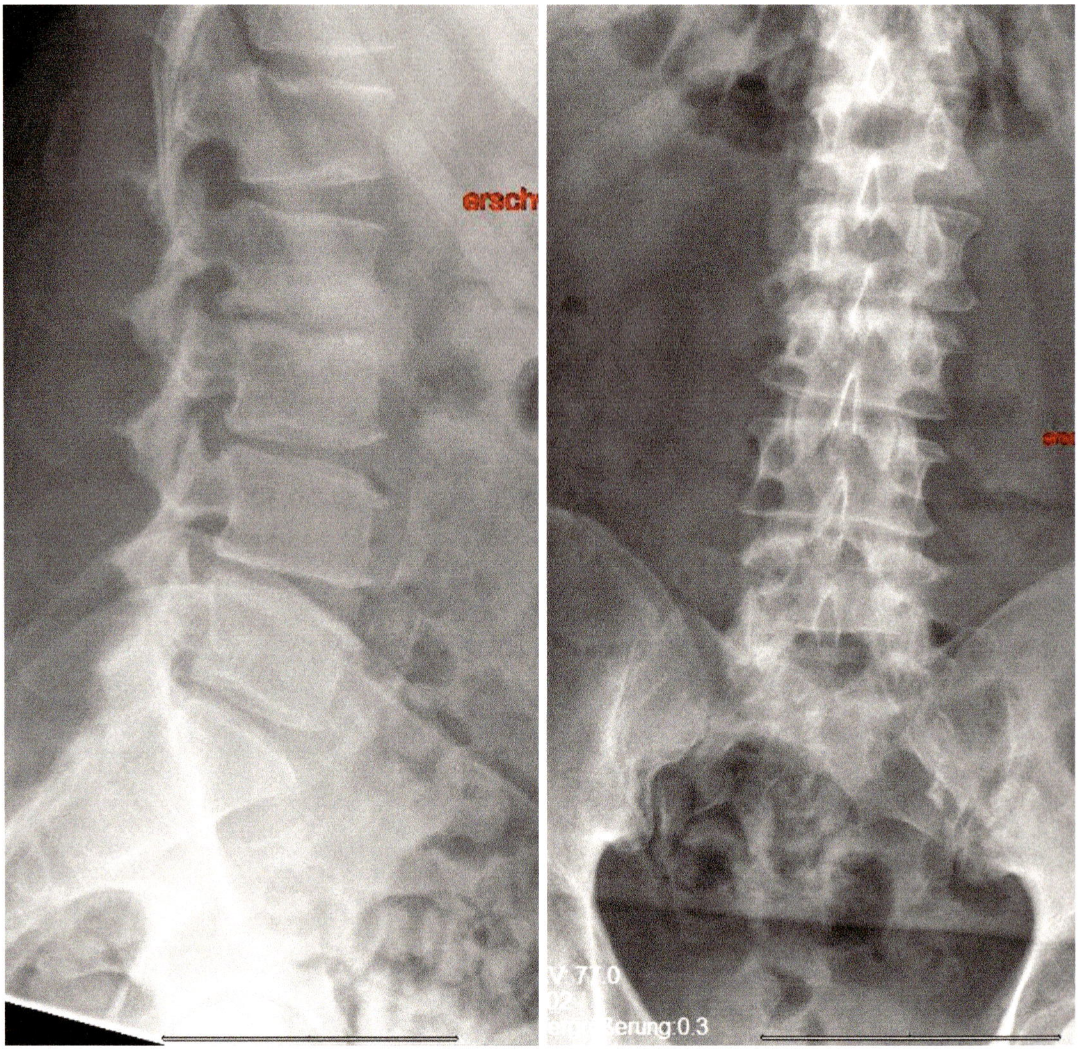

Fig. 40.3 x-ray ap and lateral view

Gram-negative pathogens such as E.coli, Proteus spp. and Pseudomonas spp. are identified as the cause of infection in immunodeficient patients [10]. Streptococci and enterococci are often associated with endocarditis and diabetes mellitus. Spondylodiscitis caused by bacteria with a primarily low virulence, such as Staphylococcus epidermidis and Streptococci, is clinically characterized by a slow progression. In clinical practice, a general increase of infections with germs that are more difficult to treat due to resistances, such as methicilin-resistant coagulase-negative staphylococci, streptococci, enterococci and gram-negative pathogens, is observed [11].

The specific spondylodiscitis is caused by the mycobacterium tuberculosis, with a noticeable increase in the rather rare infections by atypical mycobacteria (MOTT) [4]. Risk factors include poverty with malnutrition, inadequate hygiene and inadequate medical care [12].

40.3.2 Pathogenesis and Routes of Spread Symptoms

The endogenous spread of infection occurs mostly by a hematogenous scattering and only in rare cases by a continuitatem or lymphogenous way. The primary infection sites, which are often

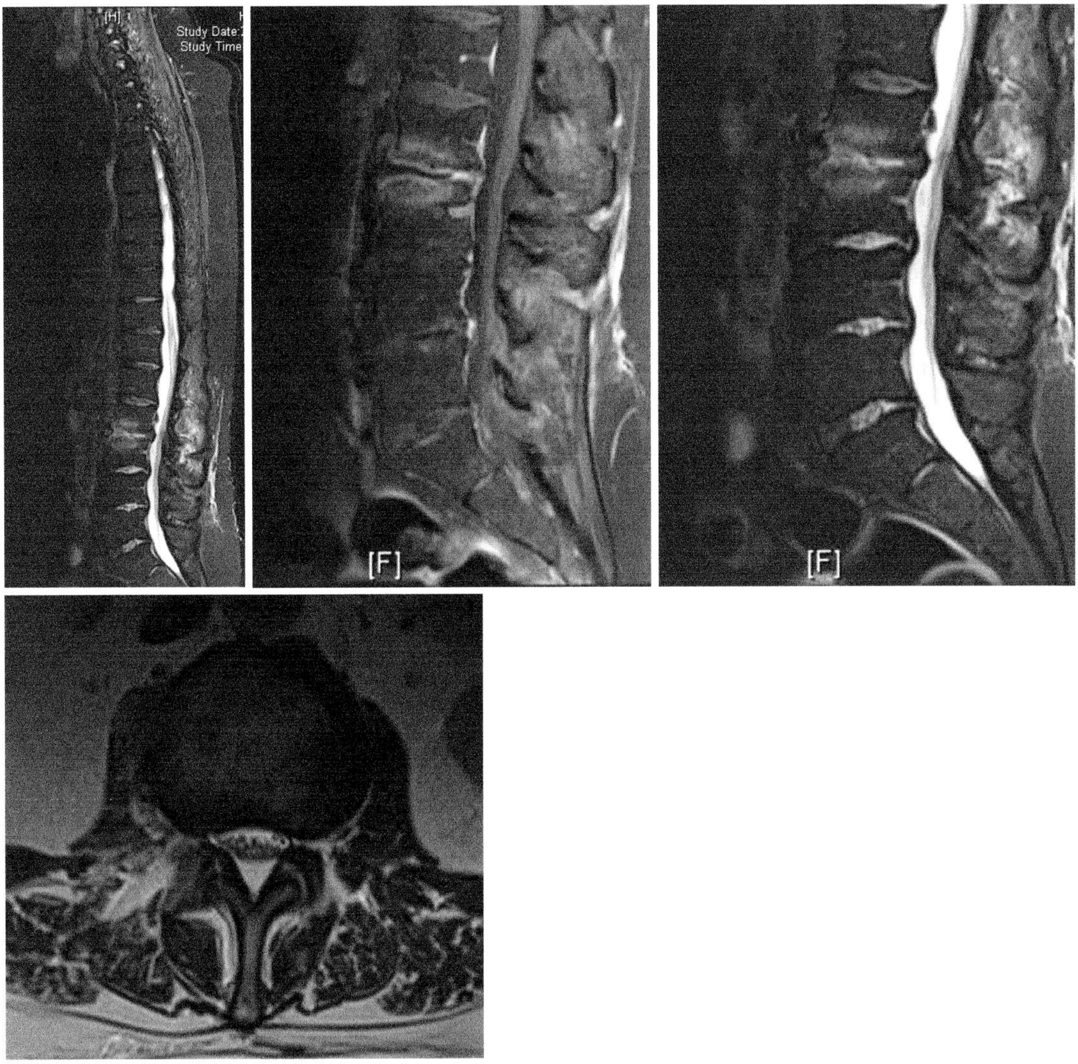

Fig. 40.4 Magnetic resonance imaging (T1, T2 and STIR) with contrast medium lumbar spine

no longer detectable at the time of diagnosis, are in the area of the pelvis, teeth or skin lacerations in the lower extremities. Anatomical particularities of the blood supply in the vertebral column may aid the hematogenous spread of infection. On the one hand, germination is aided by an arterial inoculation, which results from a rich arterial blood supply to the region of the anterior longitudinal ligament and/or infarction of the end arteries or silencing sinusoids by the bacterial embolus. On the other hand, venous scattering, caused by a valveless venous plexus connected to the organ veins of urogenital and gastrointestinal tract, increased blood flow and a long venous staging time, as well as reverse flow of intraabdominal pressure, promote colonization of the lumbar and thoracolumbar spine.

In adulthood, after hematogenous seeding, the infection begins as spondylitis and secondary, may spread to the intervertebral disc area. Studies show that many pathogens of nonspecific spondylodiscitis express collagen receptors and thus promote bone adhesion [13]. Subsequent to pathogen involvement of the terminal arterioles and development of local bone edema, local inflammatory reactions, microembolisms, and ischaemia associated with bone infarcts and necrosis can develop.

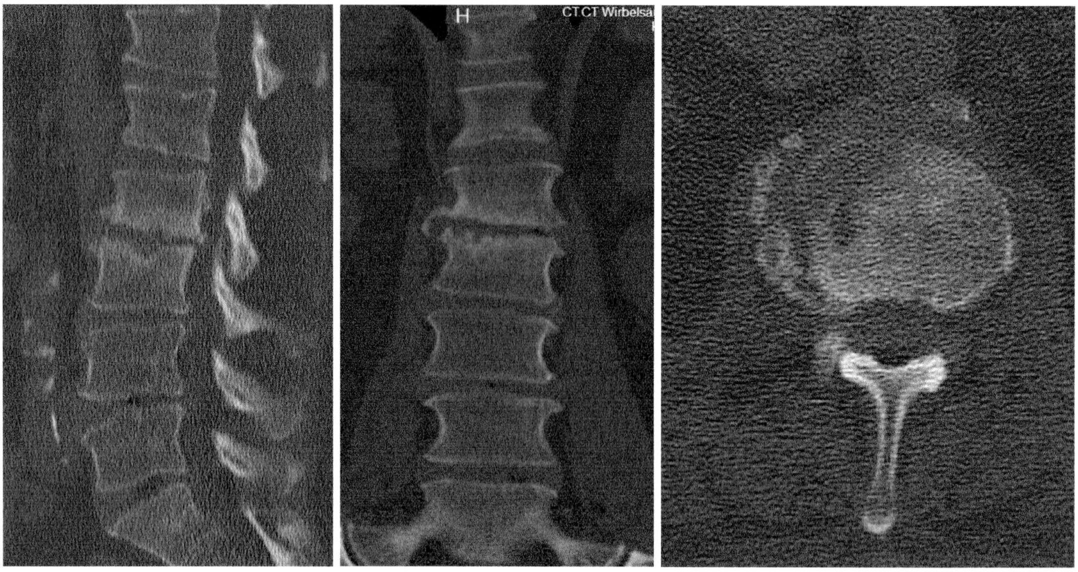

Fig. 40.5 Computer tomography of the lumbar spine

The spread of mycobacteria occurs essentially hematogenous through the arteries, with the typical picture of anterior vertebral body involvement. Spreading through the veins is also possible, via Batson's plexus with central and dorsal vertebral body involvement [12]. Finally, the granulomas characteristic for the specific spondylodiscitis may develop. Furthermore, tuberculous spondylitis typically occurs with so called "cold abscesses" which are typically huge in sice and descend along the psoas muscle to the inguinal region.

In childhood, the remaining vascularization of the intervertebral discs results in a typical kind of discitis, with the possibility to progress to the full picture of spondylodiscitis.

40.3.3 Diagnosis

The disease start's with local back pain accompanied by non-specific general symtoms, such as fever, night sweat and weight loss. Positive upsetting pain, "knocking pain" and heeldrop pain are possible. Restrictive posture, the prevention of loads of the anterior column and instability signs are further typical indicators. Just as unspecific as the clinical symptoms are the laboratory values (Leucocytes, CRP and blood sedimentation). Studies show a low sensitivity and specifity (Leucocytes 42–55%/97%, CRP 84%/71%, blood sedimentation 75–90%, 43%) [14]. In presence of an epidural abscess high leucocytes values are often noticed [10].

A crucial role in the successful treatment of spondylodiscitis is the early diagnosis and detection of the causative germ.

The early diagnosis of vertebral osteomyelitis and concomitant discitis is difficult, which may lead to a delayed diagnosis. Standard tools consist of primary imaging in patients with unclear back pain in conventional x-ray radiography in two planes with a sensitivity of 82% and specificity of 57% [15]. Because of the onset of infection in the metaphysis of the vertebral bodies, these first changes are not noticed in conventional radiological diagnostics. Signs of destruction of the corresponding endplates, especially in the ventral area, can be signs of the beginning disease. However, differentiation from erosive osteochondrosis is difficult. The destruction of spongeous bone occuring later in the course, the upper and lower endplate erosions and height reductions of the disc space are further signs that may indicate a spondylodiscitis. As the disease pro-

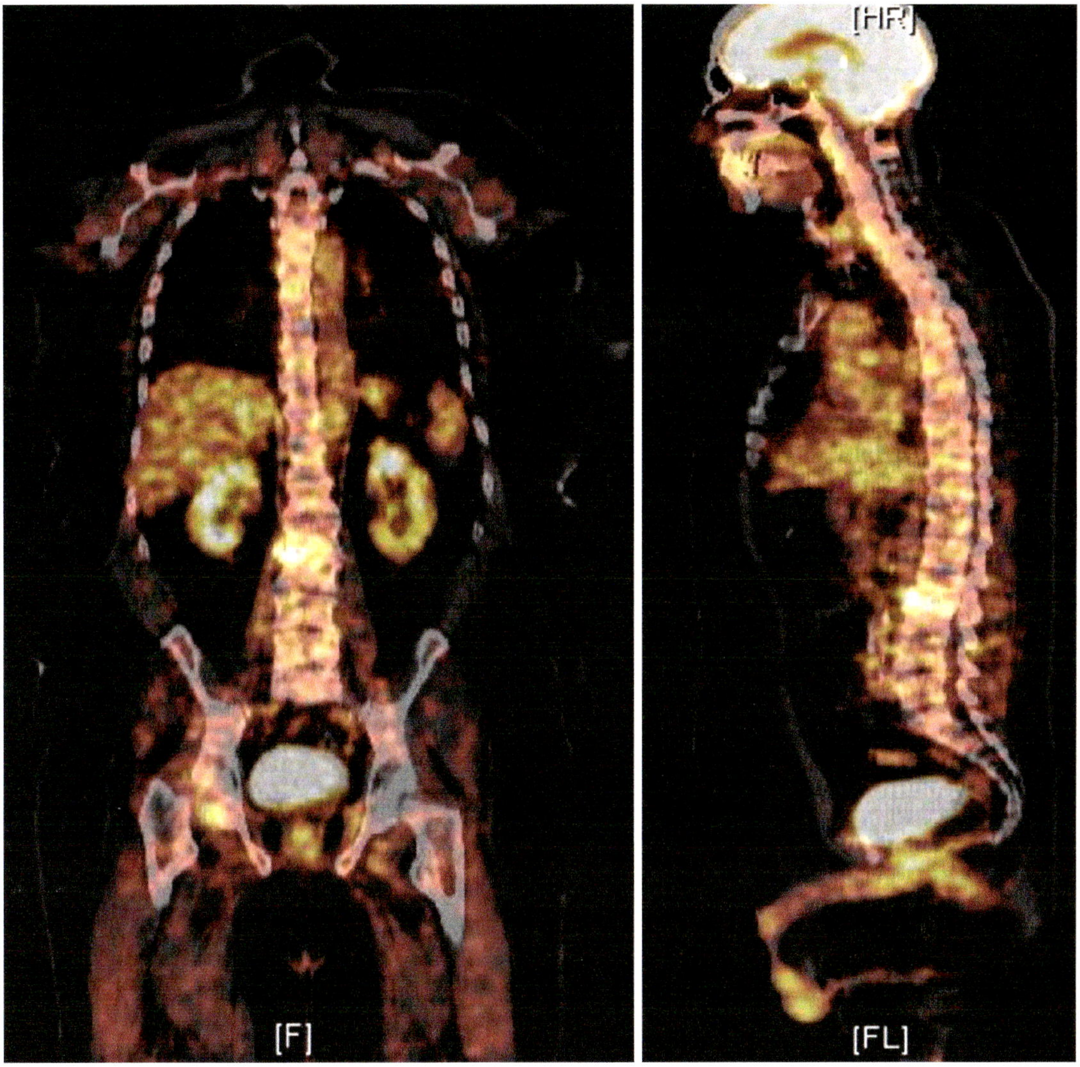

Fig. 40.6 Positron emission tomography (PET) for exclusion of further sources of infection

gresses, there is an increase in osteodestructive processes with loss of bone integrity and static malalignment of the sagittal profile. Finally, reparative processes lead to the presentation of sclerosis and bony overbridging.

Computertomography can show the bone destruction accurately and is often used as an alternative tool in cases of contraindications and in addition to MRI. The sensitivity of the examination can be increased to 83% by administering an additional contrast agent [16]. This contrast agent can also be used to differentiate between abscesses (marginal contrast agent admission) and inflammatory, pannus-like tissue (diffuse contrast agent admission). Computertomography can be helpful in differentiating between inflammatory and degenerative changes, since it shows subtile vacuum phenomena, which are mainly found in degenerative changes.

F-FDG-PET study is an alternative, especially in cases of contraindications for contrast-enhanced examinations. In evaluating the course of therapy, it is clearly superior to magnetic resonance imaging [17]. Since the scintigraphy is clearly inferior in its specificity of magnetic

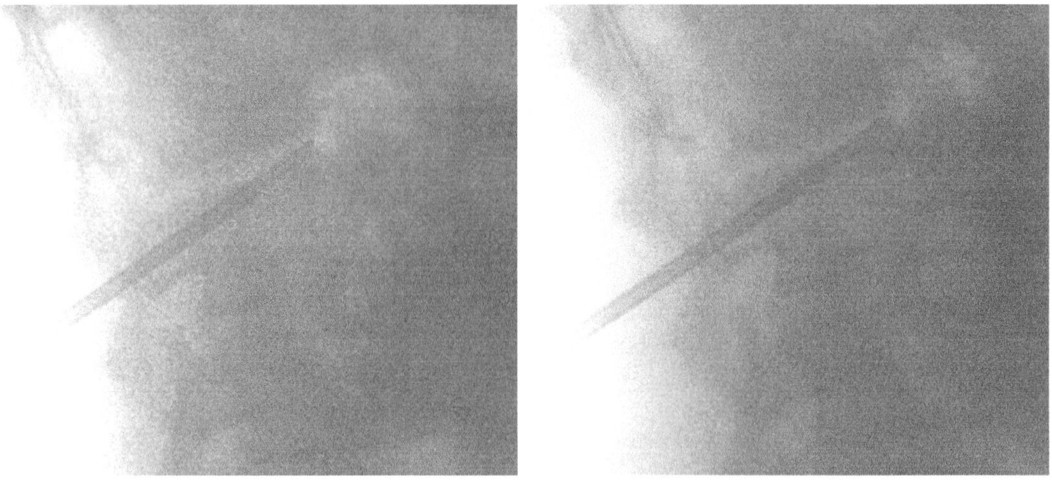

Fig. 40.7 Biopsy disc L2/3 and upper endplate L3, intraoperative x-ray documentation 2 weeks later

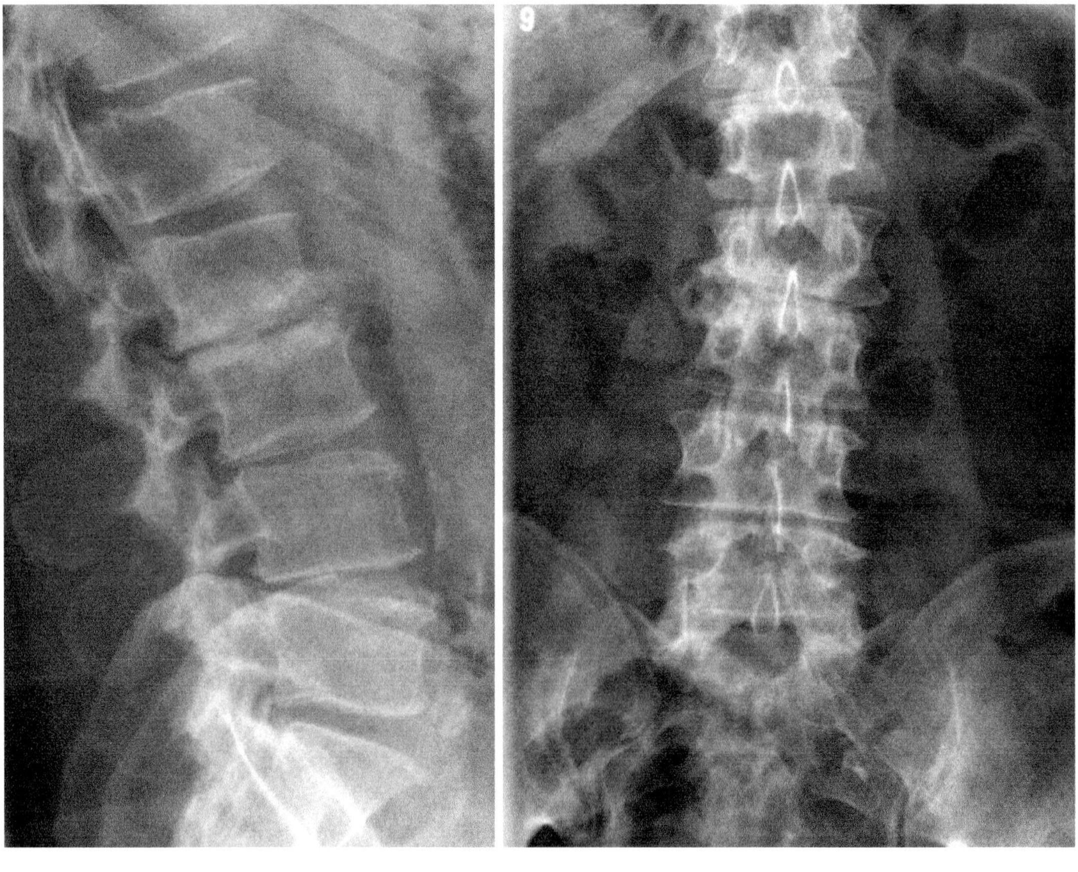

Fig. 40.8 x-ray ap and lateral view 4 month after diagnosis

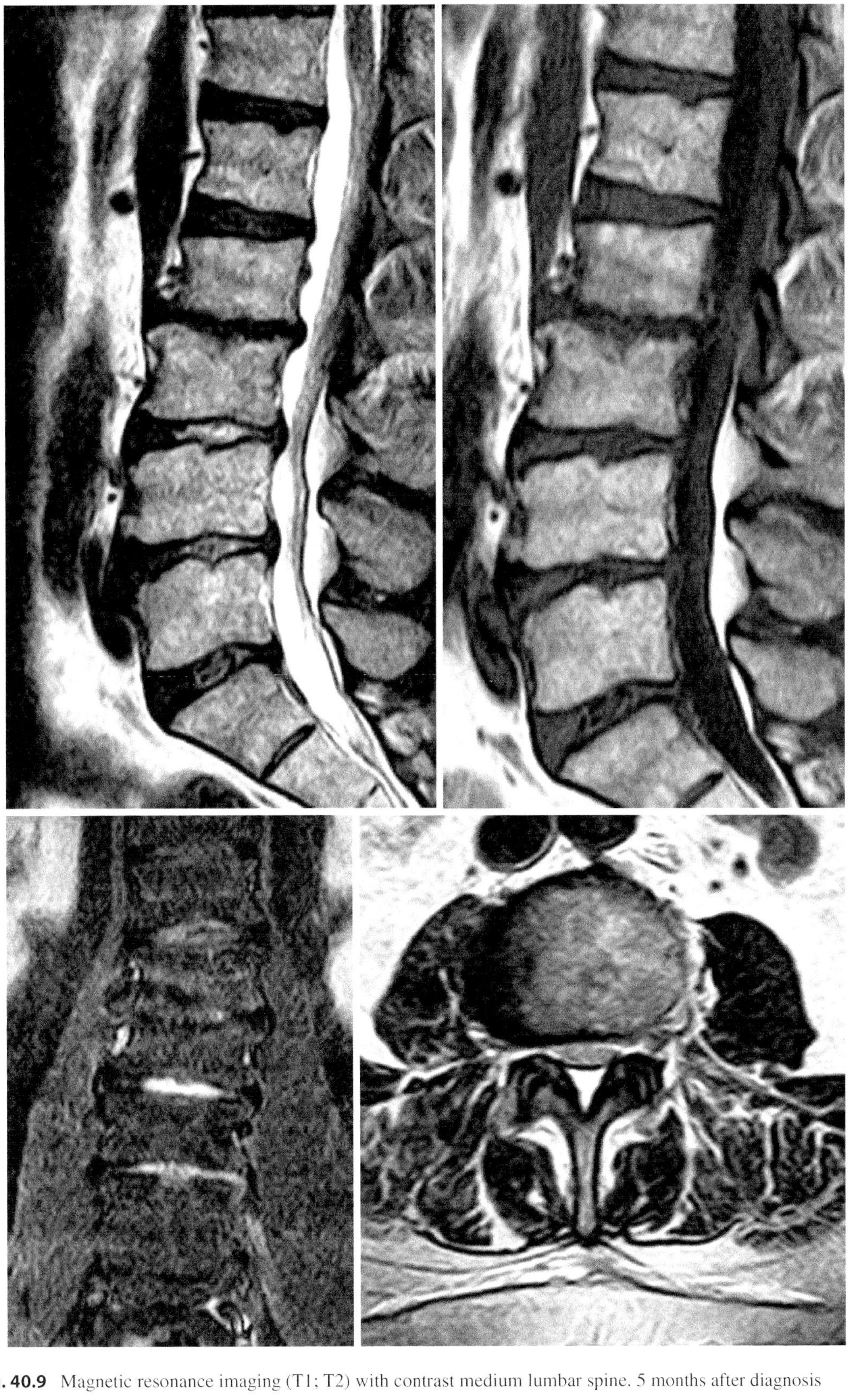

Fig. 40.9 Magnetic resonance imaging (T1; T2) with contrast medium lumbar spine. 5 months after diagnosis

resonance imaging, its main function lies in detecting multifocal infection spread.

With a sensitivity of 96% and a specificity of 92%, magnetic resonance imaging is the imaging method of choice for primary diagnosis [18]. In addition to the axial and sagittal T1 and T2 weighted sequences, a fluid-sensitive, fat-suppressing STIR sequence should be prepared. Axial and sagittal views allow the assessment of epidural abscesses, vertebral body and disc infections and provide an additional overview of the perivertebral tissue as well as the psoas muscles. In the T1-weighted sequence there is a signal reduction (hypointensity) for the affected vertebral body and the inflamed soft tissue, and a signal increase (hyperintensity) for the T2-weighted sequence. In the early phase of the disease, there is a blurring with a loss of demarcation of the endplates, which in the further course receive significant erosion. A disadvantage of magnetic resonance imaging is the poor correlation with the clinical course. A repeated MRI is probably unnecessary if clinical and laboratory outcomes are satisfactory. The persistence of bone/disc MRI findings alone does not represent therapeutic failure [19]. In this respect, the use of magnetic resonance imaging as a short-term follow-up should be viewed critically. The criteria for a healing tendency is a signal enhancement of the bone marrow in the native T1 weighting [20]. The MRI can be helpful to differentiate between inflammatory degenerative processes of osteochondrosis and a diagnosis of spondylodiscitis in clinical practice. Delineation is often possible when there is no signal enhancement of the disc in T2 weighting as well as the absence of extensive perivertebral inflammatory zones in degenerative diseases. The presence of gas inclusions in the intervertebral disc space, in the sense of a vacuum phenomenon, points to a degenerative process [21].

The detection of the causative agent plays a crucial role in the successful treatment of spondylodiscitis. Although this assumption is well established, it is not based on any evidence-based data. A retrospective study showed more positive treatment outcomes in empirically treated patients compared to patients receiving targeted therapy based on pathogen detection. The difference in the two groups of patients was, however, not significant and is limited by the assumption that negative disease pathogenicity was associated with a lower severity of the disease [22]. Several techniques are available as detection methods. Pathogen detection in cultures should be attempted primarily by preparing blood cultures. The detection through this examination method has a success rate of 40–89%. This rate is lower if antibiotic therapy has been initiated and it is higher in cases of a hematogenous pathogenesis of the infection [23–26]. An increase in the rate of positive detection can be achieved by taking of at least three blood cultures [27]. Should the results of the blood cultures be negative, even when radiological and clinical symptoms persist and the suspicion of spondylodiscitis remains, secondary pathogen detection should be done by sampling directly from the main focus of infection. Percutaneous biopsies can be performed fluoroscopically, under computerized tomography, or with magnetic resonance imaging. Studies show a superiority of computertomography-assisted biopsies with better targeting accuracy and a lower rate of complications [28]. Detection of bacteria is successful in percutaneous biopsies between 14% and 76% [26, 29, 30]. In this context, it should be remembered that local anesthetics have an antibacterial effect and may adversely affect the detection rate [31].

The French Société de Pathologie Infectieuse de Langue Francaise (SPILF), recommends percutaneous biopsies in cases of three negative blood cultures: two biopsies should be taken from the upper endplate area, two from the lower endplate area and two from the center of the disc space [32]. An increase in the yield of positive pathogens was achieved by puncture with saline injection [33]. The intraoperative sampling of inflammatory areas has the advantage of a large and safe material yield. The fact that antibiotic therapy has a negative influence on the detection rate in blood cultures has been proven [34]. However, the effect of antibiotic therapy on biopsy results is less clear. While some studies did not see any significant influence of concomitant antibiotic therapy [29, 35], others showed a significantly lower rate of detection, especially if antibiotic therapy had been administered for more than 4 days [36, 37]. In addition to the possibility of a molecular pathogen detection, the histopathological examination complements the diagnosis and provides additional information with respect to necrotic-infectious changes in cases of negative pathogen detection.

Compared to non-specific spondylodiscitis, the clinical findings in specific cases are often bland, fever is rather rare. Typical in imaging is a massive bone destruction. Decisive for the diagnosis of a specific infection is the direct detection of Myobacteria tuberculosis via biopsy.

40.4 Conclusions and Take Home Message

For a successful treatment of vertebral osteomyelitis, a knowledge of the anamnestic and clinical symptoms as well as a rapid initiation of a sufficient diagnosis are necessary. Magnetic resonance imaging is the first choice for detecting an infectious disease in the spinal column. Alternatives are available with computertomography and nuclear medicine examinations. In cases with hemodynamically and clinically stable patients without neurological deficits, primary pathogen detection should be conducted. This can be done by the preparation of several blood cultures and in the absence of pathogen detection, by a percutaneous biopsy.

Diagnostic algorithm:

1. Anamnesis and clinical examination
2. Laboratory diagnostics and microbiological diagnostics (3 blood cultures, PCR)
3. Radiological diagnostics (MRI, CT, PET)
4. Biopsy

Pearls

- Anamnestic and clinical symptoms of spondylodiscitis are often very unspecific and lead to a delayed diagnosis. **Consider this disease !!!!**
- Magnetic resonance imaging is the diagnostic gold standard
- Microbiological diagnostics by blood cultures or by percutaneous biopsy are strongly recommended

References

1. Babic M, Simpfendorfer CS. Infections of the spine. Infect Dis Clin N Am. 2017;31:279–97.
2. Jung N, Vossen S. Septische artthritis und spondylodiszitis. Z Rheumatol. 2016;75:861–8.
3. Nickerson EK, Sinha R. Vertebral osteomyelitis in adults: an update. Br Med Bull. 2016;117:121–38.
4. Zarghooni K, Röllinghoff M, Siewe J. Spondylodiszitis eine interdiszitplinäre Herausforderung. Dtsch Med Wochenschr. 2010;135:1182–5.
5. Frangen TM, Kalicke T, Gottwald M. Surgical management of spondylodiszits. An analysis of 78 cases. Unfallchirurg. 2006;109:743–53.
6. D' Agostino C, Scorzolini L, Massetti AP. A seven year prospective study on spondylodiscites; epidemiological and microbiological features. Infection. 2010;38:102–7.
7. Pricipi N, Esposito S. Infectious discitis and spondylodicitis in children. Int J Mol Sci. 2016;17:539.
8. Cottle L, Riordan T. Infectious spondylodiscitis. J Infect. 2008;56:401–12.
9. Mete B, Kurt C, Yilmaz MH, Ertan G, Ozaras R, Mert A, Tabak F, Ozturk R. Vertebral osteomyelitis: eight years experience of 100 cases. Rheumatol Int. 2011;32(11):3591–7.
10. Hadjipavlou AG, Mader JT, Nessessary JT, Muffoletto AJ. Haematogenous pyogenic spinal infections and theis surgical management. Spine. 2000;25(13):1668–79.
11. Murillo O, Grau I, Lora-Tamayo J, Gomez-Junyent J, Ribera A, Tubau F, Ariza J, Pallares R. The changing epidemiology of bacteraemic osteoarticular infections in the early 21st century. Clin Microbiol Infect. 2015;21(3):254.e1–8.
12. Garg RK, Somvanshi DS. Spinal tuberculosis: a review. J Spinal Cord Med. 2011;34:440–54.
13. Esendagly-Yilmaz G, Oluolglu O. Pathologic basis of pyogenic, non pyogenic and other spondylitis and discitis. Neuroimaging Clin N Am. 2015;25:159–61.
14. Zilkens KW, Peters KM, Schwanitz BM. New inflammation markers for early detection of spondylodiscitis Eur. Spine J. 1992;1(3):152–5.
15. Modic MT, Feiglin DH, Piraino DW. Vertebral osteomyelitis. Assessment using MR. Radiology. 1985;157:157–66.
16. Rausch VH, Bannas P, Schoen G. Diagnostic yield of multidetector computed tomography in patients with acute spondylodiscitis. Fortsch Röntgenstr. 2017;189:339–46.
17. Niccoli Asabella A, Iuele F, Simone F, Fanelli M, Lavelli V, Ferrari C, Di Palo A, Notaristefano A, Merenda NC, Rubini G. Role of 18F-FDG Pet/CT in the evaluation of response to antibiotic therapy in patients affected by infectious spondylodiscitis. Hell J Nucl Med. 2015;18(1):17–22.
18. Dagirmanjian A, Schils J, McHenry MC. MR imaging of spine infections. Magn Reson Imaging Clin N Am. 1999;7:525–38.
19. Euba G, Narvaez JA, Nolla JM, Murillo O, Narvaez J, Gomez-Vaquero C, Ariza J. Long-term clinical and

radiological magnetic rexonance imaging outcome of abscess-associated spontaneous pyogenic vertebral osteomyelitis under conservative management. Semin Arthritis Rheum. 2008;38(1):28–40.

20. Gillams AR, Chaddha B, Carter AP. MR appearances of the temporal evolution and resolution of infectious spondylitis. AJR Am J Roentgenol. 1996;166(4):903–7.
21. Stabler A, Reiser M. Imaging of spinal infection. Radiol Clin N Am. 2001;39:115–35.
22. Kim J, Kim YS, Peck KR, Kim ES, Cho SY, Ha YE, Kang CI, Chung DR, Song JH. Outcome of culture-negative pyogenic vertebral osteomyelitis: comparison with microbiologically confirmed pyogenic vertebral osteomyelitis. Semin Arthritis Rheum. 2014;44(2):246–52.
23. Sakkas LI, Davas EM, Kapsalaki E. Hematogenous spinal infection in Central Greece. Spine (Phila Pa 1976). 2009;34:E513–8.
24. Kim CJ, Song KH, Jeon JH. A comparative study of pyogenic and tuberculous spondylodiscitis. Spine (Phila Pa 1976). 2010;35:E1096.
25. Mylona E, Samarkos M, Kakalou E. Pyogenic vertebral osteomyelitis: a systematic review of clinical characteristics. Semin Arthritis Rheum. 2009;39:10–7.
26. D'Agostino C, Scorzolini L, Massetti AP. A seven year prospective study on spondylodiscitis: epidemiological and microbiological features. Infection. 2010;38:102–7.
27. Gardos F, Lescure FX, Senneville E, Flipo RM, Schmit JL, Fardellone P. Suggestions for managing pyogenic (non-tuberculous) discitis in adults. Joint Bone Spine. 2007;74(2):133–9.
28. Nourbakhsh A, Grady JJ, Garges KJ. Percutaneous spine biopsy: a meta-analysis. J Bone Joint Surg Am. 2008;90:1722–5. 49.
29. Lora-Tamayo J, Euba G, Narvaez JA. Changing trends in the epidemiology of pyogenic vertebral osteomyelitis: the impact of cases with no microbiologic diagnosis. Semin Arthritis Rheum. 2011;41:247–55.
30. Cebrian Parra JL, Saez-Arenillas Martin A, Urda Martinez-Aedo AL. Management of infectious discitis. Outcome in one hundred and eight patients in a university hospital. Int Orthop. 2012;36:239–44.
31. Lehner B, Akbar M, Rehnitz C, Omler GW, Dapunt U, Burckhardt I. Standards of microbiological diagnostics of spondylodiscitis. Orthopäde. 2012;41(9):702–10.
32. Societe de Pathologie Infectieuse de Langue Francaise (SPILF). Recommandations pour la pratique Clinique, Spondylodiscites infectieuses primitives, et secondaires a un geste intra-discal, sans mise en place de materiel. Med Mal Infect. 2007;37(9):554–72.
33. Shibayama M, Nagahara M, Kawase G. New needle biopsy technique for lumbar pyogenic spondylodiscitis. Spine (Phila Pa 1976). 2010;35:E1347–9.
34. Müller-Broich JD, Petersdorf S, Pfugmacher R. Implementation of a diagnostic-algorhythm in the treatment of unspecific spondylodiszitis – save tool for pathogen detection. Eur Spine J. 2011;20:1979–2066.
35. Marschall J, Bhavan KP, Olsen MA. The impact of prebiopsy antibiotics on pathogen recovery in hematogenous vertebral osteomyelitis. Clin Infect Dis. 2011;52:867–72.
36. de Lucas EM, Gonzalez Mandly A, Gutierrez A. CT-guided fine-needle aspiration in vertebral osteomyelitis: true usefulness of a common practice. Clin Rheumatol. 2009;28:315–20.
37. Kim CJ, Song KH, Park WB. Microbiologically and clinically diagnosed vertebral osteomyelitis: impact of prior antibiotic exposure. Antimicrob Agents Chemother. 2012;56:2122–4.

Pyogenic Infection Following Single Level Nucleotomy

41

Andrei Slavici

41.1 Introduction

Postprocedural infections of the spine are a dreaded complication putting great strain on both patients and surgeons alike. While the incidence of postoperative discitis in spine surgeries without instrumentation is often cited up to 4%, approx. 480.000 nucleotomies are performed yearly in the United States alone [1, 2]. These figures highlight the necessity for every spinal surgeon to be familiar with the diagnostics and management of postoperative infections. With the following case we will try to illustrate a typical case of postprocedural discitis managed with dorsal instrumentation and interbody fusion.

41.2 Case Description

A 49 year old patient, unable to stand or walk unaided, was urgently referred to the clinic by his general practitioner with fever and strong low back pain without radiculopathy following a right sided sequestrectomy at L4/5, 5 weeks ago. The patient had no prior illness or other prior surgical intervention and performed moderate physical labor. His GP prescribed oral second generation cephalosporins (cefaclor) for the last 2 weeks. Upon clinical examination the patient was pale and exsiccated with a fever of 39.3 °C. His lower back was mildly reddened with strong tenderness upon touch and percussion. Repetitive jarring of the examination gurney as well as heel-drop jarring (modified Markle's sign) elicited strong low back pain. The neurological examination showed intact sensory and motor functions. He was admitted, complete lab-workup and blood cultures were drawn and fluids administered over an iv-line. His bloodwork showed a leukocytosis with 20/nl and c reactive protein at 19 mg/dl albeit with procalcitonin within normal range. Urine analysis was performed as part of our admittance panel and was without pathological findings. Ap and lateral plain x-ray showed light degenerative changes as well as a light scoliosis (Figs. 41.1 and 41.2). MRI scans revealed hyperintensity in the dorsal disk space, both endplates as well as throughout the former approach on STIR sequences (Fig. 41.3) and high uptake on contrast enhanced T1 sequences (Figs. 41.4 and 41.5). The current antibiotic course was interrupted as his current condition indicated its futility. The patient was counselled that lacking other possible source this constellation had all but proven a postoperative infection. Surgical and conservative options (percutaneous biopsy followed by long double-course i.v. antibiotics) were presented to him. The monosegmental

A. Slavici (✉)
Department of Spine and Reconstructive Orthopedic Surgery, Sana Klinikum Offenbach, Offenbach am Main, Germany

B. Meyer, M. Rauschmann (eds.), *Spine Surgery*, https://doi.org/10.1007/978-3-319-98875-7_41

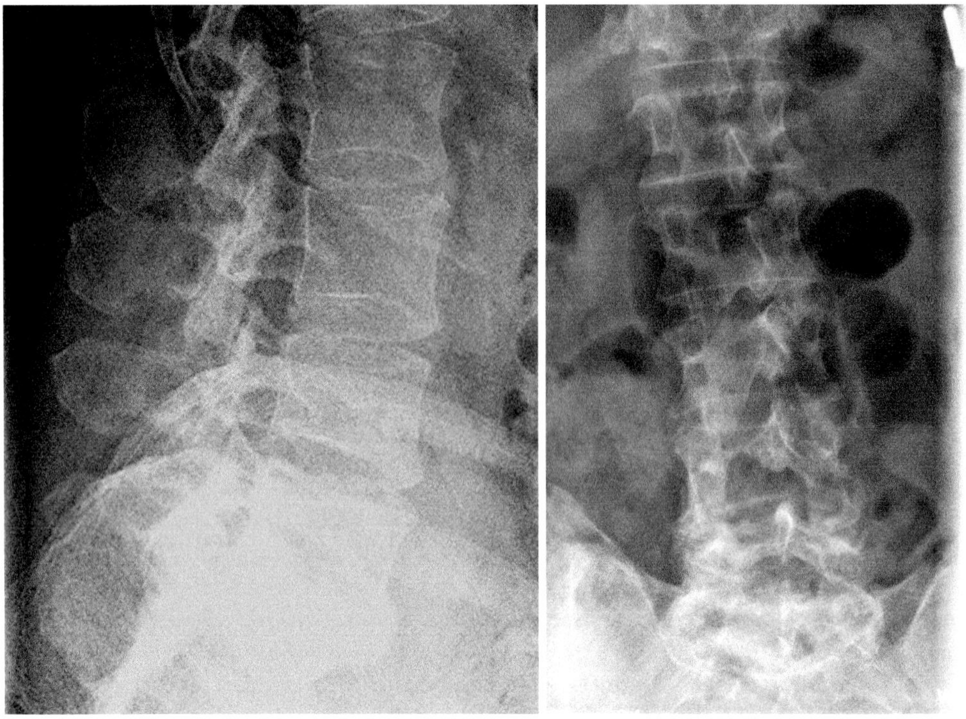

Figs. 41.1 and 41.2 Plain standing X-ray in ap (Fig. 41.1) and lateral view (Fig. 41.2) showing light degeneration of the facet joints and a light scoliosis, possibly accentuated by pain

interbody fusion, thorough debridement of the intervertebral space with dorsal instrumentation was clear recommended and accepted by the patient. A dorsal instrumentation at L4/5 in PLIF-technique with surgical titanium mesh cages loaded with bone chips and antibiotic carriers was performed (Figs. 41.6 and 41.7). On recommendation of our microbiologists he received a 14 day course of i.v. rifampicin and vancomycin followed by an oral course of rifampicin and levofloxacin for 4 weeks and levofloxacin as a mono-therapy for another 4 weeks. Pathology confirmed the diagnosis of spondylodiscitis and a cephalosporin resistant strain of *staph. epidermidis* was isolated. Ambulation was allowed directly postoperative and was aided by physiotherapists. The patient recovered well and resumed labor 5 month post-surgery. On his insistence, albeit with lacking symptoms, the patient was referred by his GP to a radiologist for a follow-up MRI without contrast. This showed no further signal hyperintensities on T2 (Fig. 41.8).

41.3 Discussion of the Case

Even with today's technological advance the start of every medical treatment remains an adequate patient history and physical examination. From the clinical presentation alone one already suspects a pyogenic infection of the spine. Following this a comprehensive bloodwork, including CBC, CRP, procalcitonin, coagulation status, liver and kidney function should be obtained. CRP naturally peaks postoperatively but normalizes quickly, making it a reliable indicator for bacterial infections with a sensitivity and specificity of 100% and 97% [3]. In clinical practice normal procalcitonin is often seen, even with microbiological findings and a small series came to the same result finding no significant differences in PCT elevation between spondylodiscitis and reoccurrence of disc herniation [4]. While often negative, it is general practice that blood cultures from all patients admitted with a suspected spinal infection, are drawn. This can facilitate the

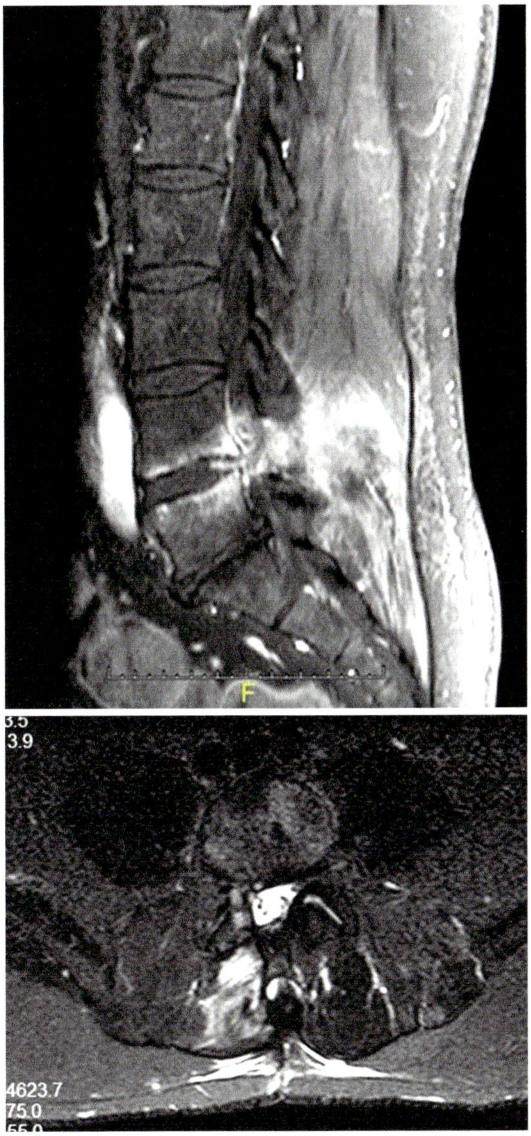

Fig. 41.3 MRI of the lumbar spine in STIR (short tau inversion recovery) sequence. Notable is the enhanced signal, indicative of edema, in the endplates as well as the paravertebral muscles along the approach in the axial view (Fig. 41.4)

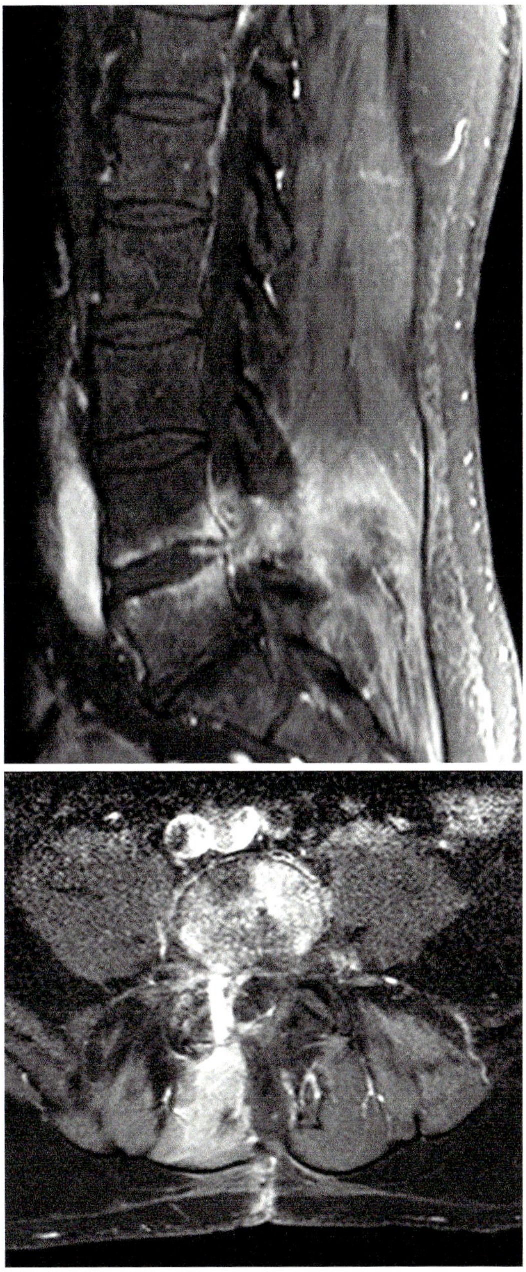

Figs. 41.4 and 41.5 MRI of the lumbar spine in contrast enhanced T1 sequence. Hypervascularization, confirming inflammation, is shown in sagittal (Fig. 41.4) and axial view (Fig. 41.5)

identification of pathogens when surgery or biopsy is delayed.

Contrast enhanced MRI should be the investigation of choice showing hyperintensity in T2/STIR, hypointensity in T1 and enhancement in the disc space and in the adjacent endplates with or without perifocal reaction. Important to mention is, to check the peridural space and the paravertebral region, concerning abscess-formations.

If the patients current condition allows antibiotics should not be started or should be paused until microbiological samples were acquired.

The segment was considered to be less then fully stabile because the patient described axial

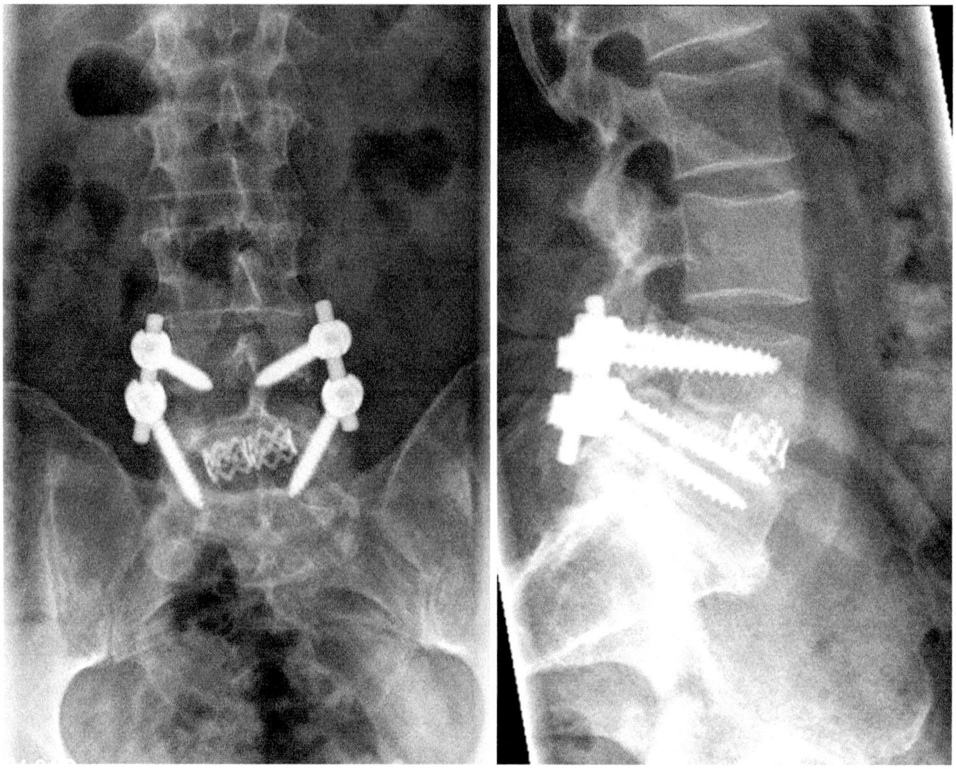

Figs. 41.6 and 41.7 Plain standing X-ray in ap (Fig. 41.7) and lateral view (Fig. 41.8) showing the post-operative status with monosegmental dorsal instrumentation (pedicle screws and rods) and interposition of 2 STM (surgical titanium mesh) –cages in PLIF technique

loading pain, pain with torsional motion while lying and ambulation only with aid of a wheeled walker, thus a stabilizing procedure with instrumentation was chosen. Due to the infected intervertebral disc-space a thorough debridement, followed by an interbody fusion to guarantee the sagittal profile in a young patient, was done. Yet it remains a controversial topic over the best approach to the surgical management with a generally scarce data and newer studies, albeit with limitations, describing no significant difference between decompression and debridement alone versus fusion [5]. If there is minimal or no damage to the anterior column, yet the patient still presents with clinical signs of instability, a dorsal instrumentation, be it percutaneous or open, can be performed with or without decompression. Bed rest under i.v. antibiotic course until CRP reduction and mobilization in stabilizing braces is a justified option. There is little evidence for a rigid brace (e.g. TLSO) versus passive assisted or semi rigid brace.

Even if a conservative treatment is convened upon a biopsy for cultures and susceptibility testing to guide the future antibiotic course is strongly advocated. When none can be obtained or cultures are negative the empirical treatment should be based on local microbial resistances, if necessary in consultation with a microbiologist. A combination therapy helps reduce the risk of resistance occurrence and fluoroquinolone + rifampicin is often recommended for staph. infections [6]. While no significant difference was reported versus a 6 week course, longer courses of up to 12 weeks should be considered in patients with present implants [7].

A follow-up with patient history, clinical examination and plain standing X-rays is recommended at 12 weeks postoperatively CT or MRI is only recommended in symptomatic patients.

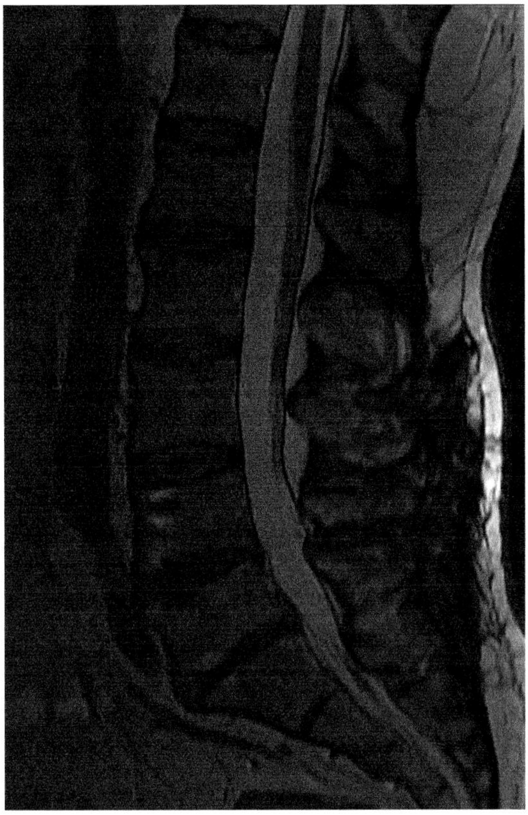

Fig. 41.8 Sagittal T2 sequence showing a free spinal canal and no edema at 5 month postoperatively

41.4 Conclusions and Take Home Message

Postprocedural spinal infections are a dreaded complication but every spinal surgeon should strive to know how to diagnose and treat, even though, unfortunately, more than just a few times the clinical presentation isn't as clear-cut as in the presented case. Whenever possible antibiotic treatment should be guided by microbial cultures and resistance testing. Surgical management with instrumentation and thorough debridement of the infected disc-space with removing almost all disc-material as well as the cartilage endplate, followed by inserting a cage, bone-substitutes in combination with local antibiotic substances is recommended. Depending on the germ, if detected, vancomycin and gentamycin are the favorite antibiotics. While titanium cages as interbody implant is prefered, there seems to be no significant difference in regard to reinfection with Polyetheretherketone (PEEK) cages [8, 9]. The main goal in treating infections is the elimination of its focus and full restoration of organ function, from conservative treatment through sole revision with decompression to instrumentation with interbody fusion. As such each case needs to be evaluated individually, guided by best clinical practice, considering stability, comorbidities and patient preference among other factors.

Pearls

- Thorough debridement of the infected disc space is the goal of treatment
- Paravertebral abscesses should be drained either surgically or through percutaneous interventions
- When MRI is not possible scintigraphy or SPECT are good alternatives

Pitfalls

- Monotherapy, especially with solely bacteriostatic agents, poses a high risk for resistance occurrence

References

1. Gray DT, Deyo RA, Kreuter W, Mirza SK, Heagerty PJ, et al. Population-based trends in volumes and rates of ambulatory lumbar spine surgery. Spine (Phila Pa 1976). 2006;31:1957–63.
2. Sherman J, Cauthen J, Schoenberg D, Burns M, Reaven NL, et al. Economic impact of improving outcomes of lumbar discectomy. Spine J Off J North Am Spine Soc. 2010;10:108–16.
3. Kang B-U, Lee S-H, Ahn Y, Choi W-C, Choi Y-G. Surgical site infection in spinal surgery: detection and management based on serial C-reactive protein measurements. J Neurosurg Spine. 2010;13:158e164.
4. Maus U, Anderega S, Gravius S, Ohnsorge JA, Miltner O. Procalcitonin (PCT) as a diagnostic tool for monitoring of spondylodiscitis. Z Orthop Unfall. 2009;147:59e64.
5. Noh S, Zhang H, Lim H, Song H, Yang K. Decompression alone versus fusion for pyogenic

spondylodiscitis. Spine J. 2017;17(8):1120–6. https://doi.org/10.1016/j.spinee.2017.04.015.
6. Legrand E, Flipo R-M, Guggenbuhl P, et al. Management of non-tuberculous infectious discitis. Treatments used in 110 patients admitted to 12 teaching hospitals in France. Joint Bone Spine. 2001;68:504e509.
7. Roblot F, Besnier JM, Juhel L, et al. Optimal duration of antibiotic therapy in vertebral osteomyelitis. Semin Arthritis Rheum. 2007;36:269e277.
8. Schomacher M, Finger T, Koeppen D, et al. Application of titanium and polyetheretherketone cages in the treatment of pyogenic spondylodiscitis. Clin Neurol Neurosur. 2014;127:65–70. https://doi.org/10.1016/j.clineuro.2014.09.027.
9. Shiban E, Janssen I, Wostrack M, et al. A retrospective study of 113 consecutive cases of surgically treated spondylodiscitis patients. A single-center experience. Acta Neurochir. 2014;156(6):1189–96. https://doi.org/10.1007/s00701-014-2058-0.

42 Diagnostics and Treatment of C1/C2-Instability in Rheumatoid Arthritis

George K. Prezerakos and Adrian T. H. Casey

42.1 Introduction

Rheumatoid arthritis is a systemic, autoimmune, inflammatory disease affecting the synovial joints, bones and ligaments. Though it mainly affects the small peripheral joints, the second most frequent disease locus is the cervical spine, as in itself comprises 32 synovial joints [1].

The prevalence of R.A is about 1–2% with cervical involvement reaching 86% as early as 2 years post diagnosis and neurological involvement up to 58% [2, 3].

42.2 Etiology

Though the exact etiology remains elusive, RA is a multifactorial disease triggered in genetically and immunologically predisposed individuals, leading to an inflammatory cascade within the synovial joint. In turn, inflammation leads to pannus formation and proteolytic and osteoclastic activity resulting in cartilage, ligament as well as bone destruction. Though the inflammatory process may be remitting, if continued usually results in progressive joint destruction, deformity, and ultimately variable degrees of incapacitation [2].

Relatively recent advances in the pharmacological arsenal are able to prevent the formation of de novo lesions in the cervical spine. However, such therapies failed to arrest the evolution of pre-existing damage [2, 4].

42.3 Pathophysiology, Clinical Manifestations and Radiological Characterisation

There are four main patho-anatomical features - and thus potential surgical targets- involved in the pathophysiology of rheumatoid disease in the cervical spine (i) atlantoaxial (AA) subluxation, (ii) peri-odontoid pannus formation, (iii) vertical translocation of the odontoid peg, (iv) sub axial subluxation .

C1–2 subluxation presents in 65% of rheumatoid patients. It results in a reduction of the space available to the cord and direct repetitive trauma. It is quantified by the anterior atlanto dental interval (AADI). The posterior atlanto dental interval (PADI) which directly measures the space available to the cord probably correlates better with neurological deterioration [5–7].

Vertical Translocation of the odontoid peg or else cranial settling stems from atlantoaxial as well

G. K. Prezerakos · A. T. H. Casey (✉)
Victor Horsley Department of Neurosurgery, The National Hospital for Neurology and Neurosurgery, Queen Square, London, UK

B. Meyer, M. Rauschmann (eds.), *Spine Surgery*, https://doi.org/10.1007/978-3-319-98875-7_42

as occipito-cervical joint destruction and results in various degrees of brainstem compression compression and vertebral artery compression [8, 9].

Vertical translocation is quantified by the Redlund-Johnell criterion, the Clarke station or Ranawat classification. None of these methods results in a satisfactory level of sensitivity. To achieve a sensitivity of more than 90%, all measurements need to be taken into consideration [10].

Subaxial subluxation is less frequent but can increase iatrogenically after occipitocervical fixation [11].

The clinical manifestations are difficult to reliably recognise and interpret, as rheumatoid patients suffer systematically and function is often impaired by the systemic and peripheral effects of the disease [12]. Cord compression results in myelopathic features including gait and manual dexterity impairment whilst compression of the C2 sensory fibers can result in neck, mastoid, ear or facial pain, as well as migraines. Vertberal artery compression as well as brainstem compression can lead to tinnitus, vertigo, diplopia, dysphagia and visual disturbances. It is important to note that a significant number of patients with AA subluxation remain asymptomatic.

42.4 Clinical Classification

Various clinical grading systems have been used to quantify the neurological (Ranawat classes I-IIIB) and functional (Steinbrocker's grades I-IV) status of patients with rheumatoid arthritis [13, 14].

The Ranawat grading system assigns patients who are asymptomatic to Class I; patients who are ambulant but exhibit subjective weakness to Class II, patients with objective weakness are assigned to Class III with those being ambulant being Class IIIA and the non-ambulant one class IIIB.

The Steinbrocker grades I-IV adopted by the American Rheumatism Association is a widely accepted score. It focuses on the functional capacity, with RA patients able to perform all everyday duties assigned to Class I, most of daily duties with some handicaps to class II, few or none daily duties and self-care class III and finally those who are heavily incapacitated bedridden or wheelchair bound assigned to Class IV.

The Ranawat classification (I-IIIB) is designed to weigh more heavily on neurological disability. It is unfortunate that both grading systems are rather crude and fail to differentiate adequately quite different levels of disability or myelopathy. Thus, the middle class myelopathic patients (Ranawat II and IIIA) are not well distinguished and significant improvements or deteriorations following surgery are "blurred" in these gradings. Whilst in the Steinbrocker grading system there is an enormous leap from Grades II to III i.e. from having function adequate for normal activities (Grade II) to being limited to little or none of the duties of self-care (Grade III).

42.5 Surgical Management

Answering questions pertaining the management of rheumatoid patients with cervical involvement (conservative vs surgical, as well as type and timing of surgery) require knowledge of the natural history, prognostic factors and surgical outcomes.

Most of the available evidence is level III as they comprise prospective or retrospective case series.

Surgery typically consists of a decompressive procedure in combination with fusion or stabilising procedure which may be performed via an anterior or posterior approach depending on the site of compression and surgeon's preference.

Anterior decompression can be achieved by a transoral odontoidectomy favored in irreducible atlantoaxial subluxation, significant peri-odontoid pannus or significant vertical translocation. It is rarely required.

Atlantoaxial instrumented fixation is the preferred option in reducible horizontal atlantoaxial subluxation with no significant vertical translocation or sub axial disease.

Occipito-cervical fusion is the treatment of choice when the atlantoaxial subluxation is complicated by vertical translocation/sub axial disease.

Finally, sub axial cervical decompression and fixation (anteriorly, posteriorly or both) is indicated in step ladder type of deformity with a reduction in the sub axial canal diameter.

42.6 Case Report

A 66 year-old woman with a previous medical history of rheumatoid arthritis and bronchectasia presented with a 3 week history of progressive tetraparesis. In particular, the patient's premorbid status was that of independent ambulation with full independence in everyday activities (Steinbrocker class II). She had been complaining of moderate sub occipital pain with a right sided dominance.

The patient had been diagnosed with rheumatoid arthritis 14 years ago, has had a metatarsophalangeal fusion and a right shoulder arthroplasty. She has been on disease modifying anti-rheumatic drugs (DMARDs) and steroid treatment.

Her neurological examination revealed signs of florid myelopathy, reduced power Medical Research Council (MRC) grade 4−/5 throughout the upper limbs with MRC 3/5 in finger grip and wrist flexion & extension bilaterally.

Hoffman's and Ono's test were positive bilaterally with brisk reflexes including pectoralis (C5), biceps (C6) and triceps (C7).

She had reduced pinprick sensation in a non-dermatomal distribution and had impaired joint position sense at the distal interphalangeal joints.

Lower limb examination revealed similar findings with proximal weakness (3/5 in hip flexion and knee extension) and 4−/5 in plantar and dorsiflexion with bilateral brisk reflexes and up going plantars. Romberg's test was positive (the patient was just able to stand up with the assistance of two).

The immediate pre-operative Ranawat grade was III(B) whilst her Steinbrocker class was IV, making it the worst possible grade.

42.7 Imaging

Dynamic, flexion-extension cervical radiographs exhibited atlanto-axial subluxation with an AADI 11 mm in flexion vs 2 mm in extension, a PADI of 12 mm in flexion vs 17 mm in extension (Fig. 42.1).

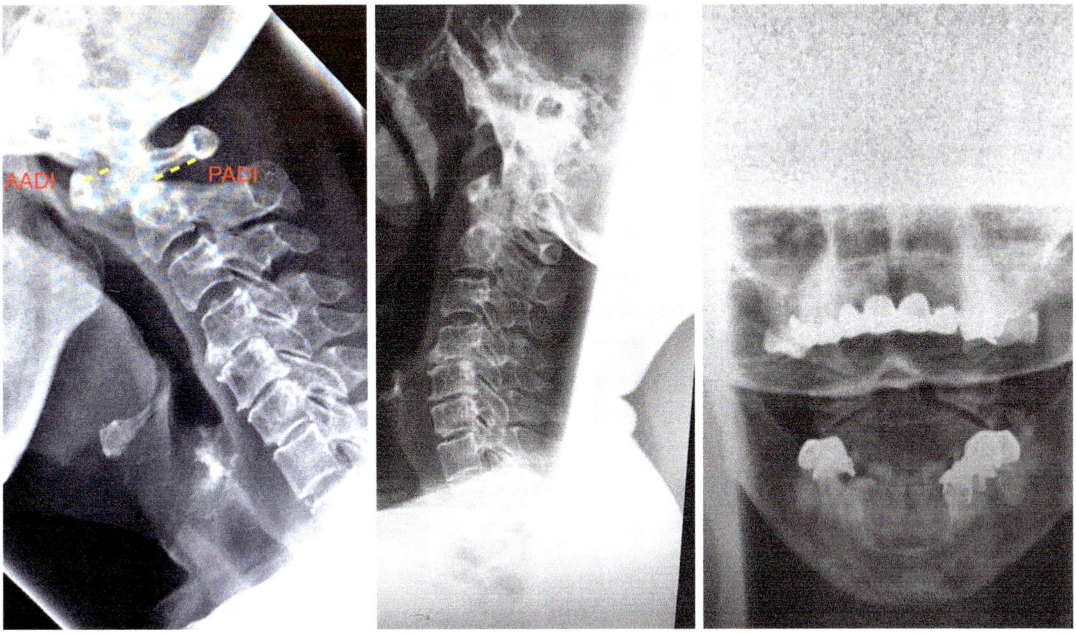

Fig. 42.1 Plain pre-operative cervical radiographs in flexion (left), extension (middle), anteroposterior (AP) (right); Atlantoaxial subluxation is demonstrated during flexion is demonstrated by the increased anterior atlanto dental interval (AADI) and the decreased posterior atlanto dental interval (PADI) which fully reduce in extension. The atlanto axial joints appear within normal limits in the AP views

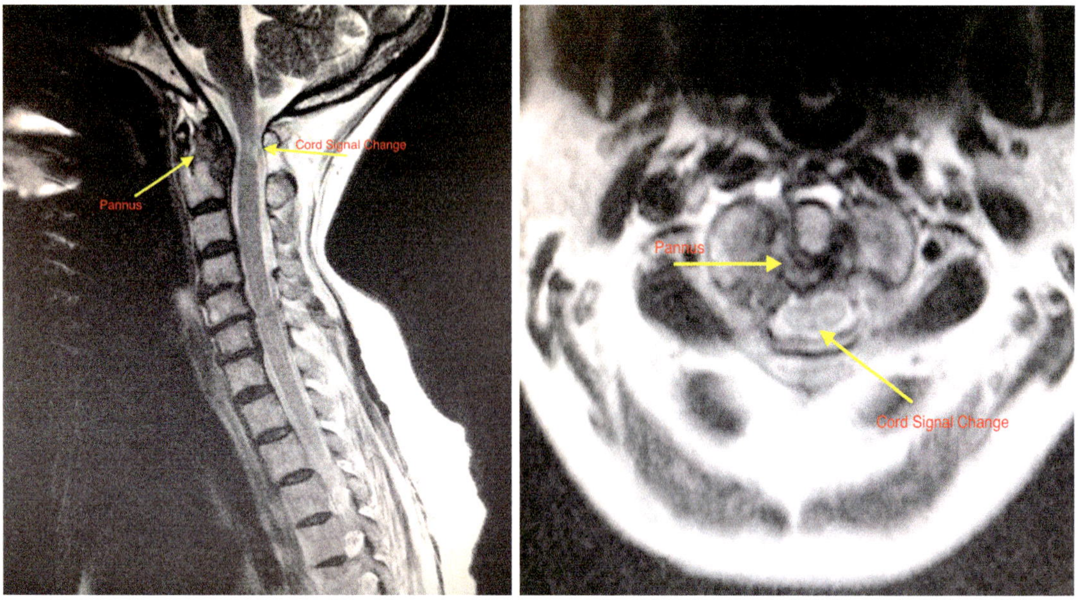

Fig. 42.2 Magnetic resonance T2 weighted mid-sagittal (left) and axial views at the C1–2 level (right) exhibit cord signal change as well as pannus presence in the retro-odontoid space. Note is made of the minimal amount of anterior compression and canal narrowing in the neutral position, suggestive of a dynamic aetiology to account for the signal change

MRI of the cervical spine in the neutral position revealed signal change within the spinal cord at the level of C1–2, with minimal narrowing of the spinal canal at this level suggestive of dynamic compression. There was also evidence of pannus formation at the peri-odontoid space resulting in minimal to moderate compression (Fig. 42.2).

42.8 Intra and Postoperative Course

The patient was offered surgical reduction, decompression with a C1 laminectomy and instrumented fusion via the Harms technique. C1 lateral mass screws were inserted, ensuring a bicortical purchase. Bilateral C2 pedicle screws incorporating pars, pedicle and 2 cortices were employed using a standard Harms technique. Reduction was achieved by tightening the C1 screw tulips onto the rod after final tightening had taken place at the C2 level with synchronous intra-operative neurophysiological monitoring. A C1 laminectomy addressed the presence of retro-odontoid pannus.

Postoperative imaging confirmed appropriate instrumentation position and good reduction of the C1-C2 complex (Fig. 42.3).

The patient was admitted to a high dependency unit postoperatively. Twenty-four hours later returned to the general neurosurgical ward. She was discharged 4 days later to a rehabilitation unit, where she remained for 2 weeks.

The patient was followed up at 6 weeks, 3 months, 6 months and 1 year. She made a spectacular neurological and functional recovery and by the initial 6 week follow-up, she was able to mobilise independently (Ranawat II). Fusion took place within 6 months.

42.9 Discussion and Evidence

A dichotomy of opinion exists as to the surgical indications for fusion and decompression in rheumatoid patients with atlanto-axial subluxation. Surgical intervention is usually recommended in

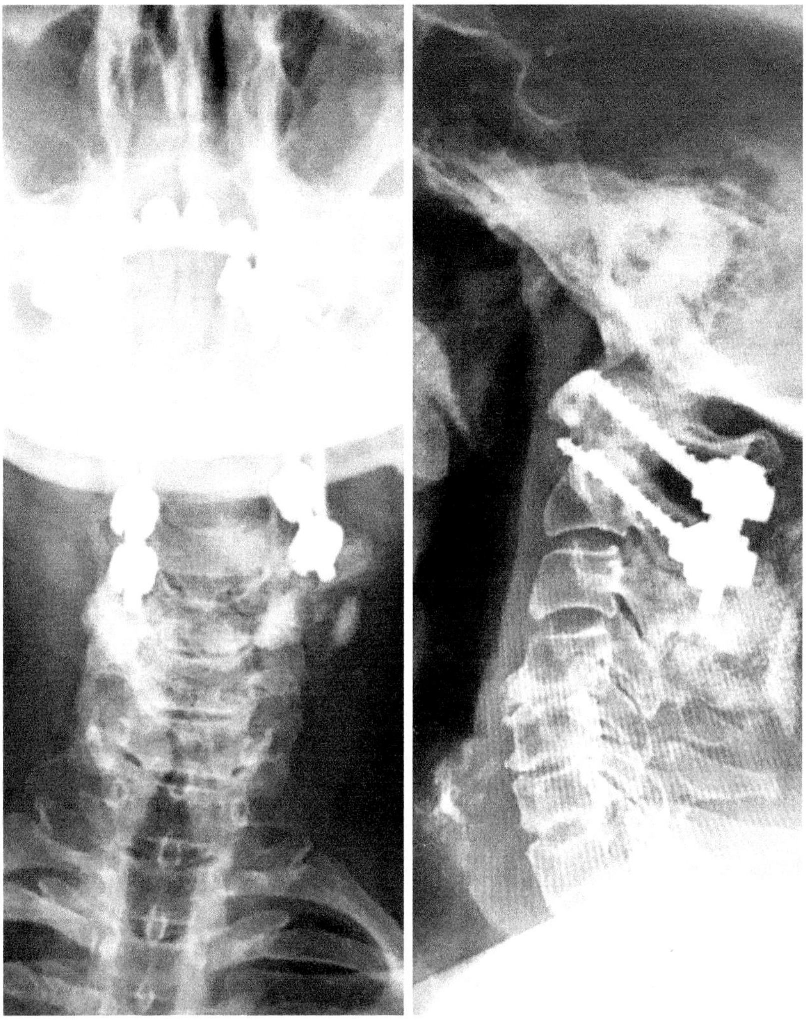

Fig. 42.3 Postoperative AP (left) and lateral (right) plain cervical radiographs demonstrating a satisfactory instrumentation positioning of C1 lateral mass and C2 pedicle screws; note is made of the complete C1-C2 reduction as well as the bicortical purchase of all four screws

the presence of myelopathy, neurological deficits or intractable cervical pain [13, 15–20].

However when recommending prophylactic surgery on the basis of an abnormal atlantodens interval in the absence of neurological signs, [16, 17, 21–26] this consensus breaks down.

The divergence of opinion, as to when surgery is appropriate, arises from the fact that radiological progression of the deformity is unpredictable [4, 5, 18, 27] and perhaps more significantly, there is a poor correlation between an increasing atlantodens interval and the development of neurological signs [5, 25, 27, 28]. This is because the compression may be dynamic or in the presence of vertical translocation the atlantodens interval actually decreases as the translocation (cranial settling) gets worse.

Conservative management is advocated by many rheumatologists [15]. This involves close clinical surveillance of the patient and subsequent referral for surgery following the development of neurological symptoms or signs. However neurological abnormalities are notoriously difficult to establish in the presence of a painful deforming arthritis with an often associated muscular atrophy or peripheral neuropathy [15] and, as a consequence, there are many such patients who do not receive surgical advice until they are tetraparetic, wheel-chair or indeed, even bed bound.

In the context of this particular case, surgical treatment was advocated in view of the recent and progressive neurological deterioration and an overall satisfactory general health. Though most available evidence supports the role of surgery in patients with neurological manifestations, outcomes in non-ambulatory patients such as this patient, have not been as encouraging [9, 12, 29].

Still, in the absence of cranial settling, a PADI of more than 10 mm as in this case carries a better chance of neurological recovery despite the preoperative poor grade [5].

With regards to the choice of surgical management, absence of significant anterior compression made a transoral odontoidectomy unnecessary. The decision is between C1-C2 instrumented fusion with decompression or occipitocervical fixation. The favorable anatomy for a C2 pedicular purchase, the absence of cranial settling and lack of sub-axial spine involvement made a Harms C1–2 instrumented fusion the preferred surgical option. On the other hand, cranial settling, subaxial involvement and prohibitive pedicular anatomy at C2 would have made an O-C fixation the preferred option.

42.10 Conclusion

The available evidence pertaining the management of cervical spine disease in patients with rheumatoid arthritis supports the surgical management in patients with neurological impairment. Nevertheless, it provides a relatively poor framework in patients who are asymptomatic or non-ambulatory. It is in these two subgroups that the surgeon's experience and patient preference play a wider role in the decision making process.

Pearls

There are certain points that a surgeon needs to take into account in order to increase the chances of a successful outcome.

From a surgical perspective, the quality of the bony stock was poor and the fusion rate in such patients is lower than usual [1]. Thus, bicortical screw placement at the maximum length anatomically allowed is advantageous. This was achieved by careful image intensifier input (true lateral films), as well as high level appreciation of the tactile feedback. Trajectory comes into play for the C1 lateral mass screws where an excessively lateral exit may result in carotid artery injury, therefore a degree a medialisation is required .

The authors have found it useful to drill away the overhanging portion of the posterior C1 arch directly above the lateral mass insertion point to ensure maximum bony purchase.

A second point is that the bone morphology is atypical secondary to the chronic inflammatory erosion. As such, careful exposure of the entirety of C2 inferior facet- lamina pars – superior C2 -C1 joint complex is necessary as described above (large size `Cobb and subperiosteal strip with cottonoids, whilst remaining soft tissue removed with bipolar cautery and a sharp Adson.) This gives a clear overview of the entry points as well as a safe medial pedicular surface palpation useful for the C2 pedicular part of the trajectory.

A third point lies with the fact that the biomechanics of the cervical spine in such patients are altered [12]. In this particular case, the unstable state of the C1–2 joint (and potentially the O-C1 joint) could result in repetitive cord injury, if significant pressure is applied to the bony structures during cortex penetration and drilling-tapping–screw insertion. Gentle maneuvers with minimal downward pressure were employed at all times.

A fourth point is that the surgeon needs to keep in mind that reduced fusion rates are seen in rheumatoid patients [1]. In order to maximize the chances of fusion, the C1–2 joint was drilled followed by the application of autologous bone graft with an osteoinductive –osteoconductive synthetic graft placed laterally to the construct. Bone morphogenic protein BMP is listed as a contraindication in rheumatoid arthritis by the manufacturers.

Finally, the general frailty of the patient and increased chances of postoperative infection and skin healing issues make a systematic, layered wound closure imperative and a high dependency cover for the immediate postoperative period essential. We also recommend an awake fiberoptic intubation in such patients, keeping in mind though that the anesthetic maneuvers during intubation are of extension nature and thus do not accentuate the AA instability.

Editorial Comment

Treating patients with RA can cause problems of woundhealing, due to the immunsupressive medication. Therefore a close cooperation with the rheumatologist should be performed, to decide, whether biologicals can be stopped early enough before the planned surgery.

References

1. Bhatia R, Haliasos N, Vergara P, et al. The surgical management of the rheumatoid spine: has the evolution of surgical intervention changed outcomes? J Craniovertebr Junction Spine. 2014;5:38–43. https://doi.org/10.4103/0974-8237.135221.
2. Wasserman BR, Moskovich R, Razi AE. Rheumatoid arthritis of the cervical spine – clinical considerations. Bull NYU Hosp Jt Dis. 2011;69:136–48.
3. Gillick JL, Wainwright J, Das K. Rheumatoid arthritis and the cervical spine: a review on the role of surgery. Int J Rheumatol. 2015; https://doi.org/10.1155/2015/252456.
4. Kaito T, Ohshima S, Fujiwara H, et al. Predictors for the progression of cervical lesion in rheumatoid arthritis under the treatment of biological agents. Spine. 2013;38:2258–63. https://doi.org/10.1097/BRS.0000000000000066.
5. Boden SD, Dodge LD, Bohlman HH, Rechtine GR. Rheumatoid arthritis of the cervical spine. A long-term analysis with predictors of paralysis and recovery. J Bone Joint Surg Am. 1993;75:1282–97.
6. Nguyen HV, Ludwig SC, Silber J, et al. Rheumatoid arthritis of the cervical spine. Spine J. 2004;4:329–34. https://doi.org/10.1016/j.spinee.2003.10.006.
7. Mallory GW, Halasz SR, Clarke MJ. Advances in the treatment of cervical rheumatoid: less surgery and less morbidity. World J Orthop. 2014;5:292–303. https://doi.org/10.5312/wjo.v5.i3.292.
8. Casey AT, Crockard HA, Geddes JF, Stevens J. Vertical translocation: the enigma of the disappearing atlantodens interval in patients with myelopathy and rheumatoid arthritis. Part I. Clinical, radiological, and neuropathological features. J Neurosurg. 1997;87:856–62. https://doi.org/10.3171/jns.1997.87.6.0856.
9. Casey AT, Crockard HA, Stevens J. Vertical translocation. Part II. Outcomes after surgical treatment of rheumatoid cervical myelopathy. J Neurosurg. 1997;87:863–9. https://doi.org/10.3171/jns.1997.87.6.0863.
10. Riew KD, Hilibrand AS, Palumbo MA, et al. Diagnosing basilar invagination in the rheumatoid patient. The reliability of radiographic criteria. J Bone Joint Surg Am. 2001;83-A:194–200.
11. Clarke MJ, Cohen-Gadol AA, Ebersold MJ, Cabanela ME. Long-term incidence of subaxial cervical spine instability following cervical arthrodesis surgery in patients with rheumatoid arthritis. Surg Neurol. 2006;66:136–40.; ; discussion 140. https://doi.org/10.1016/j.surneu.2005.12.037.
12. Casey AT, Crockard HA, Bland JM, et al. Surgery on the rheumatoid cervical spine for the non-ambulant myelopathic patient-too much, too late? Lancet. 1996;347:1004–7.
13. Ranawat CS, O'Leary P, Pellicci P, et al. Cervical spine fusion in rheumatoid arthritis. J Bone Joint Surg Am. 1979;61:1003–10.
14. Steinbrocker O, Traeger CH, Batterman RC. Therapeutic criteria in rheumatoid arthritis. J Am Med Assoc. 1949;140:659–62.
15. Agarwal AK, Peppelman WC, Kraus DR, Eisenbeis CH. The cervical spine in rheumatoid arthritis. BMJ. 1993;306:79–80.
16. Santavirta S, Slätis P, Kankaanpää U, et al. Treatment of the cervical spine in rheumatoid arthritis. J Bone Joint Surg Am. 1988;70:658–67.
17. Heywood AW, Learmonth ID, Thomas M. Cervical spine instability in rheumatoid arthritis. J Bone Joint Surg Br. 1988;70:702–7.
18. Rana NA. Natural history of atlanto-axial subluxation in rheumatoid arthritis. Spine. 1989;14:1054–6.
19. Stirrat AN, Fyfe IS. Surgery of the rheumatoid cervical spine. Correlation of the pathology and prognosis. Clin Orthop Relat Res. 1993;293:135–43.
20. Zoma A, Sturrock RD, Fisher WD, et al. Surgical stabilisation of the rheumatoid cervical spine. A review of indications and results. J Bone Joint Surg Br. 1987;69:8–12.
21. Clark CR, Goetz DD, Menezes AH. Arthrodesis of the cervical spine in rheumatoid arthritis. J Bone Joint Surg Am. 1989;71:381–92.
22. Kourtopoulos H, von Essen C. Stabilization of the unstable upper cervical spine in rheumatoid arthritis. Acta Neurochir. 1988;91:113–5.
23. McCarron RF, Robertson WW. Brooks fusion for atlantoaxial instability in rheumatoid arthritis. South Med J. 1988;81:474–6.

24. Papadopoulos SM, Dickman CA, Sonntag VK. Atlantoaxial stabilization in rheumatoid arthritis. J Neurosurg. 1991;74:1–7. https://doi.org/10.3171/jns.1991.74.1.0001.
25. Weissman BN, Aliabadi P, Weinfeld MS, et al. Prognostic features of atlantoaxial subluxation in rheumatoid arthritis patients. Radiology. 1982;144:745–51. https://doi.org/10.1148/radiology.144.4.7111719.
26. Terashima Y, Yurube T, Hirata H, et al. Predictive risk factors of cervical spine instabilities in rheumatoid arthritis: a prospective multicenter over 10-year cohort study. Spine. 2017;42:556–64. https://doi.org/10.1097/BRS.0000000000001853.
27. Pellicci PM, Ranawat CS, Tsairis P, Bryan WJ. A prospective study of the progression of rheumatoid arthritis of the cervical spine. J Bone Joint Surg Am. 1981;63:342–50.
28. Winfield J, Cooke D, Brook AS, Corbett M. A prospective study of the radiological changes in the cervical spine in early rheumatoid disease. Ann Rheum Dis. 1981;40:109–14.
29. Wolfs JFC, Kloppenburg M, Fehlings MG, et al. Neurologic outcome of surgical and conservative treatment of rheumatoid cervical spine subluxation: a systematic review. Arthritis Rheum. 2009;61:1743–52. https://doi.org/10.1002/art.25011.

43 Treatment Options in Severe Cervico-Thoracal Deformity in "Bechterew's Disease"

George K. Prezerakos and Adrian T. H. Casey

43.1 Introduction

Cervical deformity though uncommon, can result in significant limitations in physical function and everyday life activities. It usually occurs in the sagittal plane partly because of the cervical spine biomechanics (less load dispersed to the anterior column) and partly because of the nature of the underlying causes, which are usually kyphogenic [1]. The spectrum of clinical manifestations includes at one end neck pain and various levels of neurological deficit myelopathy or radiculopathy, to loss of horizontal gaze, swallowing difficulties, self-feeding and self-dressing difficulties and maintaining hygiene [2, 3].

43.2 Etiology

The causes of cervical deformity are numerous. They include trauma, infection and neoplasms (metastatic or neural tumours) where loss of the anterior column or impairment of the posterior elements can lead to sub-axial cervical and cevricothoracic deformity most commonly in the sagittal plane. As the spine column retains a degree of mobility, the reducible nature of such deformities makes them amenable to a wide spectrum of surgical correction strategies (ventral, dorsal or combination) without usually the need for extended osteotomies [4–6].

Congenital and neuromuscular pathologies, though rare can lead to imbalances most commonly in the coronal plane and scoliotic deformity.

Iatrogenic causes are one of the commonest causes of cervical deformity and include cervical laminectomy kyphosis, fusion-instrumentation failure or radiation to the paraspinal musculature resulting in atrophy and loss of posterior tension band resulting in sagittal imbalance in the drop head syndrome [7, 8].

Inflammatory and autoimmune diseases such as ankylosing spondylitis (A.S) are some of the most common causes of fixed, irreducible cervicothoracic deformities [5]. It is this type of deformity that this book chapter will mainly focus on, though the correction strategies can be applied to the previously mentioned types of deformity.

43.2.1 Ankylosing Spondylitis

Ankylosing spondylitis is an inflammatory condition of the spine associated with HLA B27. Typically, it starts in the sacro-iliac joints and

G. K. Prezerakos · A. T. H. Casey (✉)
Victor Horsley Department of Neurosurgery, The National Hospital for Neurology and Neurosurgery, Queen Square, London, UK

B. Meyer, M. Rauschmann (eds.), *Spine Surgery*, https://doi.org/10.1007/978-3-319-98875-7_43

works proximally to involve fusion of lumbar spine, then thoracic spine and rib cage and then cervical spine. It has been described by Bechterew, Strumpell and Pierre Marie. Other genes have been identified that are associated with ankylosing spondylitis, including ARTS1 and IL23R.

Ankylosing spondylitis shares many features with several other arthritis conditions, such as psoriatic arthritis, reactive arthritis (formerly called Reiter's disease), and arthritis associated with Crohn's disease and ulcerative colitis. Each of these arthritic conditions can cause disease and inflammation in the spine, other joints, eyes, skin, mouth, and various organs. In view of their similarities and tendency to cause inflammation of the spine, these medical conditions are collectively referred to as "spondyloarthropathies."

The major types of medications used to treat ankylosing spondylitis are pain-relievers and drugs aimed at stopping or slowing the progression of the disease.

The mainstay of therapy in all seronegative spondyloarthropathies are anti-inflammatory drugs, which include NSAIDs such as ibuprofen, phenylbutazone, diclofenac, indomethacin, naproxen and COX-2 inhibitors

Medications used to treat the progression of the disease include tumor necrosis factor-alpha (TNFα) blockers (antagonists), such as the biologics etanercept, infliximab, golimumab and adalimumab, as well as Interleukin-17A inhibitor secukinumab and Anti-interleukin-6 inhibitors such as tocilizumab.

Though early diagnosis and intervention with physical therapy, lifestyle modifications and pharmacological support is the mainstay of treatment, spinal involvement in the form of fixed kyphotic deformity primarily in the thoracolumbar region is frequent. A secondary site of involvement includes the cervical and cervicothoracic junction which can lead to a "chin on chest" type of deformity with all the associated physical and psychological and social problems. Cervical kyphosis is a failure of medical treatment by physicians and physiotherapists.

43.3 Radiological Evaluation

One of the most important markers of cervicothoracic deformity is the chin- brow to vertical angle (CBVA). This is an angle formed by a line drawn from the brow to the chin and a line parallel to the vertical axis of the patient (Fig 43.1). It reflects the severity of horizontal gaze loss as well as

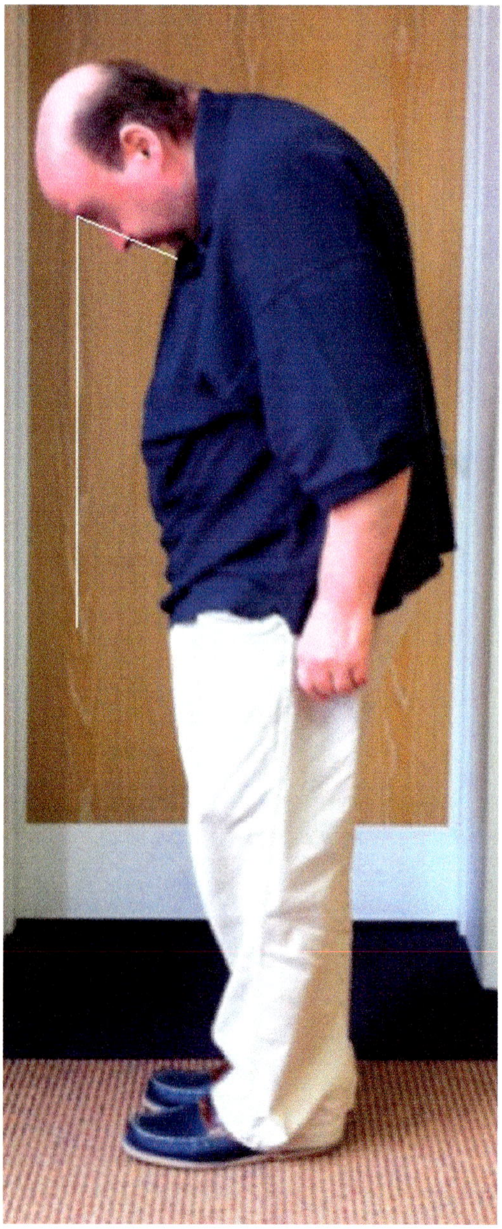

Fig. 43.1 Profile photograph with superimposed Chin Brow to Vertical Axis angle

being a measure to plan and assess the kyphotic deformity correction in ankylosing spondylitis patients [6, 9].

The cervical lordosis can be measured by the C2-C7 Cobb angle.

In severe kyphotic deformities the cervicothoracic junction can frequently form the apex of the curve and as such, the Cobb angle's distal vertebra should be modified accordingly; in the presented case, the C2-T2 angle was chosen.

Another important measure is the cervical sagittal vertical axis (cSVA). This is the horizontal distance between the plumb line from the centre of the C2 body to the posterior superior angle of C7. Again this can be modified to T2, if the CTJ forms the apex op the deformity curve. This is a significant radiological measure that not only provides clinical relevance in terms of pain, disability and quality of life scores but can also be used to plan and assess the horizontal/translational correction pre and post operatively [6, 10]. The C7 to S1 promontory sagittal vertical axis identifies misalignment in the thoracic and lumbar region, which is frequent in A.S and should be taken into consideration prior to planning corrective surgery in the CTJ.

Computed tomography is an important part of preoperative radiological assessment in order to delinate the osseous anatomy in view of instrumentation placement as well as osteotomy planning. Magnetic resonance tomography appreciates spinal cord as well as foraminal compression.

43.4 Operative Techniques

In principle, a kyphotic deformity can be corrected either by lengthening the spinal column via a ventral procedure or shortening it from the dorsal aspect or a combination of both. A significant determinant is the flexibility of the spine including the facet joint complex as well as the anterior longitudinal ligament and intervertebral discs anteriorly. In any case, the aim of surgery is to improve horizontal gaze, mobility, reduce pain and neurological disability and ultimately improve the patient's quality of life.

The overall strategies are still a matter of debate [11, 12]. Still, in fixed deformities such as in ankylosing spondylitis, surgical correction through a posterior, shortening procedure is overall a practical therapeutic choice [3, 6, 10, 13–15].

The correction can be in the form of a Smith-Petersen osteotomy (SPO) in single or more commonly multiple levels. It involves the removal of the lamina and part of the superior and inferior facet. The technique has been used extensively in its various modifications for cervicothoracic as well as thoracolumbar deformities in A.S patients [2, 16, 17].

As SPOs can be employed at many levels, advantages include evening out the stress from the correction on the neural, osseous as well as vasculature structures. There is less blood loss as bone removal is limited compared to a more extensive osteotomy. In terms of efficacy, corrections between 20° and 40° can be achieved, if multiple levels are used. Disadvantages include a high pseudoarthrosis rate, the small correction potential per SPO level, high risk of neurological injury or mortality, though this complication rate formed part of the early reports on the technique and it may not be applicable today [2, 6, 15, 18]. Furthermore, it may require a supplementary anterior approach. In the case of A.S patient, a significant limitation is the ossification of the anterior structures (including the anterior longitudinal ligament), rendering correction with a single, posterior only approach difficult.

A more effective but technically more challenging alternative is the pedicle subtraction osteotomy (PSO), whereas the amount of bone removal includes both pedicles. This procedure later evolved to include part of the posterior vertebral body, a decancellisation osteotomy, in a wedge shaped fashion or more extensively to the front of the vertebral body allowing for more corrective potential. Position evolved from sitting to prone, whereas fusion evolved from external orthosis to instrumented fixation [1, 3, 5, 10, 13–15, 19, 20].

Other variants include the "egg-shell" osteotomy and transpedicular, bivertebrae wedge osteotomy. The overall concept is to shorten the spinal column, by closing the osteotomies, thus in the literature the term "closing osteotomy" has been coined.

43.5 Case Report

We present the case of a 52-year-old man, diagnosed with ankylosing spondylitis since the age of 23. He progressively developed a "chin on chest" deformity, which rendered him, house bound and fully dependent for everyday activities. He suffered with severe neck pain with an Neck Disability Index (NDI) of 64%. He experienced significant difficulties with feeding, swallowing, self-dressing and maintaining hygiene. His mobility was significantly impaired due to almost complete loss of horizontal gaze.

His previous medical history included diabetes, hypertension and a high Body Mass Index of 36. He has been on Etanercept as well as a spectrum of anti-inflammatory medication and simple to moderate analgesics.

Pre operatively, the chin to brow angle was 68° (Fig. 43.1). A CT revealed the nose to be at the same level with heart (Figs. 43.2 and 43.3).

Cervical lordosis was 39° in kyphosis, T1 thoracic slope of 76°, cervical sagittal vertical axis −9.7 cm and thoracic slope to cervical lordosis ratio at 115°. The C2-T2 angle was 68° (Fig 43.4). The deformity was not reducible on sitting-supine dynamic radiographs.

Anteroposterior films confirmed normal alignment at the coronal plane and the C7 to sacral promontory did not reveal significant imbalance, thus thoracic and lumbar corrective surgery was deemed unnecessary.

MR imaging did not reveal cord or radicular compression (Fig 43.5).

The apex of the deformity was located at the cervicothoracic junction, in particular at C7. The patient was offered deformity correction surgery in the form of a C7 pedicle subtraction and wedge osteotomy and C2 to T4 instrumented fixation.

The patient was placed on a Mayfield 3 point fixator. The drapes were transparent to allow for visualisation of intraoperative manipulations.

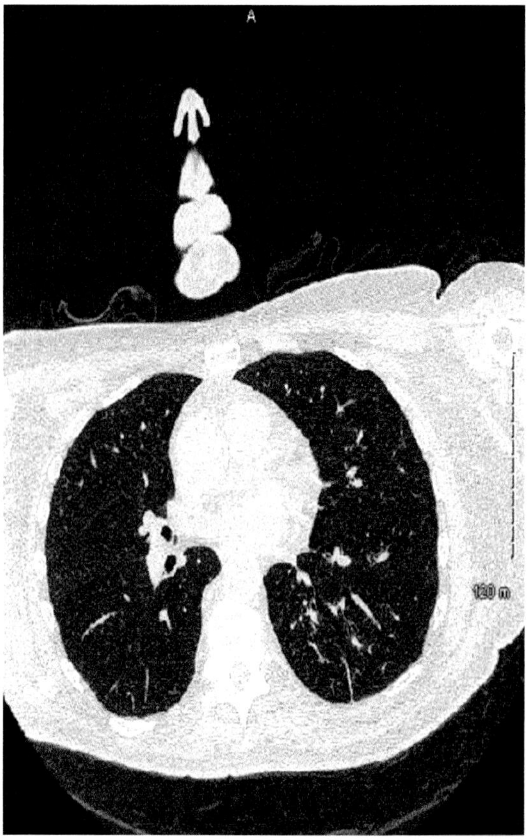

Fig. 43.2 Axial CT exhibiting the nose the heart level

Intraoperative monitoring was employed in the form of SSEPs and MEPs.

The first step was instrumentation placement with C2 bilateral pedicle screws, C3-4-5-6 lateral mass screws, and T1-2-3-4 pedicle screws.

The second step was the PSO including removal of C7 lamina, most of C6 and T1 laminae, superior and inferior facet of C7, exposure of C8 nerve roots, pedicle identification, removal of pedicles and access to C7 vertebral body.

The third step was the posterior wedge osteotomy employing ultrasonic bone cutter and lambotti osteotomes. Extra care was taken for the bone resection to be done symmetrically to avoid coronal imbalance. Finally, the posterior wall of C7 body was removed to conclude with posterior vertebral body wedge resection.

The third step was reduction under continuous image intensifier use and electrophysiological monitoring. The manipulation was done by the

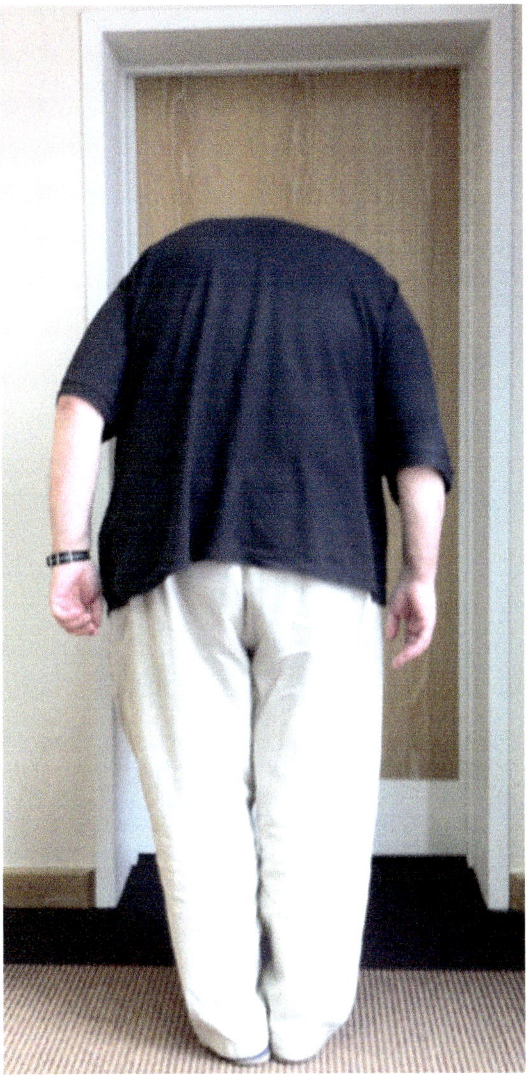

Fig. 43.3 Enface photograph

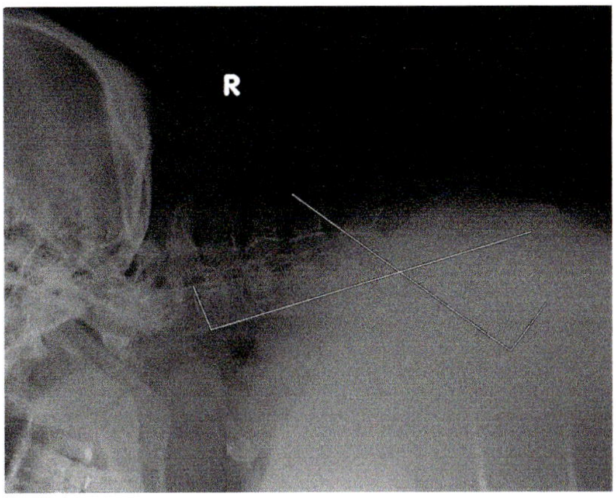

Fig. 43.4 Preoperative lateral radiograph showing a 68° angle between C2 and T2

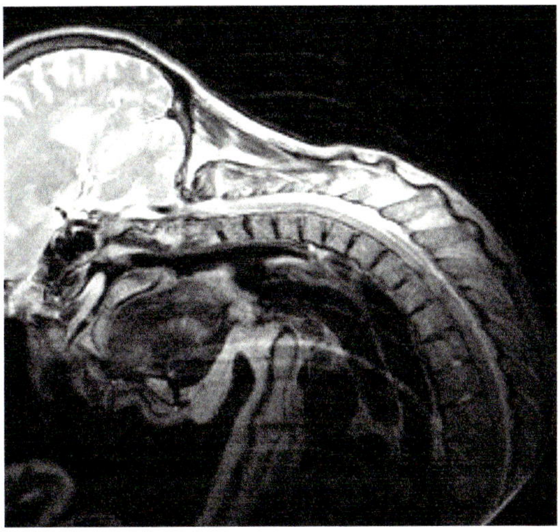

Fig. 43.5 Preoperative T2 weighted sagittal MRI of the cervicothoracic region

senior assistant, whilst the author observed the dural sac and C8 and T1 nerve roots.

The last step included application of the tapered rod.

The technique has been described elaborately elsewhere and is beyond the scope of this manuscript [10].

The patient recovered well and remained in a high dependency unit for 3 days for analgesic control optimisation and renal function management. He went on to a neurorehabilitation unit where he completed a one-month course.

Neurologically he developed a right sided adductor digiti minimi weakness (Medical Research Council grade 3/5) that persisted for 3 months only to recover fully at the 6 month postoperative point (MRC grade 4+/5).

Postoperatively, his chin to brow vertical angle was 17°. The C2-T2 angle was 13°. Cervical lordosis was positive 12° lordotic (46° improvement), thoracic slope of 73°, cervical sagittal vertical axis −5.6° cm and thoracic slope to cervical lordosis ratio at 61° (Fig. 43.6).

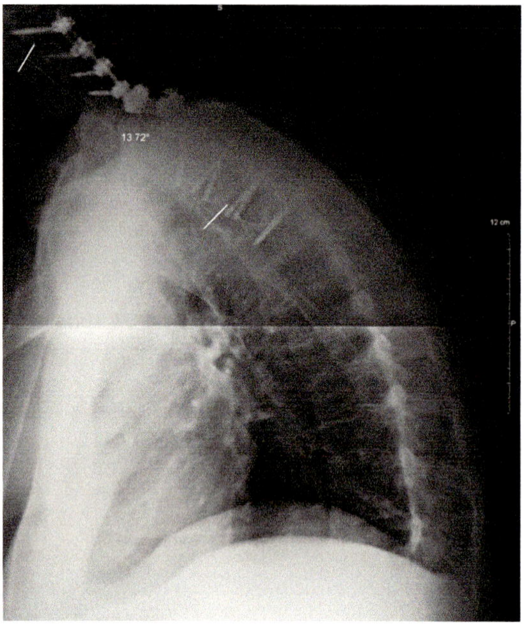

Fig. 43.6 Postoperative lateral cervicothoracic radiograph, exhibiting a C2-T2 Cobb angle of 13.7°

The osteotomy provided a correction of 55° to C2-T2 Cobb angle (Figs. 43.6 and 43.7) and 51° of correction in chin to brow (Fig. 43.8).

The correction was maintained at the final 2 year follow up.

The patient now manages daily activities independently and has even returned to part time professional activity. The NDI at the final 2 year follow up was 17%.

43.6 Discussion

Both opening/lengthening and closing/shortening osteotomies can be effective in the treatment of cervicothoracic rigid kyphosis [2]. The array of approaches includes front, back, back-front-back combinations as well as various types of SPOs and PSOs. Thus far, the studies dealing with the efficacy and safety of pedicle subtraction osteotomy in A.S patients are non-comparative, non randomised and non-prospective. As a result, there is still debate on the most optimal approach.

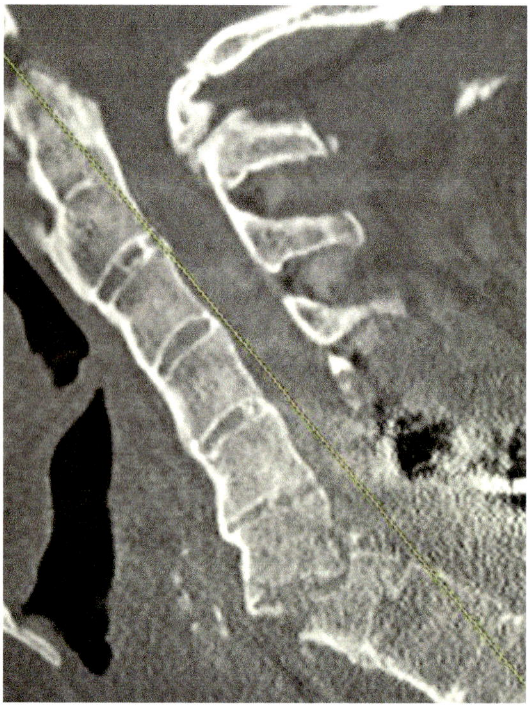

Fig. 43.7 Postoperative sagittal computed tomography exhibiting the osteotomised C7 vertebra and the associated spinal column shortening

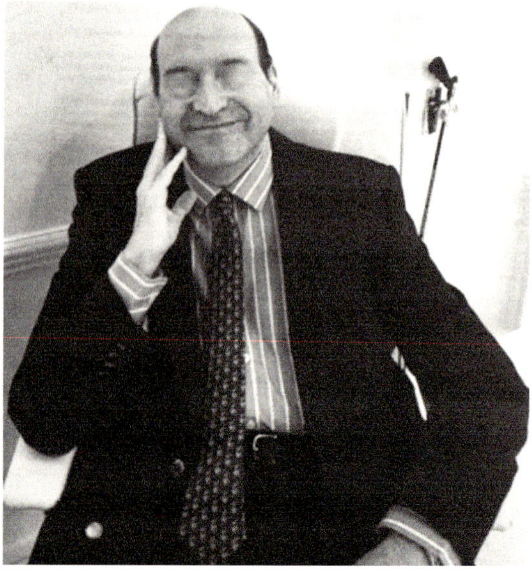

Fig. 43.8 Postoperative en face photograph

The evidence for pedicle subtraction osteotomy in fixed kyphotic deformity is derived from retrospective case series, classed as level III [21].

Simmons described the concept of a single posterior wedge shaped cervical osteotomy for the treatment of ankylosing spondylitis [22]. He performed a laminectomy and bilateral facetectomies and pedicle removal at C-7 and extended his osteotomy to include the spinous processes of C-6 and T-1. Various reasons make the C7 or T1 vertebra an attractive option. The vertebral artery enters the foramen transversarium at C6, the pedicles are wider than the rest of the sub-axial spine, the spinal canal is wider and the shape of the vertebrae is larger. Quite commonly the deformity apex is located at the cervicothoracic junction.

In the modern era, the original technique has been modified to involve a more extensive vertebral body resection with complete pedicular resection, thus creating more space for the dura, cord and C8 and T1 nerve roots. Simmons reported on his 36 years experience with 131 patients, where 17 patients underwent a modifications of the original technique with a more extensive osteotomy with halo vest orthosis. Surgery took place in the sitting position. Mean correction was 37°. Two patients developed a C8 palsy and one a hemiparesis. Three patients developed pin site infections [13]. McMaster, Belanger, Langeloo, Tokala Etame and Samudrala have all published their series on the use of PSO in subaxial deformity A.S patients [1, 3, 10, 14, 19, 20].

McMaster et al., employing a similar technique as Simmons, achieved 54° corrections. His series of 15 patients reported 1 quadraparesis, 2 transient C8 motor radiculopathies, 4 sensory C8 radiculopathies and a deep wound infection.

Belanger et al. achieved 38° of correction with a wide range between 15° and 84°. Two permanent and three sensory radiculopathies and one mortality.

Langeloo et al. published their experience with PSO for fixed cervical deformity in 16 A.S patients. 33° of kyphosis correction and 37° of CBVA improvement. They reported one death, one spinal cord injury and nine transient C8 radiculopathies.

Tokala et al. reported on their experience with decancellisation, posterior closing wedge osteotomy, a variant of a PSO with more extensive vertebral body resection. Five out of their eight patients were A.S patients. They achieved 57° of sagittal correction with 36° of CBVA improvement. Three patients developed spontaneously resolving sensory radiculopathies, two developed infections and one sustained a C6-T1 subluxation that did not warrant revision surgery [10].

Samudrala, Johnson et al. reported on eight patients that underwent C7 or T1 PSO for CTJ fixed kyphotic deformity (not of A.S aetiology) They achieved 38.67° of kyphosis correction (15–66°) with concurrent pain reduction and restoration of horizontal gaze. They report two sensorimotor radiculopathies and an upper limb weakness that required multilevel revision foraminal decompression.

Recently, Kim, Riew et al. reported on a comparative retrospective series between PSO, SPO, SPO with anterior osteotomy (ATO) [15]. They found similar corrective potential between PSOs and combined SPOs -ATOs. In particular they reported on 61 patients, 10 of which underwent PSO. The mean angular correction was 44.8° and the total mean translational correction was 2.8 cm. This was superior to SPOs, anterior osteotomy or combined, though combined ATO and SPOs provided for better translational correction (3.6 cm vs 2.8 cm). Interestingly, no neurological complications were reported in any group. There was however a C6-T1 anterior subluxation in a C7 PSO patient that required revision surgery. Furthermore, they reported one infection and one C1 screw symptomatic instrumentation misplacement [15].

Alternatives to a PSO include sequential dilatation via corpectomy as described by Mumanneni et al., achieving 24° of correction. Sixteen percent of patients required a posterior approach, only 7/100 had more than 20° of kyphosis and there were no fixed deformities or A.S patients [23]. The complication profile was overall favourable though 3 nerve root palsies and 14 cases of postoperative dysphagia were reported.

Wang, Ames et al. described an anterior only approach that achieves a 3 column correction in both sagittal and coronal planes. It involves mobilising the vertebral artery laterally and proceeds with a lateral corpectomy and facetectomy, all from a ventral access [24].

Etame et al., reviewing the aforementioned studies excluding those by Kim et al. and Samudrala et al., reported the complication rate to be high, ranging between 26.9% and 87.5% with a mortality rate of 2.6%. This is a more accurate real world figure on which to counsel patents pre operatively. Neurological morbidity accounts for 4.3%, whilst transient neurology – most commonly C8 radiculopathy- was 23.4% [1].

Nonetheless, all series report a 100% restoration of horizontal gaze in with a high degree of patient satisfaction [19]. The PSO exhibits favourable reconstructive potential, as it allows for a 3 column correction, its shortening nature avoids stress on the visceral or neural structures, it can be used in a fusion mass (as is often in previous failed cervical fusion or indeed in A.S patients), allows bone on bone contact in all three columns and most importantly exhibits a powerful corrective profile. Occasionally major kinking of the posterior dura necessitates duroplasty.

43.7 Conclusion

Pedicle subtraction osteotomy exhibits a significant deformity correction profile in fixed kyphotic deformity in A.S patients, suffering with chin on chest deformity. Its efficacy allows for improvement in the patient's functional status, quality of life and disability indices. Nevertheless, it is a surgically challenging technique and can come at a substantial cost in terms of neurological as well as non-neurological morbidity.

Editorial Comment

This presented technique of correction (PSO) in the cervicothoracic junction in patients with rheumatological disorders, is a complex surgical procedure, which should only be done by centers, who deal frequently with this type of correction. It should not be done without experience.

References

1. Etame AB, Wang AC, Than KD, et al. Outcomes after surgery for cervical spine deformity: review of the literature. Neurosurg Focus. 2010;28:E14. https://doi.org/10.3171/2010.1.FOCUS09278.
2. Hu X, Thapa AJ, Cai Z, et al. Comparison of smith-petersen osteotomy, pedicular subtraction osteotomy, and poly-segmental wedge osteotomy in treating rigid thoracolumbar kyphotic deformity in ankylosing spondylitis a systematic review and meta-analysis. BMC Surg. 2016;16:4. https://doi.org/10.1186/s12893-015-0118-x.
3. McMaster MJ. Osteotomy of the cervical spine in ankylosing spondylitis. J Bone Joint Surg Br. 1997;79:197–203.
4. Kubiak EN, Moskovich R, Errico TJ, Di Cesare PE. Orthopaedic management of ankylosing spondylitis. J Am Acad Orthop Surg. 2005;13:267–78.
5. Steinmetz MP, Stewart TJ, Kager CD, et al. Cervical deformity correction. Neurosurgery. 2007;60:S90–7. https://doi.org/10.1227/01.NEU.0000215553.49728.B0.
6. Samudrala S, Vaynman S, Thiayananthan T, et al. Cervicothoracic junction kyphosis: surgical reconstruction with pedicle subtraction osteotomy and Smith-Petersen osteotomy. Presented at the 2009 Joint Spine Section Meeting. Clinical article. J Neurosurg Spine. 2010;13:695–706. https://doi.org/10.3171/2010.5.SPINE08608.
7. Deutsch H, Haid RW, Rodts GE, Mummaneni PV. Postlaminectomy cervical deformity. Neurosurg Focus. 2003;15:E5.
8. Gerling MC, Bohlman HH. Dropped head deformity due to cervical myopathy: surgical treatment outcomes and complications spanning twenty years. Spine. 2008;33:E739–45. https://doi.org/10.1097/BRS.0b013e31817f1f8b.
9. Suk K-S, Kim K-T, Lee S-H, Kim J-M. Significance of chin-brow vertical angle in correction of kyphotic deformity of ankylosing spondylitis patients. Spine. 2003;28:2001–5. https://doi.org/10.1097/01.BRS.0000083239.06023.78.
10. Tokala DP, Lam KS, Freeman BJC, Webb JK. C7 decancellisation closing wedge osteotomy for the correction of fixed cervico-thoracic kyphosis. Eur Spine J. 2007;16:1471–8. https://doi.org/10.1007/s00586-006-0290-x.
11. Anderson DG, Silbert J, Albert TJ. Management of cervical kyphosis caused by surgery, degenerative disease, or trauma. In: The Cervical Spine, 4th ed. Lippincott Williams & Wilkins: Philadephia, PA; 2005, p. 1135–46.
12. Grosso MJ, Hwang R, Krishnaney AA, et al. Complications and outcomes for surgical approaches to cervical kyphosis. J Spinal Disord Tech. 2015;28:E385–93. https://doi.org/10.1097/BSD.0b013e318299953f.
13. Simmons ED, DiStefano RJ, Zheng Y, Simmons EH. Thirty-six years experience of cervical extension osteotomy in ankylosing spondylitis: techniques and outcomes. Spine. 2006;31:3006–12. https://doi.org/10.1097/01.brs.0000250663.12224.d9.

14. Belanger TA, Milam RAI, Roh JS, Bohlman HH. Cervicothoracic extension osteotomy for chin-on-chest deformity in ankylosing spondylitis. JBJS. 2005;87:1732.
15. Kim K-T, Park D-H, Lee S-H, Lee J-H. Results of corrective osteotomy and treatment strategy for ankylosing spondylitis with kyphotic deformity. Clin Orthop Surg. 2015;7:330–6. https://doi.org/10.4055/cios.2015.7.3.330.
16. Briggs H, Keats S, Schlesinger PT. Wedge osteotomy of the spine with bilateral intervertebral foraminotomy; correction of flexion deformity in five cases of ankylosing arthritis of the spine. J Bone Joint Surg Am. 1947;29:1075–82.
17. La Chapelle EH. Osteotomy of the lumbar spine for correction of kyphosis in a case of ankylosing spondylarthritis. J Bone Joint Surg Am. 1946;28:851–8.
18. Kim HJ, Piyaskulkaew C, Riew KD. Comparison of Smith-Petersen osteotomy versus pedicle subtraction osteotomy versus anterior-posterior osteotomy types for the correction of cervical spine deformities. Spine. 2015;40:143–6. https://doi.org/10.1097/BRS.0000000000000707.
19. Etame AB, Than KD, Wang AC, et al. Surgical management of symptomatic cervical or cervico-thoracic kyphosis due to ankylosing spondylitis. Spine. 2008;33:E559–64. https://doi.org/10.1097/BRS.0b013e31817c6c64.
20. Langeloo DD, Journee HL, Pavlov PW, de Kleuver M. Cervical osteotomy in ankylosing spondylitis: evaluation of new developments. Eur Spine J. 2006;15:493–500. https://doi.org/10.1007/s00586-005-0945-z.
21. OCEBM levels of evidence – CEBM. https://www.cebm.net/2016/05/ocebm-levels-of-evidence/. Accessed 30 Apr 2018.
22. Simmons EH. The surgical correction of flexion deformity of the cervical spine in ankylosing spondylitis. Clin Orthop Relat Res. 1972;86:132–43.
23. Lau D, Ziewacz JE, Le H, et al. A controlled anterior sequential interbody dilation technique for correction of cervical kyphosis. J Neurosurg Spine. 2015;23:263–73. https://doi.org/10.3171/2014.12.SPINE14178.
24. Wang VY, Aryan H, Ames CP. A novel anterior technique for simultaneous single-stage anterior and posterior cervical release for fixed kyphosis: technical note. J Neurosurg Spine. 2008;8:594–9. https://doi.org/10.3171/SPI/2008/8/6/594.

44 Diagnosis and Treatment of the Occipito-Atlantoaxial Complex and Subaxial Cervical Spine in Rheumatoid Diseases

Marcus Rickert

44.1 Introduction

The cervical spine involvement in rheumatoid arthritis (RA) is still of significant clinical relevance, although the clinical use of biologicals significantly reduced the incidence and severity of cervical destructions in RA.

Typically the rheumatoid destruction starts at the atlanto-axial joints and ligaments, often resulting in an atlanto-axial subluxation and may progress to cranio-cervical and subaxial instability. Due to the instability and compression of the myelon a cervical myelopathy can occur at any time and leads to a deterioration of the prognosis for the patient. The aim of the treatment in cervical spine involvement due to RA is to improve the symptoms and to prevent further progression. In case of severe instabilities an operative therapy is indicated. The clinical presentation of the rheumatoid cervical spine changed due to the increasing use of biologicals. The incidence of isolated atlanto-axial instability is reduced, whereas complex cranio-cervical and subaxial instabilities become more frequent. These patients often require longer instrumented fusions from the occiput to the upper thoracic spine. Modern operation techniques, implant systems and the availability of spinal navigation make these complex operations also possible in severely disabled patients with high comorbidities.

This chapter will outline the specifics of rheumatoid instability of the cervical spine, its typical symptomatology, mandatory preoperative imaging and surgical approaches.

At the end of this chapter the reader should be aware of the problems and pitfalls we face when treating rheumatoid instabilities of the cervical spine.

The aim of the presented case is therefore to emphasize the typical diagnostic workout and principles of operative therapy.

44.2 Case Description

A 61-year old female patient with RA since 30 years, significant involvement of the cervical spine and mutilating destruction of both hands and feet, as well as both knees and hips which recently led to bilateral total hip and knee replacement. She was under treatment with a biological (Humira, Adalimumab, TNF-α blocker) at clinical presentation. It was paused 4 weeks preoperative and 2 weeks postoperative.

M. Rickert (✉)
Spine Center, St. Josefs-Hospital,
Wiesbaden, Germany
e-mail: mrichter@joho.de

B. Meyer, M. Rauschmann (eds.), *Spine Surgery*, https://doi.org/10.1007/978-3-319-98875-7_44

The patient suffered from increasing cervical pain since 2 years and a progressive cervical myelopathy with a JOA-Score of 11. Additional she had a bilateral C8-Syndrom. The neurophysiological examination showed pathological MEP's and SSEP's as well as pathological EMG C8. The functional X-rays show a occipito-cervical instability with basilar impression. The anterior atlantodental distance was 8 mm (normal <3.5 mm). Furthermore the imaging showed a C7/Th1 rheumatoid instability with a slippage of 5 mm (normal <3.5 mm) with consecutive compression of the myelon. In rheumatoid patients the grade of instability is often very difficult to quantify using lateral x-ray images. This can be done much better with CT. The tip of the odontoid was measured 17 mm above McRae's line (odontoid not above McRae line is normal). The MRI shows an anterior compression of the medulla oblongata and the myelon down to C2 and a spinal stenosis C7-Th1 due to the instability in this level (Fig. 44.1).

The patient was admitted to the hospital and operated 3 days after the first clinical presentation. A posterior instrumentation from occiput to Th3 with open reduction of the occipito-cervical junction and the cervico-thoracic junction was performed. Due to significant destruction of the lateral masses C1 and a bilateral high riding transverse foramen C2 transarticular screws C1/2 or pedicle screws C2 could not be used. Also subaxial cervical pedicle screws were not possible due to very small cervical pedicles (Fig. 44.2).

Because of the anatomical limitations instead of transarticular screws C1/2 and subaxial pedicle screws lateral mass screws C3 and C4 were combined with pedicle screws Th1, Th2 and Th3. The pedicle screws in Th1-Th3 were placed with spinal navigation using the preoperative CT and surface matching. Posterior decompression of the cranio-cervical junction was done with resection of the posterior arch of C1 and widening of the foramen magnum. Indirect decompression of C7/Th1 was done with open reduction and fixation. For posterior fusion from the occiput down to Th3 local bone from the decompression and bone substitute (Actifuse Putty, Baxter) was used. Surgery went fine without adverse events and the preoperative neurological deficits were significantly improved postoperative. Sufficient decompression was confirmed by postoperative MRI scan on the fifth postoperative day (Fig. 44.3). Thus no anterior transoral or transnasal resection of the odontoid was necessary.

During the postoperative period the patient had wound secretion for 10 days in the cranial third of the wound which resolved without revision. Stitches were removed 16 days postopera-

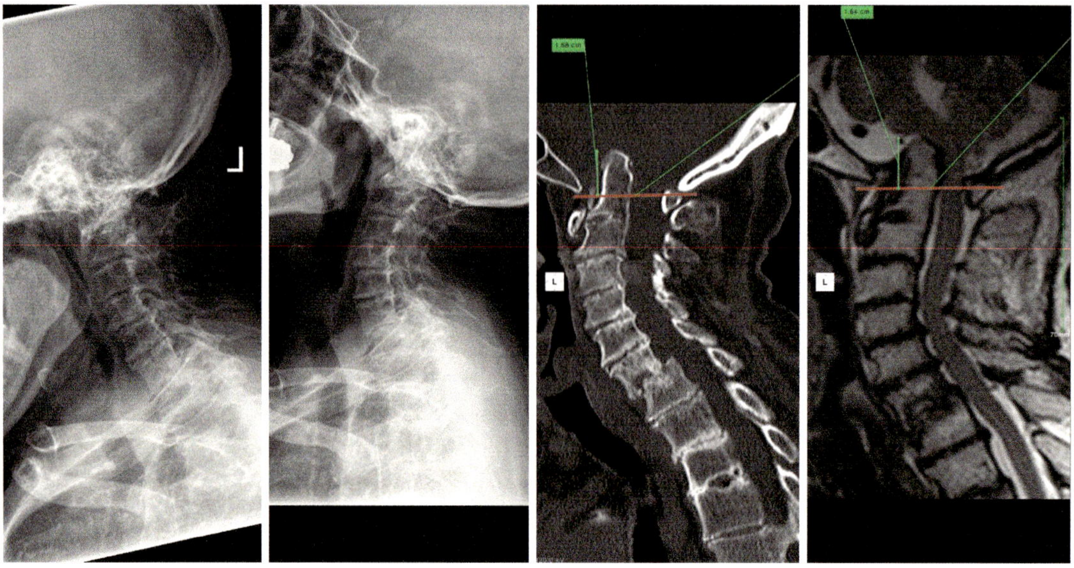

Fig. 44.1 X-Ray, CT and MRI scan on outpatient visit

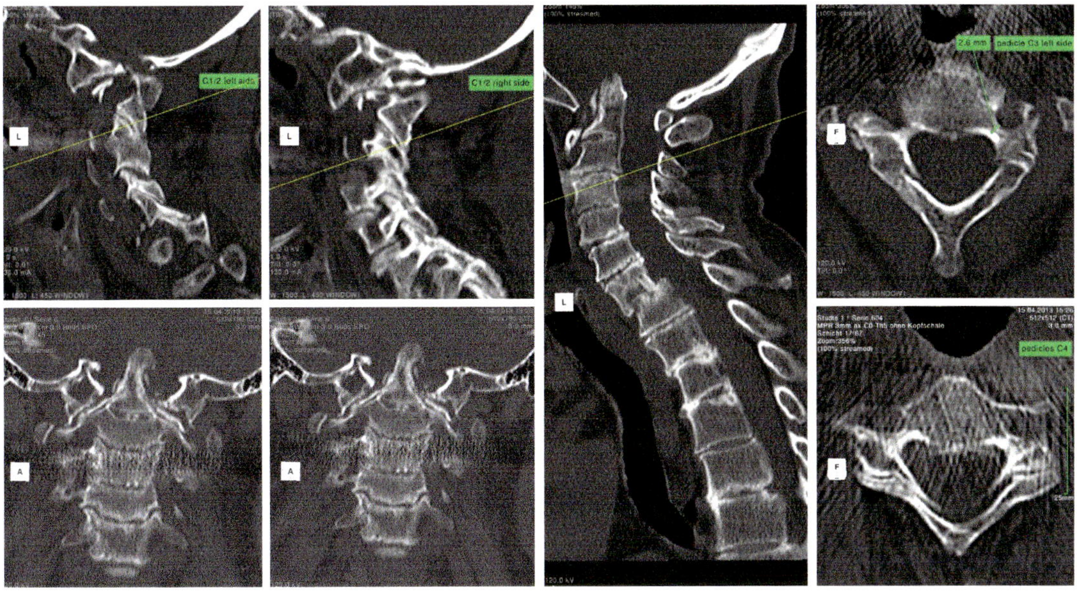

Fig. 44.2 Preoperative CT scan. Multiplanar reconstructions of the CT for preoperative screw planning show a high riding transverse foramen C2 and nearly complete destruction bilateral of the lateral masses C1 as well as small subaxial pedicles with a pedicle width <3 mm

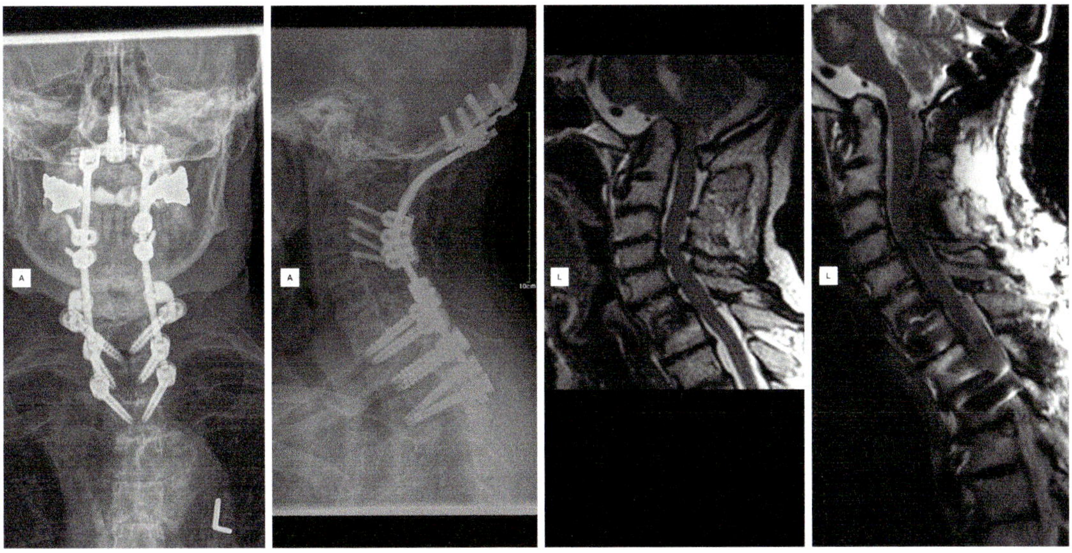

Fig. 44.3 Postoperative X-Ray and MRI. Postoperative X-ray shows good reduction of the cranio-cervical junction (**a** + **b**). The postoperative MRI (**d**) shows a good reduction and decompression of the cranio-cervical junction compared to the preoperative MRI (**c**)

tive. The patient was discharged home 20 days postoperative. At discharge the JOA-Score had significantly improved to 14 and the C8 symptoms were no more existent. The wound was healed without secretion or dehiscence.

44.3 Discussion of the Case

Indication and Techniques

The clinical symptoms of RA patients are often unspecific in the early stage. With increasing amount of the atlanto-axial instability a radiculopathy C2 is typical. Progressive bony destructions often lead to increasing neck pain and headache. With further progression of the instability and presence of a occipito-cervical instability vascular symptoms like vertigo, nystagmus and syncopes can occur. In case of myelon compression myelopathy can occur, but is more difficult to diagnose as reflexes, gait disturbance and motoric changes of the hands are difficult to examine in RA patients due to the destruction of the joints. In inclination of the head a positive Lhermitte sign is typical in occipito-cervical instability.

Indications for operative treatment in rheumatoid instability of the cervical spine are based on the amount and type of instability, compression of the myelon with myelopathy and untreatable pain.

Indications for isolated atlanto-occipital instrumented fusions are [1–3]:

- Atlanto-axial instability with anterior atlanto-dental distance >8 mm
- Symptomatic atlanto-axial arthritis (often unilateral)

An occipito-cervical instability with basilar impression or destruction of the occipito-atlantal joints should be excluded, these would be indications for occipito-cervical instrumented fusions.

The standard operative technique for rheumatoid C1/2 instabilities is the combination of transarticular screws C1/2 with a posterior three-point fixation (Galli technique with a cortical bone graft or atlas-claws connected to the C1/2 screws with bone substitute) [1–3]. The atlas-claw technique has a reduced morbidity because no cortical bone graft is needed. It is important to stabilize C1/2 in a neutral position, because the fixation in hyperextension leads to an increased risk of developing a subaxial kyphosis [4].

The alternative technique is the combination of lateral mass screws C1 with pedicle screws or isthmic screws C2, first described by Goel and Laheri [5]. The disadvantage of this technique is the possible irritation of the C2 root, especially in rheumatoid patients, the higher bloodloss and the reduced stability in flexion/extension [6, 7].

In cases where transarticular screw C1/2 are not possible due to a high riding transverse foramen or bony destructions the Goel technique is indicated.

Indications for occipito-cervical/thoracic instrumented fusion are [8]:

- Vertical instability with basilar impression due to bony destruction of the lateral masses C1 with or without atlanto-axial instability
- Destruction of the occipito-atlantal joints

The occipito-cervical fusion should be as short as possible (Occiput-C2) but not longer than C4. In case of subaxial instability should the fusion be extended to the upper thoracic spine (Th3).

The screw techniques for atlanto-axial fixation are the same as earlier described for isolated C1/2 fixation, whereas no posterior three-point fixation is necessary because of the fixation with rods to the occiput. If due to significant bony destructions a sufficient fixation in C1/2 is not possible the instrumentation should be extended to C3 with pedicle screws C3 or to C4 with lateral mass screws C3 and C4.

In patients with mutilating RA the risk of development of subaxial instabilities is significantly increased, therefore the indication of a long instrumentation down to Th3 with high thoracic pedicle screws should be discussed, even if at time of operation of an occipito-cervical instability no subaxial instability is present [9, 10].

In occipito-thoracic fusions the risk of adjacent fractures is increased, especially if the fusion is extended to Th4 or longer [11].

Indications for anterior transoral or endoscopic transnasal odontoid resection are rare:

- Persistent compression of the medulla oblongata and/or the myelon after posterior open reduction, stabilization and decompression

Due to the fact that after posterior stabilization the retrodental pannus regresses completely [2] the need for anterior transoral or endoscopic transnasal odontoid resection is very rare and it is only indicated in non-reducable dislocations of the odontoid with anterior bony compression of the medulla oblongata and/or the myelon.

Indications for isolated anterior instrumented fusions (ACDF) are rare:

- Mono- or bisegmental stenosis due to soft- and/or harddisc without instability

In case of subaxial instability at the stenotic level an additional posterior instrumentation is beneficial because of the high risk of implant failure with ACDF alone due to the very poor bone quality in RA patients. Multisegmental stenosis should be treated with posterior instrumentation and decompression.

For transarticular screws C1/2 and pedicle screws C2 -high thoracic the use of spinal navigation is benficial and reduces the implant malplacement rates significantly [12].

In the presented case based on the recommendations published the indication was given for an occipito-cervical fusion because of the occipito-cervical instability with severe basilar impression and compression of the myelon with myelopathy, significant destruction of the lateral masses C1, destruction of the occipito-atlantal joints and the atlanto-axial instability. The extension to Th3 was indicated due to the subaxial instability C7/Th1. Spinal navigation was used for the placement of the pedicle screws Th1, 2 and 3.

Without the subaxial instability C7/Th1 only a occipito-cervical instrumented fusion would have been indicated. Because of the high riding transverse foramen C2 for sufficient stability the instrumentation could not have been stopped at C2 but should be extended to C4 with lateral mass screws C3 and C4. In case of suitable pedicles the instrumentation could have been shorter ending at C3 with pedicle screws C3. The postoperative MRI showed a sufficient decompression of the medulla oblongata and the myelon due to reduction and posterior decompression. Therefore no anterior decompression was necessary.

Complications

The rate of complications after operative treatment of RA patients is higher compared to non-RA patients. Especially the risk of wound healing problems and infections is increased [13]. The main reason is the treatment with immunsupressive drugs, especially biologicals. There are guidelines published which immunsupressive drugs should be paused before an operation and how long [14].

The presented patient had a therapy with a biological (Humira, Adalimumab, TNF-α blocker) which had to be paused 4 weeks preoperatively and 2 weeks postoperatively according to the existing guidelines. Nevertheless the patient developed a wound healing problem with wound secretion for 10 days in the cranial third of the wound which resolved without revision.

Accordance with the Literature Guidelines

As discussed above, the patient was successful treated according to the existing guidelines from the literature.

Level of Evidence: A-C

The level of evidence available to date is C for the clinical data and A for the use of spinal navigation and the biomechanical data concerning the instrumentation techniques.

44.4 Conclusions and Take Home Message

Typically the rheumatoid destruction starts at the atlanto-axial joints and ligaments, often resulting in an atlanto-axial subluxation and may progress to cranio-cervical and subaxial instability. Due to the instability and compression of the myelon a cervical myelopathy can occur at any time and leads to a deterioration of the prognosis for the patient. The aim of the treatment in cervical spine involvement due to RA is to improve the symptoms and to prevent further progression. In case of severe instabilities an operative therapy is indicated. The incidence of isolated atlanto-axial instability is reduced, whereas complex cranio-cervical and subaxial instabilities become more frequent. These patients often require longer instrumented fusions from the occiput to the upper thoracic spine.

Pearls

- The incidence of operative treatment in cervical rheumatoid instabilities is reduced in the last years due to the treatment with biologicals
- In most cases a posterior approach and stabilization is indicated
- Progressive neurological deficits are rare but indications for operative therapy
- Complication rates are high, especially wound healing problems and infections, therefore biologicals should be paused according to the existing guidelines

References

1. Grob D, Luca A, Mannion A. An observational study of patient-rated outcome after atlanto-axial fusion in patients with rheumatoid arthritis and osteoarthritis. Clin Orthop Relat Res. 2011;469:702–7.
2. Grob D, Würsch R, Grauer W, et al. Atlantoaxial fusion and retrodental pannus in rheumatoid arthritis. Spine. 1997;22:1580–4.
3. Weidner A, Wähler M, Chiu ST, et al. Modification of C1-C2 transarticular screw fixation by image guided surgery. Spine. 2000;25:2668–74.
4. Iizuka H, Iizuka Y, Kobayashi R, et al. Effect of a reduction of the atlanto-axial angle on the cranio-cervical and subaxial angles following atlanto-axial arthrodesis in rheumatoid arthritis. Eur Spine J. 2013;22:1137–41.
5. Goel A, Laheri V. Plate and screw fixation for atlanto-axial subluxation. Acta Neurochir Wien. 1994;129:47–53.
6. Richter M, Schmidt R, Claes L. Posterior atlantoaxial fixation. Biomechanical comparison of six different techniques. Spine. 2002;27:1724–32.
7. Sim HB, Lee JW, Park JT, et al. Biomechanical evaluations of various C1-C2 posterior fixation techniques. Spine. 2011;36:E401–7.
8. Tanouchi T, Shimizu T, Fueki K, et al. Neurological improvement and prognosis after occipito-thoracic fusion in patients with mutilating-type rheumatoid arthritis. Eur Spine J. 2012;21:2506–11.
9. Fujiwara K, Owaki H, Fujimoto M, et al. A long-term follow-up study of cervical lesions in rheumatoid arthritis. J Spinal Disord. 2000;13:519–26.
10. Yurube T, Sumi M, Nishida K, et al. Incidence and aggravation of cervical spine instabilities in rheumatoid arthritis. Spine. 2012;37:2136–44.
11. Tanouchi T, Shimizu T, Fueki K, et al. Adjacent-level failures after occipito-thoracic fusion for rheumatoid cervical disorders. Eur Spine J. 2014;23:635–40.
12. Shin BJ, James AR, Njoku IU, et al. Pedicle screw navigation: a systematic review and meta-analysis of perforation risk for computer-navigated versus freehand insertion. J Neurosurg Spine. 2012;17:113–22.
13. Klemencsics I, Lazary A, Szoverfi Z, et al. Risk factors for surgical site infection in elective routine degenerative lumbar surgeries. Spine J. 2016;16:1377–83.
14. Kothe R. Management von immunsupprimierten Patienten. In: Börm W, Meyer F, Bullmann V, Knop C, editors. Wirbelsäule interdisiplinär: Operative und konservative Therapie. Stuttgart: Schattauer; 2017. p. 655–6.

45 Osteoporosis (Etiology, Diagnosis, Drug Therapy, Surgical Therapy)

Haiko Pape and Yu-Mi Ryang

45.1 Introduction

Patients with osteoporotic vertebral compression fractures (OVCF), both asymptomatic and symptomatic, are part of our daily routine as spine surgeons.

Despite the fact that osteoporosis is very common and widespread – with an estimated prevalence of five to six million people in Germany and an obvious surge within the next decades due to an increase in life expectancy – there is still a lack of knowledge concerning adequate diagnosis and treatment.

Osteoporosis is defined as a systemic, progressive, metabolic disease of the bones with a decreased bone mass and a reduced quality of the microarchitecture of bone tissue, consecutively leading to an increased fragility of the bones and a predisposition to fractures. The operational definition by the WHO for osteoporosis is a bone mineral density (BMD) 2.5 standard deviations below that of a young adult reference population (T-score at or below −2.5) as measured by a dual-energy x-ray absorptiometry (DXA) of the femur or lumbar spine.

H. Pape · Y.-M. Ryang (✉)
Department of Neurosurgery, Klinikum rechts der Isar, Technische Universität München, Munich, Germany
e-mail: yu.ryang@tum.de

Fractures are frequently associated with significant pain, leading to disability and a reduced quality of life and the risk to suffer from another fracture in the near future [1].

The major osteoporotic fractures (hip, proximal femur, vertebral body, forearm) are also associated with a higher mortality, especially within the first year [2, 3].

Therefore, patients need our expertise to improve their situation and it is mandatory for spine surgeons, not only to know and perform the proper diagnostic modalities to establish the diagnosis of an osteoporotic vertebral fracture, it is also essential to know about the advantages and risks of both conservative and surgical treatment options.

The aims of the case we present are:

On the one hand to illustrate a typical case of an OVCF and its adequate therapy, on the other hand to emphasize possible pitfalls regarding operative treatment and to underline that we are dealing with a systemic disease that is neither restricted to the spine nor can be treated by surgery alone.

45.2 Case Description

A 75 y/o female patient suffered from low back pain after lifting a suitcase 2 weeks prior to admission. Her family doctor suspected myo-

B. Meyer, M. Rauschmann (eds.), *Spine Surgery*, https://doi.org/10.1007/978-3-319-98875-7_45

gelosis and prescribed NSAIDs which did not alleviate pain. The patient was otherwise healthy without any known illnesses or regular medication.

Due to her severe level of pain (VAS 6–8/10) while standing, sitting or walking, she presented to the emergency room (ER). After initial clinical examination lateral and a.p. radiographs were performed showing a compression fracture of the cranial endplate of the vertebral body of L4.

On clinical examination, her gait was clearly impaired due to severe low back pain (VAS 8/10) without radiculopathy, but with significant percussion tenderness. Neurological examination showed no motor or sensory deficit or bowel and bladder dysfunction.

The patient was admitted and longstanding x-rays, CT scan and MRI were performed to give information about the BMD, the configuration of the fractured vertebral body, coronal and sagittal balance and the integrity of the ligamentous complex for the evaluation of a potential instability. There was no spinal cord compression on MRI and the STIR sequence (STIR = Short-Tau Inverse Recovery) confirmed an acute vertebral body fracture showing edema in the fractured cranial endplate.

The patient was informed about adequate treatment options, a balloon-assisted kyphoplasty was offered and performed since the patient was not willing to further prolong conservative medical therapy. She benefitted from surgery in regard to both, her pain level that was dramatically reduced to VAS 2/10 and her quality of life since she was able to increasingly mobilize herself even during the 2 days of her postoperative stay on our ward. We referred her to an osteoporosis specialist for adequate medical treatment with substitution of vitamin D, calcium and bisphosphonates as well as a standardized DXA to assess the bone mineral density in the near future. This is mandatory to have an initial assessment to be able to monitor the efficacy of the medical therapy (Figs. 45.1, 45.2, 45.3, and 45.4).

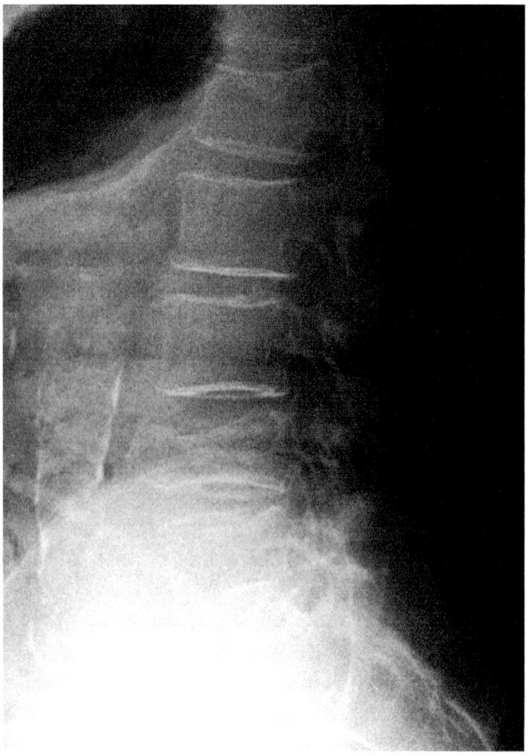

Fig. 45.1 Preoperative lateral radiography showing a fractured cranial endplate of the L4 vertebral body

45.3 Discussion of the Case

Indication

The patient suffered from severe localized back pain aggravated by axial loading.

Conservative treatment by nonsteroidal antiinflammatory drugs (NSAIDs) were not able to effectively reduce her pain level and her mobility was still dramatically impaired.

There are no guidelines as to when surgery should be considered. This is a decision that has to be made individually taking into account both, the risk of surgery and the potential risks of escalating and/or prolonging conservative treatment.

An option of intensifying the conservative regimen would be the escalation of the analgetic medication according to the WHO scheme by adding metamizol, paracetamol or opioids to

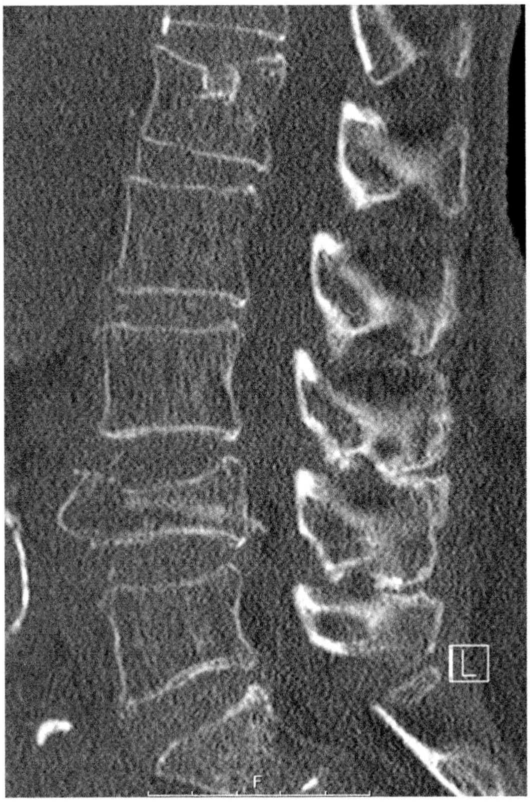

Fig. 45.2 Preoperative CT scan confirming the compression fracture of L4 with marked reduction of vertebral body height

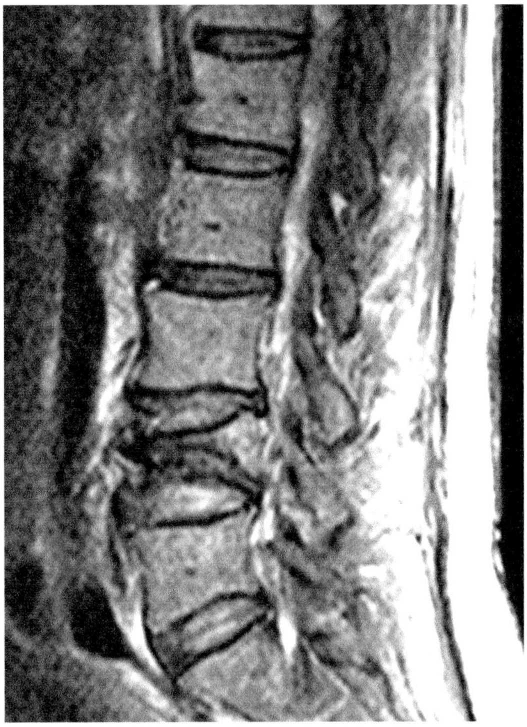

Fig. 45.3 Preoperative MRI scan showing a positive STIR signal in the fractured vertebral body of L4

avoid long-term immobility, muscular atrophy, depression, pneumonia or thrombembolic events. In addition to the medical treatment, an orthosis can improve the patient's situation.

Usually, comparable to the guidelines for the treatment of a lumbar disc herniation for patients without neurological deficit, a phase of conservative treatment of up to 6 weeks is recommended.

The treating physician should always be aware of the possible side effects of the analgetics, potential interactions with other medication and of the fact that opioid drugs lead to an increased risk for falls and consecutive fractures [4].

Surgery, with minimally-invasive vertebral augmentation procedures (VAP) should be considered in case of failure of optimal medical care, pain ≥5 on the VAS and if other pain generators have been excluded. VAPs should preferably be performed within 6–8 weeks of fracture onset, since OVCF usually heal spontaneously within this timeframe. Other indications for surgery (decompression ± instrumentation) are progressive fractures, spinal instability or deformity with sagittal and/or coronal imbalance and neural compression.

The level of evidence regarding surgical procedures for the treatment of osteoporotic vertebral fractures is not sufficient to state a clear recommendation for operative treatment yet, but there are data proving that the mortality risk is significantly reduced after a kyphoplasty or vertebroplasty in comparison to conservative treatment [5, 6]. The probability for suffering a stroke or pneumonia is also lower after surgery [5, 6].

There are some additional points to be taken into account that favor minimally-invasive surgery apart from the factors already mentioned:

- VAP result in a faster and more effective reduction of pain and an improved mobility as

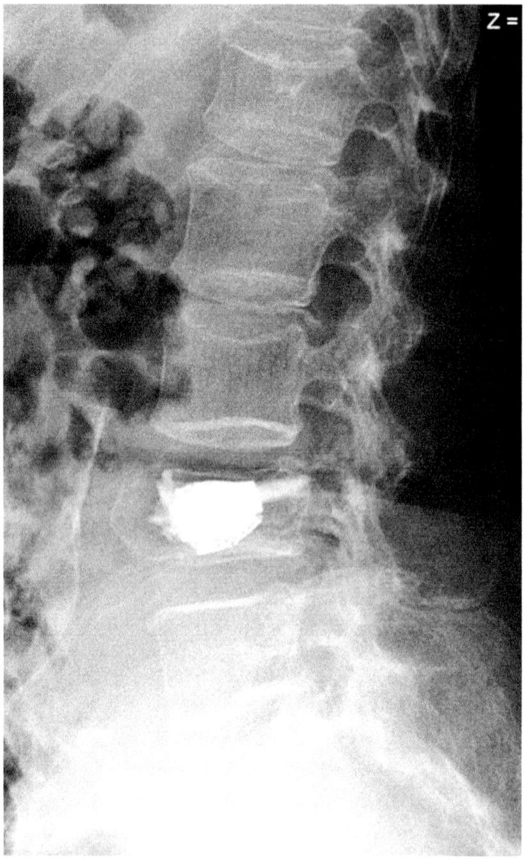

Fig. 45.4 Postoperative X-ray showing the cement distribution, no signs of cement leakage and restoration of vertebral body height

well as a better quality of life compared to conservative treatment [7, 8].

- There is no significant difference regarding the probability for the occurrence of medical complications between surgical and conservative treatment.
- VAP lead to significantly better correction of both the kyphotic deformity and vertebral body height compared to conservative treatment [9].
- The risk for additional fractures seems to be significantly higher after continued conservative treatment than after surgery [10–12].

Choice of Surgical Strategy

The standard surgical procedures, if no neural compression or instability are present, are minimally-invasive percutaneous vertebroplasty or balloon-assisted kyphoplasty. These vertebral augmentation procedures should always be performed with pulsed x-ray during the infusion of cement to be able to detect cement leakage into the disk space, the spinal canal or the venous system to stop the augmentation procedure immediately in case of cement extravasation.

Both techniques show good results regarding safety and efficacy and are superior to conservative treatment in restoring vertebral body height and correcting kyphotic deformity.

In direct comparison, kyphoplasty shows significantly superior results with regard to both the correction of the kyphotic deformity and the restoration of vertebral body height than vertebroplasty [10, 12].

Cement leakage is less frequent with kyphoplasty compared to vertebroplasty. The rate of new fractures both distant and adjacent to the augmented level shows no significant difference between kyphoplasty and vertebroplasty [13].

In general, there are no clear guidelines when to opt for a kyphoplasty or vertebroplasty.

Typically a kyphoplasty should be performed in:

- An acute or subacute fracture of less than 6 weeks
- Some degree of deformity or loss of height to be able to correct the kyphosis and restore the vertebral body height.

A vertebroplasty can be performed:

- In fractures >6 weeks of age
- In fractures without relevant deformity or height loss [14].

In case of spinal instability/deformity and/or sagittal and/or coronal imbalance or compression of neural structures, a posterior instrumentation with a PMMA(polymethylmetacrylate)-augmented pedicle screw and rod system ± decompression ± vertebral body replacement should be performed, preferably in a percutaneous minimally-invasive technique to minimize soft tissue trauma and blood loss [15].

Pedicle screw augmentation should also be performed under pulsed x-ray control in order to detect cement leakage.

If there is an indication for a corpectomy due to a significant affection of the posterior wall, severe destruction or reduced height of the vertebral body or a relevant kyphotic or scoliotic deformity, there might be the need for a dorsoventral instrumentation.

Due to the impaired quality of the bone the pedicle screws should be PMMA-augmented and it is reasonable to include at least 2 levels above and below the fractured/collapsed vertebral body. In some cases, even osteotomies are necessary to correct the kyphotic deformity.

Fortunately, only approximately 5% of patients with symptomatic osteoporotic vertebral fractures need instrumentation [16].

Accordance with the Literature Guidelines

During the last years, several RCTs and meta-analyses with inconclusive or even opposing results have been published comparing surgical procedures with either conservative treatment or SHAM procedures or comparing different surgical techniques. In 2009, two studies were published in the New England Journal of Medicine igniting a controversial debate about the potential (lack of) benefit of vertebroplasties. The study by Buchbinder et al. [17] showed a reduction of pain and an improvement of QOL in both groups with no statistically significant advantage for the vertebroplasty group within the first 24 weeks after the procedure.

In the INVEST (Investigational Vertebroplasty Safety and Efficacy Trial) study, Kallmes et al. [18] was also not able to show statistically significant differences in reduction of pain and disability. There was only a trend favoring vertebroplasty. The study had a high cross-over rate in the control group and the follow-up was only 3 months.

The statistical power of most of these studies is rather weak, due to flaws in study design, selection bias or often due to the small number of patients included.

Also, valid long-term results are lacking, even though a few studies have shown a superiority of the vertebral augmentation procedures compared to conservative treatment with regard to a faster reduction of pain, an improved mobility, shorter hospital stay and a reduced mortality with some of these effects still being statistically significant after up to 36 months [19]. For example, the VAPOUR study (Safety and Efficacy of Vertebroplasty for acute painful osteoporotic fractures) by Clark et al. [20] showed a significant advantage for the vertebroplasty group regarding pain reduction, postoperative hospital stay and consolidation of the vertebral body height both directly after the procedure as well as on follow-up after 6 months.

In patients that are not neurologically intact, there is consensus that they need surgical treatment, but so far no guideline exists regarding the specific treatment. However, a recommendation of the German Society for Orthopedics and Trauma (DGOU) was published with regard to fracture classification and treatment based on a prospective clinical cohort. An osteoporotic fracture (OF) classification-based scoring system was developed by an expert group to give specific treatment recommendations for each OF type including 7 items such as OF fracture type, bone mineral density, ongoing fracture process, pain, neurological deficit, mobilization and health status. Hence, this OF score can help in decision making concerning non-surgical vs. surgical treatment and the extent of surgery. In some non-conclusive cases an individual treatment approach is still needed [21, 22].

45.4 Conclusions and Take Home Message

A OF-score of <6 points recommends non-surgical management; a score of >6 points recommends surgery. Intermediate cases with a score of 6 need individual decision making.

In addition to the treatment of an acute symptomatic fracture, it is mandatory to ensure the patient will receive proper medical treatment to improve the bone mineral density and consecutively reduce the risk for further fractures.

Pearls and Pitfalls

- There are recommendations for the classification and treatment of OVCF. In intermediate cases the decision has to be made individually weighing the risk of surgery against the potential risks of escalating and/or prolonging conservative treatment.

- Non-surgical management is recommended for OF1 and OF2 fractures. If conservative treatment fails VAPs are indicated.
- VAP are indicated in case of failure of optimal medical care for OF1 and 2, and OF3 without an ongoing fracture process, pain ≥5 on the VAS and if other pain generators have been excluded.
- VAPs should preferably be performed within 6–8 weeks of fracture onset, since OVCF usually heal spontaneously within this timeframe.
- Other indications for surgery (decompression ± instrumentation ± vertebral body replacement ± correction of spinal imbalance) are OF types 3–5 with progressive fractures, spinal instability or deformity with spinal imbalance and neural compression.
- PMMA-augmentation should always be performed with pulsed x-ray during application to be able to detect cement leakage (pulmonary embolism, spinal canal)
- Kyphoplasty should be performed in acute or subacute fracture of <6 weeks of age and with some degree of deformity or loss of vertebral body height
- Vertebroplasty should be preferred in fractures >6 weeks of age without relevant deformity or VB height loss

Editorial Comment

Osteoporosis nowadays play a big role in fracture treatment, as mentioned in this article. Also in elective cases with degenerative findings it has to be taken in mind.

Prophlactic treatment with osteoinductive drug's (parathormone) in preparation to complex spine surgeries in osteoporotic patients can increase fusion rates and decrease complications due to weak bone quality

References

1. Delmas PD, Genant HK, Crans GG, et al. Severity of prevalent vertebral fractures and the risk of subsequent vertebral and nonvertebral fractures: results from the MORE trial. Bone. 2003;33:522–32. Level of evidence: Ib.
2. Oleksik A, Lips P, Dawson A, et al. Health-related quality of life (HRQOL) in postmenopausal women with low BMD with or without prevalent vertebral fractures. J Bone Miner Res. 2000;15:1384–92. Level of evidence: III.
3. Lau E, Ong K, Kurtz S, et al. Mortality following the diagnosis of a vertebral compression fracture in the Medicare population. J Bone Joint Surg Am. 2008;90:1479–86. Level of evidence: III.
4. Li L, Setoguchi S, Cabral H, Jick S. Opioid use for noncancer pain and risk of fracture in adults: a nested case-control study using the general practice research database. Am J Epidemiol. 2013;178(4):559–69. https://doi.org/10.1093/aje/kwt013. Epub 2013 May 2. Level of evidence: III
5. Edidin AA, Ong KL, Lau E, et al. Mortality risk for operated and nonoperated vertebral fracture patients in the medicare population. J Bone Miner Res. 2011;26:1617–26. Level of evidence: III.
6. Edidin AA, Ong KL, Lau E, et al. Life expectancy following diagnosis of a vertebral compression fracture. Osteoporos Int. 2013;24:451–8. Level of evidence: III.
7. Boonen S, Van Meirhaeghe J, Bastian L, et al. Balloon kyphoplasty for the treatment of acute vertebral compression fractures: 2-year results from a randomized trial. J Bone Miner Res. 2011;26:1627–37. Level of evidence: Ib.
8. Anderson PA, Froyshteter AB, Tontz WL Jr. Meta-analysis of vertebral augmentation compared with conservative treatment for osteoporotic spinal fractures. J Bone Miner Res. 2013;28(2):372–82. https://doi.org/10.1002/jbmr.1762. Evidenzgrad 1++ SIGN. Level of evidence: Ia.
9. Farrhoki MR, Alibai E, Maghami Z. Randomized controlled trial of percutaneous vertebroplasty versus optimal medical management for the relief of pain and disability in acute osteoporotic vertebral compression fractures. J Neurosurg Spine. 2011;14:561–9. Level of evidence: Ib.
10. Liu JT, Li CS, Chang CS, et al. Long-term follow-up study of osteoporotic vertebral compression fracture treated using balloon kyphoplasty and vertebroplasty. J Neurosurg Spine. 2015;23:94–8. Level of evidence: Ib.
11. Zou J, Mei X, Zhu X, Shi Q, Yang H. The long-term incidence of subsequent vertebral body fracture after vertebral augmentation therapy: a systemic review and meta-analysis. Pain Physician. 2012;15(4):E515–22. Level of evidence: Ia.
12. Liu JT, Liao WJ, Tan WC, et al. Balloon kyphoplasty versus vertebroplasty for treatment of osteoporotic vertebral compression fracture: a prospective, comparative, and randomized clinical trial. Osteoporos Int. 2010;21:359–64. Level of evidence: Ib.

13. Vogl TJ, Pflugmacher R, Hierholzer J, et al. Cement directed kyphoplasty reduces cement leakage as compared with vertebroplasty. Spine. 2013;38:1730–6. Level of evidence: Ib.
14. Anselmetti GC, Bernard J, Blattert T, et al. Criteria for the appropriate treatment of osteoporotic vertebral compression fractures. Pain Physician. 2013;16:E519–30. Level of evidence: IV.
15. Kashii M, Yamazaki R, Yamashita T, et al. Surgical treatment for osteoporotic vertebral collapse with neurological deficits. Eur Spine J. 2013;22:1633–42. Level of evidence: III.
16. Shen M, Kim Y. Osteoporotic vertebral compression fractures: a review of current surgical management techniques. Am J Orthop (Belle Mead NJ). 2007;36:241–8. Level of evidence: IV.
17. Buchbinder R, Osborne RH, Ebeling PR, et al. A randomized trial of vertebroplasty for painful osteoporotic vertebral fractures. N Engl J Med. 2009;361(6):557–68. https://doi.org/10.1056/NEJMoa0900429. Level of evidence: Ib.
18. Kallmes DF, Comstock BA, Heagerty PJ, et al. A randomized trial of vertebroplasty for osteoporotic spinal fractures. N Engl J Med. 2009;361(6):569–79. Level of evidence: Ib.
19. Wardlaw D, Cummings SR, Van Meirhaeghe J, et al. Efficacy and safety of balloon kyphoplasty compared with non-surgical care for vertebral compression fracture (FREE): a randomised controlled trial. Lancet. 2009;373(9668):1016–24. Level of evidence: Ib.
20. Clark W, Bird P, Gonski P, et al. Safety and efficacy of vertebroplasty for acute painful osteoporotic fractures (VAPOUR): a multicentre, randomised, double-blind, placebo-controlled trial. Lancet. 2016;388:1408–16. Level of evidence: Ib.
21. Blattert TR, Schnake KJ, Gonschorek O, et al. Nonsurgical and surgical management of osteoporotic vertebral body fractures: recommendations of the spine section of the German Society for Orthopaedics and Trauma (DGOU). Global Spine J. 2018;8(2_suppl):50S–5S. Level of evidence: II (Prospective cohort study)/V(Treatment recommendation: Expert opinion).
22. Schnake KJ, Blattert TR, Hahn P, et al. Classification of osteoporotic thoracolumbar spine fractures: recommendations of the spine section of the German Society for Orthopaedics and Trauma (DGOU). Global Spine J. 2018;8(2_suppl):46S–9S. Level of evidence: V (Expert opinion).

46 Benign Tumors and Tumor Like Lesions

Yu-Mi Ryang

46.1 Introduction

Benign tumors and tumor-like lesions of the spine are rare lesions that comprise about 10% of all extradural spine tumors.

Benign Tumors
- Vertebral hemangioma (VH)
- Osteoid osteoma (OO)
- Osteoblastoma (BOB)
- Osteochondroma (OC)
- Aneurysmal bone cyst (ABC)
- Eosinophilic granuloma (EG)

Semimalignant Tumors
- Giant cell tumor (GCT)

They show a certain predilection for age and location. While >90% of tumors occurring during the first decade of life are benign, this number decreases with age. In the fourth decade about 50% and in the seventh decade less than 10% of spinal tumors are benign [4].

Age Predilection

1.-2. decade:	Eosinophilic Granuloma (EG)
2. decade:	Osteoid Osteoma (OO)
	Aneurysmal Bone Cyst (ABC)
2.-3. decade:	Benign Osteoblastoma (BOB)
3. decade:	Osteochondroma (OC)
2.-4. decade:	semimalignant Giant Cell Tumor (GCT)
4.-6. decade:	Vertebral Hemangioma (VH)

Predilection of Location
Whereas some tumors are mainly located in the anterior vertebral body, other tumors show a predilection of the posterior elements [6, 8].

Anterior Vertebral Body
- Eospinophilic Granuloma (EG)
- Vertebral Hemangioma (VH)
- Giant Cell Tumor (GCT)

Posterior Elements
- Aneurysmal Bone Cyst (ABC)
- Benign Osteoblastoma (BOB)
- Osteoid Osteoma (OO)
- Osteochondroma (OC)

Y.-M. Ryang (✉)
Department of Neurosurgery, Klinikum rechts der Isar, Technische Universität München, Munich, Germany
e-mail: yu.ryang@tum.de

B. Meyer, M. Rauschmann (eds.), *Spine Surgery*, https://doi.org/10.1007/978-3-319-98875-7_46

Location

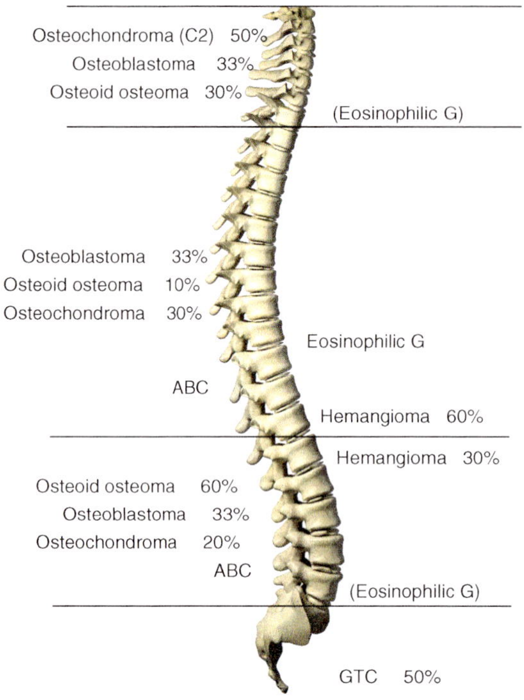

Tumor localization and percentage of benign and malignant tumors of the spine

Symptoms

The most characteristic symptom is persistent back pain unrelated to activity and typically aggravated during rest and at night.

Staging

Benign tumors are staged into three stages according to Enneking:

- Latent lesion
- Active lesion
- Aggressive lesion

Stage 1 Lesions are inactive asymptomatic slowly or non-growing with a true capsule not requiring therapy [1, 6].

Stage 2 Lesions are mildly symptomatic slowly growing lesions with enlarged tumor outlines requiring intralesional resection and show a low recurrence rate.

Stage 3 Lesions are rapidly growing with breached or absent tumor capsule and invasion of neighboring structures which require complete resection due to a high recurrence rate.

46.2 Case Description Osteoid Osteoma (OO)

2A: A 42 y/o male suffered from pain in the cervicothoracic region with diffuse irradiation into his right arm. He had no neurological deficit and reported of good response to acetylsalicylic acid (ASS), but complained of relapsing symptoms upon cessation of drug intake. CT and MRI showed a small right-sided osteoblastic lesion in the facet joint of T1/T2 with a central nidus of vascular fibrous connective tissue and a surrounding osteoid matrix (Figs. 46.1 and 46.2).

The patient did not want to take ASS or NSAIDs on a regular basis and asked for surgery. He therefore underwent CT-navigated microsurgical resection (Fig. 46.3).

The intra- and postoperative course was uneventful and the patient was discharged with complete pain relief on the fifth postoperative day.

2B. Case Description of the Aneurysmal Bone Cyst (ABC)

2B: A 16 y/o neurologically intact male juvenile presented with a 1-year history of progressive swelling and pain in the neck. CT and MRI showed a large cystic non-contrast enhancing mass lesion in the neck extending from C1 to C3 posteriorly with almost complete lysis of the posterior C2 lamina involving both vertebral arteries. Furthermore, the patient had a C2-C3 instability with subluxation (Fig. 46.4).

The patient received a planned 2-staged surgery with microsurgical removal of the tumor with posterior C1-C3 lateral mass fixation, and 1 week later an anterior C2-C3 spondylodesis with anterior discectomy and fusion with a PEEK-cage and ventral plating (Figs. 46.5 and 46.6).

The postoperative course was uneventful and the patient was discharged 4 days after the second surgery with significantly improved neck pain.

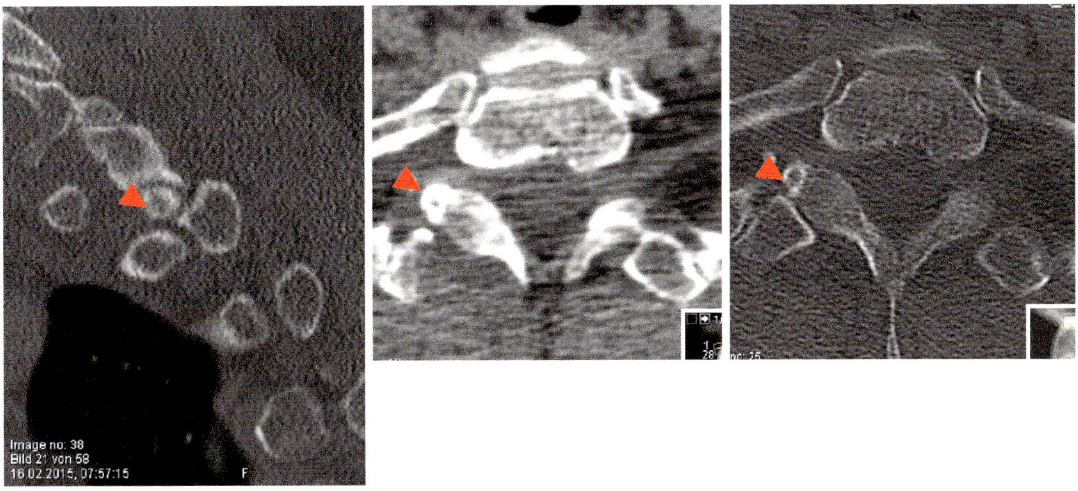

Fig. 46.1 CT-scan showing a central nidus with sclerotic margin pathognomonic for osteoid osteoma

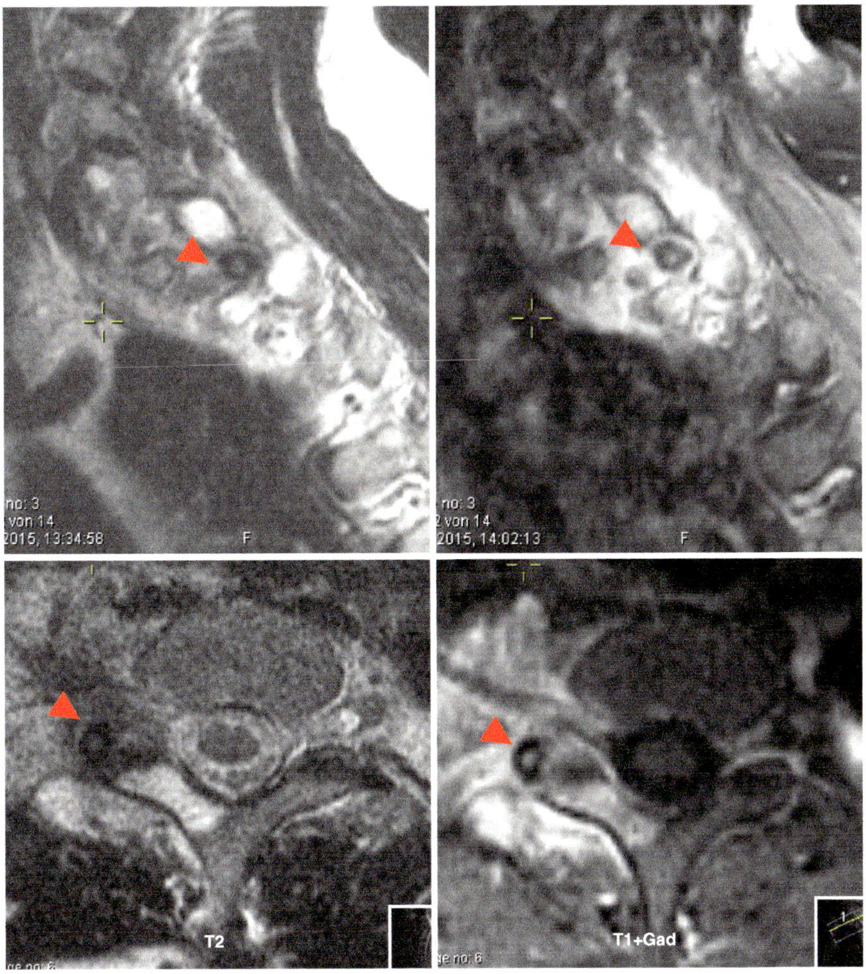

Fig. 46.2 MRI (T1+gadolinium-enhanced and T2-weighted images). The calcified margin of the nidus is T1- and T2-hypointense, whereas the non-calcified center of the nidus is hyperintense on T2- and contrast-enhanced T1-weighted images. Note the edematous changes of adjacent bone marrow and soft tissue due to nidal prostaglandin production

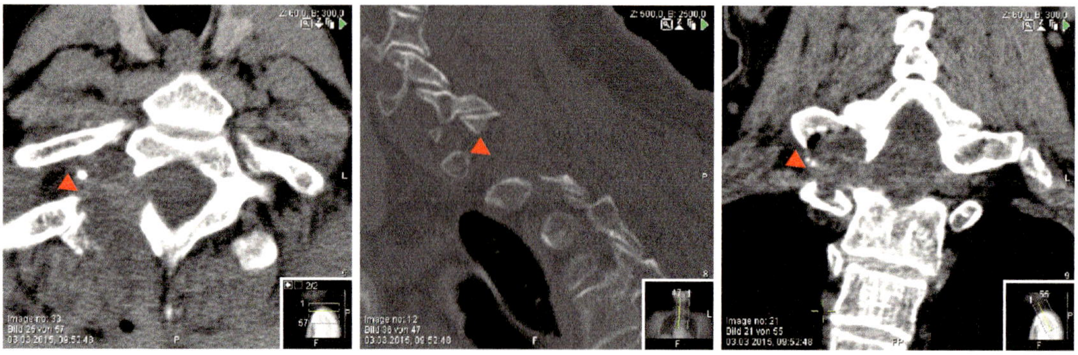

Fig. 46.3 Postoperative CT-scan showing complete removal of the nidus

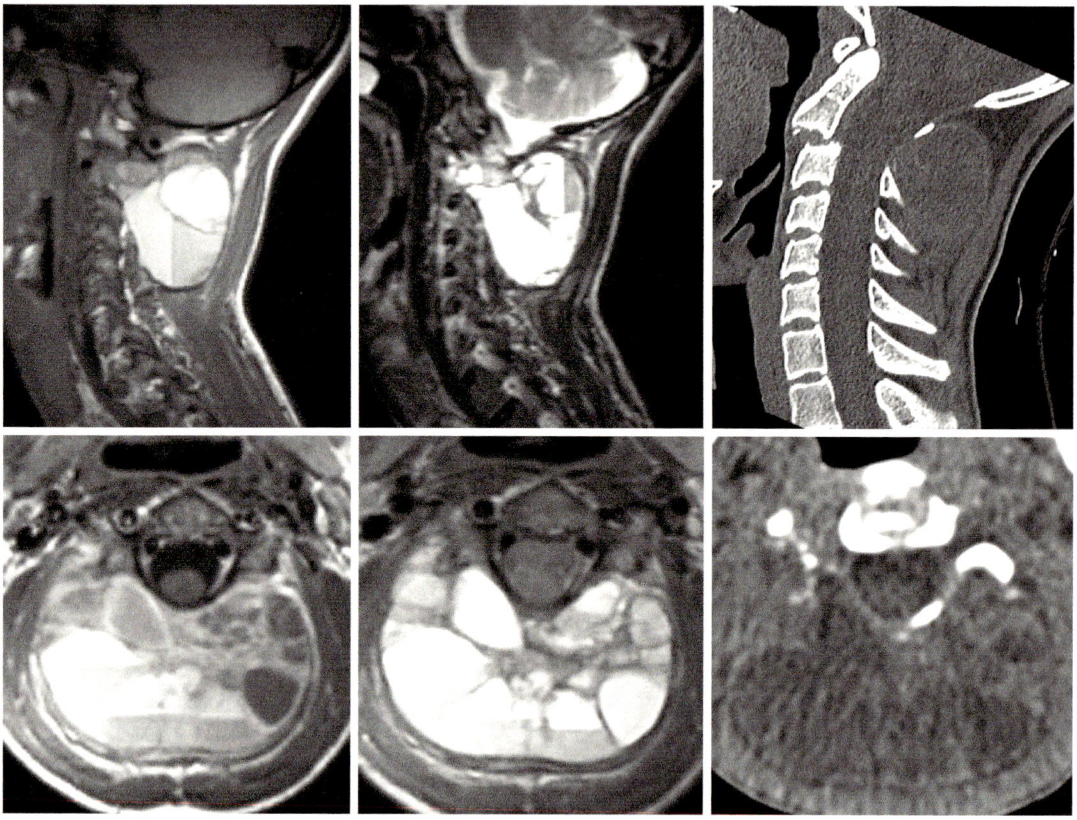

Fig. 46.4 CT scan and MRI (T1+gadolinium and T2-weighted image) showing an osteolytic expansile lesion with surrounding cortical bone and pathognomonic fluid-fluid levels

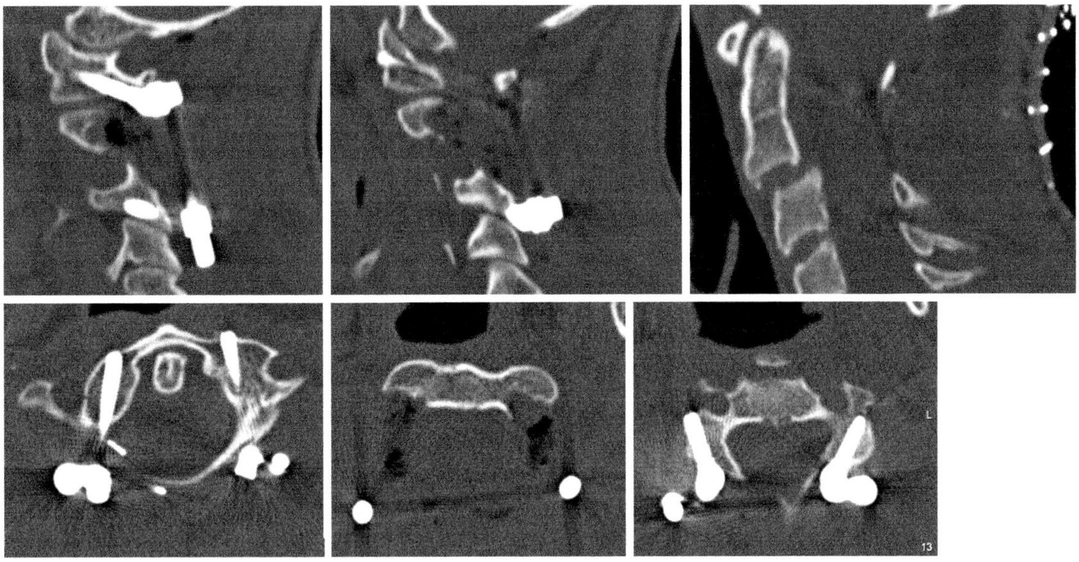

Fig. 46.5 Postoperative CT after tumor removal and posterior lateral mass screw fixation of C1-C3

Fig. 46.6 Postoperative MRI (T1+gadolinium and T2-STIR) in sagittal and axial planes showing complete tumor removal

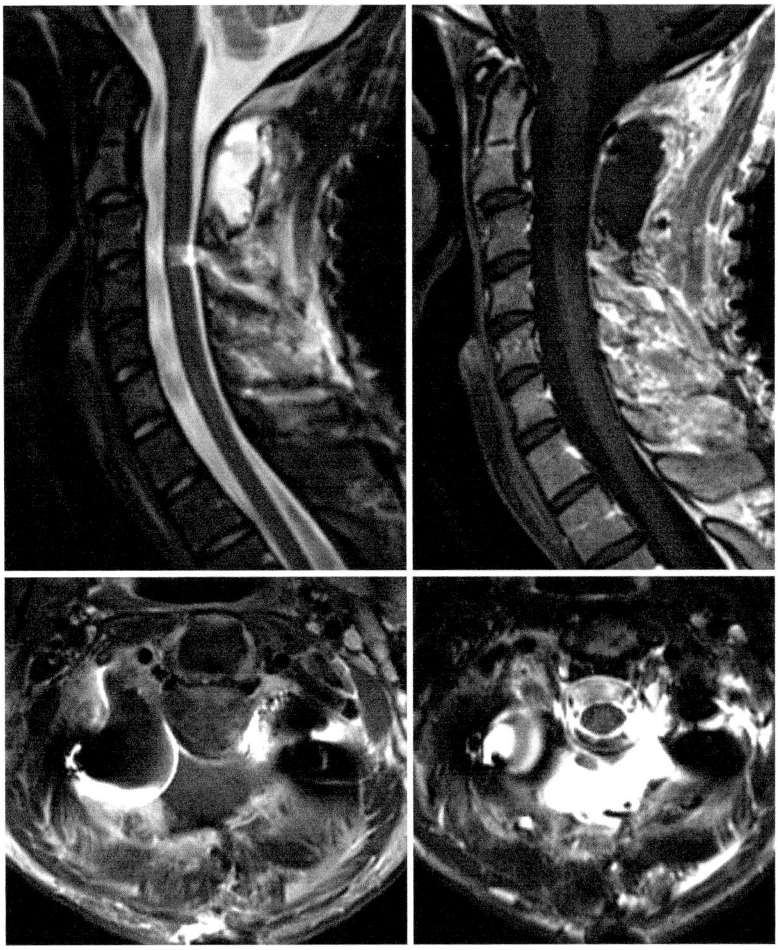

46.3 Discussion of the Cases

3A. Osteoid Osteoma (OO) OO usually occur in the second decade of life with a predilection for the posterior lamina or pedicle of the lumbar or cervical spine. This patient complained of a symptomatic OO with characteristic night pain relieved by ASS intake. Imaging-wise CT is the method of choice in these tumors, since they always show a pathognomonic central nidus surrounded by an osteoid matrix.

Since pain relapsed every time the patient seized medication, he asked for surgery. In cases of symptomatic active lesions surgery is advocated. Therefore, a CT-navigated microsurgical removal was performed. These tumors, especially OO are small in size and are hard to find and hard to differentiate visually from normal bone intraoperatively. We therefore strongly recommend navigated removal of these tumors, not to miss the tumor or risk incomplete removal.

An alternative treatment strategy is thermal nidus ablation. This minimally invasive technique is gaining increasing popularity and can be applied if neural structures are at least more than 5 mm apart from the nidus to avoid heat injury. Caution also needs to be taken in cases with absent cortical bone for the same reason. The success rate is reported to range between approx. 80–100% with recurrence and failure rates of approx. 5%, respectively. Some authors advocate this procedure as gold standard. However, the evidence on this technique is of very low quality.

Differential diagnoses for OO are osteoblastomas (BOB), which are basically histologically identical to OO, but behave differently biologically. They tend to occur slightly later in life (second to third decade) and have no predilection concerning the spinal level and their size exceeds a diameter of 1.0–1.5 cm. BOB also have a tendency to recur in 10–15%, which may rise even up to 50% if they show aggressive local growth, when excised incompletely. Other differential diagnoses are aneurysmal bone cysts (ABC) and osteosarcomas.

Concerning alternative therapies quality of evidence is also very low. Radiation therapy might be considered in cases of recurrent or incompletely resected aggressive BOB (weak recommendation). Chemotherapy might be considered in recurrent aggressive BOB (weak recommendation) [7].

3B. Aneurysmal Bone Cyst (ABC) ABCs have a predilection for the posterior elements of the lumbosacral spine and usually show extensive growth with characteristic fluid-fluid levels within the blood-filled cavities. They can lead to instability due to osteolytic lesions and involvement of contiguous vertebrae and disc spaces. Intralesional resection is recommended. If intralesional resection is incomplete, these lesions show a high recurrence rate of 20–30%. En bloc resection, however, is rarely feasible due to their expansive growth pattern.

ABC can develop secondary to preexisting other tumors, esp. osteoblastoma, hemangioma or giant cell tumor.

Alternative treatments such as stand-alone selective arterial embolization is reported with weak recommendation and very low quality evidence. However, there is a strong recommendation for preoperative embolization to reduce intraoperative blood loss. Radiation therapy should only be considered in inoperable tumors, aggressive recurrent tumor or incomplete resections (weak recommendation) [7]. There is not yet a role for Denusomab in the first line treatment of ABC (weak recommendation), but there are reports on (neo)adjuvant Denusomab use [2, 3].

Differential diagnoses of ABC are GCT and BOB.

46.4 Conclusion and Take Home Message

Benign tumors or tumor-like lesions of the spine are rare entities and mostly affect people of younger age between the first and fourth decade of life. They also show typical predilections for location in the spine. OO, BOB and ABC are -predominantly located in the posterior spinal elements. Surgery remains the treatment of choice in these tumors. Depending on their staging there are recommendations as how to treat them. Since these tumors are rare, no prospective or randomized trials exist and treatment solely relies on expert opinion only. Consequently, no level 1 evidence and no treatment guidelines are available. These tumors are curable upon complete excision. However, it is important to know that, depending on the entity and staging, these tumors show different recurrence rates requiring different surgical techniques, i.e. intralesional vs. en bloc resection and can undergo malignant transformation, such as giant cell tumors that can also metastasize, osteoblastomas which can transform to osteosarcomas and osteochondromas which can transform to chondrosarcomas.

Up to now, there is no role for alternative therapies (radiation−/chemotherapy) in the first-line treatment of BOB and ABC. Percutaneous ablation techniques in OO might be a feasible alternative to surgery.

Adjuvant radiation therapy should only be considered in aggressive recurrent BOB or ABC or in cases where complete resection is not possible. Adjuvant chemotherapy only has a limited role in aggressive recurrent BOB. There seems to be a role of (neo)adjuvant Denusomab in ABC, but evidence to support this, especially long-term results, is still lacking [2, 3].

Pearls and Pitfalls

- Complete resection should be the goal if possible, since incomplete resection is associated with varying rates of recurrence
- Intralesional excision is recommended for OO and non-aggressive BOB
- OO are easily missed during surgery and should be excised with the use of spinal navigation
- BOB are histologically identical to OO, but larger (>1.0–1.5 cm diameter)
- Non-aggressive BOB recur in 10–15%
- Aggressive BOB need en bloc resection and recur in up to 50%
- ABC may occur secondary to GCT, BOB and VH
- BOB, ABC, GCT and VH are expansive growing lesions
- GCT can be mistaken for ABC, since both show typical intracavital fluid-fluid levels
- GCT, BOB and OC have the ability to transform into malignant tumors, therefore complete excision is mandatory

References

1. Boriani S, Weinstein JN, Biagini R. Primary bone tumors of the spine. Terminology and surgical staging. Spine. 1997;22:1036–44.
2. Charest-Morin R, Boriani S, Fisher CG, Patel SR, Kawahara N, Mendel E, Bettegowda C, Rhines LD. Benign tumors of the spine: has new chemotherapy and interventional radiology changed the treatment paradigm? Spine (Phila Pa 1976). 2016;41(Suppl 20):S178–85.
3. Dubory A, Missenard G, Domont J, Charles C. Interest of Denosumab for the treatment of giant-cells tumors and aneurysmal bone cysts of the spine. About nine cases. Spine (Phila Pa 1976). 2016;41(11):E654–60.
4. Erlemann R. Imaging and differential diagnosis of primary bone tumors and tumor-like lesions of the spine. Eur J Radiol. 2006;58:48–67.
5. Enneking WF, Spanier SS, Goodman MA. A system for the surgical staging of musculoskeletal sarcoma. Clin Orthop Relat Res. 1980;153:106–20.
6. Fuchs B, Boos N. Primary tumors of the spine. In: Boos N, Aebi M, editors. Spinal disorders. Berlin, Heidelberg: Springer; 2008.
7. Harrop JS, Schmidt MH, Boriani S, Shaffrey CI. Aggressive "benign" primary spine neoplasms osteoblastoma, aneurysmal bone cyst, and giant cell tumor. Spine (Phila Pa 1976). 2009;34(22S):S39–47.
8. Ravindra VM, Eli IM, Schmidt MH, Brockmeyer DL. Primary osseous tumors of the pediatric spinal column: review of pathology and surgical decision making. Neurosurg Focus. 2016;41(2):E3.

Primary Malignant Tumors 47

Marcus Rickert and M. Rauschmann

47.1 Juvenile Sarcoma (Ewing)

47.1.1 Introduction

47.1.1.1 Epidemiology and Etiology

Primary malignant bone tumors of the spine (i.e., vertebral sarcomas, not plasmocytomas) are very rare entities and account for only 5–10% of all primary malignant bone tumors of the entire skeleton.

The primary site of predilection for spinal tumors is the thoracic spine and sacrum, followed by lumbar and cervical spine [1].

Ewing's sarcoma (EWS) of bone is a part of the Ewing's sarcoma family of tumors, which shares similar molecular and histologic findings and includes primitive neuroectodermal tumors, Ewing's soft tissue sarcomas, and Askins' tumors [2].

It was first described in detail by the pathologist James Ewing in 1921 in his first case of a teenage girl who presented with a pathologic fracture of her forearm [3].

Ewing's sarcoma accounts for 6–8% of all primary malignant bone tumors and is the second most common malignancy of the pediatric skeleton. 80% of patients are younger than 20 years, with boys being slightly more frequently affected (m: f = 1.4: 1). An average annual incidence was found of about 3 per 1 million for the US population [4].

Preferred manifestations are the meta- or metadiaphyseal portions of the long bones, the pelvis, the ribs and the spine. In up to 10% EWS originates in the spine [5, 6].

Ewing's sarcoma is the most common primary malignant bone tumor of the spine in children. Histologically, EWS is a high-grade aggressive small round blue cell tumor that most commonly originates in bone and is associated with large soft tissue masses and frequent metastases. About a quarter of Ewing's sarcomas arise in soft tissues rather than bone, and about a quarter of patients have detectable metastases at diagnosis. The lungs are the most common site for metastases (50%), followed by bone (25%) and bone marrow (20%) [2].

Most primary bone tumors are based on unknown cause. The etiology of EWS remains unclear. In general non-neoplastic changes and tumor-like bone lesions as well as benign neoplasia of the bone may favor the development of aggressive bone tumors.

M. Rickert (✉)
Orthopaedic University Hospital Friedrichsheim gGmbH Frankfurt, Frankfurt am Main, Germany
e-mail: marcus.rickert@friedrichsheim.de

M. Rauschmann
Department of Spine Surgery, Sana Klinikum Offenbach, Offenbach, Germany

B. Meyer, M. Rauschmann (eds.), *Spine Surgery*, https://doi.org/10.1007/978-3-319-98875-7_47

47.1.1.2 Pathogenesis

Molecular Pathology

Genetic factors seem to play an essential role in the development of Ewing sarcoma. The translocation t (11; 22) (q22; q24) (EWS-FLI1 fusion) is highly characteristic and present in almost 85% of all Ewing sarcoma [7].

Ewing's sarcoma cells express the 7 p30/32 MIC2 antigen encoded by the MIC2 gene, a surface glycoprotein. It can be recognized by monoclonal antibodies. The MIC2 analysis has a sensitivity of 95% in the diagnosis of Ewing sarcoma [8].

Clinical Findings

As with other primary bone sarcomas, pain is the most common initial symptom of patients with Ewing's sarcoma.

Patients with spinal/vertebral Ewing sarcomas (56–94%) are more often symptomatic with neurological deficits compared to osteosarcoma patients. Also more common than, for example, in osteosarcoma are systemic symptoms such as fever, increased lactate dehydrogenase (LDH) and leucocytes. The tumor mass is usually located in the vertebral body and often shows a large extra-osseous soft tissue portion with an expansion of the adjacent soft tissues and epidural space. The involvement of the spinal canal with compromise of neural structures can lead to neurological deficits [9].

Biopsy

The bioptic assurance of the diagnosis is always essential. Biopsy should be performed to obtain sufficient and representative tissue portions for histological evaluation and molecular biology examination. When planning the biopsy must be taken into account that the biopsy approach as well as the biopsy scar are considered to be contaminated and need to be resected or irradiated during the later local therapy.

A co-evaluation of the tissue samples by an experienced reference pathologist is strongly recommended. In general Ewing tumor is diagnosed by biopsy and then chemotherapy is initiated. For local control this may be followed by radiation and/ or surgery.

47.1.1.3 Treatment

Over the last decades the treatment and subsequent prognosis of EWS have improved dramatically especially due to the addition of systemic chemotherapy. Systemic polychemotherapy is currently the prognostically crucial step. Radiotherapy and surgery are also fundamental in particular for the local tumor control. Ewing's sarcoma responds very well to chemotherapy and radiation what helps to improve the long term survival.

The combination of this three treatment options represents the current standard of therapy. The current treatment consists of the sequential series of neoadjuvant chemotherapy, local tumor control, and subsequent adjuvant chemotherapy.

Chemotherapy

Currently, patients are being treated in accordance with a standardized polychemotherapy protocol. Initially, the patients receive 6 cycles of induction chemotherapy with VIDE (vincristine, ifosfamide, doxorubicin and etoposide). Neoadjuvant chemotherapy is performed in different therapy groups depending on the risk factors.

Local Control

Ewing's sarcoma has a good sensitivity to radiation, so that depending on the tumor localization and size for local tumor control, surgical procedures and/or radiotherapy can be used.

Due to the increased local recurrence rate with only chemo- and radiotherapy, resectable tumors should be treated with a wide tumor resection whenever possible.

Therefore the adequate treatment of spinal/vertebral Ewing sarcoma manifestations is a multimodal therapy concept from polychemotherapy and en bloc spondylectomy of the affected spinal segments followed by postoperative radiotherapy.

Adjuvant chemoradiotherapy without resection should be performed only in the case of an unfavorable anatomical position or in the case of tumors resectable only with a significant functional deficit. By means of sole radiotherapy local control rates of up to 80–85% can be achieved.

Prognosis

Significant progress has been made in the treatment of Ewing sarcoma over the past two decades. With the development of effective chemotherapy, the 5-year survival rate has improved from 5–10% to up to 75% [10]. The prognosis depends on primary tumor localization, size and volume, histological response and metastasis. In adequately locally and chemotherapeutically treated patients with a non-metastatic primary tumor, the 5-year survival rate is 50–75%. Patients with bony metastases have an unfavorable prognosis with 3–5-year survival rates of <10% to 20% [7].

About 30–40% of patients with Ewing's sarcoma experience recurrence, two thirds within the first 2 years.

47.1.2 Case Description

A 2 y/o boy was referred as an emergency case to our spinal department. The parents observed a reduced mobility and that he was whiny more often. Therefore they consulted the pediatrician regularly but no obvious focus was evaluated. After developing an unsteady and uncontrolled gait a whole spine MRI scan under sedation was performed on an emergency basis. The clinical examination was difficult due to the young patient age but an initial paraplegia was detectable. The boy was able to move the lower limbs but not able to stand or to walk anymore (Fig. 47.1).

After the images had been analyzed an emergency surgery was performed immedi-

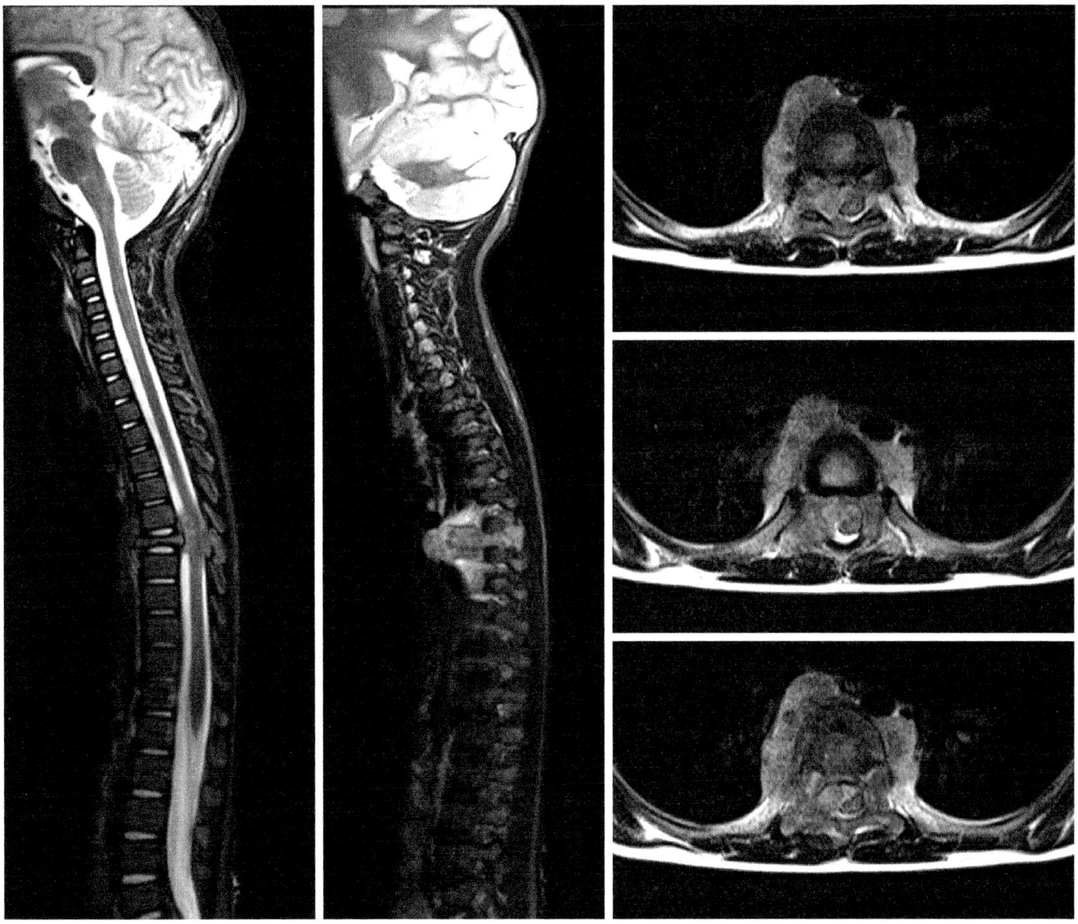

Fig. 47.1 MRI Scan at first presentation. The MRI scan shows a pathologic fracture of T 7 with tumor mass invading the spinal canal and causing spinal cord compression. Additional involvement of the paravertebral extra-osseous soft tissue

ately. The patient was treated with a posterior stabilization from T 6 to T 8 with a laminectomy T 7 and a decompression with tumordebulking via a costotransversectomy and resection of the right T 7 pedicle. Multiple samples of the tumor tissue had been collected for a detail histological and microbiological evaluation. The surgery and the postoperative course were uneventful. The neurological deficit improved and the patient was able to walk again with little assistance of his parents (Fig. 47.2).

The histological result showed a small round blue cell tumor belonging to the Ewing sarcoma family. The additional immunohistochemical examination confirmed a poorly differentiated Ewing sarcoma. A second histopathological expert opinion was ordered and concluded with the same final decision.

The further staging examination with bone scan and Positron emission tomography (PET) scan did not detect any metastasis.

For the additional oncological treatment the patient was referred to our pediatric oncology department.

Under polychemotherapy according to the VIDE combination and radiotherapy there has been no tumor progress and no onset of a metastatic spread until now. In the last clinical follow up the patient was pain free without any neuro-

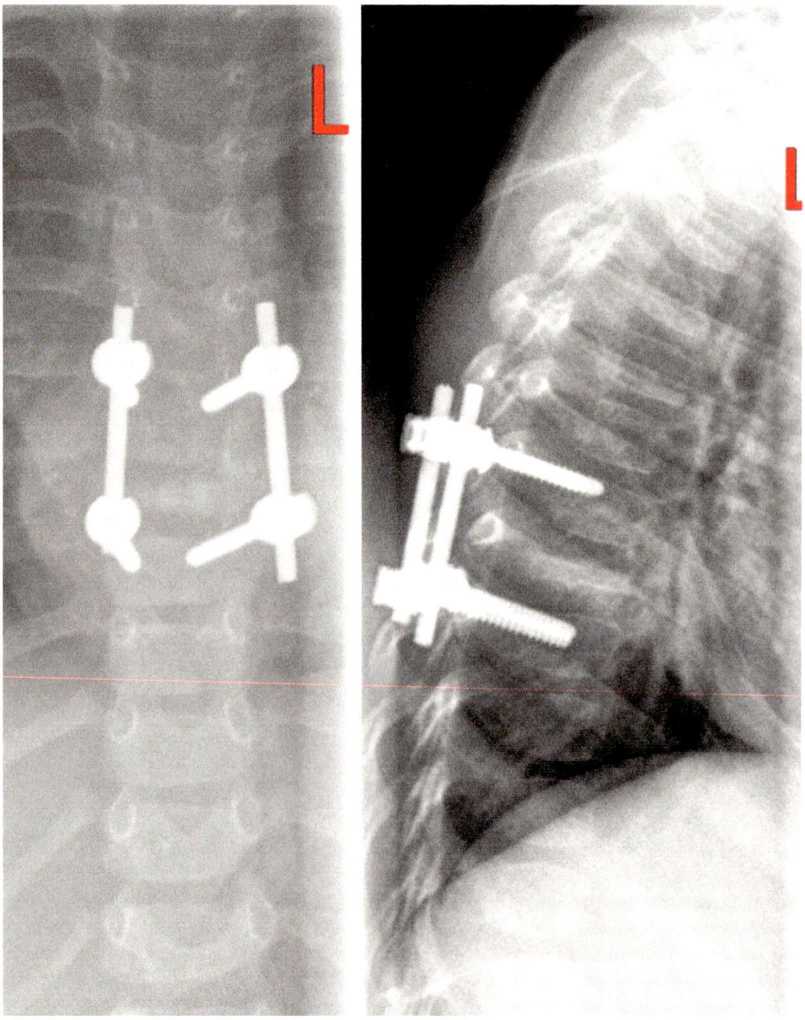

Fig. 47.2 Postoperative x-rays. Correct metalwork with adequate screw placement

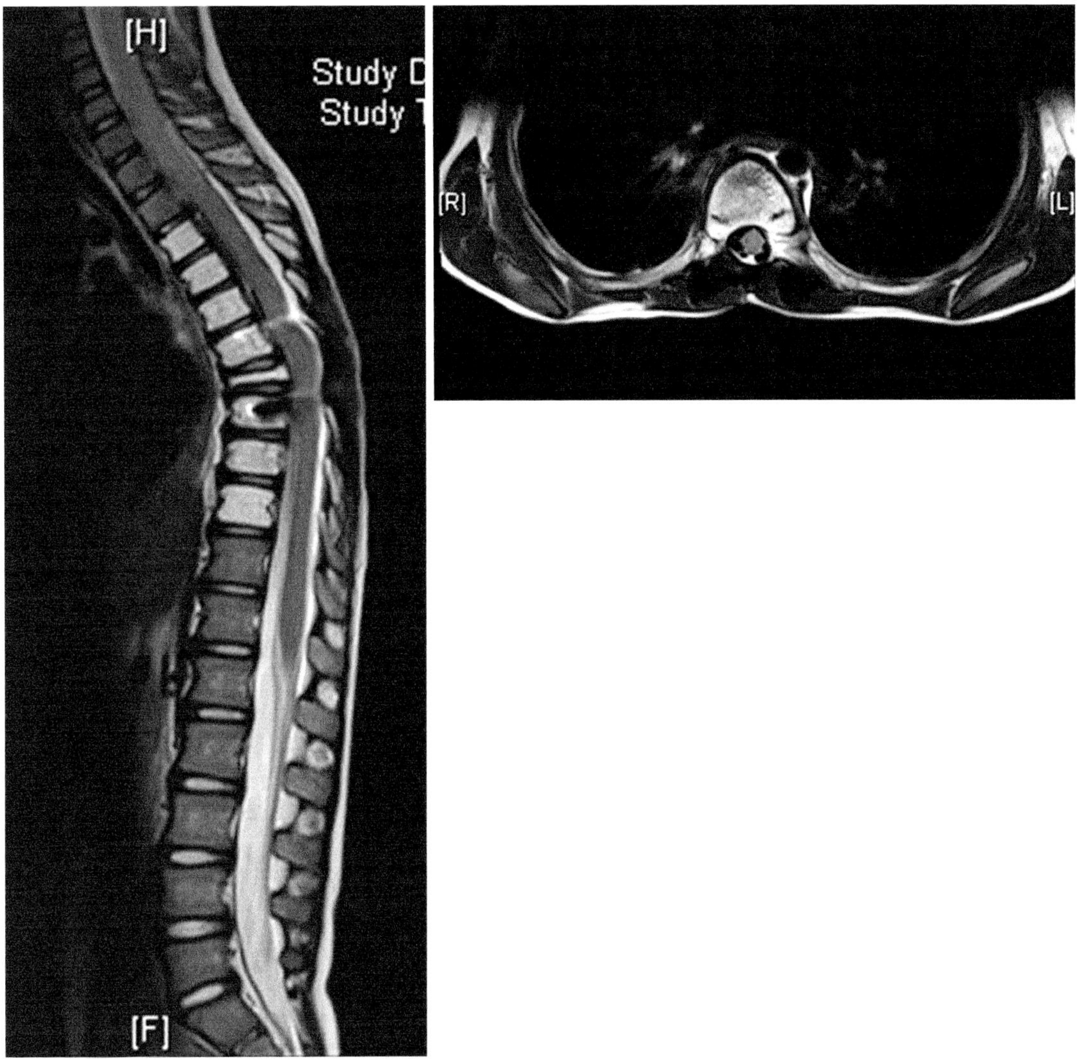

Fig. 47.3 Recent MRI Staging Scan of the thoracic spine after radio-chemotherapy. 4 years postoperatively. Reduced paravertebral tumor mass without pathological enhancement. No spinal metastasis. Post radiotherapy bone marrow changes T 3–T 10

logical deficits or any abnormal findings in the physical examination (Fig. 47.3).

For local tumor control the patient was offered a surgical plan including a wide tumor resection with a spondylectomy T 7 including T 6 + T 8 with extension of the posterior stabilization and vertebral body replacement. An additional partial resection of the thoracic aorta was discussed in the multidisciplinary tumor board as well.

A proton beam therapy was evaluated too as an alternative treatment to the surgical therapy plan.

Due to the absence of any tumor progression under the current oncological treatment and a steady clinical course the parents have not made their final decision yet.

47.1.3 Discussion of the Case

The present case does not illustrate the typical clinical pathway when dealing with pediatric primary malignant tumors. But the history of the patient with his sudden onset of paraplegia due to tumor tissue invading the spinal canal with spinal cord compression required emergency surgery. Necessary decompression and stabilization had to be the first step of treatment. The intraoperative histological samples confirmed Ewing sarcoma so that polychemotherapy und radiotherapy was added after the surgery. The patient's age was also younger than the mean age for that particular tumor entity but the case demonstrates well that especially Ewing sarcoma patients are more often symptomatic with an initial neurological deficit.

Ideally in a situation without an emergency aspect we would have taken a biopsy first and after receiving the histopathological result we had started the neoadjuvant induction chemotherapy first. Local tumor control needs to be discussed in multidisciplinary tumor board and depends on many different factors. Local control can be achieved by surgery and/or radiation therapy. Main issue for a surgical plan is the resectability of the tumor and the possibility to create tumor free resection margins. Surgery is generally the preferred approach if the lesion is resectable [11].

Radiation therapy is usually employed in patients who do not have a surgical option that preserves function and patients whose tumors have been excised but with inadequate margins. The postoperative oncological treatment was followed according to the literature guidelines with chemo- and radiotherapy and has proven its effectiveness in our case as well. The postoperative tumor staging imaging demonstrated a sufficient therapy without any tumor progress at any time of the treatment. Furthermore a suggestion for a local tumor control via resection has been made in order to improve the outcome. All surgical options were discussed with the involved disciplines. Due to the young patient age and the major surgery another option with proton beam therapy was evaluated. Currently there are promising and beneficial results for this kind of treatment especially for Ewing sarcoma in critical sites, but literature consensus reveals that more high-quality clinical research is needed to further investigate long-term effectiveness [12].

47.1.4 Conclusions and Take Home Message

Unfortunately the final result of the case cannot be reported due to an ongoing decision making. That shows as well the difficulties in treating tumor patients where the treatment plans need to be adapted frequently and to find individual solutions.

Pearls

- In the past without systemic therapy only 10% of patients could be cured
- With modern chemotherapy approaches, the 5-year survival rate has improved significantly
- The prognosis depends on primary tumor localization, size and volume, histological response and metastasis
- For local tumor control, surgical procedures and/or radiotherapy can be used

47.2 Chordoma

47.2.1 Introduction

47.2.1.1 Epidemiology and Etiology

According to current WHO classification, chordomas are called primary malignant bone tumors showing notochordal differentiation [13]. Chordomas arise from residual embryonic notochord tissue. The notochord disappears in human beings at about 8 weeks in the fetal development, and evidence suggests that chordoma develops from persistent notochordal elements.

Main localization is the os sacrum (40–50%), as well as the skull base with focus in the clivus region (35–40%) and in vertebral bodies (15–20%) [14]. Extraskeletal cases have also been reported but are very rare [15]. Chordomas account for approximately 4% of all primary malignant bone tumors.

Chordoma is most commonly diagnosed between ages 50 and 60 with an annual incidence of 1:1.000.000 for new diagnoses and a prevalence of one every 100.000. It is more common in men than women, and rare in children. Chordomas are biologically low to intermediate-grade tumors with a slow rate of proliferation. They also show locally infiltrating and bone destructive growth with frequent recurrences in up to 40% of cases. They are accompanied by a high metastatic tendency of up to 30% and a short tumor-free survival [16].

Metastases can occur in the lung, liver, bone, sub-cutis, lymph nodes, and other sites [17]. Only a minority of patients will be cured by a surgical intervention completely. The median survival is 6–7 years after diagnosis, but the range of outcome is very wide [18]. Chordomas have a pronounced tendency to recur locally; local recurrence has extremely challenging treatment and often associated with severe morbidity.

47.2.1.2 Pathology

Macroscopically chordomas are soft, gelatinous, grey to bluish-white tumors and often have a pseudocapsule. Microscopically, they show a lobular architecture with fibrous strands composed of densely packed spindle-shaped fibroblast-like cells, which encapsulate groups of highly vacuolated (physaliphorous) epithelioid tumour cells.

Chordomas can be divided into four subtypes: conventional, chondroid, dedifferentiated, and sarcomatoid [13]. Conventional (classic) chordomas are the most common entities.

Immunophenotype

To histopathologically diagnose a chordoma according to the WHO, the immunohistological evidence of EMA (epithelial membrane antigen), S100 protein and Vimentin are demanded. But their expression can vary from case to case. Brachyury is the specific immunohistochemical marker for chordomas. Brachyury, a transcription factor required for normal embryonic development, is expressed in the notochord and overexpressed in most cases of chordoma. The dedifferentiated component does not express brachyury.

Clinical Findings

The clinical symptoms in chordoma patients depend on the localization of the tumor.

Due to the slow growth sacral chordomas and lumbar spine chordomas are frequently compensated for a long time and are often clinically apparent in an advanced tumor stage. The diagnosis is often delayed because of the long standing, nonspecific initial symptoms, allowing the tumor to reach large sizes. The median time from initial symptoms to diagnosis is longer than 2 years. In contrast clivus chordomas are recognized earlier due to their neuronal symptoms. The typical symptoms of Clivus chordoma are diplopia, headache and dysphagia. Chordomas of the axial skeleton present with local pain, low back or buttocks pain, neuropathy, and/or gaits disturbance, bladder and rectal disorders if localized more caudally (sacral) [19].

47.2.1.3 Treatment

According to our case presentation the treatment options will mainly focus on the therapy of sacral chordomas.

In general the treatment of chordomas should be performed in multidisciplinary manner and in order of the global consensus published by the Chordoma Foundation in 2015 [17].

Chordomas do not respond sufficiently to conventional radiotherapy and chemotherapy. Therefore surgical treatment is the main and standard treatment option standard for limiting recurrence and maximizing survival.

Initially a preoperative biopsy is recommended. This should ideally be performed CT guided posteriorly from the midline so that the biopsy track can be involved in the approach for tumor resection.

Surgical techniques are specific to tumor site, but in general, the goal is to achieve a complete en-bloc resection with clear margins following the enneking oncologic management principles. Main target of surgery is a complete resection R0 of the tumor. The quality of surgery including the resection margins is the main factor predicting the later outcome especially the local recurrence rate. Unfortunately surgery cannot be performed with clear margins in every case due to extensive tumor infiltration involving neural structures, bladder and rectum. Complete resection would then create severe functional deficits for the patient. Sometimes surgery is even not feasible any more. Adequate margins can roughly be achieved in only 50% of the cases. To improve the resection quality a careful preoperative planning of the resection margins should be performed and to consider if extension of the resection plane for example including partial rectum or the adjacent musculature is necessary. Maybe plastic surgeons can help to deal with local soft tissue problems and inadequate wound closure because wound breakdown and infection are a major source of morbidity following sacrectomy. En-bloc resection may also lead to substantial perioperative morbidity, including bowel, bladder, and motor dysfunction. The risk of having severe functional deficits increases depending on the level of resection. Tumors arising above S3 surgery always results in a higher risk for neurologic deficits. Therefore radiotherapy needs to be discussed with the patient as a valid alternative to surgery.

Furthermore intralesional and incomplete resections are associated with higher local failure rates [17, 20].

Radiotherapy

Radiotherapy currently is performed in conjunction with en-bloc resections and that particular combination delivers high rates of local tumor control. For selected patients high dose radiation alone after biopsy can be evaluated [21].

Rotondo was treating chordoma patients with additional proton beam radiotherapy. In his study he was able to show an improved local tumor control for primary chordoma patents with combination of surgery (en-bloc resection) and pre- and postoperative radiotherapy [20].

Definitive radiation therapy alone can be considered for patients that are no candidates for surgery (medically inoperable), unresectable tumors or in patients who refuse surgery. There are encouraging reports about persistent local tumor control rates without surgery for high dose radiotherapy with protons (80% after 5 years) or carbon ions (96% after 5 years). Chen concluded that high-dose radiotherapy alone may be a reasonable alternative for patients with biopsied only, unresected chordoma, particularly in elderly patients, or high sacral levels [22, 23].

Unfortunately there is still a high risk of local recurrence that results in an even worse outcome. In all cases the final and individual treatment plan should be discussed in a multidisciplinary tumor board.

Quality of Existing Evidence

Currently there is still a lack of evidence due to the rare tumor entity. The published clinical evidence is mainly based on retrospective case series. Therefore some of uncertainty needs to be taken into account when considering clinical decision making [17].

Locoregional Relapse

Local recurrence rates are as high as 50–100% with subtotal resection compared with 0–53% with *en bloc* resection with clear margins [22].

Based on low-quality evidence, insufficient tumor resection is probably the main cause of local recurrence. Other factors that possibly influence the local recurrence have been summarized previously and include increased age, high sacral localization, lack of radiotherapy, prior resections, higher tumor grade, and increasing extent of tumor invasion [24].

Patients who recur locally are unlikely to be cured by any local salvage treatment. Treatment choice can include surgery, radiotherapy, and systemic treatment, balancing morbidity and quality of life.

Chemotherapy + Drug Therapy

Chemotherapy is often not a promising option due to the slow growth of chordomas.

Overall, not enough evidence is available to recommend chemotherapy for chordoma. Medical drug treatments for chordomas have limited efficacy [25]. To date, there have been no randomized, controlled trials in chordoma that have resulted in defined agents of clinical benefit for systemic treatment.

But recently molecular genetic pathways with the corresponding target structures have been identified in chordomas, which offer the first approach for a targeted therapy. Inhibitors of several of these targets (EGFR, Brachyury) have shown slight activity in the disease. Further studies are in progress.

47.2.2 Case Description

A 40 y/o woman was referred to our outpatient clinic. She was complaining about severe pain in the coccygeal region since a fall a few months ago. Initially the pain was under control but now she suffered from deterioration. She reported to be unable to lie on her back. She had not observed any bladder and bowel dysfunction. In here medical history no comorbidities were documented.

The clinical examination showed a tumor with pain on palpation proximal to the Rima ani with absence of any neurological deficits (Fig. 47.4).

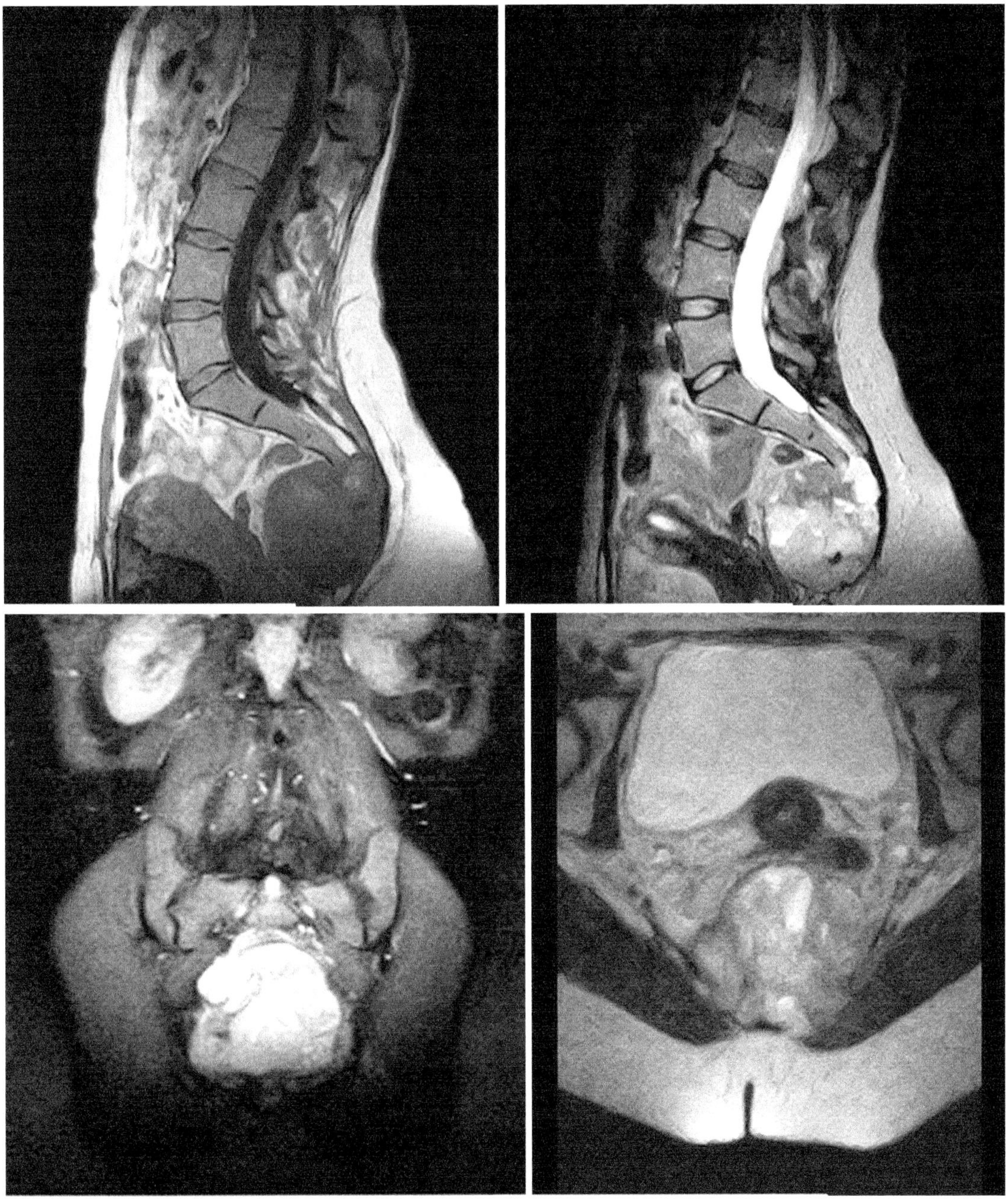

Fig. 47.4 MRI scan at first presentation. The MRI scan shows a large tumor in the distal part of the sacrum of approximately 7 cm with origin at the S4 vertebra. There is no clear margin of the tumor identifiable with extension into the pelvis suggestive for a chordoma

After the images had been analyzed we recommended a biopsy first to identify the tumor histologically and to evaluate the further treatment options. Additionally we completed the tumor staging imaging via PET CT scan. Unfortunately the PET CT detected a pulmonary metastasis (Fig. 47.5).

The biopsy was performed a few days later with a small mini-open midline incision.

The histological result showed a mesenchymal tumor in the sense of a sarcoma with residual parts of a chordoma with typical morphology. In this respect a sarcomatoid or dedifferentiated chordoma was identified whereby the proportion of a high-grade sarcoma predominates.

The patient developed a prolonged wound healing disorder after the biopsy that was treated with revision surgeries and healed properly within a few days.

Parallel the pulmonary lesion was biopsied as well with a CT guided technique and a metastasis had been confirmed.

The subsequent discussion of the case in our mulitidisciplinary tumor board recommended the tumor resection and an additional radiotherapy of the pulmonary metastasis.

After that decision and consent of the patient we performed a combined anterior-posterior tumor resection with anterior tumor release and mobilization of the rectum with help of the abdominal surgeons. From posterior a partial sacrectomy was undertaken distally sparing the right S3 nerve root and completion of the tumor release posteriorly. A partial resection of the gluteus maximus muscle bilaterally and the left piriformis muscle were added (Figs. 47.6 and 47.7).

In the early postoperative phase the patient recovered well. The postoperative neurological examination showed reduced muscle strength for the M. sphincter ani and the patient had problems to control the bladder initially without any loss of sensation. After a few days the bladder dysfunction settled. Furthermore no other neurological deficits were detectable.

In the further course the patient developed a postoperative wound infection with necrosis of the skin. That prolonged the hospitalization and required multiple wound revisions. After several revision surgeries and antibiotic treatment the final wound closure was performed (Figs. 47.8 and 47.9).

The final histological evaluation documented an aggressive Chordoma with dedifferentiated proportion with tumor cells close to the bony resection margin.

The reference pathological assessment confirmed a dedifferentiated Chordoma.

For the further oncological treatment the patient was referred to an oncological department. Due to the advanced disease a first chemotherapy was initiated with ifosfamid and doxorubicin and was continued for 3 cycles. An additional postoperative radiotherapy of the surgical site was planned as well but refused by the patient.

After the chemotherapy a re-staging examination was performed. Unfortunately the further imaging revealed an extensive local sacral, iliosacral and gluteal tumor recurrence. Additionally there was an increase of the pulmonary metastasis as well and a new metastasis in the corpus of the L4 vertebra (Fig. 47.10).

The oncologists started another drug therapy with Sorafenib which is a tyrosine kinase inhibitor.

The optimized medical treatment was not able to stop the tumor progress and due to the aggressiveness the patient died very rapidly only a few months postoperatively.

47.2.3 Discussion of the Case

The present case illustrates the unsuccessful treatment of a sacral chordoma. Due to the location of the tumor and the slow growth and with the unspecific clinical findings the definitive diagnosis is frequently delayed. Our case is demonstrating that as well with unclear symptoms and persistent pain after a fall. The diagnosis was confirmed with a biopsy and the further treatment plan was discussed in the multidisciplinary tumor board. Due to the initial wound healing problems even after only a small incision a preoperative radiotherapy was declined. Surely the patient was presenting an advanced disease

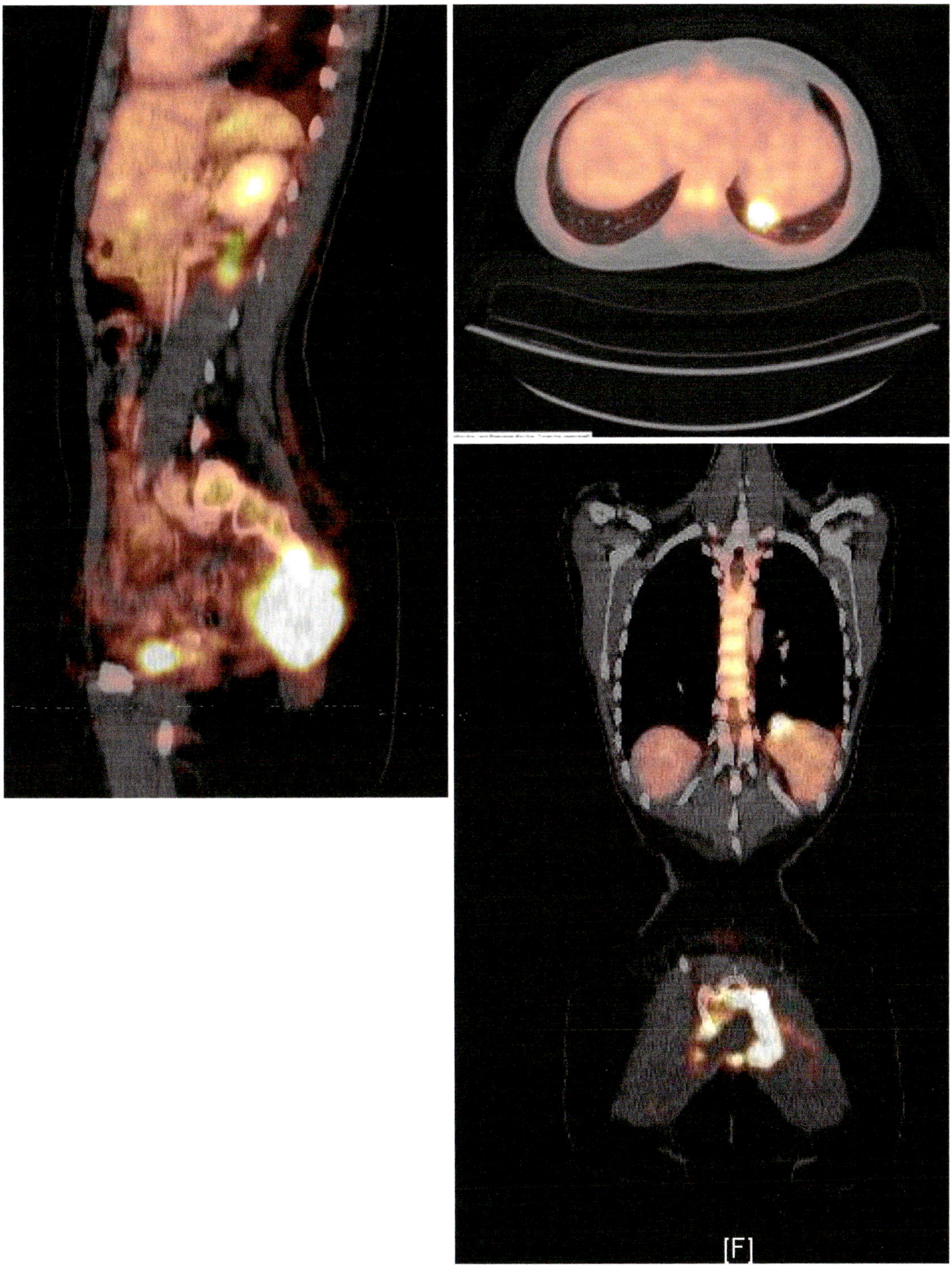

Fig. 47.5 Staging PET CT scan. Demonstration of a hypermetabolic pulmonary mass in the left lower lobe with contact to the surface of the left diaphragm consistent with a pulmonary metastasis. No evidence of hypermetabolic lymph node metastasis

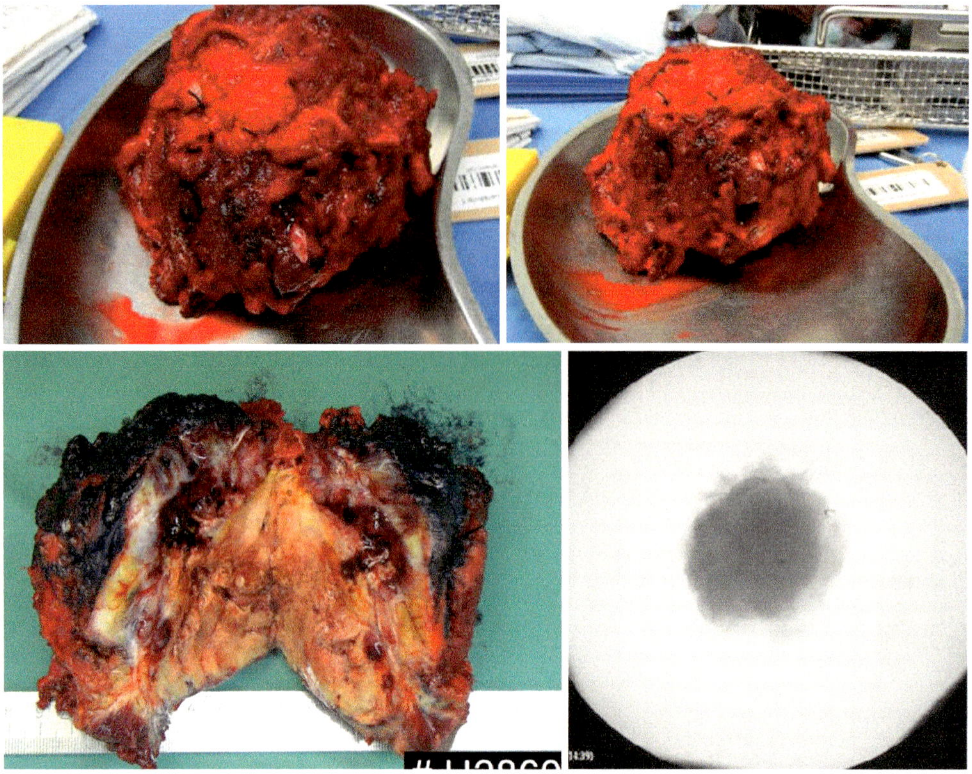

Fig. 47.6 Intraoperative result – resected tumor macroscopically and under X-ray. A 11.5 × 11 × 8.8 cm large solid tumor was resected

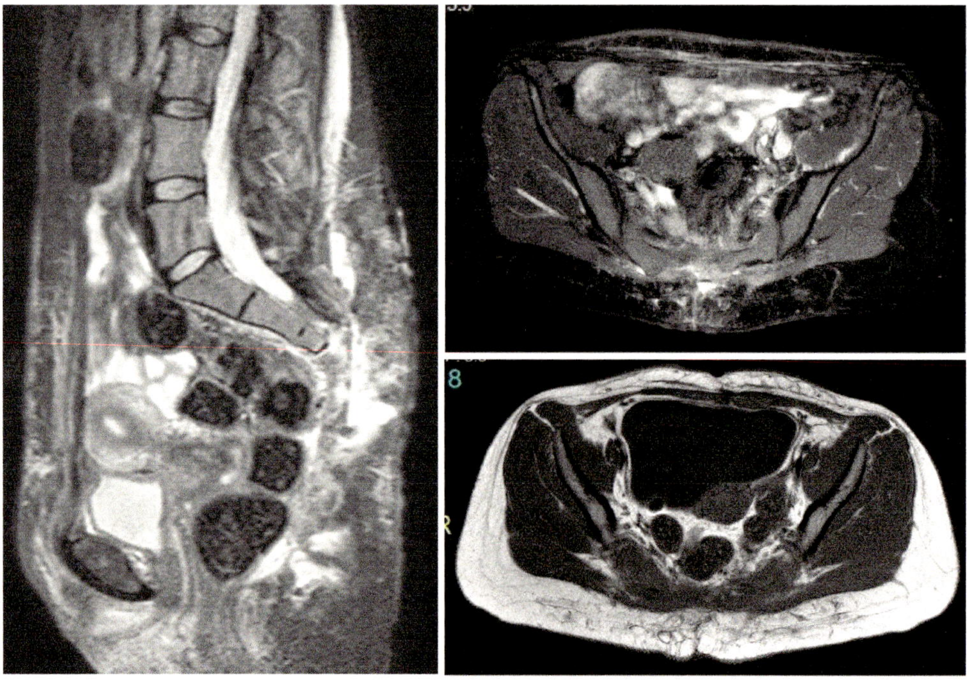

Fig. 47.7 Postoperative MRI scan. MRI scan shows the resection margins with an adequate tumor removal

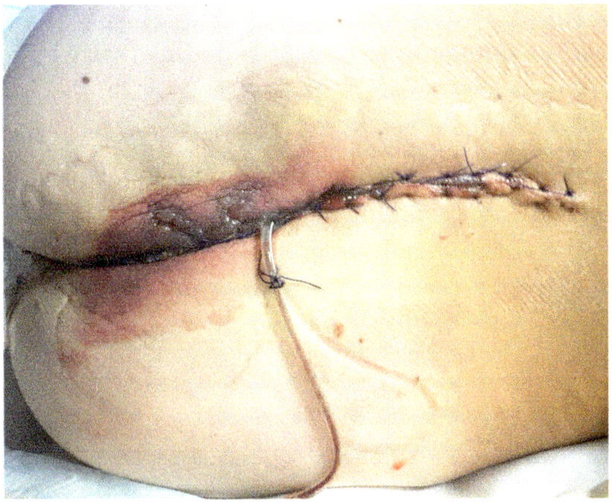

Fig. 47.8 Postoperative wound infection. The image demonstrates the local soft tissue conditions with necrosis of the skin

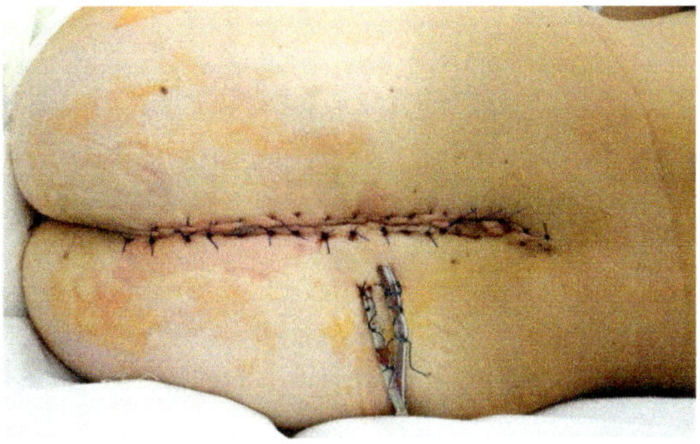

Fig. 47.9 Final result after multiple revisions. Consolidated wound conditions

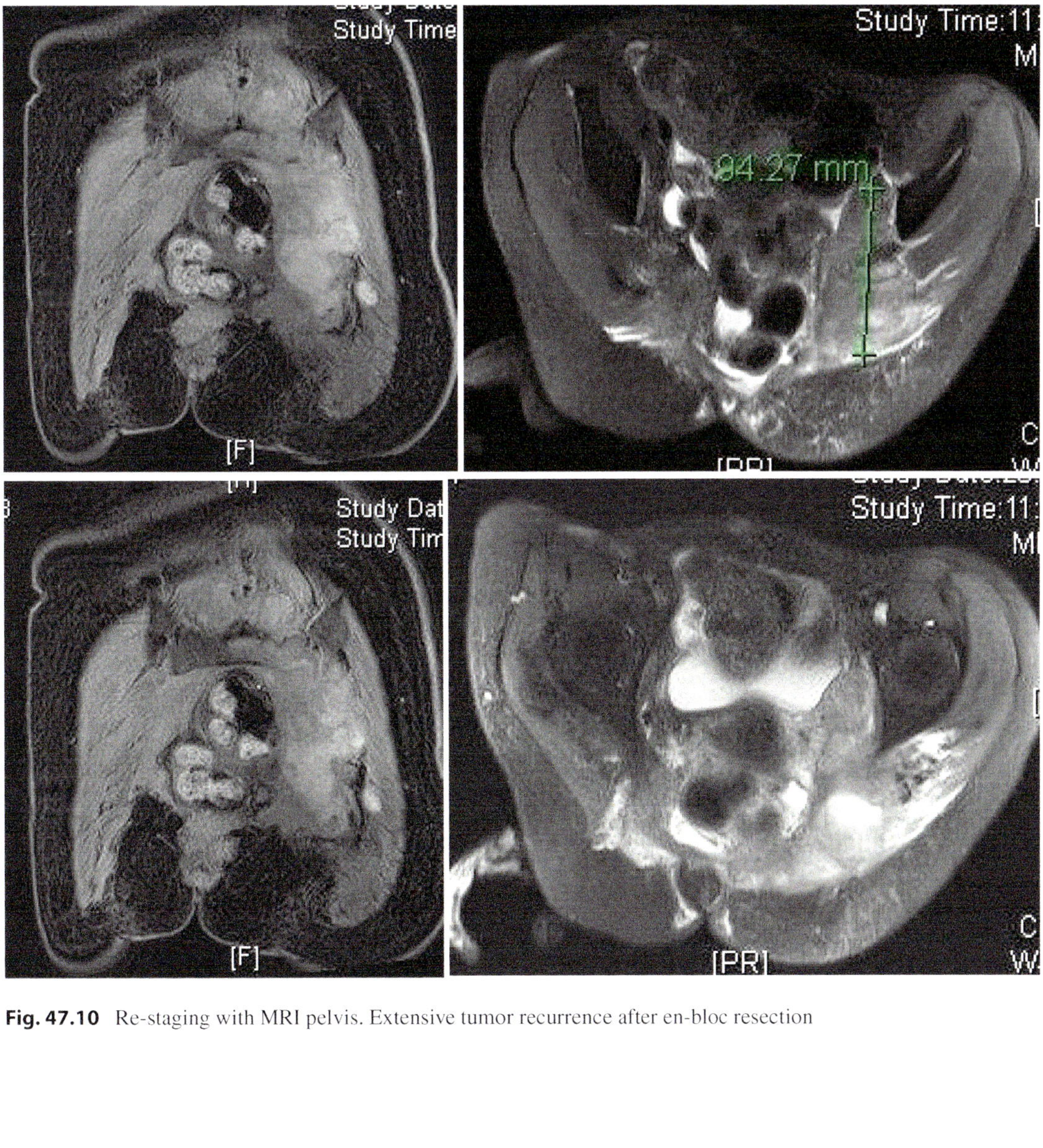

Fig. 47.10 Re-staging with MRI pelvis. Extensive tumor recurrence after en-bloc resection

with pulmonary metastasis at the point of primary diagnosis. But the treatment plan suggested tumor en-bloc resection that was performed uneventful. Even the initial neurological deficits after surgery settled in the further course an in the later follow up visits after months the patient reported of a complete bladder and bowel control again. Unfortunately the patient suffered from a serious wound infection with skin necrosis that prolonged the hospitalization and required multiple revision surgeries.

After the wound was healed properly the medical oncological treatment was initiated.

The Patient was also planned for postoperative proton beam radiotherapy but she refused so that we could not go ahead according to the recommended treatment plan [17]. The further oncological treatment showed that the tumor cells did not respond adequately to the chemotherapy. That circumstance is reported as well in the literature and shows the difficulties in treating chordomas. The second drug treatment with a tyrosine kinase inhibitor was not able to reduce the tumor progress and metastatic spread at the advanced stage was resulted in the patients' death very soon only after a few months. We were not able to hang on to the literature recommendations regarding preoperative radiotherapy due to the critical soft tissue situation. Unfortunately the patient did not accept radiotherapy postoperatively as well. If this would have changed the clinical course massively is theoretical. The further oncological treatment showed the currently very limited options for a medical treatment especially in advanced tumor cases with metastasis. No agent was able to stop the recurrence and tumor progression. The whole case shows a frustrating course and the malignancy of that tumor entity with relatively short survival rates. Nevertheless new targeted medical treatment options are under testing and delivered first results.

Radiotherapy is still improving as well and shows adequate results as an alternative to surgery for the local tumor control and fortifies its status for the neoadjuvant and adjuvant therapy.

47.2.4 Conclusions and Take Home Message

Currently only limited treatment options are available to optimize the median survival of Chordoma patients. Further studies are necessary to improve the medical treatment with new promising agents and to increase the local tumor control with combinations of radiotherapy and surgery.

Pearls

- Surgical treatment in combination with radiotherapy is the main and standard treatment option for limiting recurrence and maximizing survival.
- High-dose conformal radiotherapy should be considered for the treatment of primary (de novo) chordomas in the mobile spine and sacrum when surgery is not feasible.
- As radiation therapy continues to improve it will become a more viable option for the treatment of primary (de novo) and locally recurrent chordomas.

References

1. Kelley SP, Ashford RU, Rao AS, Dickson RA. Primary bone tumours of the spine: a 42-year survey from the Leeds Regional Bone Tumour Registry. Eur Spine J. 2007;16:405–9.
2. Moore DD. Haydon RC Ewing's sarcoma of bone. Cancer Treat Res. 2014;162:93–115.
3. Ewing J. Diffuse endothelioma of bone. Proc NY Pathol Soc. 1921;21:17–24.
4. Esiashvili N, Goodman M, Marcus RB Jr. Changes in incidence and survival of Ewing sarcoma patients over the past 3 decades: surveillance epidemiology and end results data. J Pediatr Hematol Oncol. 2008;30(6):425–30.
5. Freyschmidt J, Jundt G, Ostertag H. Knochentumoren: Klinik, Radiologie, Pathologie. Berlin/Heidelberg/New York: Springer; 2003.
6. Kim HJ, McLawhorn AS, Goldstein MJ, Boland PJ. Malignant osseous tumors of the pediatric spine. J Am Acad Orthop Surg. 2012;20(10):646–56.

7. Caudill JS, Arndt CA. Diagnosis and management of bone malignancy in adolescence. Adolesc Med State Art Rev. 2007;18(1):62–78. ix.
8. West DC. Ewing sarcoma family of tumors. Curr Opin Oncol. 2000;12(4):323–9.
9. Schaser KD, Melcher I, Druschel C, Tsitsilonis S, Disch AC. Surgical management of thoracolumbar spinal sarcoma. Orthopade. 2012;41(8):659–73.
10. Balamuth NJ, Womer RB. Ewing's sarcoma. Lancet Oncol. 2010;11(2):184–92. https://doi.org/10.1016/S1470-2045(09)70286-4.
11. Hoffmann C, Ahrens S, Dunst J, et al. Pelvic Ewing sarcoma: a retrospective analysis of 241 cases. Cancer. 1999;85(4):869–77.
12. Frisch S, Timmermann B. The evolving role of proton beam therapy for sarcomas. Clin Oncol (R Coll Radiol). 2017;29(8):500–6.
13. Flanagan AMYT. Chordoma. In: Fletcher CDM, Bridge JA, Hogendoorn PCW, Mertens F, editors. World Health Organization classification of tumours. Pathology and genetics of tumours of soft tissue and-bone. Lyon: IARC Press; 2013. p. S328–9.
14. McMaster ML, Goldstein AM, Bromley CM, Ishibe N, Parry DM. Chordoma: incidence and survival patterns in the United States, 1973–1995. Cancer Causes Control. 2001;12:1–11.
15. Lauer SR, Edgar MA, Gardner JM, Sebastian A, Weiss SW. Soft tissue chordomas: a clinicopathologic analysis of 11 cases. Am J Surg Pathol. 2013;37:719–26.
16. Bergh P, Kindblom LG, Gunterberg B, et al. Prognostic factors in chordoma of the sacrum and mobile spine: a study of 39 patients. Cancer. 2000;88:2122–34.
17. Stacchiotti S, Sommer J, Chordoma Global Consensus Group. Building a global consensus approach to chordoma: a position paper from the medical and patient community. Lancet Oncol. 2015;16(2):e71–83.
18. Stacchiotti S, Casali PG, Vullo SL. Chordoma of the mobile spine and sacrum: a retrospective analysis of a series of patients surgically treated at two referral centers. Ann Surg Oncol. 2010;17:211–9.
19. Walcott BP, Nahed BV, Mohyeldin A, Coumans JV, Kahle KT, Ferreira MJ. Chordoma: current concepts, management, and future directions. Lancet Oncol. 2012;13:e69–76.9.
20. Rotondo RL, et al. High-dose proton-based radiation therapy in the management of spine chordomas: Outcomes and clinicopathological prognostic factors. J Neurosurg Spine. 2015;23:788–97.
21. De Amorim Bernstein K, DeLaney T. Chordomas and chondrosarcomas-the role of radiation therapy. J Surg Oncol. 2016;114(5):564–9. https://doi.org/10.1002/jso.24368. Epub 2016 Oct 19.
22. Chen YL, et al. Definitive high-dose photon/proton radiotherapy for unresected mobile spine and sacral chordomas. Spine (Phila Pa 1976). 2013;38:E930–6.
23. Imai R, et al. Carbon ion radiotherapy for unresectable sacral chordomas. Clin Cancer Res. 2004;10:5741–6.
24. Varga PP, Szövérfi Z, Fisher CG, Boriani S, Gokaslan ZL, Dekutoski MB, Chou D, Quraishi NA, Reynolds JJ, Luzzati A, Williams R, Fehlings MG, Germscheid NM, Lazary A, Rhines LD. Surgical treatment of sacral chordoma: prognostic variables for local recurrence and overall survival. Eur Spine J. 2015;24(5):1092–101.
25. Stacchiotti S, Casali PG. Systemic therapy options for unresectable and metastatic chordomas. Curr Oncol Rep. 2011;13:323–30.

Secondary Malignant Tumors (Diagnosis, Staging, Surgical Treatment and Adjuvant Therapy)

48

Jens Gempt

48.1 Introduction

Spinal metastases occur in 70% of all carcinoma patients. Therefore it's a common disease today and patient numbers are constantly rising since tumor therapies are evolving and overall survival times in common tumor diseases are still increasing. In 5–15% patients suffer from epidural tumor compression.

Most common primary tumors causing spinal metastases are lung, breast, and prostate cancer. These three entities account for up to 60% of all spinal metastases. Other tumors causing frequently spinal metastasis are renal tumors, melanoma, thyroid cancer, colorectal carcinomas and lymphomas.

Therapy decisions are based on different factors like patient's neurological function, spinal stability, pain, quality of life, oncological criteria (solitary metastasis vs. multiple metastases, curative vs. palliative approach, tumor entity, life expectancy).

Therapy of spinal metastases consists of systemic therapy/chemotherapy, local radiotherapy, and of course surgical therapy. Surgical therapy options are diverse and range from decompression only to decompression and stabilization with dorsal approach combined ventral and dorsal approaches up to en bloc resection in selected cases.

The present chapter illustrates the aspects spinal metastases; frequent symptoms, preoperative imaging and surgical approaches as well as adjuvant therapy.

The aim of these cases is to illuminate important steps in treatment decision as well as surgical strategy while considering prognosis and treatment options of the underlying disease.

- Indications for surgery
- Choice of the proper approach depending on the lesion location, size and consistency
- Surgical strategy depending on tumor entity and disease staging

48.2 Case Description

48.2.1 I Case

A 55 y/o female patient suffered from strong neck pain over the last months. Her neurological examination was normal. She was treated for breast cancer for nearly 5 years with operation, paclitaxel and tamoxifen.

The staging CT and following holospinal MRI scan revealed a pathological C7 fracture as well as multiple thoracic metastases (Fig. 48.1). The interdisciplinary tumor board decided to first conduct surgery as a vertebral body replace-

J. Gempt (✉)
Department of Neurosurgery, Klinikum rechts der Isar, Technische Universität München, Munich, Germany
e-mail: Jens.Gempt@tum.de

B. Meyer, M. Rauschmann (eds.), *Spine Surgery*, https://doi.org/10.1007/978-3-319-98875-7_48

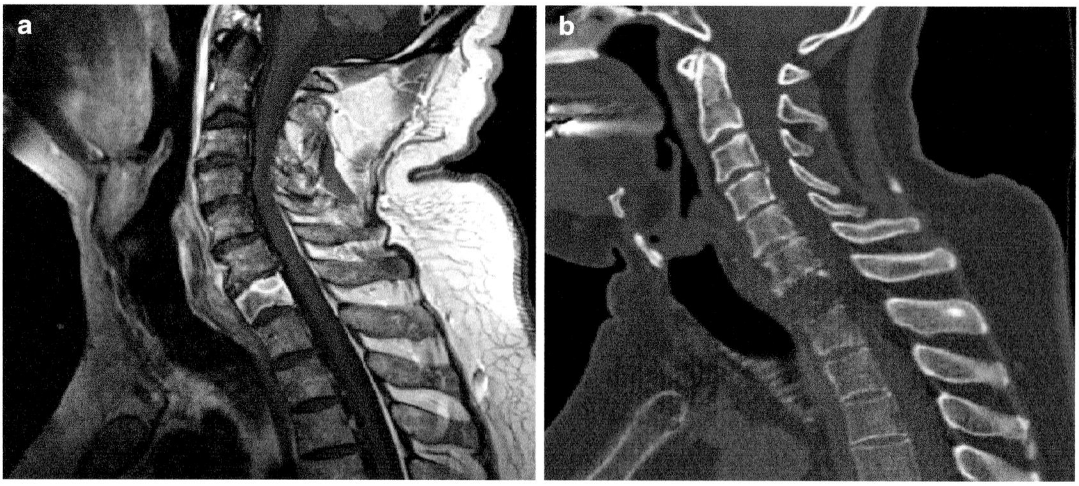

Fig. 48.1 MRI and CT scan on outpatient visit. The MRI scan (**a**) and CT scan (**b**) of a 55 y/o female patient with a pathological C7 fracture

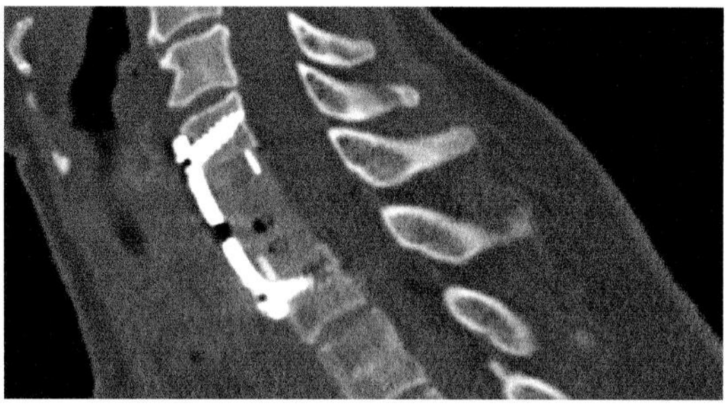

Fig. 48.2 Postoperative CT scan. The CT scan of the cervikothoracic junction shows a successful vertebral body replacement of C7 and a satisfying position of implants as well as spinal alignment

ment C7 via anterior approach. Regarding the thoracic metastasis the decision of surgical intervention and radiotherapy vs. radiotherapy only was made after the C7 vertebral body replacement. It was decided to conduct radiotherapy only (Fig. 48.2).

48.2.2 II Case

82 y/o male patient with a long history of neck and low back pain as well as a known M. Bechterew presented with a progressive thoracic pain as well as gait disturbances. The patient reported multiple falls during the last weeks due to the gait disturbances. Clinical examination revealed a spinal ataxia, hyperreflexia of the lower extremities as well as a hypoesthia below TH5.

Spinal CT imaging, which was conducted in suspect of a thoracic spinal fracture revealed a lytic TH3 vertebra as well as intraspinal tumor mass in this level and at TH4 and more spinal bony lesions at TH5 and TH6. Urine analysis was positive for Bence Jones protein. Medical history was revealed a colon carcinoma many years ago. After discussion in our interdisciplinary tumor board the patient received a dorsal stabilization TH1-2-4-5-6-7-8 via a percutaneous minimally invasive approach and a decompression and vertebral body replacement of TH3 via a dorsal midline incision. Gait disturbances as well as pain and hypoesthesia resolved 2 weeks after surgery. Histopathology revealed a plasma cell myeloma. Due to anthropic wound healing problems a wound revision was conducted 2 weeks after the initial surgery. Systemic therapy and local radiotherapy was started due to wound healing problems then 5 weeks after surgery (Figs. 48.3 and 48.4).

48.2.3 III Case

62 y/o male patient presented with weight loss during the last 3 month. He suffered from back pain as well as left sided leg pain for several

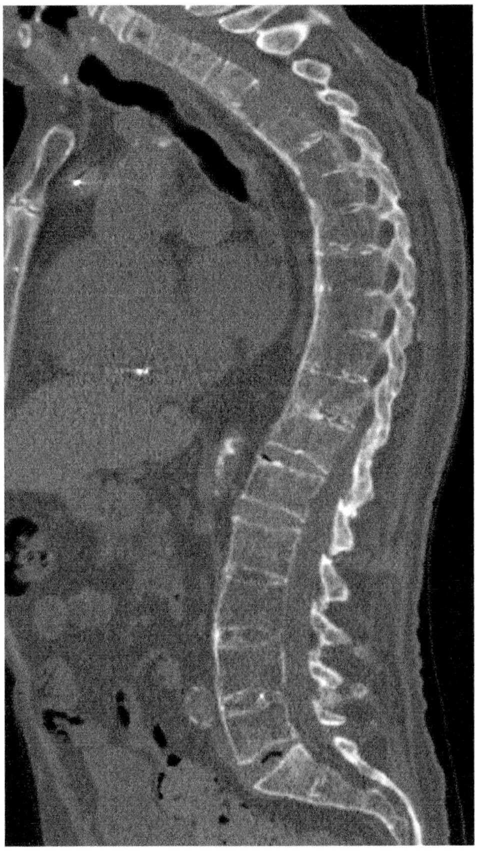

Fig. 48.3 Preoperative CT scan Case II. The CT displays a lytic TH3 vertebra as well as the M. Bechterew typical changes of the spine

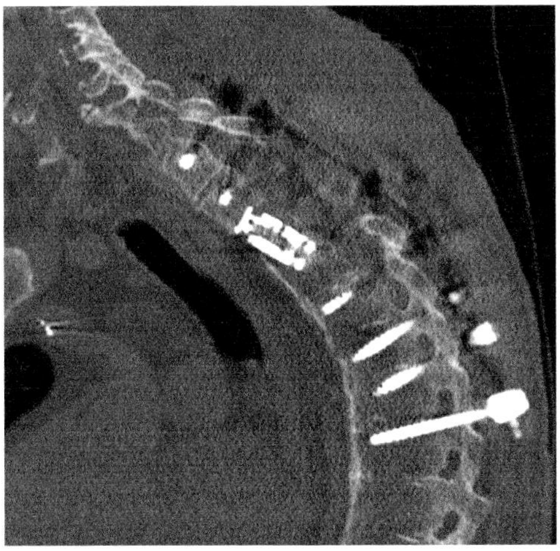

Fig. 48.4 Postoperative CT scan. The postoperative CT scan shows the dorsal stabilization with pedicle screws as well as the implant after vertebral body replacement

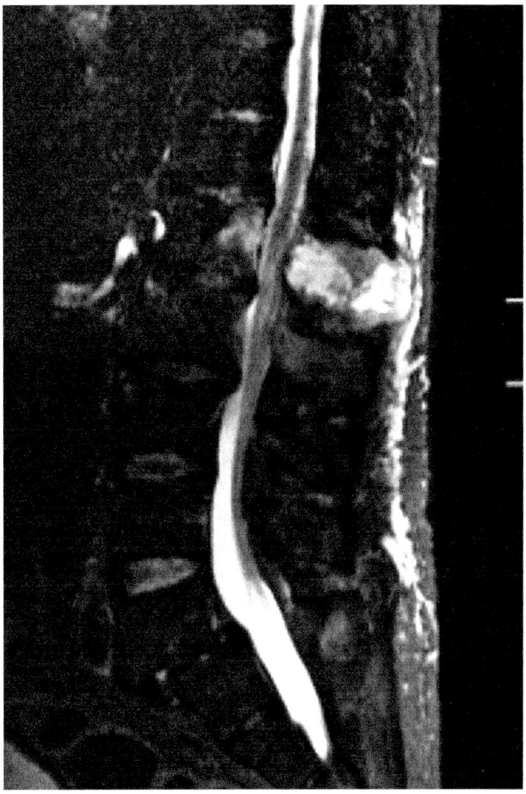

Fig. 48.5 Preoperative MRI scan with a tumor mass at level of L1 and L2

weeks. Physical examination revealed no neurological deficit.

A CT scan displayed a large lesion of the right lung suspicious for a lung carcinoma as well as of the right kidney. Additionally a metastasis of L1 with an intraspinal tumor mass was shown. Holospinal MRI scan confirmed the spinal lesion, which extends from L1 to L2.

The interdisciplinary tumor board decided for a spinal stabilization and decompression. Therefore stabilization with carbon pedicle screws from TH11-TH12-L1-L2-L3 (only one sided pedicle screws in L1 and L2) via a minimally invasive approach and decompression with tumordebulking in L1 and L2 was conducted via a midline incision. Histopathology revealed a NSCLC. Postoperative systemic therapy as well as local radiotherapy was initiated (Figs. 48.5 and 48.6).

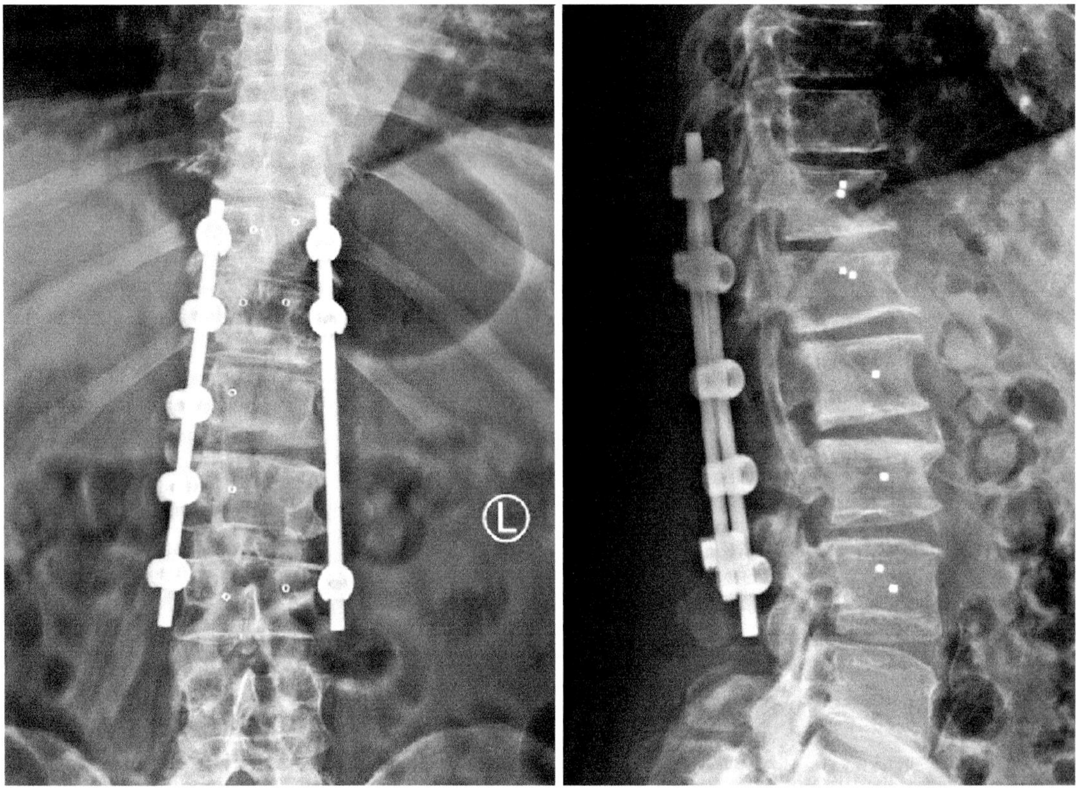

Fig. 48.6 Postoeprative x-ray with carbon pedicle screws TH11-TH12 in both pedicles and L1 and L2 one-sided as well as L3 in both pedicles

48.3 Discussion of the Cases

More or less independent from the entity of the underlying disease the decision for or against surgery is conducted while regarding the following aspects.

- Stability – is there an instability?
- Oncological – is a curative approach possible?
- Neurological function – is there a neurological deficit due to epidural spinal compression?
- Pain and quality of life – does the patient suffer from significant pain, which is difficult to control with conservative procedures?
- Histological diagnosis – Is there a need for histopathological/molecular evaluation?
- General clinical status, life expectancy – will patient survive the operation and will he recover from it to benefit from the operation?

48.3.1 Case I

The first case's patient primarily only suffers from strong neck pain. General clinical status appears good but even 5 years ago the underlying disease already qualified as metastasized which she survived in good condition until today. For breast cancer even in advanced stage disease a long survival is possible and common nowadays. HER2 receptor status should be assessed since in patients were HER2 is over-expressed it becomes more and more an important target in modern breast cancer therapy.

Neurological function in our patient is intact. There is only slight compression of the nerve roots and the tumor is mainly located in the vertebra.

From an oncological point of view we have a patient with multiple metastases and a surgical intervention will not lower the systemic tumor burden significant. Regarding spinal stability though we considered the C7 lesion as instable. The definition of stability in cases of spinal metastasis might differ though depending on different opinions. General considerations of spinal stability in case of metastatic spine lesions are summarized by the SINS-score. It incorporates lesion location, loading pain, type of bone lesion, spinal alignment, collapse of vertebral body and involvement of posterolateral structures [3]. A more pragmatic view might be to consider a lesion in patients with prevalent clear loading pain as instable.

48.3.1.1 Choice of Approach Case I

In our patient an anterior approach was used to conduct a vertebral body replacement. There are mainly retrospective case series as well as data from registers and no high class evidence, which underpins our choice of approach. Though we are in line with the recommendations of "Spine Oncology Study Group" [2]. In general for C0-C2 lesions a dorsal approach with stabilization is recommended, for C3-6 primarily a ventral approach should be considered (depending on the lesion a dorsal stabilization in addition possible), for lesions C7-T2 depending on the exact localization a ventral and/or dorsal approach are recommended with stabilization as well. A laminectomy alone without spinal stabilization is nowadays obsolete in most cases.

48.3.2 Case II

For the second cases's patient primarily a progressive neurological decline with myelopathic gait disturbances resulting from epidural spinal cord compression led to a clear decision for surgery. Spinal instability, unclear tumor entity and pain were factors in favor for a surgical intervention as well. A holospinal MRI was desired but not conducted due to cardiac pacemaker. For spinal cord compression due to metastatic lesions there is compared to other surgical aspects high-class evidence available. Comparing radiotherapy alone with surgery for circumferential decompression followed by radiotherapy results are significantly superior in patients undergoing surgery regarding the ability to walk (again) [4].

48.3.2.1 Choice of Approach Case II

A posterior approach was conducted for the stabilization and the vertebral body replacement. Stability is a major issue in this patient due to the concomitant Bechterew's disease, which necessitates a long dorsale pedicle screw construct as well as the need for vertebral body replacement anyhow. A percutaneous approach was chosen for the pedicle screws. During the postoperative course unfortunately a wound healing disorder occurred. Problems regarding wound healing and wound infections are common among patients with secondary neoplastic spine lesions. Wound infections alone might struck about 10–20% of these patients and the overall morbidity should be considered as more than 30% [1]. Therefore the approach should be as minimal as possible to avoid tissue trauma and therefore a higher risk for wound healing disorders.

48.3.3 Case III

The third case's patient presents with an already metastasized tumor disease. Though lung cancer was suspected multiple lesions were seen according to the staging CT. We observed no neurological deficit but the lesion compromised all spinal columns in the lumbar-thoracic junction. Patient has back pain, but conservative therapy was not escalated yet. Particularly in therapy naive tumor patients systemic therapy should be conducted as soon as possible. Regarding oncological considerations prognostic scores according to Tomita or Tokuhashi and others could be calculated to estimate the prognosis [6, 7]. These scores respect general condition, primary site of the cancer, number of metastases e.g.

Nowadays though due to modern immunotherapy and molecular pathology, therapy options and patient's survival experiences a quantum leap for certain patients and how long these patients we treat today might be difficult to foresee.

What has to be considered in this patient is if the systemic treatment would be significant delayed by surgery since after biopsy only time is needed for histopathological workup as well. If an operation has to be conducted under chemotherapy and radiotherapy due to progressive neurological symptoms or instability, morbidity in these patients multiplicates.

48.3.3.1 Choice of Approach Case III

Therefore we decided to go for a initial dorsal approach with decompression and stabilization via pedicle screws. Since wound healing could be a major problem in this patient as well a minimal invasive approach with as less tissue trauma as possible was aimed for.

If a vertebral body replacement is needed to spinal instability timing should depend on definite histology, pace of systemic tumor progression and available therapy options. Considering the stabilization systems materials, new radiolucent/nonmetal materials with less MR-artifacts become more and more available. Due to the novelty of these materials there are only few studies dealing with their clinical application but advantages regarding superior follow up imaging with MRI and CT as well as superior radiotherapy planning are obvious [5].

Pearls

- Major factors in treatment decision are: stability, oncological considerations, general clinical status, and life expectancy neurological function, pain and quality of life
- Treatment is always an interdisciplinary and individual patient tailored concept
- Preoperative holospinal MRI as well as staging CT should be conducted
- Predominantly surgery consist of decompression and stabilization, decompressive surgery only is the exception
- High risk of wound healing disorders necessitates as little tissue trauma as possible and therefore minimally invasive approaches

48.4 Conclusions and Take Home Message

Treatment of secondary malignant tumors of the spine is always an interdisciplinary challenge. Decision of surgery indication, timing, and extent of surgery depend on multiple factors. Due to enormous progress in therapy options regarding immunotherapy prognosis of metastasized patients increases significantly and will result in an immense increase of patients which have to be treated surgically as well. Neurological deficits in case of spinal cord compression due to epidural tumor mass as well as compromised spinal stability are against the background of the underlying disease a clear indication for surgery followed by radio- and/or chemotherapy. Depending on the urgency of surgery patients should receive staging CT as well as holospinal MRI prior to surgery.

References

1. Bakar D, Tanenbaum JE, Phan K, Alentado VJ, Steinmetz MP, Benzel EC, Mroz TE. Decompression surgery for spinal metastases: a systematic review. Neurosurg Focus. 2016;41(2):E2. https://doi.org/10.3171/2016.6.FOCUS16166.
2. Fisher CG, Andersson GB, Weinstein JN. Spine focus issue. Summary of management recommendations in spine oncology. Spine (Phila Pa 1976). 2009;34(22 Suppl):S2–6. https://doi.org/10.1097/BRS.0b013e3181baae29.
3. Fisher CG, DiPaola CP, Ryken TC, Bilsky MH, Shaffrey CI, Berven SH, Harrop JS, Fehlings MG, Boriani S, Chou D, Schmidt MH, Polly DW, Biagini R, Burch S, Dekutoski MB, Ganju A, Gerszten PC, Gokaslan ZL, Groff MW, Liebsch NJ, Mendel E, Okuno SH, Patel S, Rhines LD, Rose PS, Sciubba DM, Sundaresan N, Tomita K, Varga PP, Vialle LR, Vrionis FD, Yamada Y, Fourney DR. A novel classification system for spinal instability in neoplastic disease: an evidence-based approach and expert consensus from the Spine Oncology Study Group. Spine (Phila Pa 1976). 2010;35(22):E1221–9. https://doi.org/10.1097/BRS.0b013e3181e16ae2.
4. Patchell RA, Tibbs PA, Regine WF, Payne R, Saris S, Kryscio RJ, Mohiuddin M, Young B. Direct decompressive surgical resection in the treatment of spinal cord compression caused by metastatic cancer: a randomised trial. Lancet. 2005;366(9486):643–8. https://doi.org/10.1016/S0140-6736(05)66954-1.

5. Ringel F, Ryang YM, Kirschke JS, Muller BS, Wilkens JJ, Brodard J, Combs SE, Meyer B. Radiolucent carbon fiber-reinforced pedicle screws for treatment of spinal tumors: advantages for radiation planning and follow-up imaging. World Neurosurg. 2017;105:294–301. https://doi.org/10.1016/j.wneu.2017.04.091.
6. Tokuhashi Y, Matsuzaki H, Toriyama S, Kawano H, Ohsaka S. Scoring system for the preoperative evaluation of metastatic spine tumor prognosis. Spine (Phila Pa 1976). 1990;15(11):1110–3. Retrieved from http://www.ncbi.nlm.nih.gov/pubmed/1702559.
7. Tomita K, Kawahara N, Kobayashi T, Yoshida A, Murakami H, Akamaru T. Surgical strategy for spinal metastases. Spine (Phila Pa 1976). 2001;26(3):298–306. Retrieved from http://www.ncbi.nlm.nih.gov/pubmed/11224867.

Part VI

Advanced Module 1: Extended Indications and Advanced Operative Techniques

Indications for Craniocervical Surgery and Anterior Resection Techniques (Endonasal, Transoral)

49

Jens Gempt

49.1 Introduction

Nowadays indication for craniocervical surgery with anterior resection techniques are rare. Pathologies of the craniocervical junction with a possible need for anterior resection techniques are basilar impression/atlantoaxial subluxation and/or retrodental pannus often described in patients with rheumatoid arthritis or other non-rheumatic degeneration of the respective joints as well as infection of the craniocervical junction or rare primary or secondary malignancies.

In cases of severe rheumatoid arthritis, and long disease progression hypertrophied synovium invades and erodes cartilage and bone. Therefore it forms a tumor-like tissue, which can result in a neuro-compressive lesion at the craniocervical junction adding to the often present malalignment due to cervical joint destruction.

Since all of the possible indications are rare there is a certain lack of high level scientific evidence not only regarding which patients to treat surgically but also which approach should be used.

The aim of these cases is to illuminate important steps in surgical treatment decision as well as surgical strategy while considering the nature of the underlying disease.

- Indications for surgery
- Choice of the proper approach
- Changes in treatment strategy due to improvement in medical therapy

49.2 Case Description

49.2.1 Case I

84-year-old male patient suffering from lumbar pain for the last few years as well as progressive neck pain. He stated that he could not walk without help anymore and even then only for a few meters. His neurological examination revealed a fine motor impairment of both upper extremities and a severe myelopathic gait disturbance. Low back pain was significantly improved by lumbar facet joint infiltration. Cervical CT and MRI (Fig. 49.1) revealed massive degenerative changes as well as a malalignment of the craniocervical junction and a retro dental mass as well as a moderate spinal stenosis C5/6 and C6/7. In spite of the pronounced degeneration of the spinal joints as well as wrist- and knee joints a rheumatoid arthritis was never diagnosed for this patient and he was only treated symptomatically.

We decided to operate via a posterior approach only. The patient stabilized with bilateral C1 lateral mass screws and C2 isthmic screws (Fig. 49.2).

J. Gempt (✉)
Department of Neurosurgery, Klinikum rechts der Isar, Technische Universität München, Munich, Germany
e-mail: Jens.Gempt@tum.de

B. Meyer, M. Rauschmann (eds.), *Spine Surgery*, https://doi.org/10.1007/978-3-319-98875-7_49

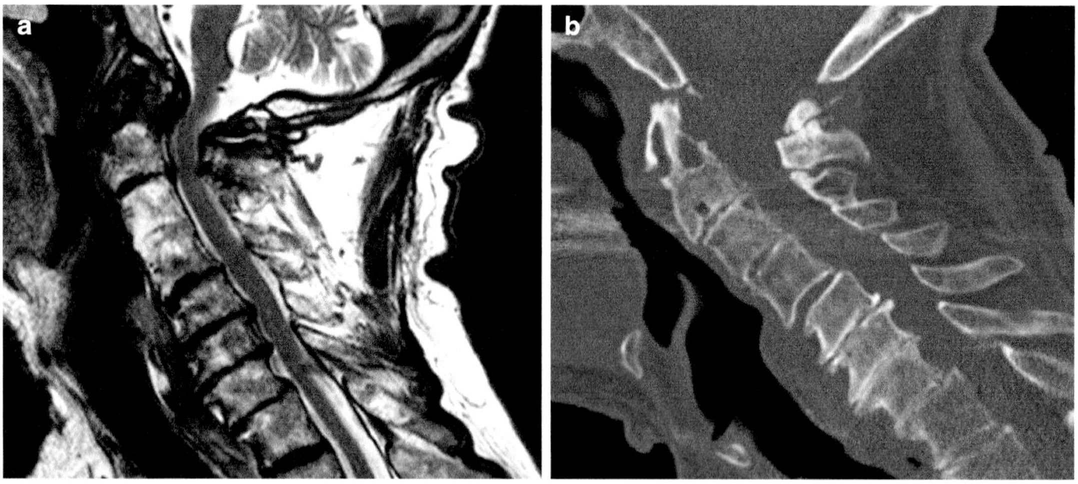

Fig. 49.1 Preoperative MRI and CT scan case I. The MRI (**a**) and CT (**b**) scan show the retro dental pannus as well as hypertrophic joints C1/2 and a cranicevical malalignment resulting altogether in a kinking and compression of the medulla oblongata/spinal cord. Also visible is a moderate spinal stenosis at the level below C5

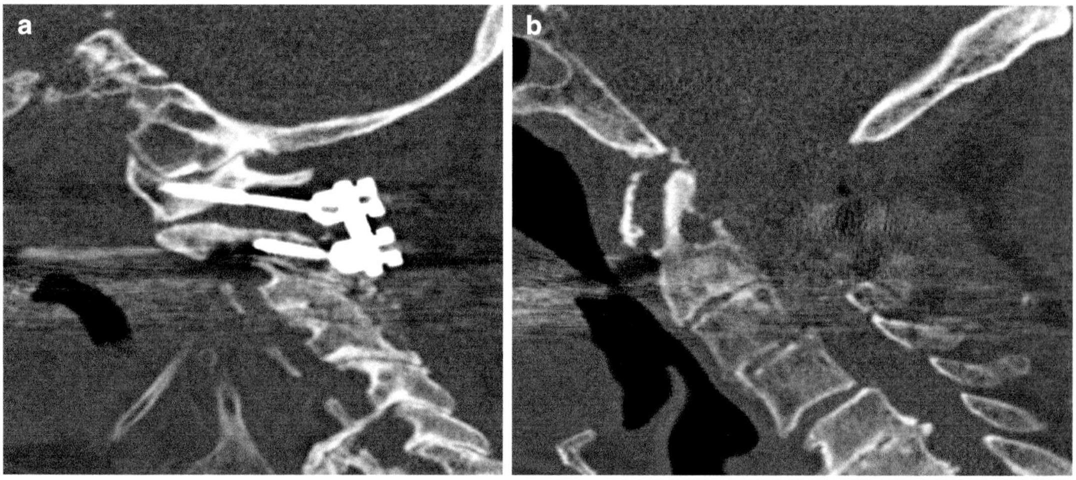

Fig. 49.2 Postoperative CT scan case I. CT scan shows the C1 lateral mass screw and C2 isthmic screw (**a**) as well as the dorsal decompression (**b**)

A laminectomy for dorsal decompression was conducted as well. During the hospital stay he improved with regards to gait disturbance and fine motor impairment and was transferred back to a rehabilitation unit.

49.2.2 Case II

85 y/o male patient suffered sensory disturbances for about 1 year of the left Arm and leg. In particular a painful sensation of cold limbs bothered him. Since a few months he had observed progressive walking problems. Now he could only walk with help. Writing with his hands had also become very difficult.

His neurological examination revealed a fine motor impairment of upper extremities and a severe myelopathic gait disturbance as well as sensory disturbances regarding his left Arm, hemithorax and left leg with a compromised sensation of cold/warm.

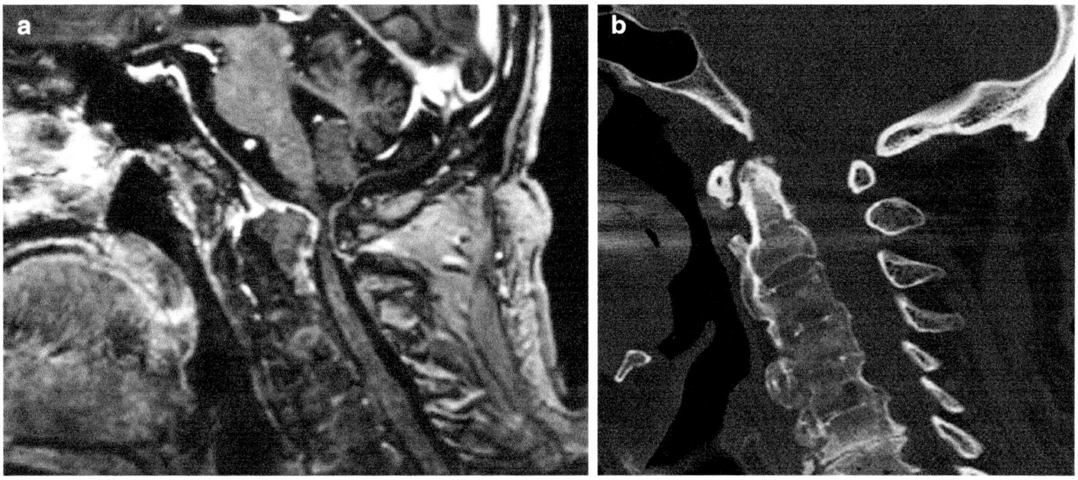

Fig. 49.3 Preoperative MRI and CT scan case II. MRI (**a**) and CT (**b**) of the craniocervical junction with changes typicall for ankylosing spondylitis of the cervical spine as well as severe degenerative changes of the craniocervical junction joints and a huge retrodental pannus formation compressing the spinal cord (**a**)

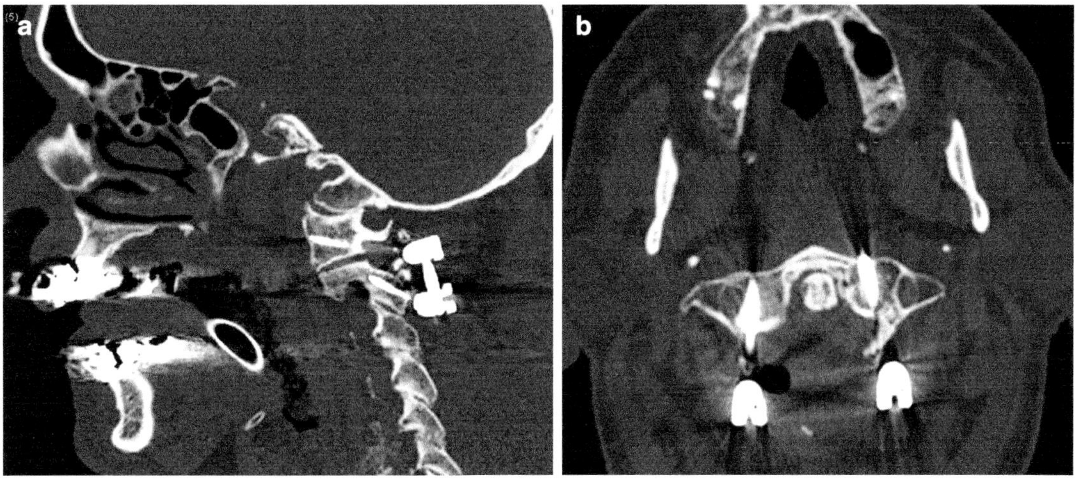

Fig. 49.4 Postperative CT scan case II, Operation 1. Postoperative CT (**a**, **b**) of the craniocervical junction following the first operation. A good position of screws (**a**), as well as the dorsal decompression is visible

CT and MRI (Fig. 49.3) was conducted and revealed changes typicall for ankylosing spondylitis of the cervical spine as well as severe degenerative changes of the craniocervical junction joints and a huge retrodental pannus formation compressing the spinal cord.

First a posterior approach was conducted with bilateral C1 lateral mass screws and bilateral C2 isthmic screws (Fig. 49.4a, b). A laminectomy for dorsal decompression was conducted as well. Surgery went without adverse events and the patient did not show further deterioration.

Due to the still present large ventral mass with compression on the spinal cord a second surgery via a transnasal endoscopic approach through both nostrils was conducted. The upper part of the C1 arch as well as the tip of the odontoid and most of the retrodental mass was resected as well to accomplish further decompression (Fig. 49.5).

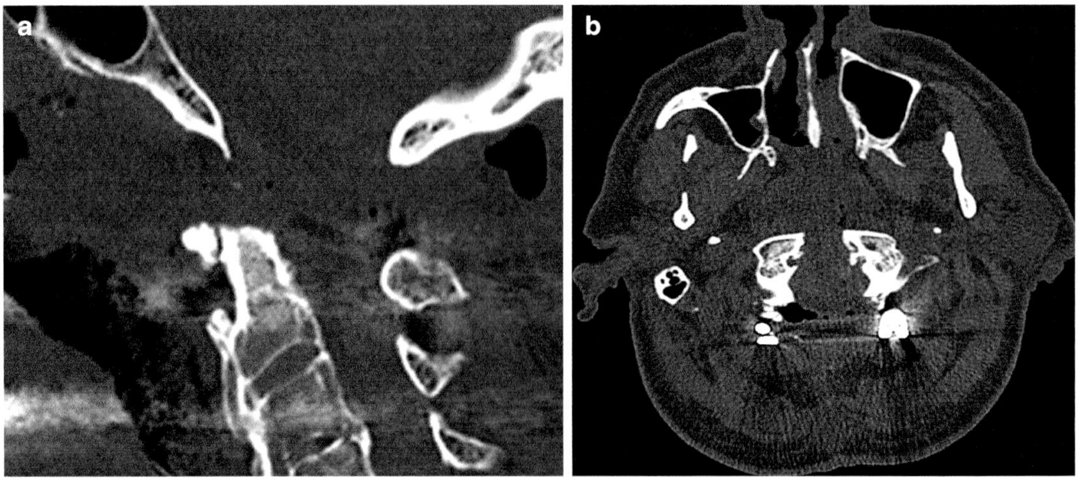

Fig. 49.5 Postoperative CT scan. The postoperative CT scan shows the resection of the odontoid tip as well as the upper part of the C1 arch therefore creating a corridor to the redtrodental mass (**a**, **b**)

49.3 Discussion of the Cases

The Indication for or against surgery and the decision regarding the proper approach is conducted while regarding the following aspects:

- Stability – is there an instability in C1-2 or in C0-1-2
- Neurological function – is there a neurological deficit due to spinal cord compression?
- Underlying disease?
- Histological diagnosis necessary?
- Posterior approach vs. combined approach – is there a significant ventral mass causing neurological deficits?

49.3.1 Case I

49.3.1.1 Indication

The first patient presented with strong neck pain as well as a malalignement of the spine of the craniocervical junction with progressive neurological symptoms. Severe gait disturbance as well as compromised fine motor function were observed. All these aspects justified the indication for surgery. Symptoms, neurological decline were caused by spinal instability and concomitant neurocompression. Therefore a stabilization procedure and decompression were indicated.

49.3.1.2 Choice of Approach

The C1-C2 joint causes instability and spinal malalignement. Therefore decision for stabilization of this segment only was made. In general the need for C0-1-2 stabilization is very rare and might be indicated for example in traumatic atlanto-occipital dislocation or cases were a fixation of C1 is not feasible [5].

Need for decompression was discussed as well. In our patient there were severe neurological deficits as well as a dorsal compression, therefore a laminectomy and dorsal decompression was indicated as well. In case of moderate neurological deficits a decompression (dorsal or ventral) might not be necessary at all since a retrodental pannus can resolve completely after fixation of the instability [3].

In our patient we considered therefore a further ventral approach to reduce the ventral mass as not necessary.

49.3.2 Case II

49.3.2.1 Indication

The second patient had a fine motor impairment of upper extremities and a severe myelopathic gait disturbance as well as sensory disturbances regarding his left Arm, hemithorax and left leg with a compromised sensation of cold/warm. In this patient symptoms, neurological decline were caused by spinal instability and concomitant large retrodental mass with severe neurocompression. Therefore a stabilization procedure and decompression was indicated.

49.3.2.2 Choice of Approach

Since also in this patient he C1-C2 joint causes instability and spinal malalignement. Therefore stabilization of this segment only was conducted. Bilateral C1 lateral mass screws and bilateral C2 isthmic screws were used. Transarticular screw fixation is the alternative and could be considered as the traditional "gold standard" in instrumented fusion of C1 and C2. We believe though C1 lateral mass screws in combination with C2 isthmic screws bear a lower risk profile [6]. Need for decompression in this patient is obvious since he suffers from severe neurological deficits. Therefore a laminectomy and dorsal decompression was indicated and conducted with the first operation as well. Due to the huge ventral mass and therefore still immanent compression a second operation with ventral decompression was indicated. Possible ventral approaches to the craniocervical junction are the transoral route, a cervicolateral approach or the transnasal endoscopic approach [1, 2, 4, 7].

Surgical site infections, as well as swallowing disturbances have to be considered the major risks of transoral spine surgery. By the transnasal route a less traumatic approach is possible [8]. In particular since the major compression in our patient was located at the tip of the odontoid and there was no need for a resection of the C2 base which might be challenging in an already fixated craniocervical junction via a transnasal approach. A pure ventrolateral cervical approach to reach the tip of the odontoid in our patient was not feasible and therefore not considered.

49.4 Conclusions and Take Home Message

Since indication for craniocervical surgery with anterior resection techniques is very rare the respective technique is custom-made. Due to advances in medical treatment of rheumatism, instability of the craniocervical junction of other causes, or other underlying diseases will be more predominant in patients receiving anterior resection techniques of the craniocervical junction compared to historical case series. In patients with moderate or absent neurological deficits a posterior approach only should be considered, in cases with severe neurological deficits due to compression of the spinal cord surgical decompression has to be conducted. Regarding possible ventral approaches the transnasal endoscopic route to the craniocervical junction is less traumatic then the transoral approach and should be the preferred approach for most pathologies.

Pearls

- Retrodental mass is generally caused by instability and might dissolve after fixation only
- In case of severe neurological deficits surgical decompression should be conducted
- Transnasal endoscopic route to the craniocervical junction is less traumatic then the transoral approach and should be the preferred approach

References and Level of Evidence (EBM)

1. Gempt J, Lehmberg J, Grams AE, Berends L, Meyer B, Stoffel M. Endoscopic transnasal resection of the odontoid: case series and clinical course. Eur Spine J. 2011;20(4):661–6. https://doi.org/10.1007/s00586-010-1629-x. **EBM V**
2. Hadley MN, Spetzler RF, Sonntag VK. The transoral approach to the superior cervical spine. A review of 53 cases of extradural cervicomedullary compression. J Neurosurg. 1989;71(1):16–23. https://doi.org/10.3171/jns.1989.71.1.0016. **EBM IV**
3. Jun BY. Complete reduction of retro-odontoid soft tissue mass in os odontoideum following the posterior C1-C2 tranarticular screw fixation. Spine (Phila Pa 1976). 1999;24(18):1961–4. **EBM V**
4. Kassam AB, Snyderman C, Gardner P, Carrau R, Spiro R. The expanded endonasal approach: a fully endoscopic transnasal approach and resection of the odontoid process: technical case report. Neurosurgery. 2005;57(1 Suppl):E213; discussion E213. **EBM IV**

5. Mendenhall SK, Sivaganesan A, Mistry A, Sivasubramaniam P, McGirt MJ, Devin CJ. Traumatic atlantooccipital dislocation: comprehensive assessment of mortality, neurologic improvement, and patient-reported outcomes at a level 1 trauma center over 15 years. Spine J. 2015;15(11):2385–95. **EBM IV**
6. Ringel F, Reinke A, Stuer C, Meyer B, Stoffel M. Posterior C1-2 fusion with C1 lateral mass and C2 isthmic screws: accuracy of screw position, alignment and patient outcome. Acta Neurochir. 2012;154(2):305–12. **EBM IV**
7. Spetzler RF, Hadley MN, Sonntag VK. The transoral approach to the anterior superior cervical spine. A review of 29 cases. Acta Neurochir Suppl (Wien). 1988;43:69–74. **EBM IV**
8. Van Abel KM, Mallory GW, Kasperbauer JL, et al. Transnasal odontoid resection: is there an anatomic explanation for differing swallowing outcomes? Neurosurg Focus. 2014;37(4):E16. **EBM V**

C0/C1/C2 Instrumentation Techniques

50

Anja Tschugg, Sebastian Hartmann, and Claudius Thomé

50.1 Introduction

The occipitocervical junction is a complex transitional zone between the cranium and the upper spine. It composes two major joints: the atlanto-occipital joint, which allows half of the overall flexion-extension motion of the cervical spine and the atlantoaxial joint, which is responsible for the majority of cervical rotation. Bilateral banding, distraction and axial loading are other important features of this region [1, 2]. Degenerative, inflammatory and tumorous lesions can cause instability of these two joints, which may require instrumentation and fusion. Since the majority of cases involve atlantoaxial instability, this chapter focusses on C1/C2 fixation, while the following chapter on basilar invagination also discusses occipitocervical instrumentation in detail.

The atlantoaxial junction dramatically differs from other spinal regions and is characterized by a very complex anatomy. An instability may be caused by trauma, inflammation, congenital malformation or tumor. In these cases, a posterior or anterior atlantoaxial fixation constitutes an effective treatment option. The so-called Magerl atlantoaxial transarticular screw technique and the screw-rod system introduced by Harms and Goel are the most widely used modern techniques for atlantoaxial fixation [3, 4]. This chapter will outline the specifics of atlantoaxial instability, its mandatory preoperative imaging and surgical approaches. Moreover, the rationale for plus both advantages and disadvantages of the different surgical approaches are discussed.

A. Tschugg (✉) · S. Hartmann · C. Thomé
Department of Neurosurgery, Medical University Innsbruck, Innsbruck, Austria
e-mail: anja.tschugg@i-med.ac.at

50.2 Case Description

A 67-year-old man presented with progressively increasing cervical pain, but without radicular pain or sensorymotor deficits in the upper extremities. Neck movements were especially associated with excruciating symptoms. Computed tomography (CT) demonstrated an osteolysis of the odontoid, which was diagnosed as an affection of the odontoid in Wegener's disease (Fig. 50.1).

50.3 Discussion

50.3.1 Indication

CT imaging suggested an inflammatory destruction and a potential instability of the atlantoaxial joint. Due to motion-dependent massive pain unresponsive to medical treatment an indication for surgery was seen.

B. Meyer, M. Rauschmann (eds.), *Spine Surgery*, https://doi.org/10.1007/978-3-319-98875-7_50

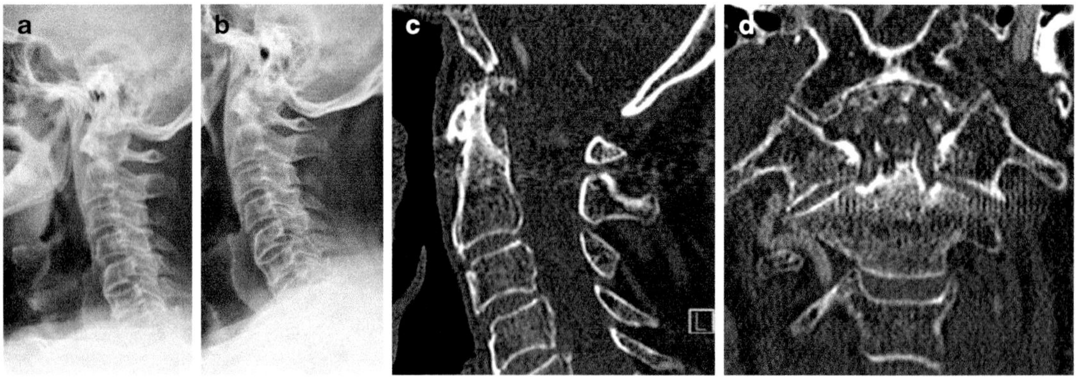

Fig. 50.1 Preoperative lateral x-ray in (**a**) flexion and (**b**) extension with limited motion due to massive pain upon motion. (**c**) Preoperative sagittal and (**d**) coronal CT demonstrating osteolysis of the odontoid and some calcification of the periodontoid ligaments

50.3.2 Choice of Approach

A posterior atlantoaxial stabilization according to Harms/Goel was performed.

50.3.3 Preoperative Preparation

The surgeon should be adequately prepared for surgery to minimize intraoperative complications and to guarantee the most favorable outcome for the patient. In case of atlantoaxial or occipitocervical instrumentation analysis of the size and course of both vertebral arteries at the craniovertebral junction is mandatory. This can be done by MRI or more precisely with depiction of bony details by preoperative computed tomographic angiography (CTA). An abnormal course is detected in approximately 10% of cases [5]. Vertebral artery injuries are most commonly reported during tapping at C2 [6].

50.3.4 Surgical Procedure

The procedure was performed in prone position with the patient's head fixed in a three-pin Mayfield head holder. The lower occiput and the upper cervical spine down to C3 were exposed. Dissection at the spinous process of C2 and the ring of C1 was carefully done. The exposure needs to be lateral enough to be able to follow and palpate the lateral aspect of the lateral masses of C1 and C2 to ensure optimal orientation. The authors commonly apply intraoperative navigation (and intraoperative CT imaging) to optimize screw trajectory. Otherwise, repeated fluoroscopy is required. In cases without navigation, the authors prefer to dissect the lateral aspects of the dural sac to identify the mediocranial aspect of the C2 pedicles and the medial aspects of the C1 lateral masses.

The entry point for the C1 screws is in the middle of the posteroinferior portion of the C1 lateral mass at its junction with the posterior arch. The lateral mass needs to be palpated and exposed in the depth adjacent to the C1/C2 joint. Venous bleeding, which is commonly encountered here, can be minimized by subperiostal dissection and an elevated head position. Various techniques have been described including screw placement through the lateral part of the posterior arch to avoid the venous plexus and blood loss. This modification of screw placement, however, is only possible if the posterior arch is "high" enough (>5 mm as depicted on CT). Otherwise the risk of injuring the vertebral artery is greatly increased. In the presented case, the C1 screws were positioned in the usual trajectory starting below the posterior arch of C1. The C1 screws are ideally placed bicortically for maximum stability, but should be pointing medially to avoid

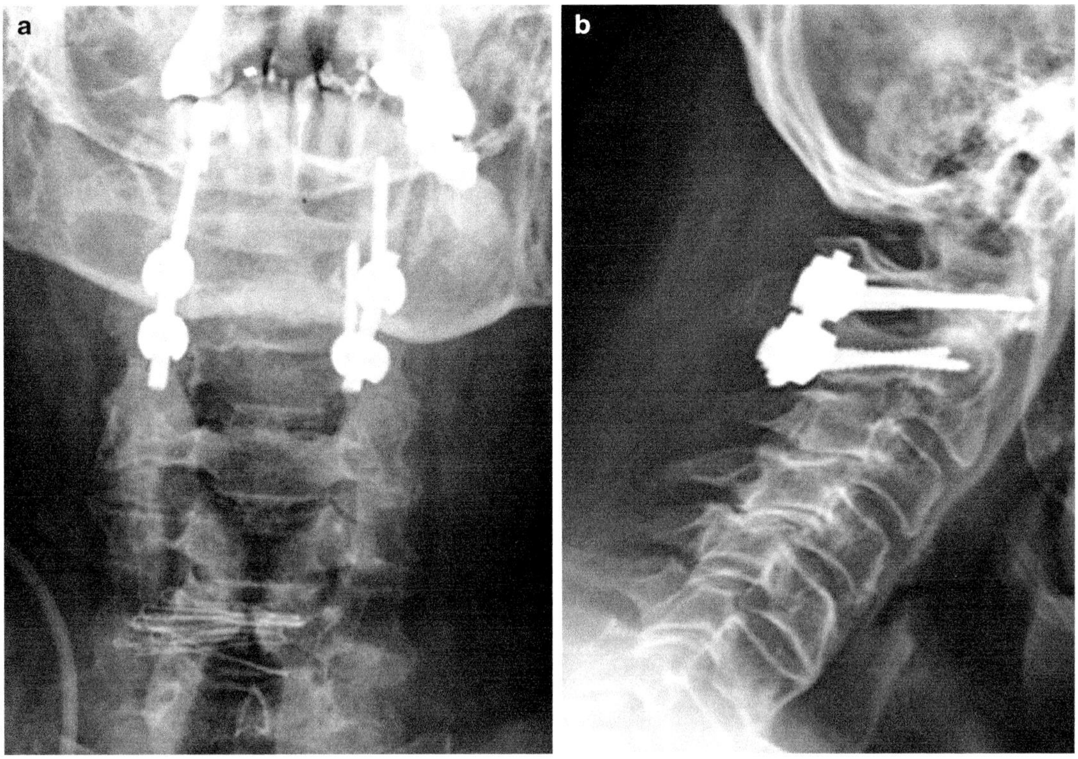

Fig. 50.2 (**a**) Postoperative X-ray in anterior-posterior and (**b**) lateral view of the atlantoaxial joint

the carotid arteries. As the tip of the anterior arch of C1 is pointing anteriorly, the screws will not reach as far anterior on fluoroscopy (see Fig. 50.2).

C2 pedicle screws were also inserted in a standard fashion followed by rod placement [3]. A postoperative x-ray is shown in Fig. 50.2. C2 can be instrumented by various techniques. A "long" pedicle screw is considered the standard in the Harms/Goel technique, but may not be possible due to a high-riding vertebral artery. Therefore, some cases require the use of "short" isthmic or pars screws. These are placed applying the same trajectory, but not fully reaching the pedicle. A 14 mm screw can usually be inserted without risk to the vertebral artery. As a further alternative, laminar screws can be placed, which cross each other at the base of the spinous process. The authors prefer the Harms/Goel technique over the transarticular screw according to Magerl (see below) mainly because of the various screw options in C2.

50.3.5 Different Surgical Techniques

Surgical treatment of C1/C2 instability may be achieved by various techniques characterized by distinct advantages and disadvantages. Historically, fixation was performed by posterior wiring and a bone graft between the arch of C1 and the spinous process of C2 (techniques according to Brooks and Dickman & Sonntag). Thereafter, transarticular fixation of the C1/C2 joint was introduced by Magerl, in which the screws are inserted in an upward angle and a straight anterior-posterior trajectory. Advantages of the transarticular screw include the possibility of percutaneous insertion and biomechanical superiority, as they traverse the joint directly plus they violate the joint surfaces, which is thought to promote fusion. Avoiding the venous plexus and the C2 roots, which may pose a problem with the Harms/Goel technique, is also appealing. On the other hand, the transarticular trajectory is rather unusual and may not be possible in patients with obesity and thoracic kyphosis. Other drawbacks include the risk to the vertebral artery upon insertion and the short purchase in C1, which may provoke screw loosening [7]. Most authors advocated additional posterior bone grafting and fusion to overcome this limitation. The Harms/Goel technique employs rather straight trajectories following the pedicles like in the rest of the spine, which most surgeons are more accustomed with. Additionally, there is more visual and tactile control of the anatomical landmarks plus a strong purchase in C1 with this technique. Many authors open the C1/C2 joint to promote fusion, while others don't deem this to be necessary, as fusion rates are high overall. The major advantages of the Harms/Goel technique are the possibility to directly reposition C1 over C2 and the various screw options for C2, which renders this technique available for basically all cases.

Anterior transarticular screws are also an option with an intuitive trajectory starting at the groove of the lateral C2 body just below the C1/C2 joint. These screws have to be rather short not to violate the C0/C1 joint. Postoperative dysphagia, however, is common, so that the authors only recommend this technique in combination with an odontoid screw or in cases, in which a posterior approach should be avoided.

In the presented case, a posterior strategy was chosen due to the straight forward access and its superior biomechanical stability [8]. For the reasons eluted to above, the Harms/Goel technique with lateral mass screws in C1 and pedicle screws in C2 was used. It has to be noted, however, that this technique requires two screw trajectories which may lead to a higher risk of vascular injuries, especially of the vertebral artery and potentially of the carotid artery as well [3, 7, 9]. To overcome this disadvantage, the authors commonly use navigation in these cases, which requires less exposure and reduces blood loss [10]. Additionally, using intraoperative CT guidance is reliable and has a high accuracy for screw placement [11].

Accordance with the literature guidelines
Level of evidence: C

50.4 Conclusion and Take Home Message

Atlantoaxial instability is mostly addressed by posterior instrumentation techniques with high biomechanical stability. Two main techniques are available: the transarticular screw according to Magerl and the Harms/Goel technique applying lateral mass screws in C1 and pedicle screws in C2. Inclusion of the occiput into these constructs can easily be performed with occipital plates.

Pearls

- The atlantoaxial fixation by Harms/Goel as well by Magerl are the most widely used techniques for atlantoaxial fixation.
- A preoperative computed tomographic angiography (CTA) of the vertebral artery should be performed.
- Intraoperative CT guidance reduces blood loss and has a high accuracy for screw placement.

References and Level of Evidence (EBM)

1. White AA, Panjabi MM. The clinical biomechanics of the occipitoatlantoaxial complex. Orthop Clin North Am. 1978;9:867–78. **EBM IV**
2. Offiah CE, Day E. The craniocervical junction: embryology, anatomy, biomechanics and imaging in blunt trauma. Insights Imaging. 2017;8:29–47. **EBM V**
3. Harms J, Melcher RP. Posterior C1-C2 fusion with polyaxial screw and rod fixation. Spine (Phila Pa 1976). 2001;26:2467–71. **EBM IV**
4. Jeanneret B, Magerl F. Primary posterior fusion C1/2 in odontoid fractures: indications, technique, and results of transarticular screw fixation. J Spinal Disord. 1992;5:464–75. **EBM IV**
5. Yamazaki M, Okawa A, Furuya T, et al. Anomalous vertebral arteries in the extra- and intraosseous regions of the craniovertebral junction visualized by 3-dimensional computed tomographic angiography: analysis of 100 consecutive surgical cases and review of the

literature. Spine (Phila Pa 1976). 2012;37:E1389–97. **EBM IV**

6. Gluf WM, Brockmeyer DL. Atlantoaxial transarticular screw fixation: a review of surgical indications, fusion rate, complications, and lessons learned in 67 pediatric patients. J Neurosurg Spine. 2005;2:164–9. **EBM IV**
7. Huang DG, Hao DJ, He BR, et al. Posterior atlantoaxial fixation: a review of all techniques. Spine J. 2015;15:2271–81. **EBM V**
8. Sim HB, Lee JW, Park JT, Mindea SA, Lim J, Park J. Biomechanical evaluations of various c1-c2 posterior fixation techniques. Spine (Phila Pa 1976). 2011;36:E401–7. **EBM V**
9. Pitzen T, Salman E, Ostrowski G, Welk T, Ruf M, Drumm J. Left-right axial rotation within C1-2 after implant removal. J Neurosurg Spine. 2013;19:688–93. **EBM IV**
10. Hitti FL, Hudgins ED, Chen HI, Malhotra NR, Zager EL, Schuster JM. Intraoperative navigation is associated with reduced blood loss during C1-C2 posterior cervical fixation. World Neurosurg. 2017;107:574–8. **EBM IV**
11. Czabanka M, Haemmerli J, Hecht N, et al. Spinal navigation for posterior instrumentation of C1-2 instability using a mobile intraoperative CT scanner. J Neurosurg Spine. 2017;27:268–75. **EBM IV**

Basilar Invagination

51

Anja Tschugg, Sebastian Hartmann,
and Claudius Thomé

51.1 Introduction

The occipitocervical junction is a complex transitional zone between the cranium and the upper spine. It composes two major joints: the atlanto-occipital and atlantoaxial joint. This region allows half of cervical flexion-extension motion in the segment C0/C1 and about half of cervical rotation at C1/C2. Bilateral banding, distraction and axial loading are other important features of this region [1, 2].

Occipitocervical fusion is indicated for various pathologic conditions like trauma, rheumatoid arthritis, tumor, congenital deformity as well as degeneration with craniocervical instability. Mostly, stabilization of the craniocervical junction is the major goal. The first operative technique was published in 1972 by Foerster who used a fibular strut graft for stabilization. Thereafter, various methods were described including pin or wire fixation, hook constructs as well as halo immobilization. Most of these techniques required prolonged immobilization with a halo vest or a Minerva jacket postoperatively or even bed rest with traction to improve fusion [3]. For faster postoperative rehabilitation and fusion, internal fixation techniques have later been developed. Occipitocervical plating with screw fixation was rapidly replaced by rod systems to eliminate disadvantages like the fixed hole-to-hole distance of plates that may not match the patient's anatomy. Screw-rod constructs were shown to have the most favorable outcome of all occipitocervical fusion techniques independent of the underlying pathology [4].

Basilar invagination is an often symptomatic anomaly of the craniocervical junction, which is characterized by the upward migration of the odontoid into the limited space of the foramen magnum. Thus, the medulla or brainstem as well as other structures of this region are displaced dorsally and compressed, potentially leading to neurological deterioration. Basilar invagination can also be a result of rheumatoid arthritis, whereas it is more common in congenital disorders and malformations (i.e. Klippel-Feil syndrome, Chiari malformation) [5]. In case of an atlantooccipital assimilation or an occipitalization of the atlas, C1/C2 instability is additionally present in approximately 50% of cases [6]. Both computed tomography (CT) and magnetic resonance imaging (MRI) are crucial for an accurate diagnosis of basilar invagination. Detailed imaging data of both bony (CT) and neural (MRI) structures in combination with the patient's clinical findings are prerequisites for determining further

A. Tschugg (✉) · S. Hartmann · C. Thomé
Department of Neurosurgery, Medical University Innsbruck, Innsbruck, Austria
e-mail: anja.tschugg@i-med.ac.at

B. Meyer, M. Rauschmann (eds.), *Spine Surgery*, https://doi.org/10.1007/978-3-319-98875-7_51

management, including surgery, if necessary. In case of an indication for surgery, preoperative cervical traction and posterior-anterior decompression with fusion has been considered the treatment of choice [7]. With modern operative techniques some authors have nowadays largely abandoned preoperative traction.

This chapter will outline the specifics of basilar invagination, its typical symptomatology, mandatory preoperative imaging and surgical approaches. Moreover, the rationale for the different surgical approaches is discussed. The general information on occipitocervical instrumentation can obviously be applied to other craniocervical junction lesions as well.

51.2 Case Description

A 47-year old woman previously diagnosed with rheumatoid arthritis presented with progressive cervicooccipital pain and bilateral hypaesthesia in the upper extremities. MRT and CT revealed basilar invagination with upward migration of the odontoid into the foramen magnum (Fig. 51.1). Conservative treatment for several months did not have a lasting beneficial effect.

51.3 Discussion of the Case

51.3.1 Indication

This patient suffered from refractory pain and early signs of myelopathy. Evoked potentials demonstrated some sensory dysfunction. Even though anterior compression of the medulla was only mild on imaging, mobility at the craniocervical junction between C2 and the cranium was considered to cause her symptoms and signs. Therefore, after failure of conservative measures surgical realignment and fusion was offered.

51.3.2 Choice of Approach

A Crutchfield-extension starting with 3 kg for 3 days followed by an instrumentation from C0 to C3 was performed (Fig. 51.2).

51.3.3 Preoperative Preparation

The surgeon should be adequately prepared for surgery to minimize intraoperative complications and to guarantee the most favorable outcome for the patient:

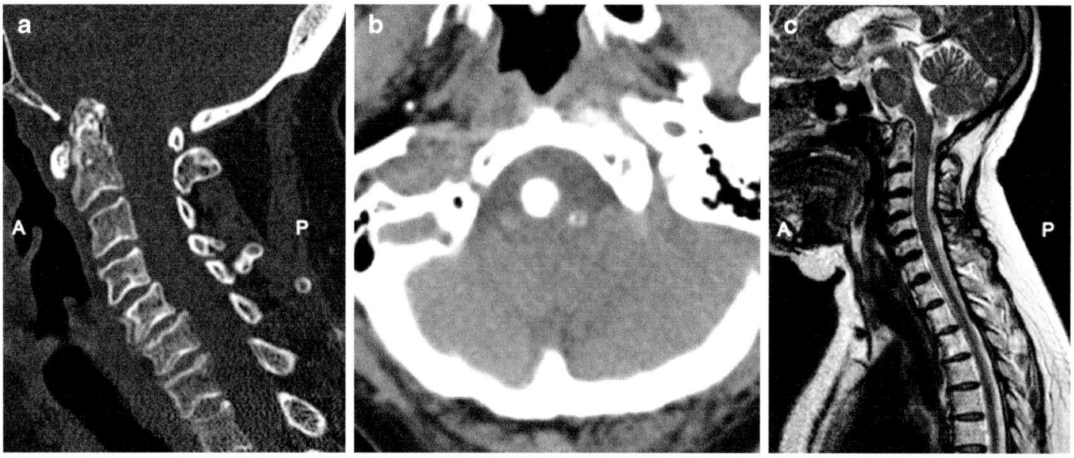

Fig. 51.1 Preoperative CT of the craniocervical junction sagittal (**a**) and axial (**b**) orientation. (**c**) Preoperative sagittal MRI. A anterior, P posterior

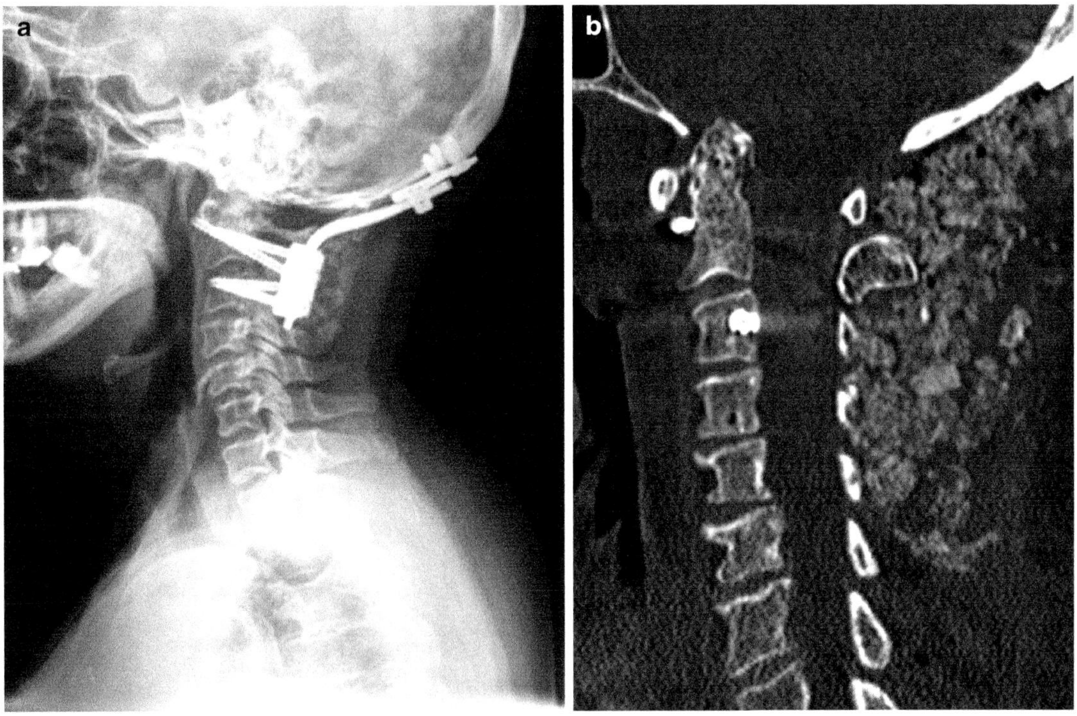

Fig. 51.2 Postoperative X-ray (**a**) and CT (**b**) of the craniocervical junction with instrumentation from the occiput down to C3 using pedicle screws. As C1 screws may be difficult to insert in basilar invagination and C2 screws alone may not be strong enough, the authors often use extra fixation in C3 by lateral mass or pedicle screws as in this case

- Before craniocervical instrumentation it is crucial to evaluate the patient's optimal head position as the patients will obviously be permanently locked in this position. This so-called neutral position is defined as the position in which the patient looks straight ahead on lateral cervical x-rays and the mandible does not overlap with C2 or C3 [8]. Various measurements on x-ray have been described with the occipitocervical inclination (OCI) as a useful method, which seems to be superior in comparison to the occipitocervical angle (OCA) and the occipitocervical distance (OCD). The OCI is specified as the angle formed by a line connecting the posterior border of the vertebral body C4 and Mc Gregor's line and amounts to $102 \pm 8°$ (for more detail see Fig. 51.3). OCA on the other hand is the angle of the junction between a line parallel to the superior endplate of C3 and McRae's line. The OCD is measured as the shortest distance between the most superior aspect of the C2 spinous process and the occipital protuberance [9].
- A preoperative computed tomography angiography (CTA) of the vertebral artery should be performed. In approximately 10% of cases an abnormal course can be detected. Especially in patients with congenital skeletal anomalies at the craniocervical junction including an os odontoideum and occipitalization of C1, a high-riding vertebral artery was commonly detected on 3D CTA [10]. Vertebral artery injuries are reported in about 3% of cases and occur most commonly during tapping at C2. In case of injury the screw should be placed through the planned pathway to tamponade bleeding [11].
- Approximately 2% of patients who undergo degenerative cervical spine surgery suffer from osteoporosis. These patients are more likely to undergo revision surgery and have a longer hospital stay than non-osteoporotic patients [12]. Therefore, it is important to con-

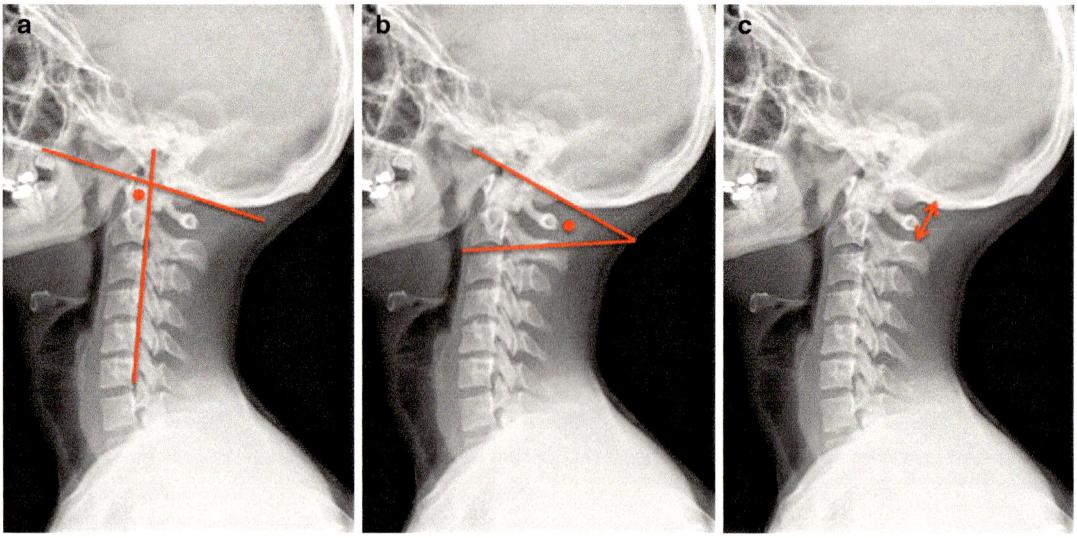

Fig. 51.3 Important parameters at the occipitocervical junction, which can be used to determine an adequate head position in occipitocervical fusion: (**a**) the occipitocervical inclination (OCI; 102 ± 8°), (**b**) the occipitocervical angle (OCA) and (**c**) the occipitocervical distance (OCD)

sider anti-osteoporotic medication as an adjuvant treatment to spine fusion. Teriparatide and also biphosphonates showed promising results for better fusion not only in in vivo studies, but also in human trials [13].

51.3.4 Surgical Procedure

The surgical technique was performed in prone position. The patient's head was fixed in a three-point Mayfield head holder. Alternatively, the patient can be placed in prone position with the head immobilized in a halo ring. The occiput and the upper cervical spine down to C5 were exposed. Dissection at the spinous process of C2 and the ring of C1 was carefully done to avoid entering the C1/2 interspace.

The occipital plate was placed in the midline. Most systems allow multiple screws to be inserted at various distances from the midline. It has to be remembered that the occipital bone is strongest in the midline and close to the occipital protuberance. If in doubt, analysis of the preoperative CT is helpful to determine optimal screw placement. The authors prefer to use the longest possible screws, which translates into completely traversing the occipital bone. If the dura is also perforated indicated by CSF or blood oozing from the screw hole, this can easily be controlled by screw insertion and does not require any additional measures.

In the presented case, C2 pedicle screws were inserted thereafter. Ideally, screws are also placed in the lateral mass of C1. In basilar invagination, however, the occiput, C1 and C2 are commonly so close together, that this may not be possible, as the screw heads interfere with each other and rod placement can be most cumbersome. As a result, the authors often use C3 lateral mass or pedicle screws for adequate lower fixation. It may even be indicated to extend the instrumentation to C4. To avoid a longer construct, C3 pedicle screws were applied in our patient. Depending on the patients anatomy C2 isthmic or laminar screws can also be used. The rods were then bent in a neutral position of the occipito-cervical junction and were connected to the occipital plate and screws [4]. Rod bending can be a challenge and rod systems employing a hinge between the occiput and C1/C2 may be helpful.

Due to the weight of the head and the resulting significant forces on the screws, screw loosening or implant failure can occur, particularly if fusion cannot be achieved in a timely manner. Thus, autologous or heterologous bone or bone substitutes need to be placed on the exposed (and prepared) bony surfaces. The authors use diamond drills to open the cortical surfaces and sometimes harvest autologous bone by burr hole trepanations laterally or cranially. Obviously, care has to be taken not to weaken the skull around the occipital plate.

Biomechanical studies recommend to terminate the occipitocervical fixation at C2, with or without the inclusion of the atlas [14, 15]. Clinically, however, this may lead to subaxial instability. Therefore, fixation more frequently includes the subaxial spine when an occipitocervical instability is present [16]. As noted above, the authors tend to rely not only on C2 screws (if C1 fixation is not possible) and extend the instrumentation caudally. With adequate screw purchase in both C1 and C2 bilaterally, however, this can be avoided. Retrospectively, there seems to be no difference in fusion rates between short or mutlilevel constructs. However, neck pain may be decreased with C2 pedicle screws only and complication rates tend to be higher when performing a multi-level fixation [3].

In summary, occipitocervical fusion can be performed with low morbidity especially when preoperative assessment of anatomic variations is conducted and perioperative complications are anticipated [11, 17, 18]. Perioperative mortality following occipitocervical fusion has been estimated at 3.75% and is mostly related to comorbid medical issues or to underlying cancer. Surgery-related mortality is less than 1% [4]. For more detail see Table 51.1.

Degenerative and rheumatoid changes of the occipitocervical junction are increasing in the elderly in parallel with the aging population. On the other hand, modern medical management of rheumatoid arthritis has greatly reduced severe affection of the craniocervical junction in recent years. In general, a worse outcome after cervical spine surgery is reported with older age, but if a neurological deficit is present, neurological function seems to improve postoperatively just as well in patients over 65 years [19]. Therefore, surgery is also indicated in elderly patients, if comorbidities can be managed.

Although most cases nowadays can be treated by posterior distraction and fusion alone, severe cases of basilar invagination may require an (additional) anterior approach. This is most commonly performed by endonasal (endoscopic) partial clivectomy and odontoidectomy in combination with posterior fixation. An anterior only transoral approach with anterior stabilization has also been described [20]. In the present case the Crutchfield extension was successful and therefore a C0/C2/C3 stabilization without anterior decompression could be chosen. Some surgeons have largely abandoned preoperative extension, as modern screw technology allows adequate intraoperative distraction or traction after induction of anesthesia is sufficient. Nevertheless, preoperative traction can provide important insights into the mobility of the deformity. Other experts have argued for "pulling" the odontoid out of the foramen magnum by distracting the C1/C2 joint. Placement of intraarticular spacers can support this maneuver, but can be associated with significant bleeding from the venous plexus.

Table 51.1 Complication rates in craniocervical fusion surgery

Total	30%	Adjacent level degeneration	7%
Wound infection	5%	Occipital neuralgia	1.7%
Pseudoarthrosis	5–7%	Vertebral artery injuries	3%

51.4 Accordance with the Literature Guidelines

Level of Evidence

C

51.5 Conclusion and Take Home Message

Basilar invagination can mostly be adequately addressed by preoperative (or intraoperative) traction and posterior instrumentation plus fusion from the occiput to C2 (or C3) applying modern screw and rod systems. Only cases with severe anterior compression of the brainstem require additional ventral decompression, which is nowadays mostly performed via an endoscopic endonasal approach. The authors generally apply posterior instrumentation and realignment first and only supplement the procedure with a later anterior decompression, if necessary.

Pearls

- In cases of craniocervical stabilization the patient's optimal head position must be evaluated.
- A preoperative computed tomography angiography (CTA) of the vertebral artery should be performed.
- If anterior decompression is not achieved by distraction and posterior fixation only, an anterior (endonasal) approach with odontoidectomy can be performed.

References and Level of Evidence (EBM)

1. White AA, Panjabi MM. The clinical biomechanics of the occipitoatlantoaxial complex. Orthop Clin North Am. 1978;9:867–78. **EBM V**
2. Offiah CE, Day E. The craniocervical junction: embryology, anatomy, biomechanics and imaging in blunt trauma. Insights Imaging. 2017;8:29–47. **EBM V**
3. Pan J, Huang D, Hao D, et al. Occipitocervical fusion: fix to C2 or C3? Clin Neurol Neurosurg. 2014;127:134–9. **EBM IV**
4. Winegar CD, Lawrence JP, Friel BC, et al. A systematic review of occipital cervical fusion: techniques and outcomes. J Neurosurg Spine. 2010;13:5–16. **EBM II**
5. Chaudhry NS, Ozpinar A, Bi WL, Chavakula V, Chi JH, Dunn IF. Basilar Invagination: Case Report and Literature Review. World Neurosurg. 2015;83:1180.e7–11. **EBM V**
6. Smith JS, Shaffrey CI, Abel MF, Menezes AH. Basilar Invagination. Neurosurgery. 2010;66:A39–47. **EBM V**
7. Goel A. Treatment of basilar invagination by atlantoaxial joint distraction and direct lateral mass fixation. J Neurosurg Spine. 2004;1:281–6. **EBM IV**
8. Wholey MH, Bruwer AJ, Baker HL. The lateral roentgenogram of the neck; with comments on the atlanto-odontoid-basion relationship. Radiology. 1958;71:350–6.
9. Yoon SD, Lee CH, Lee J, Choi JY, Min WK. Occipitocervical inclination: new radiographic parameter of neutral occipitocervical position. Eur Spine J. 2017;26:2297–302. **EBM IV**
10. Yamazaki M, Okawa A, Furuya T, et al. Anomalous vertebral arteries in the extra- and intraosseous regions of the craniovertebral junction visualized by 3-dimensional computed tomographic angiography: analysis of 100 consecutive surgical cases and review of the literature. Spine (Phila Pa 1976). 2012;37:E1389–97. **EBM III**
11. Gluf WM, Brockmeyer DL. Atlantoaxial transarticular screw fixation: a review of surgical indications, fusion rate, complications, and lessons learned in 67 pediatric patients. J Neurosurg Spine. 2005;2:164–9. **EBM IV**
12. Guzman JZ, Feldman ZM, McAnany S, Hecht AC, Qureshi SA, Cho SK. Osteoporosis in cervical spine surgery. Spine (Phila Pa 1976). 2016;41:662–8. **EBM IV**
13. Stone MA, Jakoi AM, Iorio JA, et al. Bisphosphonate's and intermittent parathyroid Hormone's effect on human spinal fusion: a systematic review of the literature. Asian Spine J. 2017;11:484–93. **EBM III**
14. Wolfla CE, Salerno SA, Yoganandan N, Pintar FA. Comparison of contemporary occipitocervical instrumentation techniques with and without C1 lateral mass screws. Neurosurgery. 2007;61:87–93. discussion 93. **EBM V**
15. Yüksel KZ, Crawford NR, Melton MS, Dickman CA. Augmentation of occipitocervical contoured rod fixation with C1-C2 transarticular screws. Spine J. 2007;7:180–7. **EBM V**
16. Abumi K, Takada T, Shono Y, Kaneda K, Fujiya M. Posterior occipitocervical reconstruction using cervical pedicle screws and plate-rod systems. Spine (Phila Pa 1976). 1999;24:1425–34. **EBM IV**
17. Lall R, Patel NJ, Resnick DK. A review of complications associated with Craniocervical fusion surgery. Neurosurgery. 2010;67:1396–403. **EBM III**
18. Deutsch H, Haid RW, Rodts GE, Mummaneni PV. Occipitocervical fixation: long-term results. Spine (Phila Pa 1976). 2005;30:530–5. **EBM IV**
19. Clarke MJ, Toussaint LG, Kumar R, Daniels DJ, Fogelson JL, Krauss WE. Occipitocervical fusion in elderly patients. World Neurosurg. 2012;78:318–25. **EBM IV**
20. Shkarubo AN, Kuleshov AA, Chernov IV, Vetrile MS. Transoral decompression and anterior stabilization of atlantoaxial joint in patients with basilar impression and Chiari Malformation Type I: a technical report of 2 clinical cases. World Neurosurg. 2017;102:181–90. **EBM V**

52 Corpectomies and Osteotomies in the Upper Thoracic Spine and Cervicothoracic Region

Nils Hecht, Marcus Czabanka, and Peter Vajkoczy

52.1 Introduction

Spine surgery in the upper thoracic and cervicothoracic region remains challenging due to difficult radiographic visualization and limited surgical accessibility. Although surgical strategies for treatment of severe deformities in this region might improve pain and disability, they remain complex and lack standardization [11]. In particular for corpectomies and vertebral column reconstruction, approaches may be anterior, posterior or combined. Further, a variety of soft tissue releases and osteotomies ranging from simple facet release (Ponte or Smith Peterson Osteotomies) to vertebral column resection (VCR) may be applied for decompression and deformity correction. Additional variability exists in the use of an increasing array for anterior and posterior instrumentation that require experience and knowledge of 360-degree (360°) approaches, in addition to the number of vertebral levels that require instrumentation to ensure biomechanical stability. Against this background, the present chapter outlines surgical approaches to the upper thoracic and cervicothoracic region, recommended imaging as well as pitfalls that may be encountered when treating spinal instabilities in this region. Specifically, the aim of the presented cases is to outline:

- Typical indications for corpectomies with vertebral body replacement
- Pre-, intra- and postoperative imaging
- Selection of anterior versus posterior versus combined approaches

52.2 Case Description

52.3 Case 1

A 60-year old female patient presented with a history of paresthesia and progressive weakness of the lower limbs over the past 12 hours. Her neurological examination revealed a decreased sensory level below Th 5 and paraplegia (ASIA B). Immediate Computed Tomography (CT) and contrast-enhanced Magnetic Resonance Imaging (MRI) revealed a lytic destruction and kyphotic deformity of Th1-3 with spinal cord compression due to a large tumor mass within the upper left thoracic cavity (Fig. 52.1).

Due to rapid neurological worsening of motor symptoms during the past 12 hours and after a detailed discussion about the requirement of surgery with the patient, she was taken to the

N. Hecht (✉) · M. Czabanka · P. Vajkoczy
Department of Neurosurgery, Charité – Universitätsmedizin Berlin, Berlin, Germany
e-mail: nils.hecht@charite.de

B. Meyer, M. Rauschmann (eds.), *Spine Surgery*, https://doi.org/10.1007/978-3-319-98875-7_52

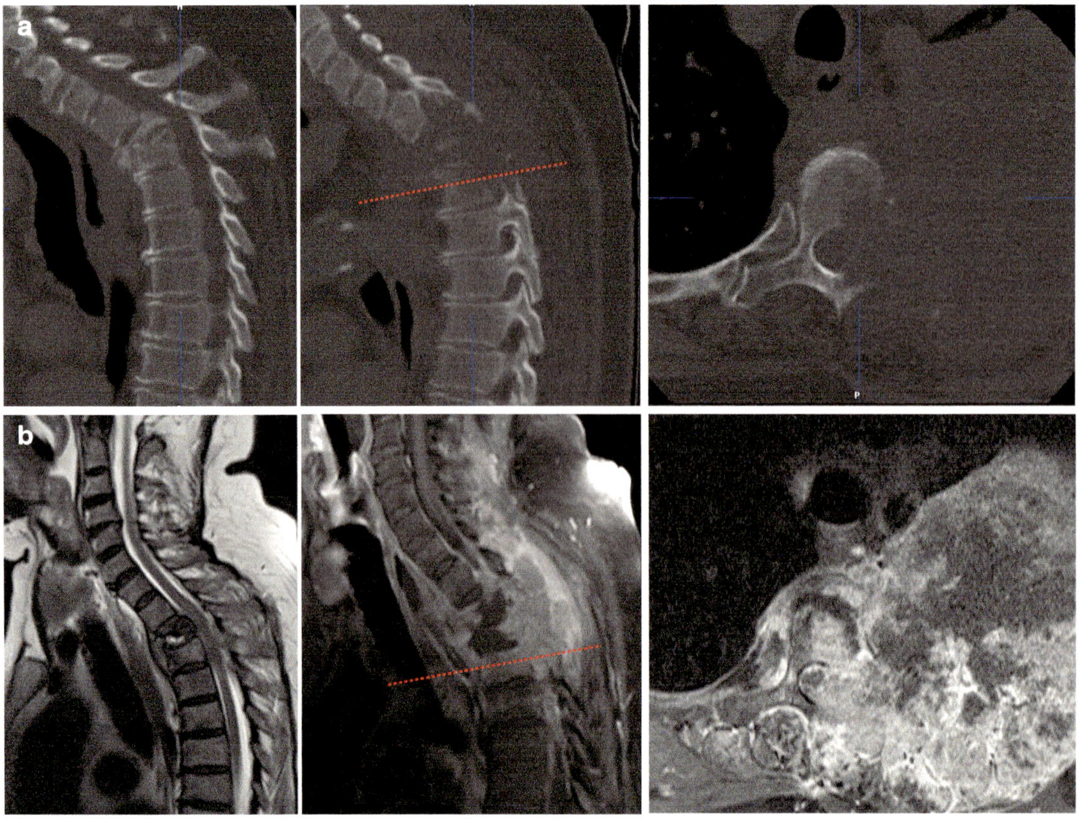

Fig. 52.1 Preoperative imaging. (**a**) CT and (**b**) MRI scans illustrate lytic destruction of Th2-4 with spinal cord compression due to a large tumor within the left apical thoracic cavity. The dashed red line indicates the corresponding transverse level

operating room for emergent circumferential decompression and navigated posterior lateral mass / pedicle screw fixation with posterior-lateral vertebral body replacement using intraoperative 3-dimensional Digital Volume Tomography (3D DVT) imaging (Fig. 52.2). After navigated screw insertion (lateral mass screws C5 and C6; pedicle screws C7, Th1, Th5, Th6 and Th7), a left-sided posterior-lateral tumor debulking and circumferential decompression with bilateral vertebral body / tumor resection from Th 2-4 and implantation of a distractible (expandable) cage was performed. Cage and screw positioning was assessed with 3D imaging (Fig. 52.2) and followed by bilateral rod fixation and cross-link connection at the level of the corpectomy (Fig. 52.3; left panels). After surgery, the patient was transferred to our intensive care unit for blood pressure maintenance and 3 days later to our regular floor, where in the course of 1 week she recovered bilateral motor function to a muscle grade < 3 in > 50% of the key muscle groups below the neurologic level of injury (ASIA C). Sufficient decompression was confirmed by a postoperative CT scan on the first postoperative day (Fig. 52.3; right panels) and the histopathological examination revealed a squamous cell carcinoma metastasis, most likely due to a previously non-diagnosed Larynx carcinoma. The patient was transferred to our oncology department for further treatment and rehabilitation.

52.4 Case 2

This 65-year old female patient had suffered a history of progressive neck pain and paresthesia in her left arm over the past month. Upon presentation, neurological examination revealed numbness and paresthesia of her left arm without clear

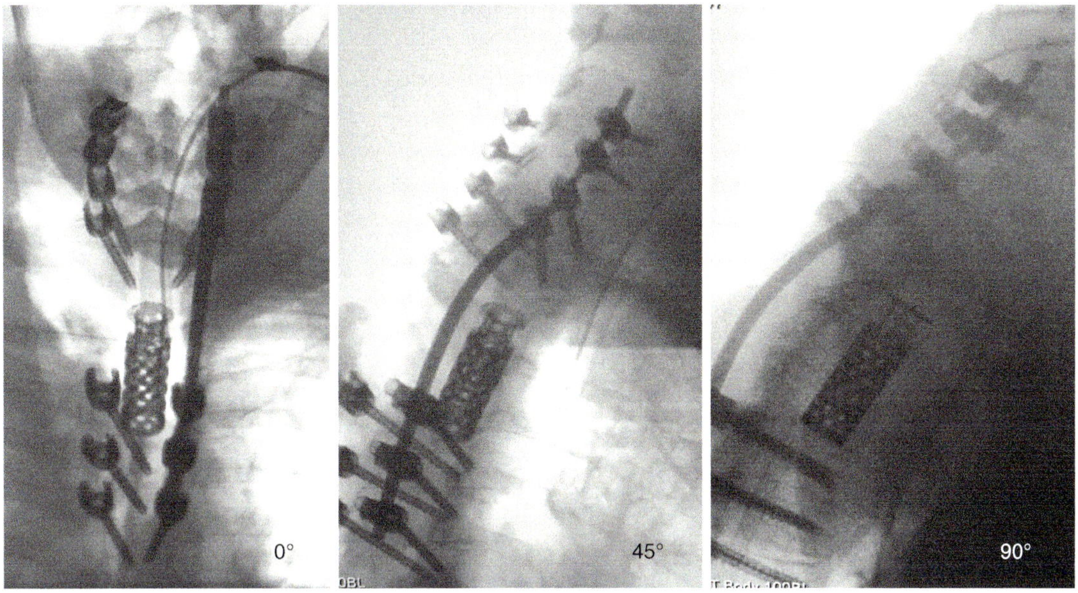

Fig. 52.2 Intraoperative imaging. Intraoperative 3D DVT rotation scan following navigated pedicle screw implantation and vertebral body replacement shows the poor lateral radiographic image quality limiting clear visualization of the anterior margin of the vertebral column at the level of the distractible cage between Th 2-4

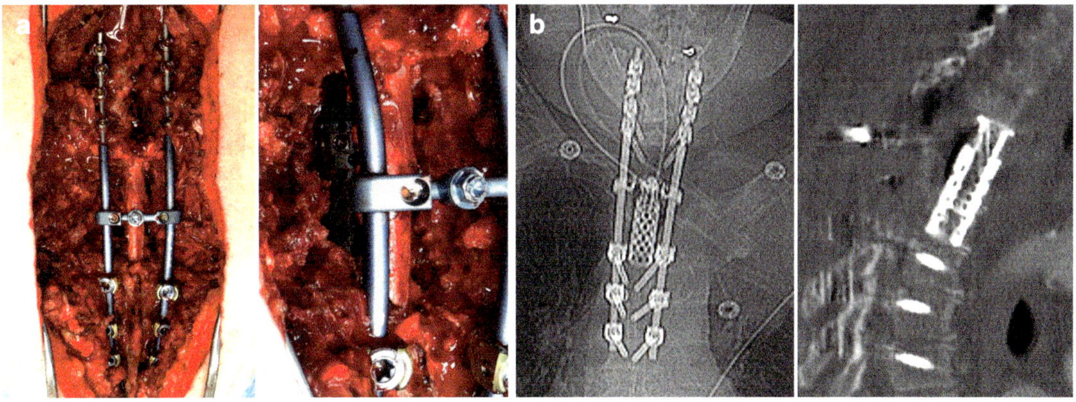

Fig. 52.3 Intraoperative view and postoperative imaging. Left panels show intraoperative final view after rod fixation and cross-link connection with posterolateral view of the vertebral body replacement after left-sided tumor debulking. The panels on the right show implant positioning on postoperative CT imaging (CT scout and sagittal reconstruction)

radiculopathy. Range-of-motion of the neck was impaired due to pain together with hypesthesia in the cervicothoracic region. Immediate MRI scanning revealed a tumor-suspicious mass lesion with lytic destruction of C7 and Th1 and kyphotic angulation at the cervicothoracic junction. In addition, there were signs of an intraspinal tumor mass with impending spinal cord compression and additional suspicious lesions in C5 and C6 (Fig. 52.4).

The patient was taken to the OR the following day and an anterior corpectomy of C7 and Th1 with vertebral body replacement and plate fixation from C6 to Th2 was performed, together with posterior decompression from C7 to Th1 and lateral mass / pedicle screw fixation from C4/C5/C6 to Th2/Th3/Th4 in a single-stage setting. Postoperatively, the patient was transferred to the recovery room. Although there were no new motor or sensory deficits with immediate subsidence of

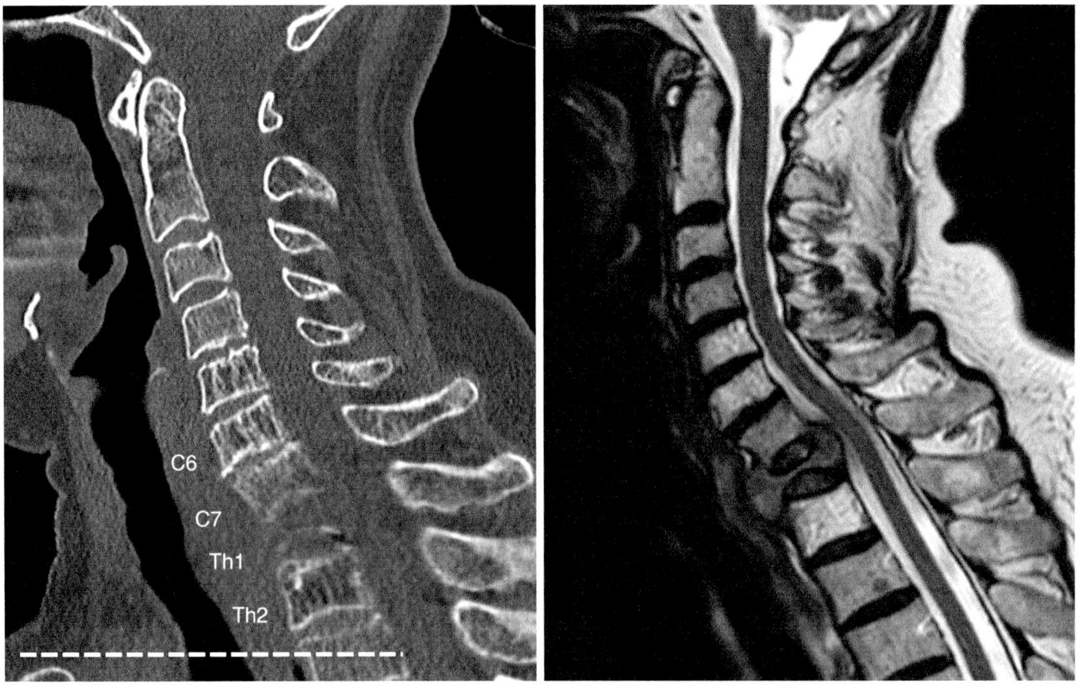

Fig. 52.4 Preoperative imaging sagittal. (**a**) CT and (**b**) MRI scans show the lytic mass lesion at the cervicothoracic junction with kyphotic deformity and spinal cord compression. The dashed white line shows the level of the sternum in relation to the cervicothoracic junction

preoperative neck pain, the patient experienced difficulties breathing in and shortness of breath. An emergent laryngoscopy revealed bilateral vocal cord paralysis and consequently, a lateral fixation of the left vocal cord according to Lichtenstein was performed. Postoperatively, the patient was transferred to our regular ward and recovered well with pain reduction and subsidence of the neurological symptoms in her arm. Postoperative imaging confirmed correct implant positioning with adequate decompression (Fig. 52.5). The histopathological examination revealed a multiple myeloma, which was treated with chemo- and radiation therapy.

52.5 Discussion of the Cases

52.5.1 Indication for Surgery

The majority of lesions in the cervicothoracic area that require decompression with at least partial vertebral body resection are metastatic tumors of the spine with destruction of osseous elements. In such cases, the paradigm of "separation surgery" has evolved, where a clear margin around the thecal sac and nerve roots is established, thereby permitting treatment with stereotactic radiosurgery and ensuring high rates of local tumor control regardless of histology [6]. Next to localized tumor control with the chance of favorable survival [3, 9], indication for surgery is determined based on instability according to the Spinal Instability Neoplasm Score (SINS) [4] and the onset or risk of suffering neurological deficits due to spinal cord compression.

In Case 1, the decision to operate was mainly influenced by the rapid onset of severe motor deficits due to tumor-induced spinal cord compression next to a kyphotic instability of the semi-rigid thoracic spine with involvement of both the anterior and posterior elements (SINS 16). In contrast, the patient in Case 2 only suffered localized pain and hypesthesia in her left arm with no severe neurological impairment, but surgery was indicated due to localized pain and high-grade instability according to imaging findings, which revealed a lytic tumor involving both vertebral bodies of the cervi-

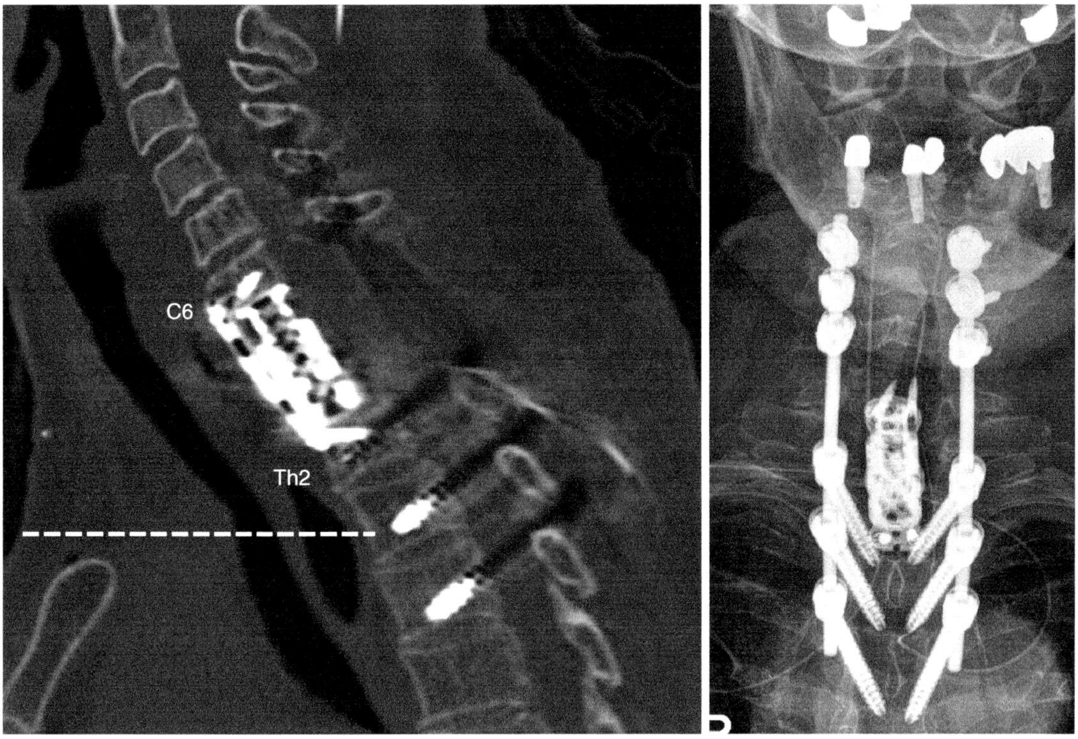

Fig. 52.5 Postoperative imaging. Postoperative CT (left) (the dashed line indicates the low level of the manubrium) and anterior-posterior radiograph (right) confirm correct implant positioning and adequate decompression

cothoracic junction with kyphosis (SINS 13) and spinal cord compression. A further argument for surgery in both cases was that both patients had a preoperative Karnofski Performance Status (KPS) of 100% and unrestricted ambulatory ability, which serve as favorable predictors of survival [1] and postoperative ambulatory status. Although the timing of decompressive surgery in such cases remains a matter of debate, both patients were operated within 24 hours of presentation, because neurological outcome – particularly in Case 1 illustrating a patient with acute neurological deficit – may improve if decompression is performed within 48 hours of presenting with symptoms instead of later [10].

52.5.2 Imaging

Preoperative imaging is necessary to determine (a) the level of the pathology, (b) the degree of deformity and (c), to assess the bone quality in order to plan the overall surgical strategy, approach and length of the construct. For this purpose, transverse, sagittal and coronal reconstructions of contrast-enhanced and non-contrast T1- and T2-weighted MRI together with CT imaging are mandatory and should be obtained immediately upon presentation. In cases with contraindication for an MRI, a CT-myelography should be performed instead.

Intraoperatively, plain radiographic imaging (C-arm imaging) in the lateral plane is difficult due to limited visibility in the cervicothoracic and upper thoracic regions. Here, an anterior-posterior projection is typically used to identify the levels of interest and perform thoracic pedicle screw implantation. In the present cases, spinal navigation with intraoperative 3D DVT imaging was used for navigated posterior instrumentation and to assess implant positioning but also to help identify the anterior margins of the Th 2-4 corpectomy in Case 1 due to limited radiographic visibility.

Postoperatively, we routinely perform a CT scan on the first postoperative day to confirm adequate decompression, correct implant positioning after rod fixation and for assessment of deformity correction, which remains limited on plain lateral radiographs. Importantly, if a patient with preoperative neurological deficit has no improvement or even neurological worsening (regardless of the preoperative motor status), an MRI is mandatory to rule out a procedure-related hemorrhage as a potentially reversible cause that requires immediate surgical evacuation.

52.5.3 Choice of Approach and Surgical Technique

While no region of the spine is easily treated, the cervicothoracic region is perhaps the least accessible. Traditional cervicothoracic approaches involve either thoracotomy or sternotomy and particularly the latter remains associated with higher complication rates compared to conventional anterior or posterior approaches to the spine.

Case 1 illustrates a lytic tumor of the upper thoracic spine requiring multilevel circumferential decompression with 360° reconstruction of the vertebral column and provides an example where the projection of the scapula and manubrium limit access to the upper thoracic spine and cervicothoracic junction via a direct lateral / transthoracic or anterior approach. In such cases, a posterolateral, transpedicular approach as shown here has the advantage of allowing spondylectomy, epidural decompression and circumferential fusion with vertebral body replacement and posterior instrumentation in a single-stage surgery that provides immediate stability while avoiding the morbidity associated with anterior / lateral and posterior approaches to this region [2, 7]. Alternatively, if the level of pathology requires midline decompression and vertebral body replacement above the level of the manubrium as shown in Case 2, an anterior approach with plate fixation followed by posterior decompression and stabilization is typically used. However, the risk profile of an anterior approach to the cervicothoracic region, particularly regarding injury to the recurrent nerve should not be underestimated, which can be seen by the bilateral vocal cord paralysis that our patient in Case 2 unfortunately suffered after the combined anterior – posterior approach. Although the opinions regarding the need for additional posterior fixation after anterior plating may vary, experimental evidence has suggested and most experts agree that additional posterior fixation resembles the standard of care for stabilization of 2- or greater-level corpectomies, even if posterior elements are not primarily involved and decompression may not be required [5].

The use of a distractible cage instead of titanium mesh has the benefit that it can be adjusted to the size of the corpectomy in situ and maintains reduction without the need for additional plate fixation. In Case 1, correction of the kyphosis was established in a single-stage posterior fashion by first achieving a 360° release and performing unilateral (right-sided) rod fixation followed by alternating cage expansion and rod reduction. In contrast, Case 2 was operated in an anterior-posterior fashion and kyphosis correction was achieved by anterior cage expansion and plate fixation with subsequent posterior instrumentation and reduction after repositioning the patient from supine to prone. Although clear evidence supporting the use of posterior cross-link fixation as we did in Case 1 but not in Case 2 is still lacking, biomechanical findings suggest that cross-link fixation at the level of a corpectomy in the cervicothoracic region could be beneficial in cases where both anterior as well as posterior elements of the spine are affected by instability, similar to Case 1 [8].

Another matter of debate concerns the number of vertebra that should be instrumented across the level of pathology. In general, we aim not to end a long construct directly at the levels of the cervicothoracic junction (C7 and Th1) but prefer to extend the posterior fixation at least 2 levels above and below (i.e. C5 to Th3) including the levels of corpectomy. In the subaxial spine (apart from C7) and depending on the quality of the bone, we generally perform lateral mass screw fixation due to the beneficial safety profile compared to cervical pedicle screw instrumentation, particularly if spinal navigation is not readily available. In both cases, the limited visualization of the cervicothoracic region on plain radiographs or C-arm imaging advocates the use of spinal navigation with high-quality intraoperative DVT or CT imaging to limit the risk of implant misplacement and allow immediate intraoperative correction, which may help reduce the incidence of secondary implant revision surgery.

52.6 Conclusions and Take-Home Message

The safety profile of surgery in the cervicothoracic and upper thoracic spine has improved due to the development of more standardized posterolateral and combined anterior-posterior approaches. Nevertheless, detailed preoperative MRI and CT imaging is necessary to plan an individual surgical strategy and approach according to anatomic considerations. In the future, safety and efficacy of spine surgery in the cervicothoracic region may further benefit from an increased implementation of spinal navigation and intraoperative 3D imaging.

Pearls

- Main factors influencing the approach are location, size and configuration of the pathology as well as the degree of potentially associated deformity
- Preoperative MRI and CT scans are mandatory
- 2- or greater-level corpectomies should include additional posterior fixation
- Spinal navigation and intraoperative 3D imaging may facilitate surgery

Levels of Evidence

Bakar II, Bilsky IV
Fehlings II
Fisher II
Koller V
Laufer III
Metcalfe IV
O'Brien V
Patchell I
Quraishi III
Smith IV

References

1. Bakar D, Tanenbaum JE, Phan K, Alentado VJ, Steinmetz MP, Benzel EC, et al. Decompression surgery for spinal metastases: a systematic review. Neurosurg Focus. 2016;41(2):E2.
2. Bilsky MH, Boland P, Lis E, Raizer JJ, Healey JH. Single-stage posterolateral transpedicle approach for spondylectomy, epidural decompression, and circumferential fusion of spinal metastases. Spine (Phila Pa 1976). 2000;25(17):2240–9. discussion250
3. Fehlings MG, Nater A, Tetreault L, Kopjar B, Arnold P, Dekutoski M, et al. Survival and clinical outcomes in surgically treated patients with metastatic epidural spinal cord compression: results of the prospective Multicenter AOSpine study. J Clin Oncol. 2016;34(3):268–76.
4. Fisher CG, Dipaola CP, Ryken TC, Bilsky MH, Shaffrey CI, Berven SH, et al. A novel classification system for spinal instability in neoplastic disease: an evidence-based approach and expert consensus from the spine oncology study group. Spine (Phila Pa 1976). 2010;35(22):E1221–9.
5. Koller H, Schmoelz W, Zenner J, Auffarth A, Resch H, Hitzl W, et al. Construct stability of an instrumented 2-level cervical corpectomy model following fatigue testing: biomechanical comparison of circumferential antero-posterior instrumentation versus a novel anterior-only transpedicular screw-plate fixation technique. Eur Spine J. 2015;24(12):2848–56.
6. Laufer I, Iorgulescu JB, Chapman T, Lis E, Shi W, Zhang Z, et al. Local disease control for spinal metastases following "separation surgery" and adjuvant hypofractionated or high-dose single-fraction stereotactic radiosurgery: outcome analysis in 186 patients. J Neurosurg Spine. 2013;18(3):207–14.
7. Metcalfe S, Gbejuade H, Patel NR. The posterior transpedicular approach for circumferential decompression and instrumented stabilization with titanium cage vertebrectomy reconstruction for spinal tumors: consecutive case series of 50 patients. Spine (Phila Pa 1976). 2012;37(16):1375–83.
8. O'Brien JR, Dmitriev AE, Yu W, Gelb D, Ludwig S. Posterior-only stabilization of 2-column and 3-column injuries at the cervicothoracic junction: a biomechanical study. J Spinal Disord Tech. 2009;22(5):340–6.

9. Patchell RA, Tibbs PA, Regine WF, Payne R, Saris S, Kryscio RJ, et al. Direct decompressive surgical resection in the treatment of spinal cord compression caused by metastatic cancer: a randomised trial. Lancet. 2005;366(9486):643–8.
10. Quraishi NA, Rajagopal TS, Manoharan SR, Elsayed S, Edwards KL, Boszczyk BM. Effect of timing of surgery on neurological outcome and survival in metastatic spinal cord compression. Eur Spine J. 2013;22(6):1383–8.
11. Smith JS, Klineberg E, Shaffrey CI, Lafage V, Schwab FJ, Protopsaltis T, et al. Assessment of surgical treatment strategies for moderate to severe cervical spinal deformity reveals marked variation in approaches, osteotomies, and fusion levels. World Neurosurg. 2016;91:228–37.

Cervicothoracic Kyphosis in Ankylosing Spondilitis

53

Bernhard Meyer and Lukas Bobinski

53.1 Introduction

Ankylosing spondylitis (AS) is a chronic inflammatory disease that particularly affects the spine. The progressive erosion of the joints is followed by ossification and consequently autofusion of the spinal column. AS affects more often males then females in age between 20–30 y/o with a prevalence of 0.1–1.4% [1]. Due to its widespread ankylosis and secondary low-density of the vertebral bodies, the radiographic appearance of AS is sometimes referred as "bamboo spine". In order to unload painful facet joints, AS patients assume a compensatory flexed posture. Patients with long-standing AS are predisposed to development of a rigid, kyphotic deformity most commonly in thoracolumbar region. However, the cervical and cervicothoracic spine can also be affected.

The kyphotic deformity in the cervicothoracic junction in its extreme form is called a chin-on-chest deformity. It presents with significant compromise of horizontal gaze, personal hygiene, swallowing and social outlook.

B. Meyer
Department of Neurosurgery, Klinikum rechts der Isar, Technische Universität München, Munich, Germany

L. Bobinski (✉)
Department of Orthopedics, Spine Unit, Umeå University Hospital, Umeå, Sweden

We describe a case of unrecognized fracture in AS patients leading to a progressive chin-on-chest deformity. The preoperative radiological evaluation highlights the technical challenges as well as clinical implications for better understanding the complexity of cervicothoracic deformities in AS patients. The applied techniques are explained with emphasizing their advantages.

The objective of this chapter is presentation of cervicothoracic deformity case in AS with rationale of its planning and surgical procedure in step-by-step fashion in order to introduce the reader to challenges of this complex pathology.

53.2 Case Description

A 82-year-old healthy (except for mild hypertension) male with known AS sustained a minor cervical trauma (fall at his home). He looked for medical attention at his primary care provider because of severe neck pain. He was advised rest, pain medication and physiotherapy. The radiological examinations were omitted. During the subsequent 6 weeks, he developed a progressive, painful cervicothoracic deformity. The patients who was previously independent deteriorated to the point he became completely dependent because of lack of horizontal gaze and difficulties with personal hygiene. At that point he was referred to the local hospital. The patient presented with severe pain in cervicothoracic region. The neurological exam according

B. Meyer, M. Rauschmann (eds.), *Spine Surgery*, https://doi.org/10.1007/978-3-319-98875-7_53

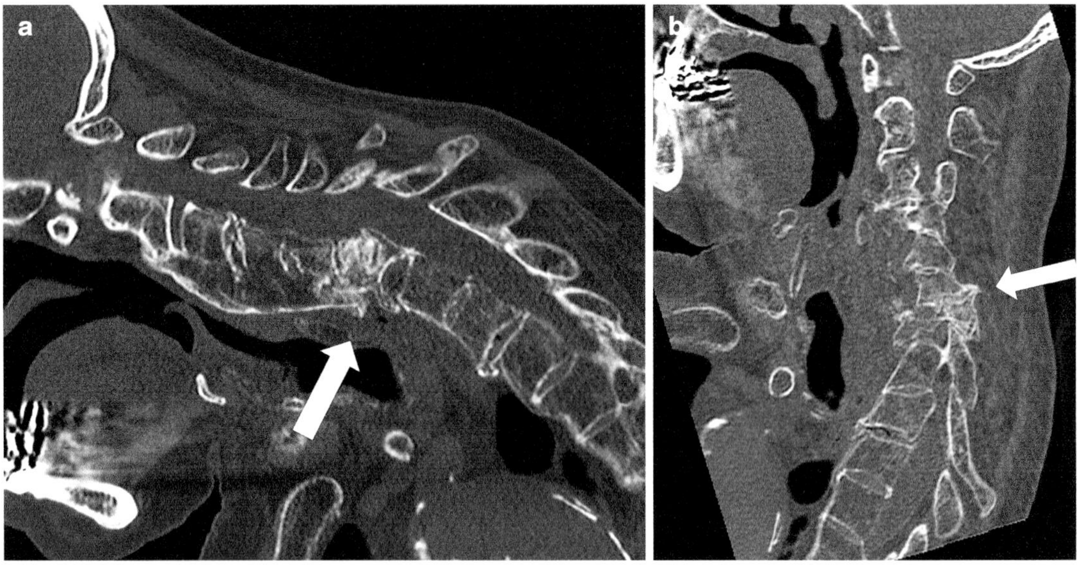

Fig. 53.1 CT scan on admission to primary hospital. The CT scan shows a subluxated cervical fracture C6/C7: B2 according to AOSpine subaxial cervical spine injury classification fracture. Typical characteristics of AS with autofusion are clearly visible. The arrows point at subluxated and partially fused fractured facets between C6 and C7 vertebrae. (**a**) midline sagittal view, (**b**) left sided sagittal view

to ASIA score was completely normal. The initial radiological evaluation with computer tomography revealed a partially healed C7 distraction fracture C6/C7: B2 in subluxation creating the cervicothoracic deformity (Fig. 53.1a, b) [2]. Patient was then referred to our spine unit at university hospital for consultation. The external immobilization was not possible due to severely advanced kyphotic deformity (Fig. 53.2). MRI was not performed because the same reason. The status at the admission revealed a chin-on-chest deformity (Fig. 53.3a, b). Due to ankylosis of the spine, the patient could not find a comfortable resting position. Furthermore, patient's relatives described a rapid deterioration of patient physical and mental health due to cervical pain, dysphagia and a loss of horizontal gaze. After receiving written consent, the patient was scheduled for corrective cervical osteotomy with a long posterior cervicothoracic fixation bridging across cervicothoracic junction (CTJ).

53.2.1 Surgery

The patient was preoperatively evaluated with transthoracic echocardiography and spirometry.

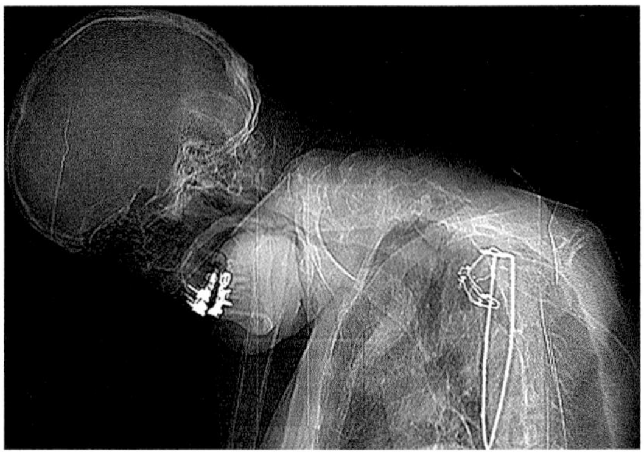

Fig. 53.2 CT scan on admission to primary hospital. The CT scan scout shows a fixed cervicothoracic chin-on-chest kyphotic deformity

The examinations did not show signs of pulmonary nor cardiac compromised function. The surgery was performed under continuous intraoperative neurophysiologic monitoring with motor evoked potentials (MEPs) and somatosensory evoked potentials (SSEPs).

After fiberoptic, awake intubation patient was gently log-rolled to prone position with his head secured in the Mayfield head holder. The positioning was very challenging due to advanced

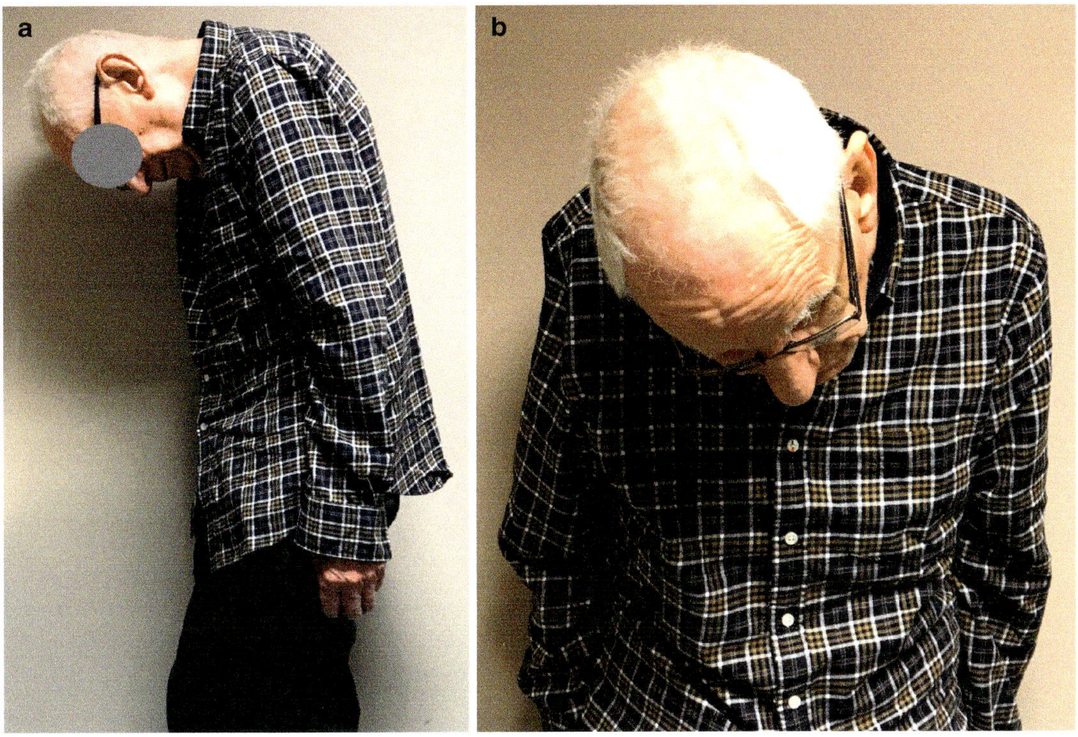

Fig. 53.3 The photography taken at admission to our unit. The images demonstrate a severe loss of horizontal gaze. (**a**) sagittal view (**b**) coronal view

deformity. It required soft, chest roll-bolster and anterior iliac crest pads for support. The abdomen was left completely free of any compression. A padded support was applied to the patient's feet and the table was then put in maximum reversed Trendelenburg position in order to minimize perioperative bleeding (Fig. 53.4a, b).

The skin incision and subperiosteal dissection of paraspinal muscles was carried out from C2 to T3 spinal segment. The presence of partially healed subluxation at C6/C7 was found intraoperatively. The site of the previous fracture was stiff enough to perform instrumentation from cranial end of cervical spine to thoracic levels T2 and T3 (C6, C7 and T1 vertebrae were not instrumented). At the lever of C2, two long Magerl screws were placed across C1/C2 joints for better bone purchase. Two temporary rods were placed in order to prevent iatrogenic spine translation during osteotomy. The modified Simmons osteotomy was then performed in sequential fashion [3].

Step 1: C6 to Th1 laminectomies, under direct visualization, short segment fixation with pedicle screws was carried out at the level of C6 and T1 bilateral.

Step 2: complete bilateral facetectomy was performed between C6/C7 and C7/T1 followed by complete removal of both C7 pedicles. This maneuver is a first step of pedicle subtraction osteotomy (PSO), which was originally planned. The PSO allowed a broad release of posterior column and decompressed completely C7 and C8 nerve roots, which were slightly impinged by subluxation. This was sufficient to access to the remaining portion of the posterior wall at the level of the disk between C6/C7, which was then opened. At the end of this step a segment C6/C7 became clearly mobile. Two short 3.0 mm lordotic titanium rods were then placed between C6 and T1 and the long rods were removed.

Step 3: Under continuous neurophysiologic monitoring the Mayfield head-holder was opened and manual correction of kyphosis was applied.

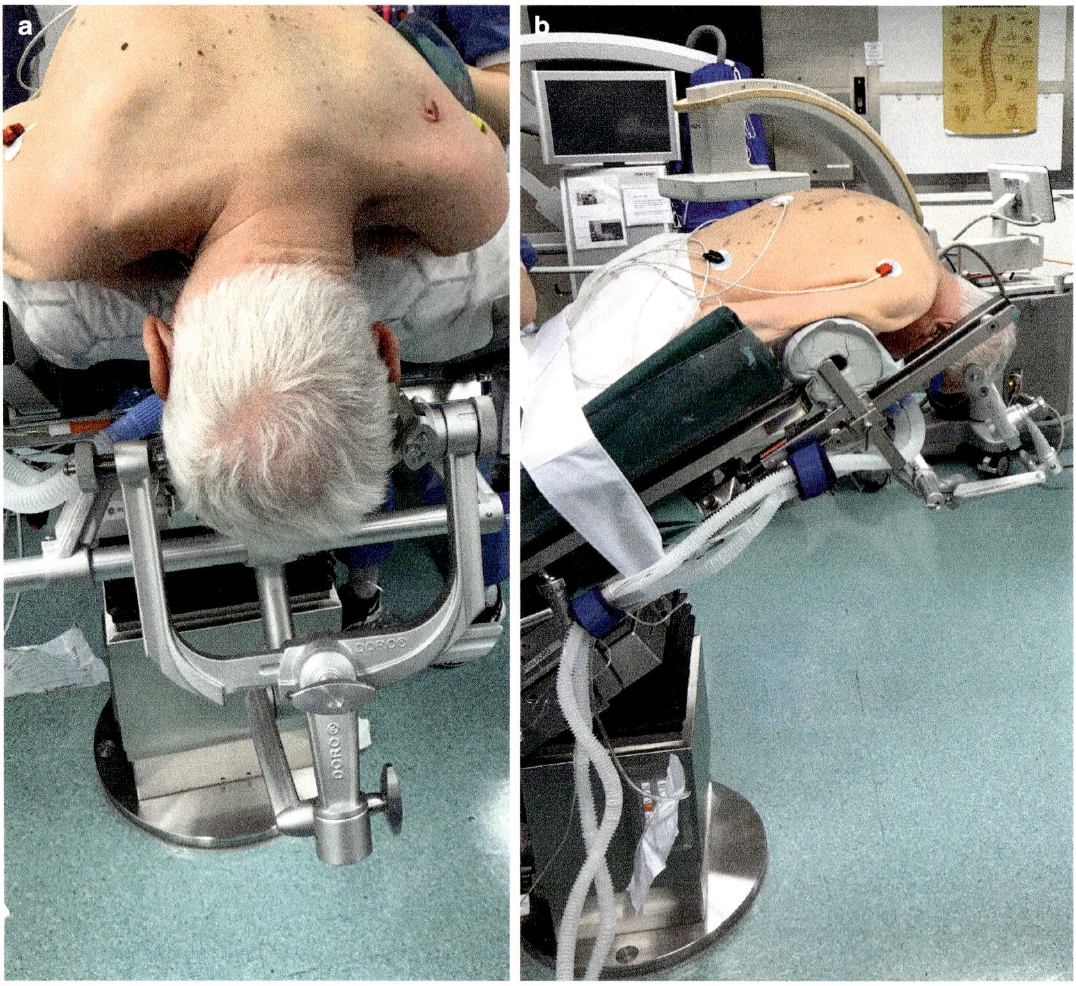

Fig. 53.4 The photography taken preoperatively after positioning. The images demonstrate a severe kyphotic deformity requiring extreme, reverse Trendelenburg position in order to get access to cervicothoracic junction. (**a**) sagittal view, (**b**) coronal view

After achieving correction short rod segment fixation was locked in place. Neither SSEP's nor MEP's changed during the correction.

Step 4: Two long rods were shaped in lordosis and placed back, creating a four-rods fixation technique followed by sequential locking of the construct. One cross-link was placed just above the short segmental fixation between the long rods.

The wound was irrigated with large amount of saline (2 L) and closed in layers in regular fashion. No drain was used.

The neurological status of the patient was unchanged after surgery. He was successfully mobilized and discharged to his local hospital for rehabilitation after a few days at our unit. Postoperative CT scans and X-rays showed a correct position of the hardware with improvement of cervicothoracic alignment (Figs. 53.5 and 53.6). The cosmetic result was also very satisfying. The patient regained the horizontal gaze and was capable to walk using walking aid (Fig. 53.7).

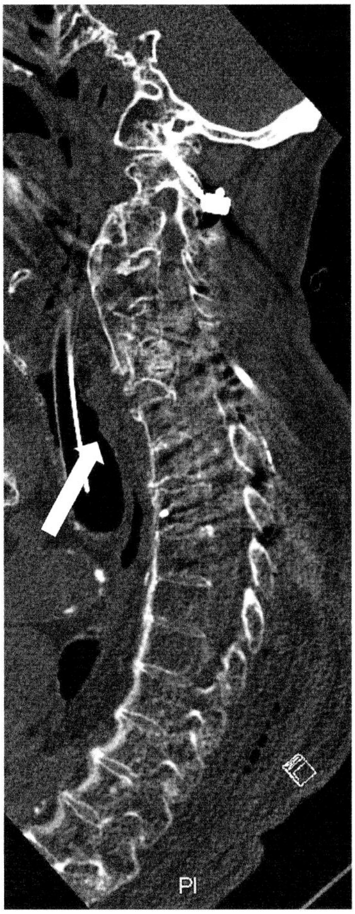

Fig. 53.5 Post-operative CT scan. The CT shows a corrected cervicothoracic alignment. The white arrows indicate wide-wedge opening of anterior column after closing of osteotomy posteriorly

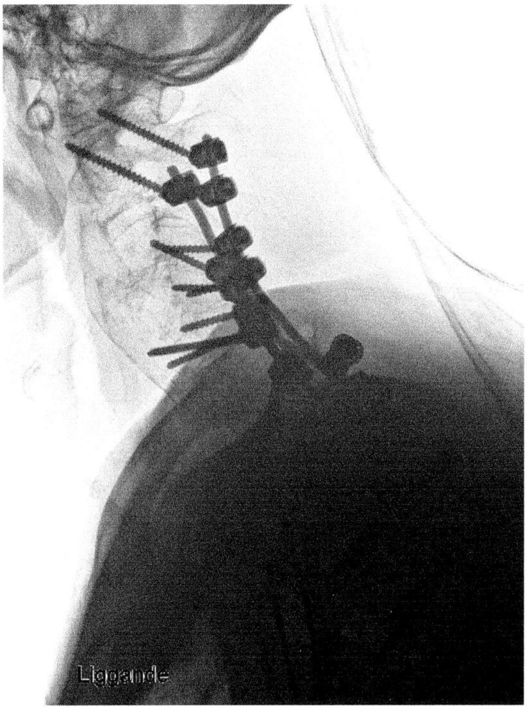

Fig. 53.6 The post-operative X-ray image demonstrates a well-aligned cervicothoracic junction

53.3 Discussion of the Case

53.3.1 Indications

Chin-on-chest deformity has become very rare because of advancement in pharmacological treatment of AS that consist of various combinations of non-steroidal, anti-inflammatory drugs (NSAIDs), analgesics, corticosteroids, synthetic and biologic disease-modifying, antirheumatic drugs (DMARDs) and continuous physiotherapy [4, 5].

Nevertheless, most of the AS patients inevitably develop rigid, brittle spinal column with secondary atrophy of the surrounding muscles and osteoporosis. That makes AS patient extremely susceptible to injuries with fourfold increased risk of fracture even with minimal trauma [6]. Patients with AS who sustained fracture, tend to deteriorate neurologically and have high morbidity and mortality rate [7]. Furthermore, similar to our presented case they can develop a chin-on-chest deformity. This usually leads to quick deterioration in their general health status with impaired horizontal gaze, dysphagia, difficulties to maintain personal hygiene and social contacts. The correction can be only achieved surgically. Surgical corrections lead to improved pain control but most importantly achieve cervicothoracic alignment [8–10].

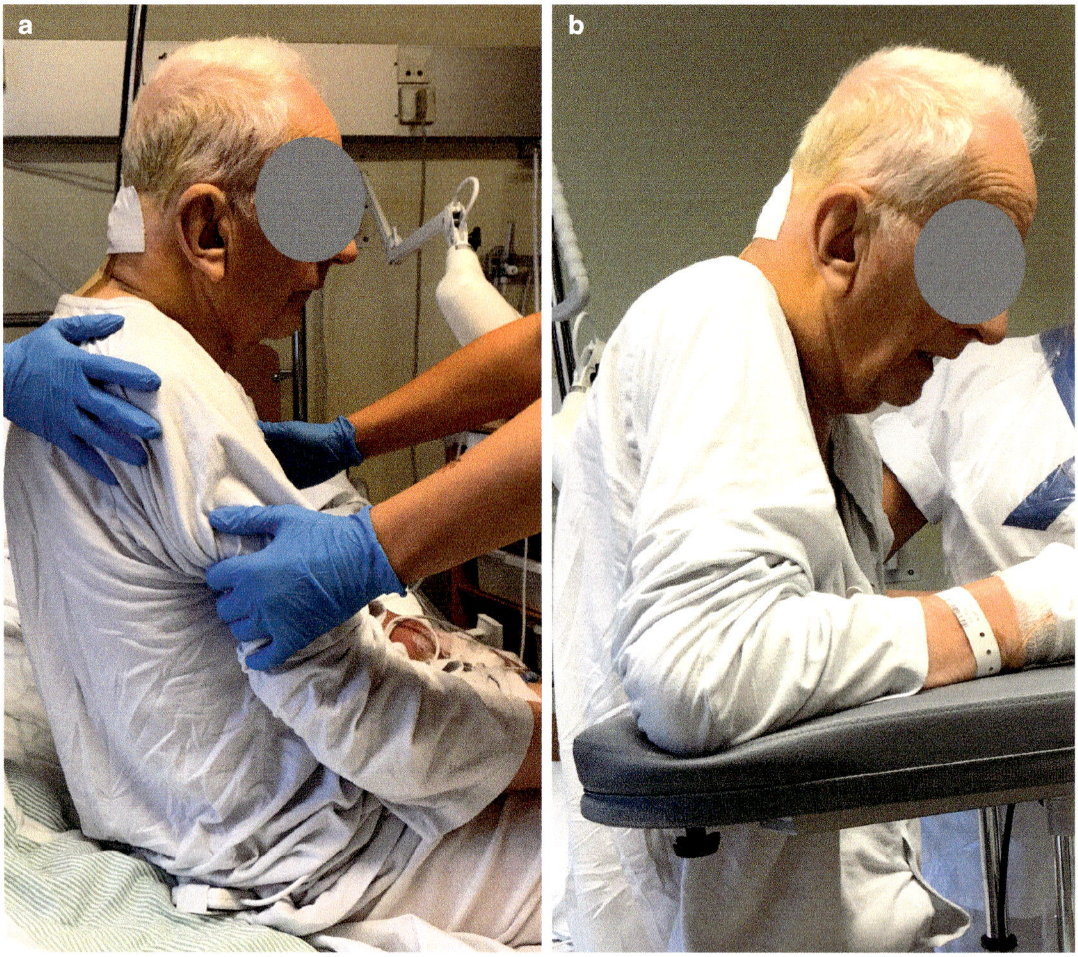

Fig. 53.7 The photography taken postoperatively at the first day during mobilization of the patient. The images demonstrate a restoration of horizontal gaze. (**a**) sagittal view sitting (**b**) sagittal view standing

53.3.2 Choice of Surgical Technique and Degree of Correction

First osteotomy for correction of kyphotic deformity in AS was described by Smith-Petersen in the lumbar spine [11]. The principles of that technique were then adopted for the cervical spine by Urist et al. [12] and Law et al. [13]. This osteotomy technique was then popularized by Simmons [14]. It is similar to the Smith-Petersen osteotomy with removal of the posterior elements at the level requiring correction with controlled fracture of anterior column at C7.

The further modification of this technique in the cervical region includes a pediculectomy to further decompress the C8 nerve roots upon closure of the osteotomy [3].

The latest technique used for correction of cervicothoracic junction is subtraction pedicle osteotomy (PSO) also known as closing wedge osteotomy [15–17]. Despite being more technical advanced it seems that it allows more extensive range of correction with a bigger fusion surface between the vertebrae.

Two parameters are mostly used in order to measure the correction:

- chin-brown vertical angle (CBVA), which can be used for assessment of horizontal gaze. It an angle measured between two lines in standing position: one drawn from the brow to the chin and a second, vertical line. In case of AS it is suggested that CBVA should be within −10° to 10° to assure a sufficient horizontal gaze [18].
- C7 Sagittal Vertical Axis (SVA) used for more global assessment of the sagittal alignment, measured as a distance between a posterior superior corner of the sacrum and a vertical line dropped from the center of C7 [19].

A rule of thumb is that patients without C0/C1 mobility have no compensating mechanism and don't tolerate overcorrection, hence require lesser correction. Patient with intact mobility between C0/C1 can tolerate overcorrection better.

Both CBVA and SVA parameters can improve regardless which osteotomy technique is used. However, perioperative measurements of correction are very restricted due to technical difficulties with fluoroscopy. Therefore, meticulous preoperative surgical planning is crucial in order to achieve a sufficient but not exaggerated correction.

53.3.3 Peri- and Postoperative Complications

The osteotomy at cervicothoracic junction, regardless the type, is technically demanding. Etame et al. [20] in their literature review described the data of osteotomy outcome based on four studies [3, 21–23]. The complication rate ranged from 26.9% to 87.5%, with a mortality rate of 2.6%. Thereby, neurological deterioration is the most feared one. The overall rate of neurologic deficits was 23.4% with vast majority due to transient C8 radiculopathy as a result of iatrogenic foraminal stenosis. The permanent neurologic complication rate was 4.3% due to C8 radiculopathy. On the other hand, medical complications include infection, dysphagia, pseudoartosis and need for tracheostomy and/or PEG tube [8, 10, 24].

53.3.4 Technical Considerations

Several technical issues must be addressed when planning corrective osteotomy in cervicothoracic kyphosis:

- C7 vertebrae is the optimal the site of the osteotomy. It is sufficiently low to provide a long laver arm for correction. It minimizes risk for vascular injuries by being above the large thoracic vessels and below vertebral arteries. Additionally, C8 nerve root injury has a lesser impact on hand function then C7 or C6 nerve roots.
- the CTJ is very difficult to visualize with fluoroscopy therefore use of the navigation is advocated to improve implant placement [25].
- surgeon should be familiar with cervical and thoracic anatomy and be experienced in both lateral mass and thoracic pedicle screw instrumentation techniques
- cranial extension of instrumentation to C2 or even C1/C2 complex can provide higher pull-out resistance
- use of continuous intraoperative neurophysiological monitoring is mandatory
- we advocate use of cell-saver because of usually extensive bleeding from spinal epidural plexus and the osteotomy

The authors personal choice is the four rod technique with cervical pedicle screws and cross-link in order to provide extremely stable fixation across the osteotomy site [26]. Short segment fixation with pedicle screws protects the spine from translating during manual correction and allows additional compression for better bone-to-bone contact after realignment. This technique may seem to be overexaggerated and can be replaced with for example hinged rods that are locked at the site of osteotomy after correction [27]. We suggest use of long posterior cervicothoracic construct crossing CTJ for solid foundation of realigned cervical spine.

53.3.5 Accordance with the Literature Guidelines

Unfortunately, there is insufficient power of evidence in the current literature to draw conclusions regarding which technique should be preferable. There was only one prospective, single institution non-randomized study suggesting that CBVA should be used for planning of correction of cervicothoracic kyphosis in AS [18]. Literature review suggest that most neurological complications are transient due to C8 nerve root compression [20]. Therefore, we cannot apply any general guidelines based on these data and decision making regarding the technique and degree of correction should be done on case-to-case bases. However, we can conclude that cervicothoracic kyphosis in AS, despite being very rare, cause tremendous suffering of the patients. Surgery should be meticulously planned and performed using modern surgical techniques and supported by neuromonitoring and image guidance instrumentation if available.

Level of Evidence: C

Most cited studies are larger retrospective single center cohort studies. Publication by Suk et al. [18], is the only cited prospective, single center, non-randomized study with a higher level of evidence.

53.4 Conclusions and Take-Home Message

Cervicothoracic deformity in AS has a great impact on patient quality of life. Currently surgical correction with osteotomy and long posterior fixation is the only valuable treatment. The surgery is challenging and requires throughout planning.

We advocate using only long posterior cervicothoracic fixation sufficient to support and sustain the re-aligned spinal column after C7 osteotomy.

Pearls

- preoperative investigation of cervical spine with CT scan and MR images (if possible), including upper thoracic levels are mandatory
- the long posterior cervical fixation can be used as only approach even with multi-segmental failure of the anterior column
- intraoperative neuromonitoring with SSEPs and MEPs is mandatory
- image guided surgery should be used if available
- C7 is preferable osteotomy site
- CBVA measured at preoperative images can be used for planning the degree of surgical correction

References

1. Braun J, Sieper J. Ankylosing spondylitis. Lancet. 2007;369(9570):1379–90.
2. Vaccaro AR, Koerner JD, Radcliff KE, et al. AOSpine subaxial cervical spine injury classification system. Eur Spine J. 2016;25(7):2173–84.
3. Simmons ED, Distefano RJ, Zheng Y, Simmons EH. Thirty-six years experience of cervical extension osteotomy in ankylosing spondylitis: techniques and outcomes. Spine (Phila Pa 1976). 2006;31(26):3006–12.
4. Maxwell LJ, Zochling J, Boonen A, et al. TNF-alpha inhibitors for ankylosing spondylitis. Cochrane Database Syst Rev. 2015;4:CD005468.
5. Tymms K, Littlejohn G, Griffiths H, et al. Treatment patterns among patients with rheumatic disease (rheumatoid arthritis (RA), ankylosing spondylitis (AS), psoriatic arthritis (PsA) and undifferentiated arthritis (UnA)) treated with subcutaneous TNF inhibitors. Clin Rheumatol. 2018;37:1617–23.
6. Finkelstein JA, Chapman JR, Mirza S. Occult vertebral fractures in ankylosing spondylitis. Spinal Cord. 1999;37(6):444–7.
7. Caron T, Bransford R, Nguyen Q, Agel J, Chapman J, Bellabarba C. Spine fractures in patients with ankylosing spinal disorders. Spine (Phila Pa 1976). 2010;35(11):E458–64.
8. Deviren V, Scheer JK, Ames CP. Technique of cervicothoracic junction pedicle subtraction osteotomy for cervical sagittal imbalance: report of 11 cases. J Neurosurg Spine. 2011;15(2):174–81.

9. Samudrala S, Vaynman S, Thiayananthan T, et al. Cervicothoracic junction kyphosis: surgical reconstruction with pedicle subtraction osteotomy and smith-Petersen osteotomy. Presented at the 2009 joint spine section meeting. Clinical article. J Neurosurg Spine. 2010;13(6):695–706.
10. Theologis AA, Tabaraee E, Funao H, et al. Three-column osteotomies of the lower cervical and upper thoracic spine: comparison of early outcomes, radiographic parameters, and peri-operative complications in 48 patients. Eur Spine J. 2015;24(Suppl 1):S23–30.
11. Smith-Petersen MN, Larson CB, Aufranc OE. Osteotomy of the spine for correction of flexion deformity in rheumatoid arthritis. Clin Orthop Relat Res. 1969;66:6–9.
12. Urist MR. Osteotomy of the cervical spine; report of a case of ankylosing rheumatoid spondylitis. J Bone Joint Surg Am. 1958;40-A(4):833–43.
13. Law WA. Osteotomy of the cervical spine. J Bone Joint Surg Br. 1959;41-B:640–1.
14. Simmons EH. The surgical correction of flexion deformity of the cervical spine in ankylosing spondylitis. Clin Orthop Relat Res. 1972;86:132–43.
15. Tokala DP, Lam KS, Freeman BJ, Webb JK. C7 decancellisation closing wedge osteotomy for the correction of fixed cervico-thoracic kyphosis. Eur Spine J. 2007;16(9):1471–8.
16. Wollowick AL, Kelly MP, Riew KD. Pedicle subtraction osteotomy in the cervical spine. Spine (Phila Pa 1976). 2012;37(5):E342–8.
17. Ames CP, Smith JS, Scheer JK, et al. A standardized nomenclature for cervical spine soft-tissue release and osteotomy for deformity correction: clinical article. J Neurosurg Spine. 2013;19(3):269–78.
18. Suk KS, Kim KT, Lee SH, Kim JM. Significance of chin-brow vertical angle in correction of kyphotic deformity of ankylosing spondylitis patients. Spine (Phila Pa 1976). 2003;28(17):2001–5.
19. Scheer JK, Tang JA, Smith JS, et al. Cervical spine alignment, sagittal deformity, and clinical implications: a review. J Neurosurg Spine. 2013;19(2):141–59.
20. Etame AB, Than KD, Wang AC, La Marca F, Park P. Surgical management of symptomatic cervical or cervicothoracic kyphosis due to ankylosing spondylitis. Spine (Phila Pa 1976). 2008;33(16):E559–64.
21. McMaster MJ. Osteotomy of the cervical spine in ankylosing spondylitis. J Bone Joint Surg Br. 1997;79(2):197–203.
22. Langeloo DD, Journee HL, Pavlov PW, de Kleuver M. Cervical osteotomy in ankylosing spondylitis: evaluation of new developments. Eur Spine J. 2006;15(4):493–500.
23. Belanger TA, Milam RA, Roh JS, Bohlman HH. Cervicothoracic extension osteotomy for chin-on-chest deformity in ankylosing spondylitis. J Bone Joint Surg Am. 2005;87(8):1732–8.
24. Hoh DJ, Khoueir P, Wang MY. Management of cervical deformity in ankylosing spondylitis. Neurosurg Focus. 2008;24(1):E9.
25. Ito Y, Sugimoto Y, Tomioka M, Hasegawa Y, Nakago K, Yagata Y. Clinical accuracy of 3D fluoroscopy-assisted cervical pedicle screw insertion. J Neurosurg Spine. 2008;9(5):450–3.
26. Johnston TL, Karaikovic EE, Lautenschlager EP, Marcu D. Cervical pedicle screws vs. lateral mass screws: uniplanar fatigue analysis and residual pullout strengths. Spine J. 2006;6(6):667–72.
27. Khoueir P, Hoh DJ, Wang MY. Use of hinged rods for controlled osteoclastic correction of a fixed cervical kyphotic deformity in ankylosing spondylitis. J Neurosurg Spine. 2008;8(6):579–83.

54 Sagittal Balance and Preoperative Planning

A. El Rahal, F. Solla, V. Fiere, Aurélie Toquart, and Cédric Y. Barrey

This chapter and theses cases will emphasize on the pre-operative planning to correct spinopelvic misalignment integrating new tools in the planning and realization of the surgery.

54.1 Context

Adult Spine Deformity (ASD) is mainly consecutive to the loss of lumbar lordosis due to degenerative changes in the lumbar spine and/or increased thoracic kyphosis, resulting into progressive non-ergonomical sagittal misalignment, imbalance and compensation mechanisms such as knee flexion and retroverted pelvis [1]. This in turn leads to progressing painful difficulties in standing upright positions [1], reduced walking distance, forward bending, often requiring support.

54.1.1 Clinical Relevance of Sagittal Alignment

The analysis of the spino-pelvic sagittal alignment constitutes a crucial key point to optimize the surgical management of ASD with spinal instrumentation as mentioned in Chap. 26 [4]. Schwab, Lafage et al. [2, 11] proposed three clinically relevant parameters to simplify the analysis and set targets for corrective surgery realignment as follows: Sagittal vertical axis (SVA) < 40 mm or 50 mm, Pelvic tilt (PT) $<20°$, and thirdly, mismatch between Pelvic Incidence and the Lumbar Lordosis (PI-LL) $<10°$. Poor postoperative alignment is correlated with significant disability and mechanical complications, such as screw pull-out, adjacent level disease or rod breakage [3, 4, 13]. Conversely, any improvement of these parameters towards normal values leads to improvement of patient's outcomes [5, 6].

Planning of spine surgery has received increasing attention in the past decades and optimization

A. El Rahal · A. Toquart · C. Y. Barrey (✉)
Department of Spine and Spinal Cord Surgery, University Hospital Pierre Wertheimer (GHE), Claude Bernard University of Lyon 1, Hospices Civils de Lyon, Lyon, France
e-mail: cedric.barrey@chu-lyon.fr

F. Solla
Department of Pediatrics Orthopedics, Lenval Hospital, Nice, France

V. Fiere
Department of Spine Surgery, Mermoz Private Hospital, Lyon, France

B. Meyer, M. Rauschmann (eds.), *Spine Surgery*, https://doi.org/10.1007/978-3-319-98875-7_54

of it with new digital tools is being developed to achieve a better spinopelvic alignment and outcome in the future. Concerning surgical planning, there are two main concerns:

1. Patient based concern with the ideal post operative spino-pelvic alignment for each patient (i.e. patient-specific sagittal alignment)
2. Surgery based concern achieving the pre-operative planning by the surgeon

54.1.2 Causes of Realignment Failure

Despite established thresholds and tools for surgical planning, adequate alignment following surgical treatment is not always achieved [2, 12], which is mainly related to either decrease or insufficient restoration of lumbar lordosis (LL).

From a pragmatic point of view, there are two main reasons for a realignment failure:

1. Poor/lack of surgical planning and/or
2. Poor execution.

The systematic analysis of the aimed alignment remains poorly implemented, despite several existing tools. This can be explained by limited formal training regarding sagittal balance and also by the historically heavier emphasis given to the coronal Cobb angle. However, a shift in perspective is in progress, as the coronal Cobb angle has been poorly correlated with clinical outcomes in ASD [7].

We can divide the successive surgical steps that influence final alignment and summarize them:

- Patient positioning
- Release of the spine
- Instrumentation strategy (mono axial screws/poly axial screws, orientation of the screws)
- Facetectomies, Osteotomies (Smith-Petersen osteotomy or Chevron (SPO), pedicle subtraction osteotomy (PSO), bone-disc-bone osteotomy (BDBO) and vertebral column resection (VCR), based on the increasing complexity of the technique)
- Screw-rod connection
- Shape of the rod with the basic concept to realign the instrumented spine along the rod
- Segmental maneuvers (compression, distraction)
- Bone grafting.

It's important to understand that each step can be a cause of failure and one of the most complex steps is the pre-operative planning. To achieve this one, we will introduce the concept of Patient Specific Rod (PSR) as a canvas for the final post-operative results. Some cases will illustrate the techniques described under mentioned.

We assume that manual bending of a rod cannot always provide the aimed shape and so this can introduce a part of operator-dependent error. Consequently, this may fail to restore the sagittal parameters as intended [8]. Actually, only 32% of patients reach neutral alignment after this kind of surgery, while 42% remain with positive sagittal misalignment and 26% are overcorrected [7]. A patient-specific rod (PSR) could be one the main advances in optimal correction and surgical realization. [14].

Some tools exist to measure the intra-operative lordosis, (Sagittal Meter App), but this provides only an approximation, not the exact spinal contour. Moreover, these measurements are performed with the patient in prone position. Thus, a new concept of patient specific rod (PSR) is proposed to decrease the inaccuracy due to unmeasured rod contouring. Based on pre-operative surgical planning, PSRs are designed to fit with each patient's unique sagittal profile.

54.2 Correction and Planning

54.2.1 Alignment Objectives

The proposed pre-operative planning is based on a full-spine (or full body) calibrated sagittal X-ray, including at least the femoral heads and preferably the knees. We consider full body Rx as mandatory for each patient before a long instrumentation and we normally use the **EOS™**

system. The current spino-pelvic parameters and the apices of kyphosis and lordosis are evaluated to characterize the spinal sagittal shape of the patient.

Then, the surgical procedures are simulated using a dedicated software to reach the following three clinically relevant parameter proposed by Schwab, Lafage et al. [2–6]:

- Sagittal vertical axis (SVA) < 40 mm or 50 mm,
- Pelvic tilt (PT) <20°
- (PI-LL) <10°

To determine the theoretical lordosis, our preference is to refer to PI classes (each 10° from class I to class VI) which are more precise compared to Schwab formula giving full account of the fact that the relation between PI and lordosis is not linear but varies according to the value of the PI, see Table 54.1.

Not only the global magnitude of the lumbar lordosis is important to consider but also the distribution of the lordosis along the lumbar spine [10]. It is important to keep in mind that 2/3 of the lordosis is given by the L4-S1 segment only and that 40% is provided by L5-S1, see Chap. 26.

The apex of the lordosis is positioned in accordance with Roussouly's "Type of Back" classification (Fig. 54.1) [9], and predefined repartition of lordosis around the apex.

For type 2, 3 and 4 morphotypes (harmonious types), distribution of lumbar lordosis should be as follows: 2/3 among L4 and S1, 1/3 among L1 and L4 [10] (Fig. 54.1). For types 1, two strategies are possible: (1) stabilize the spine as type 1 keeping the original shape of the spine with the most part of the lordosis between L4 and S1, (2) the

Table 54.1 Method to determine the theoretical lordosis according to the class of PI

PI class	PI (°)	PT_{th} (°)	LL_{th} (°)
I	<38	4	PI + 18
II	38–47	8	PI + 13
III	48–57	12	PI + 9
IV	58–67	16	PI + 6
V	68–77	20	PI + 2
VI	>78	24	PI-5

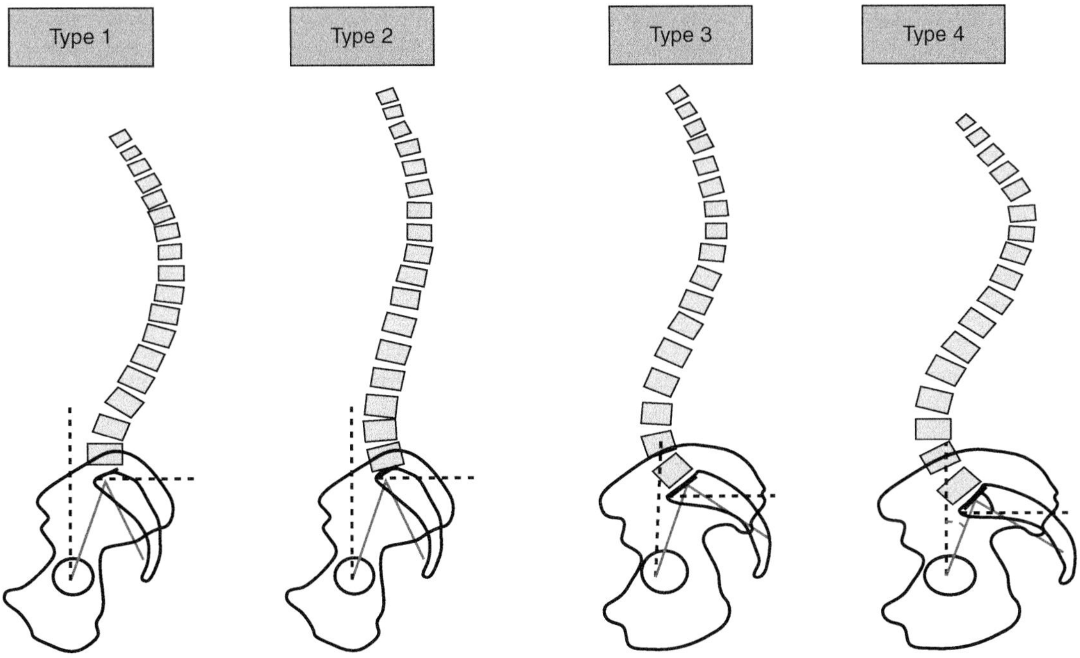

Fig. 54.1 "Type of Back" in accordance with Roussouly's classification (Fig. 54.9). The shape of lumbar lordosis depends on SS orientation. Type 1 and 2 have SS < 35°; Type 3 has 35° < SS < 45°; Type 4 has SS > 45°. Generally, Type 1 and 2 have a low PI and Type 3 and 4 have a high PI. Types 2–3-4 are considered as harmonious

second option is to transform type 1 into type 2 by reducing the lumbo-sacral hyperextension and the thoraco-lumbar kyphosis. The choice between the two strategies depends on the age of the patient, the clinical presentation and the importance of degenerative changes in lumbo-sacral segment. For anteverted type 3, diminishing of the lumbar lordosis is probably the best option. SVA should be adapted according to the age: elder patients usually accept higher values than young.

Correction has also to be adapted to the age of the patient. SVA should be <40 mm for patients under 65 y-old, SVA <55 mm is acceptable for patients between 65 and 75 y-old and SVA around 65–70 mm is enough for patients after 75 y-old. Similarly, PT around 25° is acceptable for patients after 75 y-old [10]. In case of construct below T9, the flexibility of thoracic spine should be evaluated and the post-operative behavior of the thoracic segment anticipated. If decrease of physiologic thoracic kyphosis (TK) is preoperatively suspected (e.g. TK measured around 20°), it is recommended to simulate the recovery of a more physiological value after surgery around 40° (approximately 2/3 of the LL). This is helpful to better evaluate the amount of correction that will be necessary in the lumbar segment and to better appreciate the corrective effect of the surgery on the global balance. For specific cases (e.g. multi-operated spine), a specific plan should be proposed outside the indications above.

To summarize, the four main points-based algorithm to calculate the amount of correction includes:

1. Schwab's criteria: SVA, PT and LL-PI mismatch
2. The theoretical LL of the patient (use of PI class is the preferred method to estimate the theoretical lordosis, see Table 54.1 and Chap. 26) and the natural distribution of lordosis along the lumbar spine with 2/3 between L4 and sacrum
3. The Roussouly's morphotype
4. The age of the patient

Application of just one simple formula (like the Schwab formula) without taking into consideration the other parameters may result in catastrophic post-operative outcomes with excessive correction and/or inadequate geometrical organization of the spino-pelvic complex.

54.2.2 Concept of Patient Specific Rod (PSR) and Planning

The realignment is planned in standardized phases. First, virtual correction of the sagittal alignment is simulated using posterior release techniques (from facet resections to 3-column osteotomy), inter-body cage insertion, and compression or distraction from the virtually corrected spine, the PSR's contour is defined on sagittal view. The PSR length is measured on coronal view, based on the entry points of each pedicle screw or other implant (Fig. 54.2) and the expected correction of coronal curves. Two PSRs are thus industrially manufactured and precisely bent to this specification. Landmarks on the rods (superior limit vertebra, S1 screw, sagittal line) can be laser printed to insure the correct placement of the rods during the surgical procedure [14].

54.2.2.1 Surgical Technique

After manufacturing, the two symmetrical PSR (or asymmetrical if required) are then delivered into the operating room with the predetermined shape and length, corresponding exactly to the preoperative planning, and finally inserted into the patient with no additional maneuver. PSR are currently available in titanium or cobalt-chromium, in 5.5 or 6 mm diameter (MEDICREA®, Lyon, France).

Technically, there is nothing really specific, all the surgical steps being similar as usual and corresponding to the planning. If the instrumented spine is stiffer than expected and the rods seems "too bended", an additional release procedure should be added. If the rods do not fit at all, the surgeon can use and bend standard ones. If necessary, it is also possible to bend the PSRs a little bit more or a little less and, of course, shorten them.

The pedicle screws should be placed parallel to superior endplate as that allows more accurate

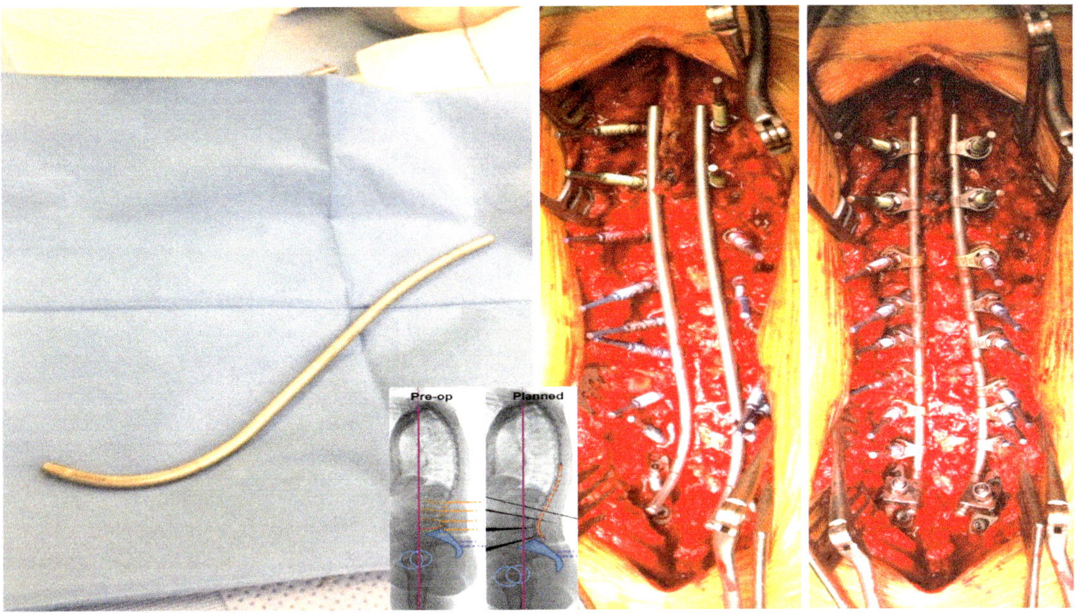

Fig. 54.2 Patient specific rod (PSR) UNID™ industrially manufactured and perfectly fits the surgical field

placement on the specific rod markings and good correspondence among the rods' contour and the final position of the vertebrae [10, 14].

In clinical practice, regarding the pre-operative planning we will illustrate this chapter with three cases.

54.3 Cases Description

54.3.1 Case 1

Patient known for a L2-S1 fusion with persistent neurogenic claudication, chronic back pain and forward bending limiting the walking distance to 40 m. Flat back with thoracic junctional kyphosis (Fig. 54.3).

Spino-pelvic parameters and the apices of kyphosis and lordosis are evaluated to characterize the spinal sagittal shape of the patient and to establish a first planning with the dedicated software.

The second step is to establish a first planning through a T4-Illiacs screws fixation + PSO: L2 (25°, Grade III according to Schwab classification) + multilevel SPO. See simulation n°1 in Fig. 54.4.

The first planning strategy was not good enough with persistent imbalance and the SVA was still >100 mm. The patient has a PI class II. The lumbar lordosis needed is PI + 13 = 51°, SVA < 50, pelvic tilt of 12°, PI-LL > 10. So, the strategy changed with a new planning. This one included a PSO of L3 (grade 4 PSO, trans-discal type) to gain 35° of lordosis and is under mentioned. See simulation n°2 in Fig. 54.5.

With this new planning the objective is to reach a SVA at 10.7 mm, LL: 41, PI-LL = 2, PT: 12 and this was done through PSO of L3 to gain 35° of lordosis (Grade IV according to Schwab classification). The use of a Patient Specific Rod shown in blue allowed achieving an optimal alignment at the end of the surgery and in this way to fit with the pre-operative planning.

This case illustrates how we establish our planning and verify it before the surgery to simulate the better strategies (Figs. 54.6 and 54.7).

54.3.2 Case 2

57-years-old patient presenting with chronic low back pain, a walking distance of 40 m and

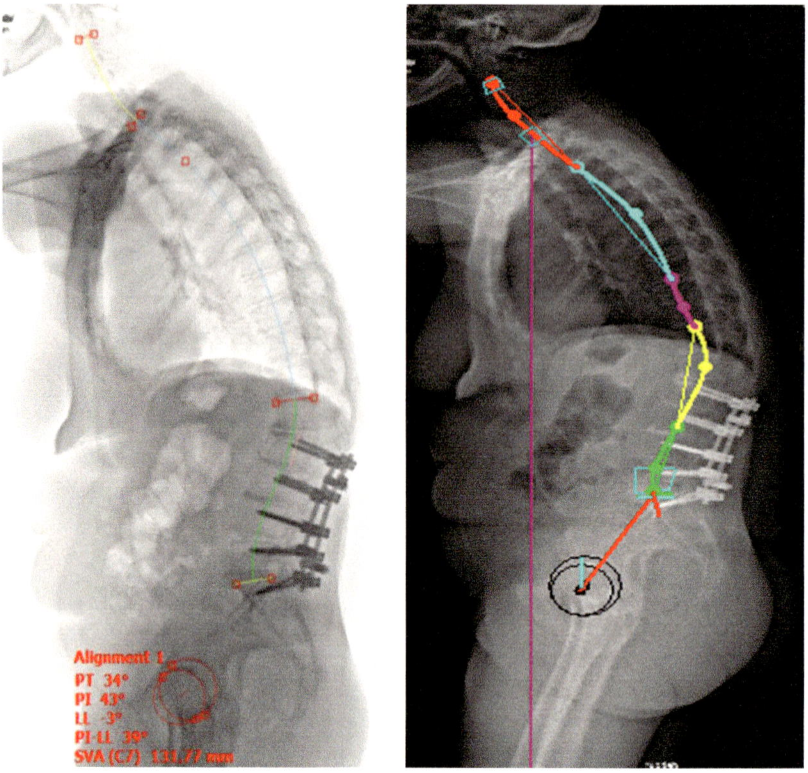

Fig. 54.3 The first step is to establish the sagittal balance parameters with the three clinically relevant parameter on a full spine EOS™ System X-Ray: PI 43°, Pelvic Tilt 34°, PI-LL: 39°, LL measured to only 3° and SVA: 131.7 mm

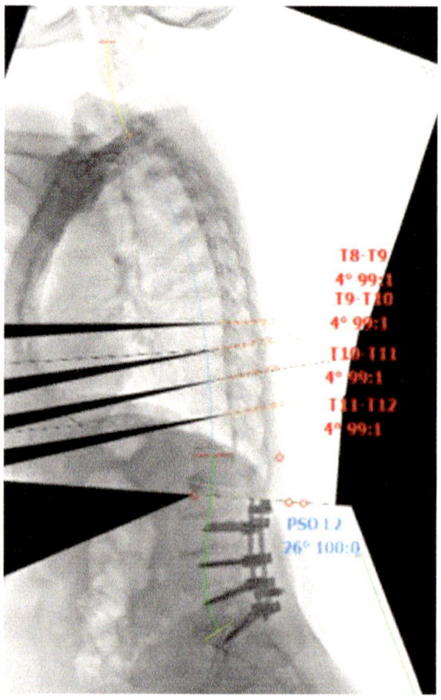

	Sagittal Vert. Alignment (mm)	Thoracic Kyphosis (°)	Pelvic Incidence PI (°)	Lumbar Lordosis LL (°)	*PI-LL (°)*	Sacral Slope (°)	Pelvic Tilt (°)
PREOPERATIVE	131.7	40	43	3	*39*	9	34
CASE PLANNING	101.8	25	43	29	*14*	31	12

Fig. 54.4 First planning strategy with a L2 PSO Grade III according to Schwab and multiples SPO's. Not enough lordosis and still a sagittal dysbalance (SVA still >100 mm)

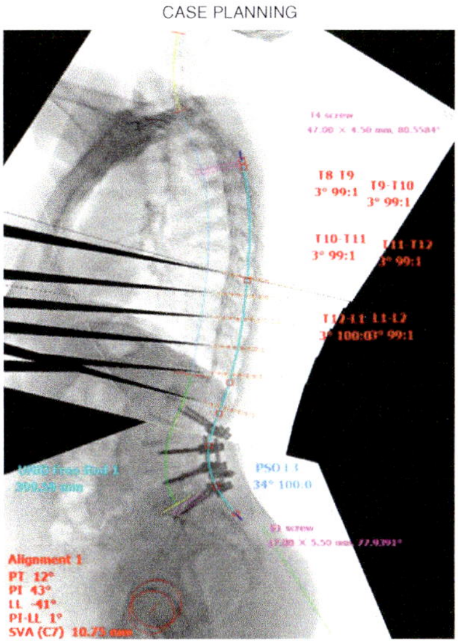

Fig. 54.5 Second planning strategy with a T4-illiac screws + L3 PSO Grade IV according to Schwab and multiples SPO's. Theoretical SVA at 10.7 mm, LL 41° and PT at 12°. The correction is now satisfying. Planning validated

	Sagittal Vert. Alignment (mm)	Thoracic Kyphosis (°)	Pelvic Incidence PI (°)	Lumbar Lorodsis LL (°)	*PI-LL (°)*	Sacral Slope (°)	Pelvic Tilt (°)
PREOPERATIVE	131.7	40	43	3	*39*	9	34
CASE PLANNING	10.7	25	43	41	*2*	31	12

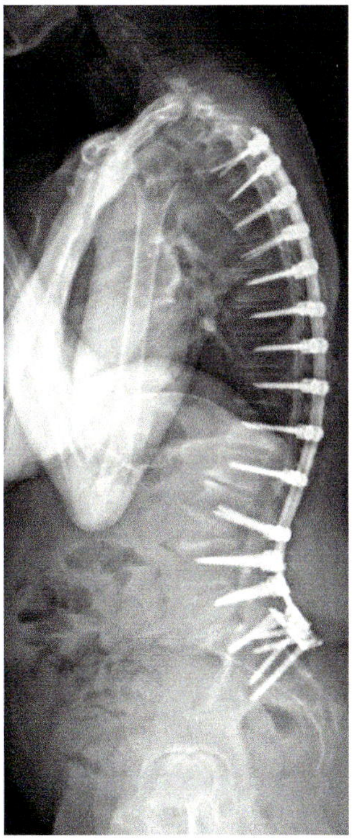

Fig. 54.6 Post-surgical result with a balanced patient. SVA at 11.1 mm, LL at 55.4°, PI-LL = −13

forward bending with a sagittal imbalance. EOS: Degenerative lumbar kyphosis with a lumbar lordosis of −8°, retroverted pelvis, ODI 52/100 and Roland-Morris score 17/24 (Figs. 54.8, 54.9, and 54.10).

54.3.3 Case 3

68-year-old female patient, history of L2-L4 arthrodesis (2005). Severe low back pain for >2 years and radicular pain on L4 and L5 territory predominant on the left with a L5 motor deficit. Walking distance estimated to 100. VAS 7, ODI 48/100, Roland Morris 12/24.

Multiples comorbidities: myocardial infarct, renal insufficiency, auricular fibrillation (Fig. 54.11).

Radiographs revealed a major rigid degenerative kypho-scoliosis in the lumbar spine. **As the patient has much comorbidity and is 68 y.o we adapted our planning to different objectives in order to shorten the surgery and to minimize the surgical risks** (Figs. 54.12 and 54.13).

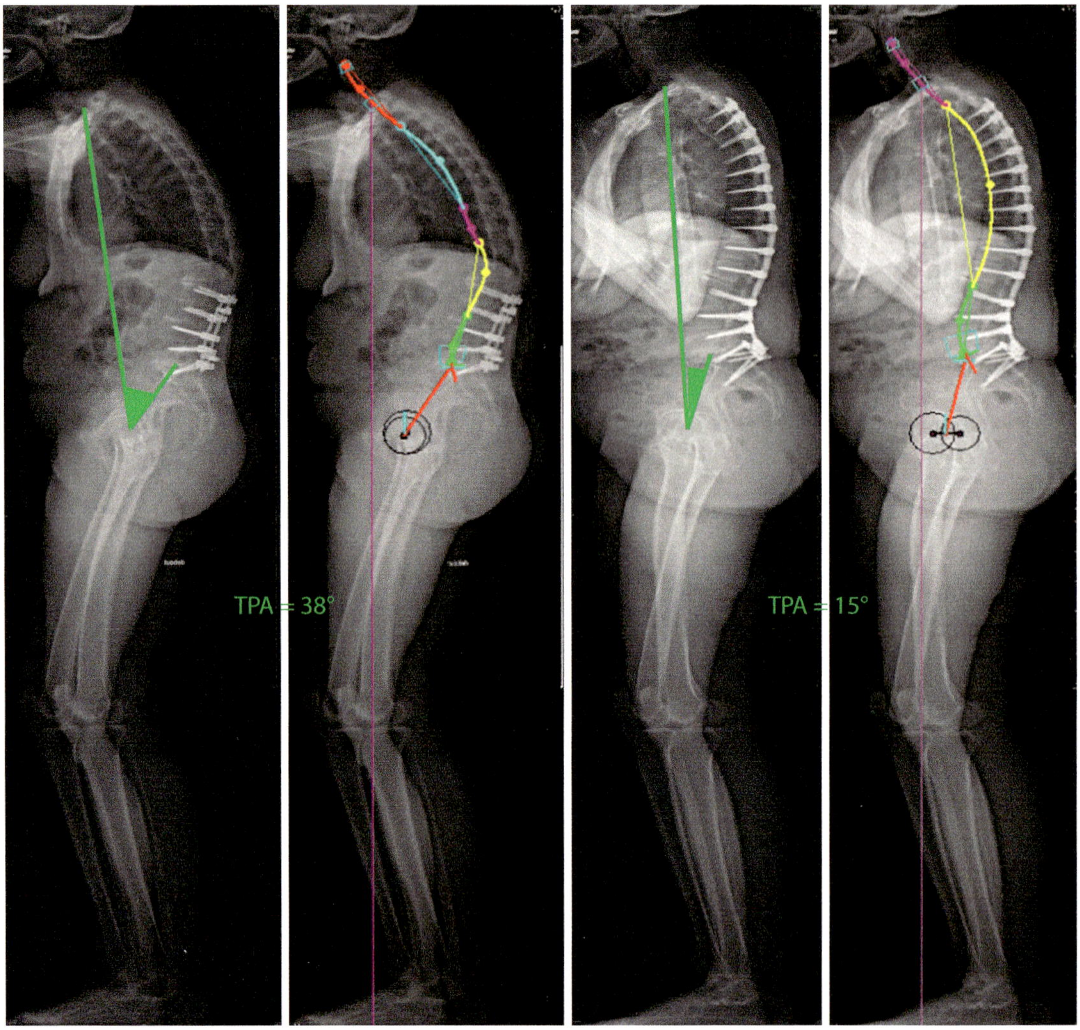

Fig. 54.7 Full body radiographs comparing pre and post surgical result with a quasi-normalization of the TPA measured at 15°, repositioning of C7 plumb line above the pelvis and decrease of the knee flexion

54.4 Discussion

This chapter had the aim to show the relevance of pre-operative planning to achieve an optimal surgical correction of sagittal balance disorders. It's mandatory to assess the spino-pelvic balance and to establish clear objectives for correction before to surgery and to try to reach them during it.

The surgical procedures can be simulated using dedicated software to reach the targets for corrective surgery realignment.

Pre-operative simulation allows a systematic attitude of all the spino-pelvic parameters and to simulate different options for surgery. It also permits a clear and concisely strategy before in order to shorten the surgical time and to avoid complications.

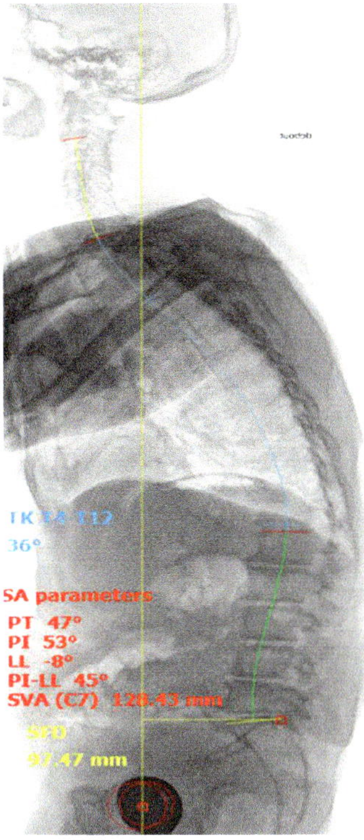

Fig. 54.8 Full spine EOS™ System X-Ray shows a flat back with degenerative lumbar kyphosis. PI: 53°, PT: 47° and LL-8°, PI-LL = 45° and SVA 128.4 mm. The theoretical LL for this patient would be PI + 9 = 61° (PI class III according to Barrey)

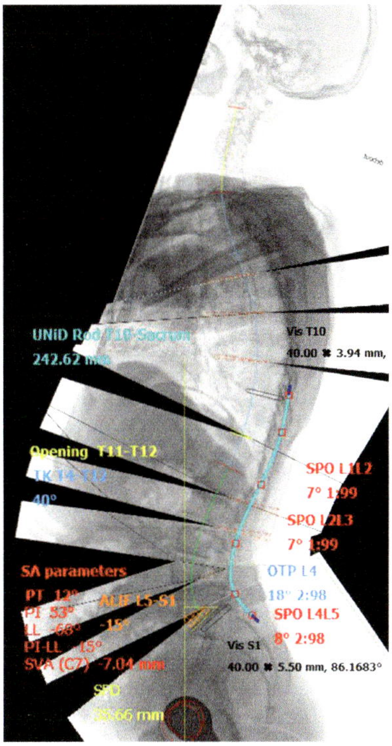

Fig. 54.9 Planning with a two steps surgery. First ALIF L5-S1 with 12° of lordosis as an objective. Second T10-Sacrum with Patient Specific Rod and PSO L4 (25° Grade III according to Schwab), PSO L1–2 L2-L3 and L4-L5, facetectomie T11-T12. Objectives: LL: 68°, SVA: -7 mm, PIO-LL: -15°, PT: 12°. The recovery of a normal TK around 40° after surgery was simulated

It is possible to plan a strategy considered as sub-optimal depending on the age and comorbidities of the patient. The objective is not always to fit the Schwab criteria's but to fit the planification criterias adapted to the condition of the patient. Different factors will be in the future a part of the pre-operative planning, for example bone quality, age, comorbidities, weight and so on. Maybe artificial intelligence can take in the future all the factors to help the surgeon in the realization of the pre-operative planning.

At the moment, the objectives have to be adapted to the age of the patient and we propose an algorithm to do it.

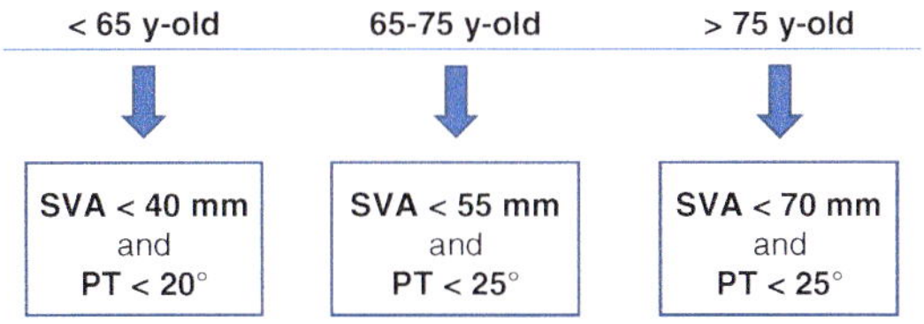

54.5 Conclusion

Pre-operative planning will be mandatory for each spine surgeon and for complex cases in the future. Many digital and informatics tools are now well developed to achieve the objectives

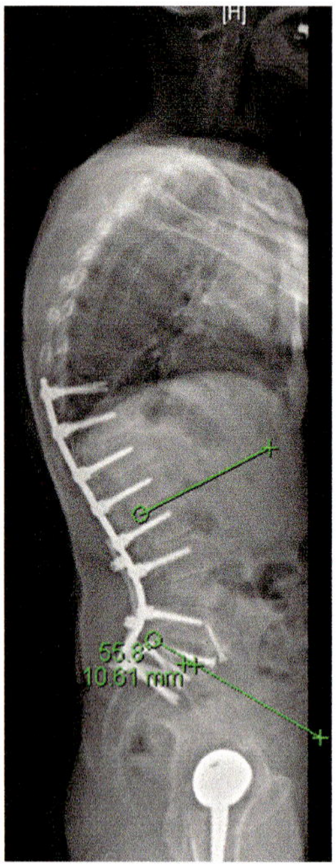

Fig. 54.10 Post-surgical result with a SVA at 10.6 mm, LL at 55.8, PI-LL = −3°, TPA 12°

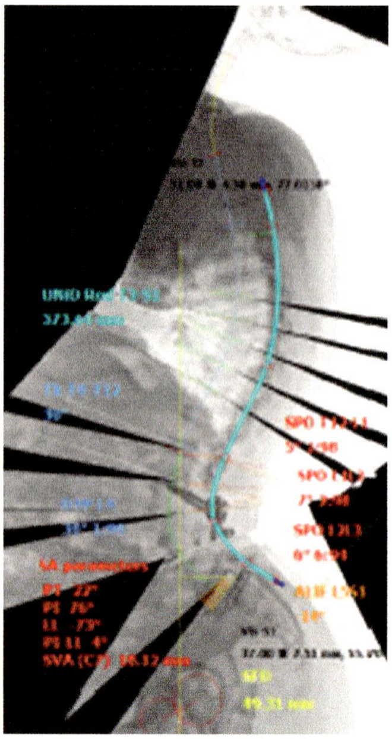

Fig. 54.12 Planning adapted to the age and to the comorbidities of the patient. SVA: 18 mm, PI-LL: 3°, PT: 22°, LL: 73° through a T3-Illiac screws fixation, asymmetrical L4 PSO (40° Grade IV according to Schwab) and multiples PSO's

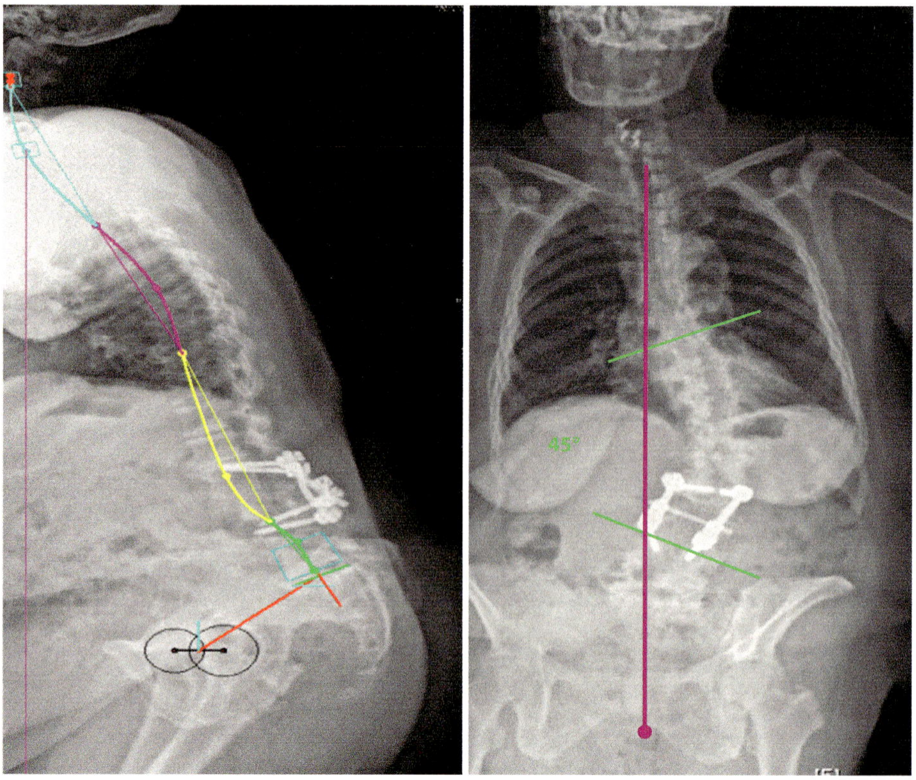

Fig. 54.11 Full spine EOS™ of a thoraco-lumbar scoliosis with spino-pelvic parameters: PI = 75°, PT = 50°, SVA = +298 mm LL L1-S1 = 8°, TK = 28° and (T4-T10) Cobb = 45°. PI Class V with a theoretical LL of PI+2 = 78

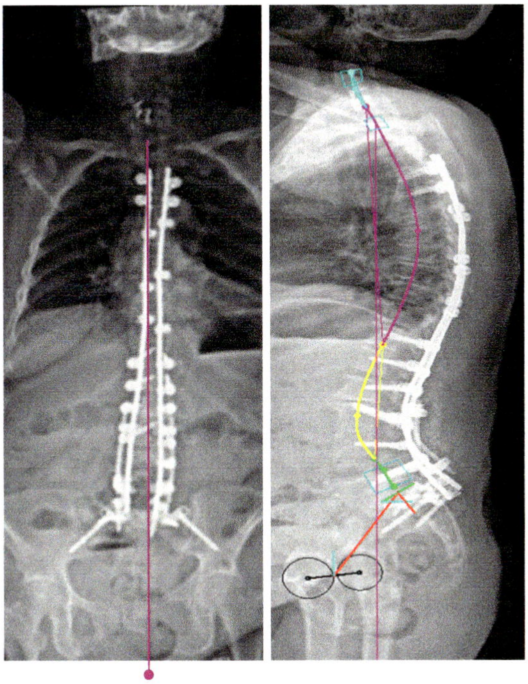

Fig. 54.13 Post-surgical EOS Full spine X Ray: Correction of the scoliosis in the coronal plane. The spino-pelvic parameters are now: PT = 30°, SVA = +32 mm L1-S1 = 56° TK = 52° Cobb = 8°. The strategy has been adapted to the condition of the patient and her age

of the surgery. These ones have to be adapted to each patient and to each type of back, artificial intelligence should be in the future a help for the planning.

Correction depends on four main criteria's:

1. Schwab and Lafage criterias
2. Roussouly's morphotypes
3. Theoretical lordosis (refer to PI classes) respecting the 2/3 rule of LL between L4-S1
4. The age of the patient and comorbidities

Patient Specific Rod are really interesting for the pre-operative planning and the final results. The is no manual rod bending and so no intra operator or inter-operator variability. Mechanically the bending is smoother and less aggressive for the rod and it also permits to shorten the surgery at the end. A multicentric study is conducted at the moment and the first results will be available in 2019 [8, 14].

Pearls

- Define the objectives for correction of sagittal balance disorders
- Define the optimal lumbar lordosis
- Achieve the pre-operative planning
- Simulate different surgical strategies

References

1. Barrey C, Roussouly P, Le Huec JC, D'Acunzi G, Perrin G. Compensatory mechanisms contributing to keep the sagittal balance of the spine. Eur Spine J. 2013;22(Suppl 6):S834–41. **EBM V**
2. Schwab F, Patel A, Ungar B, Farcy JP, Lafage V. Adult spinal deformity-postoperative standing imbalance: how much can you tolerate? An overview of key parameters in assessing alignment and planning corrective surgery. Spine (Phila Pa 1976). 2010;35:2224–31. **EBM V**
3. Le Huec JC, Cogniet A, Demezon H, Rigal J, Saddiki R, Aunoble S. Insufficient restoration of lumbar lordosis and FBI index following pedicle subtraction osteotomy is an indicator of likely mechanical complication. Eur Spine J. 2015;24(Suppl 1):S112–20. **EBM III**
4. Yagi M, Fujita N, Okada E, et al. Fine-tuning the predictive model for proximal junctional failure in surgically treated patients with adult spinal deformity. Spine (Phila Pa 1976). 2017; https://doi.org/10.1097/BRS.0000000000002415. **EBM IV**
5. Glassman SD, Berven S, Bridwell K, Horton W, Dimar JR. Correlation of radiographic parameters and clinical symptoms in adult scoliosis. Spine (Phila Pa 1976). 2005;30:682–8. **EBM IV**
6. Lafage V, Schwab F, Patel A, Hawkinson N, Farcy JP. Pelvic tilt and truncal inclination: two key radiographic parameters in the setting of adults with spinal deformity. Spine (Phila Pa 1976). 2009;34:E599–606. **EBM III**
7. Blondel B, Schwab F, Bess S, et al. Posterior global malalignment after osteotomy for sagittal plane deformity: it happens and here is why. Spine (Phila Pa 1976). 2013;38:E394–401. **EBM IV**
8. Fiere V, Armoiry X, Vital JM, Lafage V, Berthiller V, Barrey C. Preoperative planning and patient specific rods for surgical treatment of thoracolumbar sagittal imbalance. In: Van de Kelft E, editor. Surgery of the spine and spinal cord: a neurosurgical approach. Cham: Springer; 2016. p. 645–62.
9. Roussouly P, Pinheiro-Franco JL. Sagittal parameters of the spine: biomechanical approach. Eur Spine J. 2011;20(Suppl 5):578–85. **EBM V**
10. Barrey C, Darnis A. Current strategies for the restoration of adequate lordosis during lumbar fusion. World

J Orthop. 2015;6:117–26. https://doi.org/10.5312/wjo.v6.i1.117. eCollection 2015 Jan 18. **EBM V**

11. Lafage V, Schwab F, Skalli W, Hawkinson N, Gagey PM, Ondra S, Farcy JP. Standing balance and sagittal plane spinal deformity: analysis of spinopelvic and gravity line parameters. Spine (Phila Pa 1976). 2008;33:1572–8. **EBM III**
12. Smith JS, Shaffrey CI, Ames CP, et al. Assessment of symptomatic rod fracture after posterior instrumented fusion for adult spinal deformity. Neurosurgery. 2012;71:862–7. **EBM IV**
13. Lafage R, Schwab F, Glassman S, et al. Age-adjusted alignment goals have the potential to reduce PJK. Spine (Phila Pa 1976). 2017;42(17):1275–82. https://doi.org/10.1097/BRS.0000000000002146. **EBM IV**
14. Barrey C, Fiere V, Lafage V, Vital J, Armoiry X, Berthillier J, PROFILE. Surgical treatment of spinal deformity with sagittal imbalance using patient-specific rods: a multicenter, controlled, double blind randomized trial. 2014. https://clinicaltrials.gov/ct2/show/NCT02730507. Accessed 10 Nov 2017. **EBM II**

55 Technical Execution of Correction Osteotomies (SPO, PSO, etc.)

Florian Ringel

55.1 Introduction

Spinal osteotomies are gaining increasing importance and utilization during recent years. Several factors contribute to this increase.

The demographic development of many western populations towards an increasing age is associated with an increased prevalence of adult spinal deformities most of which are de novo degenerative deformities. The reduction in quality of life and the benefits of surgical treatment in comparison to conservative treatment contribute to the increased numbers of corrective osteotomies necessary. While degenerative deformities are certainly the number one indication for surgical corrections including osteotomies, deformities caused by other entities as ankylosing spondylitis, postinfectious or posttraumatic are increasingly treated with spinal osteotomies. Furthermore, the increase in utilization of osteotomies is supported by an increase in training and resulting comfort in the execution of these technical demanding procedures [4–7].

Additionally, the concept of sagittal balance and imbalance of the spine gained increasing attention in degenerative disorders of the spine [12, 13]. Increasing evidence for the relevance of this concept is accumulated leading to a further utilization of corrective procedures of the spine [11].

This chapter aims to provide an overview on the classification of osteotomies for deformity correction, the planning, the potential gain in deformity correction with the different osteotomy techniques and the surgical execution.

At the end of this chapter the reader should be aware of the different types and the classification of correction osteotomies, the attainable extent of sagittal plane correction and the technical execution.

55.2 Case Description

A 77-year-old female patient presented with low back pain and neurogenic claudication since several months. Two years earlier the patient underwent posterior fusion of the segments L2–5 with posterior decompression of L3/4 and L4/5 as well as interbody fusion of the segments L3/4 and 4/5 for a degenerative instability. The patient reported a remission of pain and pain-related immobility after initial surgery for about 1 year, until symptoms returned. Imaging revealed degeneration and a kyphotic deformity of the cranial adjacent segment, the spine was imbalanced in the sagittal plane with a sagittal vertical axis of 100 mm (Fig. 55.1).

F. Ringel (✉)
Department of Neurosurgery, Universitätsmedizin Mainz, Johannes Gutenberg Universität Mainz, Mainz, Germany
e-mail: florian.ringel@unimedizin-mainz.de

B. Meyer, M. Rauschmann (eds.), *Spine Surgery*, https://doi.org/10.1007/978-3-319-98875-7_55

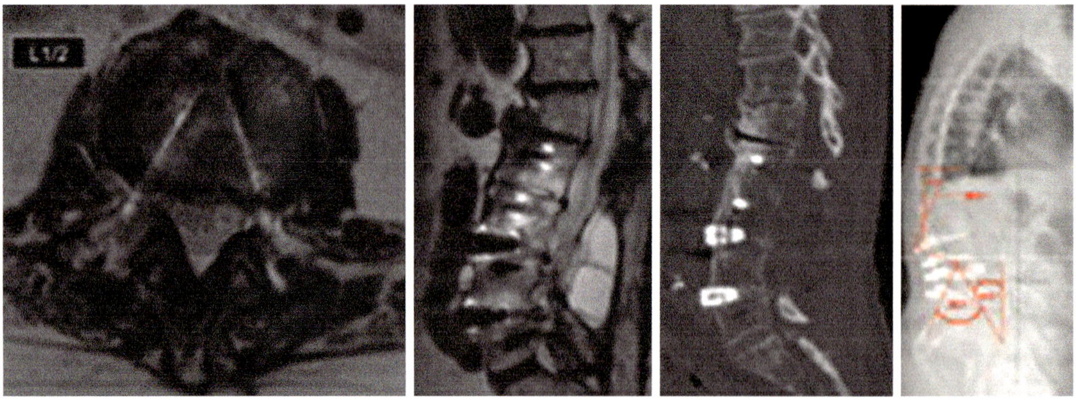

Fig. 55.1 Preoperative MRI, CT of the lumbar spine and whole standing spine x-ray with parameters of sagittal balance. Imaging data show the previous instrumentation of the lumbar spine with fusion of the segments L2/3, 3/4 and 4/5. The adjacent upper segment shows a kyphotic deformity resulting in sagittal imbalance of the spine

Due to the symptoms refractory to conservative therapy the patient consented for surgery.

The previous instrumentation was removed and posterior instrumentation above the previous fusion was implanted from T10 to L3 excluding L1. A pedicle subtraction osteotomy of L1 was performed to correct the deformity. Postoperative whole spine x-rays revealed a reduction of the sagittal deformity to a sagittal vertical axis of 44 mm.

Lumbar lordosis was increased from 28° to 44°, pelvic tilt reduced from 29° to 14° from preoperative to postoperative (Fig. 55.2).

55.3 Discussion

55.3.1 Classification of Osteotomies

Different techniques of osteotomies of the spine to achieve sagittal plane correction of varying extent have been described and classifications of these osteotomies are available and some popular techniques carry the name of its inventor [1, 8].

According to the basic principle of resection and correction, osteotomies can be differentiated in opening wedge, closing wedge and opening closing wedge techniques. A typical example of an opening wedge osteotomy would be a Smith-Peterson osteotomy (SPO), where the inferior and superior facets are resected bilaterally combined with a partial laminectomy. By closure of the posterior defect with the posterior body wall as the center of rotation an anterior wedge within the disc space is opened. The anterior spine is elongated while the posterior parts are shortened resulting in hyperlordosis of the segment. A typical closing wedge osteotomy is a pedicle subtraction osteotomy which includes resection of the posterior segmental elements, bilateral pedicles and a wedge of the vertebral body with the tip of the wedge at the anterior border of the vertebral body and the base posteriorly. By closing of the wedge posteriorly the vertebral body is lordotically deformed.

In 2014 Schwab et al. published an anatomical classification of spinal osteotomies describing 6 anatomic grades (Fig. 55.3) [15].

- Grade 1 involves a partial facet joint resection i.e. the inferior facet and joint capsule. These osteotomies allow limited amount of correction of approximately 5–10° in the sagittal plane by a posterior only approach. They are named Smith-Peterson osteotomy when generating an anterior opening wedge, Chevron osteotomy or extension osteotomy. A mobile spinal segment is a prerequisite of these osteotomies.
- Grade 2 involves a complete facet joint resection of a segment and the ligamentum flavum, potentially of further posterior elements as the

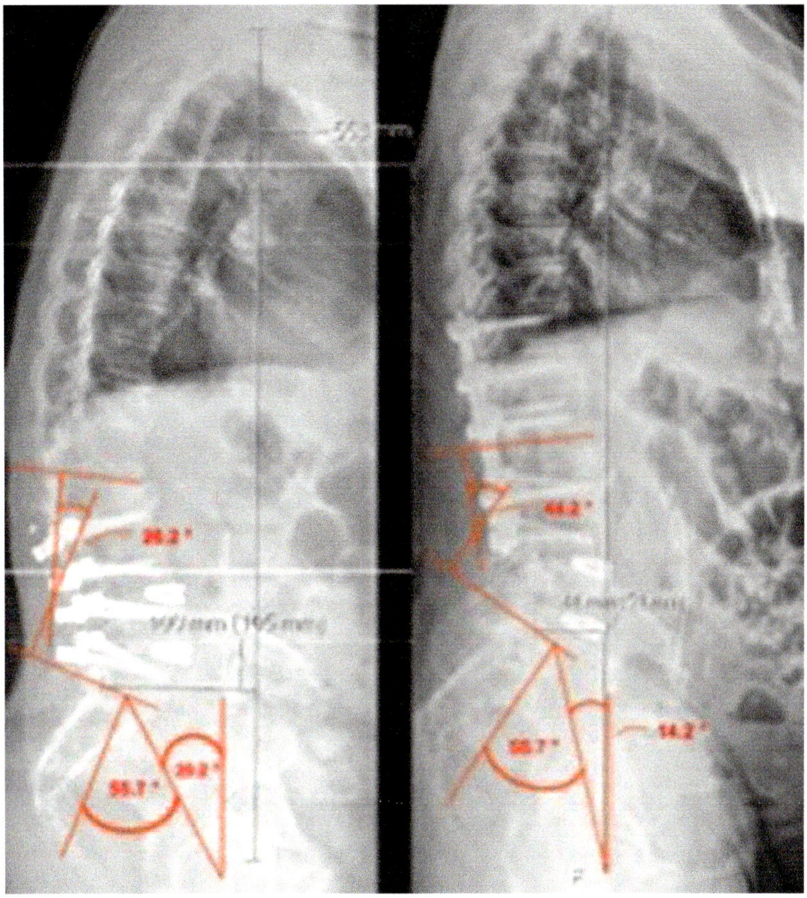

Fig. 55.2 Pre- and postoperative standing whole spine x-ray. Pre- and postoperative standing whole spine x-rays reveal a kyphotic deformity cranially to the previous instrumentation. Correction of the symptomatic deformity was performed by a L1 pedicle subtraction osteotomy. Pre- and postoperative sagittal parameters are given in the images

lamina and spinous process as well. After the bony resection the posterior defect is closed using the posterior instrumentation. The correction requires a mobile segment unless a rigid segment is released at the disc space prior to posterior closure. A typical grade 2 resection is the Ponte osteotomy.

- Grade 3 involves a pedicle and partial body resection i.e. the typical grade 3 osteotomy would be a pedicle subtraction osteotomy and its variants. These osteotomies can be performed posterior only, do not demand a mobile segment and can be performed in a rigid deformity. The degree of correction of a pedicle subtraction osteotomy is approximately 25–30° of lordosis.
- Grade 4 resection describes wider wedge resections including the superior vertebral body and cranial adjacent disc gaining 30–35° of correction.
- Grade 5 and 6 describe complete single level or multi level vertebral column resections including the vertebral bodies and discs.

These types of osteotomies allow for different extents of correction in the sagittal plane and can be modified in an asymmetrical fashion to allow for correction of coronal deformities as well [3, 14].

But prior to surgery a crucial step is the planning of required correction, the necessary osteotomies and the adequate level of osteotomies.

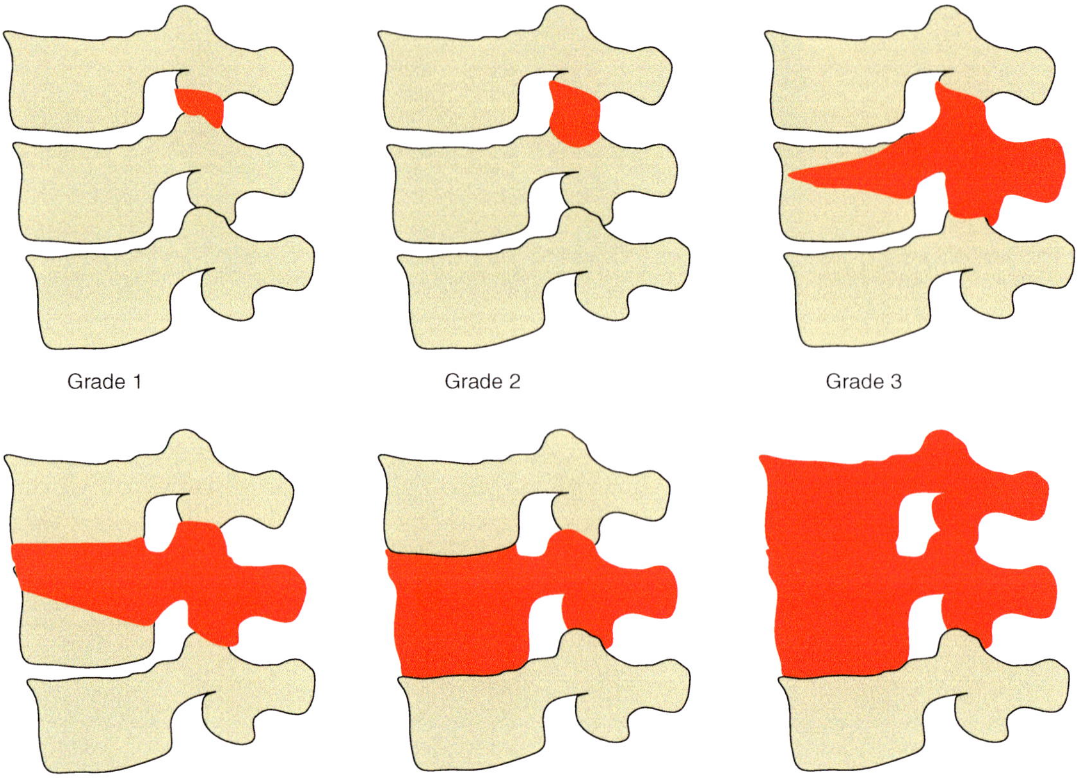

Fig. 55.3 Classification of spinal osteotomies according to Schwab et al.

55.3.2 Planning of Osteotomies

Different methods of correction planning have been described. Pragmatic target values for deformity correction have been defined by Schwab et al. as PI-LL ≤10°, PT <20°, SVA ≤4 cm. Popular approaches to plan for correction are the technique of Berjano or the ´full balance integrated method` by Le Huec [2, 10]. Furthermore, computer systems to simulate osteotomies and the expectable degree of correction are available (Surgimap, Nemaris, USA). Planning of correction should respect the SVA or C7 translation angle, compensate for the pelvic tilt and the account for the femur obliquity angle as measured in standing whole spine images including the upper femurs. The focus of correction should be in the lower lumbar spine as lower levels demand less resection to achieve the same angle of correction as more cranial osteotomies. However, despite adequate planning the positive predictive value of correction calculation has been approximately 75% in one study and over- or undercorrection occurs [9].

55.3.3 Execution of Osteotomies

For a posterior osteotomy as the pedicle subtraction osteotomy of the case described above the patient is in a prone position. Care should be taken to place sufficient cushion support to push the spine towards the correction upon bony release or to allow to break the table at the relevant level, thereby achieving correction after bony resection. A standard posterior approach to the relevant spinal levels is performed and the necessary posterior instrumentation is placed – the levels necessary to include depend on the extent of deformity and are an issue of ongoing discussion but a pedicle subtraction osteotomy should be stabilized by at least pedicle screws in two levels above and below the PSO. After posterior instrumentation a laminectomy of the respective level is performed including a partial laminectomy of the level above and below and resection of the flaval ligaments. The facet joints bilaterally superior and inferior to the level are resected, the pedicle is exposed. As a next step the pedicle is resected to the level of the posterior wall of the vertebral body. The lateral walls of the vertebral body are exposed. Next step is the resection of the posterior wall of the vertebral body as a base of the wedge. Now, either a wedge type resection or preferably in patients with poor bone quality compaction of bone is performed to the anterior wall of the vertebral body maintaining the anterior cortical bone. The lateral walls of the wedge are resected. Finally the wedge is closed via the posterior instrumentation and breaking of the table or additional cushions under the patient.

55.3.4 Complications of Osteotomies

Though complication rates of 3 column correction osteotomies decreased during the recent decade the rate of adverse events is still high. A recent study described an overall complication rate of 39% within 2 years, including 30% revisions [6]. Typical problems leading to revisions are hardware failure, pseudarthrosis, neurological deficits and proximal junctional kyphosis. An excessive intraoperative blood loss is still an intraoperative problem in about 15% of patients, as well as new neurological deficits in 10%.

55.4 Conclusions and Take Home Message

Correction osteotomies of the spine can correct for sagittal and coronal deformities. The type of osteotomy needs to be tailored to the extent of correction necessary and planning tools are available. Depending on the type of osteotomy different extents of correction can be achieved. The most common osteotomies as Smith Peterson or Ponte osteotomies gain 5–10° of correction while pedicle subtraction osteotomies allow for corrections up to 25°. With the increasing use and experience with 3 column osteotomies complication rates are decreasing although they are still at a high level. Therefore, deformity correction by osteotomies should be reserved for patients with significant reductions in quality of life.

Pearls

- Osteotomies are increasingly used to correct for sagittal and coronal deformities
- Different opening and closing wedge osteotomies are available to achieve the necessary extent of correction
- Osteotomies are associated with a high but decreasing complication rate

References and Level of Evidence (EBM)

1. Ames CP, Smith JS, Scheer JK, Shaffrey CI, Lafage V, Deviren V, Moal B, Protopsaltis T, Mummaneni PV, Mundis GM Jr, Hostin R, Klineberg E, Burton DC, Hart R, Bess S, Schwab FJ, International Spine Study Group. A standardized nomenclature for cervical spine soft-tissue release and osteotomy for deformity correction: clinical article. J Neurosurg Spine. 2013;19(3):269–78. **EBM IV**
2. Berjano P, Cecchinato R, Damilano M, Morselli C, Sansone V, Lamartina C. Preoperative calculation of the necessary correction in sagittal imbalance surgery: validation of three predictive methods. Eur Spine J. 2013;22(Suppl 6):S847–52. **EBM IV**
3. Cecchinato R, Berjano P, Aguirre MF, Lamartina C. Asymmetrical pedicle subtraction osteotomy in the lumbar spine in combined coronal and sagittal imbalance. Eur Spine J. 2015;24(Suppl 1):S66–71. **EBM V**
4. Diebo BG, Henry J, Lafage V, Berjano P. Sagittal deformities of the spine: factors influencing the outcomes and complications. Eur Spine J. 2015;24(Suppl 1):S3–15. **EBM V**
5. Diebo B, Liu S, Lafage V, Schwab F. Osteotomies in the treatment of spinal deformities: indications, classification, and surgical planning. Eur J Orthop Surg Traumatol. 2014;24(Suppl 1):S11–20. **EBM V**
6. Diebo BG, Jalai CM, Challier V, et al. Novel index to quantify the risk of surgery in the setting of adult

spinal deformity: a study on 10,912 patients from the nationwide inpatient sample. Clin Spine Surg. 2017;30(7):E993–9. **EBM III**

7. Diebo BG, Lafage V, Varghese JJ, Gupta M, Kim HJ, Ames C, Kebaish K, Shaffrey C, Hostin R, Obeid I, Burton D, Hart RA, Lafage R, Schwab FJ, International Spine Study Group (ISSG) of Denver, Colorado. After 9 years of 3-column osteotomies, are we doing better? Performance curve analysis of 573 surgeries with 2-year follow-up. Neurosurgery. 2018;83(1):69–75. **EBM III**
8. Enercan M, Ozturk C, Kahraman S, Sarıer M, Hamzaoglu A, Alanay A. Osteotomies/spinal column resections in adult deformity. Eur Spine J. 2013;22(Suppl 2):S254–64. **EBM V**
9. Lafage V, Smith JS, Bess S, Schwab FJ, Ames CP, Klineberg E, Arlet V, Hostin R, Burton DC, Shaffrey CI, International Spine Study Group. Sagittal spino-pelvic alignment failures following three column thoracic osteotomy for adult spinal deformity. Eur Spine J. 2012;21(4):698–704. **EBM IV**
10. Le Huec JC, Leijssen P, Duarte M, Aunoble S. Thoracolumbar imbalance analysis for osteotomy planification using a new method: FBI technique. Eur Spine J. 2011;20(Suppl 5):669–80. **EBM IV**
11. Le Huec JC, Faundez A, Dominguez D, Hoffmeyer P, Aunoble S. Evidence showing the relationship between sagittal balance and clinical outcomes in surgical treatment of degenerative spinal diseases: a literature review. Int Orthop. 2015;39(1):87–95. **EBM III**
12. Roussouly P, Gollogly S, Berthonnaud E, Dimnet J. Classification of the normal variation in the sagittal alignment of the human lumbar spine and pelvis in the standing position. Spine. 2005;30(3):346–53. **EBM III**
13. Roussouly P, Pinheiro-Franco JL. Sagittal parameters of the spine: biomechanical approach. Eur Spine J. 2011;20(Suppl 5):578–85. **EBM V**
14. Thambiraj S, Boszczyk BM. Asymmetric osteotomy of the spine for coronal imbalance: a technical report. Eur Spine J. 2012;21(Suppl 2):S225–9. **EBM V**
15. Schwab F, Blondel B, Chay E, et al. The comprehensive anatomical spinal osteotomy classification. Neurosurgery. 2014;74(1):112–20. **EBM III**

56 Instrumentation Techniques Including Sacral and Pelvic Fixation

Yann Philippe Charles

56.1 Introduction

Lumbar degenerative scoliosis and anterior imbalance represent common spinal deformities in the aging population. Surgical treatment might be considered if conservative treatment remains inefficient on low back and leg pain and in progressive trunk imbalance. Adult spinal deformity associated with imbalance has an impact on health-related quality of life (QoL) [1, 2]. Correction of sagittal imbalance can be performed with surgical techniques such as Smith-Petersen or Ponte osteotomies in deformities where the intersomatic space remains mobile, whereas a pedicle subtraction osteotomy (PSO) is usually indicated in severe rigid deformities [3].

Although the surgical treatment of adult spinal deformity improves QoL, the incidence of mid- and long-term mechanical complication is reported between 30% and 40% [4, 5]. These rates increase if the spinal deformity and degenerative changes require instrumentation to the sacrum. Among failures related to instrumentations including the lumbosacral junction, distal screw loosening, pseudarthrosis and rod breakage as well as proximal junctional kyphosis are the most common problems.

This case description will outline the management of a degenerative lumbar scoliosis with anterior imbalance. The aim of the presented case is to emphasize specific aspects that should help the reader in surgical planning of a posterior correction strategy. The discussion will focus on the following technical aspects:

- Posterior reduction techniques of scoliosis with instrumentation to the sacrum,
- S1 pedicle screw placement and additional iliac instrumentation with regard to risk of distal implant loosening,
- The need of a combined anterior and posterior fusion in pelvic instrumentation and the risk of pseudarthrosis,
- Planning of sagittal lumbosacral alignment according to pelvic incidence.

56.2 Case Description

A 69-year old female was referred to our outpatient clinic for a lumbar degenerative scoliosis. She was followed by a physical therapist over the last 10 years and she had been treated in a rehabilitation center twice within the last 4 years. A brace was initially indicated because of her spinal deformity and for pain relief in standing position. Her current oral pain medication comprised of paracetamol 4 g per day and tramadol 200 mg per day. Depending on her physical activities,

Y. P. Charles (✉)
Service de Chirurgie du Rachis, Hôpitaux Universitaires de Strasbourg, Strasbourg, France
e-mail: yann.philippe.charles@chru-strasbourg.fr

B. Meyer, M. Rauschmann (eds.), *Spine Surgery*, https://doi.org/10.1007/978-3-319-98875-7_56

the patient reported low back pain with a VAS score rated around 7/10. She also described a fatigue when standing with subjective anterior imbalance. Furthermore her walking distance had decreased over the last year and was estimated around 200 m. An angiologist had ruled out the hypothesis of a vascular claudication. Furthermore the past medical history revealed a mild hypertension that was treated and her cardiologist recently checked her ventricular function by echocardiography.

The clinical examination of her back and posture showed an imbalanced trunk with a left thoracolumbar rib hump of 2 cm. In the coronal plane a minor limb length discrepancy of 1 cm was measured with a slight pelvic tilt to the left. In the sagittal plane, a global anterior imbalance was partially compensated by retroversion of the pelvis and a flexion of the knees. Furthermore, the lumbar spine appeared stiff with Schober index of 10 + 1 cm. The neurologic exam revealed left leg pain and paresthesia along the L5 dermatome. There was no other peripheral sensory deficit and the motor function was intact. Her patellar reflex and Achilles tendon reflex were both symmetrically diminished. An EMG confirmed a moderate bilateral L5 root denervation.

Posterior-anterior and lateral full spine radiographs (Fig. 56.1) allowed a complete measurement of the spinal deformity. In the coronal plane, the Cobb angle was 70° between T12 and L4 with an apex at L1-L2. In the sagittal plane, a global anterior imbalance was measured by a sagittal vertical axis (SVA) of C7 at 15 cm. There was a segmental kyphosis at L1-L2 of 28°. The thoracic kyphosis T4-T12 was 65° and the lumbar lordosis L2-S1 was 55°. Spinopelvic parameters were: pelvic incidence 56°, sacral slope 23° and pelvic tilt 34°, which indicated the compensation for anterior imbalance by pelvic retroversion. Side bending films were further performed to assess curve flexibility (Fig. 56.2). The Cobb angle decreased from 70° to 48°, indicating a relatively stiff curve.

A CT scan was performed in order to analyze axial pedicle orientation and spontaneous bony fusion areas. An MRI of the entire spine ruled out spinal cord abnormalities and showed a central and lateral recess stenosis at L4-L5 (Fig. 56.3). Furthermore, a DEXA was carried out to assess bone mineral density. In the presence of spondylosis, the average lumbar T-score was −0.6, whereas the femoral neck T-score was −2.1, indicating osteopenia.

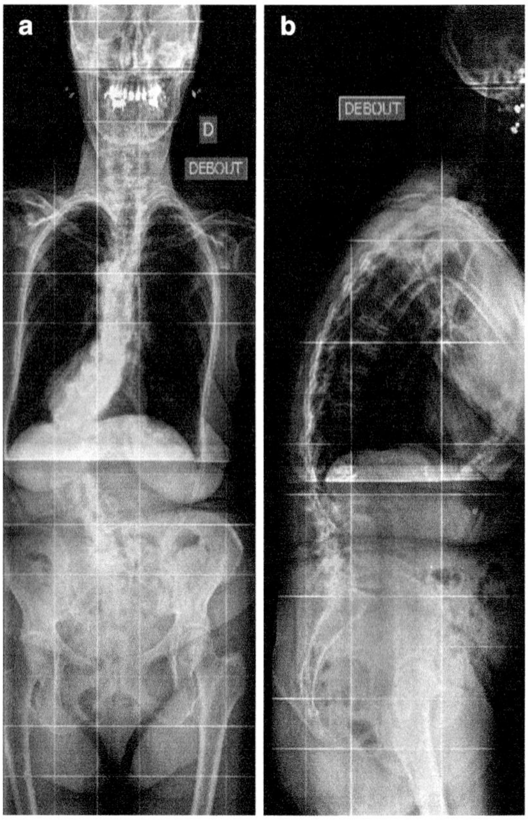

Fig. 56.1 Posterior-anterior (**a**) and lateral (**b**) full spine radiographs

After discussion with the patient, surgical treatment of her deformity and spinal stenosis was indicated under neuromonitoring control (SSEP and MEP). A posterior release was performed first from T7-T8 to L5-S1 in order to render the deformity flexible for further correction. This release was completed by Ponte osteotomies at L1-L2, L2-L3 and L3-L4 for segmental kyphosis correction. Pedicle screws were placed from T6 to S1 using a free hand technique. On the left side curve convexity, monoaxial screws were placed at L1, L2 and L3

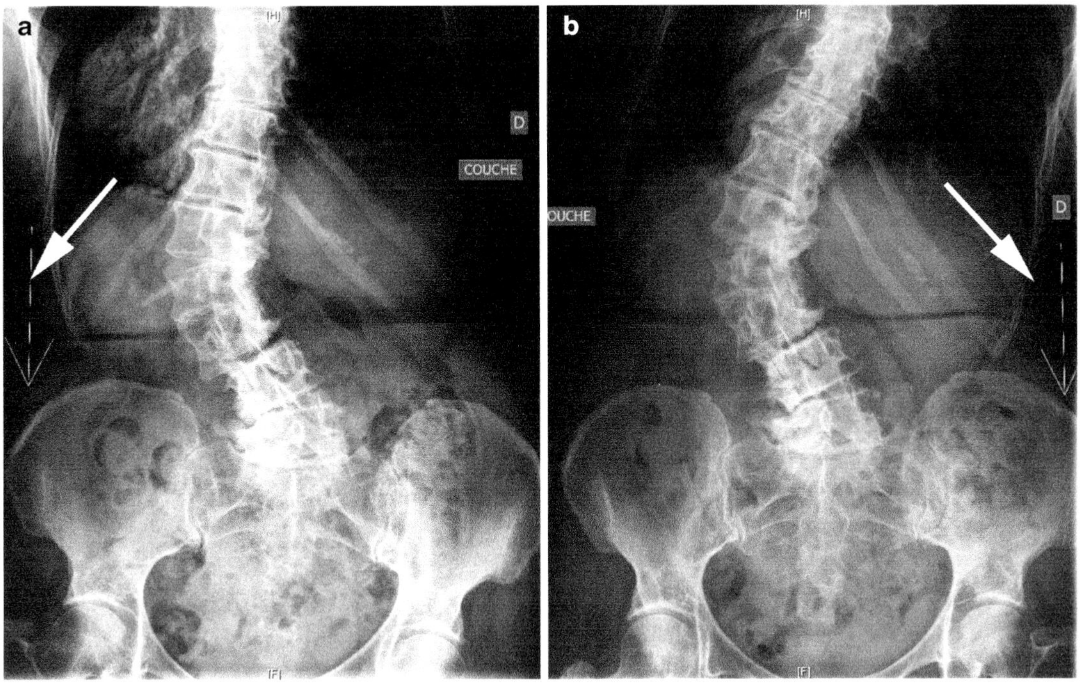

Fig. 56.2 Left (**a**) and right (**b**) side bending radiographs

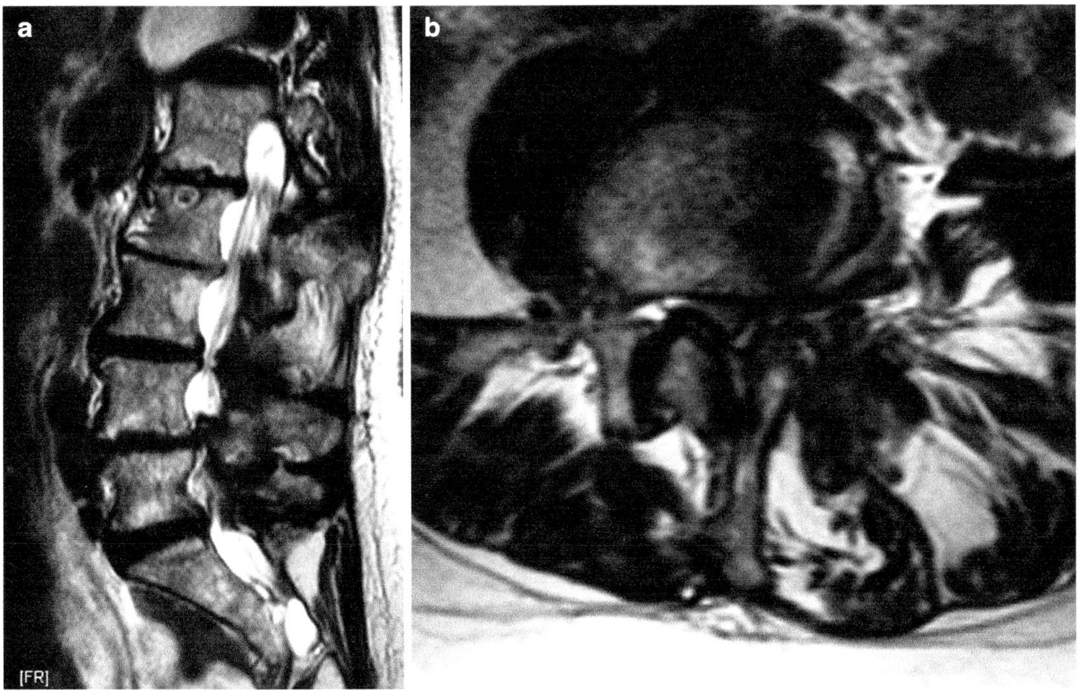

Fig. 56.3 MRI with sagittal (**a**) and axial (**b**) views showing a multiple level intervertebral disc degeneration and stenosis at L4-L5

for further derotation maneuvers of the scoliosis apex. Both posterior iliac crests were then exposed and a 2 cm superficial layer bone resection enabled bone graft harvesting in addition to spinous processes and released facets. Furthermore, this area was used as an entry point for iliac screw placement. Deformity correction was then achieved over a cobalt-chromium rod placed on the left side using several reduction techniques. The thoracic kyphosis and lumbar lordosis were pre-bent and the rod was inserted using multiple level persuaders. Derotation was then performed on monoaxial screw using specific levers, while in situ bending completed coronal curve and segmental L1-L2 kyphosis correction. The corrected spine was then locked in its final position and the contralateral right rod was inserted. The L4-L5 stenosis was then decompressed by a laminectomy, which allowed a TLIF fusion at L4-L5 and L5-S1. This intersomatic fusion was performed because of the remaining disc heights in order to prevent pseudarthrosis. The lumbar spine was additionally instrumented using 4 rods. At the levels L1-L2 and L3-L4, the discs opened up after Ponte osteotomies. The anterior intersomatic gap was fused 3 weeks after the first surgery using a minimal invasive left lateral approach and cage. The postoperative radiographic measurements were: Cobb angle 23°, SVA 0 cm, thoracic kyphosis 50°, lumbar lordosis 64°, pelvic incidence 58°, sacral slope 33° and pelvic tilt 18° (Fig. 56.4).

The patient followed a postoperative rehabilitation program in a specialized center during 4 weeks. Her pain and walking distance have improved after surgery and her QoL has progressively increased over the first postoperative year. An annual follow-up has been recommended, as mechanical alterations of the instrumented spine might occur at later stages. A CT at one-year follow-up evidenced fusion at each lumbar level. Sacral and iliac screw positioning is further demonstrated (Figs. 56.5, 56.6, and 56.7).

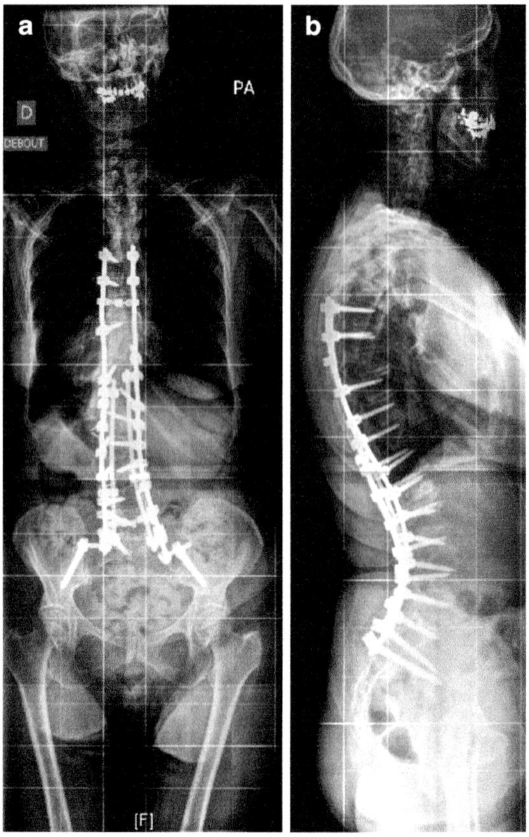

Fig. 56.4 Postoperative posterior-anterior (**a**) and lateral (**b**) full spine radiographs showing the correction of the lumbar scoliosis and sagittal imbalance

56.3 Discussion of the Case

56.3.1 Correction Strategy

A variety of instrumentations exist, aimed to obtain a balanced spine in the coronal, axial and sagittal plane. Modern approaches using segmental pedicle screw fixation act by direct vertebral derotation, rod translation and approximation with persuader systems. In situ bending uses a rod that follows the shape of the scoliotic spine, which is then bent to correct the 3D deformity sequentially [6]. Monoaxial screws are placed on most rotated vertebra on the side of the curve convexity, which is assed

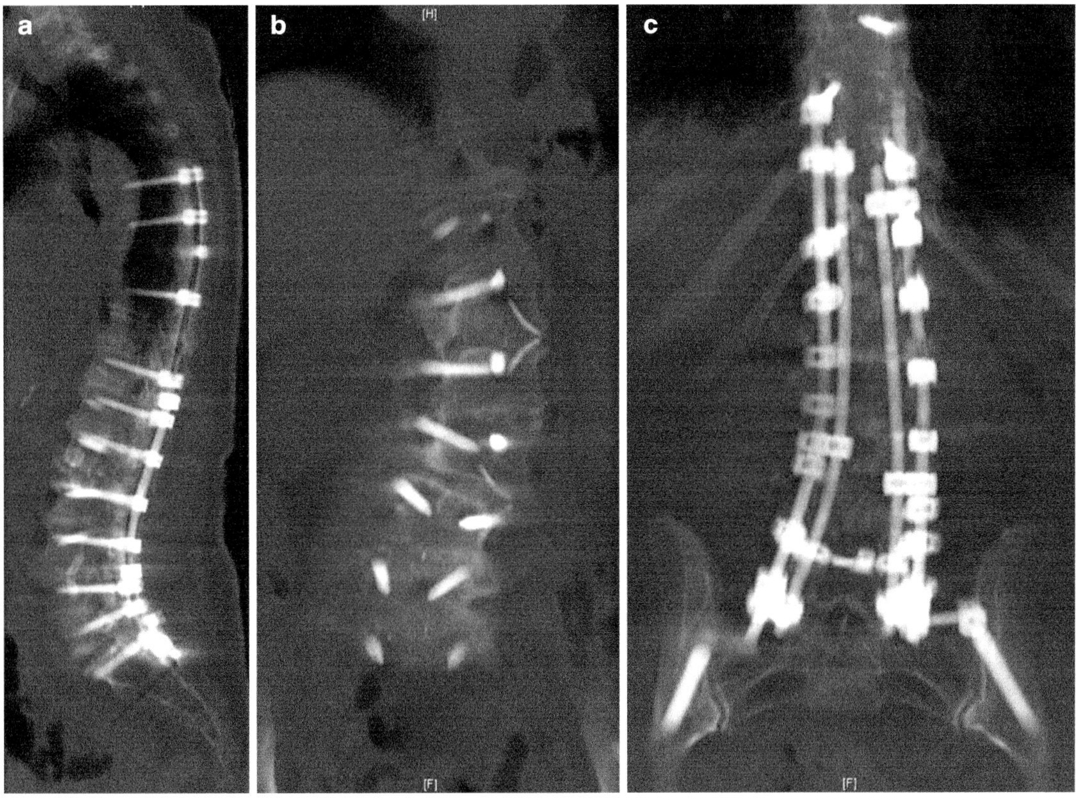

Fig. 56.5 Sagittal (**a**), anterior (**b**) and posterior (**c**) coronal CT reconstructions showing fusion and the principle of a 4-rod construct with sacral and pelvic fixation

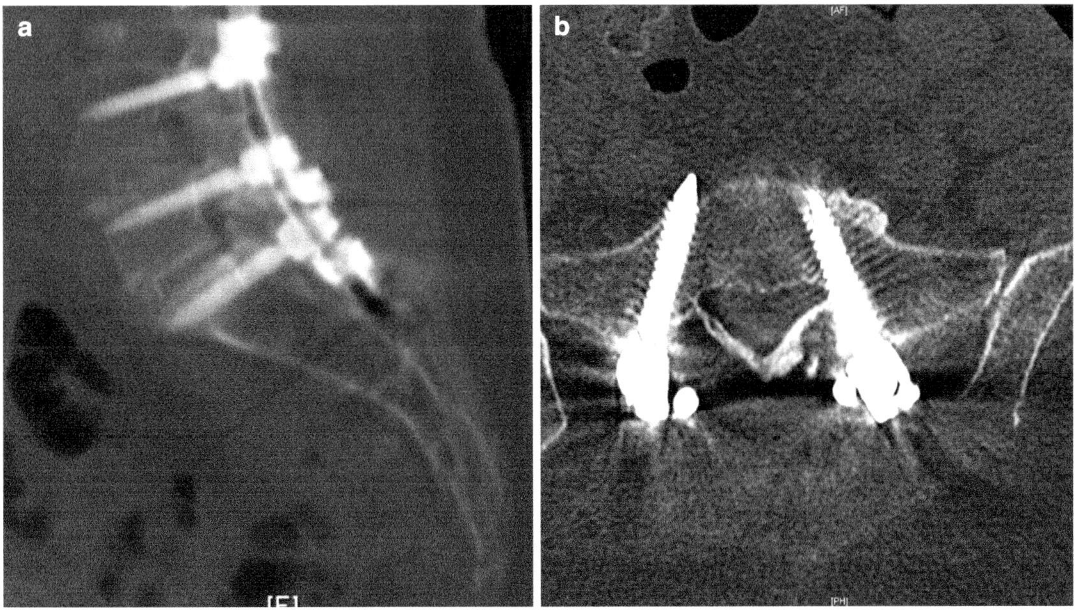

Fig. 56.6 Sagittal (**a**) and axial (**b**) orientation of S1 screws with bicortical bone purchase at the promontorium

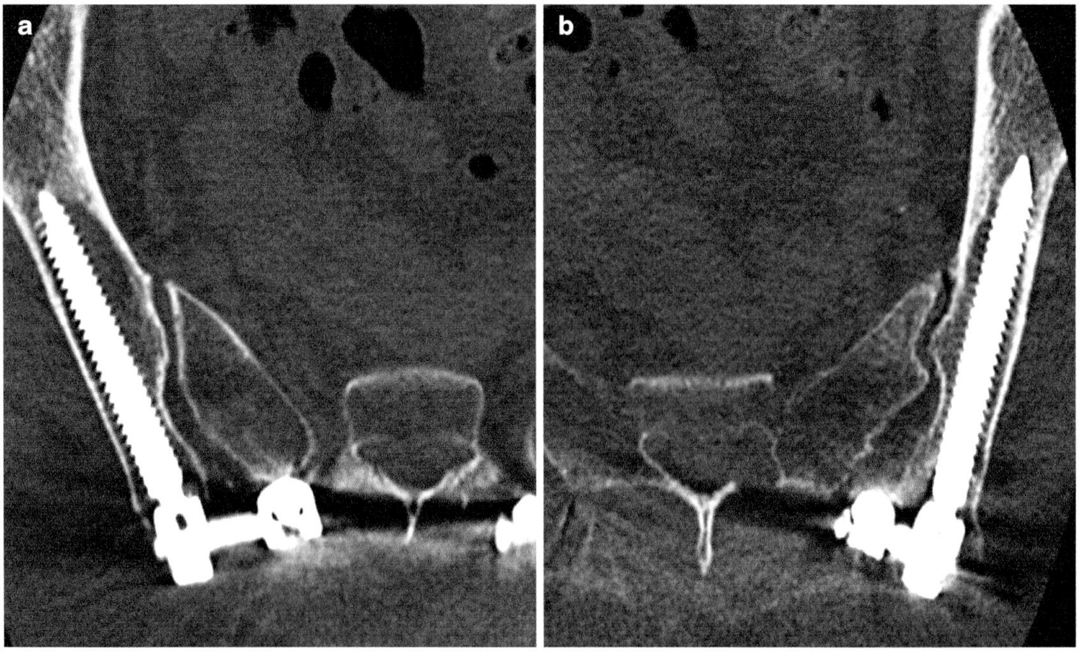

Fig. 56.7 Right (**a**) and left (**b**) iliac screws on axial CT reconstructions

on a preoperative CT or stereoradiography (EOS). This technique will allow derotating the lumbar apex using levers during sequential coronal and sagittal correction maneuvers.

Furthermore, preoperative planning requires an evaluation of residual curve flexibility on side bending radiographs. The CT analysis will further help when evaluationg interbody fusion areas by osteophytes. This aspect is crucial to achieve an adequate sagittal balance. In non-fused segments, segmental lordosis and the amount of curve correction can be enhanced by Ponte osteotomies as shown in the present case. Severe rigid deformities would either require an anterior release first, followed by posterior instrumentation, or an asymmetric PSO with a single posterior approach [3].

56.3.2 Sacral and Pelvic Instrumentation

The surgical treatment of degenerative scoliosis usually requires sacral fixation since L5-S1 disc degeneration and facet joint osteoarthritis is present in most patients. Distal screw loosening represents one major concern in long posterior instruentation [4, 5]. Setting bicortical S1 screws into the promontorium following a convergent axis enhanced the screw purchase (Fig. 56.6). The additional use of a sacropelvic fixation reduces the risk of S1 screw loosening and might be recommended [7]. In vitro biomechanical tests have demonstrated that ilium screws have the highest potential to protect the S1-anchorage [8]. Although iliac instrumentation enhances the distal fixation, risk factors leading to iliac screw failure have been reported: osteoporosis, instrumentation to the proximal thoracic spine and insufficient correction of lumbar lordosis [9]. S2-alar screws represent an alternative to ilium screws. The entry point of S2-alar screws is caudal to the posterior S1 foramen and their trajectory crosses the sacroiliac joint [10]. On long-term follow-up, a rigid pelvic fixation leads to fatigue of the lumbar instrumentation under cyclic loading (daily activities, walking, recurrent anterior imbalance) which increases the risk of pseudarthrosis and rod fractures [11].

56.3.3 Anterior Column Support

It appears that posterolateral fusion might not be sufficient when instrumenting the thoracolumbar spine including the sacrum and pelvis. Therefore, an anterior column support and fusion might be recommended to avoid pseudarthrosis and subsequent revision surgery. The lumbosacral junction might be fused by anterior approach (ALIF), which has the advantage of large cage surface and resistance under axial compression. In the present case, a posterior TLIF fusion was performed because of the concomitant L4-L5 stenosis that required decompression. In this setting, a large TLIF cage is placed anteriorly and the remaining intersomatic space posterior to the cage is filled with autologous bone graft to promote fusion.

Furthermore, the segmental kyphosis correction by posterior Ponte osteotomies will induce an anterior opening of mobile discs. It is mandatory to stabilize these segments by anterior grafting in order to prevent for loss of correction and pseudarthrosis. In the present case, mini-open left sided lumbotomy allowed the discectomy and lateral prepsoatic cage implantation at the osteotomy levels L1-L2 and L3-L4.

56.3.4 Sagittal Alignment Planning

It is crucial to take the patient specific sagittal alignment type into account when planning a posterior deformity correction. Roussouly has classified sagittal spinopelvic alignment types into 4 categories depending on the amount of pelvic incidence [12]. Type 1 has a small pelvic incidence and sacral slope; the lumbar lordosis has a short caudal arch with an apex at L5. Type 2 has a small pelvic incidence and sacral slope too, but the lordosis apex is higher at the basis of L4. Type 3 has an intermediate pelvic incidence and sacral slope; lumbar lordosis is more prominent with an apex at the center of L4. Type 4 has a high pelvic incidence and sacral slope with a large lordosis and an apex at the basis of L3. Failure of restoring the lumbar lordosis apex according to pelvic incidence was found highly predictive for proximal junctional kyphosis [13]. In practice, the theoretical apex of lumbar lordosis should not be higher than L4 if the pelvic incidence is $<55°$. Only patients with a pelvic incidence $>55°$ should be planned with an apex at the L3-L4 disc or L3. In a similar fashion, the global alignment proportion (GAP) score takes into account lordosis distribution, relative lumbar lordosis and global tilt according to pelvic incidence, relative pelvic version and age. In patients where sagittal alignment was not restored according to these proportioned indices, the mechanical failure rate increased significantly [14]. In the present case, the sagittal imbalance was corrected by apical derotation and Ponte osteotomies in the cranial lumbar spine and lordosis increase in the upper arch. Thus a balanced alignment was achieved according to Roussouly type 3 with a sagittal apex at L4.

56.4 Conclusions and Take Home Message

Degenerative scoliosis correction requires an adequate planning of deformity correction in all 3 planes. The restoration of sagittal alignment should be proportioned according to pelvic incidence, global alignment and the patient's age. Pelvic instrumentation enhanced the distal fixation of instrumentation and avoids sacral screw loosening. It should be kept in mind that the risk of pseudarthrosis and fatigue rod fractures increases with pelvic instrumentation. A circumferential fusion of the lumbosacral spine might therefore be recommended.

Pearls

- Sagittal alignment correction requires an analysis of pelvic incidence and theoretical lordosis distribution, including the patient's age, global alignment and compensation mechanisms of anterior imbalance.
- Sacral and iliac instrumentation provides a solid distal construct and should be considered in lumbar degenerative scoliosis.
- An anterior and posterior fusion might be recommended in iliac instrumentation to avoid pseudarthrosis and long-term mechanical complications.

References

1. Smith JS, Klineberg E, Schwab F, Shaffrey CI, Moal B, Ames CP, Hostin R, Fu KM, Burton D, Akbarnia B, Gupta M, Hart R, Bess S, Lafage V, International Spine Study Group. Change in classification grade by the SRS-Schwab adult spinal deformity classification predicts impact on health-related quality of life measures. Spine (Phila Pa 1976). 2013;38(19):1663–71.
2. Schwab F, Blondel B, Bess S, Hostin R, Shaffrey CI, Smith JS, Boachie-Adjei O, Burton DC, Akbarnia BA, Mundis GM, Ames CP, Kebaish K, Hart RA, Farcy JP, Lafage V, International Spine Study Group. Radiographical spinopelvic parameters and disability in the setting of adult spinal deformity. A prospective multicenter analysis. Spine (Phila Pa 1976). 2013;38(13):E803–12.
3. Enercan M, Ozturk C, Kahraman S, Sarier M, Hamzaoglu A, Alanay A. Osteotomies/spinal column resections in adult deformity. Eur Spine J. 2013;22(Suppl 2):S254–64.
4. Kelly MP, Lenke LG, Bridwell KH, Agarwal R, Godzik J, Koester L. Fate of the adult revision spinal deformity patient: a single institution experience. Spine (Phila Pa 1976). 2013;38(19):E1196–200.
5. Zhu F, Bao H, Liu Z, Bentley M, Zhu Z, Ding Y, Qiu Y. Unanticipated revision surgery in adult spinal deformity: an experience with 815 cases at one institution. Spine (Phila Pa 1976). (2014);39(26 Spec No):B36–44.
6. Steib JP, Dumas R, Mitton D, Skalli W. Surgical correction of scoliosis by in situ contouring: a detorsion analysis. Spine. 2004;29(2):193–9.
7. Finger T, Bayerl S, Onken J, Czabanka M, Woitzik J, Vajkoczy P. Sacropelvic fixation versus fusion to the sacrum for spondylodesis in multilevel degenerative spine disease. Eur Spine J. 2014;23(5):1013–20.
8. Volkheimer D, Reichel H, Wilke HJ, Lattig F. Is pelvic fixation the only option to provide additional stability to the sacral anchorage in long lumbar instrumentation? A comparative biomechanical study of new techniques. Clin Biomech (Bristol, Avon). 2017;43:34–9.
9. Banno T, Hasegawa T, Yamato Y, Kobayashi S, Togawa D, Oe S, Mihara Y, Matsuyama Y. The prevalence and risk factors of iliac screw loosening after adult spinal deformity surgery. Spine (Phila Pa 1976). 2017;42(17):E1024–30.
10. Koller H, Zenner J, Hempfing A, Ferraris L, Meier O. Reinforcement of lumbosacral instrumentation using S1-pedicle screws combined with S2-alar screws. Oper Orthop Traumatol. 2013;25(3):294–314.
11. Charles YP, Khelifi A, Schaeffer SJP. Pseudarthrosis in scoliosis instrumented to the sacrum and the pelvis. Eur Spine J. 2017;26(11):3015.
12. Roussouly P, Gollogly S, Berthonnaud E, Dimnet J. Classification of the normal variation in the sagittal alignment of the human lumbar spine and pelvis in the standing position. Spine (Phila Pa 1976). 2005;30(3):346–53.
13. Sebaaly A, Riouallon G, Obeid I, Grobost P, Rizkallah M, Laouissat F, Charles YP, Roussouly P. Proximal junctional kyphosis in adult scoliosis: comparison of four radiological predictor models. Eur Spine J. 2018;27(3):613–21.
14. Yilgor C, Sogunmez N, Boissiere L, Yavuz Y, Obeid I, Kleinstück F, FJS P-G, Acaroglu E, Haddad S, Mannion AF, Pellise F, Alanay A, European Spine Study Group (ESSG). Global alignment and proportion (GAP) score: development and validation of a new method of analyzing spinopelvic alignment to predict mechanical complications after adult spinal deformity surgery. J Bone Joint Surg Am. 2017;99(19):1661–72.

57 Degenerative Lumbar Scoliosis

Sebastian Hartmann, Anja Tschugg, and Claudius Thomé

57.1 Introduction

Treatment strategies for degenerative lumbar scoliosis (DLS) range from simple decompression of neural structures or decompression with limited fusion to invasive curve correction manoeuvres with extended fusion procedures [14]. In general, the literature demonstrates that the surgical treatment of DLS patients seems to be superior to conservative care. Nevertheless, a high rate of complications based on some neurological and predominately mechanical failures has been reported [4, 13, 15].

The scoliotic curve progresses in the fifth decade of life with a life time prevalence between 8% and 13%. Thus, the prevalence of DLS increases with age and patients in the sixth decade of life are predominantly affected [3, 5, 7, 8, 16, 17]. Therefore, the comorbidities of DLS patients associated with increased age aggravate the surgical treatment with higher complication rates, especially in case of extensive correction manoeuvres.

Approximately two-thirds of the patients suffer from an isolated and segmental coronal deformity, so that in many cases decompression with accompanied instrumented fusion seems to be sufficient. In case of additional sagittal deformity, the selection of the "appropriate" treatment strategy remains difficult. The majority of DLS patients additionally demonstrate segmental kyphosis resulting in moderate or severe sagittal imbalance [5, 8, 16].

Consequently, a classification system of degenerative disc disease based on the distribution of the degenerated symptomatic segments with regard to distinct areas of the main coronal curve (apical and end area) and the balance status of the spine has been generated to guide the treatment of DLS patients [2]. The apical area of the degenerative scoliotic curve was defined as the apex of the main curve, a vertebra or a disc level and the end area is proposed as the non-apical area adjacent to the end vertebra of the main lumbar degenerative curve. Correspondingly, four types of degenerative disease in adults with lumbar or thoracolumbar deformity were generated.

This chapter will capture the essentials of degenerative lumbar scoliosis, the clinical presentation, indications and surgical approaches, but will focus on more complex lesions with sagittal imbalance. Additionally, the clinical outcome as well as the potential complications are discussed. Pitfalls are outlined at the end of this chapter.

The presented case will detail the following problems:

S. Hartmann (✉) · A. Tschugg · C. Thomé
Department of Neurosurgery, Medical University Innsbruck, Innsbruck, Austria
e-mail: sebastian.hartmann@i-med.ac.at

B. Meyer, M. Rauschmann (eds.), *Spine Surgery*, https://doi.org/10.1007/978-3-319-98875-7_57

- Degenerative adult scoliosis with additional sagittal imbalance
- preoperative planning
- choice of approach
- complications

57.2 Case Description

This 59 year-old woman presented with severe axial low back pain (American Society of Anesthesiologists score 1 (ASA), visual analog scale (VAS) of 8/10, Oswestry disability index (ODI) of 42), but without neurological deficits. The patient suffered from neurogenic claudication with a walking distance of less than 100 meters. Preoperative imaging based on long-standing lateral and anteroposterior x-rays (Fig. 57.1), magnetic resonance imaging (MRI) (Fig. 57.2) and a high-resolution computed tomography (CT) (Fig. 57.3) showed severe degenerative lumbar scoliosis with a Cobb angle of approximately 33° and an autofused kyphoscoliotic spine from L1-L4 with a mobile collapsed segment L4/L5 and additional autofusion at L5/S1. MRI confirmed relative spinal canal stenosis at L4/L5 (Fig. 57.2). The apex of the scoliotic curve was located at the segment L2/L3 with the end vertebra L1 and L4, respectively (Fig. 57.3).

Severe sagittal imbalance with a pelvic incidence (PI) of 47°, a lumbar lordosis of 18° (LL), a SVA of 105 mm, a pelvic tilt (PT) of 42°, a T1

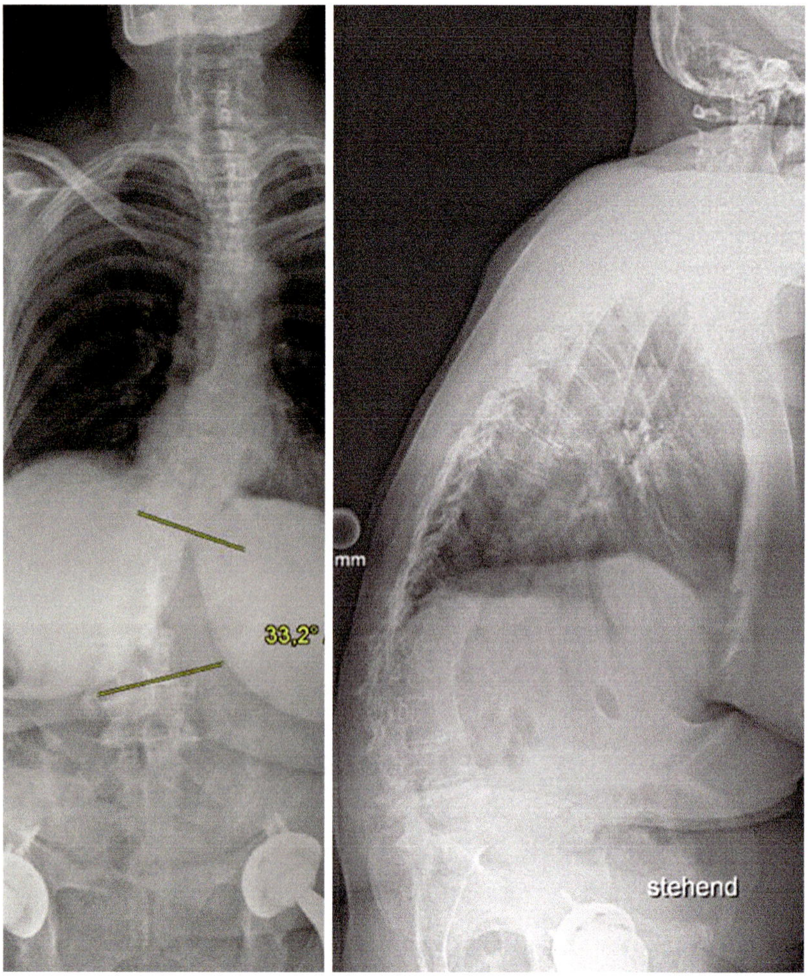

Fig. 57.1 Preoperative long-standing lateral and anteroposterior x-rays. Preoperative coronal and sagittal x-ray with a degenerative sagittal and coronal malalignment. Measurement of coronal Cobb angle revealed a degenerative lumbar scoliosis of 33°. Sagittal imbalance was defined as a decreased lumbar lordosis (LL) of 18°, a SVA of 105 mm, a pelvic tilt (PT) of 42°, a T1 pelvic angle (TPA) of 40° and a rigid lumbar kyphosis of 18°

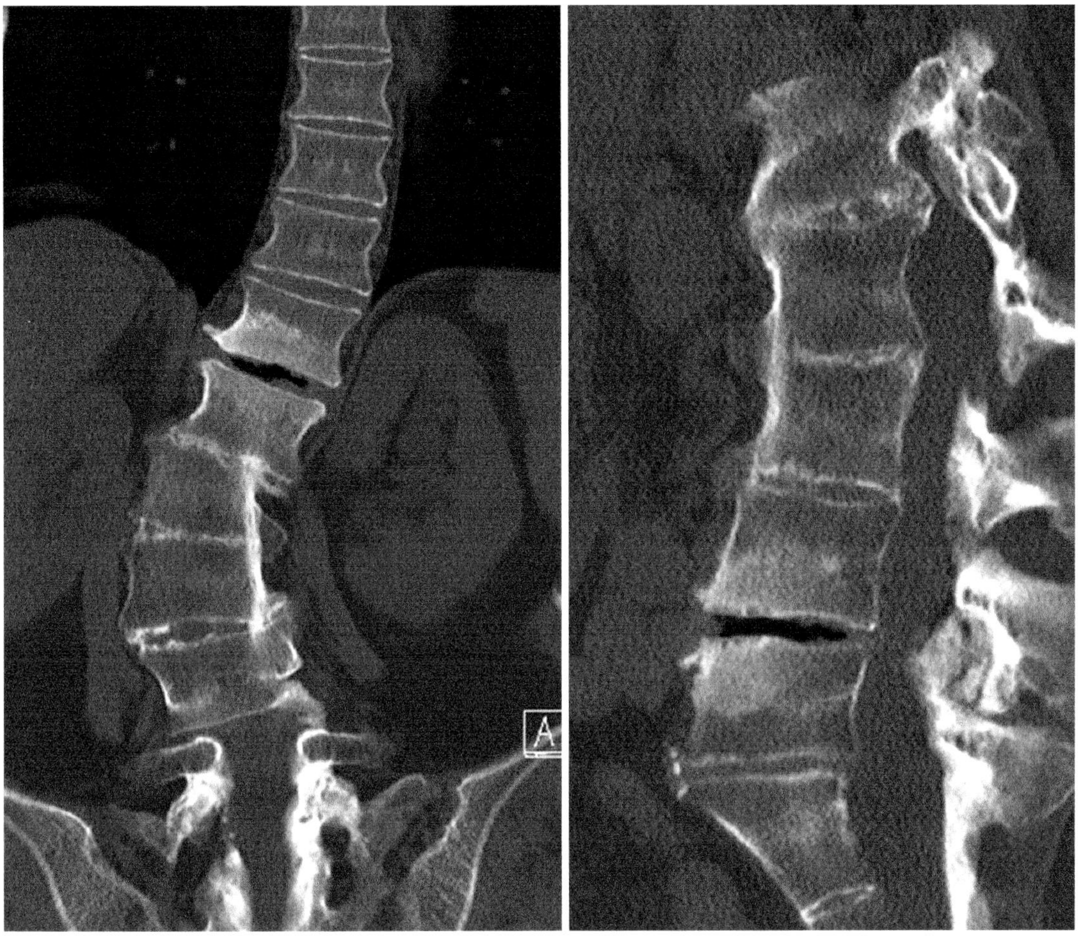

Fig. 57.2 Preoperative CT. Sagittal and coronal CT revealed a kyphoscoliotic fused malalignment at the levels L1-L4 and a severe degeneration of the segments Th12/L1 and L4/L5 with intervertebral vacuum phenomena. The apex of the scoliotic curve was located at the segment L2/L3 with the end vertebra L1 and L4, respectively

pelvic angle (TPA) of 40° and a rigid lumbar kyphosis of 18° was measured.

Surgery was performed with continuous intraoperative neuromonitoring via a dorsal approach to correct the coronal and sagittal deformity with a T12-S1 spondylodesis, asymmetric pedicle subtraction osteotomy plus (aPSOplus) of L3, a Smith Peterson osteotomy with TLIF cage implantation at L4/L5 according to the criteria of Schwab et al. [11]. The aPSOplus was chosen at the L3 vertebra with resection of the remaining L2/L3 disc to correct the apical area coronally and sagittally according to the classification system of Berjano and Lamartina (Type IVb, a severely coronally and sagittally imbalanced spine) [2].

Surgery was uneventful except for an accidental dural tear and the patient was discharged two weeks after surgery. No brace was applied. Postoperatively, the LL improved to 40°, PT to 19°, SVA to 60 mm, TPA to 22° and the coronal Cobb angle to 8°. At follow-up, VAS had improved from 8 to 3, ODI from 42 to 24 and the walking distance lengthened to 2000 m (Fig. 57.4).

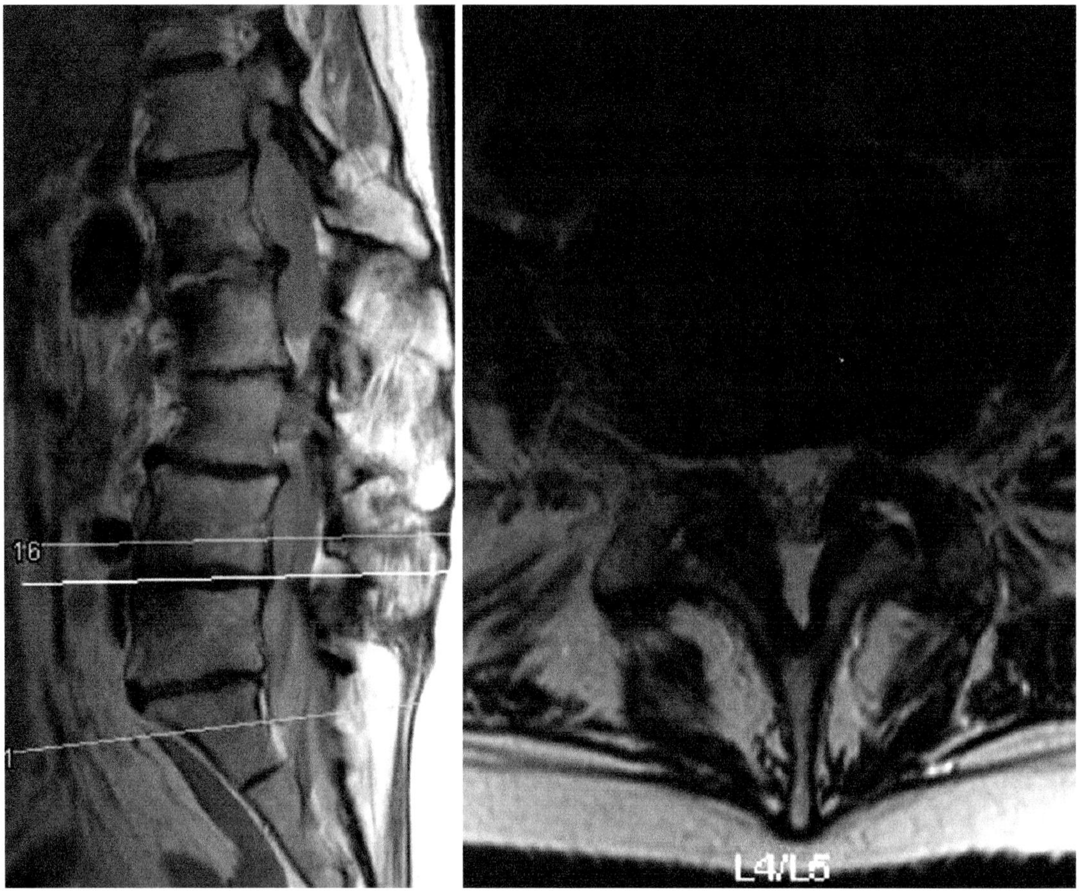

Fig. 57.3 Preoperative MRI. MRI confirmed a relative spinal canal stenosis at the level L4/L5 with effusion in the mobile joints. The clinical picture was dominated by low back pain and L5 radiculopathy in combination with spinal claudication

57.3 Discussion of the Case

Pain, disability and functional impairment represent the major symptoms prompting surgery in adult degenerative scoliosis. These complaints are a result of progressive (multi-)segmental degeneration leading to coronal and sagittal deformity with instability. In case of decreased lumbar lordosis and a compensatory reduction of thoracic kyphosis, a conventional decompression procedure may often not be appropriate. A classification system based on the distribution of the symptomatic segments and the spinal alignment was popularized by Berjano and Lamartina [2]. The apical area of the patients' degenerative scoliotic curve is described as the apex of the main curve, a vertebra or a disc level (in the presented case the vertebra L3). The end area is defined as the non-apical area adjacent to the end vertebrae of the main lumbar degenerative curve (in the case presented the vertebrae L1 and L4 cranially and caudally, respectively) [2]. Type I of that classification system represents a limited non-apical segment disease, so that the coronal deformity does not affect the symptomatic segment. In type II deformities, the symptomatic segment characterizes the limited apical segment. Type I and II might be treated by conventional decompression procedures with or without selective transpedicular instrumentation of the symptomatic segment [2]. Type III describes an extended segmental disease with apical and non-apical

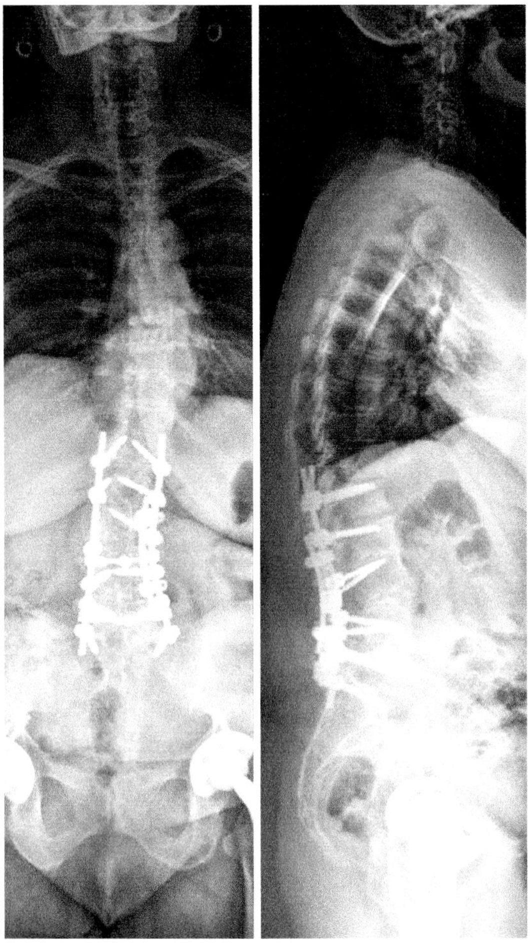

Fig. 57.4 Postoperative long-standing lateral and anteroposterior x-rays. Postoperative coronal and sagittal long-standing x-ray scans after an asymmetric pedicle subtraction osteotomy of L3 with resection of the adjacent disc (aPSOplus) and Smith-Peterson osteotomy (SPO) with TLIF L4/L5 and instrumented fusion of Th12-S1. Lumbar lordosis improved to 40°, PT to 19°, SVA to 60 mm, TPA to 22° and the coronal Cobb angle to 8°

symptomatic segments all along the coronal deformity. Instrumented fusion may be extended to include the main coronal deformity and in some cases the lumbosacral junction. Type IV is a sagittally imbalanced spine with (b) or without (a) coronal imbalance requiring an extended 3-dimensional correction procedure. According to that classification system, the case presented is defined as type IVb, a severe coronally and sagittally imbalanced spine with the apical area at the vertebra L3 and the non-apical symptomatic segments both caudally (L4/5; Fig. 57.3) and cranially (Th12/L1; Fig. 57.2) [2]. Even though the apex of the curve was located at the level L2/L3, no severe compression of neural structures was observed. Consequently, a normal decompression procedure to address the spinal canal stenosis at the symptomatic level L4/L5 would potentially have relieved the neurogenic claudication, but would most likely have led to further instability in the affected segments and thus an increment of axial symptoms. According to the literature, the major predictor of clinical outcome, complications and revision rates is sufficient improvement of sagittal malalignment, so that in the case presented an invasive operative procedure to restore the sagittal and coronal balance was chosen [9–11]. Spondylodesis was performed from Th12 to S1, so that the instrumented fusion encompasses the whole deformity including the end vertebras and not only a fusion from the sacrum to the apex of the curve [14].

As the functional outcome and the pain intensity demonstrated, the patient obviously did well after surgery despite of a reported complication rates in full curve fusions of approximately 50% [14] and in spite of a residual SVA of 60 mm. An accidental dural tear represents a common intraoperative complication, which was adequately addressed by a dural suture in the presented case and not associated with negative sequelae. In general, DLS interventions have a high rate of early complications, which mainly encompass wound healing defects, radicular deficits or paresis, and screw loosening. Many of these complications require revision surgery. Applying solely a transforaminal lumbar interbody fusion technique was particularly associated with increased early complications [12], hence two-year follow-up of the patient presented did not show any of these complications. Adjacent segment disease and proximal junctional kyphosis are late complications and occur in over 30% of the patients [12]. Additionally, anticoagulation or cardiac comorbidities were identified as possible predisposing risk factors in patients treated with fusion procedures [12]. Due to the high complication potential, the indication of surgery must be evaluated critically [6]. Nevertheless, functional outcome of surgery for DLS patients has been shown to be superior to conservative management [13], even in case of peri- or postoperative complications [1].

57.4 Accordance with the Literature Guidelines

Definitive guidelines to treat patients with DLS might be derived from the literature according to classification systems with proposed surgical strategies, but in the end, the management remains an individual patient to patient decision.

Level of evidence: B to C

The level of evidence available is poor to moderate and mostly represented by retrospective studies.

57.5 Conclusion and Take Home Message

The quality of life is significantly affected by DLS, so that this disease represents a common indication for instrumented spinal surgery. Invasive surgical options are often preferred over conservative care mostly based on the argument to ultimately prevent curve progressions. A wide variety of surgical options, ranging from simple decompressions to multisegmental instrumentations with 3D corrections are available. Due to the high prevalence of DLS in the elderly, complication and reoperation rates are high and indications should be carefully weighted. Which patient should be treated with which operative procedure is currently unclear and remains a subject of ongoing research. The mentioned classification system represents a valuable tool to choose the type of approach and the magnitude/length of the operation.

Pearls

- Acquire long-standing lateral and anteroposterior x-rays to evaluate the sagittal and the coronal alignment
- Identify of the affected segment(s)
- Consider simple decompression procedures resulting from an identified single symptomatic segment in predominantly claudicative symptoms without severe low back pain
- Consider instrumented fusion in case of severe low back pain and identification of the degenerated segments
- Consider long instrumented fusion and osteotomy procedures in case of sagittal malalignment
- The instrumentation should be done as long as necessary and as short as possible
- Anticipate high complication and reoperation rates especially in older patients
- Long-term outcome between conservative and surgically treated patients seem to favour surgery

References

1. Auerbach JD, Lenke LG, Bridwell KH, Sehn JK, Milby AH, Bumpass D, et al. Major complications and comparison between 3-column osteotomy techniques in 105 consecutive spinal deformity procedures. Spine (Phila Pa 1976). 2012;37(14):1198–210. https://doi.org/10.1097/BRS.0b013e31824fffde.
2. Berjano P, Lamartina C. Classification of degenerative segment disease in adults with deformity of the lumbar or thoracolumbar spine. Eur Spine J. 2014;23(9):1815–24. https://doi.org/10.1007/s00586-014-3219-9.
3. Carter OD, Haynes SG. Prevalence rates for scoliosis in US adults: results from the first national health and nutrition examination survey. Int J Epidemiol. 1987;16(4):537–44.
4. Charosky S, Guigui P, Blamoutier A, Roussouly P, Chopin D. Complications and risk factors of primary adult scoliosis surgery: a multicenter study of 306 patients. Spine (Phila Pa 1976). 2012;37(8):693–700. https://doi.org/10.1097/BRS.0b013e31822ff5c1.

5. Chin KR, Furey C, Bohlman HH. Risk of progression in de novo low-magnitude degenerative lumbar curves: natural history and literature review. Am J Orthop (Belle Mead NJ). 2009;38(8):404–9.
6. Faraj SSA, Haanstra TM, Martijn H, de Kleuver M, van Royen BJ. Functional outcome of non-surgical and surgical management for de novo degenerative lumbar scoliosis: a mean follow-up of 10 years. Scoliosis Spinal Disord. 2017;12:35. https://doi.org/10.1186/s13013-017-0143-x.
7. Kebaish KM, Neubauer PR, Voros GD, Khoshnevisan MA, Skolasky RL. Scoliosis in adults aged forty years and older: prevalence and relationship to age, race, and gender. Spine (Phila Pa 1976). 2011;36(9):731–6. https://doi.org/10.1097/BRS.0b013e3181e9f120.
8. Kobayashi T, Atsuta Y, Takemitsu M, Matsuno T, Takeda N. A prospective study of de novo scoliosis in a community based cohort. Spine (Phila Pa 1976). 2006;31(2):178–82.
9. Le Huec JC, Leijssen P, Duarte M, Aunoble S. Thoracolumbar imbalance analysis for osteotomy planification using a new method: FBI technique. Eur Spine J. 2011;20(Suppl 5):669–80. https://doi.org/10.1007/s00586-011-1935-y.
10. Rose PS, Bridwell KH, Lenke LG, Cronen GA, Mulconrey DS, Buchowski JM, et al. Role of pelvic incidence, thoracic kyphosis, and patient factors on sagittal plane correction following pedicle subtraction osteotomy. Spine (Phila Pa 1976). 2009;34(8):785–91. https://doi.org/10.1097/BRS.0b013e31819d0c86.
11. Schwab F, Patel A, Ungar B, Farcy JP, Lafage V. Adult spinal deformity-postoperative standing imbalance: how much can you tolerate? An overview of key parameters in assessing alignment and planning corrective surgery. Spine (Phila Pa 1976). 2010;35(25):2224–31. https://doi.org/10.1097/BRS.0b013e3181ee6bd4.
12. Simon MJK, Halm HFH, Quante M. Perioperative complications after surgical treatment in degenerative adult de novo scoliosis. BMC Musculoskelet Disord. 2018;19(1):10. https://doi.org/10.1186/s12891-017-1925-2.
13. Smith JS, Lafage V, Shaffrey CI, Schwab F, Lafage R, Hostin R, et al. Outcomes of operative and nonoperative treatment for adult spinal deformity: a prospective, multicenter, propensity-matched cohort assessment with minimum 2-year follow-up. Neurosurgery. 2016;78(6):851–61. https://doi.org/10.1227/NEU.0000000000001116.
14. Transfeldt EE, Topp R, Mehbod AA, Winter RB. Surgical outcomes of decompression, decompression with limited fusion, and decompression with full curve fusion for degenerative scoliosis with radiculopathy. Spine (Phila Pa 1976). 2010;35(20):1872–5. https://doi.org/10.1097/BRS.0b013e3181ce63a2.
15. Wang G, Hu J, Liu X, Cao Y. Surgical treatments for degenerative lumbar scoliosis: a meta analysis. Eur Spine J. 2015;24(8):1792–9. https://doi.org/10.1007/s00586-015-3942-x.
16. Watanuki A, Yamada H, Tsutsui S, En-Yo Y, Yoshida M, Yoshimura N. Radiographic features and risk of curve progression of de-novo degenerative lumbar scoliosis in the elderly: a 15-year follow-up study in a community-based cohort. J Orthop Sci. 2012;17(5):526–31. https://doi.org/10.1007/s00776-012-0253-5.
17. Xu L, Sun X, Huang S, Zhu Z, Qiao J, Zhu F, et al. Degenerative lumbar scoliosis in chinese han population: prevalence and relationship to age, gender, bone mineral density, and body mass index. Eur Spine J. 2013;22(6):1326–31. https://doi.org/10.1007/s00586-013-2678-8.

Long Versus Short Constructs

58

Sebastian Hartmann, Anja Tschugg, and Claudius Thomé

58.1 Introduction

Degenerative lumbar scoliosis (DLS) is associated with the focal development of coronal deformity due to degenerative changes in the mid portion of the lumbar spine. These degenerative changes are multifactorial and range from intervertebral disc degeneration and facet joint degeneration to changes in canal as well as pedicle morphology [11, 13]. The scoliotic curve typically progresses in the fifth decade of life with a life time prevalence of approximately 10% increasing with age. Especially older patients suffer from long curves with coronal deformity as well as abnormalities of sagittal spinopelvic parameters. Treatment strategies according to the approach (anterior, posterior, combined) as well as clear and formalized recommendations of short or long instrumentation techniques are lacking. Although single-level decompression procedures might be feasible in patients with predominantly claudicative symptoms, many patients develop multisegmental disease with long sagittally and coronally decompensated curves, so that simple decompression procedures may be expanded to "heavy metal" solutions. It is currently unclear, whether long fusion techniques with anterior, posterior or combined techniques are superior to short fusions. Due the associated complication rate, however, short fusion techniques might be favoured over long constructs, especially in older patients with comorbidities and an increased perioperative risk [8, 10]. Additionally, there is still an on-going discussion based on the distal fusion level for degenerative lumbar scoliosis. The question remains, whether the segment L5/S1 should be included in the construct or not, especially in the absence of disc degeneration at that level [3, 6]. This chapter will capture the treatment of degenerative lumbar scoliosis based on using short or long fusion constructs. Additionally, clinical outcome as well as potential complications associated with these two treatment strategies are discussed. Pitfalls are outlined at the end of the chapter.

This case will detail the following problems:

- Degenerative adult scoliosis
- Long fusion construct
- Treatment of the level L5/S1
- Complications

58.2 Case Description

This 49 year-old woman presented with severe axial low back pain and diffuse pain in the lower extremities but without neurological deficits. The

S. Hartmann (✉) · A. Tschugg · C. Thomé
Department of Neurosurgery, Medical University Innsbruck, Innsbruck, Austria
e-mail: sebastian.hartmann@i-med.ac.at

B. Meyer, M. Rauschmann (eds.), *Spine Surgery*, https://doi.org/10.1007/978-3-319-98875-7_58

patient has been suffering from these symptoms for several years without any substantial improvement in her discomfort by conservative therapy (including pain management and physiotherapy). In addition, she reported a significant deterioration in recent months. Preoperative long-standing lateral and anteroposterior x-rays revealed a degenerative lumbar scoliosis with the apex at the L3/L4 motion segment and rotatory subluxation. The upper and lower end vertebrae were defined as Th11 and L4, respectively (Fig. 58.1). The Cobb angle of this left convex curve was measured at approximately 30° (Fig. 58.1). Additionally, a compensatory curve was observed at the upper thoracic spine without any pain or discomfort at these levels. Magnetic resonance imaging (MRI) demonstrated a lateral and central spinal canal stenosis at the levels L4/L5 and L3/L4 (apex) (Fig. 58.2). The level L3/L4 revealed a collapsed neuroforamen on the right site as a result of the left convex degenerative curve with diffuse sensory abnormalities but not well-defined in the L3 dermatome. Furthermore, signs of severe on-going degeneration with disc collapse, rotatory subluxation and consecutive changes at the endplates were observed at this segment on computed tomography (CT) (Fig. 58.3).

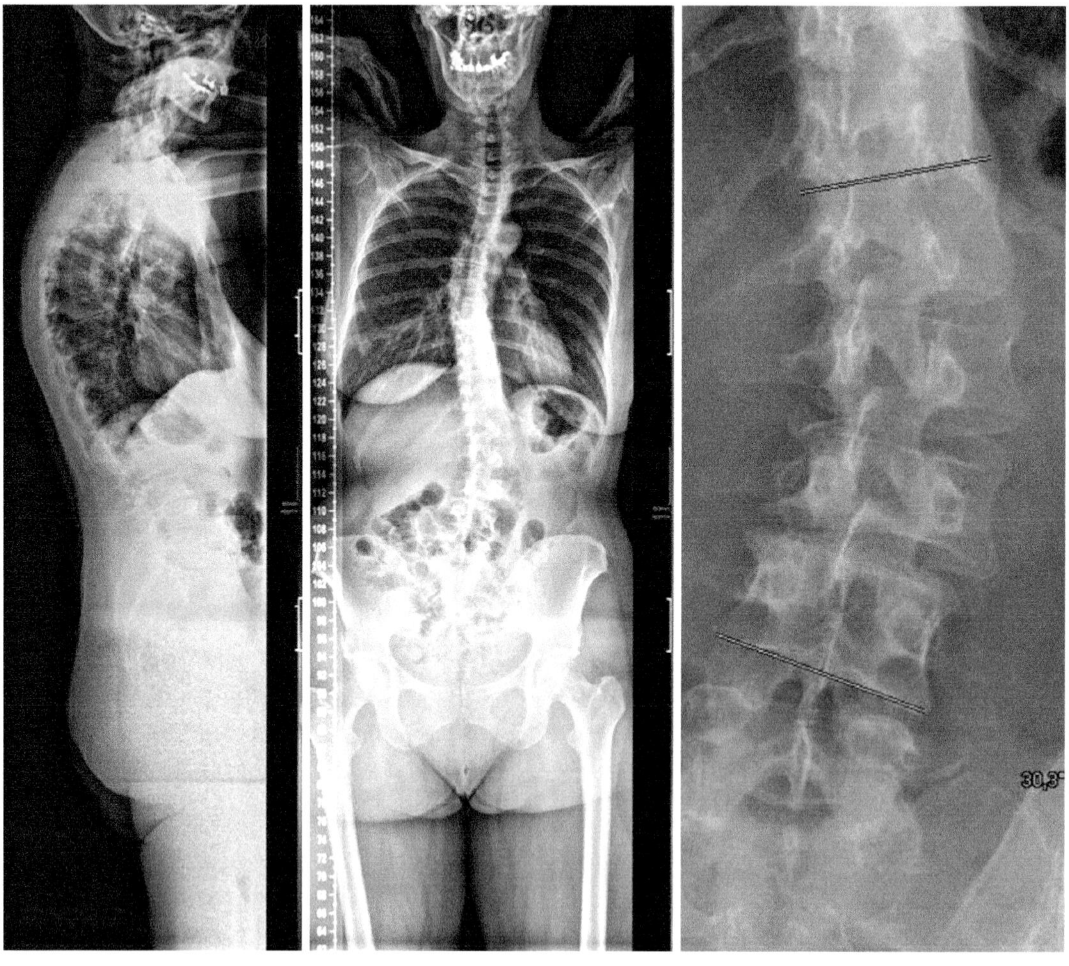

Fig. 58.1 Preoperative long-standing lateral and anteroposterior x-rays. Preoperative sagittal x-ray demonstrated no signs of severe sagittal dysbalance except a hyperkyphotic thoracic spine with a compensatory right-sided convex thoracic scoliosis. The coronal x-ray revealed a degenerative lumbar scoliosis (Cobb angle of approximately 30°) with the apex of the scoliosis at the L3/L4 motion segment and the upper and lower end vertebrae at Th11 and L4

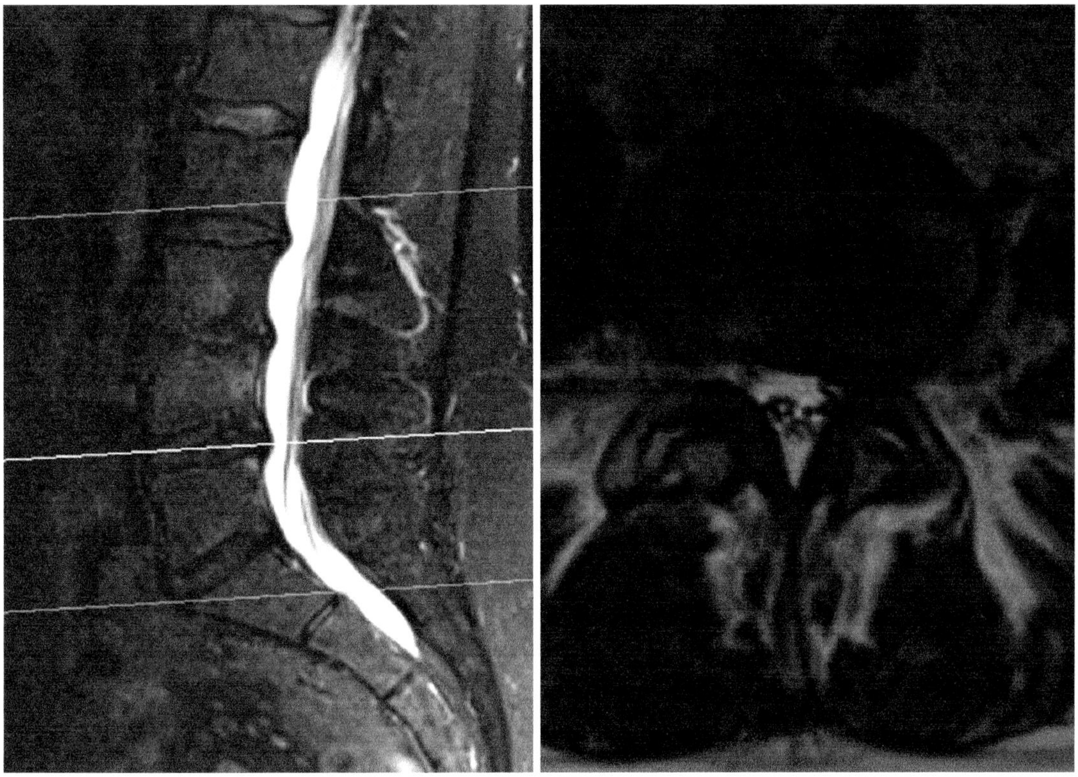

Fig. 58.2 Preoperative MRI. Sagittal and axial MRI at the level L4/L5 demonstrated a left-sided lateral recess stenosis. The apex of the lumbar scoliosis, the segment L3/L4, appeared to be collapsed and showed a relative central and lateral spinal canal stenosis

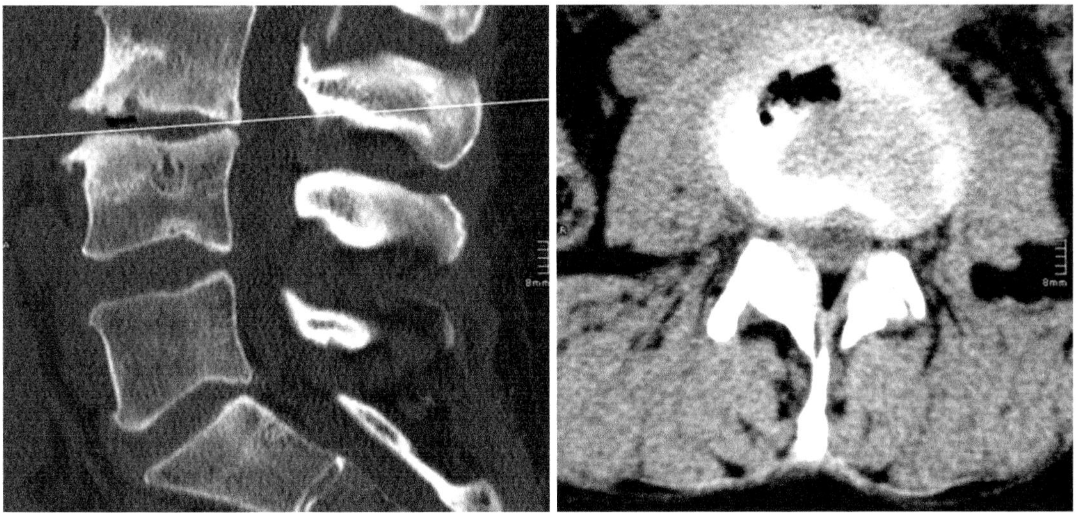

Fig. 58.3 Preoperative CT. Disc collapse and consecutive changes at the endplates of the motion segment L3/L4 with a consecutive spinal canal stenosis with rotatory subluxation were observed

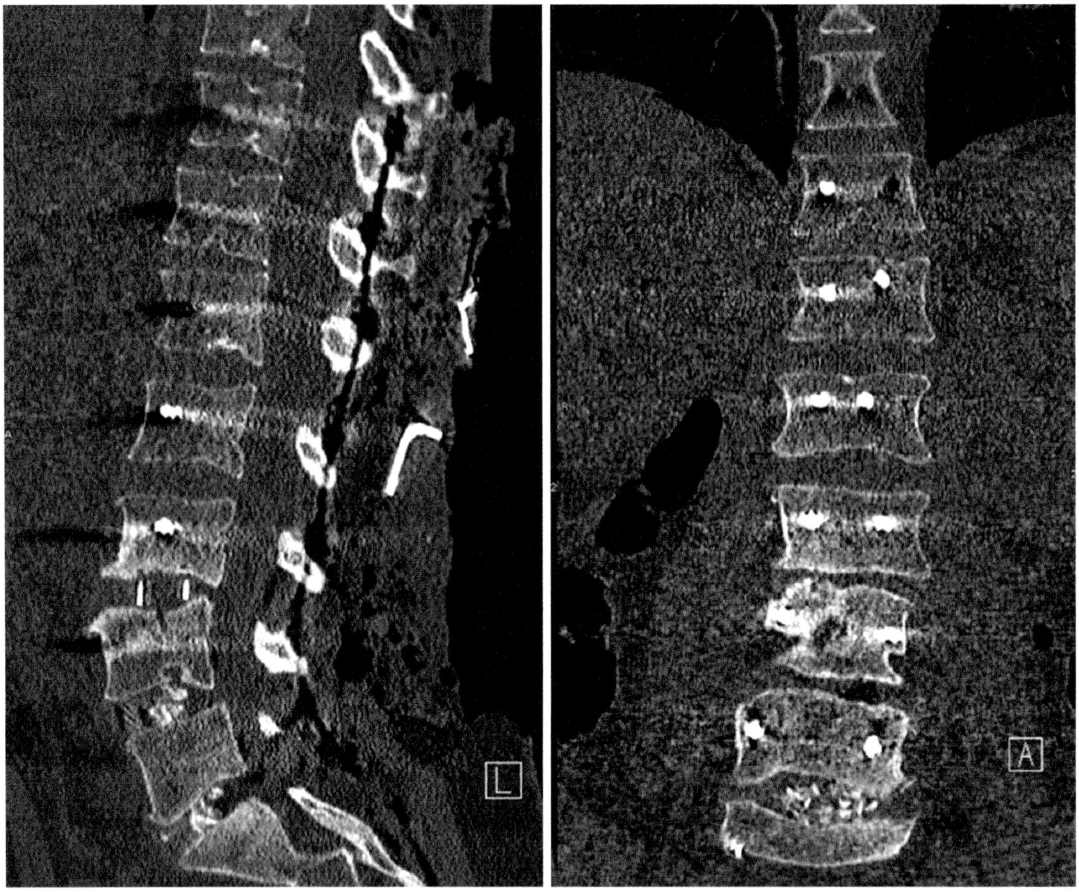

Fig. 58.4 Postoperative CT. The sagittal CT demonstrated adequate screw and cage placement at the levels L3/L4 (XLIF cage) and L4-S1 (TLIF cages). Compared to the preoperative x-rays, an appropriate correction of the coronal alignment was observed with a postoperative Cobb angle of approximately 5°

Surgery was performed in a 2-step fashion via an anterolateral approach followed by a dorsal pedicle screw instrumentation combined with transforaminal lumbar interbody fusions (TLIF) and Smith-Peterson osteotomies (SPO). First, we started with a right-sided extreme lateral interbody fusion (XLIF) at the segment L3/L4 with intraoperative neuromonitoring to protect the lumbar plexus within the psoas muscle. In the same anesthesia, we repositioned the patient in a prone position and performed a dorsal pedicle screw instrumentation from T11 to S1 with a TLIF cage implantation at the segments L4/L5 and L5/S1 and additional SPOs combined with a derotation procedure with specialized screws was performed. Additional decompression was carried out at the segment L3/L4 and at the segments with TLIF cage implantation (L4/5 and L5/S1).

Surgery was uneventful and postoperative CT revealed sufficient decompression and appropriate screw and cage placement (Fig. 58.4).

In the postoperative course, no external immobilization was necessary and the patient was sent to inpatient physiotherapy on the first day postoperatively. The patient was discharged after 9 days. Routine clinical and radiological follow-up after 3 and 12 months postoperatively showed no signs of implant-related complications, adjacent segment diseases or proximal junctional kyphosis (Fig. 58.5). A sufficient coronal realignment was observed, except for a hyperkyphotic upper thoracic spine. Nevertheless, the patient described residual low back pain without lower extremity

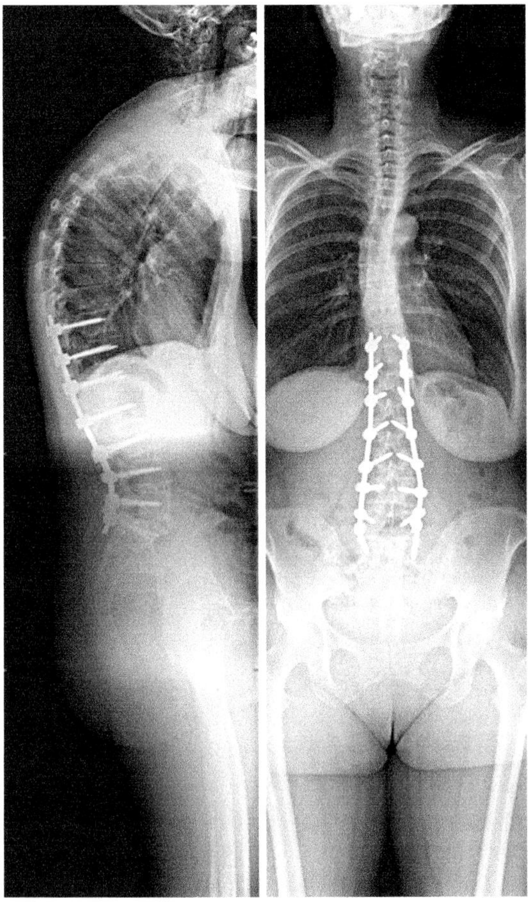

Fig. 58.5 Postoperative long-standing lateral and anteroposterior x-rays. No severe sagittal malalignment and a satisfactory coronal alignment with a remaining Cobb angle of approximately 5° were observed after 12 months. No signs of implant-related complications were noted. Compared to the preoperative lateral x-ray, a postoperative hyperkyphotic alignment of the upper thoracic spine without signs of proximal junctional kyphosis were noted

symptoms. She reported a walking distance without claudicative symptoms of more than 4000 metres, so that she was satisfied with her outcome.

58.3 Discussion of the Case

The treatment of DLS patients remains challenging and a bundle of common complications are described. The literature provides evidence that longer constructs are associated with an increased potential of complications, especially in high-risk and elderly patients [6, 10]. These complications range from neurological deterioration, infections, wound problems to the basket of implant-related complications. In contrast, short fusions may be associated with a progression of deformity and thus a worsening outcome over time. Overall, surgery appears to be effective despite the high rate of complications and revision procedures [14]. Degenerative scoliotic spinal deformities demonstrate a mean annual curvature progression in the coronal plain below 4°. The progression does not translate linearly, so that the prognosis cannot be reliably estimated. Due to the fact, that these deformities are developing spontaneously and are still progressing over time, the choice of proximal and distal fusion levels is still debated.

Short fusion approaches are often defined as instrumented fusions within the coronal deformity. In most cases the end vertebra is not included in the instrumentation. In contrast, long fusions are often characterized as procedures including the proximal and the distal end vertebrae or extending beyond them. Additionally, the question rises whether to stop distally at L5 or to extent the fusion to the sacrum (or even the ilium). Increased non-fusion rates may be associated with a higher patient age, postoperative infections, patients treated with PSO and fusions to the sacrum. In a comparative series of patients treated for adult deformities, Edwards et al. reported a pseudarthrosis rate at the level L5/S1 of over 40% in case of inclusion of the sacrum. Contrastingly, the group observed major complications in approximately 22% for fusions to the vertebral body L5 with including the sacropelvic region [7]. Charosky et al. observed a reoperation risk of 48% at 4 years for fusions to the sacrum in patients with adult degenerative scoliosis. In general, the prevalence of mechanical complications was reported at 24% and 58 patients of them needed revision surgery (19%) [5]. Accordingly, significant risk factors for mechanical or neurological complications were identified: number instrumented vertebrae, fusion to the sacrum, patients treated with PSO and an increased preoperative pelvic tilt [5].

Published classification systems aim to summarize the etiological aspects, describe the severity or deal with the cause of the deformity. However, no definitive planning based on the individual patient is possible and above all, the length of the instrumentation is difficult to estimate. Based on the distribution of the symptomatic segments and the spinal alignment, a classification system has been evaluated by Berjano and Lamartina [2]. According to these authors, the presented case is defined as type III, segmental degeneration affecting both the apical and the end area of the curve, whereas the presented spine is still balanced. In our case, the patient showed a rotatory subluxation and the apex at the segment L3/L4 with additional non-apical degeneration at L4/L5 with relative spinal canal stenosis. In preoperative planning, we were confronted with the question of the distal extent of the fusion, namely the L5 vertebra or the sacrum. With an intended long instrumentation (to T11), the subsequent degeneration of L5/S1 when stopping at L5 represents a frequent problem and may impact the whole sagittal alignment of the spine, so that the construct was extended to the sacrum [3]. In case of progressive degeneration of the L5/S1 segment after stopping a long fusion at L5, circumferential approaches are often necessary as a revision surgery to prevent pseudarthrosis which might increase the complication rate. One might argue, that fixation to L5 is feasible in short constructs, but in case of long constructs, the short and cancellous L5 pedicles might not offer sufficient fixation points for these long lever arms, especially as the lower end of the instrumentation. As a rule of thumb, a long fusion stopping at L5 may lead to screw loosening in L5 affecting the whole sagittal spinal balance and may lead to subsequent degeneration at L5/S1. Additionally, some authors describe, that a "deep-seated" L5 (pedicles of the L5 vertebra below the intercrestal line) might protect the L5/S1 segment, whereas in this special case, we were faced with a "non-deep seated" L5 vertebra [3]. The authors usually extend the instrumentation to the sacrum, if the thoracic spine is reached cranially. In these cases, an intervertebral fusion is always performed at L5/S1 and the threshold is low to strengthen the lower fixation by iliac screws, particularly in reduced bone quality. S1 screw purchase was sufficient in this case, so that no iliac fixation was performed, which is only done in a minority of patients.

Apical XLIF procedures combined with dorsal pedicle screw instrumentation represent an adequate correction technique in DLS patients. In these procedures, a bilateral annulus release with the implantation of a large cage provides a potent correction manoeuvre of coronally collapsed disc spaces [1, 12]. A pseudarthrosis rate of approximately 10% has been reported with the use of the XLIF technique and common complications are represented by lateral incisional hernias or wound infections, rupture of the anterior longitudinal ligament with cage dislocation or cage back-out in case of subtotal contralateral annulotomy [4]. Additionally, XLIF procedures tend to have higher rates of neurological deterioration due to the close relationship to the lumbar plexus. Nevertheless, XLIF procedures represent a less invasive technique to correct coronal deformities and wound complications were observed less frequently than in TLIF procedures. In combination with a spinal canal stenosis, however, an additional dorsal procedure to decompress neural structures associated with instrumented fusion may be required.

The fusion in this case was extended to the lower thoracic spine (T11) in an attempt to prevent proximal junctional kyphosis (PJK). There still is an ongoing debate whether stopping at L1 is feasible or stopping at T12 or T11 may be appropriate. Some authors argue that the instrumentation has to be extended to T10, since the stabilizing effect of the rib cage is not present below, while others recommend to go as high as the upper thoracic spine. Competence of thoracolumbar paravertebral muscles also seems to play a role.

Although the upper instrumented vertebra (UIV) at the thoracolumbar junction (TLJ) is more common to develop PJK, we did not observe sagittal malalignment at the adjacent vertebrae T9 or T10 one year after surgery [15]. Our patient was rather young without osteoporosis and a normal sagittal vertical axis, which all represent risk factors for PJK [9]. The detected postoperative hyperkyphotic alignment at the upper thoracic spine was most likely caused by the derotation procedure of the lumbar spine. In the postoperative radiographs we could thus observe a slight delordotic alignment of approximately minus 13° compared to the preoperative x-ray (Figs. 58.1 and 58.5). Consequently, the patient responded to the iatrogenic delordosation (approximately 13°) with a compensatory thoracic hyperkyphosis that matched her spinopelvic parameters postoperatively. The sagittal vertical axis postoperatively was thus within the normal range.

Although long fusions are nowadays commonly applied particularly in osteoporotic (and thus elderly) patients, it has to be kept in mind that they show more pulmonary complications ($p < 0.05$), increased blood loss and longer operative times ($p > 0.05$) plus an extended hospital stay ($p > 0.05$) [8, 10]. Patients with long fusions tend to experience an increased rate of early complications (< 3 months), whereas late complications tend to be similar in both groups [6]. The functional outcome according to the Oswestry Disability Index (ODI) was reported to be similar between long and short fusion procedures [6, 8]. Finally, the correction of the coronal Cobb angle and the lumbar lordosis tend to be equally between long and short fusion, so that a better coronal alignment correction should not be used as an argument for a more invasive procedure in DLS patients [10]. In the personal experience of the authors adjacent decompensation after fusion like PJK are most common in older (and osteoporotic) patients, so that we aim for optimal correction of sagittal dysbalance in all patients and tend to prefer long constructs in the older population and shorter constructs in younger individuals.

58.4 Accordance with the Literature Guidelines

Definitive guidelines of whether to perform short or long fusions in patients with DLS are not available. The management strategies remain an individual patient to patient decision according to comorbidities and patient characteristics.

Level of evidence: B to C
The level of evidence available is moderate

58.5 Conclusion and Take Home Message

Long fusion procedures in patients with DLS tend to exhibit a higher rate of complications compared to short fusions. The latter may provoke curve progressions, whereas this progression might be similar to that of the surgically untreated curve in patients with balanced DLS. As a general advice, short fusions should be used instead of longer fusion procedures to reduce the perioperative morbidity and complications. In patients with rotatory subluxations associated with a severe sagittal imbalanced spine, spinal osteotomy procedures may be considered a valuable alternative with acceptable clinical and radiological outcomes. In case of sagittally unbalanced DLS patients, the new classification system of Berjano and Lamartina et al. helps to plan these procedures.

Pearls

- Blood loss, general costs, operative time and length of hospital stay tend to be higher in long fusion procedures
- Perioperative outcome tends to be superior in short fusion procedures
- Short fusions should be preferred to long fusions, if biomechanically feasible
- Coronal correction after short versus long fusions are comparable
- Consider longer constructs in (elderly) patients with osteoporosis, especially when stopping at the TLJ
- XLIF approaches represent a valuable alternative to dorsal procedures with less complication rates to correct coronal deformities

References

1. Berjano P, Lamartina C. Far lateral approaches (XLIF) in adult scoliosis. Eur Spine J. 2013;22(Suppl 2):S242–53. https://doi.org/10.1007/s00586-012-2426-5.
2. Berjano P, Lamartina C. Classification of degenerative segment disease in adults with deformity of the lumbar or thoracolumbar spine. Eur Spine J. 2014;23(9):1815–24. https://doi.org/10.1007/s00586-014-3219-9.
3. Bridwell KH, Edwards CC, Lenke LG. The pros and cons to saving the L5–s1 motion segment in a long scoliosis fusion construct. Spine (Phila Pa 1976). 2003;28(20S):S234–42. https://doi.org/10.1097/01.BRS.0000092462.45111.27.
4. Caputo AM, Michael KW, Chapman TM, Jennings JM, Hubbard EW, Isaacs RE, et al. Extreme lateral interbody fusion for the treatment of adult degenerative scoliosis. J Clin Neurosci. 2013;20(11):1558–63. https://doi.org/10.1016/j.jocn.2012.12.024.
5. Charosky S, Guigui P, Blamoutier A, Roussouly P, Chopin D. Complications and risk factors of primary adult scoliosis surgery: a multicenter study of 306 patients. Spine (Phila Pa 1976). 2012;37(8):693–700. https://doi.org/10.1097/BRS.0b013e31822ff5c1.
6. Cho KJ, Suk SI, Park SR, Kim JH, Kim SS, Lee TJ, et al. Short fusion versus long fusion for degenerative lumbar scoliosis. Eur Spine J. 2008;17(5):650–6. https://doi.org/10.1007/s00586-008-0615-z.
7. Edwards CC, Bridwell KH, Patel A, Rinella AS, Berra A, Lenke LG. Long adult deformity fusions to L5 and the sacrum. A matched cohort analysis. Spine (Phila Pa 1976). 2004;29(18):1996–2005.
8. Lee C-H, Chung CK, Sohn MJ, Kim CH. Short limited fusion versus long fusion with deformity correction for spinal stenosis with balanced de novo degenerative lumbar scoliosis. Spine (Phila Pa 1976). 2017;42(19):E1126–32. https://doi.org/10.1097/BRS.0000000000002306.
9. Park SJ, Lee CS, Chung SS, Lee JY, Kang SS, Park SH. Different risk factors of proximal junctional kyphosis and proximal junctional failure following long instrumented fusion to the sacrum for adult spinal deformity: survivorship analysis of 160 patients. Neurosurgery. 2017;80(2):279–86. https://doi.org/10.1227/NEU.0000000000001240.
10. Phan K, Xu J, Maharaj MM, Li J, Kim JS, Di Capua J, et al. Outcomes of short fusion versus long fusion for adult degenerative scoliosis: a systematic review and meta-analysis. Orthop Surg. 2017;9(4):342–9. https://doi.org/10.1111/os.12357.
11. Pritchett JW, Bortel DT. Degenerative symptomatic lumbar scoliosis. Spine (Phila Pa 1976). 1993;18(6):700–3.
12. Tormenti MJ, Maserati MB, Bonfield CM, Okonkwo DO, Kanter AS. Complications and radiographic correction in adult scoliosis following combined transpsoas extreme lateral interbody fusion and posterior pedicle screw instrumentation. Neurosurg Focus. 2010;28(3):E7. https://doi.org/10.3171/2010.1.FOCUS09263.
13. Tribus CB. Degenerative lumbar scoliosis: evaluation and management. J Am Acad Orthop Surg. 2003;11(3):174–83.
14. Wang G, Hu J, Liu X, Cao Y. Surgical treatments for degenerative lumbar scoliosis: a meta analysis. Eur Spine J. 2015;24(8):1792–9. https://doi.org/10.1007/s00586-015-3942-x.
15. Wang H, Ma L, Yang D, Wang T, Yang S, Wang Y, et al. Incidence and risk factors for the progression of proximal junctional kyphosis in degenerative lumbar scoliosis following long instrumented posterior spinal fusion. Medicine (Baltimore). 2016;95(32):e4443. https://doi.org/10.1097/MD.0000000000004443.

In Situ Fusion Versus Realignment 59

Lars Wessels and Peter Vajkoczy

59.1 Introduction

Lumbar spondylolisthesis is a very common condition in the population above 50, which often results in spinal stenosis accompanied by lower back pain and neurogenic claudication. If degenerative spondylolisthesis with spinal stenosis is symptomatic surgical treatment is associated with more favorable outcome than non-surgical treatment and should be the treatment of choice [11].

In symptomatic low grade spondylolisthesis (<50%), the treatment of choice is decompression alone or decompression with fusion and realignment depending on the symptoms and on the degree of instability [1, 3].

In contrast to low grade spondylolisthesis, the treatment of high grade spondylolisthesis (>50%) is still controversial.

The two competing concepts are in situ fusion or realignment. In situ fusion encompasses postolateral fusion with decompression of the neuronal elements without correction or anterior support. In contrast, realignment aims at instrumented correction of the spinal deformity and (in-)direct decompression of the neural elements. Therefore, a posterior release is necessary with decompression of the neuronal element and postolateral fusion prior to correction of the slip. Additionally, an anterior support may be added depending on the surgical technique applied.

There is low evidence regarding superiority of one approach over the other. In high grade spondylolisthesis, both, in situ fusion and realignment, are associated with a relatively high risk for development of neurological deficit with a tendency towards an increased risk of realignment [7, 8]. Given, that in situ fusion is also less technically demanding and strenuous, its use is repeatedly propagated, especially in the case of an favorable sagittal profile.

High grade spondylolisthesis may be associated with changes in the spinopelvine parameters and, thus, may impair sagittal balance. Based on the literature, however, the anterior segmental slip in high-grade spondylolisthesis is often compensated by the global lumbar lordosis and is not necessarily leading to sagittal imbalance [8, 10]. For those cases with a maintained sagittal balance In situ fusion may be indicated. However, arguments raised against in situ fusion are: the observation that these patients carry an increased risk for developing a loss of correction with concomitant sagittal imbalance, further degeneration of adjacent segments perpetuating the loss of a harmonic lumbar profile, and a higher risk of hardware failure [7, 8].

This chapter will outline the specifics of repositioning in patients with high grade

L. Wessels (✉) · P. Vajkoczy
Department of Neurosurgery,
Charitè – Universitätsmedizin Berlin,
Berlin, Germany
e-mail: Lars.Wessels@charite.de

B. Meyer, M. Rauschmann (eds.), *Spine Surgery*, https://doi.org/10.1007/978-3-319-98875-7_59

spondylolisthesis with a special view upon the indication and preoperative considerations. At the end of the chapter the reader should be aware of the difficulties regarding the indication of realignment especially in high grade spondylolisthesis.

The aim of the presented case is therefor to outline the individual challenge in decision making in these rare cases. The key points are:

- When to operate – especially in high grade spondylolisthesis
- How to operate – Realignment vs. in situ fixation.

59.2 Case Description

A 36 year-old female patient had a car accident and suffered a posttraumatic spinal instability at L4/L5 which was treated with dorsal instrumentation 15 years ago. 6 years after the surgery, the hardware was explanted. One pedicle screw was broken and left in situ in the vertebral body L5. In the following years, the young woman developed progressive lower back pain and in the last year before presentation to our department, she experienced neurogenic claudication as well as radicular pain at L4 bilaterally. The CT and MRI scans revealed a pseudarthrosis L4/L5 with spondylolisthesis grade 3 according the Meyerding classification (Fig. 59.1). The long-standing x-ray showed no signs for sagittal imbalance (Pelvic incidence (PI) 57°, Pelvic Tilt (PT) 17°, Sacral slope (SS) 29° lumbar lordosis 48°) (Fig. 59.2).

We performed posterior instrumentation with L4/L5 pedicle screws and rods. Further, we performed neurolysis of the L4 nerve root and dorsal decompression of the neural structures via a laminectomy, as well as facetectomy for posterior release. For re-alignment, osteotomies in L4 and to a lesser extent L5 where made to achieve a realignment of the L4 and L5 vertebral bodies. The postoperative X-ray, CT (Fig. 59.3) showed good repositioning and correct placement of the screws along with sufficient decompression of the spinal canal.

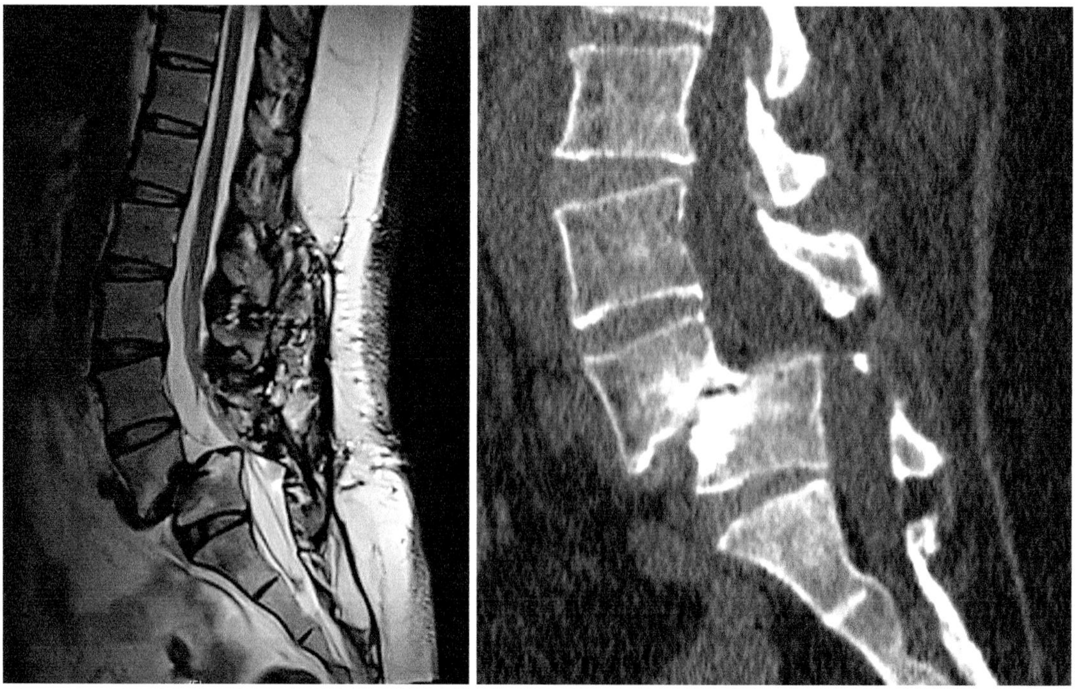

Fig. 59.1 preoperative CT and MRI scans. MRI and CT scan of the lumbar spine revealed a grade 3 spondylolisthesis L4/5 with consecutive spinal stenosis

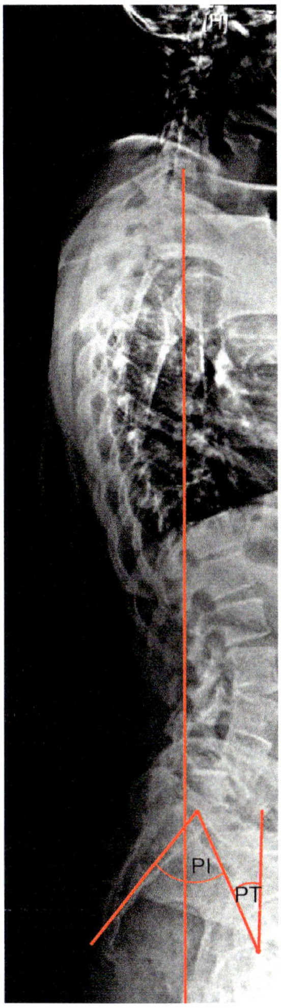

Fig. 59.2 Preoperative long-standing x-ray. The preoperative long-standing x-ray shows no signs for sagittal imbalance

Two weeks after surgery the patient was discharged home without neurological deterioration. Follow up after 3 month the patient has improved significantly regarding her pain.

59.3 Discussion of the Case

The patient suffered from radicular pain at L4 due to neuroforaminal stenosis on both sides, accompanied by symptomatic spinal canal stenosis at the level of the spondylolisthesis. In this young patient, with strong immobilizing pain, causing a huge reduction of her quality of life the indication to perform a decompression of the spinal canal and the nerve roots at this level, accompanied by dorsal instrumentation was evident. The main question is whether it was necessary to perform reduction or if in situ fusion without realignment would have been sufficient.

For high grade spondylolisthesis, only few larger series exist, indicating that realignment is feasible but associated with a higher risk for neurological deficits (increase of risk by 4–40% compared to in situ fusion) [2, 5, 9]. This wide range of reported complications for realignment strategies is the main argument against in situ fusion, although a meta-analysis fails to show a significant difference in neurological deficits between in situ fusion and realignment [7].

The degree of spondylolisthesis is associated with the prevalence of spinal sagittal imbalance. The PI has a positive correlation with the degree of the spondylolisthesis classified according to the Meyerding classification (I-II 68.5°; >III 79°) and exceeds the PI of control individuals (69°) [4, 10].

Our patient showed balanced spinopelvic parameters with a physiological SVA and PT, and no signs for spinal sagittal imbalance [6]. In this case, in situ fusion would have been a possible option with potentially lower perioperative risks for the patient and a less challenging surgical procedure by omitting the osteotomies. Nevertheless, we elected to perform realignment for the following reasons: (i) the non-union after the fracture/instrumentation, (ii) the risk for developing imbalance with aging, and (iii) further loss of a harmonic lumbar profile due to degeneration of adjacent levels (the inclination point for the sagittal profile type). The osteotomies primarily aimed at a sufficient correction of the spondylolisthesis and realignment of L4/L5 (similar to a dome resection), but also gave us the chance to re-establish segmental lordosis with a less-extensive osteotomy than a classical PSO.

To the best of our knowledge there is no data available upon a possible long-term benefit of realignment regarding a prevention for development of sagittal imbalance in patients with high grade spondylolisthesis without existing spinal sagittal imbalance.

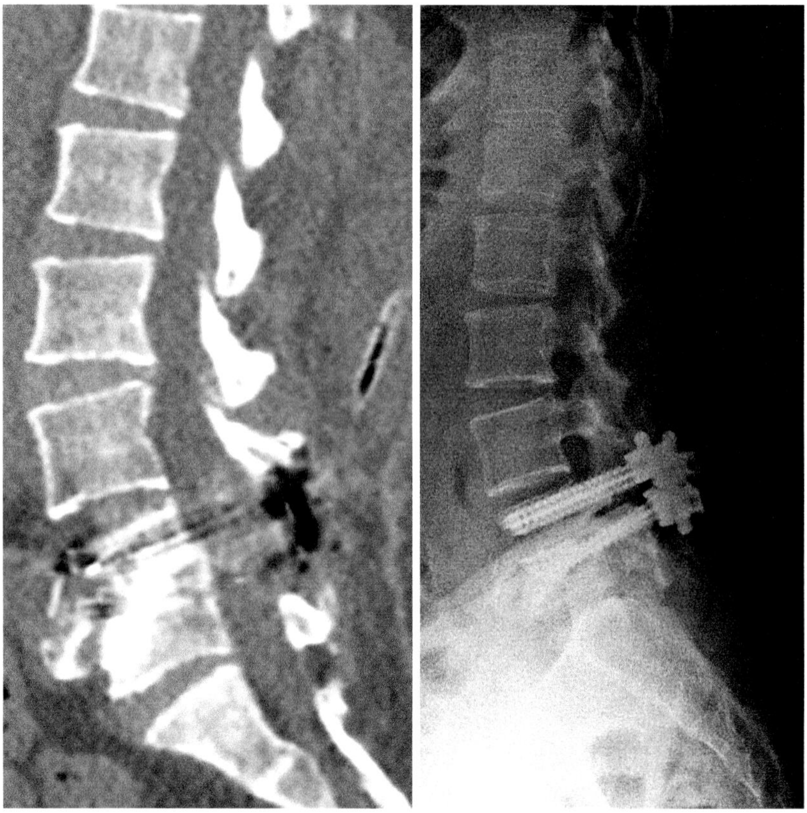

Fig. 59.3 Postoperative X-ray, CT and MRI. Postoperative X-ray and CT showing good postoperative result with sufficient decompression and correct placement of the screws as well as good repositioning

Accordance with the literature guidelines
As discussed above there is clear evidence for decompression and Fusion in patients with spondylolisthesis.
Level of evidence: A
If realignment provides a benefit in view of the long-term outcome and the sagittal balance needs further investigation.
Level of evidence: C

59.4 Conclusions and Take-Home Message

High grade spondylolisthesis remains a clinical challenge. Although realignment seems to carry a higher risk for development of neurological deficits, it should be performed in presence of spinal sagittal imbalance. If the sagittal balance is maintained it may be discussed whether realignment is necessary and whether in situ fusion should be preferred. Especially in young patient realignment should be the goal in order to avoid mid- to longterm complications.

Pearls
- In high grade spondylolisthesis Fixation is necessary.
- Realignment is a feasible procedure with a comparable complication rate as in situ fusion.
- Before decision making the spinal sagittal balance should be observed carefully.
- In patients with spondylolisthesis and compensated sagittal imbalance realignment should be the treatment of choice.
- In cases with existing imbalanced sagittal profile realignment should be the goal accompanied by correction of the sagittal profile.

References

1. Försth P, Ólafsson G, Carlsson T, Frost A, Borgström F, Fritzell P, Öhagen P, Michaëlsson K, Sandén B. A randomized, controlled trial of fusion surgery for lumbar spinal stenosis. N Engl J Med. 2016;374(15):1413–23.
2. Gandhoke GS, Kasliwal MK, Smith JS, Nieto J, Ibrahimi D, Park P, Lamarca F, Shaffrey C, Okonkwo DO, Kanter AS. A multicenter evaluation of clinical and radiographic outcomes following high-grade spondylolisthesis reduction and fusion. Clin Spine Surg. 2017;30(4):E363–9.
3. Ghogawala Z, Dziura J, Butler WE, Dai F, Terrin N, Magge SN, Coumans JV, Harrington JF, Amin-Hanjani S, Schwartz JS, Sonntag VK, Barker FG 2nd, Benzel EC. Laminectomy plus fusion versus laminectomy alone for lumbar spondylolisthesis. N Engl J Med. 2016;374(15):1424–34.
4. Hanson DS, Bridwell KH, Rhee JM, Lenke LG. Correlation of pelvic incidence with low- and high-grade isthmic spondylolisthesis. Spine. 2002;27(18):2026–9.
5. Inage K, Orita S, Yamauchi K, Suzuki M, Sakuma Y, Kubota G, Oikawa Y, Sainoh T, Sato J, Fujimoto K, Shiga Y, Abe K, Kanamoto H, Inoue M, Kinoshita H, Norimoto M, Umimura T, Takahashi K, Ohtori S. Long-term outcomes of *in situ* fusion for treating dysplastic spondylolisthesis. Asian Spine J. 2017;11(2):213–8.
6. Labelle H, Mac-Thiong J-M, Roussouly P. Spino-pelvic sagittal balance of spondylolisthesis: a review and classification. Eur Spine J. 2011;20(S5):641–6.
7. Longo UG, Loppini M, Romeo G, Maffulli N, Denaro V. Evidence-based surgical management of spondylolisthesis: reduction or arthrodesis in situ. J Bone Joint Surg Am. 2014;96(1):53–8.
8. Passias P, Poorman C, Yang S, Boniello A, Jalai C, Worley N, Lafage V. Surgical treatment strategies for high-grade spondylolisthesis: a systematic review. Int J Spine Surg. 2015;9:50.
9. Rajakumar DV, Hari A, Krishna M, Sharma A, Reddy M. Complete anatomic reduction and monosegmental fusion for lumbar spondylolisthesis of Grade II and higher: use of the minimally invasive "rocking" technique. Neurosurg Focus. 2017;43(2):E12.
10. Vialle R, Ilharreborde B, Dauzac C, Lenoir T, Rillardon L, Guigui P. Is there a sagittal imbalance of the spine in isthmic spondylolisthesis? A correlation study. Eur Spine J. 2007;16(10):1641–9.
11. Weinstein JN, Lurie JD, Tosteson TD, Hanscom B, Tosteson ANA, Blood EA, Birkmeyer NJ, Hilibrand AS, Herkowitz H, Cammisa FP, Albert TJ, Emery SE, Lenke LG, Abdu WA, Longley M, Errico TJ, Hu SS. Surgical versus nonsurgical treatment for lumbar degenerative spondylolisthesis. N Engl J Med. 2007;356(22):2257–70.

Surgical Management of Developmental High-Grade Spondylolisthesis

60

Sleiman Haddad, Kimia Rahnama Zand, and Ferran Pellisé

60.1 Introduction

Traditionally, developmental spondylolisthesis has been divided into two groups depending on the degree of slippage: low (<50% slip) and high (>50% slip) grade. These are two different clinical entities with different natural history. While low-grade spondylolisthesis is basically a painful syndrome/entity, high-grade spondylolisthesis (HGS) is a true lumbosacral deformity with significant risk of progression resulting in trunk deformity. More recent classifications take into consideration the spinopelvic alignment to further guide treatment. The objectives of surgery in HGS are to decompress the involved neural structures, correct the lumbosacral kyphosis and trunk unbalance, and stabilize the lumbosacral junction segment by fusing the least number of vertebrae. Fusion can be performed in situ or after reducing the slipped vertebra. The decision to correct high-grade slippage defects by reduction is still controversial.

60.2 Case Presentation

A 20 year-old female who presents with the chief complaints of low back pain associated to throbbing discomfort and weakness in her legs. She denies any trauma or triggering event. She reports indolent progressive back pain and trunk deformity for the past 3 years, associated for the past 2 years with leg pain, mainly over the L5 and S1 dermatomes. The patient states her symptoms worsen with activities and walking, and when standing for more than 5 min. She failed to improve with non-operative modalities including Cox-2 Inhibitors and rehabilitation and her health care provider had referred her to our clinics for surgical assessment. Past medical history is unremarkable. She does smoke regularly.

Physical examination reveals an average height female who appears to be in good health. The shoulders and pelvis are level, but she has an obvious coronal and sagittal trunk deformity associated to an abdominal crease (Fig. 60.1a–c). She is tender to palpation at the lumbosacral level. She has a limited flexion and extension of her trunk with hamstring tightness. Motor testing reveals normal strength bilaterally in both upper and lower

S. Haddad
Department of Orthopaedic Surgery, Spine Unit, University Hospital Vall d'Hebron, Barcelona, Spain

Spine Surgery, Hospital Universitari Vall d'Hebron, Spine Institute Hospital Quiron, Barcelona, Spain

K. Rahnama Zand
Clinical Neurophysiology, Intraoperative Neuromonitoring, Hospital Universitari Vall d'Hebron, Spine Institute Hospital Quiron, Barcelona, Spain

F. Pellisé (✉)
Department of Orthopaedic Surgery, Spine Unit, University Hospital Vall d'Hebron, Barcelona, Spain
e-mail:24361fpu@comb.cat

B. Meyer, M. Rauschmann (eds.), *Spine Surgery*, https://doi.org/10.1007/978-3-319-98875-7_60

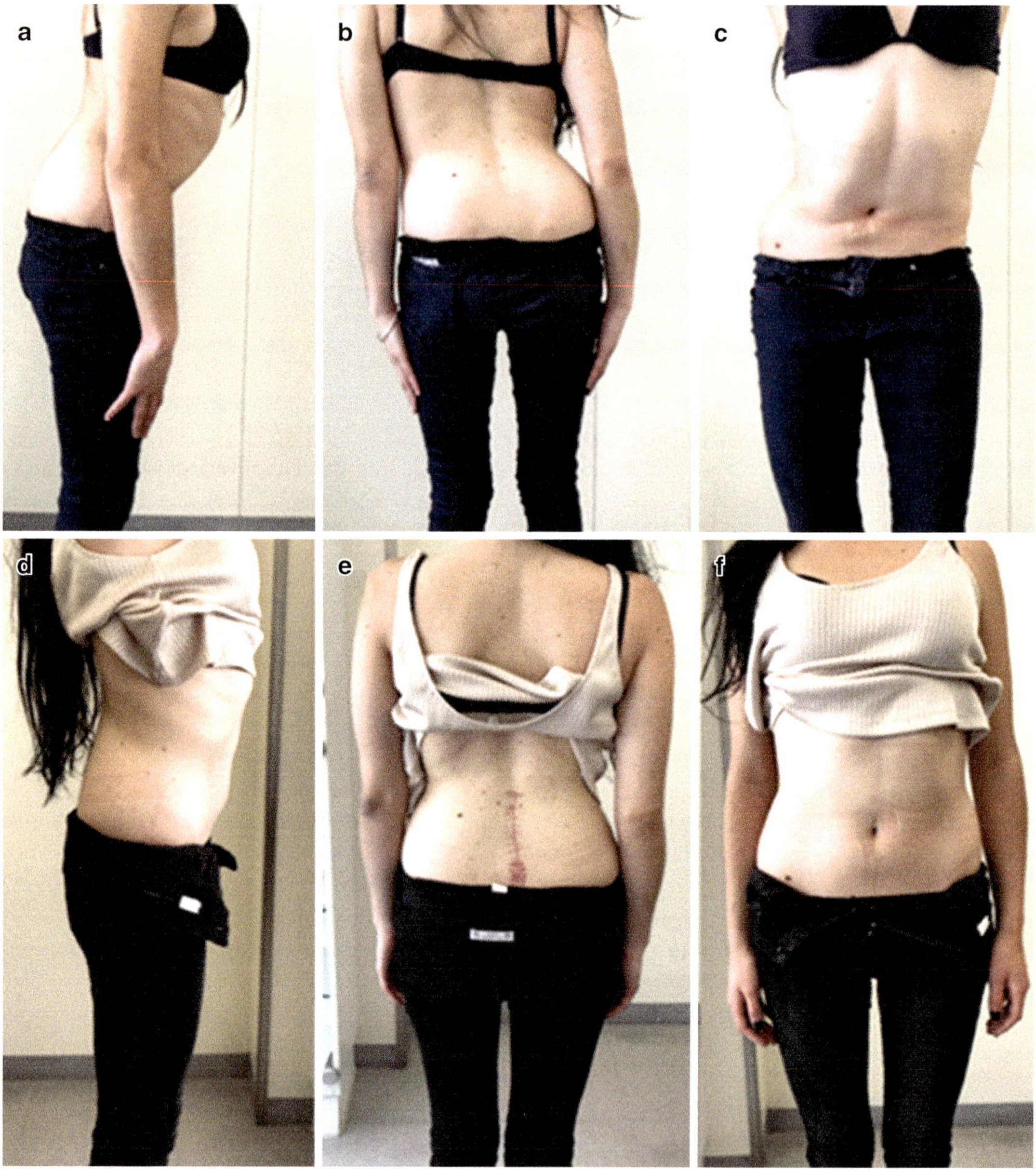

Fig. 60.1 Preoprative (**a**) Lateral, (**b**) back and (**c**) front view of a 20-year-old female with high-grade spondylolisthesis. Both coronal and sagittal deformities can be appreciated as well as an abdominal crease. Comparative postoperative views (**d**–**f**) that show correction of trunk deformity, reduction of lumbosacral kyphosis and disappearance of abdominal crease

extremities. She has an unchanged sensory exam with normal reflexes in her lower extremities. Long tract signs including Romberg's sign, Babinski, and sustained clonus were absent. There is no evidence of peripheral compression neuropathy and vascular exam was non-contributory.

Radiographic examination demonstrates spondyloptosis at the L5-S1 level, associated to a high pelvic incidence of 88°. Her lumbar Lordosis as measured from L1 to S1 is 51°. L4-S1 is kyphotic and measures 7°. Her slip angle measures 30° and Dubousset's lumbosacral angle

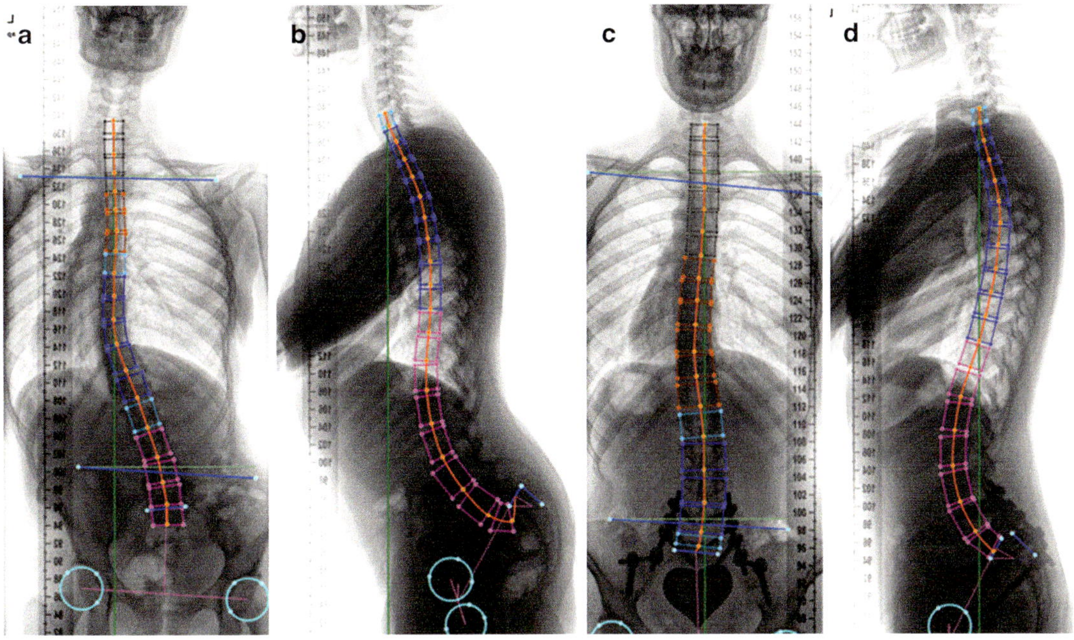

Fig. 60.2 Preoperative (**a**) coronal and (**b**) sagittal whole spine standing x-rays of a 20 year old female with HGS. She has an unbalanced pelvis (high PT and los SS) associated to an unbalanced spine (high SVA). In addition she has a scoliotic coronal deformity. Comparative ostoperative views (**c**) and (**d**) showing satisfactory biplanar reduction of the deformity and posterior L4 to Ilium instrumentation with an L5-S1 interbody cage

(Du-LSA) is significantly altered and measures 60° on standing films, partially reducing to 76° on supine scan (Figs. 60.2b and 60.4a). It further decreases to 83° when a traction fluoroscopy under general anesthesia is performed (Fig. 60.5a). She has an SVA of 16.5 cm associated to a pelvic tilt of 29° and a Global Tilt of 47° (Fig. 60.2a–c). This is associated to a coronal imbalance of 6.0 cm to the left and her L4-S1 Cobb angle is 21°. Her GAP Score is 11 denoting a severe disproportion. An MRI of her lumbosacral spine confirms a high-grade spondylolistesis with central and bilateral foraminal stenosis (Fig. 60.3a–c). A CT-Scan proves a bilateral lysis of the L5 pars and disruption of the posterior elements. She has a trapezoidal L5 associated to a domed S1. The interapophyseal joints shows significant dysplasia, the inferior articular facet of the L5 remains on the sacrum while the pedicle and the superior articular facet are dislocated anteriorly along with the lumbar spine (Fig. 60.4a–c). The L4-L5 joint was articulating over the sacral dome.

60.3 Technique Rationale

In summary, our patient had a dysplastic HGS / Spondyloptosis associated to an unbalanced spine and pelvis (Type 6 according to Labelle's classification). She had a high dysplasia and slip angles, predictive of local instability and progression. She presented with axial pain and with radicular and central symptoms due to neural compression and instability. Due to severity of clinical symptoms and radiological deformity the patient was proposed surgery. Goals of treatment in her case were to correct her biplanar deformity, stabilize the lumbosacral junction, decompress neural structures and achieve adequate axial pain relief. We opted for decompression and circumferential fusion after deformity reduction through a posterior only approach. To correct her spinopelvic unbalance, we chose to perform reduction using the technique described by Ruf et al. [1]. Due to the severe deformity as well as the dysplastic nature of both L5 and S1, we considered

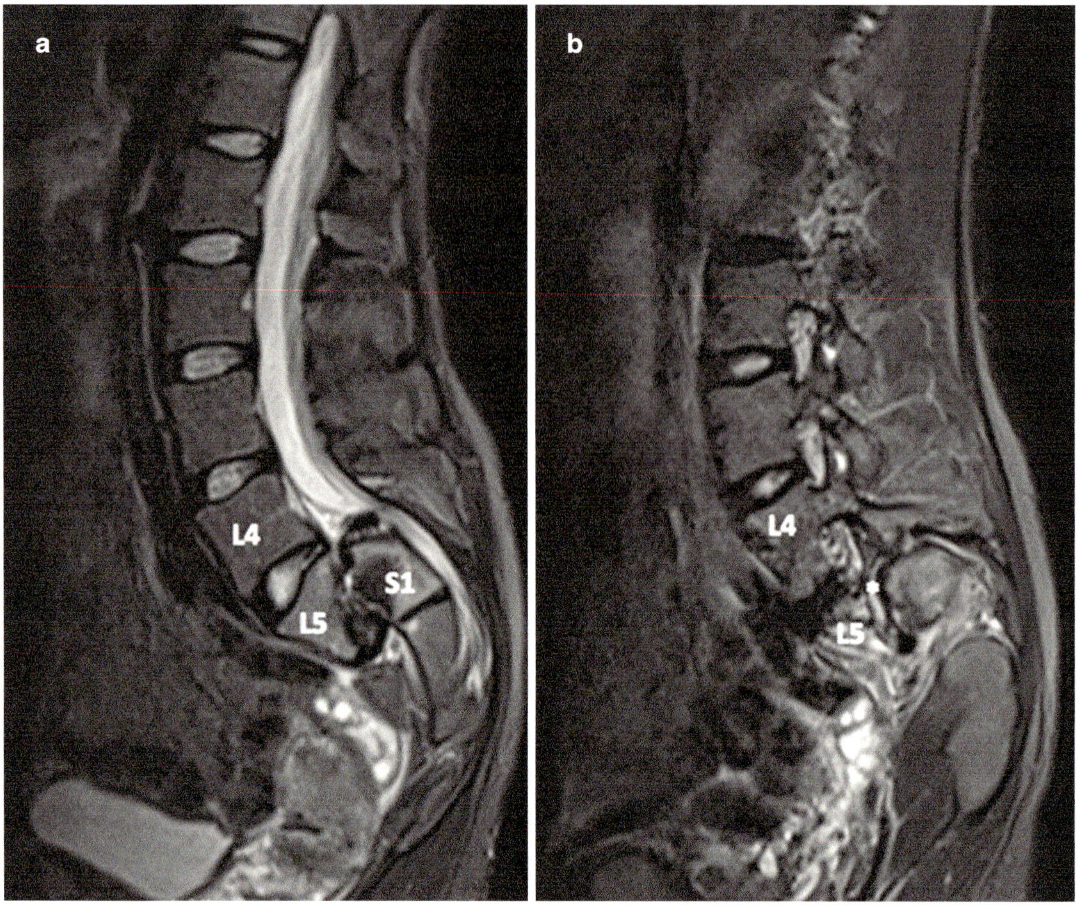

Fig. 60.3 MRI scan of the above mentioned patient. (**a**) Mid sagittal T2 sequence showing HGS and central stenosis. (**b**) Foraminal sagittal view showing obliteration of the right L5-S1 foramen (*)

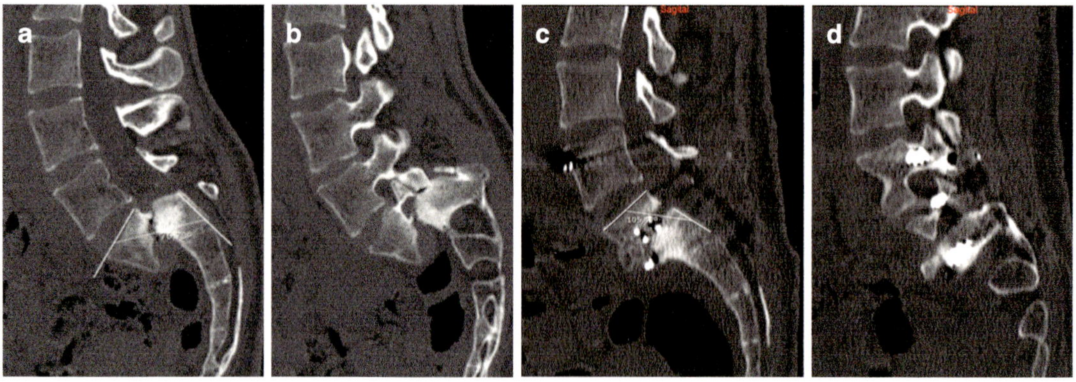

Fig. 60.4 Preoprative (**a**) mid sagittal CT scan reconstruction showing partial reduction of Dubousset's lumbosacral angle (76° Vs 60° on Standing X-ray). Note the trapezoidal L5 and dome shaped S1. (**b**) lateral sagittal sequence showing posterior elements dysplasia and lysis of the L5-S1 pars. Postoperative sagittal sequences showing lumbosacral deformity reduction with a Dubousset's LSA or 105° (**c**) and L5-S1 foramen (**d**)

performing an L4 to Iliac instrumentation initially that could be reduced to monosegmental L5-S1 at a later stage.

60.4 Surgical Technique and Outcomes

The patient is placed in a prone position over bolsters on a radiolucent table. At this stage, surgeons can assess flexibility of the deformity by performing a traction film under general anesthesia, as was performed in this case (Fig. 60.5a). The lumbosacral junction is exposed posteriorly through a midline incision. The exposure is extended laterally out to the transverse processes of L4 and L5 bilaterally. Caudally, the sacral alae and the posterior iliac spine are exposed. The intraoperative identification and exposure of L5 can be difficult in HGS. The L5/S1 facet joint is fully removed and a complete or partial L5 laminectomy is performed to identify the L5 nerve roots. The L5 nerve roots are tracked far laterally. Next, the L4 and S1 pedicles are instrumented using poliaxial screws. If the L5 pedicle is properly identified, it can be instrumented at this stage. Authors recommend longhead or extended screws to be placed in L4 and L5 to facilitate rod placement. The first stage of reduction starts by distracting between L4 and the sacrum (Fig. 60.5b). The ligamentotaxis would help reduce L5 between L4 and S1. This would in turn allow better visualization of the pedicle entry point at L5. If the L5 screw was not placed earlier due to technical difficulties, it can be placed at this stage after contralateral distraction with a temporary rod. The surgeon then proceeds to partial L5 reduction taking advantage of L5 longhead reduction screws, avoiding screw pullout. An L5-S1 discectomy with complete posterior annulotomy is performed through a bilateral approach. Under fluoroscopic guidance, the surgeon then performs a dome ostetomy of S1 (Fig. 60.5b). This shortens the sacrum, helps in the reduction and creates a flat surface for cage placement. The osteotomy is usually perpendicular to the posterior sacral wall. Further L5 reposition/reduction under IONM is then performed. In cases of severe slippage or ptosis, the anterior aspect of the trapezoidal L5 vertebral body might prevent reduction. If this is the case the addition of an L5 osteotomy, removing the antero-inferior aspect of L5 vertebral body will increase lumbosacral release and allow for a gentler reposition of the L5 vertebral body. The surgeon can proceed to the next step in reduction of L5. By tightening the nuts of the long-head screws in L5, its body is pulled posteriorly to the rod between L4 and the sacrum. During reduction, the L5 roots should be continually visualized and monitored

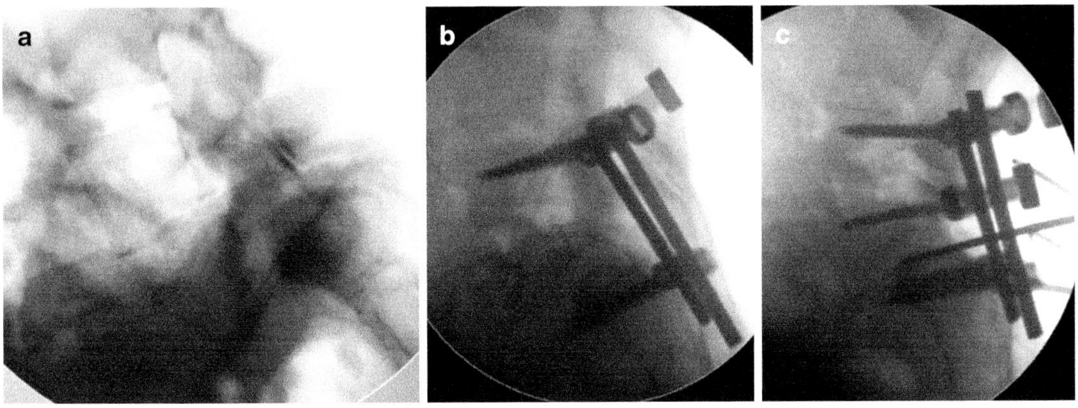

Fig. 60.5 Intraoperative fluoroscopy. (**a**) Traction film under general anesthesia showing partial reduction of the deformity. (**b**) intraoperative L4-S1 distraction to reduce the L5 vertebrae by ligamentotaxis. (**c**) Dome Osteotomy of the S1

to avoid any compression. The elongated ends of the long-headed screws can now be removed. Even though reduction of the anterior slippage of L5/S1 is now completed; some degree of lumbosacral kyphosis may still be present. The anterior part of the L5-S1 disc space can now be prepared and packed with cancellous bone chips and disc spacers. Cages do increase fusion and can also increase friction between L5-S1 and resist shear loads.

Short cages are recommended to avoid stretching the L5 roots and to allow reconstitution of lordosis. They can either be placed by a posterior (posterior lumbar interbody fusion) or by a second anterior approach (anterior lumbar interbody fusion). Authors prefer to perform a PLIF whenever possible. The third step of the reduction with correction of the segmental kyphosis is achieved by posterior compression against the anteriorly placed cages. The sacral screw is loosened, and reoriented towards the L4 and L5 screws. Loosening the polyaxial head allows for change of the angulation, and the sacrum retroversion is corrected. This kyphotic deformity correction is supported by hyperextension of the hip joints over the operative table. The sacral screws are fixed again and further compression is applied between L5 and S1. The surgeon may choose to cut the rod above L5 and remove the L4 screw at this stage or add a pelvic fixation as needed.

Autologous and allogenic bone grafts are placed over the decorticated transverse process.

A deep drain is left in situ and wound closure is performed according to surgeon's preference.

Patient is mobilized as pain allows starting the first day after surgery without any brace. Flexion of hips and knees may be needed for some days, to reduce L5 root tension in case of sciatica or radicular symptoms.

Intraoperatively IONM was performed with somatosensory evoked potentials (SEP), muscle motor evoked potentials (mMEP) as well as free-run electromyography (fEMG) and H reflex for lower extremities. During surgery we had a single IONM alert during right L5-S1 nerve root decompression that was addressed. Opening and closing baselines remained unchanged throughout the surgical procedure, for both SEP and mMEP recordings.

The patient however woke up with a right L5 partial palsy (MRC 3/5) undetected during surgery, with further electromyographic studies showing postganglionary lesion, involving the distal L5 myotomes, therefore distal to site of surgery. She recovered fully by the sixth month postoperatively.

During her last visit, 2 years after surgery, our patient was pain free and had resumed her recreational activities. She was satisfied with her physical appearance (Fig. 60.1d–f). Her Lumbar lordosis measured 70° and L4-S1 measured 38°. Global tilt was 27°, pelvic tilt was 26°, SVA 26 mm and Lumbosacral angle was 105°. Her GAP score was 0 (Fig. 60.2d–f).

60.5 Discussion and Summary of Literature

The term spondylolisthesis derives from the greek for spondylos (spine or vertebra) and listhesis (to slip or slide) and describes a pathological spinal condition characterized by the slippage or displacement of one vertebra compared to another. There are several classifications based on etiology (Wiltse, Marchetti and Bartolozzi), degree of slippage (Meyerding) or the resultant sagittal balance (Labelle). Marchetti and Bartolozzi differentiate between acquired and developmental (including isthmic and dysplastic) listhesis. They then divide developmental listhesis according to the grade of slippage, as defined by Meyerding. High-grade spondylolisthesis (HGS) is defined as greater than 50% slippage and most often affects the L5-S1 segment. Labelle et al. have proposed a classification system for developmental listhesis. It goes one step further and integrates the spinopelvic parameters. This classification was originally intended to guide the evaluation and treatment of spondylolisthesis [2]. It has high intra- and interobserver reliability. It includes six groups according to Pelvic Incidence, Pelvic retroversion and Spinal balance and can serve to better guide treatment.

It also divides spondylolisthesis to two clusters: Low and High Grade. HGS is then divided to three groups based on PT, SS and SVA. Patients with HGS are accordingly classified as having a "balanced" (low PT and high SS) or "unbalanced" pelvis (high PT and low SS). Patients with "unbalanced pelvis" are further divided to "balanced spine" (normal SVA) or "unbalanced spine" (high SVA).

Dysplastic spondylolisthesis involves congenital dysplasia of the sacrum or the L5 neural arch, with pars elongation and/ or lysis developing later. Several radiological parameters have been developed to study the lumbosacral kyphosis or the slip angle in spondylolisthesis. Boxall was the first to describe a lumbosacral slip angle (BSA) as defined by the angle subtended by the inferior end plate of L5 with a line perpendicular to the posterior aspect of S1. The inferior endplate of L5 is dysmorphic and hard to visualize in patients with severe dysplasia. This has led Dubousset to describe the "lumbosacral kyphosis angle" as the angle subtended by the superior endplate of L5 with the posterior aspect of S1 (Du-LSA). Other described angles include the Spinal Deformity Study Group's lumbosacral angle (SDSG LSA), SDSG dysplastic angle (dys-SDSG), Sagittal rotation (SR) and the Kyphotic Cobb angle (k-Cobb). These angles have been shown to be predictive of severity of deformity, poor sagittal balance and deformity progression. Du-LSA and the k-cobb are very useful as they remain unaltered by L5 or S1 endplate dysplasia and retain a high inter and intraobserver reliability. Du-LSA on the other hand has the strongest correlation with slip grade. Also, the L5-Incidence (>60°) and the proximal femoral angles (>10°) have been proposed as additional and reliable radiological measurement that could predict need for surgery.

Progressing and uncompensated high-grade developmental L5-S1 spondylolisthesis is characterized by three main pathologic hallmarks: anterior slippage of L5 against S1 superior to 50%, segmental L5/S1 kyphosis, and retroversion of the sacrum in patients with unbalanced pelvis. The sacrum gradually acquires a dome-shaped appearance as the slippage progresses and the L5 vertebra is trapezoidally deformed with a concave lower endplate. The segmental kyphosis and deformity affects the global posture of the patient. It leads to a loss of sagittal balance and gradual recruitment of compensatory mechanisms. The lumbosacral kyphosis leads to compensatory hyperlordosis of the adjacent lumbar and lower thoracic segments and retroversion of the pelvis causes hyperextension of the hip joints. The center of the lumbar lordosis is also shifted higher than L4. When these compensatory mechanisms are overcome, the gravity line is shifted anteriorly. This continuous compensatory status associated to foraminal and central stenosis is responsible for the patient's back pain and leg pain.

Nonoperative management may lead to satisfactory results in minimally symptomatic or asymptomatic patients with balanced high-grade spondylolisthesis. Surgery is indicated for high-grade slippage in patients with persistent symptoms, neurologic impairment, sagittal trunk deformity or risk of progression [3]. Slippage of >50% in itself has been considered as an indication for spinal arthrodesis in immature patients to avoid further progression.

Surgically treated patients do have good results that are maintained overtime. In a study by Lundine et al. a more kyphotic slip angle was associated with worse outcome regardless of the treatment modality (conservative vs. surgical) [4]. The slip angle was a predictor of failure of conservative treatment and crossover to surgery. In surgical patients, an older age at surgery was associated with better outcome. Joelson et al. has compared the results of patients treated with in-situ fusion to the general Swedish population 20 years after surgery and has shown that both the EQ-5 scores as well as the SF-36 scores were comparable to the general age adjusted population [5]. In another study by Bourassa-Moreau Health related Quality of Life (HRQoL) parameters improved after a surgical intervention for high-grade spondylolisthesis. Patients with lower baseline HRQOL scores were those who benefited the most from surgery [6].

The general objectives of surgery in developmental spondylolisthesis should be to correct lumbosacral kyphosis, decompress the involved neural structures and stabilize the lumbosacral junction segment to prevent slip progression, by fusing the least number of vertebrae. Fusion can be performed in situ or after reducing the slipped vertebra. In HGS the goal is to reduce lumbosacral kyphosis and restore the sagittal balance. The algorithm offered by Labelle et al. and by the SDSG might better guide the surgeon during decision-making. Based on this classification, reduction of the deformity should be considered in patients with an unbalanced pelvis, especially if they have an unbalanced spine. Reduction of the slipped vertebra may also be contemplated. Several authors advocate for reduction to improve arthrodesis rate and allow for direct neurologic decompression. The role of reduction in the operative management of spondylolisthesis is still controversial though, mainly due to historically high rates of perioperative complications, including neurologic deficits, prolonged operative time, and posterior loss of reduction. Therefore a consensus is still lacking regarding the best surgical management of high-grade developmental listhesis.

Few studies have directly compared the outcomes of arthrodesis with or without reduction in patients with HGS. In situ posterolateral spinal fusion is commonly considered safe, with good long-term results. However it can lead to progression of the deformity, especially in cases of high slip angles and if surgery does not restore physiologic alignment and balance. Slip progression despite solid non-instrumented fusion has been reported after in situ fusion in up to 26% of cases. It is a clear reminder of the shear forces remaining when the kyphotic deformity of severe lumbosacral spondylolisthesis are left uncorrected. Patients with HGS and residual lumbosacral kyphosis tend to compensate by recruiting their upper lumbar and may have persistent back pain. In addition to progression of deformity, these patients might suffer from adjacent level disease, implant failure and pseudoarthrosis. Non-fusion rates with in-situ fusion have been reported to be as high as 44%. A recent systematic review by Longo et al. showed that the rate of non-fusion was significantly higher in the in-situ fusion group compared with the reduction group (17.8% vs. 5.5%, $p = 0.004$) [7]. According to the same authors, some confounding factors might be intrinsically favoring the reduction group. Patient who had deformity reduction were more likely to have circumferential fusion (53% Vs 26%), two-level fusion (44% Vs. 33%), and to be instrumented (100% vs. 22%). Finally, the resection of the upper sacrum also favors fusion by increasing the area of cancellous bone contact.

Reduction of the slipped vertebra on the other hand can provide better alignment in the sagittal plane. Restoration of the sagittal may reduce shear forces on the lumbosacral junction, improve fusion and decrease mechanical failures. Nevertheless, aggressive reduction has been associated to great risk of neurologic deficits ranging between 10% and 50% and loss of reduction postoperatively. These findings were drawn from historical and non-comparative series. Longo.et al. showed that neurologic deficits occurring with the reduction were mainly transient, and were not higher when compared to the in-situ group (7.8% Vs. 8.9%, $p = 0.8$). The most frequently reported deficit involves the L5 nerve root and is temporary or partial as occurred in our patient. Traction is the most common cause of postoperative deficit. "Root or nerve fatigue" to continuous traction after reduction may be the origin of late neurological deficit. Some authors have also reported cases of iatrogenic cauda equina.

The importance of postoperative sagittal balance and its impact on clinical result has recently been investigated in developmental spondylolisthesis. Harroud et al. showed that an increasing positive sagittal alignment was related to a poorer SRS- 22 total score [8]. This relationship was stronger with high-grade spondylolisthesis than with low grade. This confirms the clinical importance of restoring sagittal balance and the need to eliminate compensatory mechanisms.

Regardless of the surgical approach, the addition of anterior column structural support is recommended to provide greater stability but also, more importantly, to improve fusion rates. An interbody fusion provides greater surface area for fusion to occur. Addition of an anterior interbody support will also help correct the deformity when applying posterior compression.

When planning the number of levels to be fused, surgeons must take into consideration several important aspects including the severity and extend of deformity, dysplasia and the intraoperative purchase. If reduction is performed for HGS, circumferential fusion may be supplemented with solid fixation with iliac screws to prevent slip progression and pseudarthrosis. This aspect may be particularly relevant in patients with a high PI who have additional shear forces at the lumbosacral junction. A pelvic fixation can similarly be considered in severe deformities, high lumbosacral dysplasia or in patients with poor S1 purchase. Solid posterior instrumentation combined with compression loaded interbody cages results in a very stable, shear resistant construct that would ultimately enhance fusion and decrease mechanical failure.

The L4 pedicle screw aids in L5 reduction but can be removed directly afterwards or in a subsequent surgery 3 months later. Extending the fusion proximally to L4 should be considered especially if instability is suspected at the L4-L5 segment, and if the L5 transverse processes are very small with minimal area for a fusion mass. It can also be useful when high traction forces are anticipated or in very dysplastic patients or with poor pedicle purchase. Inclusion of an L4 screw has a mechanical advantage. It creates a more vertical fusion as compared to L5-S1 and reduces shear forces.

In cases of spondyloptosis an L5 spondylectomy can be performed according to the Gaines technique. As such, the L5 vertebral body can be resected through an anterior retroperitoneal spinal approach and the vertebral body of L4, then placed directly superior to the S1 body and secured with pedicle screw-rod instrumentation.

Finally, the authors recommend for the routine use of IONM including assessment of both motor and sensory tracts, and free-run electromyography focused on L5 muscles. Nerve root testing is also advisable. SEP assess the dorsal column integrity by stimulation of the peripheral nerve. The posterior tibial nerve is used, as other nerves such as the distal plantar median nerve have showed no diagnostic value. Still, paraplegia can occur without SEP warning. mMEPs triggered by transcranial electrical stimulation evaluate the function and the flux of motor outputs from motor cortex, CT, nerve roots, and peripheral nerves to the muscle. They have a reported sensitivity of 75% to 100% and specificity of 84% to 100% for the detection of iatrogenic motor deficits in elective deformity cases. Free-run electromyography (fEMG) consists of recording spontaneous muscle activity, thus allowing the use of this technique as a monitoring tool for detecting surgically driven mechanical irritation of the peripheral nervous system. The latter depends on the integrity and function of the muscle fibers, neuromuscular junction, peripheral nerve, ventral root, alpha motor neuron, and its spinal interneuronal synapses. Patients with chronic neuropathies or radiculopathies and thus with chronic denervation may not show spontaneous activity during the reduction procedures until a severe damage is done to the nerve, therefore resulting in an uncertain test to detect radicular nerve palsies. In these circumstances, testing the conductivity of the nerve root with direct stimulation is convenient.

Whereas the role of IONM has been extensively assessed in elective deformity surgery and in decompressive tumor surgery and has been shown to decrease intraoperative neurological injuries, little is known of its utility in HGS. Up to date, there is only one prospective series of HGS cases that have been monitored intraoperatively, in addition to two case reports. In the study by Schär et al., intraoperative IONM alerts occurred in 15 out of 17 patients (88%) [9]. Only 5 patients had new onset L5 motor deficits (29.4%) after surgery, all of which with intraoperative alerts. The IONM prediction had a sensitivity of 20% and specificity of 100% with MEPs. The authors did not see any diagnostic value of dermatomal SEP monitoring for L5 radiculopathy with stimulation of the plantar medial nerve and cortical recording. Even though the authors lacked a control group and could not assess the impact of IONM on final results, IONM may have prevented further deficits by alerting the surgeon promptly, since 10 cases had intraoperative alerts that were addressed accordingly with no resultant postoperative neurologic sequelae.

References

1. Ruf M, Koch H, Melcher RP, Harms J. Anatomic reduction and monosegmental fusion in high-grade developmental spondylolisthesis. Spine. 2006;31(3):269–74.
2. Labelle H, Mac-Thiong JM, Roussouly P. Spino-pelvic sagittal balance of spondylolisthesis: a review and classification. Eur Spine J Off Publ Eur Spine Soc Eur Spinal Deform Soc Eur Sect Cerv Spine Res Soc. 2011;20(Suppl 5):641–6.
3. Kasliwal MK, Smith JS, Kanter A, Chen CJ, Mummaneni PV, Hart RA, et al. Management of high-grade spondylolisthesis. Neurosurg Clin N Am. 2013;24(2):275–91.
4. Lundine KM, Lewis SJ, Al-Aubaidi Z, Alman B, Howard AW. Patient outcomes in the operative and nonoperative management of high-grade spondylolisthesis in children. J Pediatr Orthop. 2014;34(5):483–9.
5. Joelson A, Hedlund R, Frennered K. Normal health-related quality of life and ability to work twenty-nine years after in situ arthrodesis for high-grade isthmic spondylolisthesis. J Bone Joint Surg Am. 2014;96(12):e100.
6. Bourassa-Moreau E, Mac-Thiong JM, Joncas J, Parent S, Labelle H. Quality of life of patients with high-grade spondylolisthesis: minimum 2-year follow-up after surgical and nonsurgical treatments. Spine J Off J North Am Spine Soc. 2013;13(7):770–4.
7. Longo UG, Loppini M, Romeo G, Maffulli N, Denaro V. Evidence-based surgical management of spondylolisthesis: reduction or arthrodesis in situ. J Bone Joint Surg Am. 2014;96(1):53–8.
8. Harroud A, Labelle H, Joncas J, Mac-Thiong JM. Global sagittal alignment and health-related quality of life in lumbosacral spondylolisthesis. Eur Spine J Off Publ Eur Spine Soc Eur Spinal Deform Soc Eur Sect Cerv Spine Res Soc. 2013;22(4):849–56.
9. Schar RT, Sutter M, Mannion AF, Eggspuhler A, Jeszenszky D, Fekete TF, et al. Outcome of L5 radiculopathy after reduction and instrumented transforaminal lumbar interbody fusion of high-grade L5-S1 isthmic spondylolisthesis and the role of intraoperative neurophysiological monitoring. Eur Spine J Off Publ Eur Spine Soc Eur Spinal Deform Soc Eur Sect Cerv Spine Res Soc. 2017;26(3):679–90.

61 Indications and Technique of Thoracic En Bloc Resections

Dominique A. Rothenfluh and Jeremy J. Reynolds

61.1 Introduction

En-bloc resections in the thoracic spine are mostly reserved for primary tumors of the spine. Rarely, en-bloc resections are considered for spinal metastases if the metastasis is solitary and can be removed en-bloc without a high likelihood of breaching the margins during the resection. Traditionally, it has been considered difficult to perform en-bloc resections in the thoracic spine due to the anatomic proximity of the major blood vessels and thus intralesional resections with curettage were preferred. This, however, resulted in a high risk of local recurrence and, in the case of a primary tumor, metastasis with poor survival. En bloc resection has the primary goals of gaining local control of the tumor by removing it as a whole and thereby reducing the rate of local recurrence and in primary tumors avoid tumor spread and improve survival [1, 4, 5].

The main indication for en-bloc resections are malignant primary tumors, such as chondroma, chondrosarcoma, osteosarcoma and others, or benign tumors which may be locally aggressive such as giant cell tumors or aneurysmal bone cysts for example. Especially for malignant tumors, it is important to note that the first surgery is often the most important and perhaps only chance to cure the patient. In order to plan en-bloc resection, a thorough pre-operative work up with imaging studies such as whole spine MRI, CT staging and these days often PET CT is paramount. Diagnosis is usually secured via a biopsy and upon presentation to a sarcoma board, the indication for an en-bloc resection follows an interdisciplinary discussion between oncologist, pathologist, radiologist and surgeons. A more detailed account of work up and planning of primary tumors is provided in the following chapter.

Primary tumors often become symptomatic at a more advanced stage and present with an anatomical variety which make resection and reconstruction challenging. The margin which can be achieved in surgery is relevant for outcome and particularly to reduce local recurrence. En-bloc resection strives to achieve either a wide or marginal margin [2]. In order for en-bloc resection to be feasible, the neoplastic process should not have invaded the adjacent visceral organs and it should not be adherent to the vena cava which would make mobilization of the vessels difficult, especially from posterior. In these circumstances, en-bloc resection would entail resection of the adherent visceral organs or vessels as well. In addition, a part of the vertebral ring has to be removable without breach to create a tumor-

D. A. Rothenfluh (✉) · J. J. Reynolds
Oxford University Hospitals NHS Foundation Trust, Nuffield Orthopaedic Centre, Oxford, UK
e-mail: dominique.rothenfluh@mac.com

B. Meyer, M. Rauschmann (eds.), *Spine Surgery*, https://doi.org/10.1007/978-3-319-98875-7_61

free window, a corridor, through which the spinal cord can be delivered. Delivery of the spinal cord requires that nerve roots can be reached and ligated in the epidural space but outside of the tumor margin. It is important to note that if the tumor is breached during attempted en-bloc resection, the prognosis is not better than an intralesional resection. The present case illustrates en bloc resection in an aneurysmal bone cyst, a benign but locally invasive primary bone tumor.

61.2 Case Description

61.2.1 Diagnosis and Indication

A 14-year old girl was referred to our service with pain in the thoracic spine. As the pain had not improved with physiotherapy an MRI was obtained which revealed a mass in T6 and T7. Her neurological status was normal. A fine needle biopsy was obtained at the referring institution and the patient referred to our service. The biopsy was in keeping with an aneurysmal bone cyst and no malignancy was shown. Further work up with PET-CT showed an FDG (fluorodeoxyglucose) avid expansile tumor centered on the posterior elements of T6 and T7 with adjacent rib involvement (Figs. 61.1 and 61.2). No other sites of FDG avid disease were shown. The radiological and pathological findings were discussed at the sarcoma board and given the breach into the spinal canal, a consensus was reached to consider surgical en-bloc resection. Here, en-bloc resection does not require a complete spondylectomy as the aneurysmal bone cyst is predominantly

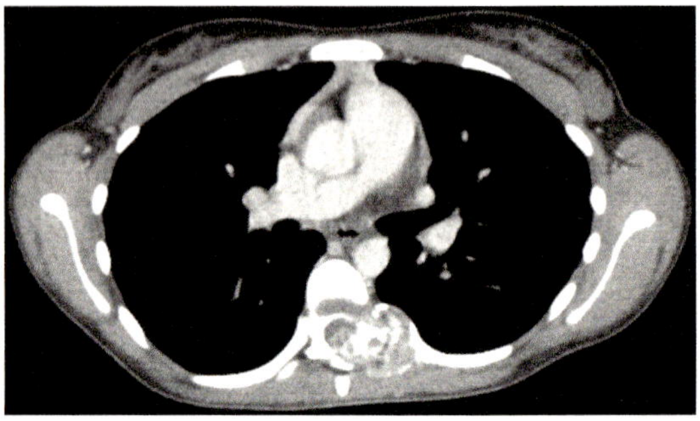

Fig. 61.1 The CT shows an expansile tumor centered on the posterior elements of T6 and T7 with adjacenty rib involvement with areas of ossification

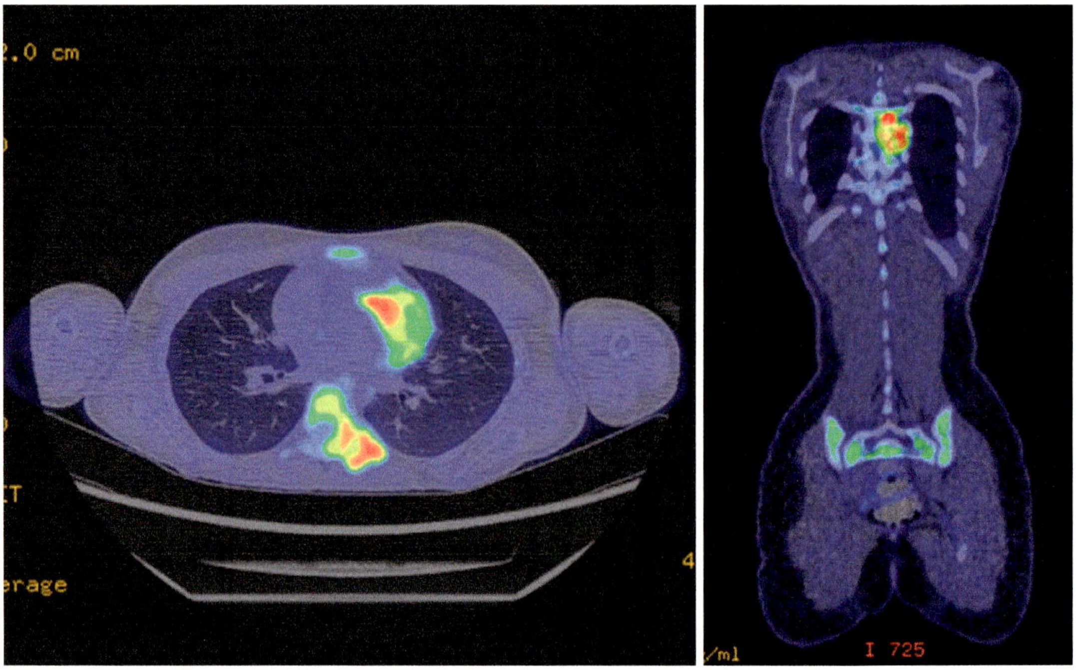

Fig. 61.2 FDG PET-CT showed the localized expansive mass and excluded other sites of FDG avid disease

located at the left costo-vertebral junction involving the left-sided pedicle and extending into the spinal canal.

Figure 61.1 shows the expansile tumor centered on the posterior elements with adjacent rib involvement and breach into the spinal canal involving the left pedicle.

61.2.2 Surgical Technique

After exposure, the spine was first instrumented from T3 to T5 and T8 to T10. The traditional technique as described by Tomita requires a bilateral pediculotomy to take off the posterior vertebral ring to allow delivery of the neural structures. As shown in the CT scan, this would have resulted into a tumor breach on the left side where the majority of the tumor is located. In order to avoid a tumor breach by a pediculotomy, a tumor-free corridor was identified as shown in Fig. 61.3 (red arrow). As it was planned not to perform a complete spondylectomy, only a part of the vertebral body needed to be resected from the healthy right side (Fig. 61.3, long dashed line). In order to do this, a costo-transversectomy of T6 and T7 on the left was performed with ligation of the respective nerve roots. In the same fashion as required in a spondylectomy, the lateral wall on the left side along the tumor capsule needed to be exposed by gently separating the parietal pleura. Segmental vessels which are encountered along the way need to be ligated. The lateral aspects of the intervertebral discs can be cut from the left side as far as possible.

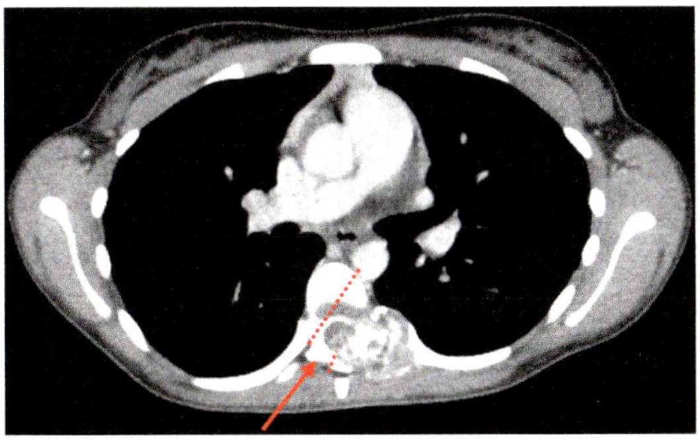

Fig. 61.3 The arrow points to the tumor-free corridor which can be used to open the posterior vertebral ring to release the spinal cord and separate it from the tumor specimen. The short dashed line illustrates the laminotomy just medial to the spinous process in order to avoid tumor breach. The long dashed line represents the right sided resection line down the vertebral bodies. This has to be carried out on both the T6 and T7 levels

At this stage now, the spinal canal can be opened by cutting the lamina just to the right of the spinous process and lateral to the pedicle, both at T6 and T7 as shown in Fig. 61.3 (short dashed line). This is done using a bone scalpel. Lateral to the dura on the right side, the vertebral body cut is performed using the bone scalpel and completed deep using an osteotome. Either a swab or a malleable retractor is inserted on the left side to protect the lung and aorta as the bony cuts are completed. The disc also need to be released on the on the right side. There are usually multiple further adhesions and tethers which have to be released before the en-bloc specimen becomes free and mobile.

Once the specimen is released, it can gradually be mobilized for delivery of the spinal canal cord through the open corridor. The specimen can now be moved to the left side and the dura gradually released. Rotating it slightly gives access to the nerve roots of T6 and T7 in the epidural space in the canal. These can now be ligated through the corridor over the top, but great care has to be taken in order not to damage the spinal cord. For theses manoeuvers, neuromonitoring with motor-evoked potentials is helpful in order to avoid any undue manipulation of the spinal cord during delivery of the tumor with potential subsequent neurologic deficit. The delivery is shown in Fig. 61.4. The specimen after resection is shown in Fig. 61.5. Reconstruction of the anterior column was then carried out by placing a PEEK expandable cage. PEEK was chosen due to its radiolucent properties which makes monitoring for recurrence using MRI available as there are very little artefacts seen. The postoperative xray is shown in Fig. 61.6.

61.2.3 Postoperative Course

The patient postoperatively made a good recovery and the specimen was examined by the

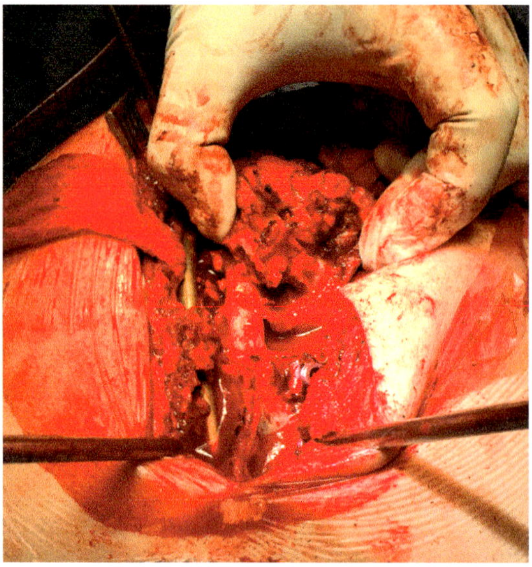

Fig. 61.4 Mobilization of the tumor en-bloc and release of the cord through the tumor-free corridor as indicated in Fig. 61.3

pathologist and the margins appeared to be tumor-free in the sections taken. On routine follow up 6 months postoperatively, cage subsidence was noted on plain radiographs and confirmed on CT imaging (Fig. 61.7). It was therefore decided and discussed with plastic surgeons to supplement the fixation with a free vascularized fibular bone graft to support the anterior column and the construct to avoid late failure. Placement of an anterior fibular strut and posterior fibular strut is seen on CT and postoperative images (Fig. 61.8).

61.3 Discussion of the Case

The present case and technique illustrates a further step in trying to get better local control from the total en-bloc spondylectomy (TES) as described by Tomita et al. [5]. In TES, a planned

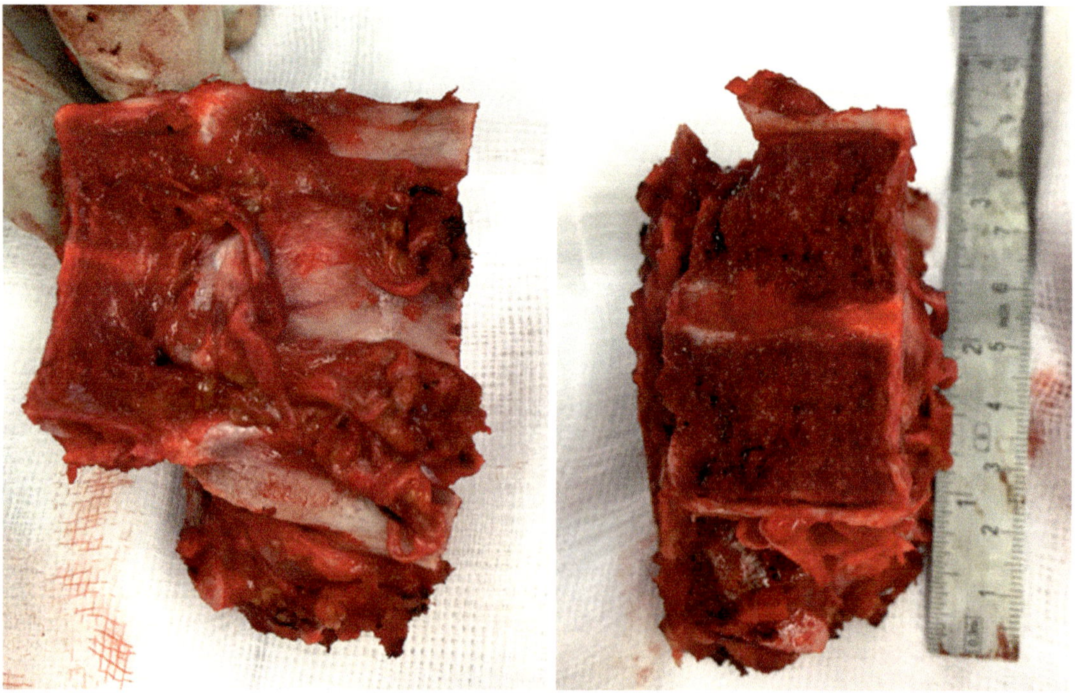

Fig. 61.5 The specimen following en-bloc resection. The split of the vertebral body is shown, the rib heads and ribs with tumor involvement are attached to the specimen

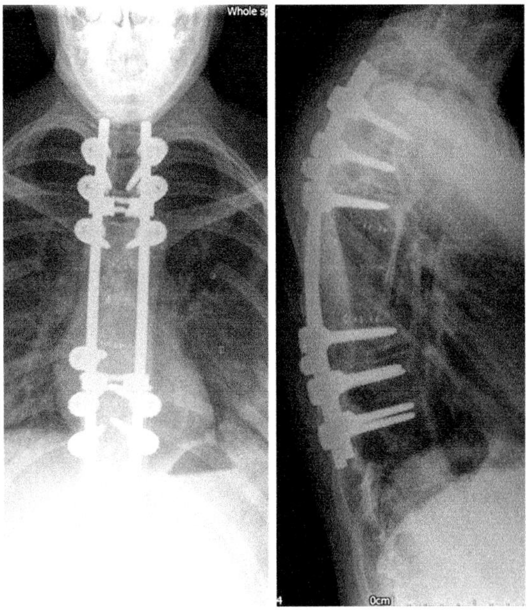

Fig. 61.6 Postoperative images following tumor en-bloc resection and posterior instrumentation T3-T10

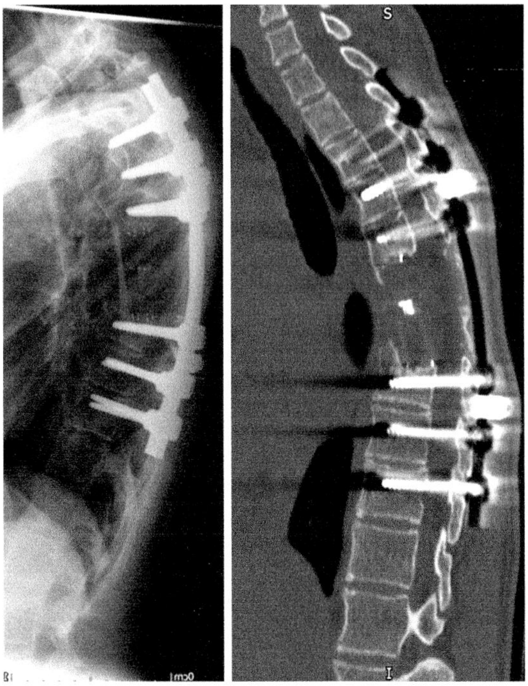

Fig. 61.7 6 months postoperatively, cage subsidence was noted. The CT scan demonstrates that bone graft has not resulted into a solid osseous fusion with subsequent cage subsidence. The instrumentation was still intact.

pediculotomy often means a breach of the tumor and therefore intralesional resection. This is avoided if a 'safe corridor' can be identified through which the neural tissues, i.e. the spinal cord, can be delivered. If a tumor-free corridor is not possible and en-bloc resection can only be achieved with a planned breach via a pediculotomy, then en-bloc resection may not be possible and its morbidity has to be weighed against the potential benefits and risk of recurrence. If a tumor-free margin cannot be achieved, en-bloc resection may not be indicated depending on the biology and oncology of the underlying tumor. In the present case of a locally aggressive benign tumor, en-bloc resection was chosen to gain local tumor control and reduce the risk of recurrence. However, for a benign tumor the sacrifice of neural tissue beyond the ligation of thoracic nerve roots and a subsequent neurologic deficit would likely not have been acceptable. The indication for an en-bloc resection therefore not only depended on the presence of a tumor-free corridor but also on the safe separation of the spinal cord from the tumor specimen.

Tumor invasion into the epidural space does not necessarily mean that en-bloc resection is not possible. There is typically a convergence of the margins if the tumor is breaching the spinal canal. Resection and isolating the tumor along the pseudocapsule results into a marginal margin but if the capsule is not breached, it does not have the local recurrence rates and poor prognosis as observed with intralesional resections. Particularly in malignant tumors, care should be taken to separate the dural sac from the tumor pseudocapsule in order to avoid breaching the tumor, which is most often possible. Resection of the dura is rarely necessary and if this seems required, it has to be considered whether en-bloc resection is possible.

A further challenge in en-bloc resections is the reconstruction of the resulting defect, particularly in terms of achieving a bony fusion. Here, while parts of the anterior column were intended to be left intact, it was not felt to be strong enough and was further supported by a cage with added

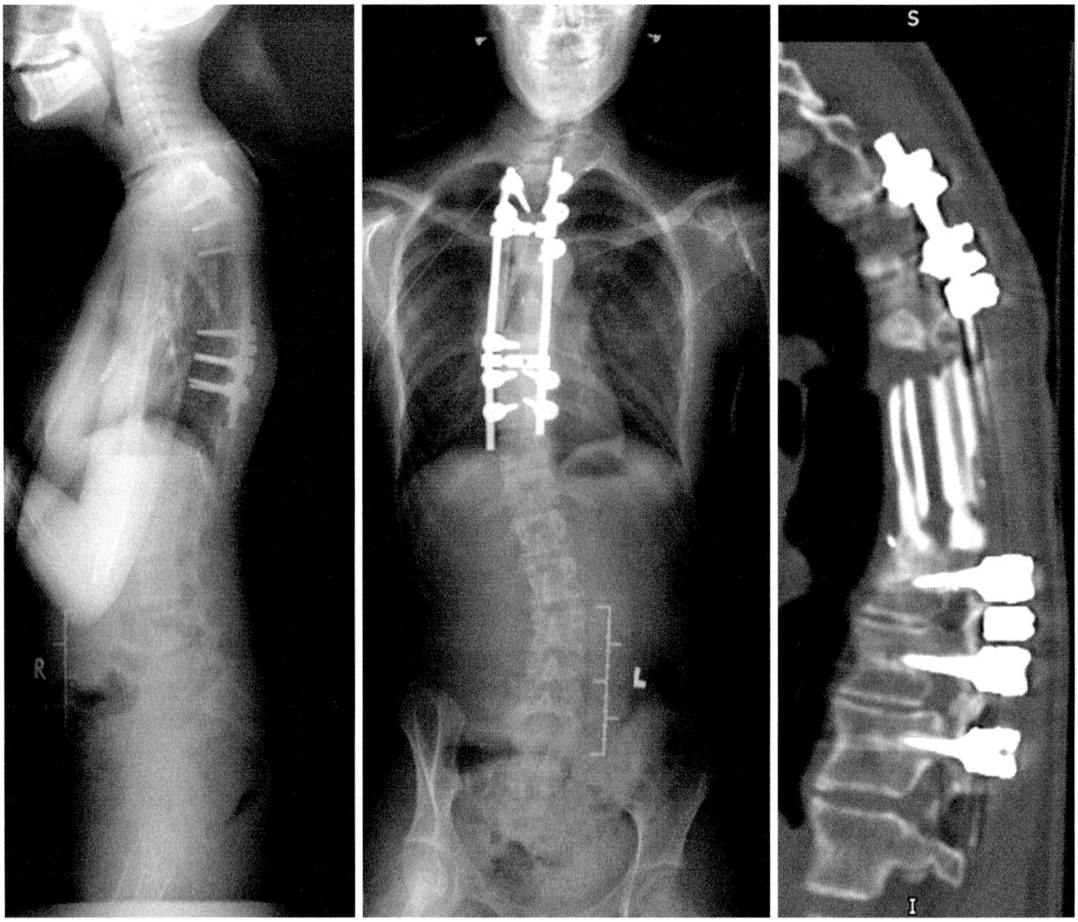

Fig. 61.8 Postoperative image following reconstruction with free vascularized fibular struts. On lateral to the right side in the anterior column and the second one bridging the posterior elements. Of note is a preoperatively existing mild scoliosis

local bone graft from the rib heads which resulted from the costo-transversectomy. Given the wide gaping defect, this strategy did not result into a good fusion resulting into cage subsidence. As the defects following resection are usually large and the surgeries often intend a surgical cure in malignant tumors, a bony fusion needs to be achieved in order to ensure long-term survival of the reconstruction and construct. If local bone graft cannot be used or the defect is too extensive, then a free vascularized fibular graft may be indicated right after resection. This has the advantage that a muscle flap can be harvested in addition on the same vascular pedicle which helps to reduce the void and soft tissue defect left after en-bloc resection. It has been shown that such reconstructions which are performed by a plastic surgeon, yield lower wound complication rates and thus long-term survival if performed immediately after resection [3]. In the present case, reconstruction with a free vascularized fibular graft had to be undertaken in order to prevent late failure.

61.4 Conclusions and Take Home Message

En-bloc resections of both benign and malignant primary tumors are some of the most challenging spinal surgeries in terms of planning, resection and reconstruction. If tumor-free margins are achieved, the local recurrence rate is low and patients with particularly malignant primary tumors are in theory cured in the absence of metastasis. Free margins can be achieved by identifying a tumor-free corridor which allow delivery of the neural tissues. Immediate soft-tissue and osseous reconstruction reduces the overall wound complication and non-union rate and improves construct survival.

Pearls

- The main goals of en-bloc resection of primary tumors in the spine are (1) to reduce the local recurrence rate and (2) improve survival.
- Whether en-bloc resection is possible depends on the presence of a tumor-free corridor through which the spinal cord or cauda equina can be separated from the tumor tissue.
- Delivery through a tumor-free corridor yields clear margins and avoids tumor breach via a planned pediculotomy.
- Depending on the biology and anatomical spread of the tumor, the morbidity of an en-bloc resection has to be weighed against the potential and desired benefits of clear tumor margins.

References

1. Boriani S, Saravanja D, Yamada Y, Varga PP, Biagini R, Fisher CG. Challenges of local recurrence and cure in low grade malignant tumors of the spine. Spine (Phila Pa 1976). 2009;34(22 Suppl):S48–57.
2. Boriani S, Weinstein JN, Biagini R. Primary bone tumors of the spine. Terminology and surgical staging. Spine (Phila Pa 1976). 1997;22(9):1036–44.
3. Dolan RT, Butler JS, Wilson-MacDonald J, Reynolds J, Cogswell L, Critchley P, Giele H. Quality of life and surgical outcomes after soft-tissue reconstruction of complex oncologic defects of the spine and sacrum. J Bone Joint Surg Am. 2016;98(2):117–26.
4. Fisher CG, Keynan O, Boyd MC, Dvorak MF. The surgical management of primary tumorsof the spine: initial results of an ongoing prospective cohort study. Spine (Phila Pa 1976). 2005;30(16):1899–908.
5. Tomita K, Kawahara N, Baba H, Tsuchiya H, Fujita T, Toribatake Y. Total en bloc spondylectomy. A new surgical technique for primary malignant vertebral tumors. Spine (Phila Pa 1976). 1997;22(3):324–33.

Primary Bone Tumour Indication and Planning of En Bloc Resection

62

Dominique A. Rothenfluh and Etienne Bourassa-Moreau

62.1 Introduction

Challenging diagnosis, complex decision making, technically demanding operative intervention and major risks for morbidity and mortality puts management of spinal primary tumour at the highest level of surgical complexity. Surgical indications and procedures must be carefully assessed and individualized for each patient with a primary spinal neoplasm.

The en-bloc resection technique involves the removal of the neoplastic lesion in one piece, as a whole, with either a cuff of normal tissue circumferentially or as a marginal resection with intact tumor pseudocapsule [1]. The aim of en-bloc resection is to remove the tumor while minimizing the risk of local recurrence and provide a chance for cure. Achievability of en-bloc resection depends on a multidisciplinary approach, careful surgical planning and a high level of surgical expertise. Proper technical execution often requires a lengthy demanding procedure but has been shown repeatedly to have a significant impact on mortality and morbidity [6].

This chapter aims to illustrate patient selection, workup and surgical planning of the en-bloc resections for primary spinal tumours.

D. A. Rothenfluh (✉) · E. Bourassa-Moreau
Oxford University Hospitals NHS Foundation Trust, Nuffield Orthopaedic Centre, Oxford, UK

62.1.1 Presentation and Clinical Workup

Patients presenting with primary spinal tumours are extremely rare with an estimated incidence of 2.5–8.5 cases per million inhabitants per year. This rarity makes initial recognition of primary spinal tumours amongst the very common degenerative spinal pain challenging. The demographic profile, pain pattern, the un-responsiveness to conservative management and history of systemic illness should trigger further investigation. Unfortunately, many patients have their diagnosis delayed or missed resulting in inappropriate management and sub-optimal outcomes. The most common presentation of patients with primary spinal tumours is pain in 76% of primary benign lesions and 95% of malignant lesions [4]. Pain patterns can be distinguished between mechanical, neurological and oncologic.

Local and systemic staging is needed to fully characterise the extent of any suspected neoplastic spinal lesion. Local staging includes standard X-ray, CT-Scan and MRI-Scan of the affected area of the spine. Standard or CT angiography should be ordered whenever the vascularity of the tumour or its relation to adjacent major vessels can possibly affect surgical planning. Systemic

B. Meyer, M. Rauschmann (eds.), *Spine Surgery*, https://doi.org/10.1007/978-3-319-98875-7_62

Histology	Local Extent	Metastasis	Stage	Margins of control
Benign				
G0	Intracompartimental (T0)	None (M0)	1	Intralesional + Local adjuvant
G0	Intracompartimental (T0)	None (M0)	2	Intra-lesional
G0	Intracompartimental (T1)	None (M0)	3	Marginal En Block excision
Malignant				
Low (G1)	Intracompartimental (T1)	None (M0)	IA	Wide (En Bloc)
Low (G1)	Extracompartimental (T2)	None (M0)	IB	Wide (En Bloc)
High (G2)	Intracompartimental (T1)	None (M0)	IIA	Wide (En Bloc) + Adjuvant
High (G2)	Extracompartimental (T2)	None (M0)	IIB	Wide (En Bloc) + Adjuvant
Any (G)	Any (T)	Regional or Distant (M1)	III	Paliative surgery, Intralesional

Fig. 62.1 The Enneking classification and suggested treatment. (Enneking et al. [5])

staging includes chest, abdominal, pelvic and brain CT-Scan looking for distant metastasis.

The last step of the work-up includes a CT-guided percutaneous biopsy. The biopsy should be done after all imaging modalities to avoid altering the radiological anatomy. It should be performed by a skilled interventional radiologist aware of the suspected diagnosis. The biopsy trajectory should ideally be excisable at the time of surgical en-bloc resection. The specimens are sent for both cultures and pathological analysis. A pathologist experienced with musculo-skeletal tumours is required to provide a final opinion on the histology of the tissue.

62.1.2 Classification and Surgical Indications

A multidisciplinary team including pathologist, medical oncologist, radiation oncologist, radiologist and a spine surgeon is required to provide the best care for primary spinal tumours. The multidisciplinary team meets at the tumour board to discuss the final diagnosis, combining the information provided by pathology, radiology and clinical assessment. The surgeon and radiologist will discuss the local extent of the tumour and the presence of systemic metastasis. The Enneking classification is used as a framework to categorize the disease and plan for surgical resection (Fig. 62.1). Although this classification was initially described for the appendicular skeleton [5], its reliability and validity for spinal tumours was demonstrated [3]. The Enneking classification dictates the most appropriate surgical margin of resection to seize the best chance of local and systemic control.

Terminology of surgical margins is essential to describe the surgical resection strategy, communicate between surgeons and report outcomes. The margins of surgical resection are described as intra-lesional, marginal or wide (Fig. 62.2) [2]. Intra-lesional margin denotes transgression of the plane between normal tissue and the lesion. It encompasses various surgical techniques including curettage, debulking and gross total removal. An intra-lesional margin is appropriate for benign lesions or known metastatic lesions. A marginal margin is accomplished in the reactive zone or pseudo capsule surrounding the tumour. Marginal margins are appropriate when benign but locally aggressive lesions are resected to prevent local recurrence. Wide margins described a dissection through a cuff of normal tissue around the tumour, beyond the reactive zone. Wide margins provide better survival and local control

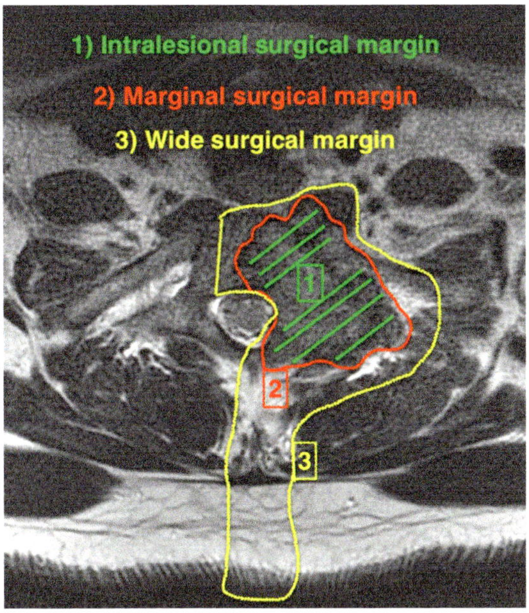

Fig. 62.2 Examples of intralesional, marginal and wide surgical margin applied the clinical case. The intralesional margins violate the plane between normal and neoplastic tissue regardless of how much of the tumour was macroscopically removed. The marginal margins refer to dissection in the reactive zone around the pseudo capsule of the tumour. Wide margin is through a cuff of normal tissue away a zone of possible micrometastasis. Note that adjacent to the epidural plane all margins converge because of the necessity to separate the tumour from the neurological tissue to avoid amputation of the spinal cord

for malignant lesions with no metastasis. However, in some cases of malignant primary spinal tumours, a wide resection can be quite morbid because it involves the resection of vascular and neurological structures. Radical resection was described for the appendicular skeleton, involves the resection of the entire bony compartment and it is almost never performed in the spine given the significant neurological morbidity. Wide and marginal margins are achieved through the en bloc resection technique.

Once the most appropriate margin is determined the execution of surgical resection can be planned using the Weinstein-Boriani-Bigiani surgical staging system. Using Axial imaging the vertebral unit is divided in twelve 30° radiating sectors numbered counter clockwise from 1 to 12 starting on the left side of the spinous process. Figure 62.3 The tissue layers are classified in alphabetical order from periphery to centre from *A* to *E*. This topographic classification helps delimitate the margin of surgical resection and formulate the surgical plan as illustrated in the following case.

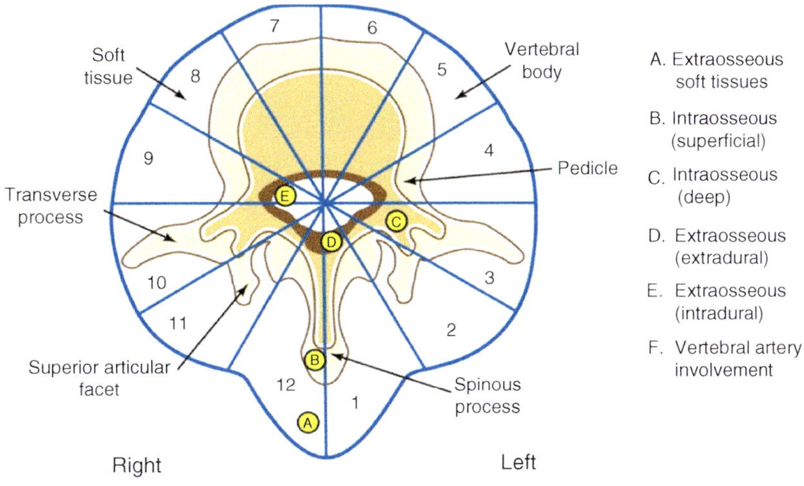

Fig. 62.3 The Weinstein-Boriani-Biagini consist in the topographical organization of the vertebra in 12 radiating sectors in the axial plane. The numbering of these sectors goes counter-clockwise from the left side of the spinous process (sector 1) to the right side of the spinous process (sector 12). Five concentric layers of tissue are ordered alphabetically from periphery to center

62.2 Case Description

62.2.1 Presentation

A 38 years old male sought medical attention after a 10 months history of low cervical pain radiating to the left middle, ring and little fingers. He denied any history of weight loss, night sweat or malignancy. The physical exam showed a positive left Spurling test, decreased left tricipital reflex, 4/5 weakness in left finger flexion and abduction. Neurological assessment was otherwise normal with no signs of myelopathy.

The CT-scan ordered by the primary physician showed a well demarcated lesion of C7 and T1 centred on the left laminae, vertebral body and transverse processes. This lesion was encasing the C8 nerve root exit foramina and into the left side of the spinal canal. An MRI-Scan confirmed the extent of the lesion and showed a relatively low T2 signal and suggested the presence of an osteoid matrix (Fig. 62.4).

Chest, abdomen and pelvis CT-scans showed no metastasis. A percutaneous biopsy was performed by the radiologist involved in the tumour board (Fig. 62.5). Dense collagen with small foci of osteoid formation, within the fibrous tissue cluster of polygonal cells with clear vacuolated cytoplasm were found and a large number of multinucleated osteoclast like giant cells with mild to moderate nuclear variability. Cultures and stains did not identify the presence of a micro-organism. The differential diagnosis included osteoblastoma, giant cell tumour or aneurysmal bone cyst. A follow-up MRI was repeated 4 month after his initial imaging to confirm the stability of the lesion.

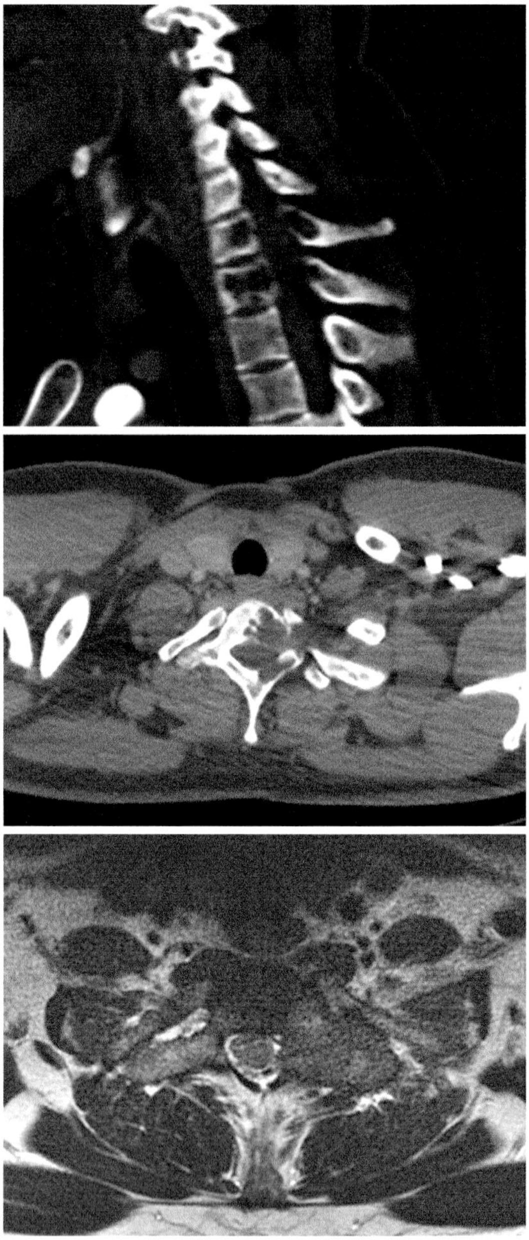

Fig. 62.4 Cervical CT-scan and showing a well demarcated lesion of C7 and T1 centred on the left lamina, vertebral body and transverse processes. Note the encasement of the left C8 nerve root and the relatively low T2 signal

62.2.2 Surgical Planning

Applying the Enneking classification to our patient, his lesion was classified as benign locally aggressive lesion with extra-compartmental involvement on the left side. WBB sectors 2 to 7 were involved in the tumour with the left C8 and possibly T1 nerve roots encroached by the tumour (Fig. 62.6). It was concluded that en-bloc resection would be feasible with the ligation of the left C8 and possibly T1 nerve root. For the planning of surgical resection, the help of a plastic, general, ENT or cardio-vascular surgeon can be useful depending on the surrounding tissues involved.

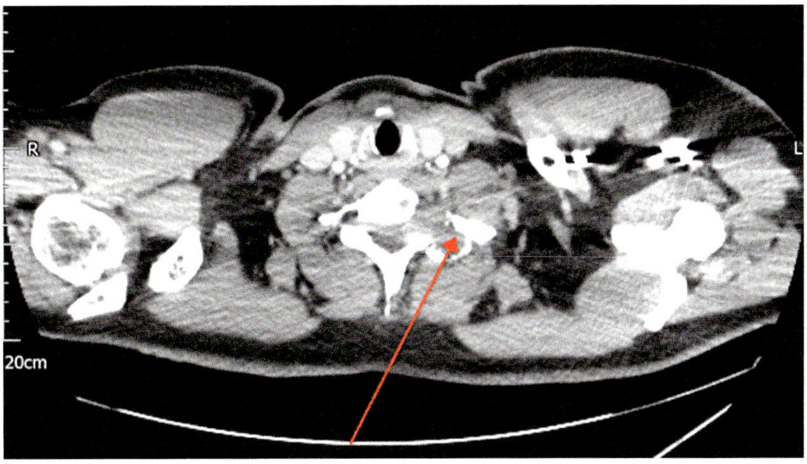

Fig. 62.5 Percutaneous trocar biopsy is performed by a skilled interventional radiologist. Specimen are sent to both microbiology and pathology. The biopsy tract is planned to be potentially included with the EnBloc specimen at the time of the resection

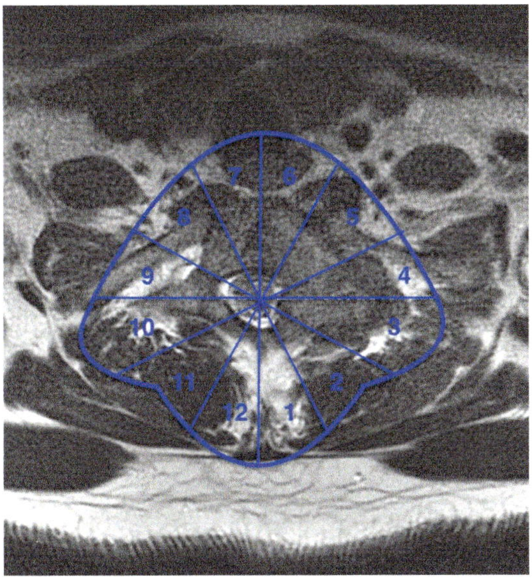

Fig. 62.6 The WBB diagram applied to a T2 MRI axial cut of our case. Note that the radiating sectors 2 to 7 are involved and sectors 11 to 1 represent the tumour free window necessary to access the epidural plane, explore the dural tissue and section the left C8 and T1 nerve roots

The critical surgical steps divided by anterior and posterior approach are presented in Figs. 62.7 and 62.8 respectively.

Anterior Approach Goals (Fig. 62.7)

1. Sub-periosteal dissection of sectors 7 to 8.
2. Wide dissection of the sectors 6 to 4.
3. Surgical ligation of the C8 nerve roots exiting the intervertebral foramen.
4. Anterior part of a sagittal osteotomy through the Sector 8.
5. Cranial and Caudal release of the C7 and T1 specimens with C6-C7 and T1-T2 discectomies and left sided T1 and T2 rib head resection (not shown on Fig. 62.7).

Posterior Approach Goals (Fig. 62.8)

1. Extra-lesional window through sectors 11, 12 and 1.
2. Wide margin dissection of the sectors 2 and 3.
3. Free the epidural plane and section of the encased C8 nerve root.
4. Sagittal osteotomy through the sector C8.
5. En-Bloc removal of the tumour.
6. Posterior instrumented fusion from C4 to T5 and reconstruction of the anterior column support (not shown on Fig. 62.8).

62.2.3 Surgical Intervention

The surgical resection was divided into anterior and posterior stages. It was planned over a single day but the option of a second day was considered.

62.2.3.1 First Stage Anterior Approach

The patient was positioned supine on a radiolucent table.

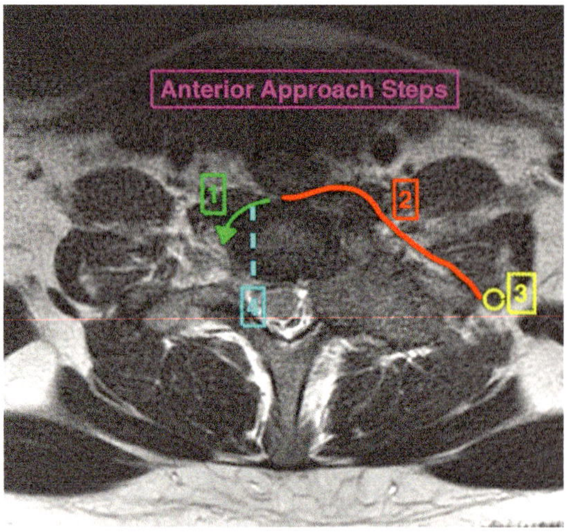

Fig. 62.7 The critical steps of En Bloc excision of C7 and T1 vertebra. The steps of the anterior approach are as follow: (1) sub-periosteal dissection (Layer B of sectors 7 and 8); (2) Wide dissection (Layer A of sectors 4 to 6); (3) Ligation and section of the left C8 nerve roots; (4) Sagittal osteotomy through the Sector 8; (5) Cranial and Caudal release of the C7 and T1 specimens with C6-C7 and T1-T2 discectomies and left sided T1 and T2 rib head resection (not shown)

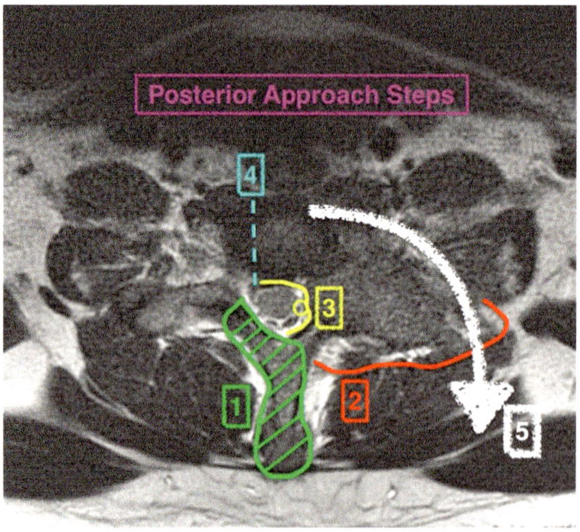

Fig. 62.8 The critical steps of En Bloc excision of C7 and T1 vertebra explained. The steps of the posterior approach are as follow: (**1**) Extra-lesional window (sectors 1, 11 and 12); (**2**) Wide margin dissection (Layer A sectors 2 and 3); (**3**) Dissection of the epidural plane (layer E setctors 2 to 7) and section of the encased C8 nerve root; (**4**) Sagittal osteotomy of C7 and T1; (**5**) En-Bloc removal of the tumour; (**6**) Posterior instrumented fusion from C4 to T5 and reconstruction of the anterior column support (not shown)

A "Z" extensile approach left sided was performed. A cardiovascular surgeon assisted the surgical approach in case a sternotomy would be needed. To achieve marginal margins, the dissection on the left side of C7 and T1 was made superficial to over the left longus colli (sectors 3 to 6) all the way to the transverse processes.

Using a bone scalpel, A sagittal osteotomy was done through the right fourth of the C6 and T1 vertebral body (Fig. 62.7). C6-C7 and T1-T2 discectomies were used to disconnect C7 and T1 cranially and caudally. The discectomies were extended laterally to resect the muscle belly of the left longus colli and resect the left T1 and T2 rib head.

An anterior cervical plate was selected to span the resected vertebra and secured to C6 and T2 vertebral bodies. The wound was then closed over a drain and the patient was turned prone.

62.2.3.2 Second Stage Posterior Approach

A posterior midline incision was performed from C5 to T4. Posterior dissection followed a wide surgical margin. Sub-periosteal dissection was carried out on the right side (sectors 9 to 12) and trans-muscular dissection (through sectors 1 to 3) was carried out on the left side (Fig. 62.8). The left dissection was extended laterally all the way to the left T1 and T2 ribs, which were exposed further laterally. The release of posterior elements started with the disconnection of the left T1 and T2 ribs. The first rib was divided and a portion of the second rib was removed as a strut graft.

Than the caudal part of C6 Lamina and cranial part of T2 Lamina were removed followed by a right hemi-laminectomy through C7 and T1. Right sided C5 and C6 lateral mass screws and T2, T3 pedicle screws were inserted and a rod inserted.

At that time-point, in light of copious amount of epidural bleeding and transient change in neuro-monitoring, the decision was made to postpone the remainder of the procedure.

The patient was brought back to the operating room at a later stage to finish the posterior part of the procedure. The posterior wound was reopened and washed-out.

The epidural plane was carefully released circumferentially without any retraction on the spinal cord. Using the bone scalpel, the sagittal osteotomy was completed through the posterior wall to reach the sagittal osteotomy line performed from the anterior approach. The C7 and T1 left nerve roots were unroofed from their foramen and mobilized laterally. The left C8 nerve root was ligated and sectioned in the epidural plane as planned. At that point the whole lesion was released from all attachments and entirely free to be delivered. The delivery was carried through gentle rolling movement to the left with greatest care to avoid excessive traction on the spinal cord, C7 and T1 nerve roots.

The specimen was carefully inspected and no macroscopic margin violation was noted. The vertebral defect was filled with an expanding PEEK cage and with some bone autograft. The posterior instrumentation was completed. Biplanar x-rays confirmed the appropriate position of the surgical implants (Fig. 62.9). The wound was irrigated and closed.

62.2.3.3 Post-operative Course

As expected, the post-operative neurological assessment revealed a left C8 sensory-motor deficit with insensate ulnar border of the left hand, flickers (1/5) of long finger flexors and abductors. Otherwise the post-operative course went uneventfully.

Postoperatively, the pathology team reviewed the intra-operative specimen. Successful C7 and T1 en -bloc resection without violation of the tumour margins was confirmed. However, after molecular studies, the diagnosis was changed from osteoblastoma to low grade osteogenic osteosarcoma.

The 2-year follow-up demonstrated absence of local recurrence or systemic metastasis (Figs. 62.9 and 62.10). The patient will still be followed up every year with MRI (Fig. 62.11).

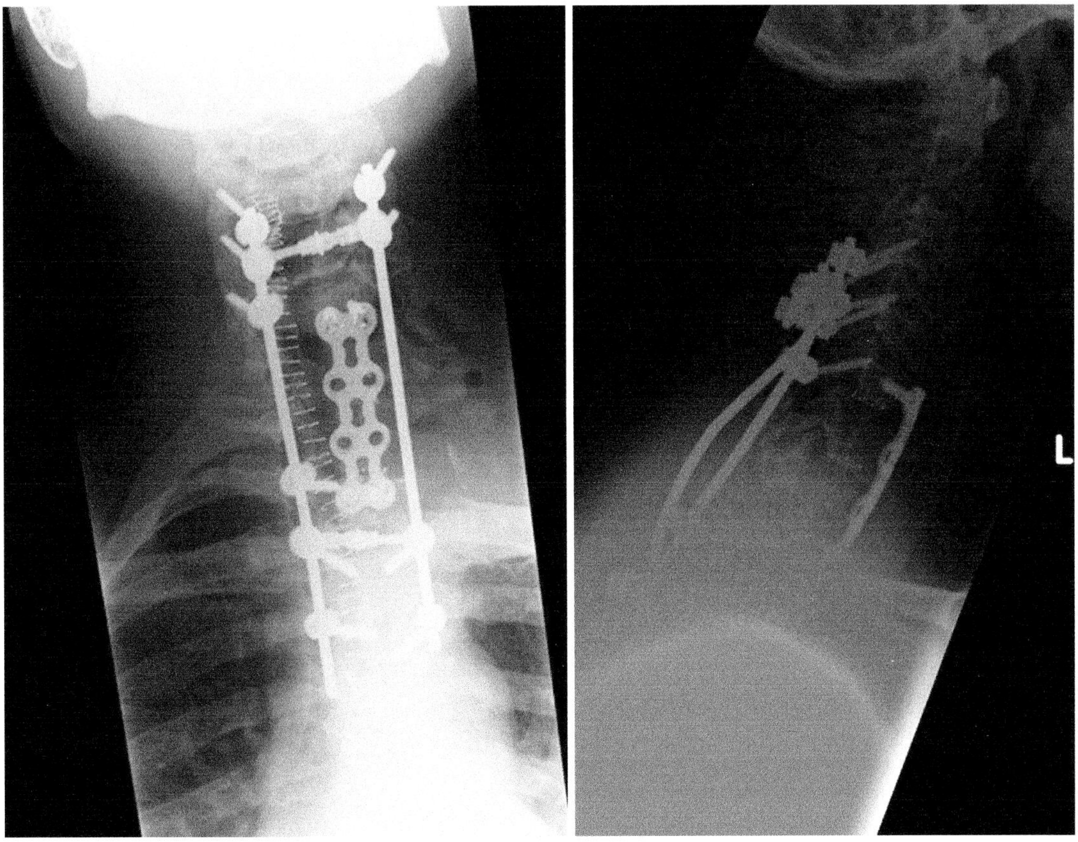

Fig. 62.9 Early post-operative imaging of C7-T1 En-Bloc resection and reconstruction of cervico-thoracic spine

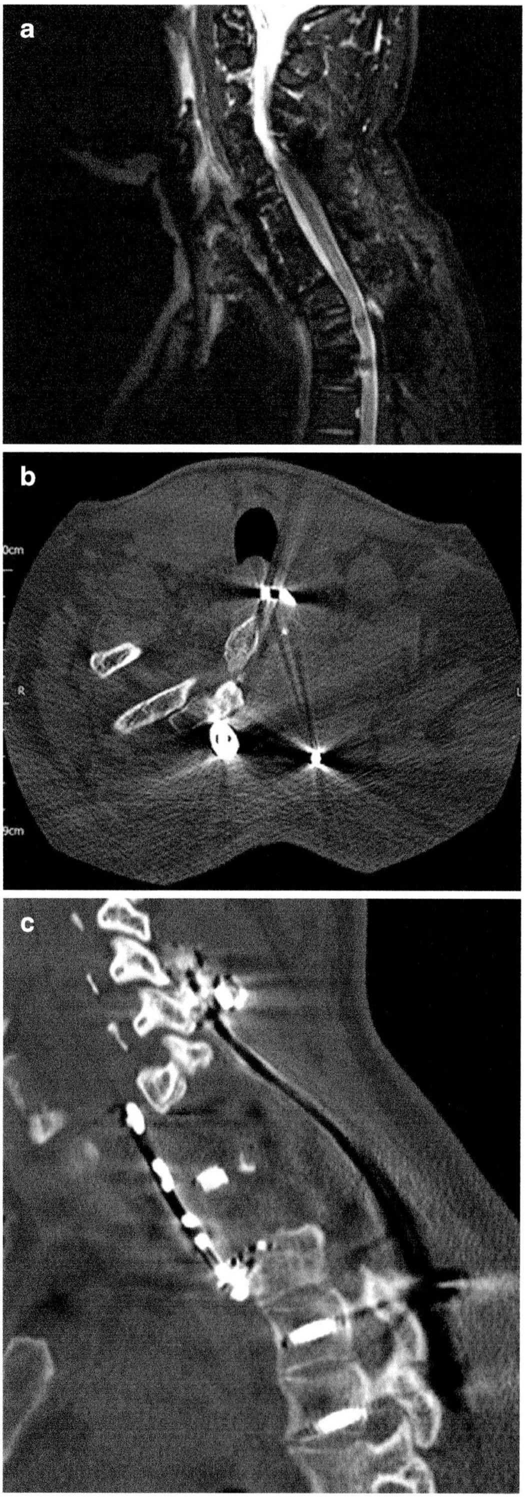

Fig. 62.10 Ct scan and MRI demonstrating the absence of local recurrence. Note the radiolucent peek cage that minimizes artefacts around the zone at risk of local recurrence

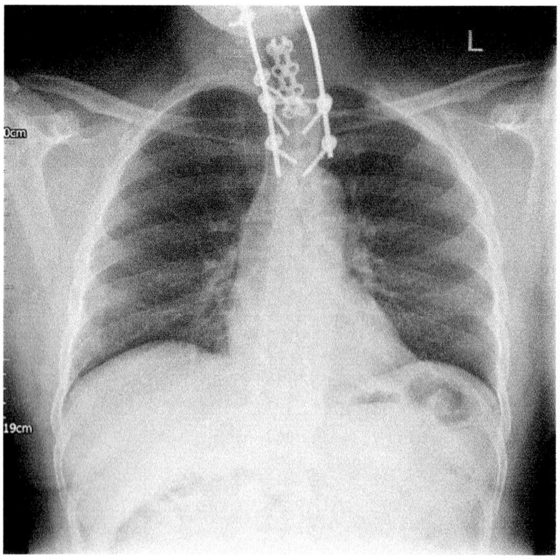

Fig. 62.11 Chest X-ray demonstrating the absence of pulmonary metastasis 2 year after enbloc resection of the primary spinal tumor

62.2.4 Discussion

En-bloc resection requires a tremendous amount of resources at the surgical, medical and patient level. Appropriate indications for en-bloc resection are rare and, even when indicated, it comes at the cost of significant morbidity and at the risk of major complications. This case demonstrates two different indications of en-bloc resection. Although initially the goal of the en-bloc resection was mainly that of local control for a benign locally aggressive tumour, interestingly, the shift in diagnosis towards a malignant pathology suggested that the en-bloc resection was also beneficial for improved survival of the patient. While an intra-lesional resection may have been justified given the initial differential diagnosis, the size and potential causes prompted an en-bloc resection as it was deemed feasible. This was retrospectively the right decision, as an intra-lesional resection of even a low-grade osteosarcoma would have most likely lead to local recurrence and would have been associated with a poor prognosis.

The rationale for en-bloc resection is to obtain the best local control of the growing tumour with a single surgical intervention. With such a benign locally aggressive lesion (Enneking Stage 3) intra-lesional resection entails local recurrence and potentially multiple revision surgery. Revision surgeries for primary tumour are associated with higher complication and higher recurrence rate.

It was explained to the patient that to obtain the best control of local recurrence, sacrifice of the left C8 and T1 nerve roots would be needed. Only after a thorough discussion about the expected morbidity, the potential benefits and risks of an en-bloc excision of C7 and T1, the patient consented for the procedure.

En-bloc resection is not always feasible without compromising neurological function significantly. For en-bloc resection to be achievable without significant neurological morbidity two conditions have to be met:

1. A sector of the vertebral ring can be removed outside the tumor margins to create a tumour-free window. This window should be wide enough to allow delivery of the tumor without traction on the spinal cord or cauda equina.
2. Any nerve roots involved with the tumour can be reached outside the tumor margin to be tied off at the epidural space and ligated.

Additionally, in the cervical spine the vertebral artery might have to be sacrificed to respect the oncological surgical margin. The consequence of unilateral vertebral artery sacrifice depends on the anatomy of the variable anatomy of the basilar artery system. A pre-operative angiogram and balloon-occlusion test can help to predict the ischemic consequences of scarifying the vertebral artery [7].

Very importantly, the patient must be involved in the surgical decision making. The amount of morbidity associated with the proposed procedure has to be explained to the patient and his family. Ultimately, the patient decides if the potentially improved survival outweigh the surgical risks and morbidity with often associated loss of neurological function.

For the planning of surgical resection, the help of plastic surgeon, general surgeon, ENT surgeon and cardio-vascular surgeon can also be useful depending on the surrounding tissues involved.

62.2.5 Conclusions and Take Home Message

Primary spinal tumours are challenging to diagnose and treat. Experienced, dedicated multidisciplinary teams deliver the most appropriate care for these rare patients.

The Enneking classification is used to determine the oncological surgical margins and the Weinstein-Boriani-Biagini classification is of help to plan the feasibility of the resection.

En-Bloc resection technique is among the most complex and challenging surgical interventions. However, despite the invasiveness and morbidity associated with en-bloc resection, there are numerous reports to support its benefits in improving local control and survival in primary spinal tumours. Even in seemingly benign tumours, en-bloc resection may be indicated if feasible, as the diagnosis can change particularly in larger and invasive benign tumours. If intralesional resection had been carried out in this case, then the only chance of a surgical cure would have been missed.

References

1. Boriani S, Gasbarrini A, Bandiera S, Ghermandi R, Lador R. En bloc resections in the spine: the experience of 220 patients during 25 years. World Neurosurg. 2017;98:217–29.
2. Boriani S, Weinstein JN, Biagini R. Primary bone tumors of the spine. Terminology and surgical staging. Spine (Phila Pa 1976). 1997;22(9):1036–44.
3. Chan P, Boriani S, Fourney DR, Biagini R, Dekutoski MB, Fehlings MG, Ryken TC, Gokaslan ZL, Vrionis FD, Harrop JS, Schmidt MH, Vialle LR, Gerszten PC, Rhines LD, Ondra SL, Pratt SR, Fisher CG. An assessment of the reliability of the Enneking and Weinstein-Boriani-Biagini classifications for staging of primary spinal tumors by the Spine Oncology Study Group. Spine (Phila Pa 1976). 2009;34(4):384–91.
4. Dreghorn CR, Newman RJ, Hardy GJ, Dickson RA. Primary tumors of the axial skeleton. Experience of the Leeds Regional Bone Tumor Registry. Spine (Phila Pa 1976). 1990;15(2):137–40.
5. Enneking WF, Spanier SS, Goodman MA. A system for the surgical staging of musculoskeletal sarcoma. Clin Orthop Relat Res. 1980;(153):106–20.
6. Fisher CG, Saravanja DD, Dvorak MF, Rampersaud YR, Clarkson PW, Hurlbert J, Fox R, Zhang H,

Lewis S, Riaz S, Ferguson PC, Boyd MC. Surgical management of primary bone tumors of the spine: validation of an approach to enhance cure and reduce local recurrence. Spine (Phila Pa 1976). 2011;36(10):830–6.

7. Ogungbemi A, Elwell V, Choi D, Robertson F. Permanent endovascular balloon occlusion of the vertebral artery as an adjunct to the surgical resection of selected cervical spine tumors: a single center experience. Interv Neuroradiol. 2015;21(4):532–7.

63 Minimally Invasive (Long) Dorsal Instrumentation Including Augmentation for Metastasis

Ehab Shiban and Bernhard Meyer

63.1 Introduction

The Spine is the most common osseous site for metastatic disease. In the past, because of the overall limited survival, a simple palliative approach was advocated for the majority of those patients. However, with the on-going improvements in oncology patients are now living much longer, therefore there have been a paradigm shift towards more aggressive treatment regimes. For spinal metastases with epidural compression standard of care has become decompression and instrumentation of the affected level. Thereby minimal invasive surgery (MIS) is being successfully utilized in order to reduce operative morbidity, hospital stay and soft tissue trauma. Thereby postoperative chemotherapy and radiotherapy can be initiated more rapidly.

This chapter will illustrate the various MIS techniques with emphasis on their efficacy and level of evidence for the treatment of spinal metastases. At the end of this chapter the readers should be able to describe the various minimal invasive techniques used for spinal metastases and well as discuss their benefits over the standard open approaches.

E. Shiban (✉) · B. Meyer
Department of Neurosurgery, Klinikum rechts der Isar, Technische Universität München, Munich, Germany
e-mail: Ehab.shiban@tum.de

The aim of the presented case is to illustrate a case of MIS instrumentation for metastatic spine disease.

63.2 Case Description

63.2.1 Case I

A 54 year-old female patient with a known breast cancer presented abroad with a 2 months history of persisting mid thoracic back pain. Magnetic resonance imaging (MRI) and computer tomography (CT) scans of the thoracic spine revealed a fracture to the 8th thoracic vertebrae (Figs. 63.1 and 63.2). Presumably a pathologic fracture due to the known history of breast cancer the patient underwent cement augmentation via vertebroplasty and biopsy of the 8th thoracic vertebrae. Thereafter she was relieved of her symptoms for 4 months. Biopsy did not reveal any cancer cells. Therefore there was no adjuvant treatment. 5 months thereafter she presented to out department with a 1 months history of mid thoracic back pain once more. Plan radiographs and CT scan showed local kyphosis of the thoracic spine at the vertebroplasty level (Fig. 63.3). We then performed percutaneous stabilization above and below the index level (cement augmented pedicle

B. Meyer, M. Rauschmann (eds.), *Spine Surgery*, https://doi.org/10.1007/978-3-319-98875-7_63

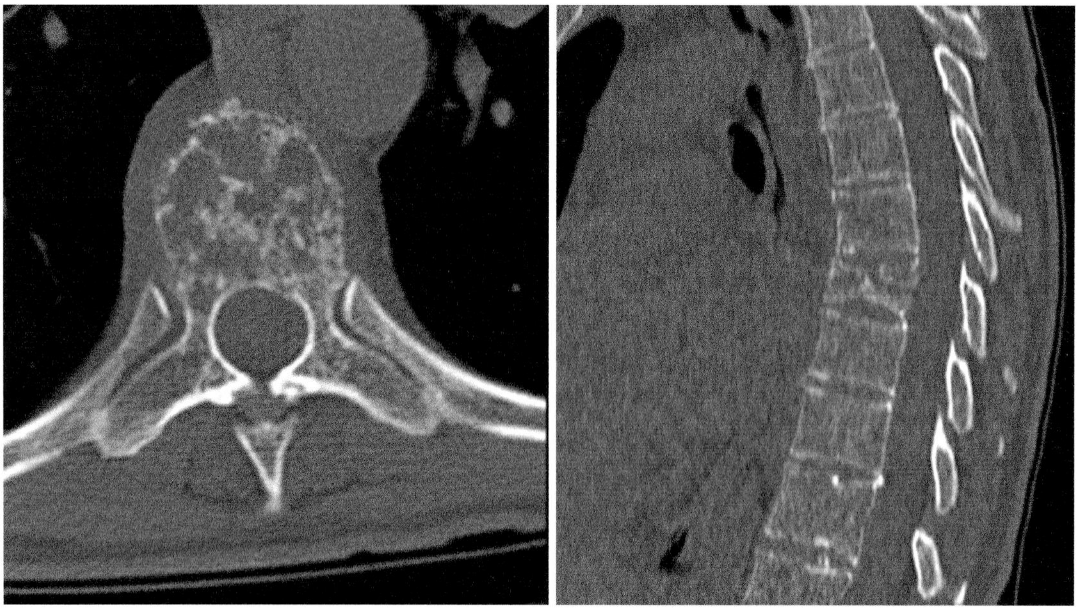

Fig. 63.1 CT scan to the thoracic spine illustrating an osteolytic lesion of the 8th thoracic vertebrae with a slight vertebral body collapse

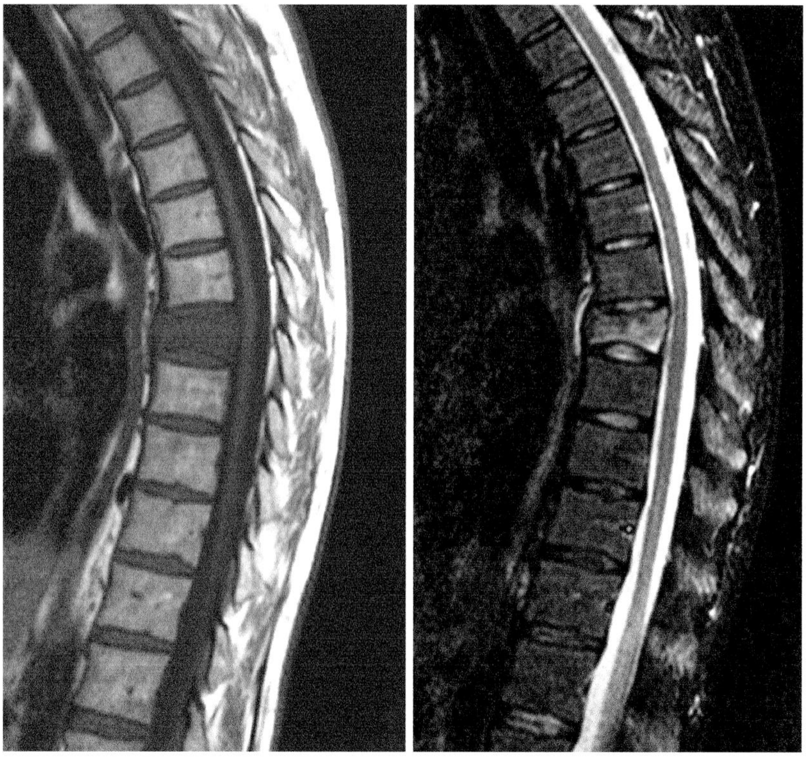

Fig. 63.2 MRI scan to the thoracic spine illustrating a gadolinium enhancing lesion to the 8th thoracic vertebrae

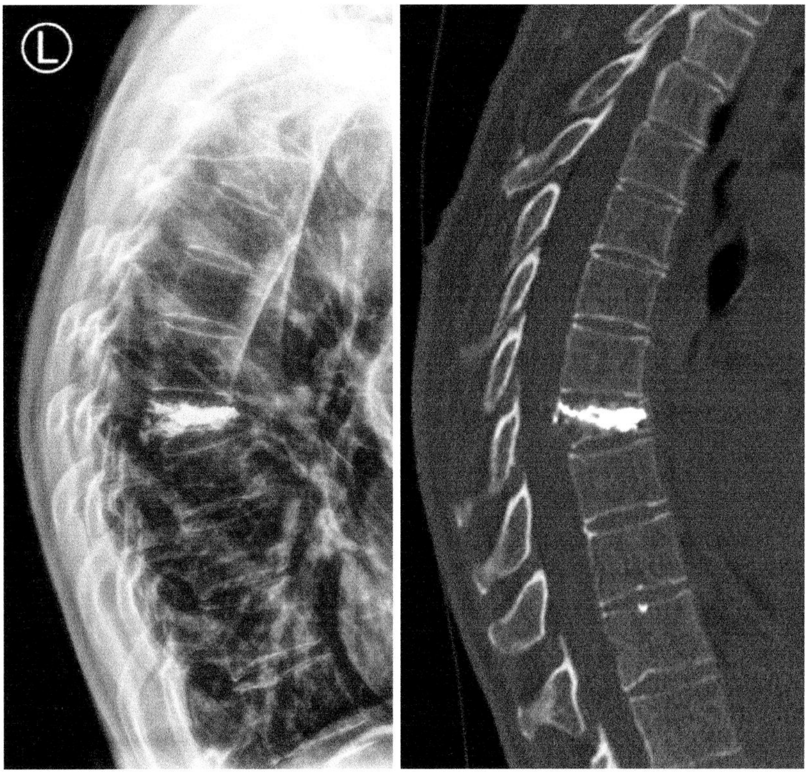

Fig. 63.3 (Left) plain radiograph (right) CT scan demonstrating local kyphosis to the thoracic spine following vertebroplasty to the 8th vertebrae

screws th6-th7-th9-th10; Fig. 63.4) followed by corpectomy and expandable titanium cage placement through a mini-open transthoracic approach (Fig. 63.5). Histopathology from the second surgery was positive for cancer. The patients had an uneventful postoperative recovery and underwent radiotherapy 3 weeks postoperatively.

63.2.2 Case II

A 53 year-old male patient with a known history of malignant melanoma presented with 3 weeks history of persisting mid thoracic back pain. Magnetic resonance imaging (MRI) and computer tomography (CT) scans of the thoracic spine revealed a fracture to the 5th thoracic vertebrae (Fig. 63.6). He had a SINS score of 11. We performed minimal invasive pedicle screw instrumentation using carbon/PEEK screws and corpectomy and replacement via a posterior approach with a PEEK cage all in one surgery (Figs. 63.7 and 63.8). 3 weeks thereafter, she underwent stereotactic radiosurgery.

63.3 Discussion of the Cases

63.3.1 Why Were Things Done This Way

63.3.1.1 Case I

At initial presentation abroad the patient presented with pain and an osteolytic lesion in a semirigid segment of the spine (3rd – 10th Thoracic vertebra) with vertebral body collapse less than 50% without deformity or posterior element involvement. Ergo the patient had a Spinal Instability Neoplastic Score (SINS) [2] score of 8 (Table 63.1). Stabilization could have been recommended initially however cement augmentation for this suspected pathologic fracture with intermediate instability (SINS score 7–12) might also be performed. At presentation in our department the patient had already failed this minimal invasive approach and had developed pain but also a local kyphosis. Therefore stabilization was needed. In order to facilitate for rapid postoperative radiotherapy by reducing the surgical wound

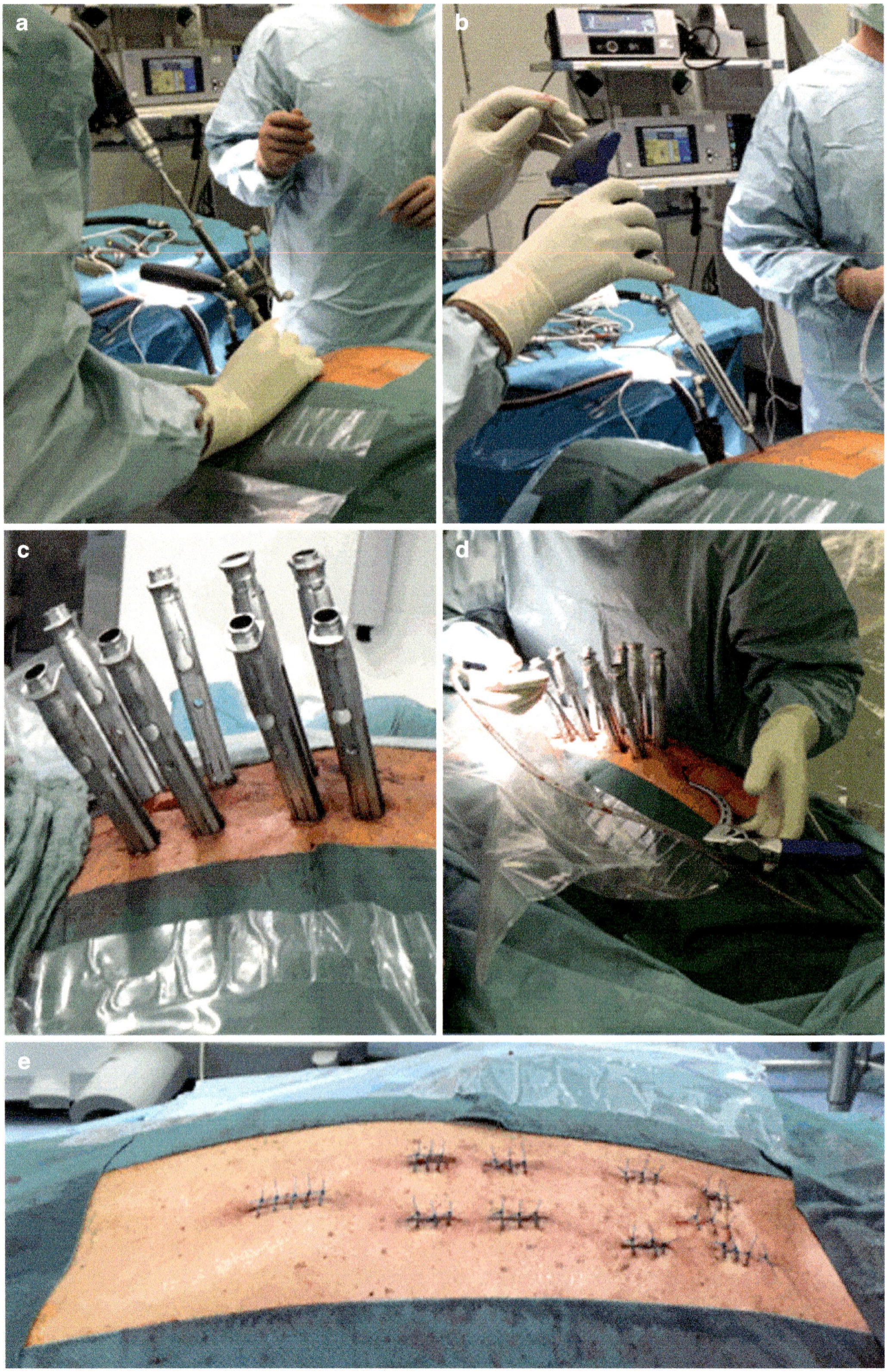

Fig. 63.4 Operative picture of percutaneous pedicle screw placement (**a**) navigation assisted K-Wire placement (**b**, **c**) pedicle screw placement (**d**) percutaneous rod insertion (**e**) the multiple small incisions needed

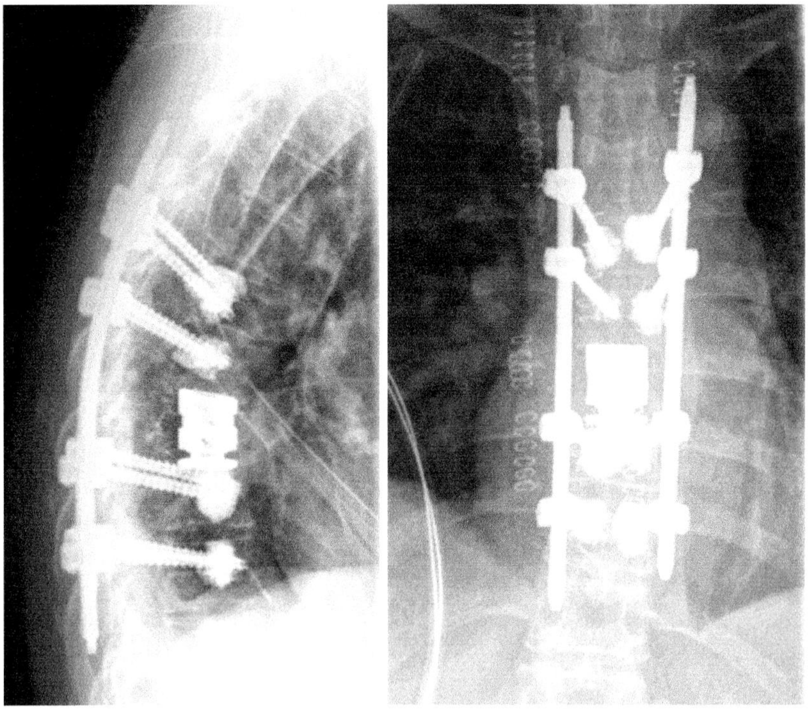

Fig. 63.5 Postoperative plan radiograph demonstrating the cement augmented pedicle scew stabilisation and vertebral body replacement with an expandable titanium cage

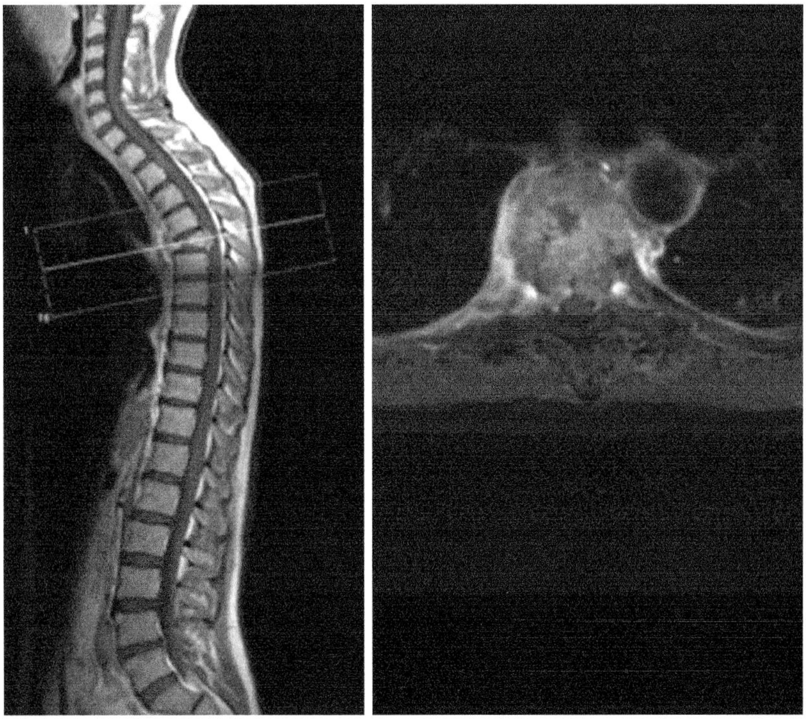

Fig. 63.6 MRI scan to the thoracic spine illustrating a gadolinium enhancing lesion to the 8th thoracic vertebrae with epidural spinal cord compression

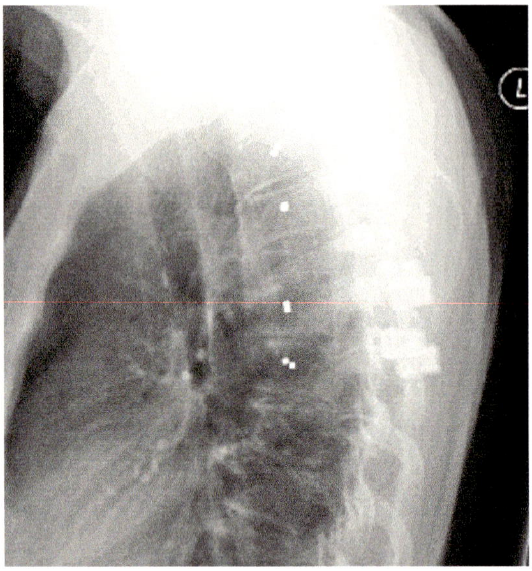

Fig. 63.7 Postoperative plan radiograph demonstrating the Carbon/PEEK pedicle scews and vertebral body replacement with a PEEK cage

and hospital stay duration, percutaneous stabilisation followed by corpectomy and replacement via a mini-open approach 3 days thereafter were performed. Radiotherapy ensued 3 weeks postoperatively because the diagnosis of metastatic disease was confirmed.

63.3.1.2 Case II

He presented with a painful metastases with a SINS score of 11 with an otherwise stable disease and good clinical status. Therefore Instrumentation was deemed necessary. To facilitate for long-term stability a 360° instrumentation was planned. Because this was the upper thoracic region, making an anterolateral approach due to the great vessels very demanding, a single step surgical approach was most appropriate. The usage of radiolucent PEEK/carbon composite implants is believed to better than titanium implants because of better postoperative imaging and to facilitate for more accurate radiosurgical planning.

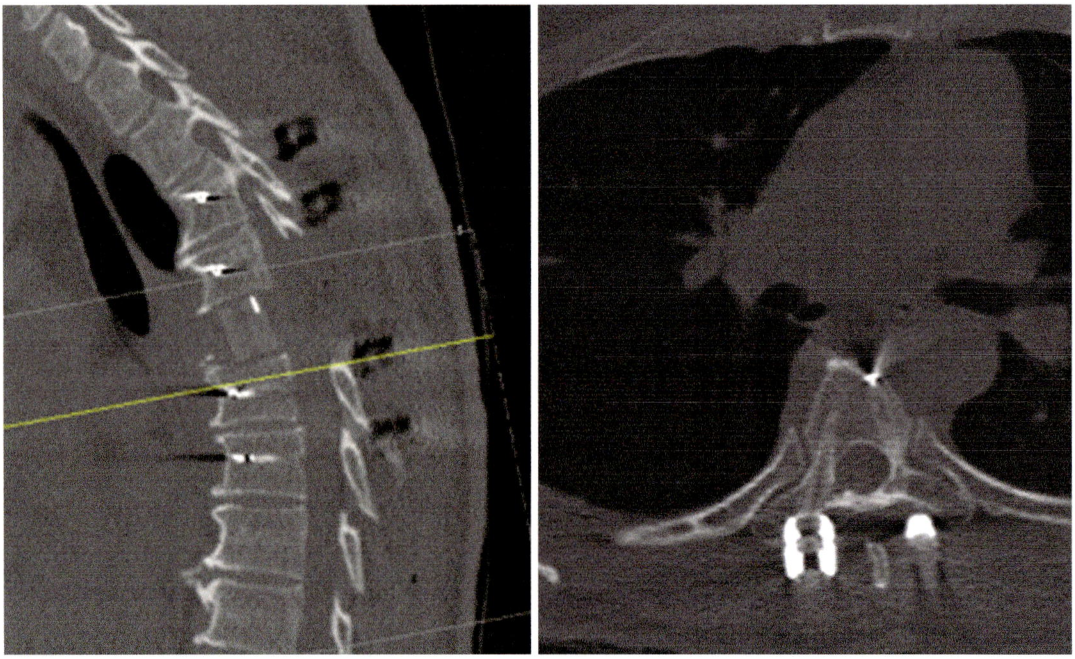

Fig. 63.8 Postoperative CT scan demonstrating the Carbon/PEEK pedicle scews and vertebral body replacement with a PEEK cage

63.3.2 Were They in Accordance with the Literature Guidelines

The main indications for surgical treatment are epidural spinal cord compression or spinal instability. To access spinal instability the Spine Oncology Study Group introduced the 18-point Spinal Instability Neoplastic Score (SINS) [2]. Spinal metastases with high scores (13–18) are considered unstable and require surgical intervention (Table 63.1). For patients with epidural spinal cord compression and neurological deficits the role of surgery was made clear more than two decades ago. The seminal publication by Patchell et. could clearly show that surgical decompression followed by radiotherapy resulted in significantly higher ambulatory rates in comparison to radiotherapy alone [6].

For patients without spinal instability presenting with refractory pain, cement augmentation via kyphoplasty or vertebroplasty may also be recommended [1]. In a randomised multicenter study comparing kyphoplasty to non-surgical treatment (CAFE Study) for patients with painful spinal metastases the superiority of kyphoplasty was evident. The patients had a statistically significant superior outcome at 1 and 6 months postoperatively [1].

MIS has recently gained much popularity for the treatment of spinal metastases. Due to the reduced invasiveness of surgery recovery time is markedly reduced and postoperative chemotherapy and radiotherapy can begin much sooner. To date only the previously mentioned CAFE study [1] is providing high-level evidence for the use of MIS in spinal metastases. There are numerous low-level evidence publications illustrating the use of percutaneous pedicle screw stabilization, tubular retractors, mini-open approaches and thoracoscopy/endoscopy for spinal metastases [8].

Most spine MIS publications in general as well as for the metastatic spine illustrate the benefits of percutaneous stabilization. There are two low-level single center studies comparing open approaches to MIS [3, 4]. In an analysis of 42 patients with thoracic spinal metastasis and myelopathy MIS was compared to the traditional open approach [4]. 23 prospectively enrolled patients undergoing MIS decompression and percutaneous stabilization were compared to retrospectively collected data from 19 patients following laminectomy and traditional open stabilization. There were no significant differences in neurological recovery rates or in complication rates. However, the MIS group illustrated a clear reduction of blood loss, operation time, bed rest length, postoperative pain and postoperative

Table 63.1 18-point Spinal Instability Neoplastic Score (SINS)

	Score
Location	
Junctional (Occiput-C2,C7-T2, T11-L1, L5-S1)	3
Mobile spine (C3-C6,L2-L4)	2
Semirigid (T3-T10)	1
Rigid (S2-S5)	0
Pain	
Yes	3
Occasional pain but not mechanical	1
Pain-free lesion	0
Bone lesion	
Lytic	2
Mixed (lytic/blastic)	1
Blastic	0
Radiographic spinal alignment	
Subluxation/translation present	4
De novo deformity (kyphosis/scoliosis)	2
Normal alignment	0
Vertebral body collapse	
>50% collapse	3
<50% collapse	2
No collapse with >50% body involvement	1
None of the above	0
Posteriolateral involvement of spinal elements	
Bilateral	3
Unilateral	1
None of the above	0
Total score	
Stable	0–6
Intermediate	7–12
Unstable	13–18

Modified from Fisher et al. [2]

opioid use [4]. In a retrospective analysis of 49 patients with thoracic metastasis MIS was also compared to a traditional open approach. 21 patients underwent a mini-open transpedicular corpectomy and percutaneous stabilization and 28 patients underwent traditional open transpedicular corpectomy and stabilization. There were no statistically significant differences in operation time, complication rates or neurological recovery. The MIS group had a significant reduction of blood loss and hospital stay duration [3].

For the additional use of cement augmentation in the metastatic spine there is also no high-level evidence. In a multicenter retrospective analysis of 101 patients following percutaneous pedicle screw stabilization and cement augmentation 87% of patients were ambulatory within 3 days after surgery. 18 patients experienced a postoperative complication but most (9/18) were not directly related to the surgical technique (e.g. delirium, urinary tract infection). Also, none of the complications was related to the cement augmentation (e.g. cement embolism). Prolonged operating time was the only factor significantly associated with the development of a complication [7]. In a second retrospective single center study, the safety and efficacy of cement-augmented short-segment percutaneous stabilization was analysed in 44 patients. The rate of patients reporting severe pain was reduced from 86% to 0% after surgery. On patient developed an adjacent-level fracture and in one case there was an asymptomatic screw pullout. Two patients required secondary decompression due to tumor progression despite radiotherapy [5].

All other current publications on the use of MIS in metastatic spine disease were restricted to a relatively small number of patients providing low-level evidence [8].

63.4 Conclusions and Take Home Message

- Patients with metastatic disease are living longer so that management of spine instability due to spinal metastasis comes more into focus.
- To access spinal instability the 18-point Spinal Instability Neoplastic Score (SINS) should be used.
- Decompression with Stabilization followed by radiotherapy has become the gold standard in most cases.
- Although without high-level evidence the benefits of MIS techniques in spinal metastases surgery are clear. Reduction of soft tissue trauma, blood loss and hospital stay facilitate a more rapid initiation of adjuvant treatments.
- For the additional use of cement augmentation in the metastatic spine there is also no high-level evidence. However in oncologic patients poor bone quality is very frequent and cement augmentation can therefore be recommended in selected cases.
- The use of radiolucent implants in the metastatic spine disease may be beneficial with regards to postoperative follow-up imaging and more accurate radiotherapy planning and delivery. However, there are still to data on this subject.

References

1. Berenson J, Pflugmacher R, Jarzem P, Zonder J, Schechtman K, Tillman JB et al. Cancer Patient Fracture Evaluation (CAFE) Investigators. Balloon kyphoplasty versus non-surgical fracture management for treatment of painful vertebral body compression fractures in patients with cancer: a multicentre, randomised controlled trial. Lancet Oncol. 2011;12(3):225–35. EBM 1b.
2. Fisher CG, DiPaola CP, Ryken TC, et al. A novel classification system for spinal instability in neoplastic disease: an evidence-based approach and expert consensus from the Spine Oncology Study Group. Spine. 2010;35:E1221–9. EBM 2a.
3. Lau D, Chou D. Posterior thoracic corpectomy with cage reconstruction for metastatic spinal tumors: comparing the mini-open approach to the open approach. J Neurosurg Spine. 2015;23(2):217–27. EBM 3b.
4. Miscusi M, Polli FM, Forcato S, Ricciardi L, Frati A, Cimatti M, De Martino L, Ramieri A, Raco A. Comparison of minimally invasive surgery with standard open surgery for vertebral thoracic metastases causing acute myelopathy in patients with short- or mid-term life expectancy: surgical technique and early clinical results. J Neurosurg Spine. 2015;22(5):518–25. EBM 3b.

5. Moussazadeh N, Rubin DG, McLaughlin L, Lis E, Bilsky MH, Laufer I. Short-segment percutaneous pedicle screw fixation with cement augmentation for tumor-induced spinal instability. Spine J. 2015;15(7):1609–17. EBM 3b.
6. Patchell RA, Tibbs PA, Regine WF, et al. Direct decompressive surgical resection in the treatment of Spinal cord compression caused by metastatic cancer: a randomised trial. Lancet. 2005;366:643–8. EBM 1b.
7. Versteeg AL, Verlaan JJ, de Baat P, Jiya TU, Stadhouder A, Diekerhof CH, van Solinge GB, Oner FC. Complications after percutaneous pedicle screw fixation for the treatment of unstable spinal metastases. Ann Surg Oncol. 2016;23(7):2343–9. EBM 4.
8. Zuckerman SL, Laufer I, Sahgal A, Yamada YJ, Schmidt MH, Chou D, Shin JH, Kumar N, Sciubba DM. When less is more: the indications for MIS techniques and separation surgery in metastatic spine disease. Spine (Phila Pa 1976). 2016;41(Suppl 20):S246–53. EBM 2a.

En Bloc Resection for Metastatic Disease

64

Ulf Liljenqvist

64.1 Introduction

This case will detail the aspects of en bloc resection in metastatic disease of the spine. It is indicated in very rare cases of solitary metastases or oligometastatic patients with primary tumors of good prognosis or highly likelyhood of local recurrence in case of intralesional resection.

64.2 Case Description

43 year old woman and wife of an orthopedic surgeon with history of breast cancer diagnosed and treated successfully 5 years earlier with breast amputation, lympdadenectomy and local radiation. On routine postoperative staging a solitary lesion of L5 was diagnosed. CT-guided biopsy revealed metastatic disease of breast cancer. Clinically, neurologically intact, only mild low back pain. Preop. MRI, CT and PET-CT showing the lesion of L5 with affection of the left pedicle and only minor soft tissue involvement (Fig. 64.1a–c).

Both tumor board and patient opted for complete resection. First, the non-affected posterior elements of L5 (lamina, articular processes, right transverse process and pedicle) were resected to create a corridor for the dural sac. The nerve roots L4 and L5 were released bilaterally and the discs L4/5 and L5/S1 incised and partially resected. Pedicle screw instrumentation was carried out from L3 to S1, backed up with S2 ala screws. Finally, the defect was covered with an autologous cortical iliac crest graft that had been harvested at the beginning of the procedure. It was pressfitted between the spinous processes of L4 and S1 and secured with a transverse connector.

Patient was placed supine and a team of two vascular surgeons visualized and controlled the great abdominal and iliac vessels via a transperitoenal approach (Fig. 64.2). The disc resection L4/5 and L5/S1 was completed and the remaining psoas attachments were released and the fifth lumbar vertebra was removed en bloc (Fig. 64.3). Anterior column reconstruction with a distractable titanium vertebral body replacement, filled with cancellous bone graft (Figs. 64.4 and 64.5a, b). Total OR time was 8.5 h. Early postoperative recovery was uneventful except for a left sided foot extensor weakness of 3/5 which was attributed to the intraoperative retraction of the lumbar plexus. Histological examination showed a contaminated margin at the left pedicle.

Six weeks postoperatively abdominal revision surgery due to intraabdominal adhesions. Postoperative radiation of the lower lumbar spine

U. Liljenqvist (✉)
Department for Spine Surgery,
St. Franziskus Hospital, Münster, Germany
e-mail: ulf.liljenqvist@sfh-muenster.de

B. Meyer, M. Rauschmann (eds.), *Spine Surgery*, https://doi.org/10.1007/978-3-319-98875-7_64

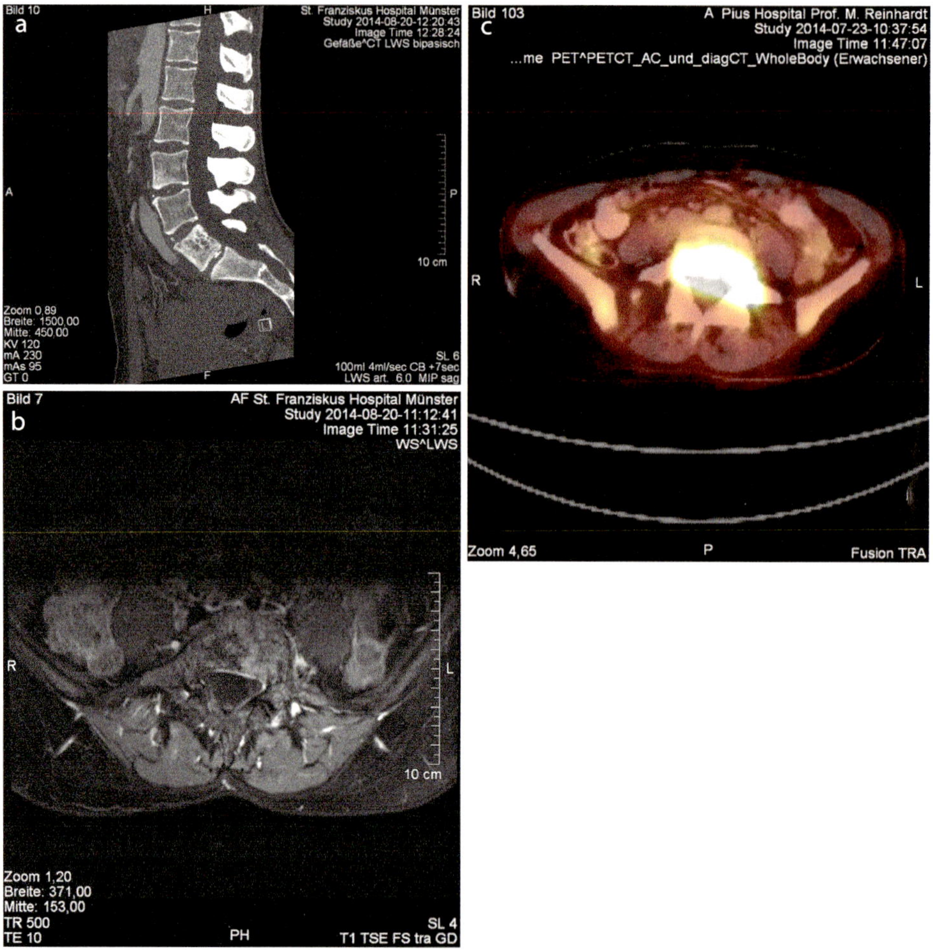

Fig. 64.1 (**a**–**c**) CT (**a**), MRI (**b**) and PET CT (**c**) demonstrating the lesion of L5

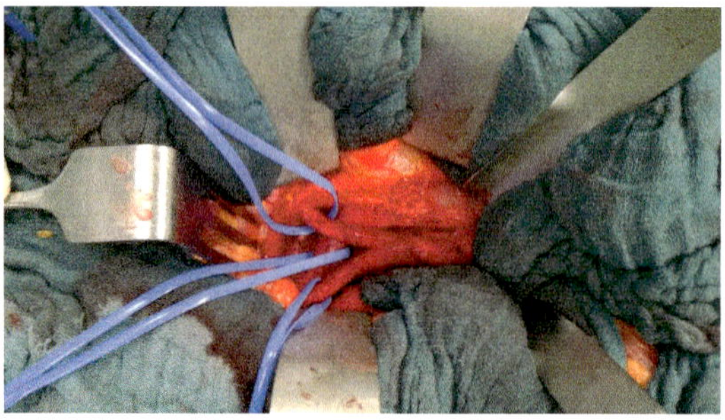

Fig. 64.2 Intraoperative picture of the transperitoneal approach with preparation of the great vessels (aorta, vena cava, left common iliac vein, both common iliac arteries)

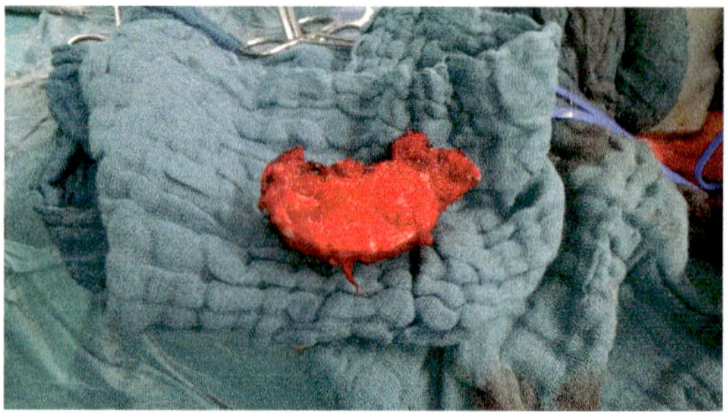

Fig. 64.3 Resected corpus vertebrae L5 including left pedicle and transverse process

with 44 Gy was perfomed. Continuous medication with Denusomab. Two years postoperatively, removal of the prominent S2 screws was done. CT scan demonstrates fusion of both cage and the posterior iliac crest graft (Figs. 64.6a, b and 64.7).

Four years postoperatively she is in complete remission without any evidence of disease and works part time as a lawyer with still some weakness of the left foot (4/5). The medication with Denusomab is continued and she is in regular oncological control.

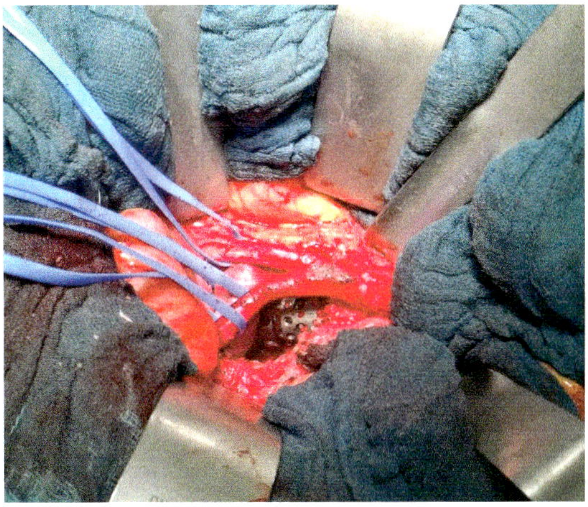

Fig. 64.4 Intraoperative picture with the vertebral body replacement cage in-situ

64.3 Discussion

Primary goal in metastatic spine surgery is local control. In the literature the clinically relevant local recurrence rate ranges between 5% and 15%. Risk factors were found to be posterior only surgery (intralesional resection) and thyroid or kidney metastases [1–3]. The overall local recurrence rate after intralesional resection of spinal kidney metastases ranges between even 20% and 50%. Up to 50% of all revisions due to local recurrence are found in kidney metastases [1, 2]. Jansson and Bauer [3] found an increase in the local recurrence rate to 20% if the patient survived longer than 1 year.

En bloc resection with clear margins almost eliminates the risk local recurrence due to the complete tumor removal [4]. In thyroid metastases en bloc spondylectomy reduced the local recurrence rate from 57% after intralesional

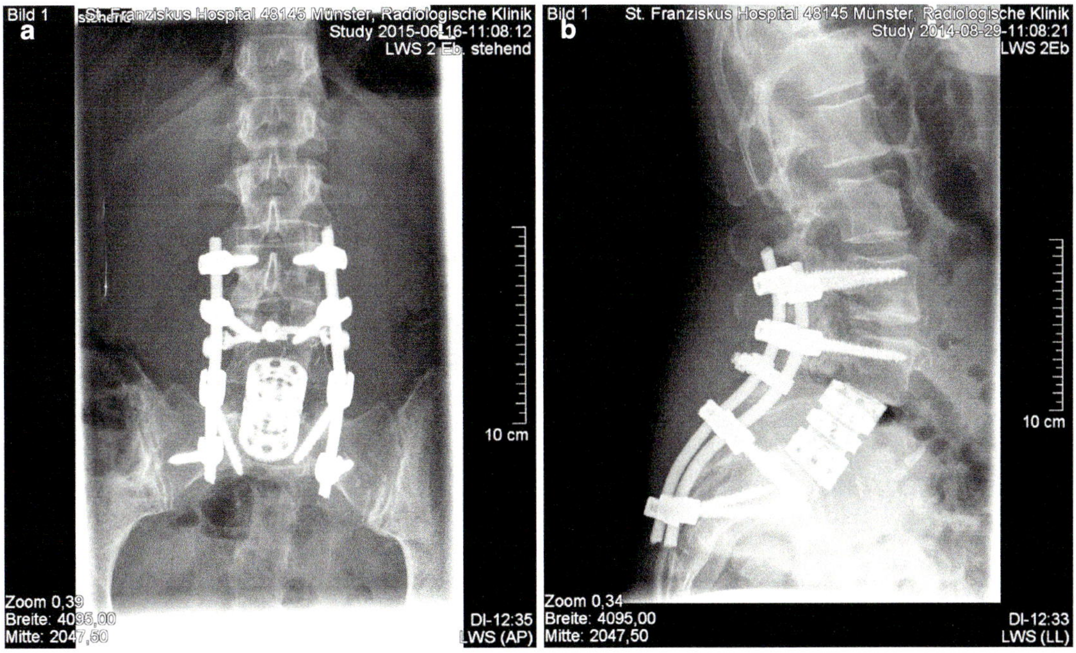

Fig. 64.5 (**a**, **b**) Postoperative ap and lateral lumbar X-rays

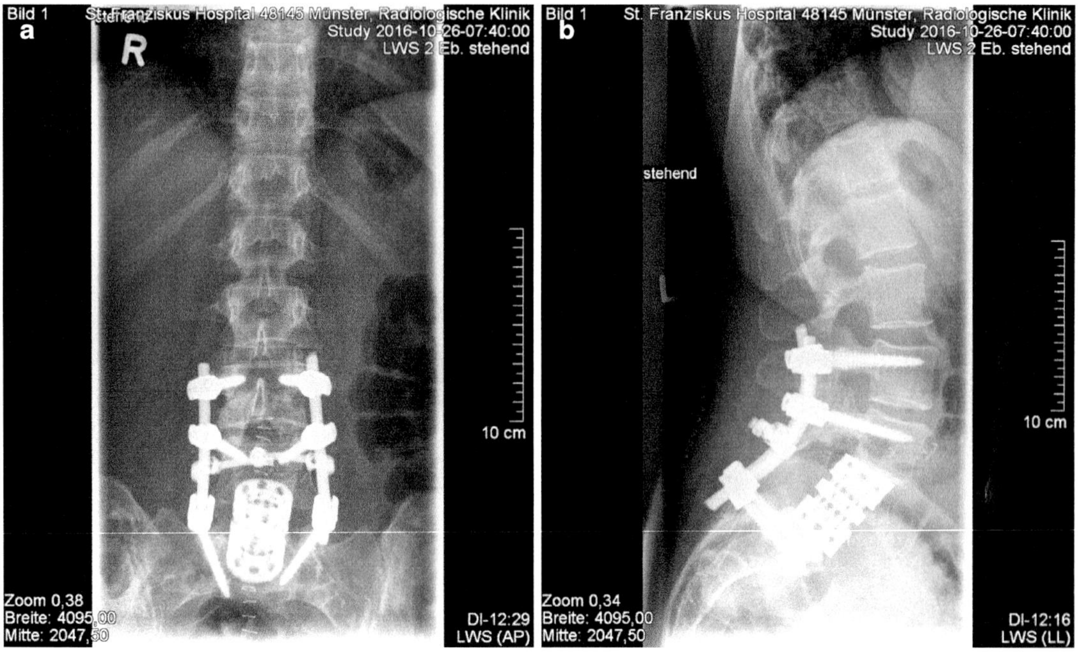

Fig. 64.6 (**a**, **b**) X-rays 2 years postop. with removal of prominent S2 screws

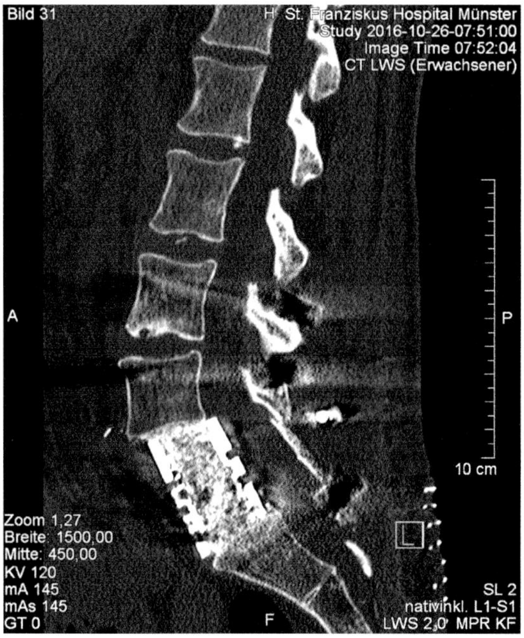

Fig. 64.7 CT scan 2 years postop. showing fusion of both the cage and the posterior iliac graft

resection to 10% [5]. Matsumoto et al. [6] recommend total en bloc spondylectomy in thyroid metastases to optimize local control. In a long-term study on 8 patients they found a complete remission in 5 patients and only 2 local recurrences.

Concerning the technique of en bloc spondylectomy, a combined posteroanterior approach allows full control of both neural and vascular structures and increases safety of the procedure [7]. Prerequisite for extralesional en bloc resection is a tumorfree area around the lamina and one pedicle. Thus a tumorfree corridor can be created to release the dural tube sac and its contents. Disadvantages of an all posterior approach with bilateral pediculotomies are limited control of anterior vital structures, the necessity of far lateral bilateral rib osteotomies and tumor spillage in case of tumor involvement of the pedicle(s).

64.4 Conclusions and Take Home Message

- In solitary metastases or oligometastatic patients with thyroid or renal cancer en bloc resection reduces the local recurrence rate.
- In late solitary breast metastases with good prognosis en bloc resection may improve local control.
- A posteroanterior approach for en bloc spondylectomy increases the safety of the procedure.

References

1. Chataigner H, Onimus M. Surgery in spinal metastasis without spinal cord compression: indications and strategy related to the risk of recurrence. Eur Spine J. 2000;9:523–7.
2. Polly D, Chou D, Sembrano J, et al. An analysis of decision making and treatment in thoracolumbar metastases. Spine. 2009;15:S118–27.
3. Jansson K, Bauer H. Survival, complications and outome in 282 patients operated for neurological deficit due to thoracic or lumbar spinal metastases. Eur Spine J. 2006;15:196–202.
4. Fang T, Dong J, Zhou X, et al. Comparison of mini-open anterior corpectomy and posterior total en bloc spondylectomy für solitary metastases of the thoracolumbar spine. J Neurosurg Spine. 2012;17:271–9.
5. Demura S, Kawahara N, Murakami H, et al. Total en bloc spondylectomy for spinal metastases in thyroid carcinoma. J Neurosurg Spine. 2011;14:172–6.
6. Matsumoto M, Tsuji T, Iwanami A, et al. Total en bloc spondylectomy for spinal metastases of differentiated thyroid cancer: a long-term follow-up. J Spinal Disord Tech. 2013;26:E137–42.
7. Liljenqvist U, Lerner T, Halm H, et al. En bloc spondylectomy in malignant tumors of the spine. Eur Spine J. 2008;17:600–9.

Principles of Posterior Surgery in Adolescent Idiopathic Scoliosis

65

R. Emre Acaroglu and Michael E. Doany

65.1 Introduction

This is a typical case of Adolescent Idiopathic Scoliosis (AIS) who has had a trial of conservative treatment with a rigid brace that was not necessarily indicated before surgery. Based on her case;

- Surgical indications in AIS,
- Use and application of Lenke classification in surgical decision making,
- Uses, advantages and disadvantages of surgical correction maneuvers, and
- Priorities in surgical treatment of AIS will be discussed.

65.2 Case Description

A 14 year old female patient who was diagnosed with AIS 1 year ago and was referred for surgical treatment is presented. She has had her menarche 1 year before her referral and had a trial of brace treatment with a rigid custom made TLSO over the past year. Treating physician states the Cobb measurements of her curves as 35° and 42° (for thoracic and lumbar curves respectively) at the time of the commencement of the brace treatment (no X-rays were available). Braced was discontinued upon demonstrated progression to 44° and 49° respectively and she was referred for surgical treatment.

At presentation, she has right thoracic and left lumbar humps of pretty much equal sizes and 1–2 cm elevation at her right shoulder. Her leg lengths are equal and her neurological examination including abdominal reflexes are normal. Presentation X-rays are notable for left sided upper thoracic (UT) (T1-T4) curve of 21.5°, right sided thoracic (T) (T5-T12) curve of 45.8° and left sided lumbar (L) (L1-L4) curve of 51.1° on the AP view (Fig. 65.1a). These curves would correct down to 18°, 38° and 29° respectively on left and right side bending X-rays. Her coronal balance is shifted to left by 32 mm, her right shoulder is higher by 18 mm. Her Risser status at the time was Grade II. Her sagittal curves on the lateral x-ray were measured as 44° of thoracic kyphosis (TK) and 57° for lumbar lordosis (LL) (Fig. 65.1b). She is perfectly balanced in the sagittal plane (SVA = 0 mm).

Based on these, she was classified as type VI (or III) C (+) by Lenke classification.

Surgery was planned to cover both major curves (T and L) in the coronal plane from the upper end vertebra of the T (T4) to the lower end vertebra of the L (L4) curves. Although the

R. E. Acaroglu (✉)
Ankara Spine Center, Ankara, Turkey

M. E. Doany
Department of Orthopedics, Stony Brook University, Stony Brook, NY, USA

B. Meyer, M. Rauschmann (eds.), *Spine Surgery*, https://doi.org/10.1007/978-3-319-98875-7_65

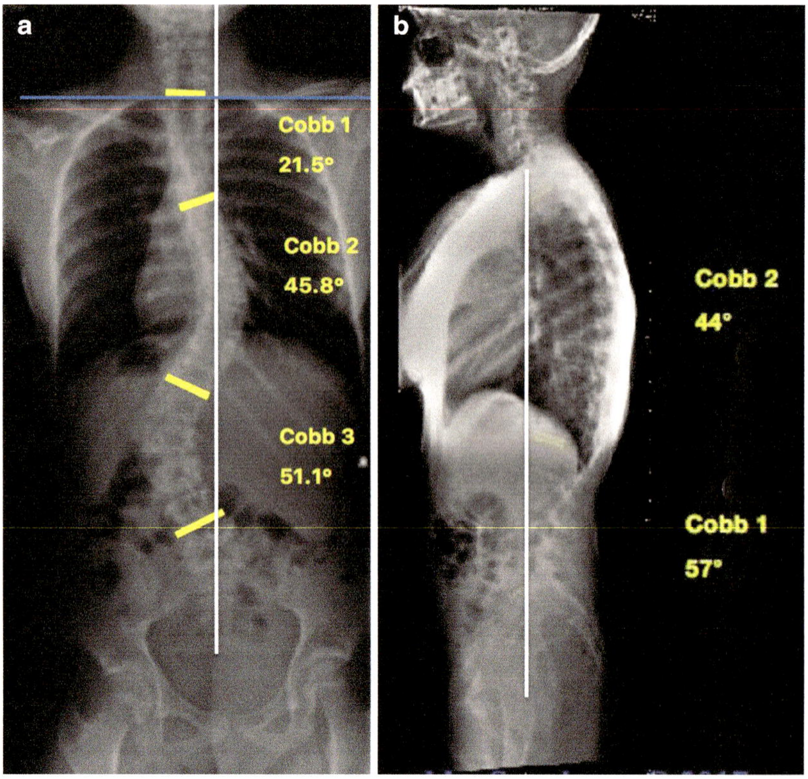

Fig. 65.1 (**a**) Pre-operative PA X-ray of the patient. Cobb measurements 1 to 3 are for UT, T and L curves respectively. White line is the Central Sacral Vertical Line, and the Blue line is the shoulder balance line. (**b**) Pre-operative lateral X-ray. Cobb measurements 1 and 2 are for TK and LL respectively. White line is the Sagittal Vertical Axis from C7

original plan was to use pedicle screws on both sides for every level (the accepted norm at that time), three pedicles T 6, 7 and 10 was not instrumented on the right side due to technical difficulties. Surgical correction was achieved by double rod rotation maneuver starting with the insertion of the convex rod (see below for description and discussion) which was followed by bilateral Harrington distraction/compression maneuvers (see below for description and discussion) so as to adjust coronal balance. Her x-rays on the post-operative day 3 can be seen in Fig. 65.2a, b. Her coronal curves were corrected down to 14.3°, 16.3° and 15.6° for the UT, T, and L curves respectively. Her coronal balance is 3 mm to right and her shoulder are balanced. On the sagittal plane, her TK measures 21.8°, her LL measures 48.7° and her sagittal balance is seen to be deteriorated to SVA = 76 mm. She was discharged from the hospital in that alignment on the 4th post-op day, following an uncomplicated clinical course.

Her 2 year follow-up x-rays can be seen in Fig. 65.3a, b. Her coronal measurements at this time are 14.4°, 16.9° and 13.7° for UT, T and L curves; her coronal balance is 2 mm to left and her right shoulder is 8 mm lower. On the sagittal view, her TK is 26.8°, her LL has increased to 55.1° and her sagittal balance has become (−) (SVA = −12 mm). Both the patient and her family expressed satisfaction (less than complete due to persisting minor asymmetry) with the end result and she was discharged from scheduled controls.

65.3 Discussion of the Case

A. A brief note on brace treatment:

Treatment recommendations in AIS are based on the fairly well documented natural history of the disease [1] and delineated in several guidelines including those by the Scoliosis Research Society

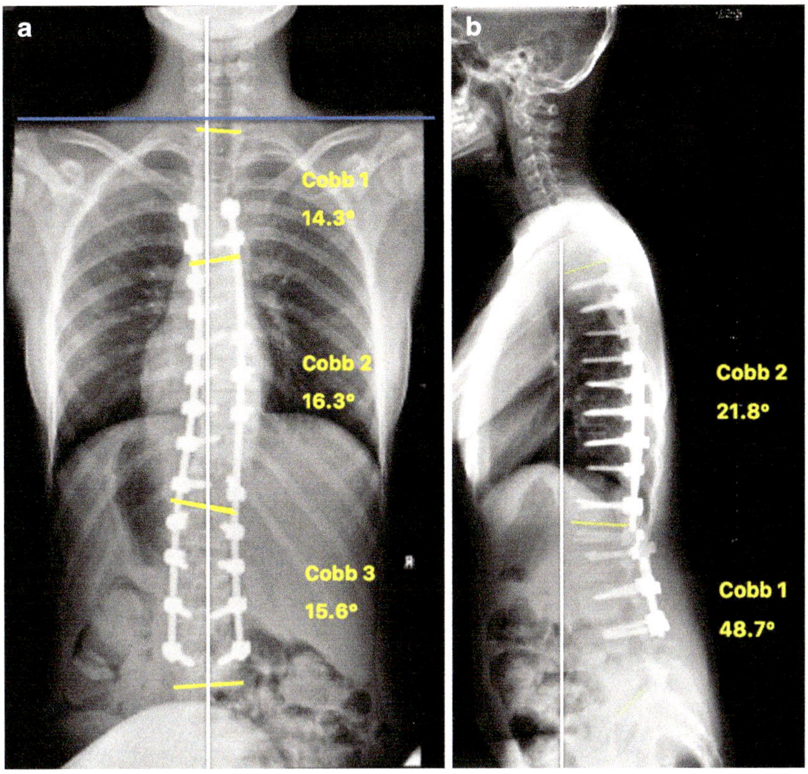

Fig. 65.2 (**a**) PA X-ray at the 3rd post-operative day. Cobb measurements 1 to 3 are for UT, T and L curves respectively. White line is the Central Sacral Vertical Line, and the Blue line is the shoulder balance line. (**b**) Lateral X-ray at the 3rd post-operative day. Cobb measurements 1 and 2 are for TK and LL respectively. White line is the Sagittal Vertical Axis from C7

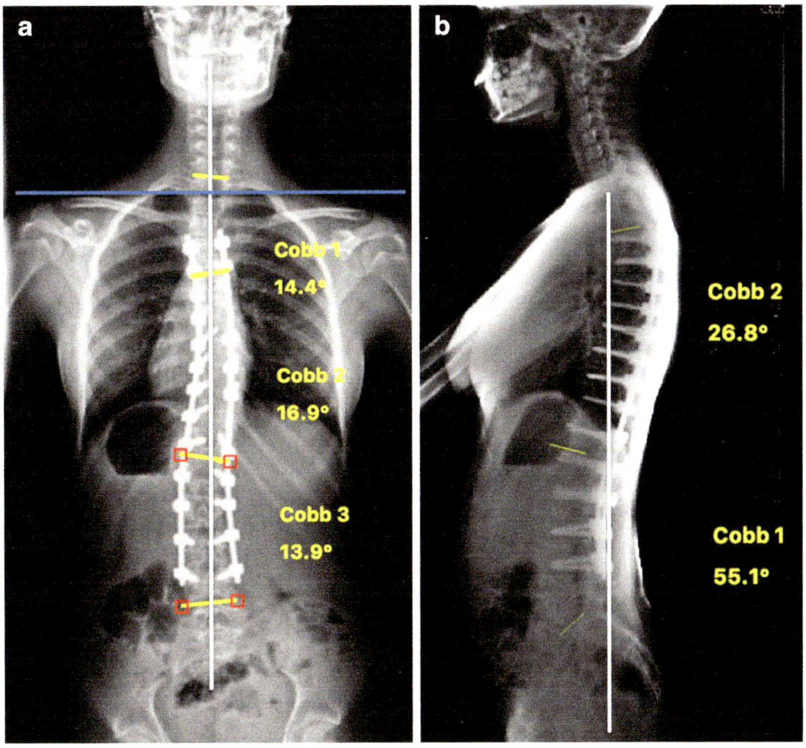

Fig. 65.3 (**a**) PA X-ray at the end of the 2nd post-operative year. Cobb measurements 1 to 3 are for UT, T and L curves respectively. White line is the Central Sacral Vertical Line, and the Blue line is the shoulder balance line. (**b**) Lateral X-ray at the end of the 2nd post-operative year. Cobb measurements 1 and 2 are for TK and LL respectively. White line is the Sagittal Vertical Axis from C7

(SRS) [2]. SRS suggests that brace treatment is indicated for curves between 25° and 40° in immature patients. In this regard, an argument on the appropriateness of bracing in this patient (with a T curve of 44°) may be questioned. On the other hand, this decision was probably based on her immaturity at the time (just at menarche and probably Risser 0), and the physician who had started brace treatment deserves commend for recognizing the failure of her prescription at an early period and referring the patient for surgery.

B. Selection of fusion levels:

Guidance in the selection of is the main clinical application of Lenke classification (for any AIS classification for that matter). Classification calls for an identification of major curves (that does not correct to below 25° on bending and/or is associated with junctional kyphosis >20°) to be included in surgical fusion [3]. The present case was classified as Type VI (double major with L > T) or III (double major with T > L; based on the flexibility of the L curve). As can be seen, these two types are essentially the same with only minor (if any) changes in the selection of fusion levels. The UT curve was not included in the fusion levels based on the same classification.

C. The choice of correction maneuver:

Several corrective maneuvers may be used in AIS surgery, individually or (more frequently) in combination. These may be listed as follows:

(i) Harrington Forces (Fig. 65.4a): Described originally to be utilized with Harrington instrumentation, these forces comprise of distraction (of the concave/short side) and compression (of the convex/long side). They are still extremely useful in conjunction with all other correction maneuvers. Their usefulness is not limited to correction in the coronal plane, but even more pronounced in the sagittal plane, in which *'compression in the posterior column decreases kyphosis and increases lordosis; whereas distraction increases kyphosis and decreases lordosis'*.

(ii) Translation (Fig. 65.4b): First introduced by the use sublaminar wires, consists of aligning and stabilizing the rod(s) in the desired sagittal and coronal alignment and pulling the spine to the rod(s) by means of wires, bands, pedicle screws etc. By this, deformity is corrected not only by translating the apex towards the concavity in coronal and sagittal planes, but also, in the presence of axial rotation, by derotation as the posterior/concave corner of the rotated level(s) is pulled in the posterior direction. Translation is much easier to be used on the concave side of the deformity, a similar maneuver perform from the convex side (pushing) is called cantilevering (see below).

(iii) Cantilevering (Fig. 65.4c): Is the act of attaching the to the upper or lower end of the (kyphotic, by definition) deformity and achieving correction by pushing the free end towards the spine and fixing. By this, deformity is corrected not only by translating the apex towards the concavity in coronal and sagittal planes, but also, in the presence of axial rotation, by derotation as the posterior/convex corner of the rotated level(s) is pushed in the anterior direction.

(iv) Single rod rotation (Fig. 65.4d): Introduced and popularized as a part of CD instrumentation, this maneuver consists of the application of the contoured concave rod first, rotation of this rod in the correction direction by 90°, and application of the convex rod after that for stabilization and partial derotation. Although credited as a derotation maneuver at the time of its introduction, this maneuver is now considered as a modification of translation.

(v) Double rod rotation (Fig. 65.4e): This is the rod rotation performed with both rods in place. Its advantages are less rod deformation, better control convex side of the deformity thereby (theoretically) affording better rotational correction and better (demonstrated) preservation/control of the T kyphosis. Main disadvantage is the relative

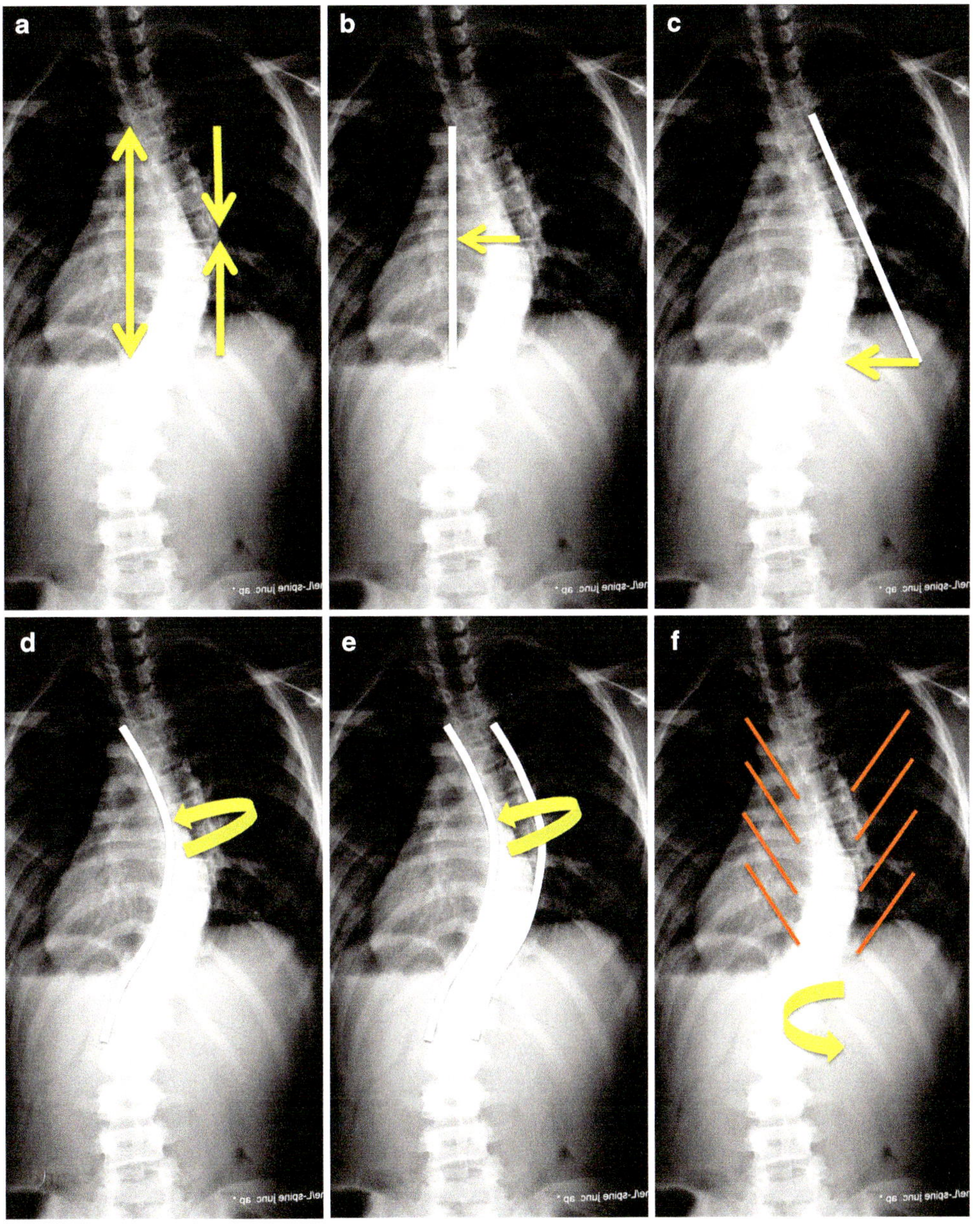

Fig. 65.4 (**a**) Harrington forces (compression and distraction) as a correction maneuver. (**b**) Translation as a correction maneuver. The concave rod is contoured and aligned in the desired sagittal alignment. The deformed spinal segment is then pulled towards that rod (towards midline and posteriorly) by means of wires, cables, bands or pedicle screws. (**c**) Cantilevering as a correction maneuver. The convex rod is contoured and fixed to the upper (or lower) half of the deformed segment in the desired sagittal alignment. Pushing the free end of the rod towards the lower (or upper) half of the curve translates the apex towards the concavity as well as anteriorly. (**d**) Single rod rotation as a correction maneuver. The rod is contoured into the desired sagittal alignment, fixed to the anchors on the concave side and rotated in a direction that would translate the coronal curve into a sagittal one. Insertion of the convex rod follows. (**e**) Double rod rotation as a correction maneuver. Both rods are contoured into the desired sagittal alignment, fixed to the anchors on both sides and rotated in a direction that would translate the coronal curve into a sagittal one. (**f**) Direct vertebral rotation as a (complementary) correction maneuver. Following correction of the coronal (and sagittal) plane deformities by means of the maneuvers described above, the apically located pedicle screws are loaded with tubes or sticks to allow for the manipulation of these vertebrae in the axial plane, thereby affording for a better correction of rotation in that plane

difficulty of rotating both rods due to an increased rigidity of the spinal column that is fixed on both sides, resulting in (theoretically) lesser coronal correction rates.

(vi) Direct vertebral rotation (Fig. 65.4f): This is the procedure of attaching sticks or towers to the pedicle screws at and around the apex and using these as joysticks to correct axial rotation of these segments. This maneuver is associated with the highest axial and coronal plane correction rates whereas the main disadvantage being its lordosing effect of the derotated T spine.

Of these, a combination of cantilevering (introduction and complete insertion of the convex rod first), double rod rotation and Harrington forces (to adjust the coronal plane balance) was used for this case. The choice of cantilevering is far from being arbitrary; it was based on the (+) TK designation of the curve in Lenke classification. Correction of a kyphotic segment should always be performed starting from the convexity of the scoliotic curve (see discussion above).

Of interest, it is extremely important to emphasize and understand that the maximum amount of coronal plane correction was not sought for nor achieved in any of the curves of this patient. This is the main point in using Harrington forces to adjust the coronal plane balance as the last maneuver in surgery; one or both curves may need to be uncorrected to various extents in order to achieve an optimally balanced alignment (of both the spinal column and shoulders). The risk for imbalance, especially in shoulder levels is unacceptably high if this final tuning is not performed. Of note again, as to our knowledge, there is no such described maneuver that can tune the sagittal alignment during surgery; we have to rely on the patients' own capacity to correct themselves in the sagittal plane as evidenced by the case described here.

D. Pedicle screw instrumentation and density:

Pedicle screws afford the ability to perform truly segmental instrumentation in scoliosis surgery. They have better intrinsic stability (that is, being stable by itself) compared to other anchors (hooks, wires, bands etc.) and as they may be at all levels of TL instrumentation, they are very useful in distributing the loads and corrective forces throughout the involved region. In this regard, it is also important to understand that the use of pedicle screws do not necessarily mandate the use of a certain correction maneuver, pedicle screws may be used successfully in all correction maneuvers described above, a major advantage and reason for their widespread use in scoliosis surgery.

Recent evidence on pedicle screw density in posterior surgery for AIS suggests that higher densities (i.e., using screws closer to the potential number possible, that is, number of levels*2) are not necessarily associated with improved patient outcomes but with significantly higher surgical costs [4, 5]. As mentioned above, this patient was operated at a time when this information was not available and the accepted norm, based on an understanding that higher screw densities may allow for better correction rates.

E. The status of evidence in posterior AIS surgery:

Evidence on surgical management of AIS needs to be considered from two different perspectives:

(i) Evidence on deformity correction; which is abundant. There is no doubt that surgery affords very satisfactory correction rates in coronal and lately, in axial planes. Sagittal plane correction (i.e., restoration of TK when needed) is less predictable as evidenced by a recent literature review by us in Table 65.1.

Table 65.1 Pooled sagittal plane correction data from 53 papers reporting sagittal correction data in posterior AIS surgery

Pooled sagittal plane deformity correction [N = 3780]	
Avg. Pre-op Sagittal Cobb (°)	22.1
Avg. Post-op Sagittal Cobb (°)	22.6
Avg. Correction (°)	0.5 [−13.9 to +20]

Unpublished literature review by Acaroglu and Doany (2018)

The evidence level of the available literature is level III at best, but there is a demonstrable consistency of these trends from a very large number of reports.

(ii) Evidence on long term patient well-being and quality of life; which is far less than abundant [6, 7]. There is some level IV evidence suggesting better rates of coronal correction are associated with better satisfaction and SRS 22 scores but the longevity of this trend is virtually unknown [8].

65.4 Conclusions and Take Home Message

Through this case we wanted to emphasize the need for a complete deformity analysis and accurate classification as the first and foremost step in AIS surgery. This is also true for an absolute command on the tools (i.e., screws, rods, wires etc.) and correction maneuvers. Without a proper understanding of each individual deformity in all planes and that of the surgical options, achieving consistent, acceptable and tailored results may virtually be impossible.

References

1. Lonstein JE, Carlson JM. The prediction of curve progression in untreated idiopathic scoliosis during growth. J Bone Joint Surg Am. 1984;66(7):1061–71. PubMed PMID: 6480635. Evidence level: 3.
2. Rowe DE. Adolescent idiopathic scoliosis. In: SRS bracing manual. Available at: http://www.srs.org/UserFiles/file/bracing-manual/section1.pdf. Accessed 16 Apr 2018. Evidence level: 5.
3. Lenke LG, Edwards CC 2nd, Bridwell KH. The Lenke classification of adolescent idiopathic scoliosis: how it organizes curve patterns as a template to perform selective fusions of the spine. Spine (Phila Pa 1976). 2003;28(20):S199–207. PubMed PMID: 14560193. Evidence level: 4.
4. Bharucha NJ, Lonner BS, Auerbach JD, Kean KE, Trobisch PD. Low-density versus high-density thoracic pedicle screw constructs in adolescent idiopathic scoliosis: do more screws lead to a better outcome? Spine J. 2013;13(4):375–81. https://doi.org/10.1016/j.spinee.2012.05.029. Epub 2012 Aug 15. PubMed PMID: 22901787. Evidence level: 3.
5. Larson AN, Polly DW Jr, Diamond B, Ledonio C, Richards BS 3rd, Emans JB, Sucato DJ, Johnston CE, Minimize Implants Maximize Outcomes Study Group. Does higher anchor density result in increased curve correction and improved clinical outcomes in adolescent idiopathic scoliosis? Spine (Phila Pa 1976). 2014;39(7):571–8. https://doi.org/10.1097/BRS.0000000000000204. PubMed PMID: 24430717.
6. Mariconda M, Andolfi C, Cerbasi S, Servodidio V. Effect of surgical correction of adolescent idiopathic scoliosis on the quality of life: a prospective study with a minimum 5-year follow-up. Eur Spine J. 2016;25(10):3331–40. Epub2016 Mar 16. PubMed PMID: 26984879. Evidence level: 3.
7. Takayama K, Nakamura H, Matsuda H. Quality of life in patients treated surgically for scoliosis: longer than sixteen-year follow-up. Spine (Phila Pa 1976). 2009;34(20):2179–84. https://doi.org/10.1097/BRS.0b013e3181abf684. PubMed PMID: 19713874. Evidence level: 4.
8. Sanders JO, Carreon LY, Sucato DJ, Sturm PF, Diab M, Spinal Deformity Study Group, et al. Spine (Phila Pa 1976). 2010;35(20):1867–71. https://doi.org/10.1097/BRS.0b013e3181efa6f5. PubMed PMID: 20802382. Evidence level: 4.

Tumors of the Sacrum

66

Sandro M. Krieg and Bernhard Meyer

66.1 Introduction

Sacral tumors can be metastases or primary tumors. The latter represent an uncommon entity, only accounting for approximately 7% of all primary tumors of the spine. While giant cell tumors and chordomas are the most frequent tumor type, they are also considerably resistant to chemo- and radiotherapy [1]. Along with their slow speed of growth sacral tumors most commonly induce only minor symptoms resulting in large tumors when the patients present in our clinics [16]. Moreover, many sacral tumors, such as chordomas and chondrosarcomas are proved to have a better oncological outcome if resected en bloc; yet, this is not possible in a large protion of cases [15]. This, however, is surgically demanding considering the critical biomechanical role, complex anatomy, interdisciplinary involvement, and frequently large anterior tumor mass.

This chapter therefore aims on elucidating the three most crucial aspects of surgery to the sacrum:

1. Indication and techniques of sacral tumor resections
2. Sacrectomy in particular
3. Fixation and reconstruction techniques following resection

The two illustrative cases will help to better understand the clinical implications, potential complications, and considerations which need to be taken when consulting patients with such tumors.

66.2 Case Description

66.2.1 Case 1

A 50 year-old male patient presented with right-sided local pain in the sacrum, without any sciatica or neurological deficits. CT and MRI were performed showing a tumor in the right sacrum (Figs. 66.1 and 66.2).

A needle biopsy was performed showing a chondrosarcoma and the tumor board recommended lumbopelvic instrumentation L4-L5 to Os Ileum, complete en bloc tumor resection via hemisacrectomy and excision of the biopsy trajectory. Tumor resection went as planned: lumbopelvic instrumentation L4-L5 to Os Ileum (plus S1 in the left side) and complete en bloc tumor resection via hemisacrectomy. After surgery, no new deficit occurred and the patient was able to walk without help at the first postoperative day. Tumorboard recommended adjuvant radiotherapy (Fig. 66.3).

S. M. Krieg (✉) · B. Meyer
Department of Neurosurgery, Klinikum rechts der Isar, Technische Universität München, Munich, Germany
e-mail: Sandro.Krieg@tum.de

B. Meyer, M. Rauschmann (eds.), *Spine Surgery*, https://doi.org/10.1007/978-3-319-98875-7_66

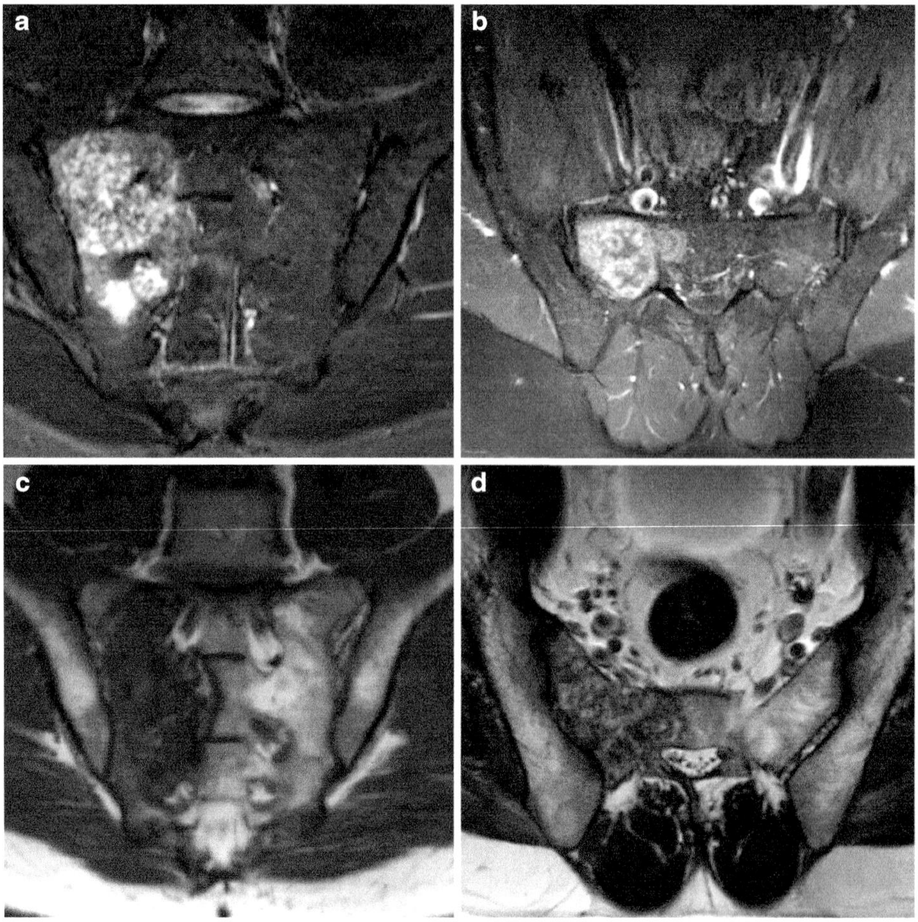

Fig. 66.1 MRI scan of a tumor in the right sacrum. This MRI scan shows the coronal (**a**, **c**) and axial (**b**, **d**) slices of a right-sided sacral tumor with inhomogenous contrast-enhancement (**a**, **b**)

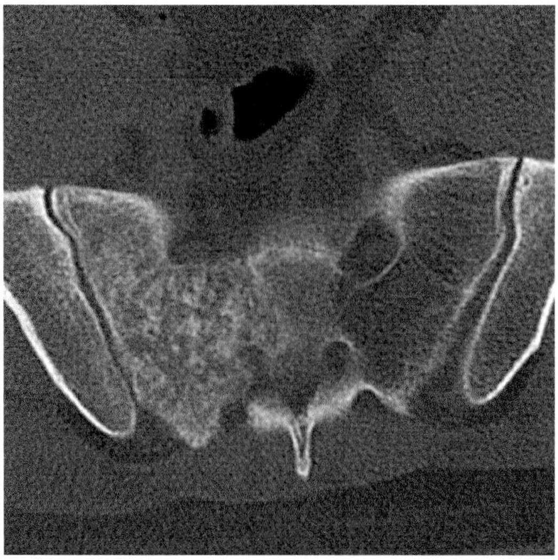

Fig. 66.2 CT scan of a tumor in the right sacrum. This CT scan shows the axial slice of a right-sided sacral tumor with inhomogenous osteoblastic components

66.2.2 Case 2

A 66 year-old male patient came to our department with a sacral chordoma biopsied in another hospital already (Fig. 66.4). His previous medical history contains a prostate cancer with prostatectomy performed the year before. Since then, he had perineal and genital hypaesthesia as well as bladder and bowel dysfunction.

The patient only suffered from pain in the sacral region and therefore refused surgery. For the next year the patient experienced progressive weakness of the lower limbs and for another 9 months he required a wheel chair. 2 years after the initial presentation in our department he came back with paraparesis of both lower limbs (BMRC 1/5), hypesthesia of lower limbs, perineal and genital hypaesthesia as well as bladder and bowel dysfunction. Due to urinary retention

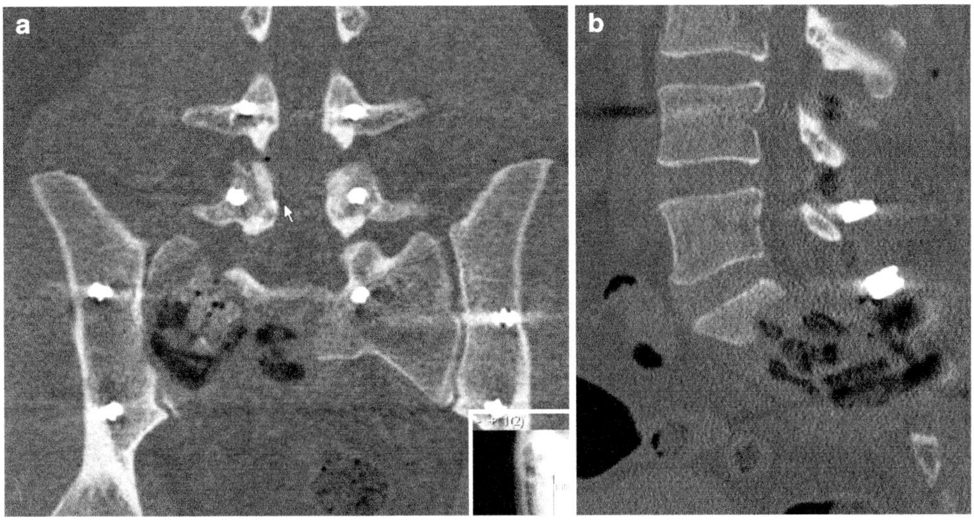

Fig. 66.3 Postoperative CT scan. This CT scan shows the coronal (**a**) and sagittal (**b**) slice of the postoperative resection control. No residual tumor

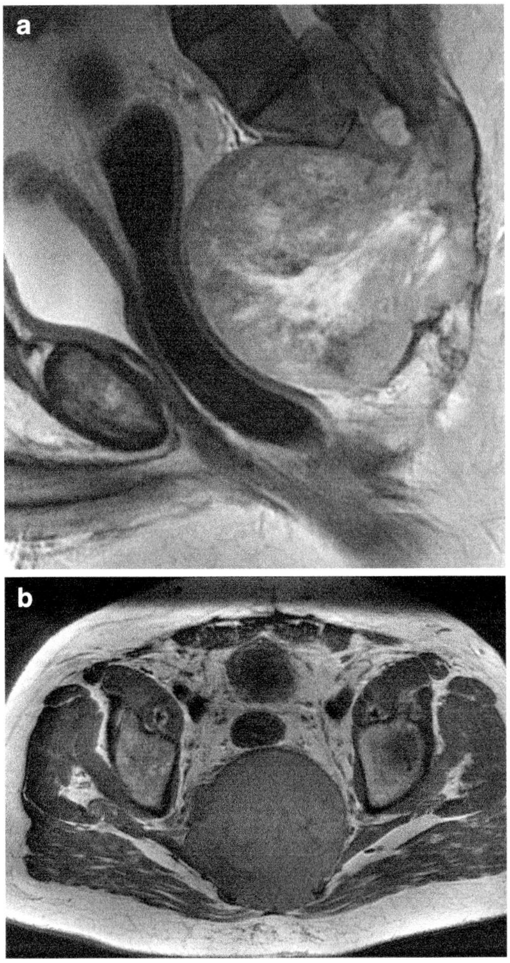

Fig. 66.4 Initial MRI scan. This MRI scan shows sagittal (**a**) and axial (**b**) slices in T2 sequences of a large sacral chordoma with large anterior and intradural extension

he now suffered from urosepsis, which was treated by iv antibiotics and a new suprapubic catheter. He then developed an obstructive ileus requiring colostomy. A new CT scan showed a large tumor progression including liver metastases (Fig. 66.5).

The patient recovered quickly and further discussion about the tumor was brought up and the patient and his family finally decided for surgery in a multistaged approach:

1st surgery:

- Posterior approach
- lumbopelvic instrumentation L4-L5 to Os Ileum
- Laminectomie L4 and Cauda equina resection at L4 with watertight suture of the thekal sac
- Resection of L5 and sacrum
- Tumordebulking in the soft tissue lateral to the femur

The patient recovered quickly and very well with no new neurological deficit (Fig. 66.6).

He had no pain anymore and the 2nd surgery was scheduled 1 week afterwards:

2nd surgery (1 week later):

- Abdominal approach
- Interdisciplinary team including abdominal surgeon, urologist, and neurosurgeon
- Abdominoperineal rectum extirpation (Miles)

- Colostoma
- Partial sacral tumor resection
- Resection of the bladder and ileum conduit

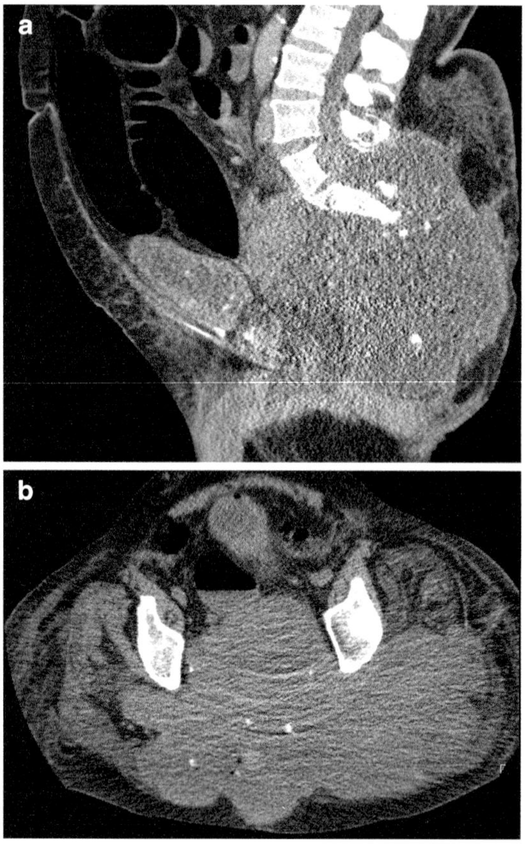

Fig. 66.5 Preoperative CT scan. This CT scan performed 2 years after the initial presentation shows a heavily increased sacral tumor in sagittal (**a**) and axial (**b**) slices with large anterior tumor mass and osteolysis

- Reconstruction of pelvic floor via pig skin xenograft
- Biopsy of hepatic lesions
- Reconstruction of the space left by the sacral resection via an omentum graft failed due to omentum hypoperfusion

The liver biopsy proved chordoma metastases in the liver but the patient again recovered very quickly. Thus, a third surgery with further tumor resection around the iliac bone was scheduled:

3rd surgery (2 weeks after 1st surgery):

- Posterior approach
- Tumor resection around the iliac bone
- Microbiology biopsies

The patient recovered again very quickly and suffered from no pain. The CT scan showed an almost complete resection of the tumor mass (Fig. 66.7).

Microbiology biopsies proved E. coli and Candida species in the situs this leading to antibiotic and antifungal medication plus vacuum treatment of the dorsal approach requiring another 2 surgeries (4th and 5th surgery). The 6th surgery was then scheduled 5 weeks after the initial surgery to reconstruct the space left by the sacral resection via a bilobed femoro-gluteal flap gaining skin from the left thigh which was then rotated in the resection cavity after de-epithelilization (Fig. 66.8).

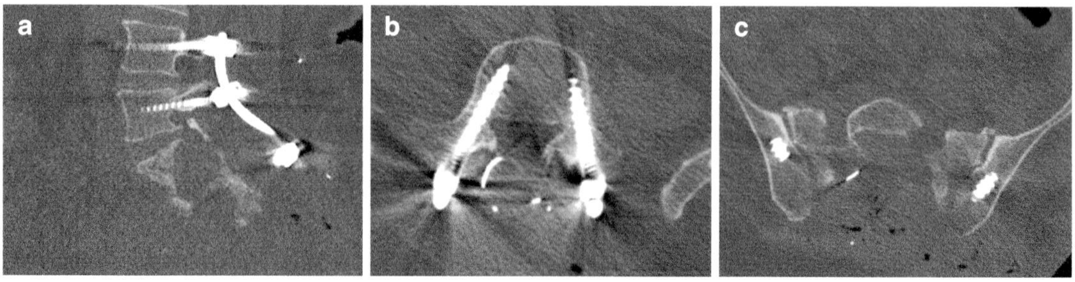

Fig. 66.6 Postoperative CT scan after the first surgery. This CT scan performed after the 1st surgery shows the bony resection as well as the lumbopelvic instrumentation L4-L5 to Os Ileum in sagittal (**a**) and axial slices in L4 (**b**) and Os ilium (**c**)

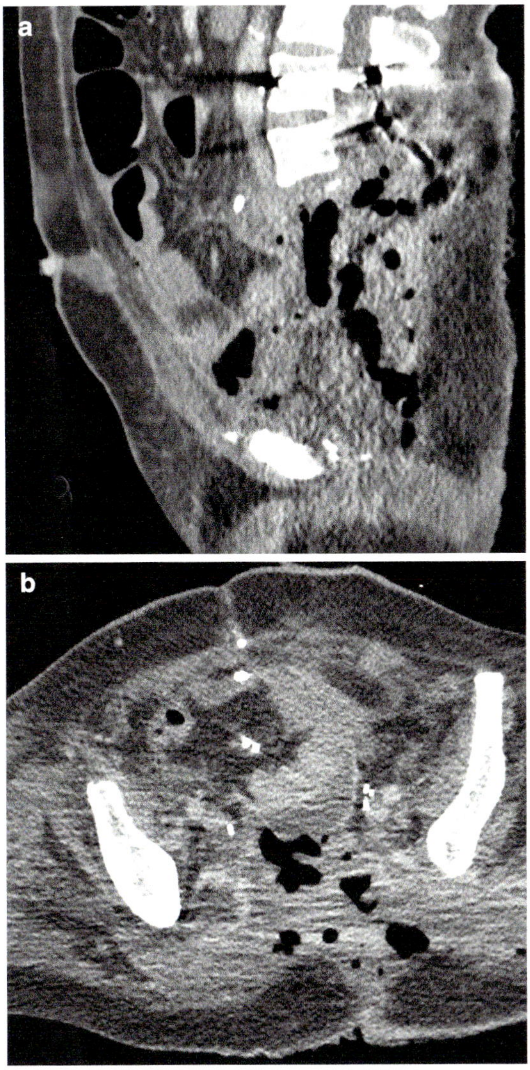

Fig. 66.7 Postoperative CT scan after the 3rd surgery. This CT scan performed after the 3rd tumor resection shows the resection of the tumor, bladder and rectum in sagittal (**a**) and axial (**b**) slices

After these surgeries, the patient was in a good mood, has no pain, ASI A down from L4, and colostoma plus ileum conduit make the care much easier for nurses and the patient himself.

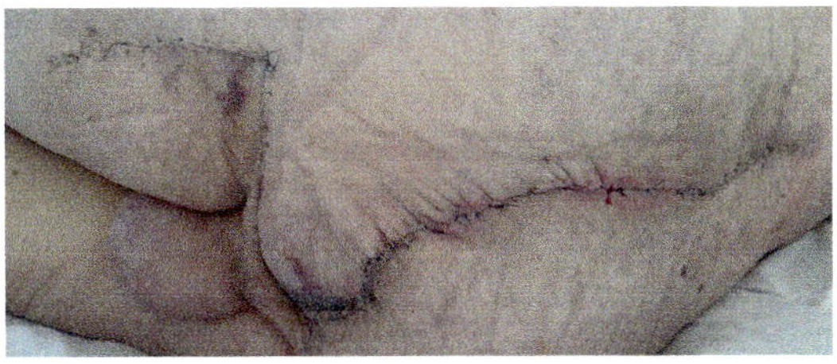

Fig. 66.8 Bilobed gluteal flap. This picture shows the bilobed femoro-gluteal flap which was used to gain skin from the left thigh, which was then rotated in the resection cavity after de-epithelilization in a two-step manner. The femoral site was closed primarily

The patient was then scheduled for local radiotherapy and radiotherapy of the liver and retroperitoneum.

66.3 Discussion of the Cases

66.3.1 Anatomy of the Sacrum

The osseos part of the sacrum consists of five fused vertebrae with the sacral canal opening posteriorly at the lower end at S5. From posterior, the sacrum is convex and opens in four right- and left-sided anterior and posterior foramina. The spinous processes of S1 to S4 fuse to the median sacral crest. At the cranial end, the S1 endplate neigbours the L5/S1 disc which – togehter with the two facet articulations allow flexion–extension of 10–15° and 5° of rotation to each side. The sacrococcygeal as well as the sacroiliac joints (SIJ) are amphiarthroses with no actual movement [16]. Many ligaments hold the sacrum in place and do not allow too much movement: sacrotuberous and sacrospinous ligaments to the ischial tuberosity and ischial spine, interosseous sacroiliac ligaments within SIJ, anterior sacroiliac ligament, and dorsal sacroiliac ligament to the SIJ. Musclewise, the multifidus and erector spinae muscles, gluteus maximus, and the pyriform muscle an insert at the sacrum. Concerning nerve structures, the dural sac end at S2 containing the terminal filum (a continuation of the pia) leads from the conus medullaris to the dural sac's end attaching to the dura and further down to the periosteum of the first coccygeal segment. The nerve roots of the sacrum enter anteriorily through the 4 foramina with their ventral rami anterior and the dorsal one posterior while S5 exits at the sacral ends. The lumbosacral plexus is formed by the L4 to S4 roots bilaterally. Concerning the autonomous system, the inferior hypogastric anterior of the lower sacrum surrounds pelvic organs while the superior hypogastric plexus surrounds the bifurcation of the aorty and the anterior side the body of L5 vertebra and upper sacral part. The sympathetic trunks go down to the anterior sacral side including ganglia and terminate by fusing at the coccyx as ganglion impar [16]. Surgically, the adjacent structures are also crucial to know, including.

66.3.2 Indication and Techniques of Sacral Tumor Resections Including Sacrectomy

While partial sacrectomy is well tolerated and does not require instrumentation, extensive tumor expansion – which is quite common due to the long and unspecific symptoms causing large tumor sizes upon diagnosis – requires lumbopelvic instrumentation as shown in our cases.

Concerning the extent of resection, sacrum resection should be supramarginal – if possible – meaning approximately one sacral segment above the tumor [17].

Low sacrectomy down from S3 does not involve the SIJ and can be performed comparably easily from a dorsal approach (Fig. 66.9). Depending on the involvement of anterior structures, an abdominosacral approach can still be necessary, however [17]. Since the S3 nerve root is not affected, low sacrectomy usually does not cause bowel and bladder dysfunction.

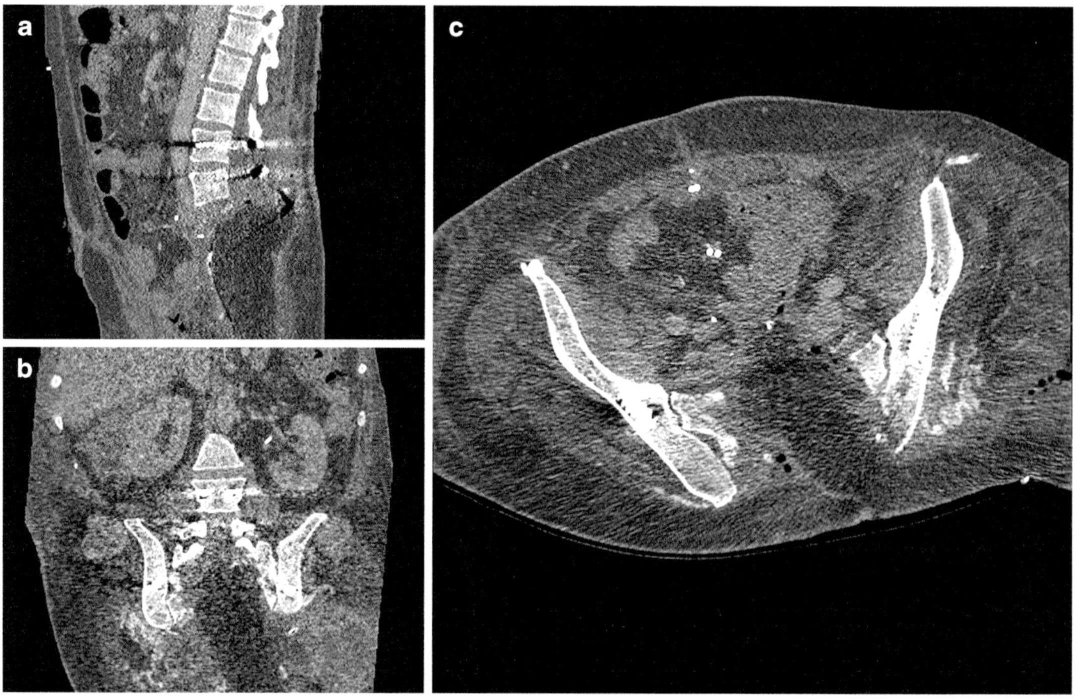

Fig. 66.9 Postoperative CT scan after the 6th and last surgery. This CT scan shows the previous tumor space after resection and after reconstruction via the bilobed gluteal flap in sagittal (**a**), coronal (**b**), and axial (**c**) slices. The hypodense structure filling the resection cavity is the de-epithelialized cutaneous flap and its subcutaneous fatty tissue

More extensive sacral resection goes along with a higher risk of sequelae. High blood loss during bony resection, affection of the sacral nerve roots but also the large resection cavity that is difficult to fill can cause considerable wound complications as in our case 2. In this case, the first attempt using an omentum majus graft failed due to omental ischemia after mobilization. Since a large resection cavity is also more prone to develop infection, we then first treated this complication by vaccum draping and by a consecutive large skin flap, which was rotated into the resection cavity after the upper dermal layers were removed.

Additionally, high sacrectomy can necessitate the resection and closure of the dural sac, which can result in CSF leakage if not watertight.

Concerning the preservation of neurological function, some authors recommend the preservation of the S2 root in order to potentially preserve rectal and bladder control. Yet, although each nerve root should be preserved if possible, this should not affect tumor free margins. Preservation of all roots was possible in case 1 but not case 2, since this patient already had intradural tumor mass up to L5 and no neurological function below L4 (Fig. 66.4). Important to mention that despite complete sacral resection, lower extremity function is only affected to a minor extent if gluteal and sciatic nerves are preserved [17].

Considering Fig. 66.10, it is worth mentioning that a subtotal sacrectomy preserving the S1 roots maintains the spinopelvic continuity, thus making instrumentation not necessary.

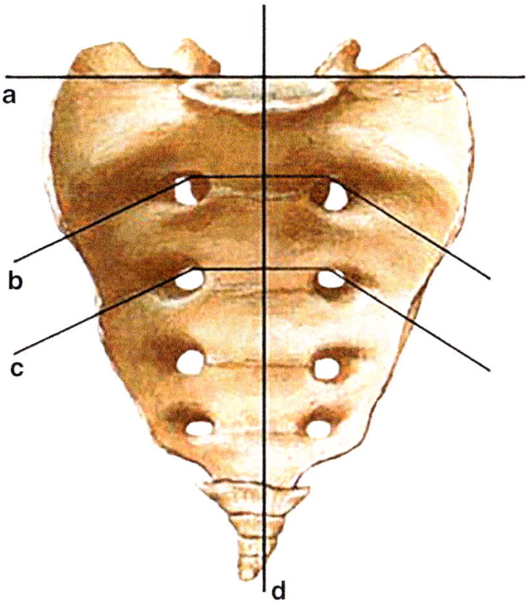

Fig. 66.10 Levels of sacrectomy. This is Fig. 11 from Ramamurthy et al. [17] showing the different levels of secrectomy: A = total (upper margin at L5/S1), B = subtotal (S1 roots preserved), C = partial sacrectomy (S2 roots preserved), and D = hemisacrectomy [17]

66.3.3 Fixation and Bony Reconstruction Techniques Following Resection

Both our cases required spinopelvic instrumentation due to the resection of 1 (case 1) or 2 (case 2) sacral alae including S1 thus causing spinopelvic discontinuation. Usually, subtotal sacral resection caudal of S1 does not cause any instability since the oblique SIJ can take over the weight from the spine; some authors even define the remaining upper half of S1 as being stable. Total sacrectomy including S1, however, requires instrumentation in order to reconstruct the pelvic ring and any connection between the lumbar spine and pelvis [17]. Nowadays, lumbar pedicle screws to the lowest non-infiltrated vertebrae (L4&5 in case 1, L3&4 in case 2) plus iliac screws are the treatment of choice if instrumentation is required. Yet, other approaches have been used over the last decades, including Galveston rods, Harrington compression plates, sacral bars, and anterior instrumentation (Tables 66.1 and 66.2) [1, 17].

Depending on the type of tumor and further treatment, additional bone grafts are recommended. In our cases, however, immediate radiotherapy 4 weeks after surgery lead to not using bone grafts in order to avoid additional risk of infection and considering the minimal chance of bony fusion due to radiotherapy. Concerning implant failure, a larger series investigated instrumentation complications in sacral tumor patients and found a rate of revision surgery due to implant failure by 16.1% [1].

Given this high rate of severe complications, there is a considerable number of authors reporting no instrumentation after total sacrectomy at all. They argue that scar formation, ligaments and muscles bridging between spine and pelvis provide a flexible "sling" which frequently admitting ambulation [1]. The furthermost described reconstruction strategies are anterior spinal column fixation (ASCF), spinopelvic fixation (SPF), and posterior pelvic ring fixation (PPRF) which are mostly used in a combined fashion [17]. Yet, an general failure rate of instrumentation by 16.1% is frequently reported [1]. Concerning outcome, many authors favor very radical approached including resection of the S1 to S5 nerve roots leading to total bowel and badder dysfunction. Concerning the instrumentation failure, this is reported to be more common if no anterior spinal column support is provided.

While traditionally Galveston L-rods and transiliac bars were used for spinopelvic fusion and pelvic ring fixation most recent approaches favor lumbar pedicle screw systems, cross conectors and iliac screws.

66.3.4 Management of Sacral Defect

Sacrectomy is associated with a high rate of wound dehiscence or skin necrosis as we experienced it in case 2 (Tables 66.1 and 66.2) [1, 17]. Several reasons make this course obvious: large defects are created, the situs is close to the anus, and vessels important for local perfusion such as branches of the iliac arteries are closed. Thus, in order to avoid complications, it is crucial to avoid wound dehiscence, hematoma, and dead space at any circumstances. Besides omentum flaps, a primary transabdominal vertical rectus abdominis myocutaneous flap (VRAM flap), and gluteal advancement flaps (as in case 2) provide the most straightforward options. Free flaps can be an option but are lacking sufficient blood supply if the tumor already infiltrated major glutal vessels and are usually more prone to complications than the options above. General surgical complications in sacral tumor resections are common due to the extensive surgeries. A larger series by Bederman et al. reported the use of soft tissue flaps in 72.1% of cases and an average blood loss of 9.3 L per patient (range 1.5–21.7 L).

66.3.5 General Outcome

After surgery, complications included vascular complications in 30.4%, infections in 30.4%, wound dehiscence in 17.4%, and GI complications in 30.4% of cases [1]. The same series reported long-term outcomes showing that 56% of patients had no recurrence 37 months after surgery while 24% had local and 20% had metastastic disease due to osteosarcoma, chondrosarcoma, and chordoma (Table 66.2). From a functional point of view, 89.7% of patients were still ambulatory if they were before surgery.

Our 2 cases nicely outline the major aspects of sacral resection: while the first case did not show any deficit after resection of this still circumscribed tumor, the larger resection of the gigantic tumor in case 2 lead to a variety of complications which are quite typical and frequent in the literature.

66.3.6 Accordance with the Literature Guidelines

Due to the rarity of the diseases and the surgeries, there are no guidelines available. There is only one comprehensive review which outlines the surgical therapy and reconstruction for patients with sacral tumors [1].

Level of Evidence: C
The level of evidence available to date is still poor with only case reports and small series being available.

66.4 Conclusions and Take Home Message

The surgical treatment of sacral tumors is a large and complexe endeavor and patient need to be made aware of the chances but also the high rate of complications and morbidity such surgeries might cause.

Table 66.1 Reconstruction and complications

Author	Year	# Pts	Extra sacral resection	Nerve sacrifice	Spinopelvic fixation (cephalad level)	Posterior pelvic ring fixation	Anterior spinal column support	Soft tissue flaps	Blood loss (mL)	Operative complications?
Humphries et al. [8]	2010	1	No	S1–S5	PS (L3). connected to transverse rod between IS	(1) TI bar (2) IS with transverse rod (3) Titanium mesh cage between ilia	–	VRAM	NR	*S. epidemidis* abscess, ischial decubitus ulcer
Gallia et al. [6]	2010	1	(B) ilia, L5	L5–S5	PS (LI), connected to transverse rod between IS	(1) 2 TI bars (2) IS with transverse rod (3) TI femoral graft	(1) Vertical rod through L2–L4 bodies (2) DiSractable cage between L4 endplate and TI bar	Paraspinal and partial LD	800 (stage 1). 8,500 (stage 2)	Abdominal hematoma, wound dehiscence, DVT
Varga et al. [25]	2010	1	No	S1–S5	PS (L2), connected to IS with U-shaped rod	(1) Bone graft between ilium and L5	–	GM	NR	NR
Newman et al. [13]	2009	1	(L) ilium	S1–S5	PS (LI), connected to transverse rod between IS	(1) IS with two transverse rods (2) Stacked, carbon-fiber cages	–	RAM + (R) GM	1,500	Flap hematoma
McLoughlin et al. [10]	2008	1	(B) ilia	S1–S5	PS (L3), connected to IS: two vertical rods connected to PS rod and TI bar	(1) TI bar (2) TI femoral graft	–	Alloderm sling	6,000	NR
Shen el al. [20]	2006	1	No	NR	PS (L2), connected to IS–two rods/side	–	(1) Bilateral titanium mesh cages from L5 to SI joint	(R) RAM	1,100 (stage 1). 2,900 (stage 2)	Ileus

(continued)

Table 66.1 (continued)

Author	Year	# Pts	Extra sacral resection	Nerve sacrifice	Spinopelvic fixation (cephalad level)	Posterior pelvic ring fixation	Anterior spinal column support	Soft tissue flaps	Blood loss (mL)	Operative complications?
Gallia et al. [5]	2005	1	(B) ilia	S1–S5	PS (L3), connected to transverse rod between IS	(1) TI bar (2) IS with transverse rod (3) TI femoral graft	–	RAM	NR	Ileus, vocal cord paralysis. UTI, infection (8 mo)
Foumey et al. [4]	2005	3	No	S1–S5	PS (L3), connected to Galveston rods	(1) TI bar (2) TI tibial graft	–	RAM	NR	SB injury, upper GI hemorrhage and major wound dehiscence
								GM		NR
								RAM		NR
Dickey et al. [2]	2005	6	L5 (some cases)	SI–S5	PS (L3 or L4), connected to IS	(1) 2 TI bars	(1) Two oblique, fibular grafts	RAM RAM RAM None None RAM	NR	None None NR None None Wound infection
Min et al. [11]	2005	1	(B) ilia	SI–S4	PS (L4), connected to IS	(1) Two TI tibial grafts	–	NR	4,300	Wound dehiscence
Zileli et al. [27]	2003	1	No	SI–S5	PS (L2 or L3). connected to custom iliac plate	(1) Custom iliac plate	–	Myocutaneous	3,400	Instrument infection
		2			PS (L2 or L3), connected to TI bar	(1) Two TI bars		NR	NR	NR
Ohata et al. [14]	2004	1	(B) ilia	(L) L5 and S1–S5	PS (L3), connected to IS	(1) TI bar (2) Two TI fibular grafts	–	GM	12,000	UTI, instrument infection

Doita et al. [3]	2003	3	No (B) ilia No	SI–S5 (R) sciatic, S1–S5	PS (L5), connected to TI bar PS (L3), connected to IS; fibular graft between posterolateral spine and ilia	(1) TI bar (1) TI bar	– –	NR NR NR	9250 7,500 9,600	NR NR Wound infections (debridement)
Mooney et al. [12]	1999	1	No	SI–S5	PS (L3), connected to Galveston rods	(1) TI bar (2) TI fibular graft	(1) Two oblique, iliolumbar screws	GM	NR	NR
Sar et al. [19]	2002	3	NR	SI–S4	PS (L3), connected to Galveston rods or IS	(1) one or two TI fibular graft	–	NR	NR	NR Deep wound infection NR
Wuisman et al. [26]	2001	1	(B) ilia	SI–S5	PS (L2), connected to custom plate	(1) Custom iliac plate	–	GM	8,500	Right lateral wound dehiscence
Jackson et al. [9]	2000	5	NR	NR	PS (L3), connected to Galveston rods	(1) TI bar	–	RAM RAM RAM	NR NR NR	None Seizures and UTI Small intestinal perforation, sepsis, coagulopathy, *C difficile*
								GM	NR	*C. difficile*
								RAM	NR	UTI
Spiegel et al. [23]	1999	1	(R) ilia	S1–S5	PS (L3), connected to Galveston rods	(1) Pelvic reconstruction place	–	NR	NR	NR
Gokaslan et al. [7]	1997	2	No	SI–S5	PS (L3), connected to Galveston rods	(1) TI bar	–	RAM	21,500 21,700	NR
Santi et al. [18]	1993	1	No	SI–S5	Hooks and CD rods, connected to TI bar (LA)	(l) Two TI bars	–	NR	6,500	NR
Shikata et al. [22]	1992	1	(B) ilia	L5–S5	Two compression rods. connected to TI bar (L3)	(1) Two TI bars	–	NR	6,300	NR

(continued)

Table 66.1 (continued)

Author	Year	# Pts	Extra sacral resection	Nerve sacrifice	Spinopelvic fixation (cephalad level)	Posterior pelvic ring fixation	Anterior spinal column support	Soft tissue flaps	Blood loss (mL)	Operative complications?
Tomita et al. [24]	1990	2	No	S1–S5	2 Harrington rods; fibular grafts between L4 pedicles and ipsilateral ilium (NR)	(1) TI bar	_	NR	7,500	NR
			No	(R) L5, S1–S5	CD Instrumentation (T12)	(1) AO 16-hole broad plate (2) AO Recon ante lion plate	_	NR	17,000	Tom iliac vein
Shikata et al. [21]	1988	2	(B) ilia	S1–S5	Two Harrington rods (L3); fibular grafts between L3, L4, and ipsilateral ilium	(1) Two TI bars	_	NR	10,000	NR

This is Table 2 from Bedermann et a. (2014) providing an overview on the reconstruction and the concomitant complications [1]
B bilateral, *L* left, *R* right, *N* no, *N/A* not applicable, *NR* not reported, *PS* pedicle screw, *IS* iliac screw, *TI* transiliac, *CD* Cotrel–Dubousset, *RAM* rectus abdominis myocutaneous, *LD* latissimus dorsi, *CM* gluteus maximus

Table 66.2 Reconstruction and long-term outcome

Author	Year	SPF	PSF	PPRF	ASF	Follow up (months)	Ambulation	Bowel/bladder deficit	Revision instrumentation	Pain at final follow up	Tumor recurrence
Humphries et al. [8]	2010	N	Y	Y	N	12	Yes (R-AFO)	NR	None	None	None
Gallia et at. [6]	2010	N	Y	Y	Y	5	No	Yes	None	Metastasis	Metastasis
Varga et al. [25]	2010	N	Y	Y	N	NR	Yes (cane)	NR	None[a]	None[a]	None[a]
Newman et al. [13]	2009	N	Y	Y	N	6	Yes (Walker)	Partial	None[a]	NR	NR
McLoughlin et al. [10]	2008	N	Y	Y	N	24	Yes	Yes	None	None	NR
Shen et al. [20]	2006	N	Y	N	Y	9	No	Yes	None	NR	NR
Gallia et al. [5]	2005	N	Y	Y	N	12	Yes	Yes	None	Due to metastasis	Local + Metastasis
Fourney et al. [4]	2005	O	Y	Y	N	83	Yes	Yes	NR	NR	Local
						58	NR		NR	NR	Local + Metastasis
						33	Yes		NR	NR	Local
Dickey et al. [2]	2005	N	Y	Y	Y	8	Yes	Yes	None	Improved	None
						7	Yes		None		None
						38	Yes		Revision instrumentation (6 and 29 months)		None
						42	No		None		Local
						36	Yes		None		None
						14	No		None		Local
Min et al. [11]	2005	N	Y	Y	N	60	Yes (crutches)	Yes	Lumbar rod breakage at 4 months (rods replaced)	Improved4	None
Zileli et al. [27]	2003	N	Y	Y	N	Mean 28 (range 18-42)	Yes (crutches)	NR	None		Local + Metastasis
							Yes (crutches)	NR	Revision instrumentation at 7 years		None
							Yes (crutches)	NR	None	None	None
Ohara et al. [14]	2004	N	Y	Y	N	60	Yes (crutches)	Yes	None	NR	None

(continued)

Table 66.2 (continued)

Author	Year	SPF	PSF	PPRF	ASF	Follow up (months)	Ambulation	Bowel/ bladder deficit	Revision instrumentation	Pain at final follow up	Tumor recurrence
Doita et al. [3]	2003	N	Y	Y	N	36	Yes (cane)	Partial	None	Improved	NR
						36	Yes (crutches)	Yes	None	NR	Local
						36	Yes (crutches)	Partial	None	NR	NR
Mooney et al. [12]	1999	O	Y	Y	Y	8	Yes (walker + R- AFO)	Yes	NR	NR	Metastasis
Sar et al. [19]	2002	O	Y	Y	N	49	NR	Yes	None	NR	None
						33	NR	Yes	None	NR	Local
						47	NR	Yes	None	NR	None
Wuisman et al. [26]	2001	N	Y	Y	N	36	Yes (cane + AFO)	Yes	None	None	None
Jackson et al. [9]	2000	O	Y	Y	N	50	Yes (walker)	NR	NR	Improved	NR
						47	Yes				
						31	Yes (walker)				
						11	Yes				
						8	Yes (cane)				
Spiegel et al. [23]	1999	O	Y	Y	N	74	Yes (AFO)	Yes	Ilial rod and pelvic ptate breakage (no operation–patient asymptomatic)	Occasional	None
Gokaslan et al. [7]	1997	O	Y	Y	N	12	Yes (cane)	Yes	NR	NR	NR
							Yes	Yes	NR	NR	NR
Santi et al. [18]	1993	O	Y	Y	N	33	Yes (AFO)	NR	Hardware removed due to discomfort (7 months)	None	None
Shikala et al. [22]	1992	O	Y	Y	N	72	Yes (cane)	Partial	None	NR	NR
Tomita et al. [24]	1990	O	Y	Y	N	69	Yes	Yes	None	NR	None
			Y	Y	N	10	Yes (AFO)	Partial	NR	NR	None
Shikala et al. [21]	1988	O	Y	Y	N	24	Yes (brace)	Partial	None	NR	NR
			Y	Y	N	14	Yes (cane)	Partial	None	NR	NR

This is Table 3 from Bedermann et a. (2014) providing an overview on the reconstruction method and the long-term outcome [1]
NR not reported, *AFO* ankle foot orthosis
[a]Based on email correspondence

Pearls

- Sacral tumors should mostly be resected with safe margins
- The risk of deficits is high especially for bowel and bladder function
- Considering the load in the instrumentation, hardware failure rates of 16% are actually lower than expected
- No dead space should be left after sacrectomy

Level of Evidence

Bederman: III, B

Ozaki: III, B

Payer: III, B

Ramamurthy: III, C

References

1. Bederman SS, Shah KN, Hassan JM, Hoang BH, Kiester PD, Bhatia NN. Surgical techniques for spinopelvic reconstruction following total sacrectomy: a systematic review. Eur Spine J. 2014;23(2):305–19. https://doi.org/10.1007/s00586-013-3075-z.
2. Dickey ID, Hugate RR Jr, Fuchs B, et al. Reconstruction after total sacrectomy: early experience with a new surgical technique. Clin Orthop Relat Res. 2005;438:42–50. pii:00003086-200509000-00010.
3. Doita M, Harada T, Iguchi T, et al. Total sacrectomy and reconstruction for sacral tumors. Spine (Phila Pa 1976). 2003;28:E296–301. https://doi.org/10.1097/01.BRS.0000083230.12704.E3.
4. Fourney DR, Rhines LD, Hentschel SJ, et al. En bloc resection of primary sacral tumors: classification of surgical approaches and outcome. J Neurosurg Spine. 2005;3:111–22. https://doi.org/10.3171/spi.2005.3.2.0111.
5. Gallia GL, Haque R, Garonzik I, et al. Spinal pelvic reconstruction after total sacrectomy for en bloc resection of a giant sacral chordoma: technical note. J Neurosurg Spine. 2005;3:501–6. https://doi.org/10.3171/spi.2005.3.6.0501.
6. Gallia GL, Suk I, Witham TF, et al. Lumbopelvic reconstruction after combined L5 spondylectomy and total sacrectomy for en bloc resection of a malignant fibrous histiocytoma. Neurosurgery. 2010;67:E498–502. https://doi.org/10.1227/01.NEU.0000382972 15422.10.
7. Gokaslan ZL, Romsdahl MM, Kroll SS, et al. Total sacrectomy and Galveston L-rod reconstruction for malignant neoplasms. Technical note. J Neurosurg. 1997;87:781–7. https://doi.org/10.3171/jns.1997.87.5.0781.
8. Humphries WE 3rd, Satyan KB, Relyea K, et al. Low-grade myofibroblastic sarcoma of the sacrum. J Neurosurg Pediatr. 2010;6:286–90. https://doi.org/10.3171/2010.5.PEDS09289.
9. Jackson RJ, Gokaslan ZL. Spinal-pelvic fixation in patients with lumbosacral neoplasms. J Neurosurg. 2000;92:61–70.
10. McLoughlin GS, Sciubba DM, Suk I, et al. En bloc total sacrectomy performed in a single stage through a posterior approach. Neurosurgery. 2008;63:ONS115–20. https://doi.org/10.1227/01.neu.0000335025.93026.68. (discussion ONS120).
11. Min K, Espinosa N, Bode B, Exner GU. Total sacrectomy and reconstruction with structural allografts for neurofibrosarcoma of the sacrum. A case report. J Bone Joint Surg Am. 2005;87:864–9. https://doi.org/10.2106/JBJS.D.02299.
12. Mooney JF 3rd, Glazier SS, Turner CS, DeFranzo AJ Jr. Fibrosarcoma of the sacrum in a child: management by sacral resection and reconstruction. J South Orthop Assoc. 1999;8:218–21.
13. Newman CB, Keshavarzi S, Aryan HE. En bloc sacrectomy and reconstruction: technique modification for pelvic fixation. Surg Neurol. 2009;72:752–6. https://doi.org/10.1016/j.surneu.2009.02.008. (discussion 756).
14. Ohata N, Ozaki T, Kunisada T, et al. Extended total sacrectomy and reconstruction for sacral tumor. Spine (Phila Pa 1976). 2004;29:E123–6. pii:00007632-200403150-00021.
15. Ozaki T, Flege S, Liljenqvist U, Hillmann A, Delling G, Salzer-Kuntschik M, et al. Osteosarcoma of the spine: experience of the Cooperative Osteosarcoma Study Group. Cancer. 2002;94(4):1069–77.
16. Payer M. Neurological manifestation of sacral tumors. Neurosurg Focus. 2003;15(2):E1. https://doi.org/10.3171/foc.2003.15.2.1.
17. Ramamurthy R, Bose JC, Muthusamy V, Natarajan M, Kunjithapatham D. Staged sacrectomy – an adaptive approach. J Neurosurg Spine. 2009;11(3):285–94. https://doi.org/10.3171/2009.3.SPINE08824.
18. Santi MD, Mitsunaga MM, Lockett JL. Total sacrectomy for a giant sacral schwannoma. A case report. Clin Orthop Relat Res. 1993;294:285–9.
19. Sar C, Eralp L. Surgical treatment of primary tumors of the sacrum. Arch Orthop Trauma Surg. 2002;122:148–55. https://doi.org/10.1007/s00402-001-0356-5.
20. Shen FH, Harper M, Foster WC, et al. A novel "four-rod technique" for lumbo-pelvic reconstruction: theory and technical considerations. Spine (Phila Pa 1976). 2006;31:1395–401. https://doi.org/10.1097/01.brs.0000219527.64180.95.
21. Shikata J, Yamamuro T, Kotoura Y, et al. Total sacrectomy and reconstruction for primary tumors. Report of two cases. J Bone Joint Surg Am. 1988;70:122–5.

22. Shikata J, Yamamuro T, Shimizu K, Kotoura Y. Surgical treatment of giant-cell tumors of the spine. Clin Orthop Relat Res. 1992;278:29–36.
23. Spiegel DA, Richardson WJ, Scully SP, Harrelson JM. Long-term survival following total sacrectomy with reconstruction for the treatment of primary osteosarcoma of the sacrum. A case report. J Bone Joint Surg Am. 1999;81:848–55.
24. Tomita K, Tsuchiya H. Total sacrectomy and reconstruction for huge sacral tumors. Spine (Phila Pa 1976). 1990;15:1223–7.
25. Varga PP, Lazary A. Chordoma of the sacrum: "en bloc"total sacrectomy and lumbopelvic reconstruction. Eur Spine J. 2010;19:1039–40. https://doi.org/10.1007/s00586-010-1460-4.
26. Wuisman P, Lieshout O, Van Dijk M, Van Diest P. Reconstruction after total en bloc sacrectomy for osteosarcoma using a custom-made prosthesis: a technical note. Spine (Phila Pa1976). 2001;26:431–9.
27. Zileli M, Hoscoskun C, Brastianos P, Sabah D. Surgical treatment of primary sacral tumors: complications associated with sacrectomy. Neurosurg Focus. 2003;15:E9 (pii:150509).

67 Radical Excision Is Beneficial for Chordoma?

Martin Gehrchen

67.1 Introduction

Sacral chordomas are rare tumors associated with a poor long-term prognosis mainly caused by local recurrence. Furthermore, resection in this anatomical region is often associated with loss of neural function. The present case illustrates the use of resection with wide surgical margin (R0).

67.2 Case Description

Fifty-two year old female referred to our hospital due to sacral lesion as depicted on MRI (Fig. 67.1). Symptoms started 7 years prior with nonspecific noncontinues discomfort from the sacral and coccygeal region. The last year before examination the pain has become constant. Clinically only tenderness of the lower sacral bone and coccygeal

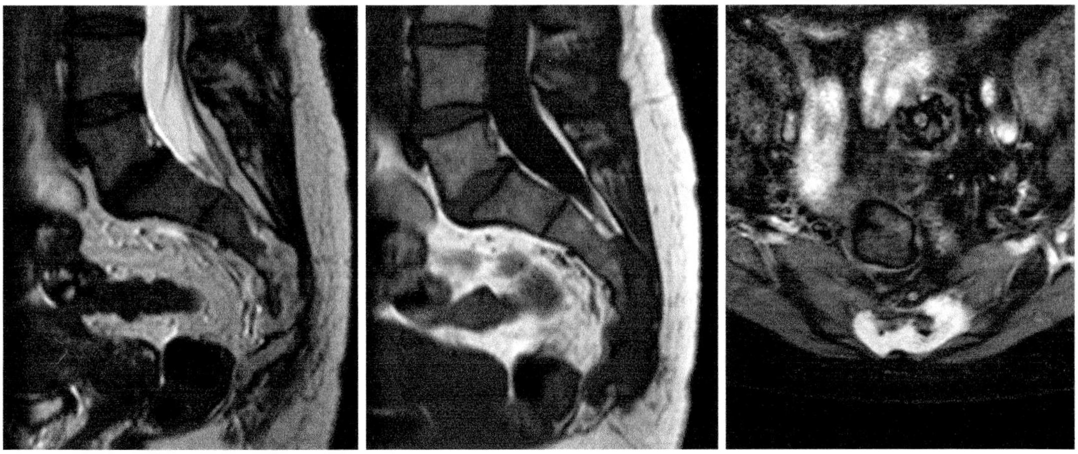

Fig. 67.1 T1 and T2 weighted sagittal and an axial sections showing the chroma from S2 and distally

M. Gehrchen (✉)
Spine Unit, Department of Orthopaedic Surgery, Rigshospitalet, University of Copenhagen, Copenhagen, Denmark

B. Meyer, M. Rauschmann (eds.), *Spine Surgery*, https://doi.org/10.1007/978-3-319-98875-7_67

bone was found and altered consistence of the tissue at the tumor site. Tumor cannot be palpated with certainty. The patient had no relevant comorbidities. Posterior biopsy confirms the diagnosis and surgery was planned based on MRI and PET-CT demonstrating the chordoma reaching the S2 level from distally making it possible to spare the S1 and S2 nerve roots (Fig. 67.2). A R0 resection was performed and histology confirms the wide resection. The patient had a postoperative bleed that was evacuated succesfully. Minor micturion problems evolved, therefore abdominal pressure was used when voiding. No incontinence. Patient has been followed now for 7 years with MRI and CT with no signs of local recurrence or metastasis (Fig. 67.3).

67.3 Discussion of the Case

The wide resection in this case is a good choice because due to the level of involvement it was possible to save the S2 nerve roots and above. This leaves minor sequelae compared to more proximal levels and the possibility of neurological recovery (Level of evidence IV, Recommendation A). In chordomas arising above level S3, surgery will always result in severe neurological deficits including bowel, bladder and motor impairment. In all cases of sacral chordomas, thorough information to the patient and relatives are necessary since some patients without preoperatively neurological impairment would prefer radiation therapy alone accepting a higher risk of recurrence.

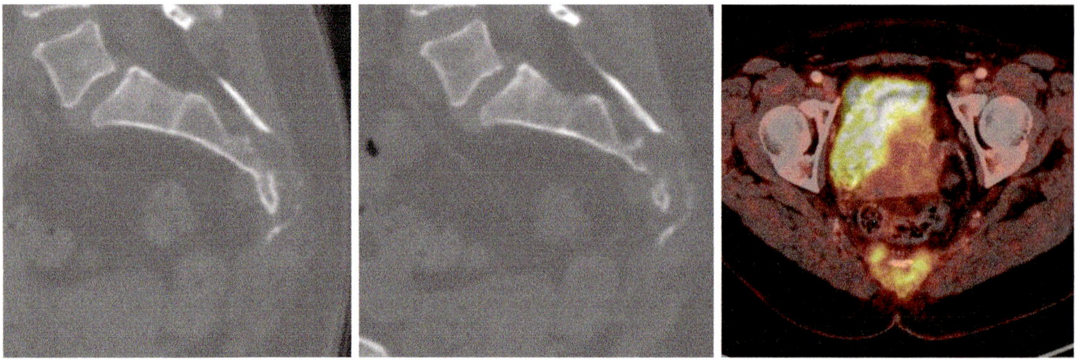

Fig. 67.2 CT demonstrating a bone lesion and PET CT illustrating uptake on the right

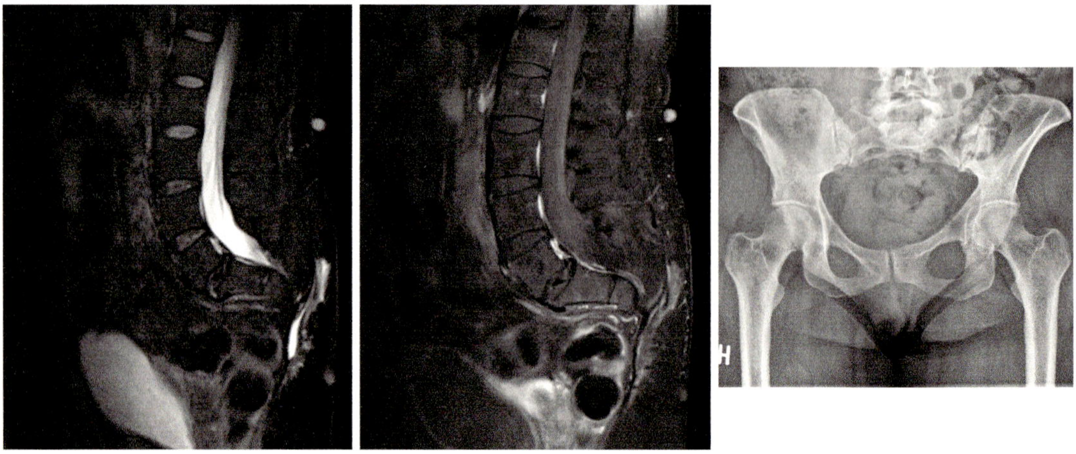

Fig. 67.3 Seven year postoperative T1 and T2 weighted sagittal imaging and an x-ray

The patients should be made aware however of the potential toxic effect of high dose definitive radiation therapy. Radiation therapy should be considered a valid alternative to surgery in patients with intact neurological function (Level of evidence V, Recommendation A).

Instead of radiation therapy, particle therapy (carbon ion therapy (CIT) and proton beam therapy (PBT)) has shown very promising results on both local recurrence rate and rate of metastases. This technique can especially enhance the treatment of sacral chordomas originating above S3 reducing severe neurological affection in these patients. Furthermore, the toxic effect off radiation therapy is also reduced and in combination with debulging of tumors it's a very promising option. To reduce toxic effect of particle therapy spacers can be inserted between tumor and rectum.

67.4 Conclusions and Take Home Message

The most important thing in evaluation of sacral chordomas is to differentiate the origin of the tumor above or below S3 due to the impact on neural structures at risk when performing wide surgical resection and thus reducing postoperative morbidity. Particle therapy is a valid and durable option, maybe even in tumors originating below S2 and revision cases.

References

1. Radaelli S, et al. Sacral chordoma: long-term outcome of a large series of patients surgically treated at two reference centers. Spine. 2017;41(12):1049–57.
2. Stacchiotti S, et al. Best practices for the management of local-regional recurrent chordoma: a position paper by the Chordoma Global Concensus Group. Ann Oncol. 2017;28:1230–42.
3. Stacchiotti S, Sommer J. Building a global consensus approach to chordoma: a position paper from the medical and patient community. Lancet Oncol. 2015;16:e71–83.
4. Aibe N, et al. Outcomes of patients with primary sacral chordoma treated with definitive proton beam therapy. Int J Radiat Oncol Phys. 2018;100(4):972–9.
5. Mima M, et al. Particle therapy using carbon ion or protons as a definitive therapy for patients with primary sacral chordoma. Br J Radiol. 2014;87(1033):20130512.

Intradural Extramedullary Lesions

68

Anna Zdunczyk and Peter Vajkoczy

68.1 Introduction

Intradural extramedullary lesions are tumors arising within the dura but outside the actual spinal cord and account for 40% of all spinal tumors. Among these, meningeomas (33%) and tumors of spinal nerves (27%) are the most common [1]. Spinal meningeomas most frequently occur in the posterior or lateral thoracic region, followed by anterior cervical region and lumbosacral region. Nerve sheath tumors may occur sporadic or associated with neurofibromatosis type 1 or neurofibromatosis type 2. By the WHO grading, these tumors include schwannomas, neurofibromas, and malignant nerve sheath tumors. Rarely, other extramedullary tumors may occur including myxopapillary ependymomas, hemangiopericytomas, lipomas, paragangliomas, epidermoid and dermoid cysts [2].

Clinical symptoms develop through an impairment of neural elements and pathways, producing both local and distal effects. Noctural pain is one of the most frequent symptoms followed by dysesthesias and muscular weakness. Once a tumor reaches a critical mass, signs and symptoms of myelopathy may occur [3].

Early diagnosis and adequacy of surgical intervention are the key determinants for the best long-term prognosis and preservation of neurological integrity [3, 4].

Traditionally, open surgical techniques have been used. These include a dorsal midline incision, subperiostal dissection of the paraspinal muscles and a wide laminectomy. In the recent years, minimally invasive approaches have become increasingly popular due to the reduced soft tissue dissection and disruption of midline structures. Studies comparing the traditional open versus minimally invasive approach have shown a nearly identical rate of gross total resection while reducing the risk for postoperative spinal instability. Furthemore, minimally invasive procedures were associated with significantly decreased operative blood loss, diminished narcotic use, shorter postoperative stay, and lower costs of hospitalization [5].

In tumors located anterior to the dentate ligament and/or severe tumor calcifications an anterior or anterlateral approach via an anterior corporectomy and spinal reconstruction have been discussed as an alternative to the common posterior or posterolateral approaches. These more complex procedures, however, need to be weighted against the surgical/neurological risks and increased operative morbidity [6].

A. Zdunczyk · P. Vajkoczy (✉)
Department of Neurosurgery,
Charitè – Universitätsmedizin Berlin,
Berlin, Germany
e-mail: anna.zdunczyk@charite.de;
peter.vajkoczy@charite.de

B. Meyer, M. Rauschmann (eds.), *Spine Surgery*, https://doi.org/10.1007/978-3-319-98875-7_68

The intent of this chapter is to present the clinical characteristics of intradural extramedullary lesions, preoperative physical examination, recommended imaging techniques and specifics of the different surgical techniques. In particular, we will discuss posterior and anterior approaches and the advantages of open and minimally invasive surgery.

By the end of this chapter the reader should develop an understanding of the problems and pitfalls we face when treating intradural extramedullary lesions and be aware of the factors influencing surgical decision-making.

These are:

- Prolonged history and large tumor size until diagnosis
- Technical consideration in choosing the surgical approach depending on tumor location and compression of surrounding structures, calcifications and adhesion site
- Postoperative complications including spinal instability, CSF leakage and wound infections

68.2 Case Description

Here we present the medical history of a 59-years old female patient who presented with a progressive back pain between both scapulae with aggravation during coughing. The patient also described a numbness starting below the umbilicus including both legs and a subjective loss of motor strength in the lower extremity. The physical examination revealed a sensory deficit below the level of T12 and dysesthesia in both feet, however motor strength was not reduced. The patient presented with a mild spinal ataxia and impaired blind – and straight-line walking. MR-imaging of the spinal column detected an isointense, intradural-extramedullary lesion on both T1- and T2-weighted images between C7 and T1 with compression of the spinal cord ventrally and a homogeneous contrast enhancement after the administration of gadolinium (Figs. 68.1 and 68.2).

Due to the patients' progressive clinical symptoms and newly detected homogeneous mass lesion on the level of C7 and T1 with consecutive compression of the spinal cord surgical resection was recommended. Since the tumor adhesion to the dura was localized anterior to the dentate ligament the tumor was categorized as an anterior meningioma.

Surgical procedure

The patient was in a prone position with the head in a Mayfield clamp. Despite the anterior origin of the tumor resection was performed through a dorsal approach with a left sided hemilaminectomy of C7 and T1, under continuous intraoperative MEP monitoring. The dura was opened paramedially. As a next step, the denticulate ligament was identified as the bilateral triangular extension of the pia mater connecting laterally to the dura mater and dividing the spinal canal in an anterior compartment with the ventral nerve root and a posterior with the dorsal nerve root. After transection of the denticulate ligament further mobility was gained through a gentle rotation of the spinal cord. Then the tumor could be distinguished clearly from the surrounding structures. The lesion presented with a strong ventral adhesion. Consequently, the lateral tumor margins were identified and dissected primarily, followed by the ventral and finally cranio-caudal part. After tumor resection, the dura was closed-up water tight, followed by suture of the muscle fascia and skin layers.

Postoperatively, the patient presented with a moderate hypesthesia in the left C8 dermatome but without any new motor deficit. The preoperatively described dorsal pain resolved within a few weeks.

68.3 Discussion of the Case

68.3.1 Indication

Microsurgical resection was performed though a dorsal minimally-invasive approach with hemilaminectomy of C7 and T1. The surgical indication was based upon the progressive clinical symptomatology with pain and dysfunction of the lower motor pathways. The preoperative planning was based upon the spinal MRI with

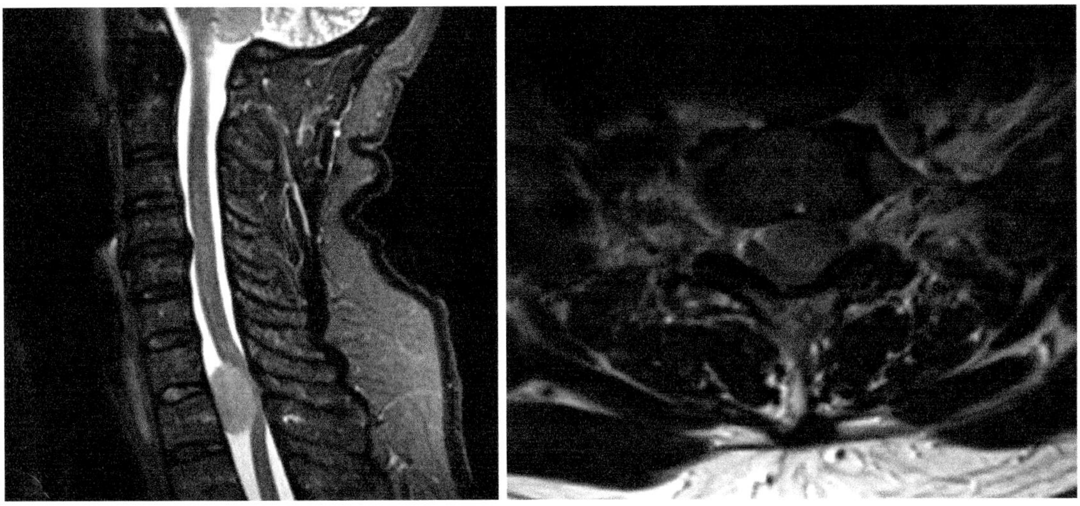

Fig. 68.1 Preoperative T2 weighted MRI

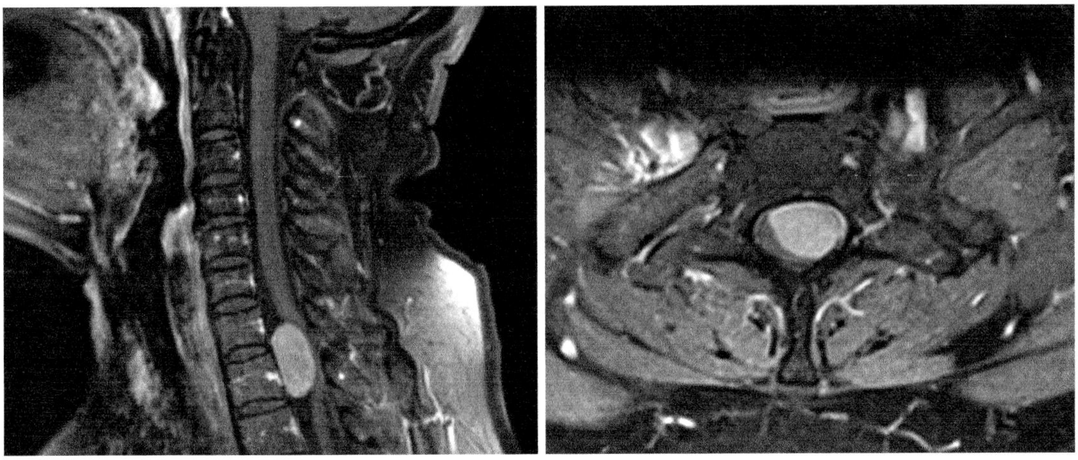

Fig. 68.2 Preoperative T1 weighted MRI with contrast fluid

contrast media application defining the tumor boundaries and extension in relationship to the spinal cord and surrounding neural and vascular structures. Although MRI has become the diagnostic modality of choice for intradural, extramedullary pathologies [7], preoperative CT or Myelo-CT might better appreciate boney intricacies or calcifications and delineate an alternative when MRI is contraindicated.

The surgical goal was a (gross total) resection of the tumor with identification and coagulation of the dural adhesion sites (Simpson II). This is in accordance with the actual guidelines for the management of spinal meningeomas [3, evidence level II, recommendation level B], where surgery is the treatment option of choice to provide the best long-term results and lowest recurrence rates [8]. In spinal meningioma, recent studies failed to demonstrate an advantage for radical Simpson I resections (gross total resection of tumor, excision of dural attachment, and abnormal bone) versus Simpson II in terms of local tumor control and recurrence rate. In contrast, Simpson I resections are associated with a higher complication rate [9]. Therefore a Simpson I resection is recommended only for higher grade, i.e. malignant, lesions. For benign spinal meningioma, a Simpson II resection is recommended by most authors due to comparable long term results and a lower risk for CSF leckage [9].

68.3.2 Choice of Approach

In this illustrative case, a dorsolateral approach through a hemilaminectomy of C7 and T1 was chosen, although the tumor presented with a ventral adhesion site with dorsal displacement of the spinal cord. Tumor resection was accomplished by identification and transsection of the denticulate ligament, mobilization of the tumor mass and further ventral and cranio-caudal dissection.

A complete and safe tumor removal and decompression of the spinal cord are the primary goals of surgery. Standard minimally-invasive posterior or posterolateral approaches provide an adequate exposure for a safe tumor removal in the majority of patients without causing spinal instability by facet joint violation or pedicle resection. Dorsal stabilization should be considered, however, in tumors located at the cervicothoracic or thoracolumbar junction, if there is a previous deformity, 3 or more levels of laminectomy, facetectomy ≥50% (unilateral or bilateral, C2 laminectomy), in "young adults" (<40 years) and persistence of deformity after 1 year of the surgery [10]. This may in particular apply to large intraforaminal neurinoma, where a large bony corridor is needed to achieve complete tumor resection.

When utilizing the posterior approach, a standard longitudinal mid-line incision is followed by dissection of muscular and ligamentous tissue and bony removal one level above and below the targeted lesion [11, 12]. Today, most surgeons would advocate for a unilateral hemilaminectomy or foraminotomy. Some authors also advocate for minimally invasive transmuscular approaches using tubular retractors [8]. After opening the dura and visualization of the tumor, the arachnoid is opened directly over it and detachment of the tumor is started from its dural adhesion site dorsal, lateral or ventrolateral. In the case of primarily ventral attachment, the dorsal approach may be extended more laterally to gain a more oblique approach to the tumor and its attachment without the risk of substantial spinal cord displacement. Using microscissors, bipolar cauterization, ultrasonic cavitation aspirator [8, 13] or less frequently pituitary rongeurs a central tumor debulking is performed. Importantly, In ventral tumors, denticulate ligament division should be the first maneuver following dural opening. Only then, the spinal cord may be gently rotated, followed by a piecemeal tumor resection. The dural attachment is then cauterized, in order to obtain a Simpson II resection [3, 13].

Since most of intradural extramedullary tumors present with some degree of lateralization and spinal cord displacement, a dorsal approach offers a sufficient direct corridor to the tumor surface. If the lesion arises purely ventral or with a vast bilateral extension without spinal cord displacement a safe resection might be challenging. This might also be the case in heavily calcified or dense fibrotic lesions. In these situations, some authors consider an anterior cervical corporectomy with instrumented reconstruction in the cervical spine or retropleural thoracotomy on a thoracic level [6]. The advantage of a large bony window of access, extradural coagulation of anterior blood supply and fewer manipulation of the spinal cord however needs to weighed against the disadvantages. These include a deep and thus less secure surgical field, problematic ventral epidural bleeding, limited lateral access, risk and consequences of CSF fistulas, and the requirement for spinal reconstruction and stabilization [6]. The use of anterior approaches is, therefore, associated with an approach-related increase in surgical risks and morbidity when compared to pure posterior mid- line approaches. Due to this fact most authors strongly support a dorsal approach even in purely ventrally located lesions through a minimally invasive approach with following the surgical principles mentioned above (recommendation level: good practice point).

Postoperative complications include CSF leak and wound infection, occurring in up to 4% and 6%, respectively. Other less frequent complications are meningitis, epidural hematoma, permanent neurologic deficit and pulmonary embolism, as the major cause of death [8, 10, 14, 15]. Electrophysiological monitoring in the form of MEPs and SSEPs is used routinely in some institutions and may improve safety of resection and limit postoperative complications [8].

Radiosurgery as an adjuvant therapy is recommended in en plaque or recurrent meningeomas, subtotal resections, surgically inaccessible lesions or preexisting comorbidities [2, 13].

68.3.3 Accordance with the Literature Guidelines

Comparing to malignant lesions, the level of evidence to provide recommendations for the treatment of intradural extramedullary lesions is low. Surgery is recommended in the presence of clinical symptoms or radiologically confirmed tumor growth (evidence level II, recommendation level B). Standard posterior approaches allow for a safe and complete resection in the majority of spinal meningeomas (evidence level III, recommendation level B). Radiotherapy might be an option in elderly patients, surgically inaccessible tumors, after incomplete resection or tumor recurrence (evidence level III, recommendation level B).

68.4 Conclusions and Take Home Message

Spinal meningeomas and peripheral nerve sheath tumors are the most common intradural extramedullary tumors. MRI of the spinal column with contrast media application is the imaging technique of choice, however spinal CT might add up for information concerning calcification of the tumor or bony destruction. The preferred treatment for intradural extramedullary tumors is resection to assure best oncological outcome and preserve neural function. In meningeomas, the dural origin is generally cauterized and occasionally resected. Postoperative complications include CSF leak, wound infection, meningitis, epidural hematoma and permanent neurologic deficit.

Pearls

- Surgical resection is the treatment of choice in intradural extramedullary lesion
- The vast majority of lesions can safely be removed through standard dorsal or dorsolateral approaches
- Anterior approaches with instrumented reconstruction should be considered in purely ventral lesions, bilateral tumor extension or heavy calcifications
- The most common postoperative complications are CSF leak, wound infection, meningitis, epidural hematoma and permanent neurologic deficit

Editorial Comment

According to us even ventrally located meningiomas or other tumors should exclusively treated by posterior approaches.

References

1. Duong LM, et al. Descriptive epidemiology of malignant and nonmalignant primary spinal cord, spinal meninges, and cauda equina tumors, United States, 2004–2007. Cancer. 2012;118(17):4220–7. (EBM level: III).
2. Traul DE, Shaffrey ME, Schiff D. Part I: spinal-cord neoplasms–intradural neo-plasms. Lancet Oncol. 2007;8(1):35–45. (Evidence level II, recommendation level B).
3. Solero CL, et al. Spinal meningiomas: review of 174 operated cases. Neurosurgery. 1989;25(2):153–60. (EBM level: III, recommendation level C).
4. Goldbrunner R, Minniti G, Preusser M, et al. EANO guidelines for the diagnosis and treatment of meningiomas. Lancet Oncol. 2016;17(9):e383–91. (Evidence level II, recommendation level B).
5. Wong A, Lall R, Dahdaleh N, et al. Comparison of open and minimally invasive surgery for intradural-extramedullary spine tumors. Neurosurg Focus. 2015;39:E11. (EBM level: III, recommendation level C).
6. Angevine PD, Kellner C, Haque RM, McCormick PC. Surgical management of ventral intradural spinal lesions. J Neurosurg Spine. 2011;15(1):28–37. (EBM level: III, recommendation level C).

7. Lee RR. MR Imaging of intradural tumors of the cervical spine. Magn Reson Imaging Clin N Am. 2000;8(3):529–40. (EBM level: III, recommendation level C).
8. Gottfried ON, Gluf W, Quinones-Hinojosa A, Kan P, Schmidt MH, et al. Spinal meningiomas: surgical management and outcome. Neurosurg Focus. 2003;14(6):1–7. (EBM level: III, recommendation level B).
9. Tsuda K, Akutsu H, Yamamoto T, Nakai K, Ishikawa E, Matsumura A. Is Simpson grade I removal necessary in all cases of spinal meningioma? Assessment of postoperative recurrence during long-term follow-up. Neurol Med Chir. 2014;54:907–13. (EBM level: III, recommendation level B).
10. Avila MJ, Walter CM, Skoch J, Abbasifard S, Patel AS. Fusion after intradural spine tumor resection in adults: a review of evidence and practices. Clin Neurol Neurosurg. 2015;138:169–73. (EBM level: III, recommendation level C).
11. Tredway TL, Santiago P, Hrubes MR, Song JK, Christie SD, Fessler RG, et al. Minimally invasive resection of intradural extramedullary spinal neoplasms. Oper Neurosurg. 2006;58(1):52–7. (EBM level: II, recommendation level B).
12. Parsa AT, Lee J, Parney IF, Weinstein P, McCormick P, Ames C. Spinal cord and intradural-extraparenchymal spinal tumors: current best care practices and strategies. J Neuro-Oncol. 2004;69:291–318. (EBM level: II, recommendation level B).
13. Roux FX, Nataf F, Pinaudeau M, Borne G, Devaux B, Mender JF, et al. Intraspinal meningiomas: review of 54 cases with discussion of poor prognosis factors and modern therapeutic management. Surg Neurol. 1996;46:458–64. (EBM level: III, recommendation level C).
14. Klekamp J, Samii M. Surgical results for spinal meningiomas. Surg Neurol. 1999;52:552–62. (EBM level: III, recommendation level C).
15. McCormick PC, Post KD, Stein BM. Intradural extramedullary tumors in adults. Neurosurg Clin N Am. 1990;1(3):591–608. (EBM level: III, recommendation level C).

Indications and Technique for Intradural Intramedullary Lesions

69

Maria Wostrack

69.1 Introduction

Intradural intramedullary neoplasms are extremely rare. Only 5–10% of all spinal and 2–4% of all CNS tumors are located intramedullary.

The most common entities are spinal cord gliomas-intramedullary ependymomas (WHO grade I-III) and astrocytomas (WHO grade I-IV) – with approximately 80–90% of all intramedullary tumors [1–3]. Their incidence is higher in childhood [4]. Men are affected more often. The majority are benign or low grade lesions, whereas the incidence of higher graded tumors is higher in children. Due to the benign natural history and slow growing patterns, especially of ependymomas, the clinical signs are usually mild and non-specific, which delay the correct diagnosis. The average duration of symptoms up to the first diagnosis is more than 2 years [5], but less than 1 year for astrocytomas [6].

Other less common entities are hemangioblastomas (5–10%), metastatic lesions (<5%), and cavernomas (5–10%) [1, 7, 8].

Prospective data and thus clear evidence for optimal treatment are missing.

69.2 Case Description

69.2.1 Case 1

A 28 year-old female patient presented with neck and diffuse arm pain, bilateral distal arm paresis and mild gait ataxia. The symptoms were quickly progressing over the last 2 weeks. The next day after the hospitalization the patient showed an acute worsening of her symptoms developing tetraparesis, pronounced gait ataxia and bladder dysfunction (ASIA C).

MRI showed an intramedullary contrast enhanced tumor at C5/6 with an extensive edema of the cervical spinal cord (Fig. 69.1).

Resection of the contrast enhanced tumor resection was urgently performed under neuromonitoring (motor and sensor evoked potentials) via a right-sided hemilaminectomy C5 and partly C4 and C6, durotomy and myelotomy at the dorsal root entry zone C6, as the tumor reached the cord surface at this point.

After the surgery, the patient showed a partial improvement of the motor and vegetative dysfunction. The postoperative MRI confirmed the gross total resection (Fig. 69.2). Histological examination revealed an astrocytoma WHO

M. Wostrack (✉)
Department of Neurosurgery, Klinikum rechts der Isar, Technische Universität München, Munich, Germany
e-mail: maria.wostrack@tum.de

B. Meyer, M. Rauschmann (eds.), *Spine Surgery*, https://doi.org/10.1007/978-3-319-98875-7_69

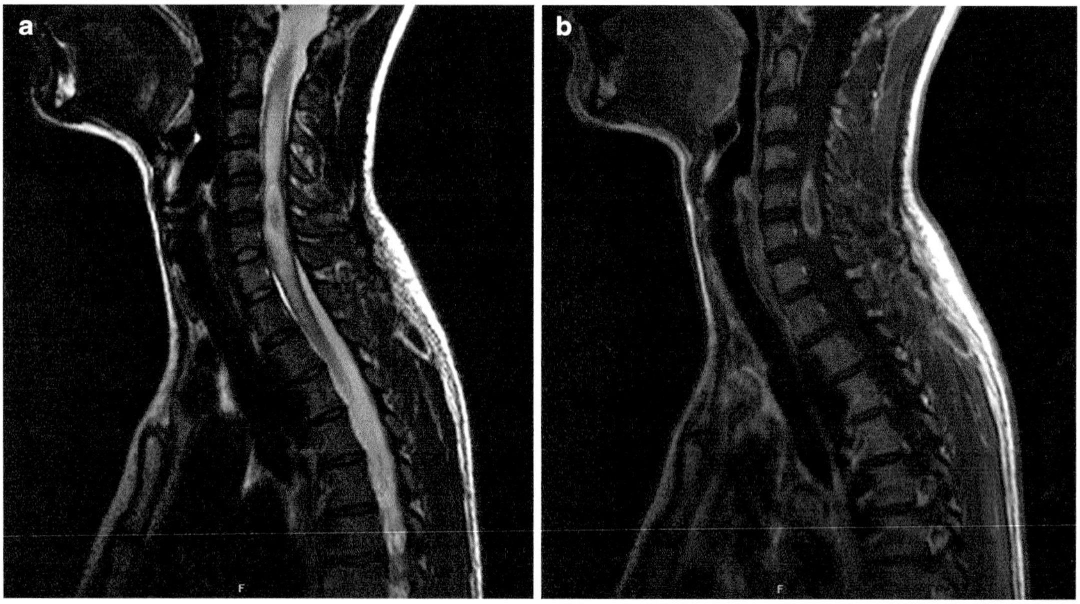

Fig. 69.1 Initial MRI scan. The MRI scan shows an intramedullary astrocytoma at C5/6. Sagittal T2 (**a**) and contrast T1 (**b**)

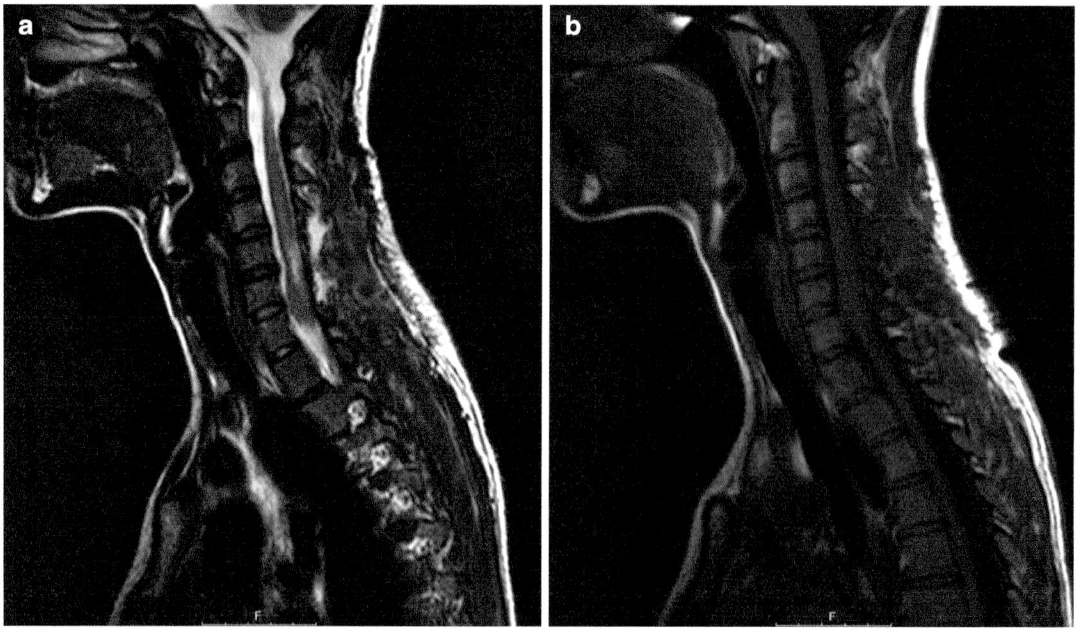

Fig. 69.2 Postoperative MRI scan I. The MRI scan shows postoperative sagittal T2 (**a**) and contrast T1 (**b**) rendering gros total tumor resection

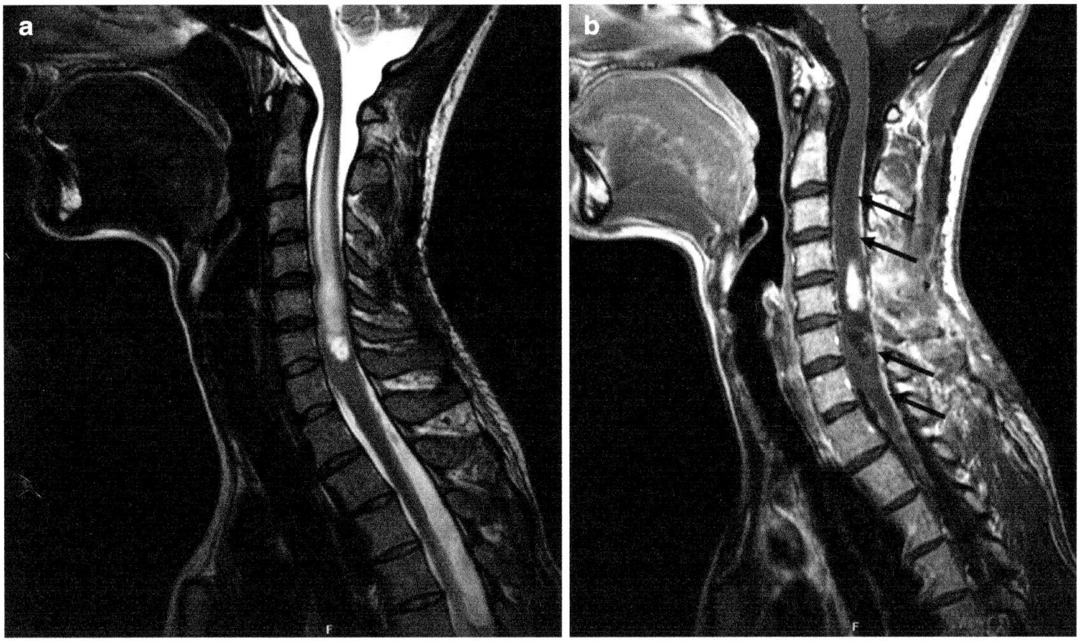

Fig. 69.3 Follow up MRI scan 6 weeks after surgery. The MRI scan shows postoperative sagittal T2 showing progressive edema of the cervical spinal cord (**a**) and contrast T1 (**b**) showing local tumor recurrence and diffuse pial enhancement along the cervical spine (arrows)

grade II. Holospinal MRI and CSF cytology were negative for tumor dissemination. The patient was assigned to receive adjuvant radiation therapy after the neurorehabilitation.

Six weeks later the patient was transferred back emergently to our department from the rehabilitation clinic because of secondary worsening of the right sided hemiparesis. The new MRI revealed a recurrent contrast enhanced lesion at the initial tumor site, additionally diffuse pial enhancement along the cervical spine (Fig. 69.3). The tumor was subtotally re-resected (Fig. 69.4), the histology was anaplastic astrocytoma WHO grade 3. Additional holospinal and cerebral MRI confirmed the suspected leptomeningeal tumor spread (Fig. 69.5).

The patient was referred to radiation oncology center for palliative radiation therapy. The patient died 5 months after the last surgery.

69.2.2 Case 2

A 44 year-old man presented with neck pain and a mild myelopathy involving slightly impaired fine motor skills, hypesthesia of the right hand and foot, and gait ataxia. Initially misdiagnosed as suffering from polyneuropathy, the patient was treated by his neurologist with Vitamin B12 without any success. The symptoms were slowly progressive over the last 3 years. A finally performed MRI revealed a large intramedullary tumor of the craniocervical junction (Fig. 69.6).

The tumor was gross totally resected via laminectomy C1–3, durotomy and median myelotomy under neuromonitoring with motor and sensory evoked potentials.

Immediately after the surgery the patient was transferred for 1 week to the intensive care unit due to the transiently impaired tetraparesis, difficulties with swallowing and ventilation. Over the

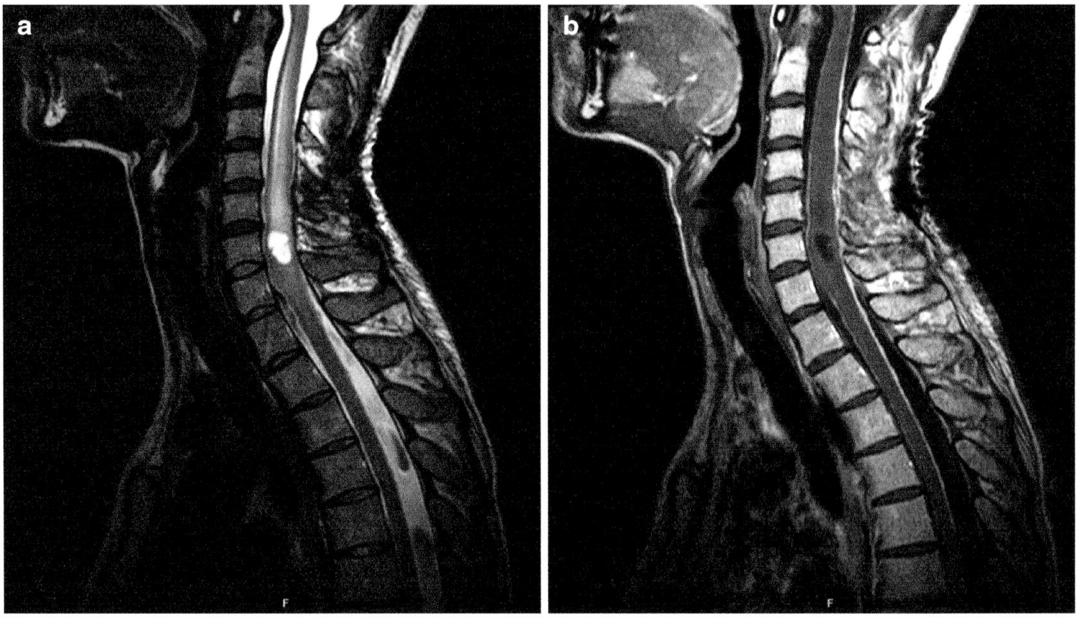

Fig. 69.4 Postoperative MRI scan II. The MRI scan shows sagittal T2 (**a**) and contrast T1 (**b**) after the subtotal resection of the recurrent astrocytoma

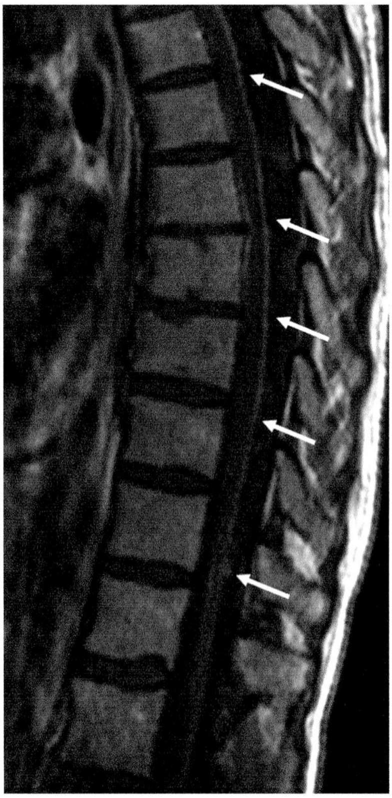

Fig. 69.5 Holospinal MRI. The holospinal contrast T1 MRI scan (here shown: thoracic spine) demonstrates diffuse contrast enhancement along the whole spinal axis corresponding to leptomeningeal tumor spread (arrows)

next 2 weeks the new deficits were fully recurrent and at discharge his clinical status was unchanged to that before surgery. Over the next 3 months the symptoms improved. The patient walks without assistance. He is back to his full-time job as sales manager with a slight residual gait ataxia and hypesthesia of his right hand.

The histological examination revealed a WHO grade II ependymoma. The postoperative holospinal MRI showed no residual tumor (Fig. 69.7). The CSF cytology and cranial MRI were negative for tumor dissemination. According to the tumor board decision the patient received no adjuvant radiotherapy. The follow up examinations proceeded every year. The patient is progression-free for almost 10 years now after the surgery (Fig. 69.8).

69.3 Discussion of the Cases

69.3.1 Indication

Due to the rare occurrence of intramedullary gliomas and a predominantly benign behavioral pattern of the majority of them, there are no randomized data available regarding the optimal therapy. The largest retrospective

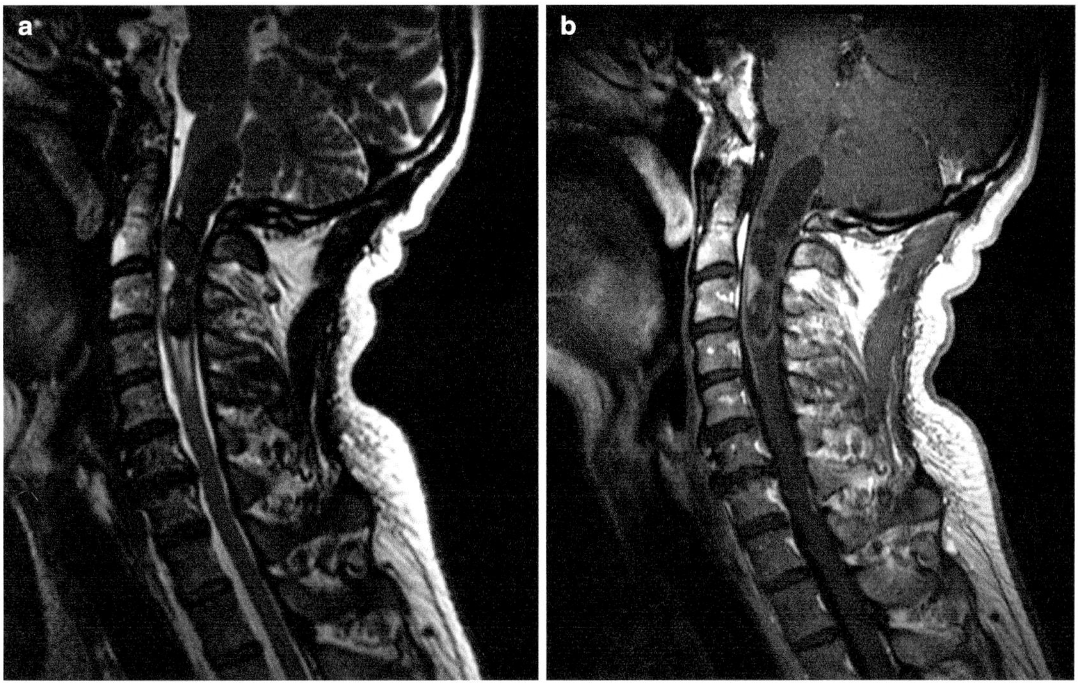

Fig. 69.6 Initial MRI scan: Preoperative MRI showing a contrast enhanced spinal cord tumor between the medulla oblongata and the C3 level with an associated syrinx formation (Sagittal T2 in **a**, sagittal contrast T1 in **b**)

series included maximum 100–150 cases [6, 9–12]. Therefore, there are no clear guidelines for the indication of the specific therapeutic modality.

According to the results of larger clinical series and expert opinions, a gross tumor resection represents the gold standard in the treatment of spinal ependymomas and [9, 10] pilocytic astrocytomas [13].

Higher-grade infiltrative astrocytomas cannot be treated by surgical treatment alone. As demonstrated by our first case, even the complete resection of the contrast enhanced tumor mass appears to be not sufficiently effective due to the tumor infiltration of the surrounding spinal cord tissue and a high tendency of these tumors to recur. Some authors find that surgical resection is associated with a poorer neurological outcome and poorer overall survival [6, 11, 14]. Only few series show an advantage of radical tumor removal in terms of oncological prognosis, even in malignant astrocytomas [15]. In any case, operative debulking to reduce the space-occupying effect and to obtain histological samples plays an important role in the treatment of infiltrative spinal astrocytomas.

Regarding the optimal timing of surgery, the majority is convinced that early resection should be attempted when symptoms are mild, because of a then clearly better prognosis for a neurological recovery and a lower risk for new postoperative deterioration [1, 16, 17]. Opinions vary as to the timing of the operation of inicidental findings, but the majority tends to follow up these patients first at close intervals and to proceed with surgery in cases of tumor progression and/or a development of a neurological deficit.

Spinal gliomas occasionally show drop metatases or disseminated manfestation at the first diagnosis. In such cases, the operation should focus primarily on the resection of the main tumor, since no additional benefits appear from the resection of the metastatic lesions [18]. Due to the ability of spinal cord glioma cells to spread along the neural axis, the perioperative diagnostics should include holospinal and cerebral MRI as well as CSF cytology.

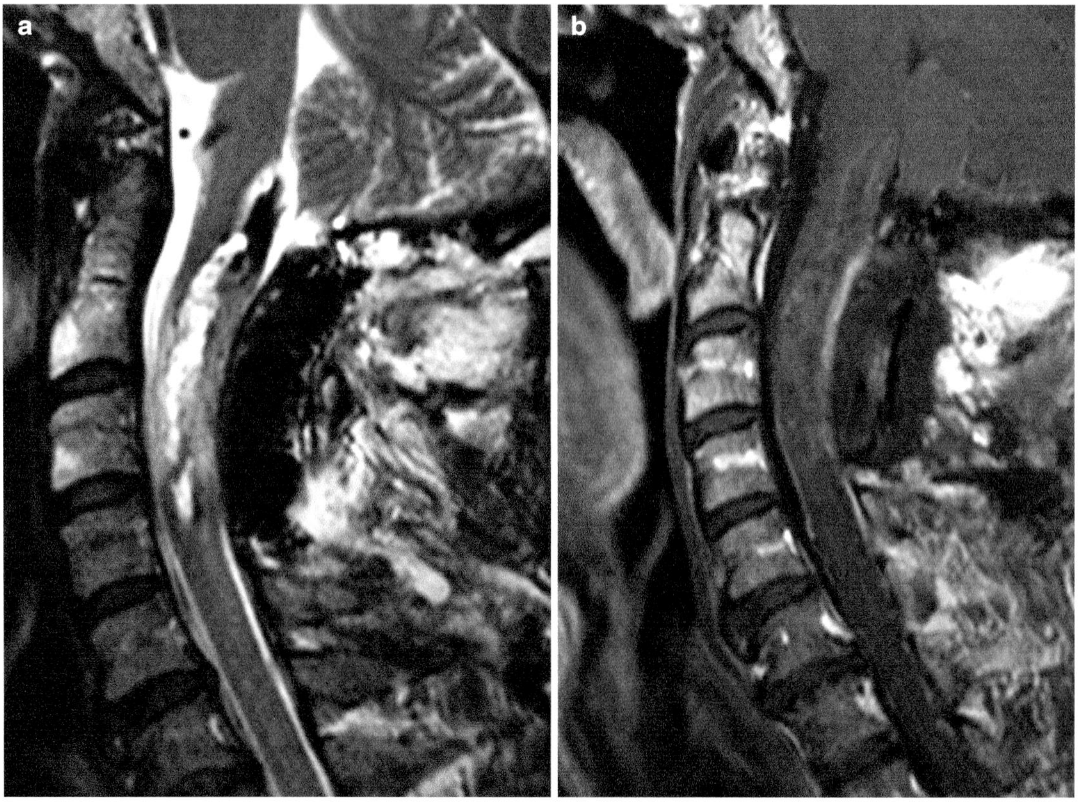

Fig. 69.7 Postoperative MRI scan. The MRI scan shows postoperative sagittal T2 (**a**) and contrast T1 (**b**) rendering gros total resection of the ependymoma

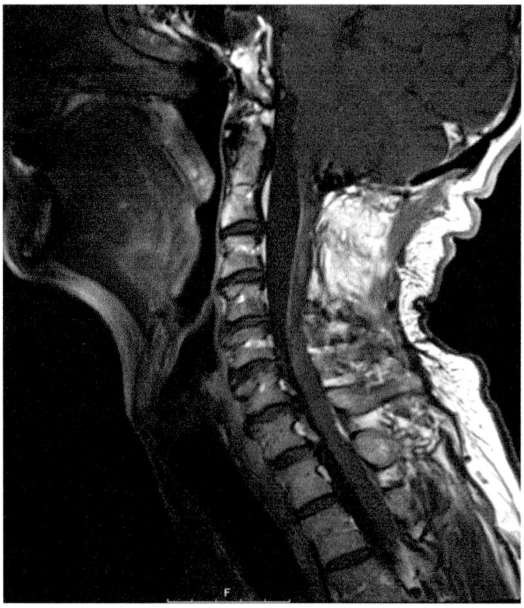

Fig. 69.8 Follow up MRI 9 years after surgery. The contrast T1 MRI 9 years after surgery shows no signs of a local tumor recurrence

69.3.2 Surgical Aspects

For the resection of most intramedullary tumors, a mono- or multi-segment laminotomy/laminectomy is suitable. For circumscribed pathologies with a side-emphasis, hemilaminectomy is often sufficient. The risk of secondary postoperative instability of the spine after removal of intradural tumors varies between 10% in adults and up to more than 50% in pediatric series [19–21]. Therefore, laminoplasty is often thought to prevent secondary deformity, especially in childhood. However, no statistically clear evidence for benefits of this approach to secondary stability exists [22].

In cases with multi-segmental laminectomies for large intramedullary tumors additional stabilization with internal fixation may be considered. However, difficulties would occur in assessment of the follow up MRIs.

For the resection of spinal gliomas, the median myelotomy is usually chosen. After opening the dura in the midline, the edges are held apart with sutures (Fig. 69.9a). After the opening of the pia, the myelon is opened between the posterior branches. The degree of resection is determined by the demarcation of the tumor against the surrounding spinal cord tissue, the histological findings and any changes to the IONM. In infiltrative higher graded astrocytomas a complete resection can rarely be achieved. Rather, it is a debulking operation for decompression, relief of syrinx and recovery of histological samples. In contrast, in benign processes a gros total resection should be attemptes, provided there is no permanent neurological damage. Since almost 40% of postoperative deficits are due to surgical manipulation before or after tumor resection [23], ultrasonic aspirator debulking of the central parts of the tumor is performed as the first step to prevent further spinal cord injury due to the traction of larger tumor masses (Fig. 69.9b). Subsequently, tumor-supplying vessels are coagulated and severed; the capsule and remaining tumor tissue are removed in toto if possible. After the adaptation of the Pia a watertight dural closure takes place.

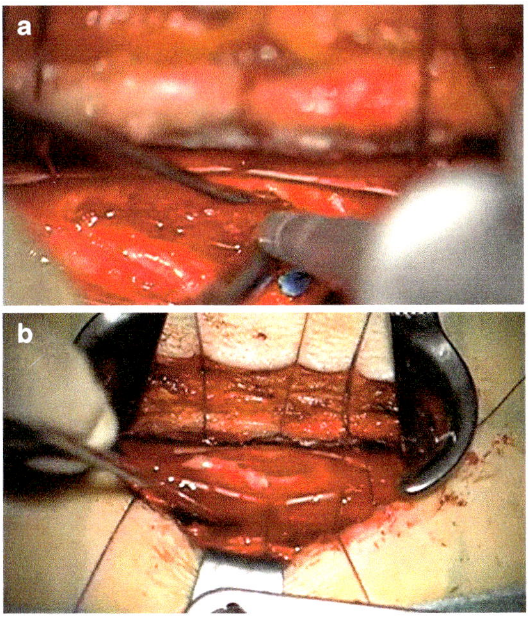

Fig. 69.9 Intraoperative photographs of ependymoma resection. Midline approach with the dura being held apart by tenting sutures (**a**); tumor mass reduction by an ultrasonic aspirator to prevent additional traction during the further resection (**b**)

Surgery of intramedullary pathology without the use of IONM is obsolete. With the introduction of the IONM, the extent of resection of the tumors was significantly increased, while the rates of postoperative new deficits were reduced by continuous monitoring of the motor and sensory pathways [24]. The standard IONM includes cortical derivation of SEP after peripheral stimulation, and MEP monitoring after transcranial electrical stimulation. In recent years, more and more attention has been drawn to the benefits of direct epidural MEP derivation in terms of the D wave as the strongest predictor of the occurrence of postoperative neurological deterioration [25]. When resecting the ependymomas in the area of the conus medullaris or cauda equina, an intraoperative electromyography for monitoring the sphincter function and individual nerve roots may be used.

69.3.3 Outcome and the Role of the Adjuvant Treatment

Diffuse and malignant astrocytomas of the spinal cord grow infiltratively, which limits the resectability and surgical safety of postoperative deficits: while gros total resection can be achieved in maximum 15% of cases, new permanent deficits are expected in up to 50% [6]. In contrast, pilocytic astrocytomas and ependymomas are well circumscribed, and thus, are well operable tumors with a rate of complete removal of 70–90% and a likelihood of severe residual deficiency of <10% [10]. The oncological prognosis of ependymomas is generally favorable: the median progression-free survival after a gros total resection is about 7 years on average (6 years for grade I, 15 years for grade II and 4 years for grade III ependymomas) [12, 26, 27]. In terms of overall survival, ependymomas and pilocytic astrocytomas also have a good prognosis with a 10-year survival of about 80% [11, 28]. Higher-grade astrocytomas have a significantly worse prognosis with a median survival of 17 months in anaplastic astrocytomas and 9–10 months in patients with spinal glioblastomas [6, 15].

Adjuvant radiotherapy is not recommended following gross total resection of grade I-II ependymomas and spinal pilocytic astrocytomas [10, 11, 17]. In cases of partial tumor resection, recurrence, disseminated and anaplastic ependymomas, as well as in cases of astrocytomas grade II-IV, a fractionated radiotherapy is recommended [11, 29], although there is no clear evidence for that either, and decisions for the radiotherapy are usually made on a case-by-case basis.

69.3.4 Accordance with the Literature Guidelines

As discussed above, guidelines cannot be derived from the literature. However, the indication for treatment as well as the surgical approach were most probably not in accordance with the current common consensus of the majority of peers. Yet the same accounts for the authors' preferred method.

Level of Evidence: C

The level of evidence available to date is low. Only several large restrospective series of more than 50 cases (cited above) are available on surgical and adjuvant treatment of intramedullary tumors.

69.4 Conclusions and Take Home Message

Primary spinal cord tumors are extremely rare with about 3% of all primary CNS tumors. Prospective data and thus clear evidence for optimal treatment are missing. The most common entites are intramedullary ependymomas (> 60% in adults) and astrocytomas (15–20% in adults, >50% in children). The majority of intramedullary tumors are benign or low grade (WHO grades I-II). Diffuse and malignant astrocytomas of the spinal cord grow infiltratively, which limits the resectability and surgical safety of postoperative deficits: at a complete resection rate of maximum 15%, new permanent deficits are expected in up to 50%. In contrast, pilocytic astrocytomas and ependymomas are well circumscribed, and thus, are well operable tumors at a rate of complete removal of 70–90% and a likelihood of a severe persistent deficiency of <10%. Therefore, a complete resection represents the gold standard in the therapy of the latter entities. In terms of overall survival, ependymomas and pilocytic astrocytomas have a good prognosis with a 10-year survival rate of more than 80% after a gros total resection. Higher-graded astrocytomas have a significantly worse median survival with 17 months in anaplastic astrocytomas and 9–10 months in patients with spinal glioblastomas. Adjuvant radiotherapy is not recommended following gross total resection resection of grade I-II ependymomas and spinal pilocytic astrocytomas. In cases of recurrence, disseminated and anaplastic ependymomas, as well as after any surgical treatment of spinal astrocytomas grade II-IV, a fractionated radiotherapy should be performed.

Pearls

- Ependymomas and pilocytic astrocytoma: go for a gross total resection
- Infiltrative or malignant astrocytoma: go for a biopsy
- Intraoperative IONM is mandatory resp. highly recommended
- Radiation therapy for grade II-IV astrocytomas and grade III ependymomas

Editorial Comment

Intramedullary tumors are an orphan disease and should therefore be treated in specialized centers only according to us. It is a benign disease in unsually younger patients with a high probability of "cure" and a potential for devastating operative complications.

References

1. Bostrom A, Kanther NC, Grote A, Bostrom J. Management and outcome in adult intramedullary spinal cord tumours: a 20-year single institution experience. BMC Res Notes. 2014;7:908.
2. Slooff JL, Kernohan JW, MacCarty CS. Primary intramedullary tumors of the spinal cord and filum terminale. Philadelphia-London: WB Saunders Company; 1964. p. 124–9.
3. Yang S, Yang X, Hong G. Surgical treatment of one hundred seventy-four intramedullary spinal cord tumors. Spine. 2009;34:2705–10.
4. Parsa AT, Lee J, Parney IF, Weinstein P, McCormick PC, Ames C. Spinal cord and intradural-extraparenchymal spinal tumors: current best care practices and strategies. J Neuro-Oncol. 2004;69:291–318.
5. McCormick PC, Stein BM. Intramedullary tumors in adults. Neurosurg Clin N Am. 1990;1:609–30.
6. Babu R, Karikari IO, Owens TR, Bagley CA. Spinal cord astrocytomas: a modern 20-year experience at a single institution. Spine. 2014;39:533–40.
7. Duong LM, McCarthy BJ, McLendon RE, Dolecek TA, Kruchko C, Douglas LL, Ajani UA. Descriptive epidemiology of malignant and nonmalignant primary spinal cord, spinal meninges, and cauda equina tumors, United States, 2004–2007. Cancer. 2012;118:4220–7.
8. Manzano G, Green BA, Vanni S, Levi AD. Contemporary management of adult intramedullary spinal tumors-pathology and neurological outcomes related to surgical resection. Spinal Cord. 2008;46:540–6.
9. Bostrom A, von Lehe M, Hartmann W, Pietsch T, Feuss M, Bostrom JP, Schramm J, Simon M. Surgery for spinal cord ependymomas: outcome and prognostic factors. Neurosurgery. 2011;68:302–8; discussion 309.
10. Brotchi J, Fischer G. Spinal cord ependymomas. Neurosurg Focus. 1998;4:e2.
11. Minehan KJ, Shaw EG, Scheithauer BW, Davis DL, Onofrio BM. Spinal cord astrocytoma: pathological and treatment considerations. J Neurosurg. 1995;83:590–5.
12. Tarapore PE, Modera P, Naujokas A, Oh MC, Amin B, Tihan T, Parsa AT, Ames CP, Chou D, Mummaneni PV, Weinstein PR. Pathology of spinal ependymomas: an institutional experience over 25 years in 134 patients. Neurosurgery. 2013;73:247–55. discussion 255
13. Fakhreddine MH, Mahajan A, Penas-Prado M, Weinberg J, McCutcheon IE, Puduvalli V, Brown PD. Treatment, prognostic factors, and outcomes in spinal cord astrocytomas. Neuro-Oncology. 2013;15:406–12.
14. Garces-Ambrossi GL, McGirt MJ, Mehta VA, Sciubba DM, Witham TF, Bydon A, Wolinksy JP, Jallo GI, Gokaslan ZL. Factors associated with progression-free survival and long-term neurological outcome after resection of intramedullary spinal cord tumors: analysis of 101 consecutive cases. J Neurosurg Spine. 2009;11:591–9.
15. Adams H, Avendano J, Raza SM, Gokaslan ZL, Jallo GI, Quinones-Hinojosa A. Prognostic factors and survival in primary malignant astrocytomas of the spinal cord: a population-based analysis from 1973 to 2007. Spine. 2012;37:E727–35.
16. Chang UK, Choe WJ, Chung SK, Chung CK, Kim HJ. Surgical outcome and prognostic factors of spinal intramedullary ependymomas in adults. J Neuro-Oncol. 2002;57:133–9.
17. Lee SH, Chung CK, Kim CH, Yoon SH, Hyun SJ, Kim KJ, Kim ES, Eoh W, Kim HJ. Long-term outcomes of surgical resection with or without adjuvant radiation therapy for treatment of spinal ependymoma: a retrospective multicenter study by the Korea Spinal Oncology Research Group. Neuro-Oncology. 2013;15:921–9.
18. Pencovich N, Bot G, Lidar Z, Korn A, Wostrack M, Meyer B, Bydon M, Jallo G, Constantini S. Spinal ependymoma with regional metastasis at presentation. Acta Neurochir. 2014;156:1215–22.
19. Ahmed R, Menezes AH, Awe OO, Mahaney KB, Torner JC, Weinstein SL. Long-term incidence and risk factors for development of spinal deformity following resection of pediatric intramedullary spinal cord tumors. J Neurosurg Pediatr. 2014;13:613–21.
20. McGirt MJ, Chaichana KL, Atiba A, Bydon A, Witham TF, Yao KC, Jallo GI. Incidence of spinal deformity after resection of intramedullary spinal cord tumors in children who underwent laminectomy compared with laminoplasty. J Neurosurg Pediatr. 2008;1:57–62.
21. Yao KC, McGirt MJ, Chaichana KL, Constantini S, Jallo GI. Risk factors for progressive spinal deformity following resection of intramedullary spinal cord tumors in children: an analysis of 161 consecutive cases. J Neurosurg. 2007;107:463–8.
22. McGirt MJ, Garces-Ambrossi GL, Parker SL, Sciubba DM, Bydon A, Wolinksy JP, Gokaslan ZL, Jallo G, Witham TF. Short-term progressive spinal deformity following laminoplasty versus laminectomy for resection of intradural spinal tumors: analysis of 238 patients. Neurosurgery. 2010;66:1005–12.
23. Forster MT, Marquardt G, Seifert V, Szelenyi A. Spinal cord tumor surgery–importance of continuous intraoperative neurophysiological monitoring after tumor resection. Spine. 2012;37:E1001–8.
24. Sala F, Bricolo A, Faccioli F, Lanteri P, Gerosa M. Surgery for intramedullary spinal cord tumors: the role of intraoperative (neurophysiological) monitoring. Eur Spine J. 2007;16(Suppl 2):S130–9.
25. Costa P, Peretta P, Faccani G. Relevance of intraoperative D wave in spine and spinal cord surgeries. Eur Spine J. 2013;22:840–8.

26. Oh MC, Kim JM, Kaur G, Safaee M, Sun MZ, Singh A, Aranda D, Molinaro AM, Parsa AT. Prognosis by tumor location in adults with spinal ependymomas. J Neurosurg Spine. 2013;18:226–35.
27. Oh MC, Tarapore PE, Kim JM, Sun MZ, Safaee M, Kaur G, Aranda DM, Parsa AT. Spinal ependymomas: benefits of extent of resection for different histological grades. J Clin Neurosci. 2013;20:1390–7.
28. Lin Y, Smith ZA, Wong AP, Melkonian S, Harris DA, Lam S. Predictors of survival in patients with spinal ependymoma. Neurol Res. 2015;37:650–5.
29. Oh MC, Ivan ME, Sun MZ, Kaur G, Safaee M, Kim JM, Sayegh ET, Aranda D, Parsa AT. Adjuvant radiotherapy delays recurrence following subtotal resection of spinal cord ependymomas. Neuro-Oncology. 2013;15:208–15.

Part VII

Advanced Module 2: Complications and Management

Safety Checklist for Spine Patients

70

Sandro M. Krieg

70.1 Introduction

Errors are human. Nonetheless, we all pursue the aim not to produce errors at all and if they occur, not to harm the patient at least. Yet, with nowadays' patient volume and critical time schedule, avoiding errors requires an ever-increasing level of attention. Operating a patient on the wrong level or wrong side is a nightmare mistake for surgeons, but however happens quite frequently. In a recent survey spine surgeons answered that 50% already performed wrong-level, and in 10% wrong-side surgery at least once [1, 2].

Mostly originating from the aviation industry, the use of checklists gained acceptance among surgeons as well in the last decade. Starting with personal checklists in various hospitals all over the globe and finally received evidence by evaluating the influence of a newly developed WHO patient-safety checklist on surgical outcomes [3]. When starting to create today's WHO Surgical Safety Checklist, the authors stated that "There is little guidance in the literature regarding methods for creating a medical checklist. The airline industry, however, has more than 70 years of experience in developing and using checklists." [4]. The authors therefore approached the aviation industry in order to develop this checklist by reviewing charts, getting interviews and pure observation.

Such checklists were then proven to support us in further eliminating human error by considerably simple methods like a checklist. Those checklists not only focus on the surgical part but also on general issues, such as proper oxygenation measurements, expected blood loss, available implants, recent imaging, prophylactic antibiotics, and: correct patient (Fig. 70.1).

The first comprehensive study on the use of surgical checklists proved a considerable impact. Mortality was reduced from 1.5% to 0.7% and in-hospital complications diminished from 11% to 7% [3]. With regard to these impressive data, checklists more focused on spine procedures were reported in the last years [6].

The aim of this chapter is to underline the importance of using surgical checklists prior to surgery by presenting cases in which surgical checklists prevented further harm to the patient and by providing an overview on the existing scientific evidence on surgical checklists per se.

S. M. Krieg (✉)
Department of Neurosurgery, Klinikum rechts der Isar, Technische Universität München, Munich, Germany
e-mail: Sandro.Krieg@tum.de

B. Meyer, M. Rauschmann (eds.), *Spine Surgery*, https://doi.org/10.1007/978-3-319-98875-7_70

Surgical Safety Checklist

World Health Organization | Patient Safety
A World Alliance for Safer Health Care

Before induction of anaesthesia

(with at least nurse and anaesthetist)

Has the patient confirmed his/her identity, site, procedure, and consent?
- ☐ Yes

Is the site marked?
- ☐ Yes
- ☐ Not applicable

Is the anaesthesia machine and medication check complete?
- ☐ Yes

Is the pulse oximeter on the patient and functioning?
- ☐ Yes

Does the patient have a:

Known allergy?
- ☐ No
- ☐ Yes

Difficult airway or aspiration risk?
- ☐ No
- ☐ Yes, and equipment/assistance available

Risk of >500ml blood loss (7ml/kg in children)?
- ☐ No
- ☐ Yes, and two IVs/central access and fluids planned

Before skin incision

(with nurse, anaesthetist and surgeon)

- ☐ **Confirm all team members have introduced themselves by name and role.**
- ☐ **Confirm the patient's name, procedure, and where the incision will be made.**

Has antibiotic prophylaxis been given within the last 60 minutes?
- ☐ Yes
- ☐ Not applicable

Anticipated Critical Events

To Surgeon:
- ☐ What are the critical or non-routine steps?
- ☐ How long will the case take?
- ☐ What is the anticipated blood loss?

To Anaesthetist:
- ☐ Are there any patient-specific concerns?

To Nursing Team:
- ☐ Has sterility (including indicator results) been confirmed?
- ☐ Are there equipment issues or any concerns?

Is essential imaging displayed?
- ☐ Yes
- ☐ Not applicable

Before patient leaves operating room

(with nurse, anaesthetist and surgeon)

Nurse Verbally Confirms:
- ☐ The name of the procedure
- ☐ Completion of instrument, sponge and needle counts
- ☐ Specimen labelling (read specimen labels aloud, including patient name)
- ☐ Whether there are any equipment problems to be addressed

To Surgeon, Anaesthetist and Nurse:
- ☐ What are the key concerns for recovery and management of this patient?

This checklist is not intended to be comprehensive. Additions and modifications to fit local practice are encouraged.

Revised 1/2009

Fig. 70.1 WHO Surgical Safety Checklist. This is the WHO Surgical Safety Checklist published and evaluated for its clinical impact in 2009. Various steps before anesthesia, before incision, and after surgery need to be checked and help all participating professionals in avoiding human errors [5]

70.2 Case Description

70.2.1 Case 1: Indication and Planning

A 76 y/o female patient was seen in our outpatient department with severe spinal claudication causing a significant reduction in quality of life for the patient. MRI from 3 months ago showed multisegmental lumbar instability and consecutive spinal stenosis from L2 to S1 (Fig. 70.2).

Due to the severe symptoms of the patient, including reduced quality of life, surgery with fusion and decompression from L2 to S1 was recommended by the outpatient physician. Due to other disease, the appointment for surgery was delayed for 3 months. Clinical symptoms, however, were unchanged since 3 years. Due to the 6 months old imaging, the attending board reviewing all surgical patients for the next day recommended a new lumbar MRI scan for the upcoming morning before surgery. The next morning, the patient underwent the MRI scan and was directly taken to the OR where she was put under general anesthesia. The new MRI scan was then reviewed by the surgeon in charge in the context of our presurgical checklist. It showed a new spinal stenosis at L1/2 plus new vertebral body fractures of T12, L1, and L2 (Fig. 70.3).

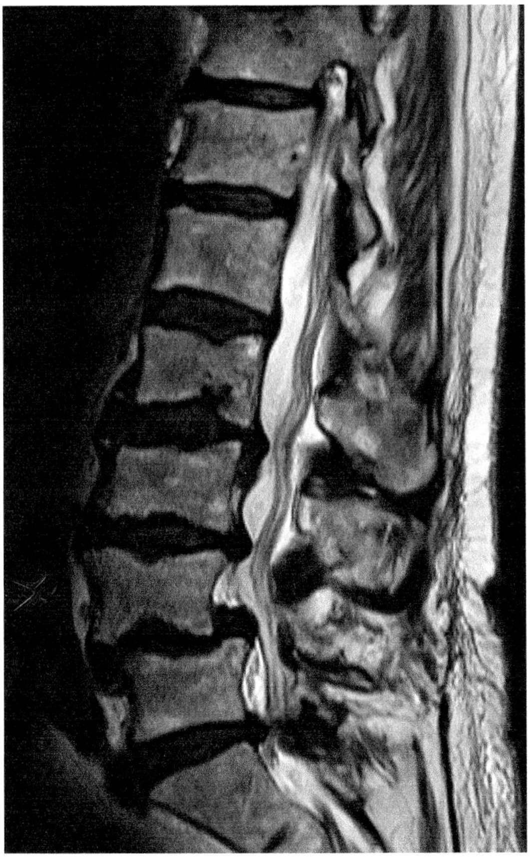

Fig. 70.2 Initial MRI scan. This is the sagittal view of the MRI scan performed from 3 months before the patient presented in the outpatient department. It shows multisegmental lumbar instability and consecutive spinal stenosis from L2 to S1

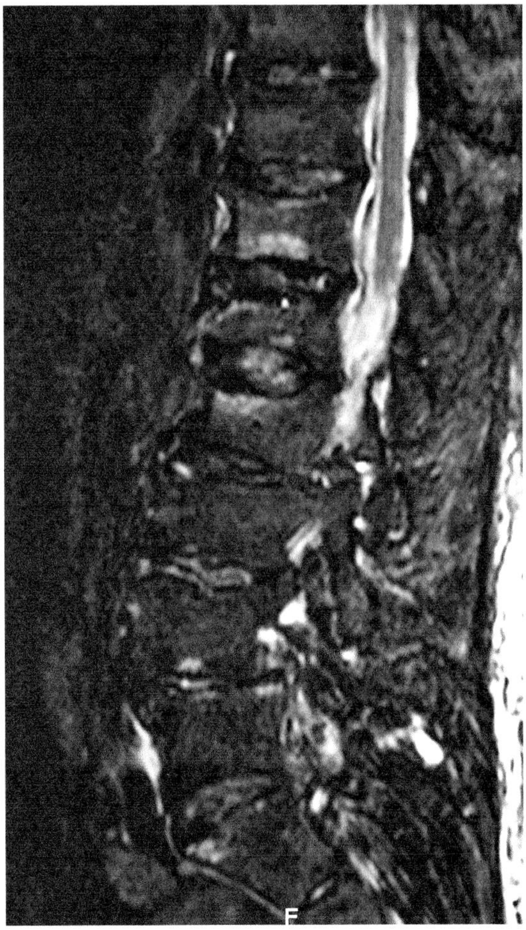

Fig. 70.3 Preoperative MRI scan. This is the sagittal view of the MRI scan performed 3 months after the patient presented in the outpatient department. It now shows a new spinal stenosis at L1/2 plus new vertebral body fractures of T12, L1, and L2

After the case was discussed among the attendings and the department chair, indication for a long dorsal instrumentation from T9 to S2 (alariliac) was set. The patient was taken out of anesthesia and the new results and treatment recommendations were discussed with her. She decided for the long fusion, which was then done 2 weeks later without adverse events.

70.2.2 Case 2: Side and Level

A 69 y/o male patient presented with sciatica of L2 and L3 on the right side since 5 months. Conservative management did not result in any improvement and the patient decided for surgical therapy. MRI showed recessal stenosis at L2/3 and right-sided foraminal stenosis of L3/4 (Fig. 70.4). Surgical decompression via hemilaminectomy L3 plus foraminal decompression via a lateral approach L3/4 was recommended and scheduled accordingly.

Before surgery, the resident in charge, anesthesiologist, scrub nurse and circulating nurse performed not only the preoperative in-room checklist but also a team time-out before incision (Fig. 70.5).

Incision was done and the resident prepared the lamina of L3, which was confirmed via intraoperative X-ray (Fig. 70.6a). When the surgeon joined the surgery, he did his preoperative checklist himself and then asked the resident again for the side of the pain (right side). Contralateral (wrong side) preparation was then stopped, the other – then right side – was prepared and the supposed level L2/3 was decompressed via an interlaminar fenestration first. After decompressing this level, another X-ray was performed showing L3/4 instead of the supposed level L2/3 (Fig. 70.6b).

Surgery was then continued by the L3 hemilaminectomy and lateral approach at L3/4 as planned. The patient woke up without any sciatica and was cleared about the left-sided fasciatomy.

70.3 Discussion of the Cases

In both cases the patients did not suffer from any harm. Also in both cases, the presurgical checklist was the major factor leading to the reanalysis of the case. In case 1, the newly performed imaging was reevaluated since the checklist requires a) the date of the last imaging and b) the conformity between indication planning and the latest imaging (Fig. 70.5).

70.3.1 Case 1: Indication and Planning

In the meeting the day before surgery, the attendings correctly requested new imaging. However, the time between imaging and surgery was too small to neither discuss the new data properly nor to receive informed consent from the patient. If we expect new and changing data, there needs to be enough time to evaluate it with colleagues and the patient. However, the current WHO checklist would not protect us from such an error.

70.3.2 Case 2: Side and Level

This case has three aspects, which need to be discussed:

1. As you can see in the picture taken after surgery (Fig. 70.5), the resident did do the presurgical checklists. Nonetheless, when scrubbing in on this prone patient, he chose the wrong side.
2. The second surgeon did the checklist as well and recognized the mistake
3. After preparation, an intraoperative X-ray was performed

Most colleagues among spine surgeons agree that wrong-side surgery cannot be fully avoided by checklists [1]. There are many factors which can lead to operating the wrong side, such as changed patient orientation that day, triggering by scrub

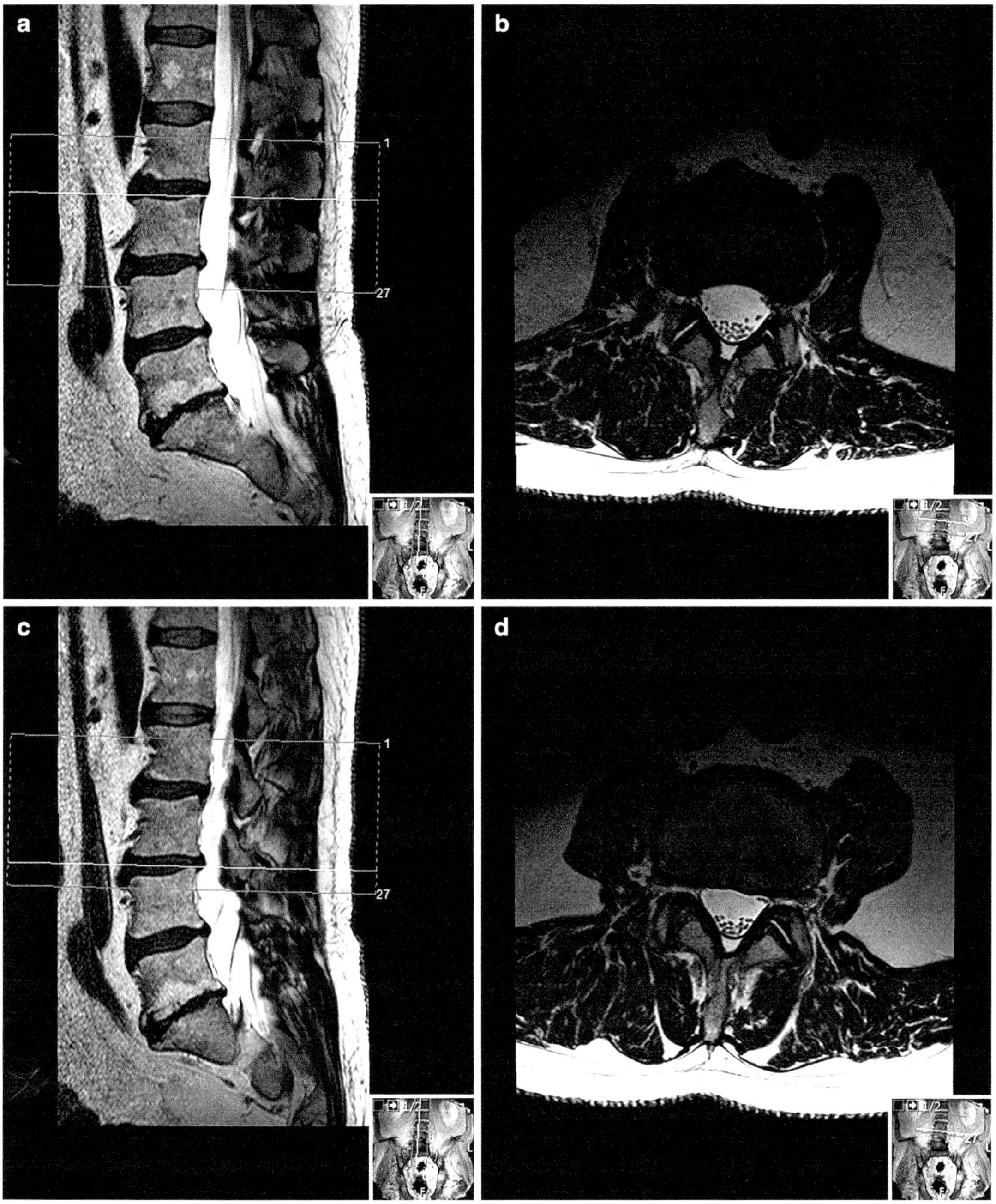

Fig. 70.4 Preoperative MRI scan. This MRI scan shows recessal stenosis at L2/3 (**a**: sagittal, **b**: axial) and right-sided foraminal stenosis of L3/4 (**c**: sagittal, **d**: axial)

nurse putting suction or bipolar on the other side, placement of devices, or the whole OR setup changed, thus implying surgery on the other side. Since we all are quite used to our regular setup, which many of us use in each case the same way, any irregular change to this setup by others could cause us to stand on the wrong side and then also operate the wrong side. Marking the side of surgery on the awake patient the day before could maybe prevent this issue. However, then fully relying on

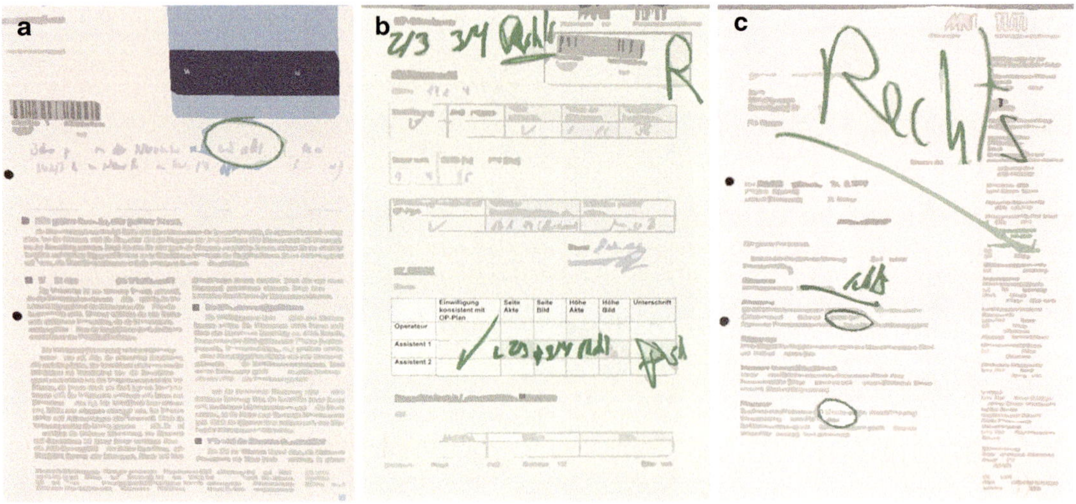

Fig. 70.5 Patient charts and preoperative checklist. This image shows the preoperatively performed surgical check using the informed consent form (**a**), the outpatient department letter with disease and indication (**c**) and the preoperative surgical checklist of our department (**b**). All items indicate L2/3 and L3/4 on the right side

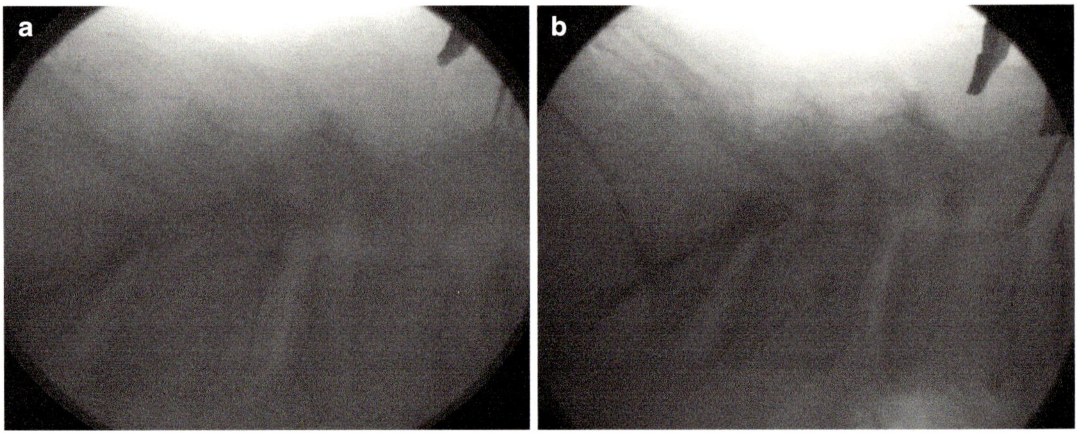

Fig. 70.6 Intraoperative X-rays. These images show the intraoperative X-rays performed after the first preparation of the L3 lamina on the left side (**a**) and after decompression of the supposed level L2/3 on the – then correct – right side (**b**)

this marking could also create other problems and mistakes. Secondy, the second surgeon also performed the checklist and recognized the mistake made by the first one which nicely shows us two things: checklists can help in preventing further harm; but only if every participating professional does them instead on relying on checks, other colleagues did. Third, the second surgeon insisted on performing an intraoperative X-ray since out of experience he always does it to double-check himself; although it is not on any checklist or standard operating procedure of his institution. Moreover, from a litigation point of view, it is quite reasonable to perform a final intraoperative X-ray before removing bone. And take special care that the imaging is stored and saved. So, double-checking yourself and your colleague significantly helps in preventing such actually avoidable errors.

70.3.3 General Discussion

In our department, we use three different checklists until a patient undergoes surgery:

1. On the ward, including
   (a) Anesthesia approval,
   (b) Available imaging and date of last imaging,
   (c) Laboratory tests including coagulation system,
   (d) Blood preservation ordered,
   (e) Patient approved spine registry participation,
   (f) Indication by,
   (g) Approved by the presurgical meeting the day before, and
   (h) Consistency of informed consent with planned surgery.
2. In the OR before positioning, including
   (a) Level according to chart,
   (b) Side according to chart,
   (c) Level according to imaging,
   (d) Side according to imaging, and
   (e) Consistency with informed consent form.
3. In the OR, right before the incision, including
   (a) Identitiy,
   (b) Side of surgery,
   (c) Type of surgery,
   (d) Expected blood loss,
   (e) Implants availability,
   (f) Prophylactic antibiotics, and
   (g) Expected postoperative ICU stay.

Yet, as seen in this case, even such an elaborate setup does not avoid 100% of errors. Maybe, too many checklists even reduce sensitivity to the importance of using these checklists. This is also why many surgeons still believe that time out and checklist do not avoid these errors per se [1]. And this might even be true in many cases. One problem is of course that a lot of people are involved in preparing, scheduling and operating the patient. Data from anesthesiologists show us that handovers during surgery, even when using checklists, correlate with an increased in-hospital mortality, infection as well as further complications of cardiac, respiratory, or infectious nature [7]. The authors found an odds ratio of up to 1.48 (CI 1.22–1.79) for these complications when investigating a cohort of 138,932 patients even after adjusting for sex, race, ASA status, etc. Although comparable data do not exist for surgical teams, the reasons and consequences of missing information when involving more and more people in one case are obvious.

Concerning neurosurgical applications, there are checklists available which were already evaluated and published in the last years (Table 70.1).

Although the number of wrong-side or wrong-level surgeries were too small for further statistical analysis, the author stated that "... all team members appreciate the chance to focus on the patient, the surgical procedure, and expected difficulties." [8]. Important to say that checklists do not only reduce the already small number of severe mistakes, such as wrong-side or wrong-level surgery. They also help us to improve or care significantly thus not only reducing worst-case scenarios but also daily care, in-hospital morbidity, and minor errors [9] (Table 70.2).

After now having learned to use checklists from aviation in order to reduce complications and errors, we should further try to learn from aviation experience. Both fields are highly complex, events are time-critical and unpredictable, they require considerable training and in most cases, specialists in both perform routine procedures with very little deviation [4].

Yet, maybe they differences between both are what we can learn from: hierarchy vs. team approach, litigation only vs. personal risk upon errors, little/no mandatory training after certification vs. surveillance and regular performance evaluations, and minor vs. very strictly regulated working hours.

Beyond the pure check of facts, checklists such as the WHO checklist also create further positive influence on the procedures. By forcing the team to introduce themselves and to talk about the case before incision, mutual communication is enhanced and a team feeling is built. And by providing a structured check of crucial facts, a safety culture is promoted.

Important to say that the WHO Surgical Safety Checklist is not meant to be used manda-

Table 70.1 Literature on neurosurgical checklists and corresponding impact

Authors and year	Specialty	Aims	Outcomes
Fargen et al. [25]	Vascular	Standardize unique demands of neurointerventional procedures	After checklist implementation, total no. of adverse events was reduced by 35%, & 95% of staff championed checklist continuation
Kramer et al. [27]	Stereotactic & functional neurosurgery	Assess improvement in no. of errors w/ long-term checklist use	Reduction in no. of errors after 1 year of use, from 3.2 to 0.8 total errors per case
Da Silva-Freitas et al. [18]	General neurosurgery	Evaluate a modified WFIO surgical safety checklist on the safety & quality of care of neurosurgical pts	Identification of 51 events in 44 ops; correction of 88% of errors prior to initiation of surgery
Matsumae et al. [31]	General neurosurgery	Evaluate effect on surgical quality & communication	NA
Chen [14]	Vascular	Design endovascular checklists in the event of aneurysm perforation & thromboembolic event	NA
Lyons [30]	General neurosurgery	Prevent rare errors, ensure correct imaging studies, & ensure antibiotic prophylaxis	No wrong-site, wrong-procedure, or wrong- patient error in 8 years of study; initiation of safety culture
Taussky et al. [40]	Vascular	Design endovascular checklist in event of aneurysm perforation during coil insertion	NA
Connolly et al. [17]	Stereotactic & functional neurosurgery	Detect & remediate procedural errors	No change in no. of errors; decreased time to complete checklist
NASS [33]	Spine	Prevent wrong-site, wrong-level surgery	NA

This is Table 2 from Zuckerman et al. [6], showing available neurosurgical studies on the use of checklists and the resulting impact on patient treatment and outcome [6]
NA not assessed

torily in the published form [5]. It is meant to be modified depending on the local processes, staff, culture, etc. Yet, it should be done with a critical eye and tested for some weeks until final approval.

When using these checklists during time outs in the OR, it is important that all staff members in the room participate and get the feeling that every person in the room is in charge and responsible for preventing avoidable harm to this patient. In daily practice, surgeon and anesthetist are performing the time out and checklist while the nurses use this time to sort out cables, instruments, foot pedals or whatever. It is important, however, to insist on the participation of each team member. With this culture, even the youngest team member should be motivated to mention any observed error instead of being hesitant to mention such observations due to a too hierarchic culture.

Culture, likewise, is another important aspect for the prevention of avoidable errors, which also differ between surgery and aviation. The quote of unknown but neither less discussed origin "Culture eats strategy for breakfast every day" is well-known and tells us to reduce hierarchy at least in occasions where harm to our patients could be avoided easily by such simple measures. This is also true when creating checklists. They should not take longer than 1 min and the amount of checklists in a department should not be overwhelming in order to allow the staff to fully concentrate on each one and recognize its importance at the same time.

Table 70.2 Literature on surgical checklist and corresponding impact

Authors and year	Specialty	Aims	Outcomes
Robb et al. [36]	GI surgery	Assess performance of laparoscopic cholecystectomies	Decreased conversion to open cholecystectomy in females & pts w/ Grade III & IV gallbladder disease
de Vries et al. [22]	General surgery	Assess no., nature, & timing of incidents intercepted by use of the SURPASS	≥1 incidents were intercepted in 2563 checklists (40.6%), w/ majority of Incidents Intercepted In preop & postop stages
Berrisford et al. [10]	Cardlothoracic surgery	Audit errors captured by an extended surgical time-out checklist	VTE prophylaxis, blood products, & clerical & Imaging errors were captured, in addition to reduction In VTE prophylaxis errors after checklist
Calland et al. [13]	GI surgery	assess Improvement In teamwork, situation awareness, & error catching	No difference in pt outcomes, case time, or proficiency; less satisfactory subjective comfort, team efficiency, & communication
deVries et al. [20]	General surgery	Assess prevention of malpractice claims using a surgical safety checklist (SURPASS)	29% of malpractice claims may have been intercepted by SURPASS checklist; may have prevented 40% of deaths & 29% of permanent damage
Nilsson et al. [32]	Anesthesiology	Assess personnel attitudes toward preop time-out checklist	93% noted contribution to increased pt safety; 86% noted opportunity to identify & solve problems; factors considered important by 78-84% were pt identity, correct procedure, correct side, allergy checking, contagious disease
Peyré et al. [34]	General surgery	Determine reliability of laparoscopic Nissen fundoplication procedural checklist as a measurement of advanced technical skill	Higher degree of surgical reliability w/ Nissen procedural checklist
Buzink et al. [11]	Surgical endoscopy	Investigate digital checklists in the no. & type of equipment- & instrument-related RSEs during laparoscopic cholecystectomies	At least 1 RSE Initially Identified in 87% of procedures; digital checklist reduced RSEs to 47%; overall reduction in no. of RSEs by 65%
deVries et al. [19, 23]	General surgery	Determine effect of SURPASS checklist on timing of antibiotic prophylaxis	Increased interval between administration of antibiotic prophylaxis & incision ranged from 23.9 min to 29.9 min (32.9 min in procedures In which the checklist was used); significant decrease In no. of pts who did not receive antibiotics until incision
Semel et al. [38]	Multiple surgical specialities	Decision analysis comparing implementation of WHO surgical safety checklist to existing practice in US hospitals	In hospitals w/ baseline complication rates of at least 3%, implementation generated cost savings after prevention of at least 5 major complications
Chua et al. [15]	Trauma surgery	Determine adherence to Infection protocols & Impact on infection & complications	Cases of central line infections, urinary tract infections, & ventilator-associated pneumonia decreased by 100%, 26%, & 82%, respectively, during study period
Peyre et al. [35]	Surgical endoscopy	Develop a procedural checklist for laparoscopic Nissen fundoplication	65-step procedural checklist created; subjective Improvement in learning model for resident education

(continued)

Table 70.2 (continued)

Authors and year	Specialty	Aims	Outcomes
de Vries et al. [21]	General surgery	Develop SURPASS checklist	In 171 high-risk procedures, 593 process deviations observed; 96% corresponded to a checklist item
Byrnes et al. [12]	Critical care	Assess effect of checklist on consideration of ICU protocols	Verbal consideration improved from 90.9% to 99.7% in the following: DVT prophylaxis, stress ulcer prophylaxis, oral care for pts undergoing ventilation, electrolyte repletion, initiation of physical therapy, & documentation of restraint orders; Increased pt transfer out of ICU on telemetry & Initiation of physical therapy
DuBose et al. [24]	Trauma surgery	Examine effectiveness of Quality Rounds Checklist (QRC) tool to increase prophylaxis	Improvement In 16 measures w/ <95% compliance initially identified
Lingard et al. [28]	Anesthesiology	Assess whether structured briefings Improve OR communication	Mean no. of failures per procedure declined from 3.95 to 1.31; 34% of briefings identified problems, resolved critical knowledge gaps, & resulted in follow-up actions
Verdaasdonk et al. [41]	Surgical endoscopy	Determine reduction In no. of incidents w/ technical laparoscopic equipment	53% reduction in total no. of Incidents vs control; overall reduction In problems w/ laparoscopic equipment
Clark et al. [16]	Obstetrics & gynecology	Examine effects of checklist-based protocol for oxytocin administration on maternal & fetal outcome	Improvement In indices of newborn outcome; system-wide decline In rate of cesarean section deliveries (from 23.6% to 21%) in 1-year period
Lingard et al. [29]	Anesthesiology	Assess feasibility of checklist use in OR & perceived functions of the checklist discussion	Respondents saw subjective value in checklist discussion; however, it impeded work flow patterns
Romagnuolo et al. [37]	Gastroenterology & hepatology	Examine effect of improved communication on hospital stay for upper GI bleeding	Checklist reduced in-patient stay from median 7 days to 3.5 days
Hart and Owen [26]	Anesthesiology	Create checklist to Improve general endotracheal anesthesia for cesarean section delivery	95% of respondents assessed checklist as useful; 80% support use in simulations
Soyer et al. [39]	Dermatology	Evaluate diagnostic performance of nonexperts by using a 3-polnt checklist based on a simplified dermoscopic pattern analysis	Improvement in diagnosis of melanoma In nonexperts compared to experts

This is Table 1 from Zuckerman et al. [6], showing available studies on the use of surgical checklists and the resulting impact on patient treatment and outcome across surgical specialties [6]
DVT deep vein thrombosis, *GI* gastrointestinal, *pt* patient, *RSE* risk-sensitive event, *VTE* venous thromboembolism

70.3.4 Accordance with the Literature Guidelines

The only guidelines for the improvement of surgery are the WHO Guidelines for Safe Surgery 2009. They not only summarize the development and required parts to make surgical intervantions safer, they also provide multicentric strong study data on the impact of using the WHO Safe Surgery Checklist [5].

Level of Evidence: A

The level of evidence available to date is considerably good for using checklists.

70.4 Conclusions and Take Home Message

Today we have considerably good scientific evidence for using surgical checklists before, during and after surgery. The WHO Safe Surgery Checklist provides us a good template which can be carefully customized to different hospitals and specialties in order to not only reduce fatal errors or stupid mistakes but also to optimizing care via various nuances thus reducing morbidity and improving outcome.

Pearls

- Today we have considerably fair scientific evidence for using surgical checklists
- They improve outcome in general and but also reduce fatal errors
- Numbers are often too small to prove efficacy in clinical trials
- Culture plays an important role in preventing potentially avoidable errors

References

1. Groff MW, Heller JE, Potts EA, Mummaneni PV, Shaffrey CI, Smith JS. A survey-based study of wrong-level lumbar spine surgery: the scope of the problem and current practices in place to help avoid these errors. World Neurosurg. 2013;79(3–4):585–92. https://doi.org/10.1016/j.wneu.2012.03.017.
2. Mody MG, Nourbakhsh A, Stahl DL, Gibbs M, Alfawareh M, Garges KJ. The prevalence of wrong level surgery among spine surgeons. Spine (Phila Pa 1976). 2008;33(2):194–8. https://doi.org/10.1097/BRS.0b013e31816043d1.
3. Haynes AB, Weiser TG, Berry WR, Lipsitz SR, Breizat AH, Dellinger EP, et al. A surgical safety checklist to reduce morbidity and mortality in a global population. N Engl J Med. 2009;360(5):491–9. https://doi.org/10.1056/NEJMsa0810119.
4. Weiser TG, Haynes AB, Lashoher A, Dziekan G, Boorman DJ, Berry WR, et al. Perspectives in quality: designing the WHO Surgical Safety Checklist. Int J Qual Health Care. 2010;22(5):365–70. https://doi.org/10.1093/intqhc/mzq039.
5. In: WHO guidelines for safe surgery 2009: safe surgery saves lives (WHO guidelines approved by the guidelines review committee). Geneva: World Health Organization.
6. Zuckerman SL, Green CS, Carr KR, Dewan MC, Morone PJ, Mocco J. Neurosurgical checklists: a review. Neurosurg Focus. 2012;33(5):E2. https://doi.org/10.3171/2012.9.FOCUS12257.
7. Saager L, Hesler BD, You J, Turan A, Mascha EJ, Sessler DI, et al. Intraoperative transitions of anesthesia care and postoperative adverse outcomes. Anesthesiology. 2014;121(4):695–706. https://doi.org/10.1097/ALN.0000000000000401.
8. Oszvald A, Vatter H, Byhahn C, Seifert V, Guresir E. "Team time-out" and surgical safety-experiences in 12,390 neurosurgical patients. Neurosurg Focus. 2012;33(5):E6. https://doi.org/10.3171/2012.8.FOCUS12261.
9. Wong JM, Bader AM, Laws ER, Popp AJ, Gawande AA. Patterns in neurosurgical adverse events and proposed strategies for reduction. Neurosurg Focus. 2012;33(5):E1. https://doi.org/10.3171/2012.9.FOCUS12184.
10. Berrisford RG, Wilson IH, Davidge M, Sanders D. Surgical time out checklist with debriefing and multidisciplinary feedback improves venous thromboembolism prophylaxis in thoracic surgery: a prospective audit. Eur J Cardiothorac Surg. 2012;41:1326–9.

11. Buzink SN, van Lier L, de Hingh IH, Jakimowicz JJ. Risksensitive events during laparoscopic cholecystectomy: the influence of the integrated operating room and a preoperative checklist tool. Surg Endosc. 2010;24:1990–5.
12. Byrnes MC, Schuerer DJ, Schallom ME, Sona CS, Mazuski JE, Taylor BE, et al. Implementation of a mandatory checklist of protocols and objectives improves compliance with a wide range of evidence-based intensive care unit practices. Crit Care Med. 2009;37:2775–81.
13. Calland JF, Turrentine FE, Guerlain S, Bovbjerg V, Poole GR, Lebeau K, et al. The surgical safety checklist: lessons learned during implementation. Am Surg. 2011;77:1131–7.
14. Chen M. A checklist for cerebral aneurysm embolization complications. J Neurointerv Surg. 2011. [epub ahead of print].
15. Chua C, Wisniewski T, Ramos A, Schlepp M, Fildes JJ, Kuhls DA. Multidisciplinary trauma intensive care unit checklist: impact on infection rates. J Trauma Nurs. 2010;17:163–6.
16. Clark S, Belfort M, Saade G, Hankins G, Miller D, Frye D, et al. Implementation of a conservative checklist-based protocol for oxytocin administration: maternal and newborn outcomes. Am J Obstet Gynecol. 2007;197:480.e1–5.
17. Connolly PJ, Kilpatrick M, Jaggi JL, Church E, Baltuch GH. Feasibility of an operational standardized checklist for movement disorder surgery. A pilot study. Stereotact Funct Neurosurg. 2009;87:94–100.
18. Da Silva-Freitas R, Martín-Laez R, Madrazo-Leal CB, Villena-Martin M, Valduvieco-Juaristi I, Martínez-Agüeros JA, et al. Establishment of a modified surgical safety checklist for the neurosurgical patient: initial experience in 400 cases. Neurocirugia (Astur). 2012;23:60–9. (Span).
19. de Vries EN, Dijkstra L, Smorenburg SM, Meijer RP, Boermeester MA. The SURgical PAtient Safety System (SURPASS) checklist optimizes timing of antibiotic prophylaxis. Patient Saf Surg. 2010;4:6.
20. de Vries EN, Eikens-Jansen MP, Hamersma AM, Smorenburg SM, Gouma DJ, Boermeester MA. Prevention of surgical malpractice claims by use of a surgical safety checklist. Ann Surg. 2011;253:624–8.
21. de Vries EN, Hollmann MW, Smorenburg SM, Gouma DJ, Boermeester MA. Development and validation of the SURgical PAtient Safety System (SURPASS) checklist. Qual Saf Health Care. 2009;18:121–6.
22. de Vries EN, Prins HA, Bennink MC, Neijenhuis P, van Stijn I, van Helden SH, et al. Nature and timing of incidents intercepted by the SURPASS checklist in surgical patients. BMJ Qual Saf. 2012;21:503–8.
23. de Vries EN, Prins HA, Crolla RM, den Outer AJ, van Andel G, van Helden SH, et al. Effect of a comprehensive surgical safety system on patient outcomes. N Engl J Med. 2010;363:1928–37.
24. DuBose JJ, Inaba K, Shiflett A, Trankiem C, Teixeira PG, Salim A, et al. Measurable outcomes of quality improvement in the trauma intensive care unit: the impact of a daily quality rounding checklist. J Trauma. 2008;64:22–9.
25. Fargen KM, Velat GJ, Lawson MF, Firment CS, Mocco J, Hoh BL. Enhanced staff communication and reduced near-miss errors with a neurointerventional procedural checklist. J Neurointerv Surg. 2012. [epub ahead of print].
26. Hart EM, Owen H. Errors and omissions in anesthesia: a pilot study using a pilot's checklist. Anesth Analg. 2005;101:246–50.
27. Kramer DR, Halpern CH, Connolly PJ, Jaggi JL, Baltuch GH. Error reduction with routine checklist use during deep brain stimulation surgery. Stereotact Funct Neurosurg. 2012;90:255–9.
28. Lingard L, Regehr G, Orser B, Reznick R, Baker GR, Doran D, et al. Evaluation of a preoperative checklist and team briefing among surgeons, nurses, and anesthesiologists to reduce failures in communication. Arch Surg. 2008;143:12–8.
29. Lingard L, Whyte S, Espin S, Baker GR, Orser B, Doran D. Towards safer interprofessional communication: constructing a model of "utility" from preoperative team briefings. J Interprof Care. 2006;20:471–83.
30. Lyons MK. Eight-year experience with a neurosurgical checklist. Am J Med Qual. 2010;25:285–8.
31. Matsumae M, Nakajima Y, Morikawa E, Nishiyama J, Atsumi H, Tominaga J, et al. Improving patient safety in the intra-operative MRI suite using an on-duty safety nurse, safety manual and checklist. Acta Neurochir Suppl. 2011;109:219–22.
32. Nilsson L, Lindberget O, Gupta A, Vegfors M. Implementing a pre-operative checklist to increase patient safety: a 1-year follow-up of personnel attitudes. Acta Anaesthesiol Scand. 2010;54:176–82.
33. North American Spine Society. Sign, mark & x-ray (SMaX): prevent wrong-site surgery. (http://www.spine.org/Pages/PracticePolicy/ClinicalCare/SMAX/Default.aspx). [Accessed 25 Sept 2012].
34. Peyré SE, Peyré CG, Hagen JA, Sullivan ME. Reliability of a procedural checklist as a high-stakes measurement of advanced technical skill. Am J Surg. 2010;199:110–4.
35. Peyre SE, Peyre CG, Hagen JA, Sullivan ME, Lipham JC, Demeester SR, et al. Laparoscopic Nissen fundoplication assessment: task analysis as a model for the development of a procedural checklist. Surg Endosc. 2009;23:1227–32.
36. Robb WB, Falk GA, Larkin JO, Waldron R Jr, Waldron RP. A 10-step intraoperative surgical checklist (ISC) for laparoscopic cholecystectomy-can it really reduce conversion rates to open cholecystectomy? J Gastrointest Surg. 2012;16:1318–23.
37. Romagnuolo J, Flemons WW, Perkins L, Lutz L, Jamieson PC, Hiscock CA, et al. Post-endoscopy checklist reduces length of stay for non-variceal upper

gastrointestinal bleeding. Int J Qual Health Care. 2005;17:249–54.
38. Semel ME, Resch S, Haynes AB, Funk LM, Bader A, Berry WR, et al. Adopting a surgical safety checklist could save money and improve the quality of care in U.S. hospitals. Health Aff (Millwood). 2010;29:1593–9.
39. Soyer HP, Argenziano G, Zalaudek I, Corona R, Sera F, Talamini R, et al. Three-point checklist of dermoscopy. A new screening method for early detection of melanoma. Dermatology. 2004;208:27–31.
40. Taussky P, Lanzino G, Cloft H, Kallmes D. A checklist in the event of aneurysm perforation during coiling. AJNR Am J Neuroradiol. 2010;31:E59.
41. Verdaasdonk EG, Stassen LP, Hoffmann WF, van der Elst M, Dankelman J. Can a structured checklist prevent problems with laparoscopic equipment? Surg Endosc. 2008;22:2238–43.
42. Yu H, Neimat JS. The treatment of movement disorders by deep brain stimulation. Neurotherapeutics. 2008;5:26–36.

Positioning of the Patient and Related Complications

71

Florian Ringel and Jens Conrad

71.1 Introduction

Optimal positioning of patients for spine surgery is crucial for ideal surgical conditions and operative-site exposure. During surgery of the spine patients are placed in non-physiological conditions already in anesthesia which lead to complications as patients are not able react to an unpleasant tissue damaging position. The factors duration of a surgical procedure, mechanical pressure and immobility increase the risk for positioning related complications and rare complications such as postoperative visual loss (POVL) or perioperative peripheral nerve injury (PPNI) result in significant patient disability and functional restrictions [8, 16].

For adequate exposure of the spine a variety of intraoperative positions of the patient are possible as: prone (Wilson, Concorde), kneeling, knee-chest, knee-elbow, lateral decubitus, supine (French, Da Vinci, cervical spine reclined), lateral and sitting. However, each of these different positions has specific risks for positioning-related complications. While some complications are transient, others can result in a permanent deficit. Thus, surgeons, anesthesiologists and nurses as a team must be aware of intraoperative patient positioning to relieve potentially harmful pressure upon susceptible structures [14].

71.2 Case Description

A 46 y/o male patient suffered from significant lower back pain refractory to conservative therapy since many years. MRI of the lumbar spine revealed a L4/5 disc degeneration with a black disc and Pfirrmann grade 3 disc degeneration and Modic type I changes in the endplates of L4 and 5. Following negative facet joint infiltrations of L4/5 a lumbar total disc replacement was indicated. For surgery the patient was placed in a supine so called French or DaVinci position (Fig. 71.1). The legs were placed slightly flexed at the pelvis and the knees in order to relax the iliopsoas muscle. Special attention was placed to the pressure-free positioning of the knees. The patient underwent eventless total disc replacement at the level L4/5 (Fig. 71.2). After waking up from surgery he had a paralysis of the left dorsiflexion of the foot, no pain, a sensory deficit according to the peroneal nerve. He underwent immediate electrophysiological examination of the peroneal nerve and a conduction block at the fibular head was diagnosed. I.e. the patient had a peroneal nerve palsy from pressure or stretch of the peroneal nerve at the fibular head. During the following days the motor and sensory deficit

F. Ringel (✉) · J. Conrad
Department of Neurosurgery, Universitätsmedizin Mainz, Johannes Gutenberg Universität Mainz, Mainz, Germany
e-mail: florian.ringel@unimedizin-mainz.de

B. Meyer, M. Rauschmann (eds.), *Spine Surgery*, https://doi.org/10.1007/978-3-319-98875-7_71

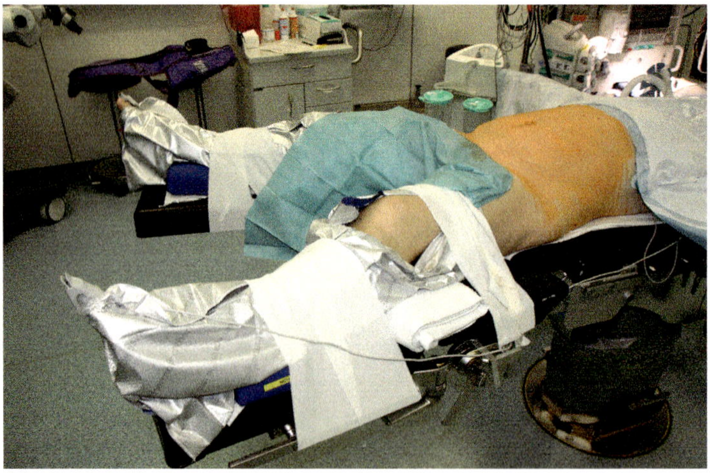

Fig. 71.1 Intraoperative positioning of the patient. The image shows the pressure-free positioning of the knee especially at the fibular head

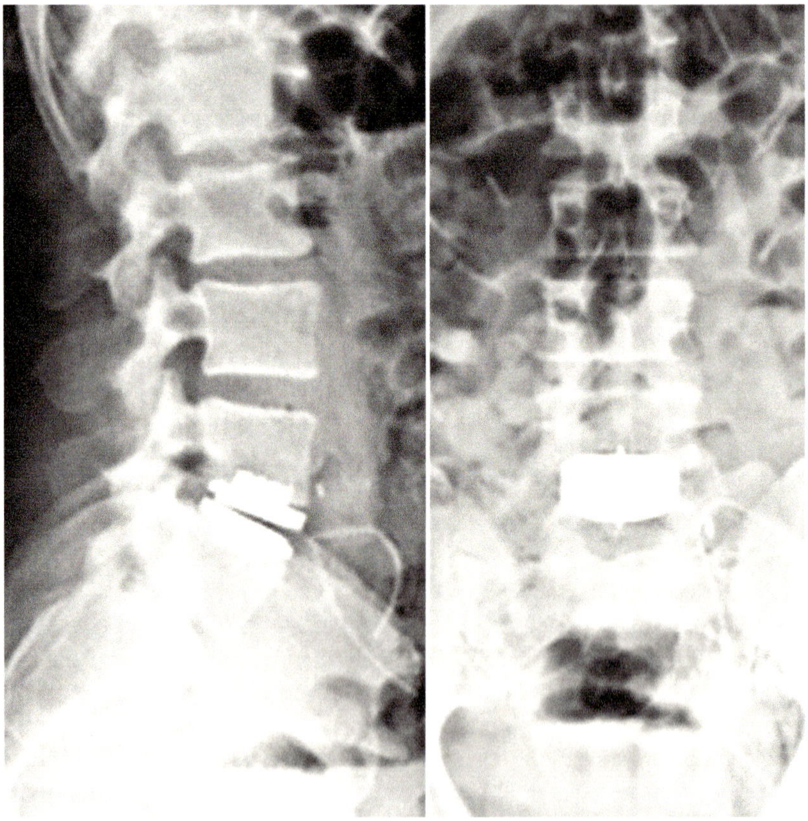

Fig. 71.2 Postoperative lateral and ap X-rays of the lumbar spine. Postoperative images of the lumbar spine with disc prosthesis in L4/5 showing a correct position of the implant

recovered fast. Upon discharge 6 days later, the weakness in foot dorsiflexion was apparent during one legged standing with dorsiflexed foot, only. During further follow-up it recovered completely.

71.3 Discussion

71.3.1 Discussion of the Case

The patient was positioned in a supine so-called Trendelenburg, French or DaVinci position. Special care was taken with regards to tissues at risk for damage from patient positioning. The arms were placed on arm rests in an angle not exceeding 90° to the torso in order to avoid any stretch injury to the brachial plexus. Attention was paid to the ulnar nerve in the cubital tunnel. At the lower extremities special attention was given to the position of the knee and the peroneal nerve at the fibular head. Additionally the heels were positioned pressure-free.

However, despite these precautions a damage to the peroneal nerve at the fibular head occurred, the reason remains unclear. The functional deficit recovered fast during follow-up.

This case illustrates, that positioning-related complications can be reduced to a minimum by careful placement of the patient but it is not 100% controllable despite all efforts.

71.3.2 Common Patient Positions in Spine Surgery

The ***supine position*** is used for anterior approaches to the spine and therefore most commonly for anterior cervical procedures. In contrast to all other patient positions it allows the awake patient to actively move to the OR table under his/her own control finding an adequate position. Prior to induction of anesthesia most of the patient positioning can be accomplished.

Great care needs to be taken to ensure physiological alignment of the head and neck. The head should be straight to prevent brachial plexus injury or vascular injury of the neck. A physiological position of the cervical spine should be chosen while in some cases of anterior cervical surgery the cervical spine is often positioned in a hyperextended position.

In the supine position the arms either rest on an arm board or at the side of the patient supported by an arm protector. In cases where the arms need to be elevated the angle in the shoulder should be below 90° to avoid stretch injury of the brachial plexus of the ulnar nerve or a compression or occlusion injury of the axillar and subclavian arteries. Any pressure to the cubital tunnel needs to be prevented. Pronation and extension of the arm can compress the ulnar nerve between the cubital tunnel and the OR table and should be avoided.

To protect the common peroneal and tibial nerves from stretch injuries upon hyperextension of the knee, pillows are placed under the back of the patient's knees to maintain mild flexion. The patient's heels are slightly elevated from the surface or a gel pad should be placed under the heel to avoid pressure damage.

The Trendelenburg position (French, Da Vinci) is a variation of the supine position where patient's legs are spread and might be elevated. It is used for anterior approaches to the lumbar especially the lumbosacral spine. Prolonged positioning in the Trendelenburg position can be associated with venous pooling in the upper extremities, head and neck edema formation has been described. Therefore, elevation of the lower extremities should be limited and avoided where possible. A posterior ischemic optic neuropathy (PION) has been reported as a complication of this position while the mechanism remains unclear [12, 23].

The ***prone position*** (position on a Wilson frame or Concorde position as variances) is the most common position in spine surgery which allows for posterior approaches to the whole spine from the occipitocervical junction to the sacrum [10]. Special attention needs to be paid to the positioning of the head to avoid pressure to the face which can result in pressure ulcers and pressure to the eyes. Usually the head is positioned in a cushion with a cut-out for the face. But depending on the length of surgery and the patient's facial anatomy, some surgeons decide the fixation of the head in a three-point head clamp. The headrest avoids pressure to the eyes and prevents ocular compression and reduces the risk of perioperative central retinal artery occlusion. Again, arms, elbows and hands should be positioned in a physiological alignment in a neutral position. Upper arms should be protected from pressure to the radial nerves [7]. The preferred arm position is adducted at the patients' side. In surgeries with abducted arms it is necessary to place the arms on arm boards. Again, abduction should be less than 90° to avoid stretch to the brachial plexus. Elbows are flexed and palms should face downwards.

For posterior cervical approaches the patient in a prone position is usually placed on a slightly tilted plane with the head elevated. This positioning can reduce the venous filling in the upper body and thereby avoid approach-related venous bleeding.

A disadvantage of the prone position is the abdominal compression with associated reduced venous drainage from epidural veins. Therefore as a modification of the prone position the position on a Wilson frame can be used. It does lead to a delordosed position of the lumbar spine easing interlaminar approaches and to an uncompressed position of the abdomen avoiding an increase of epidural venous pressure. However, the Wilson frame does not allow for ap fluoroscopy imaging and therefore needs to be avoided in cases where biplanar imaging is necessary.

An alternative to the position on the Wilson frame is the ***knee-chest position*** used for lumbar posterior approaches. Even less abdominal compression than on a Wilson frame is the advantage of the knee-chest position. However, it does not delordose the lumbar spine it rather leads to a hyperlordosis. For this position ocular injury has been reported as well as perioperative central retinal artery occlusion [16]. Shriver et al. [14] analyzed seven studies reporting the use of the knee-chest position. Acute renal failure, rhabdomyolysis, insecure endotracheal intubation and quadriplegia were only reported among studies using the knee-chest position.

A **lateral position** is necessary for anterolateral thoracic or lumbar approaches, rarely for lateral cervical approaches. For this position a vacuum-device to stabilize the torso is helpful. To relieve pressure to the nerves and vessels of the brachial plexus and axilla a round cushion should be placed below the downsided axilla. The downsided arm is positioned in a 90° angle to the body. The upsided arm is usually elevated, an angle above 90° should be avoided for this arm as well. A cushion needs to be placed between both legs. Critical structures of this position are the brachial plexus, ulnar nerve, ear and peroneal nerve.

This **semisitting position** provides access to the posterior cervical spine. It improves cerebral venous drainage but remains controversial because of the potential for serious complications such as venous air embolism, hemodynamic instability and compressive peripheral neuropathy.

71.3.3 Position-Related Complications

Perioperative peripheral nerve injury (PPNI) is a rare but significant positioning-related complication. The reported incidence is between 0.03% and 0.1% [2, 24]. Direct trauma to a peripheral nerve can be the cause of PPNI, but one of the main and crucial mechanisms of PPNI is the ischemia of nerve fibers with focal demyelination [9, 17, 20, 22]. Stretch of peripheral nerves is another mechanism of PPNI and occurs if nerves are stretched beyond 5–15% of their resting length [11, 18, 19]. In lumbar spine surgery positioning-related damage of peripheral nerves was reported following prone, knee-elbow and lateral decubitus positioning of the patient.

Causes for **peroneal nerve injury** are often compressive straps used to restrain the legs in the Trendelenburg position. Both stretch and external compression are possible mechanisms, especially during long durations of surgery (>6 h). Positioning devices should not involve fixation of the leg at the level of the knee or ankle. About half of the patients suffering from peroneal nerve injury recover within 1 year, the other half might be corrected surgical and/or treated by casts [20, 22]. The most common PPNI (28% of all neuropathies) is the **ulnar neuropathy** with an incidence of 0.5% of all surgically treated patients [21]. It is the neuropathy most commonly associated with supine positioning [1, 4]. Perioperative ulnar nerve injury can have a delayed onset, most cases manifest within 2–7 days after surgery [8]. Compression of the ulnar nerve in the cubital tunnel from externally is associated with the development of a nerve injury. At this location the nerve is superficial and often unprotected by soft tissue. Extreme flexion of the elbow (>90°) tightens the arcuate ligament and shrinks the cubital tunnel. Supination and padding of the extended arm reduce the risk of external compression. Ulnar nerve injuries have a less favorable outcome compared to other nerve injuries. Regularly, ulnar nerve decompression or transposition surgery is required. The second most common PPNI is **brachial plexus injury** (20% of all neuropathies) with a reported incidence of 0.02% [6]. The main mechanisms of positioning-related brachial plexus injury are stretch and compression. Stretching is typically caused by shoulder abduction greater than 90°, external rotation of the arm and posterior shoulder displacement. In the supine position extension and lateral flexion of the head may stretch the brachial plexus on the contralateral side. Brachial plexus positioning injuries present as a typically painless motor dysfunction referable to the upper and middle trunks. Less commonly the lower trunk can be affected. Careful positioning is required in the prone position to avoid brachial plexus injury. Excessive intraoperative shoulder abduction (>90°) can injure the plexus. Therefore, arm positioning at the sides of the patient can prevent these injuries. In the lateral decubitus position compression of the dependent arm and axilla should be avoided using an appropriately placed axillary roll. **Median nerve neuropathy** is with 4% of PPNI a rare complication, stretching the main mechanism. Hanging the unpadded pronated arm off the table can compress the median nerve. **Radial nerve injury** (3% of PPNI) is mainly caused by direct compression at the spiral grove of the humerus [8], especially when the posterior aspect of the arm is pushed against a rigid structure. Radial nerve injuries usually recover over several months dependent on the length of the nerve. [5] reported neuropathy of the **lateral femoral cutaneus nerve** at the level of the anterior superior iliac spine following PLIF-surgery.

Isolated **axillary nerve injury** is rare but has been reported in the prone position.

Overall, intraoperative positioning-related nerve injuries are rare, however they continue to occur. To avoid perioperative nerve injuries surgeons must maintain high attention to avoid excessive stretching of the nerves and intraoperative pressure near key peripheral nerve locations, especially in thin patients. Nerve injuries have to be recognized and diagnosed.

Perioperative visual loss (POVL) The prevalence of POVL after spine surgery is 0.0028–0.2% [3, 13]. POVL can result in bi- or unilateral visual loss. Risk factors are prolonged duration of surgery, prone position, posterior lumbar fusion and correction of scoliosis. The most common cause of POVL in cases of spine surgery is ischemic optic neuropathy (ION) and central retinal artery (CRA) occlusion. ION is divided into an anterior ION (AION) and a posterior ION (PION) which is the most common cause of POVL after spine surgery [8]. Spine surgeons should be aware of POVL and participate in safe perioperative care of patients positioned in the prone position. The prone position has been shown to increase the intraocular pressure (IOP) under general anesthesia. As a result IOP may become the critical factor in perfusion of the anterior optic nerve in the presence of decreased hematocrit and mean arterial blood pressure.

Patient with head-neutral positioning compared with the head-down position had a lower incidence of **chemosis (conjunctival swelling)** in prone position. Additionally increased duration of surgery and a positive fluid balance correlated with an increased incidence of postoperative chemosis [14].

Bite Injury, oropharyngeal swelling and macroglossia are potential further positioning-related injuries. A neutral head position and also bite blockers minimize the risk for intraoperative tongue displacement and swelling and also decrease bite injuries. A case of oropharyngeal swelling and macroglossia after cervical spine surgery in the prone position is reported by Sinha et al. [15]. Maneuvers to avoid these complications are the use of a transtracheal ventilation, bite block, no extreme flexion of the head against the chest and an hourly check of the swelling of the tongue, head and neck while surgery in risky positions.

Thromboembolic complications are a further problem. Intraoperative positioning plays a crucial role in the rate of deep vein thrombosis and pulmonary embolism. Reported rates following spine surgery are between 0.3% and 12%.

71.4 Conclusions and Take Home Message

Positioning-related complications are rare problems as they can be prevented by carful positioning of the patient. However, despite all care in placement of the patient, positioning-related complications cannot be controlled completely and occur in a very low frequency.

Pearls

Avoid

- Pressure at areas with superficial nerve position.
- Stretching of peripheral nerves by unphysiological positions of extremities.

References

1. Akhavan A, Gainsburg DM, Stock JA. Complications associated with patient positioning in urologic surgery. Urology. 2010;76:1309–16.
2. Cassoria L, Lee JW. Patient positioning in anesthesia (2009). In: Miller RD, editor. Miller's anesthesia. 7th ed. Philadelphia: Elsevier; 2009. p. 1151–70.
3. Chang SH, Miller NR. The incidence of vision loss due to perioperative ischemic optic neuropathy associated with spinesurgery: the Johns Hopkins Hospital Experience. Spine (Phila Pa 1976). 2005;30(11):1299–302.
4. Cheney FW, Domino KB, Caplan RA, Posner KL. Nerve injury associated with anesthesia: a closed claims analysis. Anesthesiology. 1999;90(4):1062–9.
5. Cho KT, Lee HJ. Prone position-related meralgia paresthetica after lumbar spinal surgery: a case report and review of the literature. J Korean Neurosurg Soc. 2008;44:392–5.
6. Cooper DE, Jenkins RS, Bready L, Rockwood CA. The prevention of injuries of the brachial plexus secondary to malposition of the patient during surgery. Clin Orhop Relat Res. 1988;228:33–41.
7. Heizenroth PA. Positioning the patient for surgery. In: Rothrock JC, editor. Alexander's care of the patient in surgery. 13th ed. St Louis: Mosby; 2007. p. 130–57.
8. Kamel I, Barnette R. Positioning patients for spine surgery: avoiding uncommon position-related complications. World J Orthop. 2014;5(4):425–43.
9. Myers RR, Yamamoto T, Yaksh TL, Powell HC. The role of focal nerve ischemia and Wallerian degeneration in peripheral nerve injury producing hyperesthesia. Anesthesiology. 1993;78:308–16.
10. O'Connell P. Positioning impact on the surgical patient. Nurs Clin North Am. 2006;41(3):173–92.
11. Ogata K, Naito M. Blood flow of peripheral nerve effects of dissection, stretching and compression. J Hand Surg Br. 1986;11:10–4.
12. Phong SV, Koh LK. Anaesthesia for robotic-assisted radical prostatectomy: considerations for laparoscopy in the Trendelenburg position. Anaesth Intensive Care. 2007;35:281–5.
13. Shen Y, Drum M, Roth S. The prevalence of perioperative visual loss in the United States: a 10-year study from 1996 to 2005 of spinal, orthopedic, cardiac, and general surgery. Anesth Analg. 2009;109(5):1534–45.
14. Shriver MF, Zeer V, Alentado VJ, Mroz TE, Benzel EC, Steinmetz MP. Lumbar spine surgery positioning complications: a systematic review. Neurosurg Focus. 2015;39(4):E16.
15. Sinha A, Agarwal A, Gaur A, Pandey CK. Oropharyngeal swelling and macroglossia after cervical spine surgery in the prone position. J Neurosurg Anesthesiol. 2001;13(3):237–9.
16. St-Arnaud D, Paquin MJ. Safe positioning for neurosurgical patients. AORN J. 2008;87(6):1156–68; quiz 1169–1172.
17. Sunderland S. The intraneural topography of the radial, median and ulnar nerves. Brain. 1945;68:243–99.
18. Tanoue M, Yamaga M, Ide J, Takagi K. Acute stretching of peripheral nerves inhibits retrograde axonal transport. J Hand Surg Br. 1996;21:358–63.
19. Wall EJ, Massie JB, Kwan MK, Rydevik BL, Myers RR, Garfin SR. Experimental stretch neuropathy. Changes in nerve conduction unter tension. J Bone Joint Surg Br. 1992;74:126–9.
20. Warner MA, Martin JT, Schroeder DR, Offord KP, Chute CG. Lower-extremity motor neuropathy associated with surgery performed on patients

in a lithotomy position. Anesthesiology. 1994a;81: 6–12.
21. Warner MA, Warner DO, Matsumoto JY, Harper CM, Schroeder DR, Maxson PM. Ulnar neuropathy in surgical patients. Anesthesiology. 1999;90:54–9.
22. Warner MA, Warner ME, Martin JT. Ulnar neuropathy. Incidence, outcome, and risk factors in sedated or anesthetized patients. Anesthesiology. 1994b;81:1332–40.
23. Weber ED, Colyer MH, Lesser RL, Subramanian PS. Posterior ischemic optic neuropathy after minimally invasive prostatectomy. J Neuroophthalmol. 2007;27(4):285–7.
24. Welch MB, Brummett CM, Welch TD, Tremper KK, Shanks AM, Guglani P, Mashour GA. Perioperative peripheral nerve injuries: a retrospective study of 380,680 cases during a 10-year period at a single institution. Anesthesiology. 2009;111:490–7.

Post-laminectomy Kyphosis 72

Hanno S. Meyer

72.1 Introduction

Spinal column deformity is a well-known musculoskeletal complication following laminectomies for various spinal pathologies, such as intraspinal tumors, degenerative disease, or traumatic spinal injury. Post-laminectomy kyphosis is the most common deformity.

The most important risk factors are young patient age and site of laminectomy. It has long been known that children, adolescents and young adults are at a particular risk for post-laminectomy deformity [1]. This is due to the ongoing development of the spine. The most common site is the cervical spine, where virtually all children and young adults develop post-laminectomy kyphosis. The reported risk is lower for the thoracic (36%) and for the thoracolumbar/lumbar (0–28%) spine in this age group [2, 3]. At the cervical spine, even adults are at a significant risk. In cervical spondylotic myelopathy (CSM), e.g., kyphosis may develop in approximately 20% of patients [5], with even higher rates in patients with ossification of the posterior longitudinal ligament (OPLL) [7].

Post-laminectomy cervical kyphosis may progress over time and can be associated with severe pain and even neurological deterioration, requiring surgical correction performed via an anterior, posterior, or combined approach [6].

The following case will illustrate that failure to take post-laminectomy deformity into account can lead to severe consequences for the patient and how to deal with it surgically.

72.2 Case Description

A 21-year-old male had a motor vehicle accident in Russia and was transferred to a hospital. He suffered from bilateral upper extremity weakness. A fracture of the fourth cervical vertebra was diagnosed. He underwent dorsal decompression via a C4 laminectomy and was provided with a cervical collar.

He presented 2 weeks later. After initial incomplete recovery, the upper extremity weakness had deteriorated (right upper extremity: 1–2/5 proximal, 3–4/5 distal; left upper extremity: 2–3/5 proximal, 4+/5 distal), and he had severe gait ataxia and bilateral plantar hypesthesia.

A CT scan showed a translation injury of C4 vs. C3 and C5 with bilaterally dislocated facets and a combined burst/sagittal split fracture of C4 [AO type: C3–4-5: C (C4: A4, F4, N3, M2)]. The kyphosis had progressed since the first CT after laminectomy (Figs. 72.1 and 72.2).

H. S. Meyer (✉)
Department of Neurosurgery, Klinikum rechts der Isar, Technische Universität München, Munich, Germany
e-mail: Hanno.Meyer@tum.de

B. Meyer, M. Rauschmann (eds.), *Spine Surgery*, https://doi.org/10.1007/978-3-319-98875-7_72

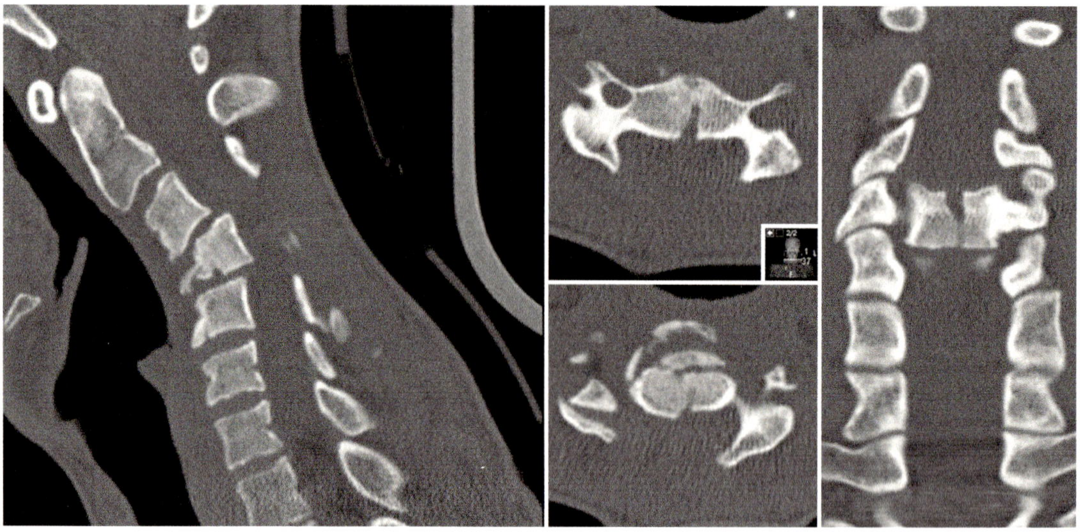

Fig. 72.1 CT. Sagittal (left panel), axial (middle panels) and coronal (right panel) CT slices. There is substantial dislocation in C3–4 and C4–5, resulting in kyphotic deformity of the cervical spine (left panel). The vertebral body of C4 has suffered a split (upper middle panel and right panel) and a burst fracture (lower middle panel). The lamina of C4 has been removed during the initial surgery

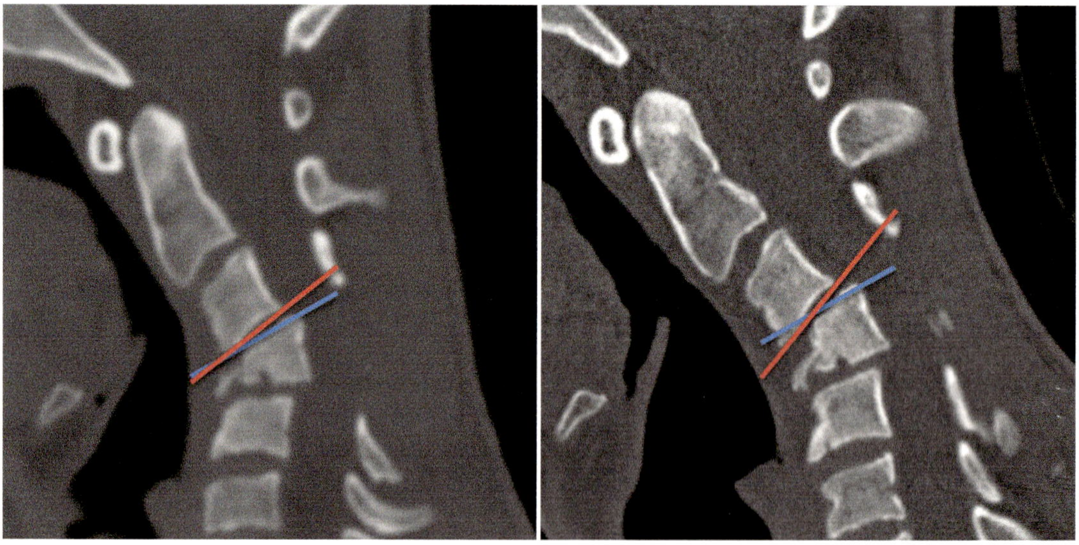

Fig. 72.2 CT. Comparison of a CT scan obtained immediately after (left panel) and 2 weeks after (right panel) C4 laminectomy. The kyphotic deformity has progressed (blue vs. red lines in left vs. right panel)

The patient was operated immediately employing a two-staged anterior-posterior approach. As a first step, anterior open reduction was performed using a caspar cervical distractor and by means of a neck support roll. The vertebral body of C4 was removed and replaced by a PEEK-based graft. A titanium screw-plate-graft was placed from C3 to C5. The postoperative X-ray is shown in Fig. 72.3.

The next day, the instrumentation was completed via a dorsal approach. A screw-rod-fixation was put in place using lateral mass screws. The postoperative X-ray is shown in Fig. 72.4.

After surgery, the patient's condition improved rapidly. Upon discharge, there was much less gait ataxia, and the pareses had diminished (right upper extremity: proximal 3–4/5, distal 4+/5; left upper extremity: proximal 3–4/5, distal 4+/5).

72.3 Discussion of the Case

We present an extreme case of post-laminectomy cervical kyphosis. The patient had a highly unstable dislocated cervical fracture with primary neurological injury due to spinal cord compression. In principle, aiming at a decompression of the spinal cord is correct. The first surgery in the present case, however, jeopardized this goal by making an unstable fracture even more prone to dislocation by performing a laminectomy alone and by forgoing primary stabilization, risking further neurological deterioration.

In other diseases potentially treatable by cervical laminectomy, such as multi-level CSM or OPLL, the indication for concurrent stabilization aiming at preventing post-laminectomy kyphosis is often less clear. There is much data, but not much high-quality evidence in the literature on the subject. Laminectomy was initially regarded as the gold standard treatment of multilevel CSM. When surgeons realized, based on retrospective studies, that this may lead to progressive (instable) post-laminectomy deformity/kyphosis and delayed clinical deterioration, they introduced fusion procedures performed in addition to decompression. Retrospective series reported relatively low complication rates, good outcome, and a low incidence of late deterioration using these techniques, leading surgeons to abandon standalone laminectomies in favor of instrumentation-augmented fusion for these conditions [4–7]. Studies reporting direct comparisons of the two methods are scarce. The various drawbacks associated with instrumented

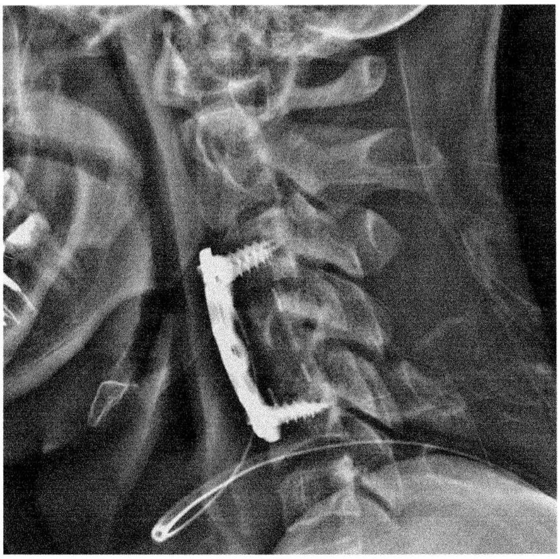

Fig. 72.3 X-Ray. Lateral X-ray image acquired after reduction, replacement of C4 with a PEEK graft and ventral plating. Note the reduction of the kyphotic deformity (cf. Figs. 72.3 and 72.4)

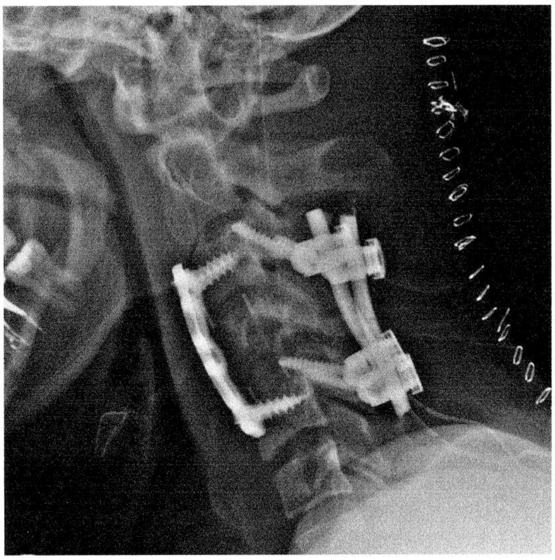

Fig. 72.4 X-Ray. Lateral X-ray image acquired after dorsal instrumentation using lateral mass screws in C3 and C5

fusion, such as addition of time and morbidity to the operation as well as reduced spinal mobility, led to the development of laminoplasty [6]. Comparing the long-term follow-up results of laminoplasty vs. laminectomy for cervical spondylotic myelopathy with regards to kyphotic deformity, however, there appears to be no significant difference [7]. The comparison of laminoplasty vs. laminectomy and fusion provides no evidence supporting one method over the other as well, as shown by two meta-analyses involving mostly observational studies and one randomized controlled trial [8, 9]. Finally, procedures based on an anterior approach, such as anterior cervical discectomy/corpectomy and fusion, have been employed in the treatment of both CSM and OPLL as well. Comparisons with laminoplasty have remained elusive, and there is no clear evidence supporting one over the other. In summary, while dorsal approaches might be associated with less complications, there might be less late deformity with anterior surgery [10, 11].

The data on cervical kyphosis after resection of spinal intradural tumors is even scarcer. These patients are, on average, younger than those with CSM or OPLL. Young age is an important risk factor for post-laminectomy deformity, especially in children and adolescents whose spine is still developing [1, 2, 6]. This patient group is prone to post-laminectomy deformity even at the thoracolumbar spine [3]. However, placement of extensive instrumentation is generally avoided in children to avoid growth-related sagittal deformity and degeneration of adjacent segments. In this population, instrumentation is primarily considered in cases involving extensive bone removal or in those with other risk factors for postoperative instability.

In general, the decision for a surgical strategy with or without instrumentation should be based on the individual case and take all risk factors for post-laminectomy deformity into account. Apart from patient age and site of laminectomy, this includes extent of laminectomy, facet capsule destruction,

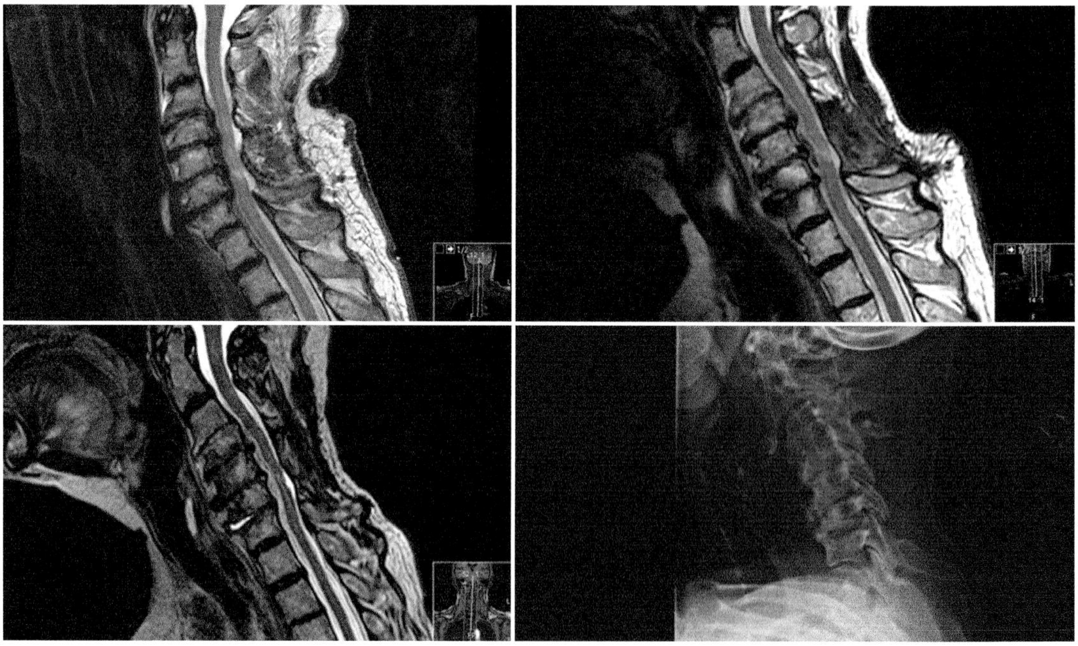

Fig. 72.5 Swan neck deformity after cervical laminectomy. Series of cervical spine images illustrating development of swan neck deformity in an 80 year old female. The patient suffered from CSM (top left panel: initial sagittal MRI). She was treated with a laminectomy of C5 and C6. Afterwards, she complained of increasing neck pain and a perceived cervical instability. The imaging shows that, over the course of 20 months, she developed both kyphotic deformity as well as a compensatory lordotic malalignment of the cervical spine (top right: sagittal MRI, 6 months after surgery; bottom left: sagittal MRI, 17 months after surgery; bottom right: lateral X-ray, 20 months after surgery)

tumor as a primary diagnosis, additional irradiation, and preoperative deformity/lordosis [6, 7].

The present case represents an acute form of a focal post-laminectomy kyphosis. However, both focal kyphosis as well as more complex deformities, such as swan neck deformity (the simultaneous development of both abnormal kyphosis and hyperlordotic malalignments), can develop over time (Fig. 72.5).

Once post-laminectomy cervical kyphosis has developed, there are several treatment options. When pain is the only clinical problem, conservative treatment may be sufficient. In patients with progressive deformity, intractable pain, functional loss, or even neurological decline, surgical treatment strategies have to be considered. They depend on the individual pathology. If possible, reduction is achieved via anterior approaches including discectomies and disc interspace distraction to restore cervical lordosis, as was done in the presented trauma case. When multi-level procedures or corpectomies have to be performed to achieve sufficient reduction, or when the spine is especially unstable (as in the presented case), a subsequent posterior instrumentation can be necessary. Lateral mass screws may often be sufficient in these cases. A limited degree of additional correction can be achieved by posterior Smith-Peterson osteotomies. Pedicle subtraction osteotomies provide a greater degree of reduction. However, they are associated with high morbidity and should be limited to extreme cases where anterior approaches are not feasible [6].

Sometimes, deformity correction is not necessary. If the goal is to just prevent progression of a complex multi-level deformity, as was the case with the 80 year-old patient suffering from swan neck deformity, a stand-alone posterior stabilization may be sufficient. In these cases, pedicle screws should be considered, providing more stability than lateral mass screws.

72.4 Conclusions and Take Home Message

Spinal column deformity can occur after decompression surgery for various spinal pathologies. Post-laminectomy kyphosis of the cervical spine is the most common form. It can be focal or more complex (swan neck deformity, or combined kyphosis and scoliosis). Children, adolescents and young adults are at particular risk. Risk factors, such as patient age, site and extent of laminectomy, existing preoperative deformity, and presumed postoperative stability must be taken into account when considering decompressive spinal surgery. Stabilization surgery may be required in the first place, especially in spinal trauma, but also when extensive bone removal is required or when preoperative loss of lordosis is present. Patients should be followed up to recognize progressive late deformity in time and to prevent possible neurological injury by performing secondary stabilization surgery. Symptomatic cervical post-laminectomy kyphosis can be treated surgically, primarily via anterior or combined anterior-posterior approaches. The evidence on strategies aiming at preventing and treating post-laminectomy kyphosis is low.

Pearls

- Spinal column deformity can occur after decompressive surgery
- Post-laminectomy kyphosis of the cervical spine is the most common form
- Risk factors include young patient age, decompression at the cervical spine, extent of laminectomy, tumor as a primary diagnosis, preoperative deformity, and postoperative irradiation
- For any decompressive spinal surgery, the individual risk for postoperative spinal column deformity must be taken into account
- In high - risk patients, primary stabilization may be required
- Symptomatic cervical post-laminectomy kyphosis can be treated surgically, primarily via anterior or combined anterior-posterior approaches

References

1. Haft H, Ransohoff J, Carter S. Spinal cord tumors in children. Pediatrics. 1959;23:1152–9.
2. Yasuoka S, Peterson HA, MacCarty CS. Incidence of spinal column deformity after multilevel laminectomy in children and adults. J Neurosurg. 1982;57:441–5.
3. Papagelopoulos PJ, Peterson HA, Ebersold MJ, Emmanuel PR, Choudhury SN, Quast LM. Spinal column deformity and instability after lumbar or thoracolumbar laminectomy for intraspinal tumors in children and young adults. Spine (Phila Pa 1976). 1997;22:442–51.
4. Kumar VG, Rea GL, Mervis LJ, McGregor JM. Cervical spondylotic myelopathy: functional and radiographic long-term outcome after laminectomy and posterior fusion. Neurosurgery. 1999;44:771–7; discussion 777–8.
5. Kaptain GJ, Simmons NE, Replogle RE, Pobereskin L. Incidence and outcome of kyphotic deformity following laminectomy for cervical spondylotic myelopathy. J Neurosurg. 2000;93:199–204.
6. Deutsch H, Haid RW, Rodts GE, Mummaneni PV. Postlaminectomy cervical deformity. Neurosurg Focus. 2003;15:E5.
7. Cho WS, Chung CK, Jahng TA, Kim HJ. Post-laminectomy kyphosis in patients with cervical ossification of the posterior longitudinal ligament: does it cause neurological deterioration? J Korean Neurosurg Soc. 2008;43:259–64.
8. Lee CH, Lee J, Kang JD, Hyun SJ, Kim KJ, Jahng TA, Kim HJ. Laminoplasty versus laminectomy and fusion for multilevel cervical myelopathy: a meta-analysis of clinical and radiological outcomes. J Neurosurg Spine. 2015;22:589–95.
9. Liu FY, Yang SD, Huo LS, Wang T, Yang DL, Ding WY. Laminoplasty versus laminectomy and fusion for multilevel cervical compressive myelopathy: a meta-analysis. Medicine (Baltimore). 2016;95:e3588.
10. Xu L, Sun H, Li Z, Liu X, Xu G. Anterior cervical discectomy and fusion versus posterior laminoplasty for multilevel cervical myelopathy: a meta-analysis. Int J Surg. 2017;48:247–53.
11. Qin R, Chen X, Zhou P, Li M, Hao J, Zhang F. Anterior cervical corpectomy and fusion versus posterior laminoplasty for the treatment of oppressive myelopathy owing to cervical ossification of posterior longitudinal ligament: a meta-analysis. Eur Spine J. 2018;27:1375–87.

Failed Back Surgery Syndrome: The Scar Is a Myth

73

Sebastian Ille, Sandro M. Krieg, and Bernhard Meyer

73.1 Introduction

The term "failed back surgery syndrome" (FBSS) is wide-ranged and includes any sequelae following surgery of a lumbar disc herniation. Symptoms might be variable and multiple reasons exist, which can lead to a FBSS. Both the axial lumbar back pain as well as the persistent radiculopathy after surgery are symptoms of the FBSS. A large-scaled study could show that the FBSS depends on a recessal stenosis in 58% of cases, on a spinal stenosis in 7–14% of cases, on a new disc herniation in 12–16% of cases, on an arachnoiditis in 6–16% of cases, and on epidural scars in 6–8% of patients [1]. As described later, the latter must be questioned. In most cases the pain occurs under stress and differs from the preoperative symptoms. Multiple operative and nonoperative strategies can be chosen for the therapy of FBSS, but they only lead to a satisfying result if they are adapted to the underlying reason. Hence, making the diagnosis and the right indication particularly for the operative therapy of the FBSS is complex.

The chapter will outline the variable symptoms of the FBSS, the necessity of diagnostics, underlying pathologies of the postoperative symptoms, and according surgical options. Most importantly, the chapter will highlight that the term FBSS is an umbrella term without being a real syndrome, which should be ruled out after the appropriate diagnostics. Moreover, it will show that the rationale of a postoperative scar as a reason for persistent or new pain after surgery and thereby for the FBSS is unlikely and describes a myth in spine surgery since the scar itself does not gain size and therefore does not create any pressure on the dural sac or roots.

At the end of this chapter the reader should be familiar with the underlying pathologies of the FBSS and should choose the according diagnostics and if necessary the appropriate surgical approaches. Additionally, we outline that the term FBSS choose should be used with care.

73.2 Case Description

A 36 y/o male patient presented at our department after he underwent a sequesterectomy of a left-sided lumbar disc herniation L4/5 2 months before at another department. Initially, his preoperative left-sided L5 radicular pain was gone for a few days. Afterwards, he suffered from a predominant lower back pain, a pain correlating to parts of the dermatome L5 as well as a pain correlating to parts of the dermatome L4 on the left

S. Ille · S. M. Krieg (✉) · B. Meyer
Department of Neurosurgery, Klinikum rechts der Isar, Technische Universität München, Munich, Germany
e-mail: Sandro.Krieg@tum.de

B. Meyer, M. Rauschmann (eds.), *Spine Surgery*, https://doi.org/10.1007/978-3-319-98875-7_73

side. The treating center stated a normal postoperative pain and prescribed pain medication. Another colleague from a private practice interpreted the predominant lumbar back pain as a FBSS and referred the patient to a rehabilitation clinic in order to get him treated by a multimodal pain therapy. Yet, the patient presented at our department for a third opinion. We performed a new MRI scan, which showed a recurrent lumbar disc herniation at the operated level L4/5 and an intraforaminal disc herniation (Fig. 73.1). Apart from the above-mentioned, he did not suffer from any neurological deficits.

The intraforaminal disc herniation was assumed to be asymptomatic when the indication for the first operation was made. Since the patient suffered from a pain which partially correlated with the dermatome L4, we performed a sequential diagnostic *periradicular* infiltration of the spinal nerve roots L4 and L5 on the left side.

The patient showed a complete pain relief after the infiltration of the spinal nerve root L4, but no pain relief after the infiltration of the spinal nerve root of L5. Due to the results of the *periradicular* infiltrations in combination with the MRI scan, we performed a re-operation of the level L4/5 for the purpose of an extended interlaminar fenestration, sequestrectomy, and complete decompression of the left-sided L4 root including a foraminotomy L4/5 on the left side. The view of the situs confirmed that the intraforaminal disc herniation was assumed to be asymptomatic during the first operation, since we could not find a lateral approach. Postoperatively, the patient was free of any complaints and could be discharged 2 days after surgery.

One and a half months postoperatively the patient again presented at our outpatient clinic with an immobilizing lower back pain combined with a bilateral pain to the groin. The neurological examination showed a slight, pain-related, bilateral hip flexor paresis without any further deficit. Inflammation parameters were normal and wound conditions were plain. The patient also showed a bilateral facet joint pain, so we performed a diagnostic facet joint infiltration. Since the diagnostic facet joint infiltration did not show any pain relief we conducted a new MRI scan (Fig. 73.2).

Since an infection could at least not be ruled out by the new MRI scan and the patient did still not show signs of inflammation, we performed a CT-controlled biopsy of the operated level L4/5 (Fig. 73.3). At this point of time, the patient reported a decreasing pain intensity under oral pain medication.

Microbiological results showed an infection with Staphylococcus epidermidis, hence, as a result of this examination, the clinical symptoms,

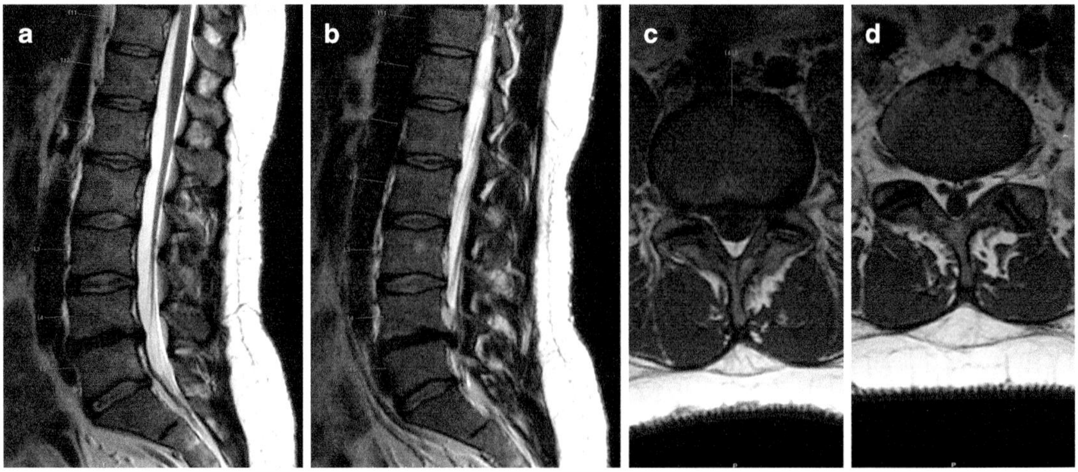

Fig. 73.1 Postoperative MRI after left-sided sequestrectomy L4/5. The MRI scan at first presentation in our outpatient clinic shows a recurrent lumbar disc herniation at the operated level L4/5 as well as an intraforaminal disc herniation (**a**–**c**). The axial slice of (**d**) shows the level L5/S1

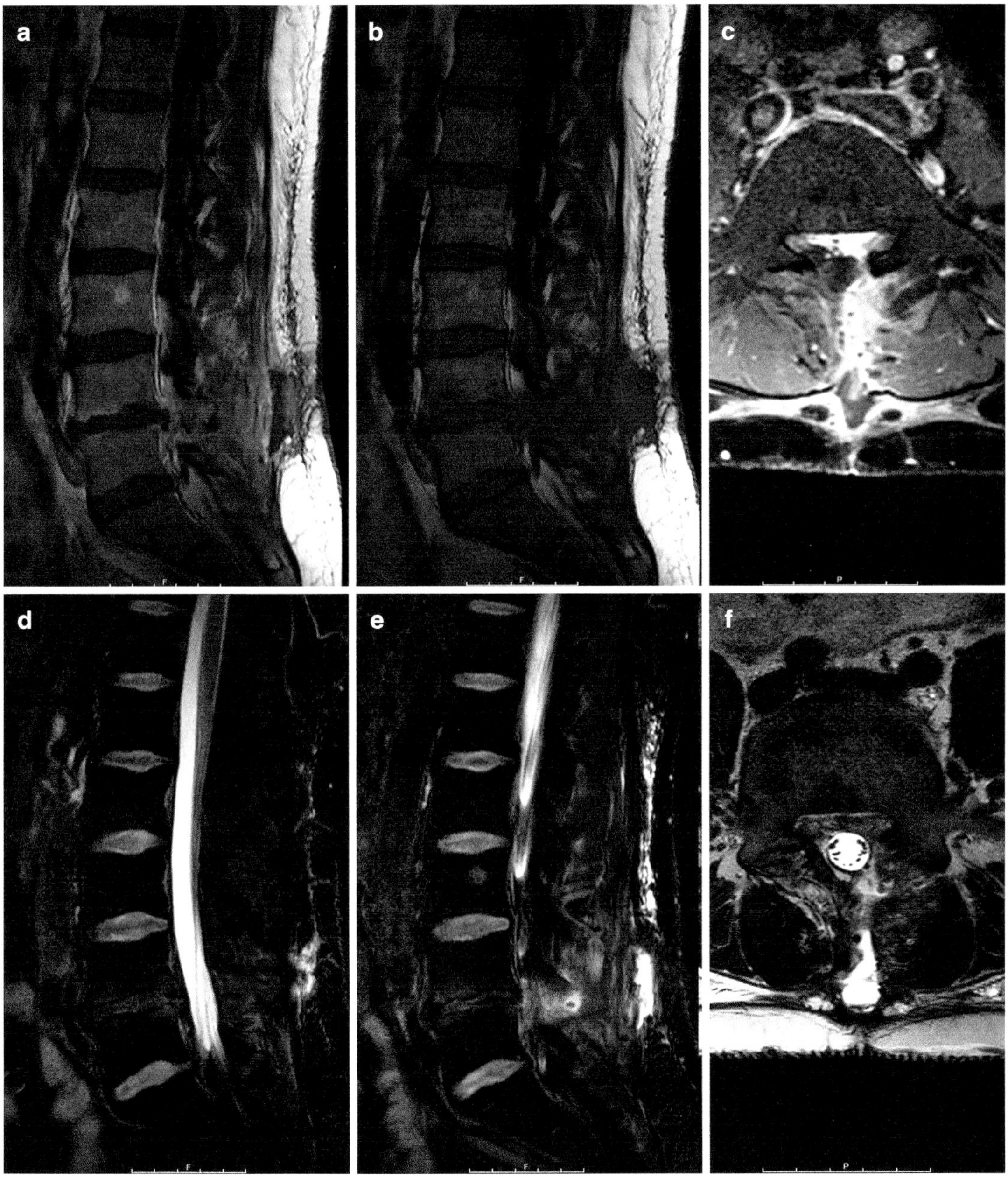

Fig. 73.2 New MRI scan 1.5 months after re-operation. The new MRI scan after the re-operation shows doubtful signs of a postoperative infection or an early spondylodiscitis and postoperative scar tissue at level L4/5 (T1 with (**a**, **c**) and without (**b**) contrast agent; T2 (**d**–**f**) and T2 STIR (**d** and **e**))

and the MRI scan, we made the indication for a second re-operation of the level L4/5, including discectomy with an augmentation with autologous bone, and a dorsal instrumentation L4/5 (Fig. 73.4). Intraoperatively, the surgical field did not show clear signs of infection, but microbiological results of intraoperative smears again showed Staphylococcus epidermidis and the histopathological examination of the intraoperative samples showed signs of an inflammation.

Finally, the patient could be discharged without any complaints after an intravenous antibiotic therapy for 2 weeks. Oral antibiotic therapy was continued for another 10 weeks.

73.3 Discussion of the Case

73.3.1 Indication and Diagnostics

We chose this case, since it showed two possible reasons for a FBSS. Basically, the indication for re-operation of a FBSS, particularly in case of a mono-segmental pathology and a definite clinical correlation, should be clear. In the presented case the initial first postoperative MRI scan showed a recurrent disc herniation and an intraforaminal disc herniation. Furthermore, the patient reported that he initially benefited from the first surgery. Hence, he presented with new symptoms after being free of complaints; such a course always reasons a new MRI scan. A recurrent disc herniation or an already existing intraforaminal disc herniation which has been interpreted as asymptomatic, is probably one of the most common reasons for a FBSS [2]. Recurrent disc herniation occurs especially due to the increase of pure sequestrectomy without performing nucleotomy. A randomized and well-designed trial could show that the pure sequestrectomy without nucleotomy leads to an increased rate of recurrent disc herniation on the one hand, but on the other hand also lowers the rate of postoperative axial pain significantly [3, 4]. Furthermore, Modic changes were reduced from 47% to 14% after 2 years of follow-up. Hence, this surgical approach and strategy must be seen as preventive in such cases, particularly regarding the FBSS as a complication. On the other hand, the rate of intraforaminal disc herniation, which was misinterpreted as asymptomatic when the first indication for surgery was made is of course lower. However, this

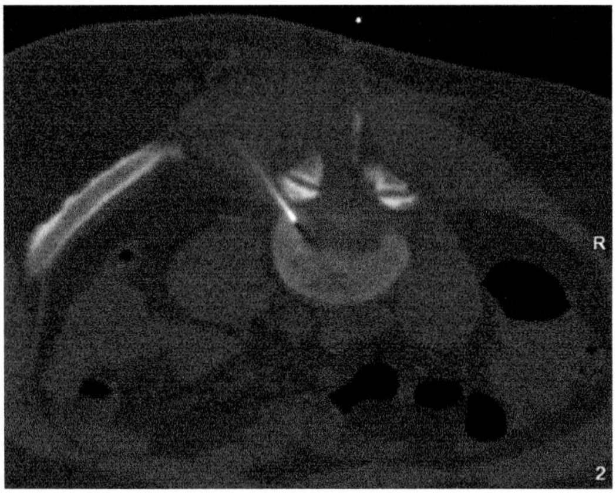

Fig. 73.3 CT-controlled biopsy of disc L4/5. The scan shows the CT-controlled biopsy of the operated level L4/5

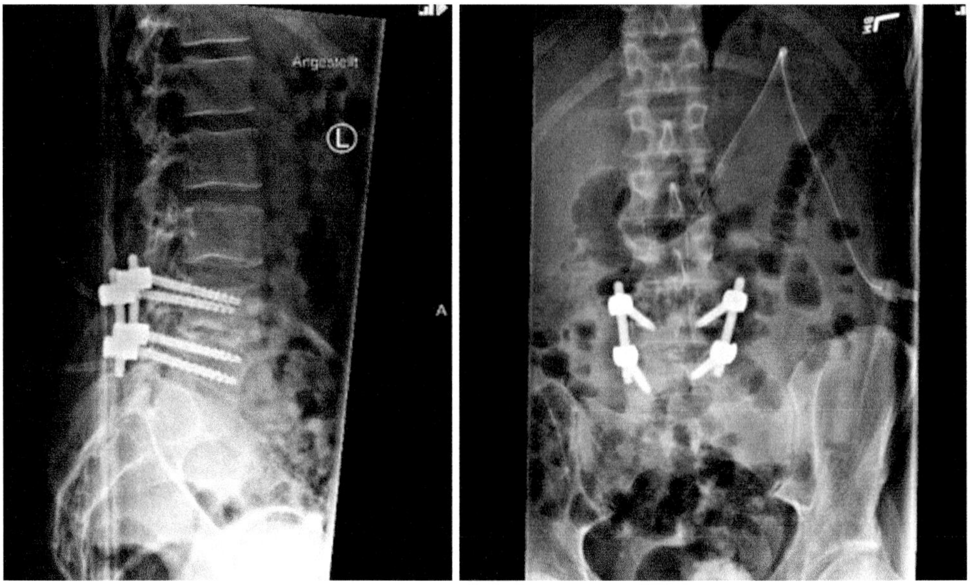

Fig. 73.4 Postoperative X-ray. The figure shows the postoperative X-ray after dorsal instrumentation L4/5

possible reason for a FBSS must also be considered, particularly in case of persistent radiculopathy after surgery. The postoperative MRI scan also showed epidural scar tissue. This was also confirmed intraoperatively. A recently published study identified epidural scar formations in 12.3% of patients with a diagnosed FBSS [2]. Further studies even treated epidural scars by adhesiolysis, partially, with controversial results [5, 6]. By experience of the authors, and confirmed by the presented case, scar tissue does not apply pressure to the dura and neural structures. It must be banned from the people's minds that scar tissue is a reason of FBSS. It is present on MRI scans after spinal decompression, but against all radiological myths scar tissue does not cause neuronal compression.

Meanwhile, we know that a new postoperative radiculopathy must not have a correlate in standard imaging [7]. New MRI scans in case of persistent or new pain after the operation of lumbar disc herniation are only useful in a few of these patients. Hence, in these cases additional diagnostics is needed and indicated such as periradicular infiltrations with local anesthetics or even a myelography.

When the patient presented for the second time at our department reporting an immobilizing lower back pain combined with a bilateral pain to the groin, the decision-making was more difficult. Since the patient did not show clinical or laboratory signs of inflammation, the initial diagnostic facet joint infiltration was justified. The partial resection of the facet joints and the ligaments might lead to an instability within the operated level. Possible symptoms are pseudoradicular pain, axial pain under stress, or even a new disc herniation [8]. The postoperative facet joint syndrome might be another reason for FBSS. A well-designed study, which examined the postoperative facet joint syndrome showed that this complication occurred in 8.4% of patients who underwent the resection of a lumbar disc herniation [9]. Apart from others, the study identified discectomies and an older age as risk factors for a facet joint syndrome. Two options are available for the conservative treatment of the lumbar facet joint syndrome: the intraarticular injection and the ablation of the Ramus medialis nerve. However, the patient did not benefit from the diagnostic facet joint infiltration. Hence, the new MRI scan was indicated. The result of the new MRI scan was not clear regarding a postoperative infection or an early spondylodiscitis. Due to this dilemma we performed a CT-controlled biopsy of the operated level L4/5. Although the patient's clinical symptoms were declining under oral pain medication and he did not show inflammation parameters in the laboratory examinations, an infection as the reason for a FBSS always has to be ruled out if suspected.

73.3.2 Choice of Approach

Since the microbiological results showed the growth of Staphylococcus epidermidis, the indication for re-operation on the one hand, and for instrumentation on the other hand, was clear.

The implantation of a lumbar disc arthroplasty is basically indicated in young patients suffering from osteochondrosis and an axial lumbar pain without a degeneration of the facet joints but a degenerated disc as confirmed by imaging. Well-designed studies are available comparing the pure anterior lumbar interbody fusion (ALIF) with the implantation of a lumbar disc arthroplasty. Regarding the therapeutic effect both the ALIF as well as the implantation of a lumbar disc arthroplasty could show a significant improvement of pain and quality of life [10]. However, the two procedures significantly differ regarding the degeneration of the neighbored levels after 5 years (ALIF: 28.6%, lumbar disc arthroplasty: 9.2%) [11]. Nevertheless, in case of osteoporosis, the affected level should be immobilized by a stand-alone cage and the use of a lumbar disc arthroplasty is not recommended. Furthermore, although it is often performed, the use of a lumbar disc arthroplasty for the treatment of a FBSS is usually not indicated, since it does not solve the underlying problem of the FBSS. Usually, when recurrent or intraforaminal disc herniations can be ruled out, lumbar instability is the reason for the FBSS in many cases. Stress on the facet joints has therefore to be reduced. This status will not be obtained by an arthroplasty but by the immobilization of the according level, i.e. stabilization.

In case of lumbar instability as a reason for the FBSS a dorsal stabilization is indicated especially in case of recurrent disc herniation. A dorsal stabilization should also be considered in case of a intraforaminal disc herniation, which was assumed to be asymptomatic during the resection of an intraspinal disc herniation and now reasons a FBSS. The partial resection of the facet joint, which must usually be performed in order to decompress the nerve root, might lead to a destabilization of the operated level and thereby could make a dorsal stabilization necessary. For the operative therapy of the FBSS, based on osteochondrosis, lumbar instability, or recurrent disc herniation, dynamic, semi-rigid, and rigid instrumentation are options [8].

The dynamic stabilization is especially used to prevent the painful rotation and to take the pressure off the facet joints. Similarly, by enabling a slight grade of motion, the possible complications of a dorsal stabilization should be reduced [12]. Although we do not yet have long-term results of comparison studies, prospective cohort studies show a significant pain relief, an improvement of psychological health, and of mobility [13]. Two years postoperatively, rigid and dynamic stabilizations showed comparable results regarding instabilities of neighbored levels and hardware failures [14, 15]. However, the dynamic stabilization should only be applied up to two levels.

The semi-rigid stabilization shares the load between the screw-rod-system and the ventral cages (so-called "load-sharing") which is thought to promote anterior fusion [16]. However, previous studies showed comparable results in comparison to studies examining rigid or dynamic stabilizations [15, 17].

As a last operative option for the treatment of the FBSS, after ruling out structural reasons eligible for direct surgical therapy, the implantation of a spinal cord stimulator (SCS) must be considered. Meanwhile, reliable data of meta-analyses showed a significant pain reduction of lower back and leg pain [18, 19]. Furthermore, a randomized trial showed superiority of SCS over pain medications. However, this trial also showed at least one device-related complication in 32% of patients, such as electrode migration, infection, or wound issues. Due to complications, 24% of patients had to undergo a re-operation [20]. Today, reliable high-quality data exists regarding the use of SCS in patients suffering from FBSS [21]. Nevertheless, its application in FBSS patients is controversially discussed [22, 23]. Hence, the indication for SCS in such patients must be made very carefully.

73.3.3 Accordance with the Literature Guidelines

Concerning the presented case, our strategy was according to current literature guidelines [8]. However, it has to be mentioned that apart from studies examining the influence of SCS implantation in FBSS patients, high-quality data for the treatment of these patients are not available.

Level of Evidence
C

73.4 Conclusions and Take Home Message

Postoperative epidural scar is often mentioned to be the reason of a FBSS. The chapter describes the opposite, in particular that obvious reasons for the FBSS can be detected and treated after an appropriate diagnostic management. Empirically, scar tissue does not apply pressure to the dura and neural structures. Hence, epidural scar tissue as the reason for FBSS must be banned from the people's minds. It's a myth. After appropriate diagnostics and the according treatment strategy the FBSS can be treated successfully.

Pearls

- especially new symptoms after surgery indicate a new MRI scan
- yet, MRI scans are of limited value in already operated levels
- the indication for re-surgery must be made carefully and the appropriate strategy is essential
- carefully rule out intraforaminal disc protrusion; in doubtful cases use periradicular infiltration of local anesthetics to confirm the affected root
- the application of SCS is only indicated in very selected FBSS patients
- postoperative scar tissue as the reason for FBSS is a myth

References

1. Onesti ST. Failed back syndrome. Neurologist. 2004;10(5):259–64.
2. Bokov A, Isrelov A, Skorodumov A, Aleynik A, Simonov A, Mlyavykh S. An analysis of reasons for failed back surgery syndrome and partial results after different types of surgical lumbar nerve root decompression. Pain Physician. 2011;14(6):545–57.
3. Barth M, Diepers M, Weiss C, Thome C. Two-year outcome after lumbar microdiscectomy versus microscopic sequestrectomy: part 2: radiographic evaluation and correlation with clinical outcome. Spine (Phila Pa 1976). 2008a;33(3):273–9. https://doi.org/10.1097/BRS.0b013e31816201a6.
4. Barth M, Weiss C, Thome C. Two-year outcome after lumbar microdiscectomy versus microscopic sequestrectomy: part 1: evaluation of clinical outcome. Spine (Phila Pa 1976). 2008b;33(3):265–72. https://doi.org/10.1097/BRS.0b013e318162018c.
5. Hossieni B, Dadkhah P, Moradi S, Hashemi SM, Safdari F. The results of treating failed back surgery syndrome by adhesiolysis: comparing the one- and three-day protocols. Anesth Pain Med. 2017;7(5):e60271. https://doi.org/10.5812/aapm.60271.
6. Manchikanti L, Singh V, Cash KA, Pampati V, Datta S. A comparative effectiveness evaluation of percutaneous adhesiolysis and epidural steroid injections in managing lumbar post surgery syndrome: a randomized, equivalence controlled trial. Pain Physician. 2009;12(6):E355–68.
7. el Barzouhi A, Vleggeert-Lankamp CL, Lycklama a Nijeholt GJ, Van der Kallen BF, van den Hout WB, Jacobs WC, et al. Magnetic resonance imaging in follow-up assessment of sciatica. N Engl J Med. 2013;368(11):999–1007. https://doi.org/10.1056/NEJMoa1209250.
8. Wang JC, Dailey AT, Mummaneni PV, Ghogawala Z, Resnick DK, Watters WC 3rd, et al. Guideline update for the performance of fusion procedures for degenerative disease of the lumbar spine. Part 8: lumbar fusion for disc herniation and radiculopathy. J Neurosurg Spine. 2014;21(1):48–53. https://doi.org/10.3171/2014.4.SPINE14271.
9. Steib K, Proescholdt M, Brawanski A, Lange M, Schlaier J, Schebesch KM. Predictors of facet joint syndrome after lumbar disc surgery. J Clin Neurosci. 2012;19(3):418–22. https://doi.org/10.1016/j.jocn.2011.05.039.
10. Gornet MF, Burkus JK, Dryer RF, Peloza JH. Lumbar disc arthroplasty with Maverick disc versus standalone interbody fusion: a prospective, randomized, controlled, multicenter investigational device exemption trial. Spine (Phila Pa 1976). 2011;36(25):E1600–11. https://doi.org/10.1097/BRS.0b013e318217668f.
11. Zigler JE, Delamarter RB. Five-year results of the prospective, randomized, multicenter, Food and Drug Administration investigational device exemption study of the ProDisc-L total disc replacement versus circumferential arthrodesis for the treatment of single-level degenerative disc disease. J Neurosurg Spine. 2012;17(6):493–501. https://doi.org/10.3171/2012.9.SPINE11498.
12. Jahng TA, Kim YE, Moon KY. Comparison of the biomechanical effect of pedicle-based dynamic stabilization: a study using finite element analysis. Spine J. 2013;13(1):85–94. https://doi.org/10.1016/j.spinee.2012.11.014.
13. von Strempel A. Dynamic posterior stabilization with the cosmic system. Oper Orthop Traumatol. 2010;22(5–6):561–72. https://doi.org/10.1007/s00064-010-9016-7.
14. Chou D, Lau D, Skelly A, Ecker E. Dynamic stabilization versus fusion for treatment of degenerative spine conditions. Evid Based Spine Care J. 2011;2(3):33–42. https://doi.org/10.1055/s-0030-1267111.
15. Korovessis P, Papazisis Z, Koureas G, Lambiris E. Rigid, semirigid versus dynamic instrumentation for degenerative lumbar spinal stenosis: a correlative radiological and clinical analysis of short-term results. Spine (Phila Pa 1976). 2004;29(7):735–42.
16. Rickert M, Rauschmann M, Fleege C, Behrbalk E, Harms J. Interbody fusion procedures. Orthopade. 2015;44(2):104–13. https://doi.org/10.1007/s00132-015-3076-1.
17. Liu HY, Zhou J, Wang B, Wang HM, Jin ZH, Zhu ZQ, et al. Comparison of topping-off and posterior lumbar interbody fusion surgery in lumbar degen-

erative disease: a retrospective study. Chin Med J. 2012;125(22):3942–6.
18. Taylor RS, Van Buyten JP, Buchser E. Spinal cord stimulation for chronic back and leg pain and failed back surgery syndrome: a systematic review and analysis of prognostic factors. Spine (Phila Pa 1976). 2005;30(1):152–60.
19. Taylor RS, Desai MJ, Rigoard P, Taylor RJ. Predictors of pain relief following spinal cord stimulation in chronic back and leg pain and failed back surgery syndrome: a systematic review and meta-regression analysis. Pain Pract. 2014;14(6):489–505. https://doi.org/10.1111/papr.12095.
20. Kumar K, Taylor RS, Jacques L, Eldabe S, Meglio M, Molet J, et al. Spinal cord stimulation versus conventional medical management for neuropathic pain: a multicentre randomised controlled trial in patients with failed back surgery syndrome. Pain. 2007;132(1–2):179–88. https://doi.org/10.1016/j.pain.2007.07.028.
21. Al-Kaisy A, Palmisani S, Pang D, Sanderson K, Wesley S, Tan Y, et al. Prospective, randomized, sham-control, double blind, crossover trial of subthreshold spinal cord stimulation at various kilohertz frequencies in subjects suffering from failed back surgery syndrome (SCS frequency study). Neuromodulation. 2018. https://doi.org/10.1111/ner.12771.
22. Sengupta DK. Is spinal cord stimulation a viable therapy for failed back surgery syndrome? No! Spine (Phila Pa 1976). 2018;43(7S Suppl 1):S15–s16. https://doi.org/10.1097/brs.0000000000002551.
23. Veizi E. Integration of spinal cord stimulation in treatment of failed back surgery syndrome. Spine (Phila Pa 1976). 2018;43(7S Suppl 1):S19–21. https://doi.org/10.1097/brs.0000000000002552.

Adjacent Segment Disease with 13 Years Follow Up and Five Operations

74

Jörg Franke and S. Michalitsis

74.1 Introduction

Adjacent segment degeneration (ASD) is defined as radiographic degenerative changes at a spinal level immediately cranial or caudal to the site of a previous fusion procedure. ASD can progress to adjacent segment disease (ASDis) a clinical phenomenon characterized by the presentation of new symptoms referable to the adjacent level, presumably related to the degenerative changes [1].

This case will describe in detail the problem of ASDis on a course of a patient over 13 years and five operations. Special attention will be paid to potential contributing factors to the natural history of degenerative disc disease (DDD) and possible strategies to avoid additional stressors for the adjacent segments of a fusion. Secondary, the presented case will demonstrate the necessity of a detailed indication management in order to avoid unnecessary inclusion of non-symptomatic segments.

J. Franke (✉) · S. Michalitsis
Department of Orthopedics, Klinikum Magdeburg, Magdeburg, Germany
e-mail: Joerg.franke@klinikum-magdeburg.de

74.2 Case Description

This report is about a 1950 born female patient suffering from rheumatoid arthritis in addition to her back and leg pain. Her major complaint in 2005 was mechanical axial back pain (VAS 8/10) combined with a left sided radicular pain component on the left (VAS 6/10) especially worsening after walking of more than 1000 meter. The identified problem was disc degeneration worse on the left side with a kyphotic position of the segment L3/4 and a central as well as a foraminal stenosis in the segment L3/4. There was no permanent neurological deficit (Figs. 74.1, 74.2, and 74.3).

The decision was made to perform a PLIF procedure L3/4 (Figs. 74.4 and 74.5).

The procedure was performed uneventful. Please pay attention to the resorbable cage which was used and the positioning of the segment in the lateral radiograph in a more or less neutral position. Clinically the patient had a quick recovery an th pain level dropped to 2/10 on the VAS (back pain) quickly. The referred pain to the legs resolved immediately. After 1 year the patient developed neurogenic claudication again after 300 meters and referred leg pain following the root of L4. Right more than left. The axial back pain increased to VAS 7/10. Still, the neurologic examination did not reveal any formal deficits (see Figs. 74.6, 74.7, 74.8, 74.9, and 74.10).

B. Meyer, M. Rauschmann (eds.), *Spine Surgery*, https://doi.org/10.1007/978-3-319-98875-7_74

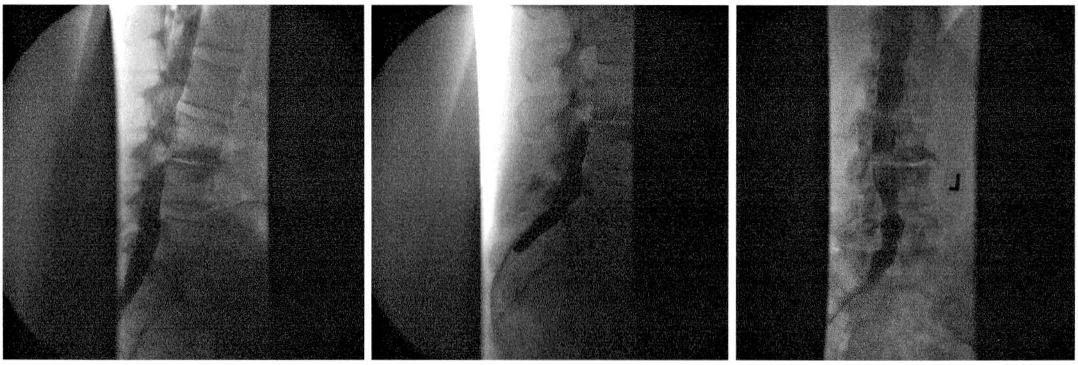

Figs. 74.1, 74.2, and 74.3 Lumbar myelography 2005 ap and lateral (in flection left and extension middle picture)

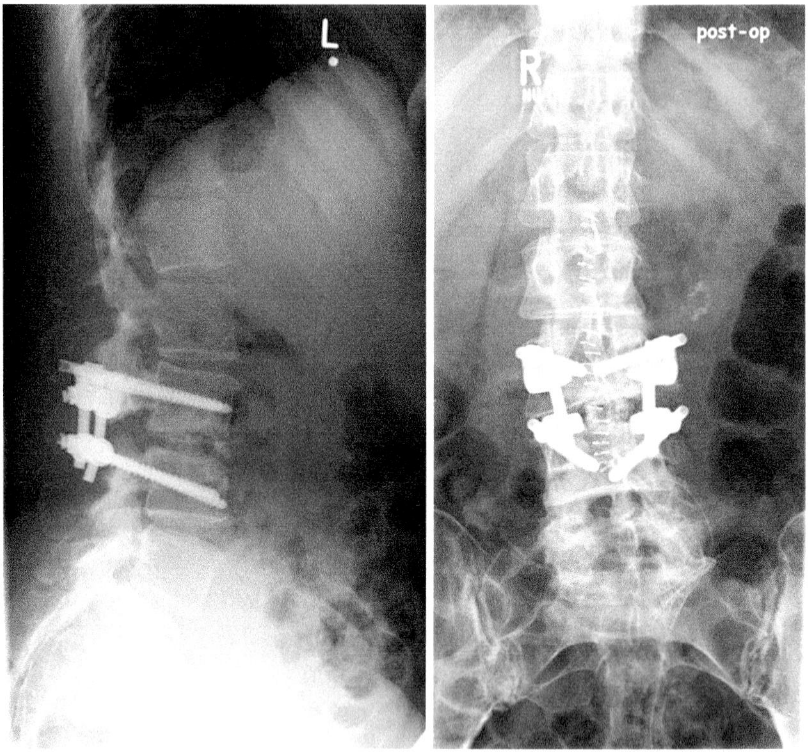

Figs. 74.4 and 74.5 Ap and lateral view postoperatively in 2005 with titanium internal fixateur and two resorbable cages and local bone plus bone graft extenders (hydroxyapatit nanostructure)

The decision was made to extend the fusion to L2–5 with PLIF in L2/3 und L4/5 with a better sagittal correction in order to improve her sagittal profile of her lumbar spine (Figs. 74.11 and 74.12).

The patient recovered without an postoperative problems rather quick and the VAS for back pain dropped to 2/10. Patient was not restricted in walking distance 8 weeks after the operation. The patient was seen till 1 year postoperatively. The VAS for back pain stayed at the 2/10 level. The patient was fully ambulatory and not restricted from her back in her walking distance keeping in mind, that the patient suffered from rheumatoid arthritis and therefore there were several lower and upper

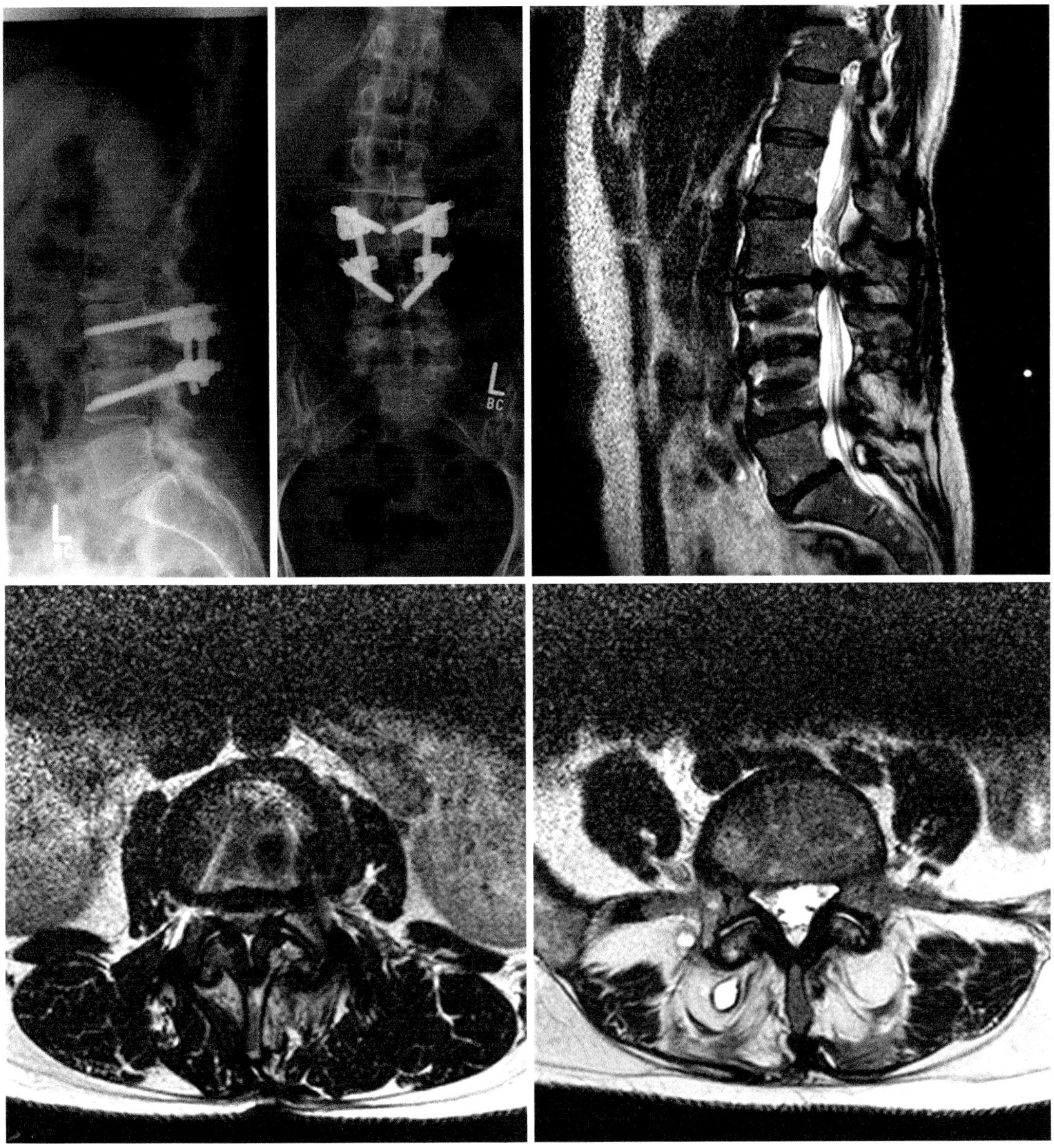

Figs. 74.6, 74.7, 74.8, 74.9, and 74.10 In 2006, the left X-ray (standing position show the ASD in L2/3 and L4/5). The middle MRI demonstrates the stenosis and ASD in both segments the upper right figure shows the type D stenosis in L2/3 and the lower figure the wider central canal whereas with the retrolisthetic position seen on the X-ray on the most left picture represents a functional foraminal stenosis

limp joint problems in addition. The next visit from the patient was in 2010. She complained about recurrent back pain in the lower lumbar spine VAS 8/10 and after 200 meters increasing leg pain on a L5 distribution without a formal motor deficit. X-ray and MRI were taken (Figs. 74.13, 74.14, and 74.15).

The decision was made to extend the fusion to S1 and not to L1 as the pain pattern showed a clear focus on the lumbar sacral region in addition with the dynamic L5 component and the absence of a positive pain reduction of a L1/2 facet infiltration. Figures 74.16 and 74.17 show the direct postoperative ap and lateral x-rays.

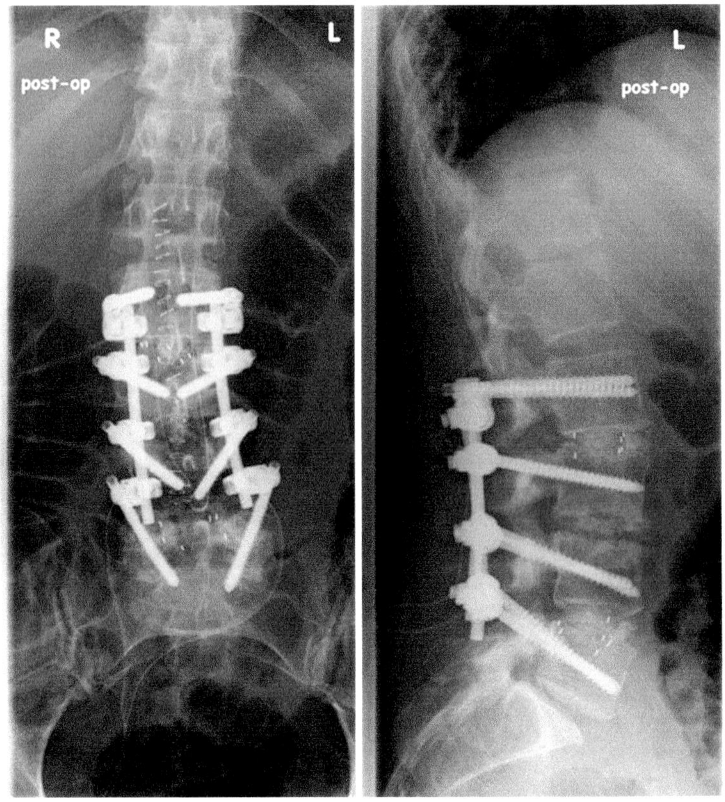

Figs. 74.11 and 74.12 2006, direct postoperative X-ray images show a much better overall sagittal alignment and a full correction in ap view especially in the L2/ 3 level. The cage material was PEEK and again local bone and Hydroxyapatit nanostructure as extender was used

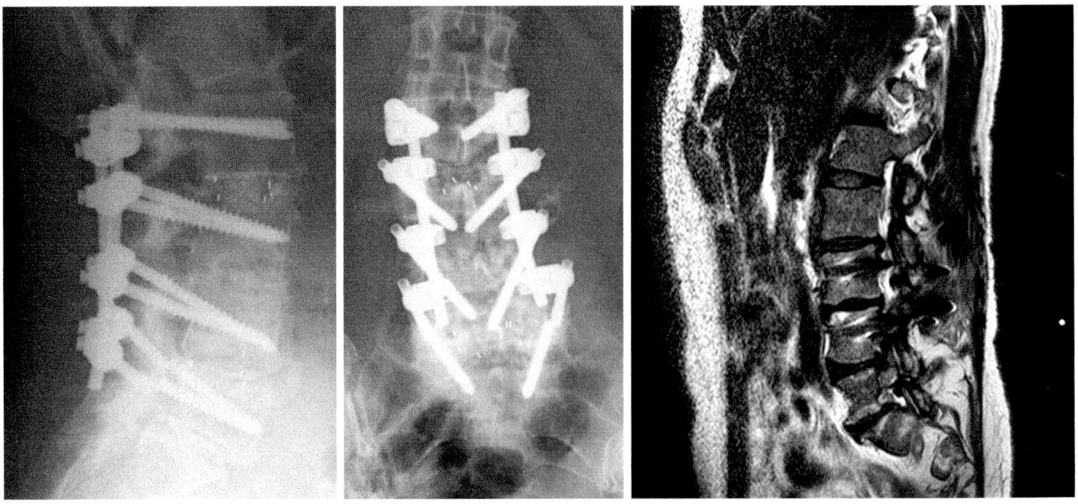

Figs. 74.13, 74.14, and 74.15 2010 on the left lateral x-ray broken screws in L5 as a sign for pseudoarthrosis and on the lateral MRI clear modic signs as an indication for adjacent segment disease in L5/S1. The ap view revealed in addition a lateral instability on L1/2 with a beginning scoliotic deformation

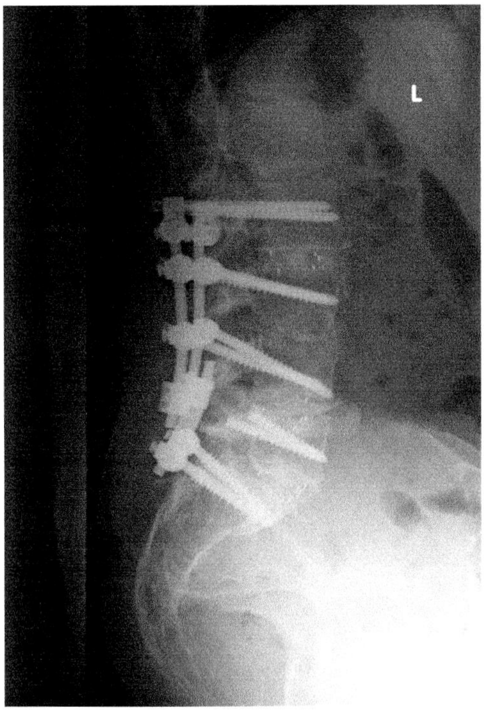

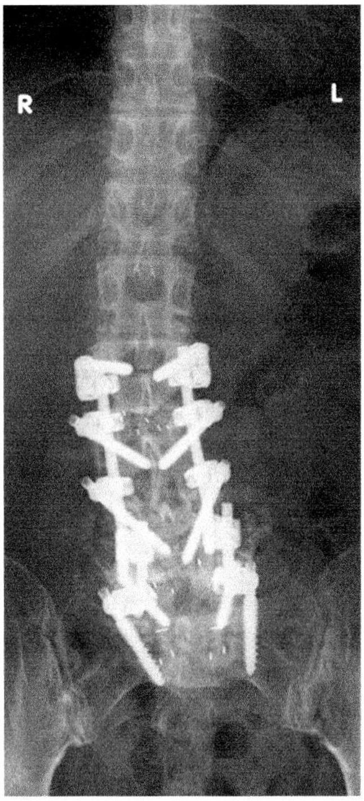

Figs. 74.16 and 74.17 Ap and lateral X-Ray after revision in 2010 and extension of the fusion to L5/S1 with a PLIF Procedure

Again, there was an uneventful quick recovery. The walking distance became free, the back and right sided L5 problem resolved again. The VAS for back pain dropped to 2 again and the referred L5 pain was gone. The postoperative control up 1 year showed bony fusion of L5/S1 and no complication after the last revision whatsoever. The next visit of the patient in the department was then in 2013 experiencing left sided lumbar sacral pain with some radiation to the posterior left leg above the knee. On examination there was no neurological deficit. A clear SI joint pain pattern with a positive Mennell sign. The X-ray and CT Scan (Figs. 74.18, 74.19, and 74.20) demonstrate a mild arthrosis within both Si joints and a bony fusion L2-S1 no screw loosening and and moderate increase in the ASD in L1/2 with an increased scoliotic deformation compared to 2010. Additional SI joint injection showed a major pain reduction after the injection on the left side.

On the basis of the current radiological findings and the fact of a clear and recurrent pain reduction of the left sided SI joint injection the patient was sent elsewhere in order to get an MIS SI fusion on the left side. This was to my knowledge performed in 2013 and led to a sufficient pain reduction to her know level of 2/10 for her back pain till 2017. The patient contacted the department with an increased level of right sided back pain. A EOS imaging was done and CT of the lumbar spine and the SI joint (Figs. 74.6, 74.7, 74.8, 74.9, 74.10, 74.11, 74.12, 74.13, 74.14, 74.15, 74.16, 74.17, 74.18, 74.19, and 74.20). There was a positive Mennell sign of the right SI joint. There was no neurological deficit nor positive straight leg rise test. There was virtually no pain in the thoracolumbar region (Figs. 74.21 and 74.22).

The EOS and the CT scan revealed an increase of the ASD with osteochondrosis for the level L1/2 and lateral instability with a consecutive increasing scoliotic deformation of the thoracolumbar junction. The SI joint injection generated a full pain reduction for 1 week. On this basis the conclusion was drawn that the indication is given for the SI fusion on the right side.

This was performed in November 2017 (Figs. 74.23, 74.24, 74.25, and 74.26).

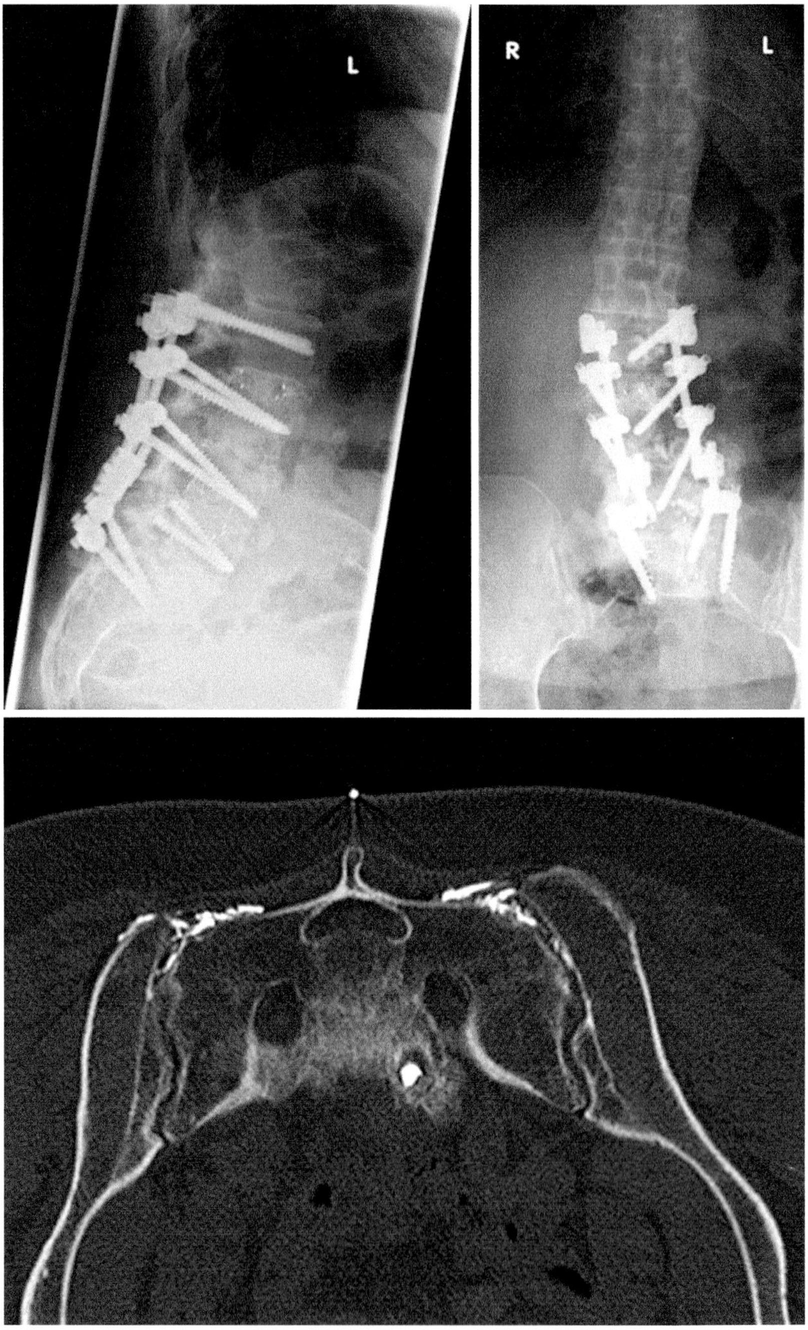

Figs. 74.18, 74.19, and 74.20 2013 ap and lateral X-ray showing a full anterior fusion L2-S1 and mild arthrosis on both SI joints (Fig. 74.20) as well as an increased scoliotic deformation and lateral instability of L1/2

The patient was discharged on day 4 after the operation with a drop in her VAS for back pain 3/10 with any pain medication. Her rheumatoid arthritis is currently more or less worn out. The recovery was uneventful. As the patient now lives 600 kilometers away from our department I had a last phone call follow-up with her in April 2018 and she was more or less back to normal with the back pain level of VAS Score of 2/10. The next on- site visit is scheduled for 1 year after the last operation in November 2018.

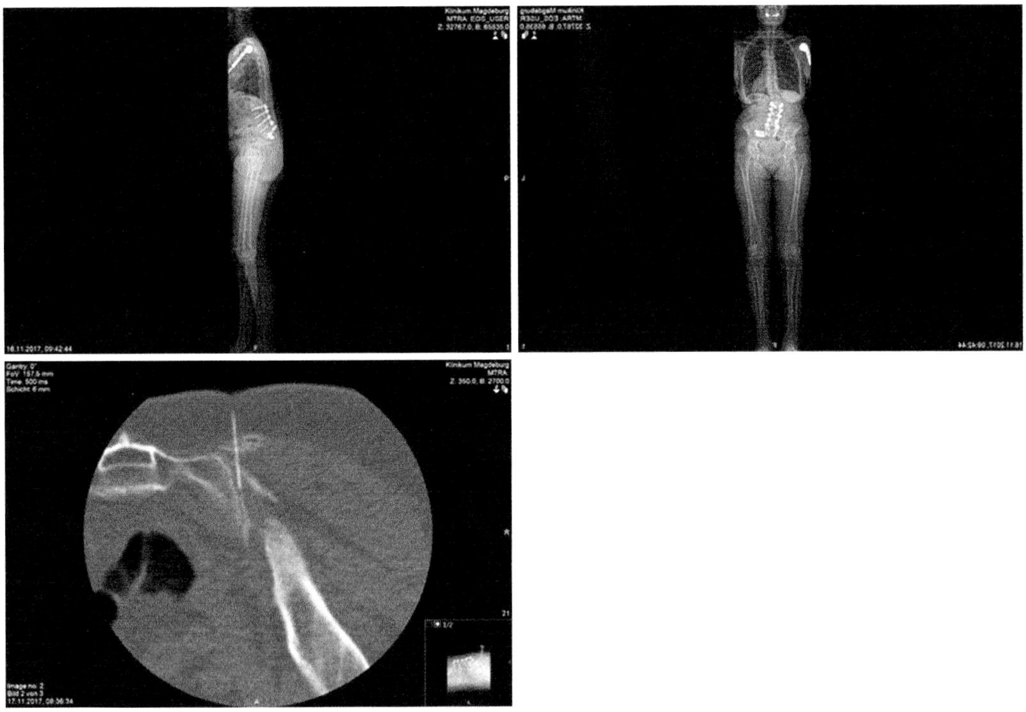

Figs. 74.21, 74.22, and 74.23 2017 EOS Imaging lateral and AP and SI joint injection on the right side

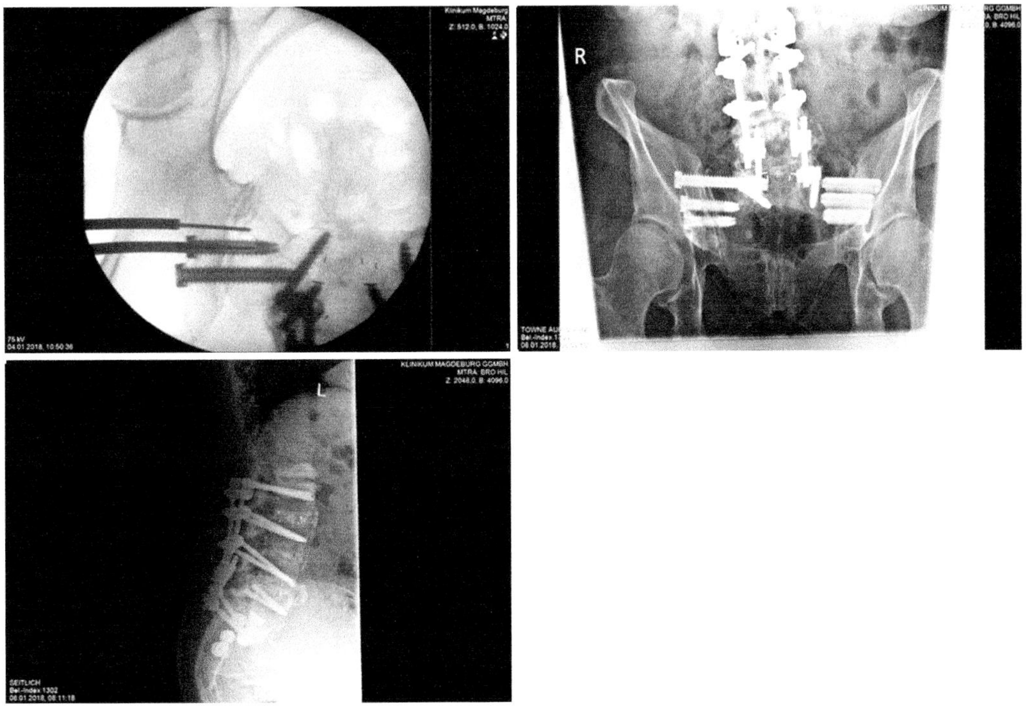

Figs. 74.24, 74.25, and 74.26 2017 Fig. 74.24 shows and intraoperative positioning of the last of three Screw crossing the SI joint from lateral to medial for the SI fusion. Figures 74.25 and 74.26 show ap and lateral X-ray images 3 days postoperatively with well-positioned SI screws and especially on the lateral X-ray Fig. 74.26 the increasing sclerosis of the Level L1/2

74.3 Discussion of the Case

One theory holds that adjacent segment pathologies, like ASD and the clinically more relevant ASDis, are simply reflections of the natural history of lumbar degenerative disease. Others argue that prior fusion results in increased motion, intradiscal pressure, and strain adjacent to the fusion, leading to an increased risk of ASD [2].

Although spinal fusion is an established and exceedingly common procedure, the steady evolution of surgical techniques and the availability of a myriad of graft materials, cage designs, and plate fixation systems have given rise to considerable variability between treatment methods. In addition, the current literature on adjacent segment pathology suffers from the absence of a universally accepted radiographic modality for diagnosis of ASD or validated outcome instrument for diagnosis of ASDis [3, 4]. Because of this heterogeneity, estimates of ASD incidence after lumbar fusion range from 0% to 36% [5]. For the cervical spine A. Hilibrand [6] could demonstrate a annual incidence of 2.9% for ASDis.

For the lumbar spine there is no such study existing with the exeption of the limited investigation of Ghiselli [7]. Figure 74.27 shows this "annual" incidence of symptomatic ASD (ASDis) according to the Ghiselli paper with the results of other studies more or less matching this line. This in turn means that something like an annual incidence for ASDis exists for the lumbar spine as in the demonstrated case, too.

Obviously, there is a rate of given natural segment degeneration regardless of an adjacent segment fusion or not. Therefore, having the necessity of a fusion or moreover a needed operative indication to a spinal segment, the surgeon should simply try to avoid additional stressors not to boost the degenerative process of the cranial or caudal segments.

This leads to the search of risk factor for an increased incidence of ASD and ASDis after those spinal procedures. For this specific case there will be a focus on risk factors for lumbar spinal fusions.

There are many proposed risk factors for ASD, including age, instrumentation, fusion type, fusion length, and the degree of lumbar lordosis.

Although there is only limited evidence a 2–3 times higher risk for multilevel fusion could be demonstrated for example by the studies from Sears [8].

In addition, we get more evidence that a mismatch of the lordosis of the fused segments even in short level fusions might contribute to the natural occurrence of segment degeneration [9].

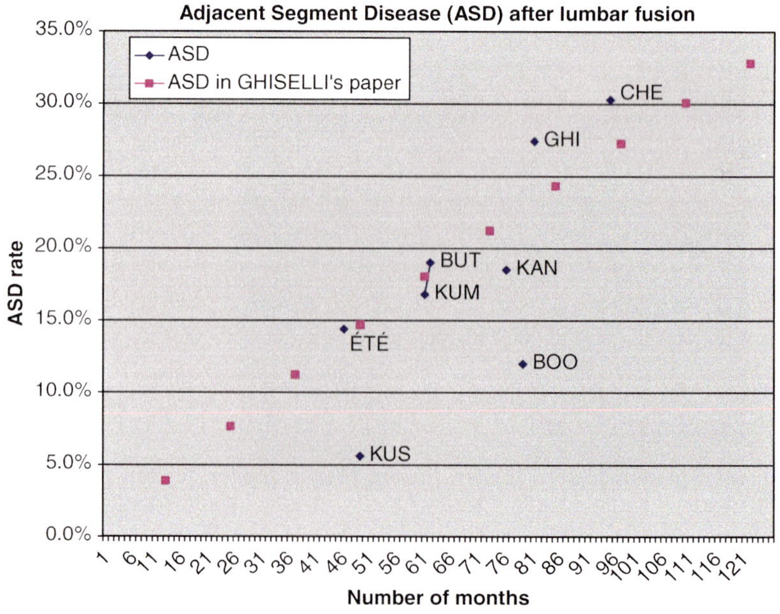

Fig. 74.27 Symptomatic ASD rate (ASDis) according to the Ghiselli paper with the results of several other ASD studies plotted on the proposed percentage line per months

Particularly for this case there was another potential risk factor for the development of ASD with the existence of rheumatoid arthritis. Park et al. could show that for this patient population the risk of developing ASD is 4,5 times higher compared to the normal population [10].

Looking at this case there were two mistakes with the first operation. First the use of resorbable cage, which showed too fast degradation and therefore anterior height loss with additional loss of lordosis. This in addition to the fixation of the segment and a almost kyphotic position may have led to the very quick development of the ASDis in both adjacent segments with 1 year. Having been a little more wise in 2005 concerning the necessity of matching the sagittal balance parameter better even in case of a short fusion, such a fast ASD may have not happened as early as 2006. But especially the paper from Rothenfluh et al. was not published before 2015 [9].

After the Fusion extension to L2–5 with a much better sagittal alignment the patient was fine for almost 4 years. Keeping in mind the factors: three level fusion, age over 60 now, rheumatoid arthritis the occurrence of an ASD neglecting the fact of the broken screws with a radiologically fused segment L4/5, this seems to be a rather "normal" event in the course of a patient with a degenerative history. In contrast to some of the available literature this patient always came back to an almost normal VAS for back pain and life. This is may be due to the fact the we always addressed a "new" problem of her lumbar spine as compared to a revision for the same pathology and segment.

For the fourth and fifth operation (SI fusion left and right in 2013 and 2017) there was a clear indicative workout by several injections that the pain generator was the SI joint. Looking at the radiological imaging, one could have the idea that the radiological evident increasing degeneration and deformation of the L1/2 level may contribute to the pain level. This was not affirmed by the diagnostic injections. Actually, we can confess that according to the pain level reduction by both SI joint fusions, this could have been the main pain generator in 2013 and 2017. Therefore, it is a perfect example that a clear radiologic ASD of L1/2 does not necessarily needs to be a symptomatic ASDis. At the end we hope that the patient does not need a further operation at least for the next 4 years.

74.4 Conclusions and Take Home Message

ASD is a phenomenon which occurs naturally by an obviously genetically influenced process called degenerative disc disease. There are obvious risk factors like age, fusion length additional disease (e.g. rheumatoid arthritis) which we are not able to changes while fusing a patient for an ideal indication. On the other hand there are known factors for ASD development where we are able to not contribute to the naturally given rate of ASD which is segmental lordosis, soft tissue handling aso. Paying attention to those factors and optimizing the fusion procedure for this could prevent the development of ASD as much as possible.

Pearls

- The transformation of ASD into ASDis is a combination of natural progressive degeneration and potential suboptimal treatment solutions
- Always treat the actual problem
- A good clinical outcome is achievable several times

Editorial Comment

One needs to acknowledge that ASD is inevitable, because it relates to the very nature of a degenerative disease. Fusing a segment will also inevitably increase the risk for its development, irrespective of the biomechanical quality of the construct. This is known and also underscored by numbers from high class recent studies. Whether a "suboptimal" solution further increases the risk for it is not proven to the same extent. One should be careful to think that an ideal construct will prevent ASD.

References

1. Radcliff KE, et al. Adjacent segment disease in the lumbar spine following different treatment interventions. Spine J. 2013;13(10):1339–49.
2. Abode-Iyamah K, et al. Spinal motion and intradiscal pressure measurements before and after lumbar spine instrumentation with titanium or PEEK rods. J Clin Neurosci. 2014;21(4):651–5.
3. Lee CS, et al. Risk factors for adjacent segment disease after lumbar fusion. Eur Spine J. 2009;18(11):1637–43.
4. Kraemer P, et al. A systematic review of definitions and classification systems of adjacent segment pathology. Spine (Phila Pa 1976). 2012;37(22 Suppl):S31–9.
5. Harrop JS, et al. Lumbar adjacent segment degeneration and disease after arthrodesis and total disc arthroplasty. Spine (Phila Pa 1976). 2008;33(15):1701–7.
6. Hilibrand AS, et al. Radiculopathy and myelopathy at segments adjacent to the site of a previous anterior cervical arthrodesis. J Bone Joint Surg Am. 1999;81(4):519–28.
7. Ghiselli G, et al. Adjacent segment degeneration in the lumbar spine. J Bone Joint Surg Am. 2004;86-A(7):1497–503.
8. Sears WR, et al. Incidence and prevalence of surgery at segments adjacent to a previous posterior lumbar arthrodesis. Spine J. 2011;11(1):11–20.
9. Rothenfluh DA, et al. Pelvic incidence-lumbar lordosis mismatch predisposes to adjacent segment disease after lumbar spinal fusion. Eur Spine J. 2015;24(6):1251–8.
10. Park JS, et al. Risk-factor analysis of adjacent segment disease requiring surgery after short lumbar fusion: the influence of rheumatoid arthritis. Spine J. 2018;18(9):1578–83.

Management of Postoperative Infections

75

Marcus Rickert

75.1 Introduction

Postoperative wound infection after instrumented spinal surgery is still one of the most common complication in spine surgery. It affects the clinical outcome negatively, makes operative debridement necessary and often even multiple revisions may be required, can lead to chronic pain and deformity, extends hospitalization and is therefore also responsible for higher treatment costs [1].

As the most frequent causative agent of postoperative wound infections the literature highlights Staphylococcus aureus and Staphylococcus epidermidis [2].

The incidence of post-operative spinal infection varies widely from 0.7% to 16%. The main reason for this wide range is that different types of interventions have different risks for postoperative infections. Therefore less invasive procedures present with a reduced infection rate compared to surgeries with additional instrumentation showing the highest risk for a postoperative surgical site infection.

M. Rickert (✉)
Orthopaedic University Hospital Friedrichsheim gGmbH Frankfurt, Frankfurt am Main, Germany
e-mail: marcus.rickert@friedrichsheim.de

Numerous influences on the development of postoperative infections have been identified and can be divided into subgroups [3, 4]:

75.1.1 Patient Related Risk Factors

- Age (>65 yrs)
- Obesity (BMI >35 kg/m^2)
- Previous spine surgery
- Hyperglycaemia (perioperative (stress) hyperglycaemia in non-diabetics)
- Diabetes mellitus
- Malnutrition
- Nicotine abuse
- Steroid use
- Chronic obstructive pulmonary disease
- Osteoporosis

75.1.2 Procedure-Related Risk Factors

- Implants/instrumentation
- Posterior approach
- Tumor surgery (resection)
- Multilevel spondylodesis with inclusion of the sacrum
- Extended operating time
- Blood loss

B. Meyer, M. Rauschmann (eds.), *Spine Surgery*, https://doi.org/10.1007/978-3-319-98875-7_75

Postoperative wound infections can be classified into early and late infections. The exact onset of a late infection is not defined clearly. Some authors describe a late or delayed infection after more than 4 weeks postoperatively. But generally most of the literature accepts the detection of an infection after >3 months postoperatively as late infection [5]. In late (low-grade) infections the classical signs of infection like fever, night sweats, high white blood cell counts and elevated C-reactive protein can be absent. More often low virulence organisms like Propionibacteria are cultured in low-grade infections [6].

Regarding the therapy of wound infections, there are no uniform guidelines due to lack of reasonable studies. Often several revisions are necessary until a wound infection has been treated successfully. A national multicenter survey of spinal surgeons showed that 55% of the colleagues do not apply a fixed therapy standard to eradicate postoperative infections of the spine [7].

Therefore the next two following cases will demonstrate the different treatment options in an early and a late postoperative infection after spinal fusion surgery and will emphasize the potential problems and lack of evidence in the treatment of this disease.

75.2 Case Description

75.2.1 Early Infection

A 42 y/o male without any relevant comorbidities suffered from severe bilateral leg pain with a reduced walking distance due to ataxia. He presented a mild weakness of the right ankle extensors 4/5. Apart from numbness at the calves bilaterally there was a normal neurological status without any upper motor neuron signs. His MRI demonstrated a disc herniation at the level T11/T12 with spinal cord compression and myelopathy.

The patient was treated surgically and a single level TLIF fusion at T11/T12 with decompression was performed. There haven't been any intraoperative complications and the patient was well after the procedure and mobilized immediately (Figs. 75.1 and 75.2).

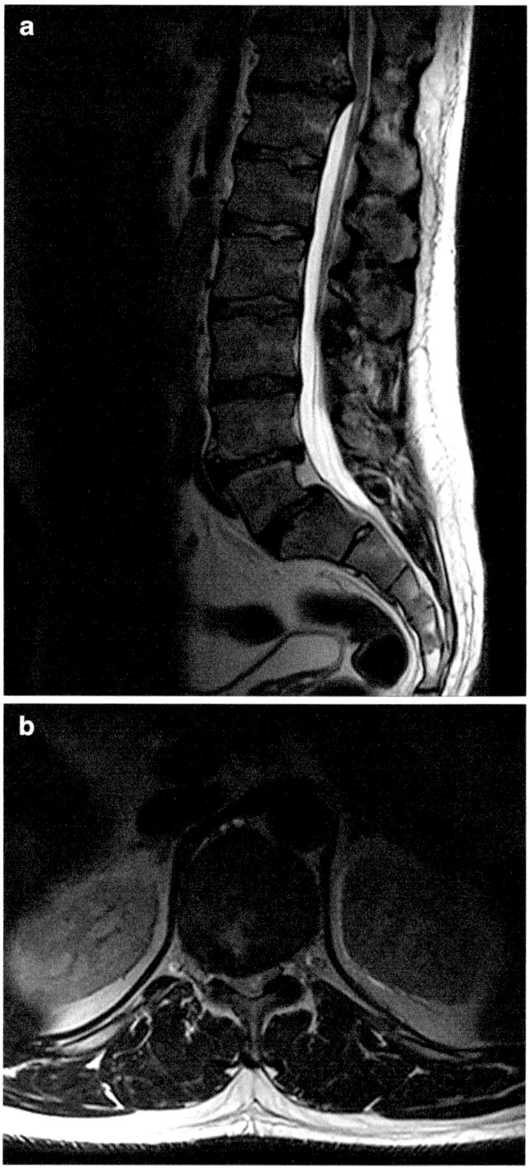

Fig. 75.1 MRI scan on outpatient visit. The MRI scan shows a right sided disc herniation T11/T12 with spinal cord compression and a myelopathy. Secondary finding was a spondylolisthesis L5/S1 (untreated). Sagittal (**a**) and, axial slices (**b**)

After 15 days postoperatively the patient returned to our outpatient clinic without any deterioration of pain but with subfebrile temperature and a leaking wound of the middle/distal part. The wound was covered with a fibrin layer but still attached. The collected blood showed only a

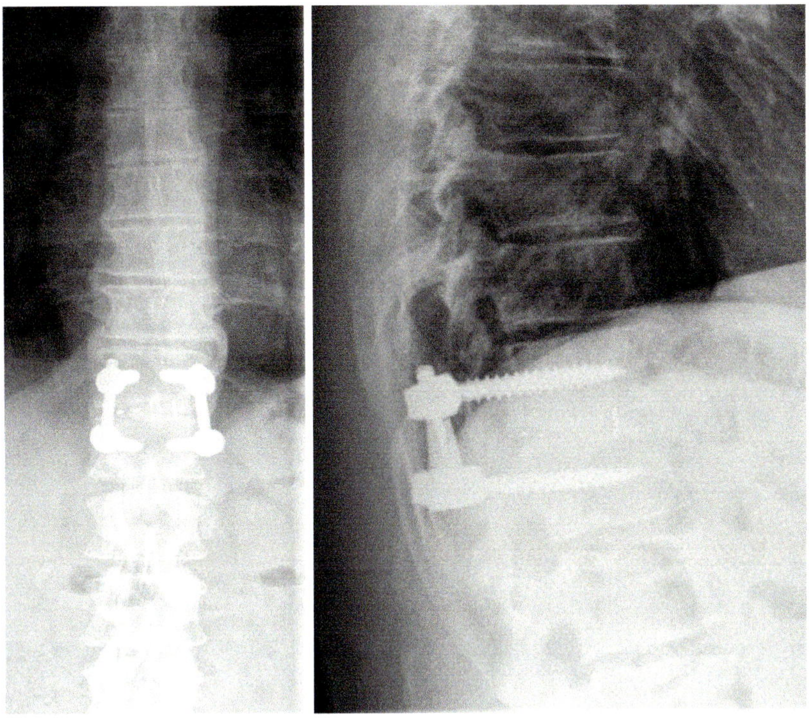

Fig. 75.2 Postoperative standing X-rays. Correct implants with adequate screw and cage placement

mild increase of the white blood cells and the CRP value.

An additional MRI scan was ordered and the patient prepared for revision surgery.

The wound revision with debridement and wash out was performed the next day (Figs. 75.3 and 75.4).

The intraoperative finding was an extensive infection with pus involving the deep soft tissue layers and the metalwork but without any severe muscle necrosis. After thorough debridement and extensive wash with betadine and Ringer's solution including pulsed lavage two deep drains had been inserted.

The multiple microbiological wound swabs confirmed the infection caused by Staphylococcus aureus. The antibiotic treatment (Rifampicin/Levofloxacin – i.v. as an inpatient) was decided according to the resistogram and after discussion with the microbiologists and continued for 4 weeks (orally) postoperatively.

The postoperative wound infection was resolved with a single wound revision and without any further complications.

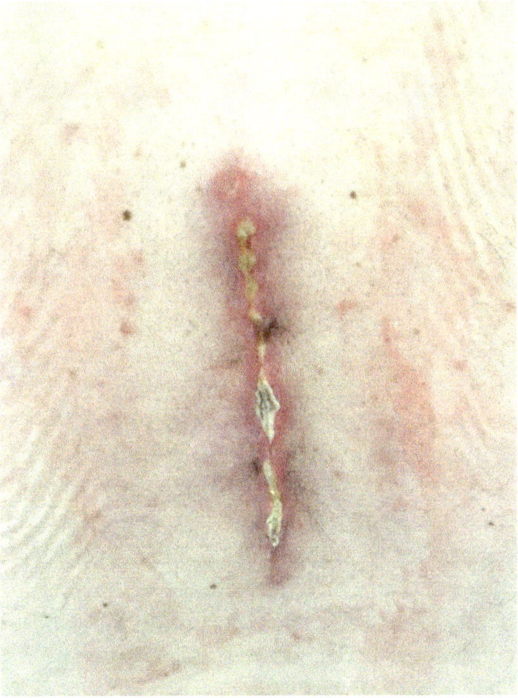

Fig. 75.3 Postoperative wound status after 15 days. Postoperative wound infection with wound leakage. Sutures are removed already

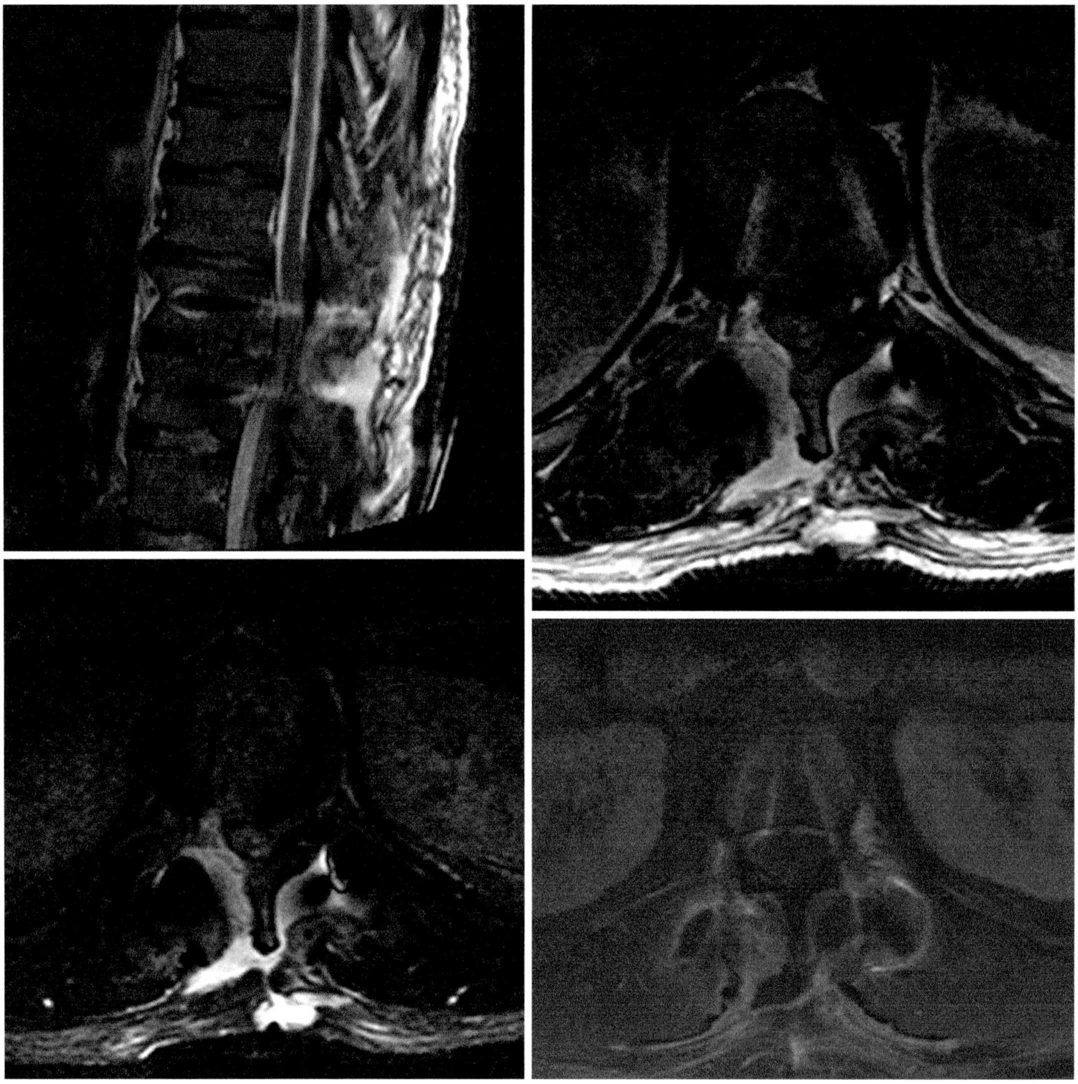

Fig. 75.4 MRI scan prior to revision surgery. MRI confirms a deep fluid collection at the fused segment involving the paraspinal muscles with contrast enhancement

75.2.2 Delayed/Late Infection

A 59 y/o male was referred to our department with a history of a prostate cancer and acute deterioration of a formerly diagnosed metastatic disease involving lungs and liver. Clinically he complained about a progressive unsteady gait and increasing weakness of his left leg (3/5) since weeks. The imaging (X-ray, CT and MRI) demonstrated multiple bony metastases with a maximum at T11 and osteolysis. The tumor mass was invading the spinal canal causing a severe spinal stenosis with spinal cord compression (Fig. 75.5).

The patient was treated surgically from posterior only with stabilization from T9 to L1 with cementaugmented screws, wide decompression and a vertebral body replacement after corpectomy of T11 via costotransversectomy. The postoperative course was uneventful with a normal wound healing without any signs of infection (Fig. 75.6).

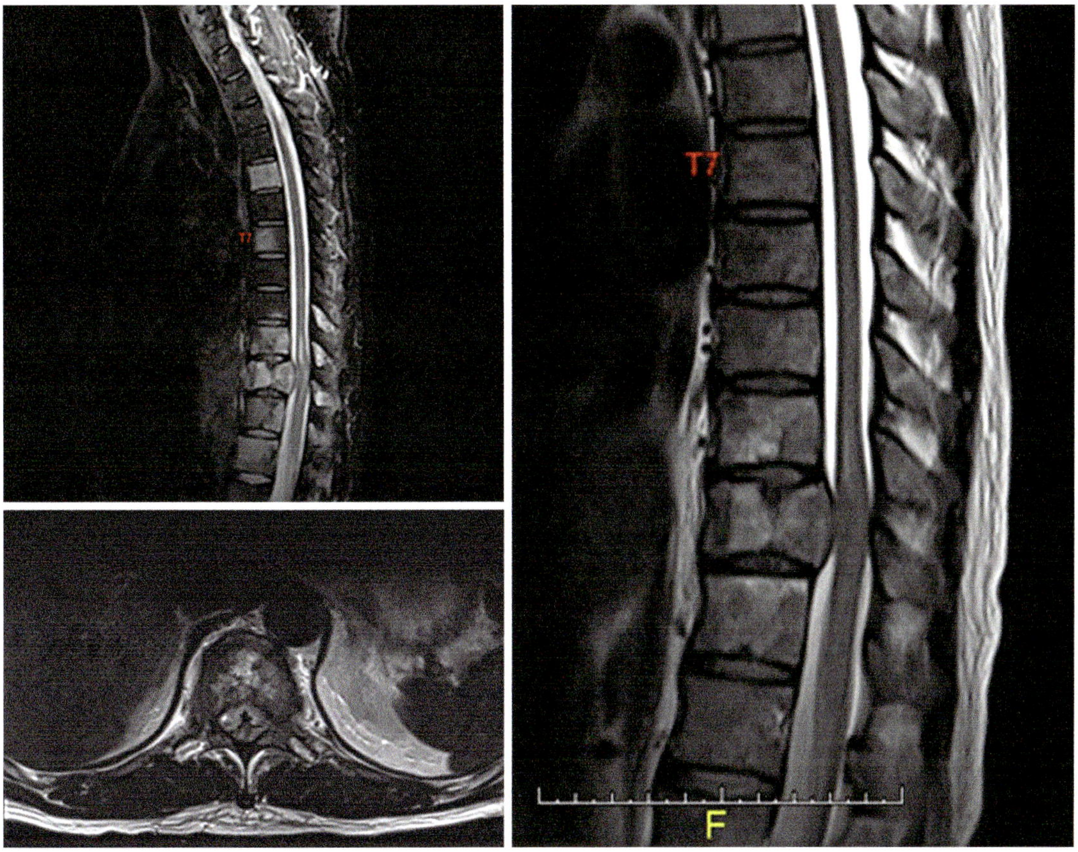

Fig. 75.5 MRI scan before admittance. T11 prostate metastasis invading the spinal canal and causing spinal cord compression with myelopathy. Pathological fracture of T11

After 6 weeks postoperatively the patient was sent back to our clinic by his oncologist due to raised laboratory inflammation markers (white blood cells, CRP) and a leaking wound that was healed initially. The neurological status was unchanged (Fig. 75.7).

Due to the wound condition and clinical findings the patient was treated with revision surgery. The intraoperative situation proved a deep purulent infection including thesubfascial soft tissue and metalwork. There were also extensive muscle and soft-tissue necrosis involving the fascia. With these findings the decision was made to insert a deep VAC system first and to consolidate the soft tissue with a staged strategy and a planned re-revision surgery. Before applying the VAC therapy a thorough debridement and irrigation was performed. Then the VAC sponge was positioned bilaterally close to the screws and rods underneath the fascia. Then the wound was closed completely. The VAC therapy was applied with a negative pressure of 125 mm/Hg continuously (Fig. 75.8).

The microbiological results identified a Staphylococcus aureus infection and the antibiotics have been adapted selectively (Cefuroxime). The microbiological recommendation was continuation of antibiotics for 6–8 weeks postoperatively.

The second look revision was performed 5 days later and demonstrated much better local wound conditions but still mild signs of infection so that we repeated the VAC therapy once more in the same manner. The third look revision showed a macroscopic clean wound which allowed the end of the VAC treatment. Before wound closure

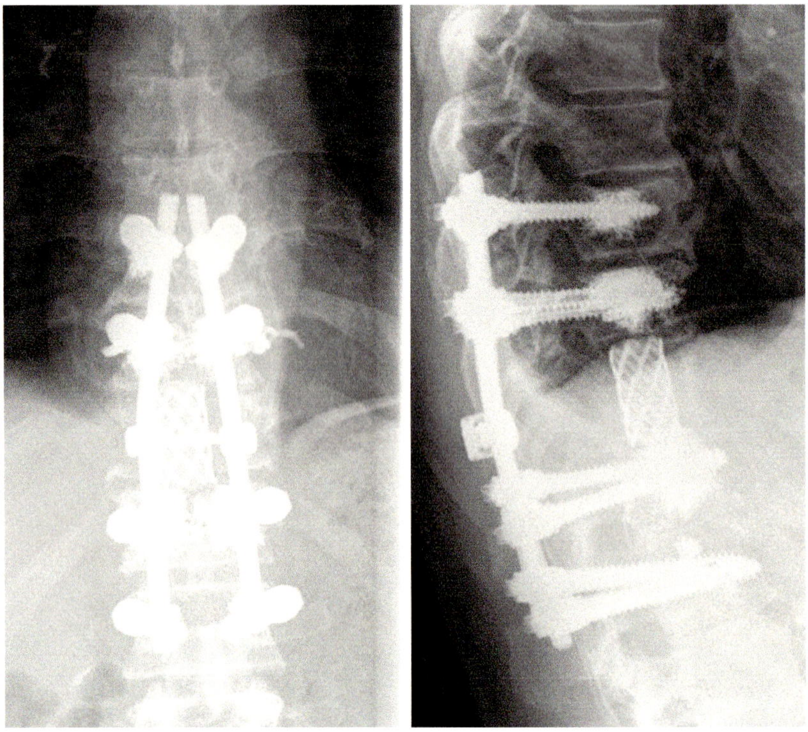

Fig. 75.6 Postoperative standing X-rays. Correct metalwork with adequate screw and cage placement

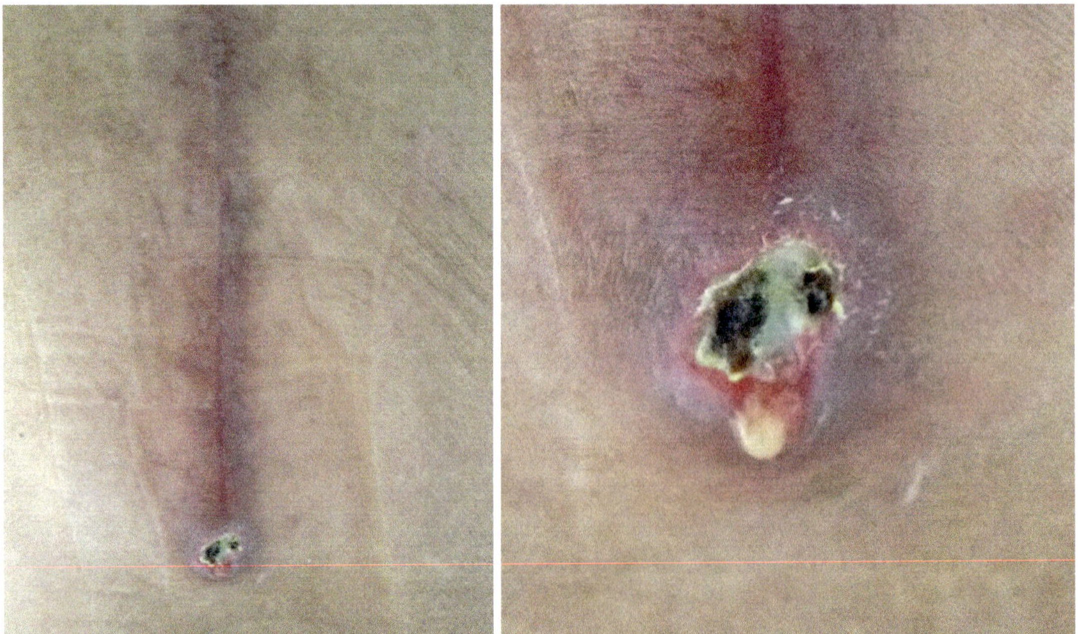

Fig. 75.7 Postoperative wound status after 6 weeks. Postoperative wound infection with wound leakage. Wound healing disorder distally with pus

two deep drains were inlaid finally. The wound healed nicely without irritations in the further postoperative period. Chemotherapy was restricted for another 4 weeks (Fig. 75.9).

75.3 Discussion of the Case

The first case presenting the early postoperative wound infection was treated with revision surgery, debridement, wash out and drains. An immediate surgical treatment with a thorough debridement is widely accepted and standard of care in the literature [8]. Main indicator for wound revision is the local wound condition. Persistent leaking wounds, necrosis of the wound edges with a fibrin film and dehiscence may require surgical treatment. The authors prefer an immediate revision and no "wait and see" strategy to reduce the extent of infection with concomitant complications (sepsis) and to shorten the hospitalization.

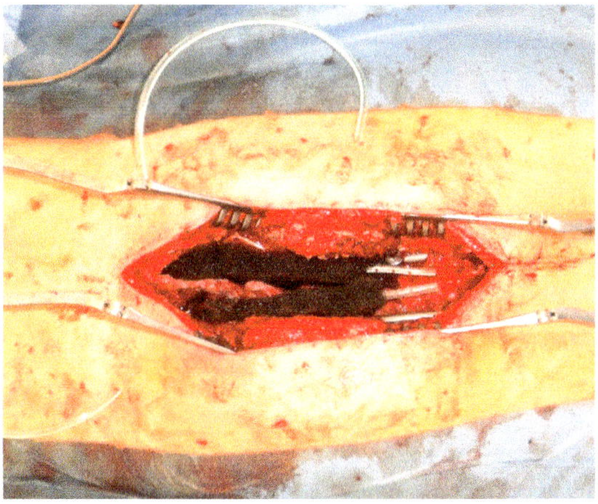

Fig. 75.8 Intraoperative VAC application. The VAC foams are positioned bilaterally close to the screws and rods underneath the fascia

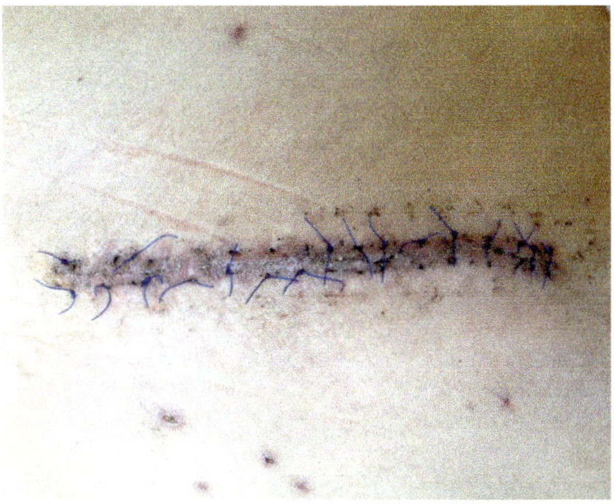

Fig. 75.9 Result after VAC therapy. After three wound revisions the wound has healed nicely

The identification of Staphylococcus aureus as pathogen confirms the statement to be the most prevalent bacteria causing postoperative infection. In some cases it is necessary to repeat the revisions until the wound and soft tissue is consolidated. Rickert et al. showed in their survey which included also wound infections after decompression and microsdiscectomy that on average approximately two revisions are necessary to heal the wound completely. Unfortunately there is no clear evidence for the efficacy of any supportive treatment strategy like antibiotic adjuncts, pulsed lavage or specific wash solutions [7]. For example in case of the pulsed irrigation there are trends in the literature to be more effective in the dorsal muscle layers than the conventional irrigation [9]. But the current literature does not suggest any clear standards of care in case of a wound infection and often there is no detailed treatment algorithm in spinal units [7]. But there is broad agreement that in early infections the implants should be preserved and not removed to maintain the stability of the spine. That is also beneficial for the patient's mobility [8, 10].

The second case demonstrates a delayed or late infection after a tumor surgery with instrumentation, debulking and vertebral body replacement in an immune compromised patient with a metastatic disease. Firstly, due to the late onset and dimension of the infection with extensive muscle and soft tissue necrosis the decision was made to utilize an additional VAC therapy. Secondly there are positive considerations in the literature that VAC with negative pressure therapy leads to advantageous results regarding implant preservation. Especially in that case removal of implants would have led to an unstable spine and was hence no option. Therefore one of the targets was to eradicate the infection and to leave the implants in place. The VAC therapy leads to a permanent drainage of the wound helps to stimulate wound granulation and to reduce the bacterial load. It also improves the blood supply in terms of microcirculation and neovascularization (vascular endothelial growth factor) [11]. In the authors experience when using VAC it is important to always close the wound completely above the polyurethane foam to avoid retraction of the wound edges. Otherwise this can lead to serious problems for the definitive and final wound closure and can make a plastic surgery necessary. When a patient is treated with a staged strategy and multiple revisions it is mandatory to take microbiological samples each revision so that changes of the pathogens can be detected. Implant removal especially in late infection is still a topic of discussion. There are different opinions in the literature but without any clear evidence from large clinical studies a helpful answer cannot be given. Some authors suggest implant removal only in rare cases with late (>3 months) and recurrent infections when a solid fusion is verified and the implants are suspicious to maintain the infection caused by bacteria living in a biofilm [5].

In both cases the antibiotic treatment was decided in collaboration with the microbiologists and according to the resistograms. For deep wound infections with involvement of the metalwork usually a long term antibiotic treatment up to 6–12 weeks is recommended. If the wound infection is classified to be superficial (only subcutaneous layer involved – fascia intact), antibiotic treatment for 2 weeks postoperative is sufficient [12].

75.4 Conclusions and Take Home Message

Wound infections are an upcoming problem and therefore it is crucial to optimize risk factors preoperatively especially in older patients. As the first case shows wound healing problems are not only concerning the older population with multiple comorbidities even young healthy patients can be affected. Routinely a surgical treatment is necessary for deep postoperative infections to eradicate the infection and achieve an adequate wound healing. In severe cases sometimes multiple revision surgery is required and VAC therapy might be helpful. In times of multiresistent pathogens the antibiotic treatment should be advised by the microbiologists. Postoperative wound infections prolong the patient's suffering, impair the clinical outcome and present a great challenge for the entire treatment team. Therefore all efforts for the avoidance should be made.

Pearls

- Preoperative reduction of risk factors is mandatory
- No "wait and see strategy" early revision and wound exploration
- Surgical treatment with debridement and wash out is accepted as standard of care
- For implant preservation VAC therapy can be helpful
- When using VAC it is important to always close the wound completely above the polyurethane foam

References

1. Mok JM, Guillaume TJ, Talu U, et al. Clinical outcome of deep wound infection after instrumented posterior spinal fusion: a matched cohort analysis. Spine (Phila Pa 1976). 2009;34:578–83.
2. Parchi PD, Evangelisti G, Andreani L, et al. Postoperative spine infections. Orthop Rev (Pavia). 2015;7:5900.
3. Fang A, Hu SS, Endres N, et al. Risk factors for infection after spinal surgery. Spine (Phila Pa 1976). 2005;30:1460–5.
4. Koutsoumbelis S, Hughes AP, Girardi FP, et al. Risk factors for postoperative infection following posterior lumbar instrumented arthrodesis. J Bone Joint Surg Am. 2011;93:1627–33.
5. Hedequist D, Haugen A, Hresko T, et al. Failure of attempted implant retention in spinal deformity

delayed surgical site infections. Spine (PhilaPa1986). 2009;34:60–4.
6. Collins I, Wilson-MacDonald J, Chami G, Burgoyne W, Vineyakam P, Berendt T, Fairbank J. The diagnosis and management of infection following instrumented spinal fusion. Eur Spine J. 2008;17:445–50.
7. Rickert M, Schleicher P, Fleege C, et al. Management of postoperative wound infections following spine surgery: first results of a multicenter study. Orthopade. 2016;45:780–8.
8. Lee JS, Ahn DK, Chang BK, Lee JI. Treatment of surgical site infection in posterior lumbar interbody fusion. Asian Spine J. 2015;9(6):841–8. https://doi.org/10.4184/asj.2015.9.6.841.
9. Ahn DK, Lee S, Moon SH, et al. Bulb syringe and pulsed irrigation: which is more effective to remove bacteria in spine surgeries? Clin Spine Surg. 2016;29:34–7.
10. Ahmed R, Greenlee JD, Traynelis VC. Preservation of spinal instrumentation after development of postoperative bacterial infections in patients undergoing spinal arthrodesis. J Spinal Disord Tech. 2012;25(6):299–302.
11. Ousey KJ, Atkinson RA, Williamson JB, et al. Negative pressure wound therapy (NPWT) for spinal wounds: a systematic review. Spine J. 2013;13:1393–405.
12. Rickert M, Fleege C, Rauschmann M. Algorithm for treatment of spinal infections and first results of a retrospective analysis of postoperative wound infection and application of a vacuum system for infection treatment. Die Wirbelsäule. 2017;4:265–72.

76 Management of Pseudarthrosis with Implant Failure

Christoph Fleege

76.1 Introduction

The degeneration of the intervertebral disc and the associated segmental instability is one of the most common causes of specific back pain. The currently most effective surgical treatment with spinal fusion performed by dorsal instrumentation and intercorporal interposition of cages and bone or bone replacement material shows satisfactory radiographic and clinical results. However, 9–45% of the operated patients undergo revision surgery [1]. The reasons for the need for surgical revision in the early phase are technical errors or postoperative complications. In the further course, the non-union with pseudarthrosis and adjacent segment disease are predominate [1, 2]. In addition to the poorer results of the revision surgeries [3], they are an additional burden for the patient and a particular challenge for the surgeon. The number of pseudoarthrosis given in the literature vary according to surgical procedures and evaluation criteria and reach levels below 10% in the recent literature.

This chapter describes risk factors that may favor the lack of a bony fusion and it's consequences. In addition, solution strategies of the case are presented. The characteristic case was selected in order to show that existing risk factors can have a significant influence on the postoperative result of spinal fusion and if necessary an adaptation of the surgical procedure in special case constellations are necessary.

C. Fleege (✉)
Spine Department, Orthopaedic University Hospital Friedrichsheim, Frankfurt, Germany
e-mail: c.fleege@friedrichsheim.de

76.2 Case Description

39-year-old female patient, monosegmental spondylodesis L5/S1 with dorsal instrumentation and interposition of a cage in TLIF technique ex domo, March 2013 suffering of an isthmic spondylolysis. Secondary diseases: obesity BMI 36.2 kg/m^2, nicotine abuse, diabetes mellitus type II (Figs. 76.1 and 76.2).

Subsequently, repeated conservative treatment with infiltration of the facet joints L4/5 and the sacroiliac joint, multimodal pain therapy for pain processing disorder, was performed. The lumbalgiform symptoms with pseudoradicular spreading into the lower extremities could not be influenced by the conservative treatment (Figs. 76.3 and 76.4).

Posterior-anterior revision surgery was performed in August 2017, with extirpation of the right broken screw in S1 and replacement of the remaining 6 mm screws with new 8 mm diameter screws. Anterior revision with removal of the loose TLIF cage and interposition of an ALIF cage filled with homologous cancellous bone graft was done (Figs. 76.5 and 76.6).

B. Meyer, M. Rauschmann (eds.), *Spine Surgery*, https://doi.org/10.1007/978-3-319-98875-7_76

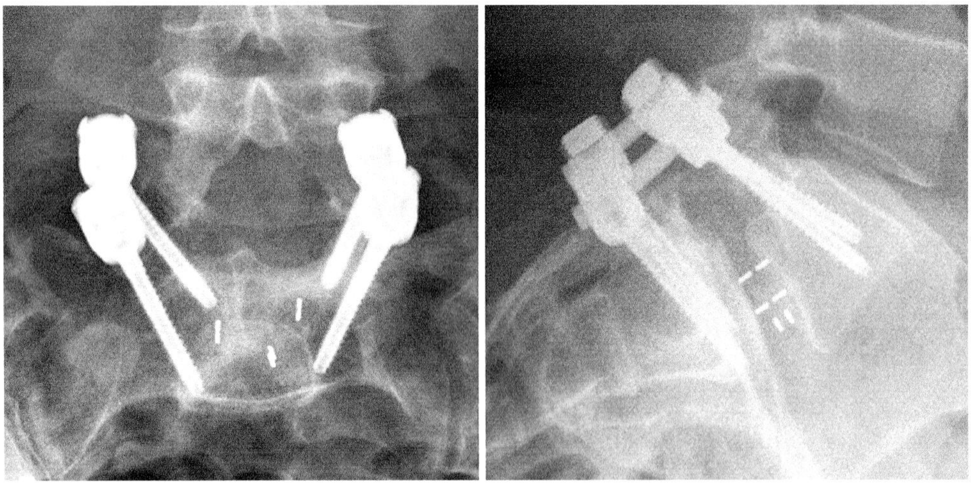

Fig. 76.1 Conventional X-rays ap. and laterally lumbar spine April 2015. The X-rays show a correct implant position (pedicle screws and TLIF-cage) without signs of loosening and without signs of bony fusion

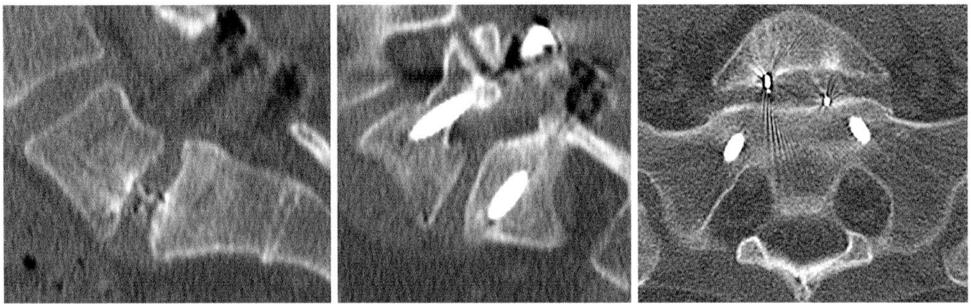

Fig. 76.2 CT scan lumbar spine September 2015. In the transverse CT-investigation, aswell in the sagittal reconstruction, a regular implant position without signs of loosening and without signs of bone union, can be observed. Only a little additive bone material in the disc space can be detected

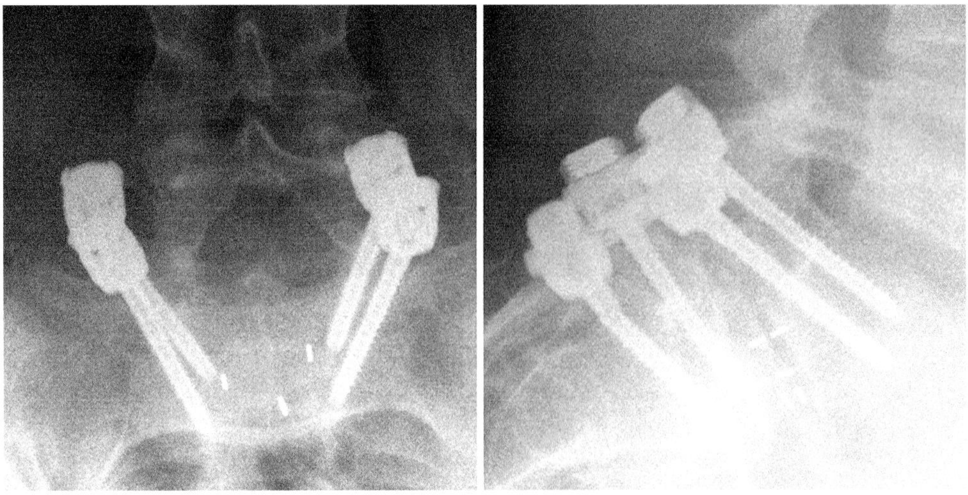

Fig. 76.3 Conventional X-rays of the lumbosacral junction in ap. and lateral direction, January 2017. The x-rays show a screw breakage S1 on the right, no bone fusion and loss of correction L5/S1

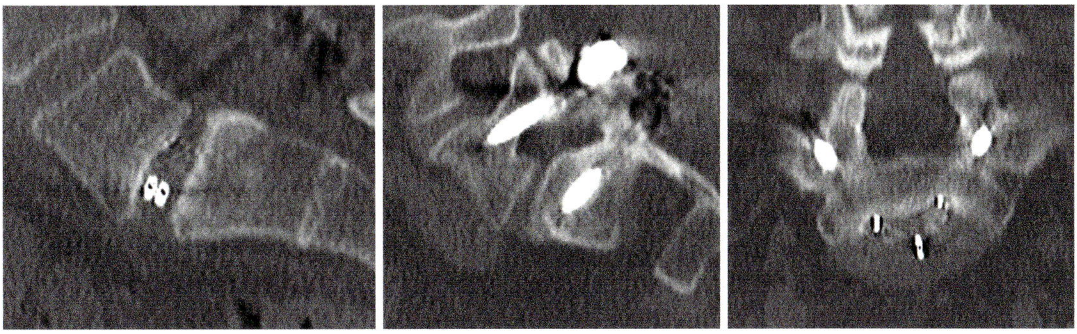

Fig. 76.4 CT scan lumbar spine March 2017. The transverse CT-scan and the sagittal reconstruction show a proper implant position and no bone fusion

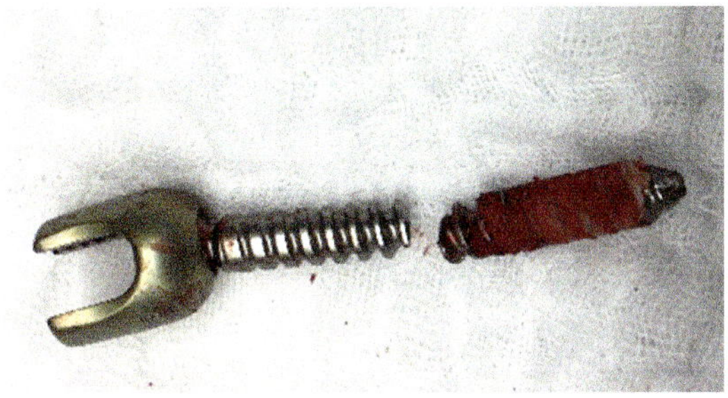

Fig. 76.5 Illustration of the intraoperative salvaged material. Presentation of the broken screw

Afterwords, the patient was completely pain free, no analgetics were used and she was able to return to work as a geriatric nurse.

76.3 Discussion of the Cases

At the beginning of the introduction of posterior instrumentation and interposition of intervertebral implants in the 1980's, pseudarthrosis rates of up to 40% were observed. Due to the development of better implants and an optimization of the surgical techniques, the incidence of non-fusion after instrumentation and cage interposition in the lumbar spine, depending on the selected surgical technique and the underlying disease, is mostly below 10%. However, patient-related factors can significantly increase this value.

76.3.1 Nicotine

In 1986, a radomized study showed a significantly different pseudarthrosis rate of 8% in non-smokers and 40% in smokers [4], although postoperative weaning can reduce the negative influence [5]. A confirmation of the significantly lower fusion rate (69.6% vs. 85.1%) is also evident in cases with ALIF fusion technique [6]. The use of rhBMP-2 (76.2% vs. 95.2%) leads to an improvement in the fusion rate in smokers, although the clinical outcome is still adversely affected by nicotine use [7]. The most important recommendation is smoking cessation for four weeks after surgery. In addition, patients may be treated with certain surgical techniques, including the use of BMPs [8].

76.3.2 Obesity

Scientific research suggests that in the field of lumbar fusion, obesity may have a negative impact on duration of surgery, blood loss, intraoperative dura injuries, postoperative wound healing, length of hospital stay and adjacent segment diseases, but pain and functional outcome are similar to non-obese patients [9]. In ALIF-technique spondylodesis, there are significant differences in the rates of fusion for obesity (60%), overweight (76%) and normal weight (88.2%) patients, with no negative impact on

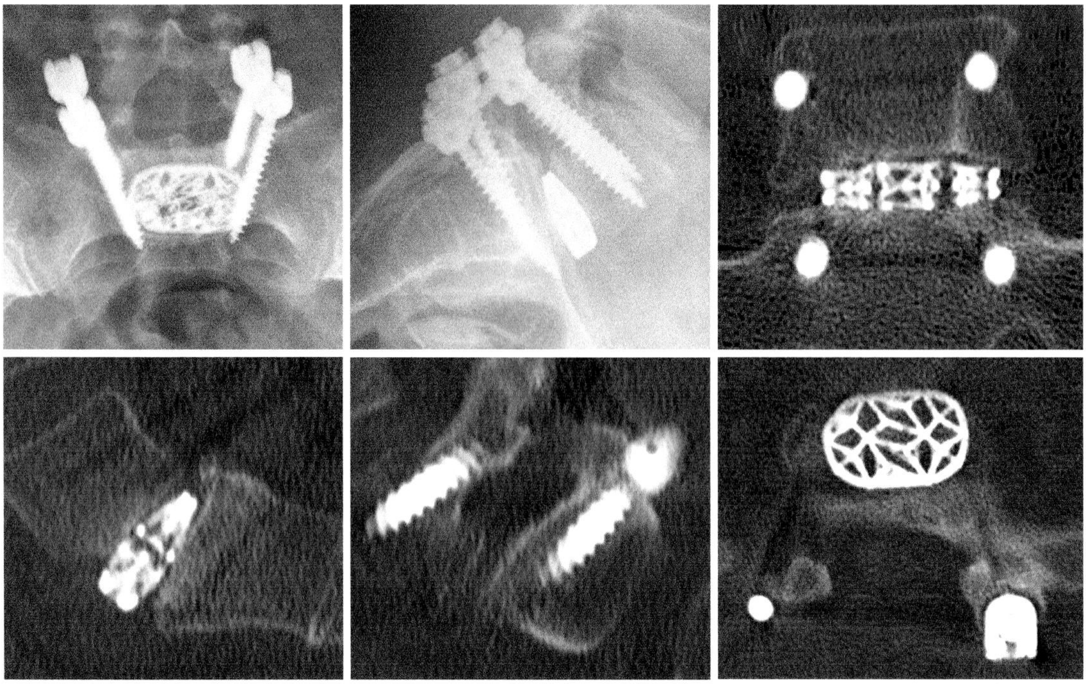

Fig. 76.6 Postoperative X-ray and CT examination December 2017. The conventional X-rays and the 12 weeks postop. CT scans show a correct implant position of pedicle screws and the ALIF-Cage (4 Web)

postoperative functional outcomes [10]. Studies investigating the influence of obesity on posterior fusion rates are lacking.

76.3.3 Steroid Use

Studies on animal models have shown an inhibitory effect of corticosteroids on bone fusion [11]. Although patients with rheumatoid arthritis show slightly higher complication rates compared to the normal population, the pseudarthrosis rates are not affected (11% vs. 16%) [12].

76.3.4 Osteoporosis

Although recent studies have shown that zoledronic acid accelerates bone fusion after lumbar spondylodesis in osteoporotic bone structure, it does not significantly increase the fusion rate [13]. Similar results are shown by comparative studies between teriparatide and bisphosphonate applications. Teriparatide increases the time to fusion, but not the total fusion rate [14]. Injection therapy with teriparatide is significantly superior to oral treatment with bisphosphonates in terms of fusion rate (92% vs. 70%) [15].

Low serum vitamin D levels can affect the incidence of nonunions and the time to fusion [16]. Through an additive postoperative administration of vitamin D3, the fusion rate in patients with osteoporosis can be significantly increased (96.2% vs. 65.2%) [17].

76.3.5 Diabetes Mellitus

In 2003, a negative influence of diabetes mellitus on the pseudarthrosis rate was shown (IDDM 26%, NIDDM 22%, control group 5%) [18]. No further specific studies on the relationship between lumbar fusion and diabetes mellitus have been published. A correlation between an increased postoperative wound infection and an increased HbA1c value has been confirmed several times.

76.3.6 Different Surgical Techniques (ALIF, PLIF, TLIF)

The fusion rate between the listed surgical techniques varies. A study comparing the three established fusion techniques show differences in fusion rates without being able to demonstrate significant superiority of a surgical technique on CT scan and segmental ROM (ALIF 69.2%, PLIF 64.3%, TLIF 72.7%) [19]. ALIF was associated with better restoration of segmental lordosis. TLIF was associated with a better postoperative pain on visual analogue scale. PLIF showed the lowest cage subsidence rate [19]. Also identical fusion rates for the TLIF and PLIF restorations are shown in another study [20]. A review and meta-analysis descripes that the available evidence suggests that both TLIF and PLIF could achieve similar clinical satisfaction and fusion rate in the management of degenerative lumbar diseases. However, TLIF was superior to PLIF with shorter operation time, less blood loss, and lower incidence of nerve root injury and dural tear [21]. Influences of the segment level on the fusion rate has not been examined in detail. A two-level posterior lumbar interbody fusion study, with patients treated in PLIF technique, observed all non-unions at the caudal level, concentrated at the level L5/S1 [22]. This observation can be explained by the increased shear forces at this segment and leads to the consideration of applying the largest possible cage surface. In non-union cases a revision surgery in ALIF technique achieved good clinical and radiologic outcomes with low complication rates [23].

76.3.7 Cage Materials (Titanium Versus PEEK)

Although in clinical practice it appears that the rate of fusion seems to be higher for titanium or titanium-coated cages, clinical studies cannot confirm this impression. A review and meta-analysis found that Titanium and PEEK cages are associated with a similar rate of fusion, with an increased rate of subsidence by titanium cage-treated cases at all parts of spinal fusion [24]. Another study from 2014 demonstrates different fusion rates, titanium 96% – PEEK 64% at 12 month and titanium 100% – PEEK 76% at 24 month follow up [25]. PEEK cages with or without titanium coating showed no differences with a similar fusion rate of 91.7% in both groups after 3 month [26]. However, both studies included only about 50 patients and can therefore be assessed to a limited extent.

76.3.8 Sagittal Alignement

Initial data suggest that postoperative sagittal imbalance may increase the rate of pseudarthrosis after lumbar fusion [27].

76.3.9 Bone Morphogenetic Proteins or Bone Substitutes

After evaluation by a systematic review, rhBMP-2 has only a positive effect on the fusion rate when using the ALIF technique and posterolateral fusion [28]. Hydroxyapatite demineralized bone matrix and autograft taken from the lamina show equivalent effects on bone fusion [29].

76.4 Conclusions and Take Home Message

The risk factors listed above, have an influence on the rate of fusion in lumbar spinal surgery. Therefore, a special preoperative assessment of the risks should be performed. In addition to an optimal performed surgical technique with careful dissection of the intervertebral disc space and impaction of autologous bone or bone substitute material, the use of BMP, the administration of vitamin D supplements, improved diabetes adjustment, can increase bone fusion and reduce revisions. In cases with proven non-union and/or implant failure, careful revision is required posterior and anterior. Important are stable situations and no complete stress shielding due to Wolffs law to support a bony healing in the intervertebral disc space. Due to the variety of diseases and the inadequate study situation with low cases at the field of cage materials and fusion technique, evidence-based therapy recommendations are difficult to give.

Pearls
- Screening of preoperative risk factors
- Surgical technique using the optimized material and bone substitutes to increase bony fusion after instrumentation
- In cases with a higher risk of non-unions, additional measures such as the application of BMP are possible

References

1. Kelly MP, Lenke LG, Bridwell KH, Agarwal R, Godzik J, Koester L. Fate of the adult revision spinal deformity patient: a single institution experience. Spine. 2013;38:E1196–200.
2. Deyo RA, Martin BI, Kreuter W, Jarvik JG, Angier H, Mirza SK. Revision surgery following operations for lumbar stenosis. J Bone Joint Surg Am. 2011;93:1979–86.
3. Djurasovic M, Glassman SD, Howard JM, Copay AG, Carreon LY. Health-related quality of life improvements in patients undergoing lumbar spinal fusion as a revision surgery. Spine. 2011;36:269–76.
4. Brown CW, Orme TJ, Rickardson HD. The rate of pseudarthrosis (surgical nonunion) in patients who are smokers and patients who are nonsmokers: a comparison study. Spine. 1986;11(9):942–3.
5. Glassmann SD, Anagnost SC, Parker A, Burke D, Johnson JR, Dimar JR. The effect of cigarette smoking and smoking cessation on spinal fusion. Spine. 2000;25(20):2608–15.
6. Phan K, Fadhil M, Chang N, Giang G, Gragnaniello C, Mobbs RJ. Effect of smoking status on successful arthrodesis, clinical outcome, and complications after anterior lumbar interbody fusion (ALIF). World Neurosurg. 2017;110:e998–e1003.
7. Glassmann SD, Dimar JR, Burkus K, Hardacker JW, Pryor PW, Boden SD, Carreon LY. The efficacy of rh BMP-2 for posterolateral lumbar fusion in smokers. Spine. 2007;32(15):1693–8.
8. Berman D, Oren JH, Bendo J, Spivek J. The effect of smoking on spinal fusion. Int J Spine Surg. 2017;28:1129.
9. Lingutla KK, Pollock R, Benomran E, Purushothaman B, Kasis A, Bhatia CK, Krishna M, Friesem T. Outcome of lumbar spinal fusion surguryin obese patients; A systematic review and meta-analysis. Bone Joint J. 2015;97-(B):1395–404.
10. Phan K, Rogers P, Rao PJ, Mobbs RJ. Influence of obesity on complications, clinical outcome and subsidence after anterior lumbar interbody fusion (ALIF) Prospective observational study. World Neurosurg. 2017;107:334–41.
11. Sawin PD, Dickman CA, Crawford NR, Melton MS, Bichard WD, Sonntag VK. The effects of dexamethasone on bone fusion in an experimental model of posterolateral lumbar spinal arthrodesis. J Neursurg. 2001;94:76–81.
12. Crawford CH, Carreon LY, Djurasovic M, Glassmann SD. Lumbar fusion outcomes in patients with rheumatoid arthritis. Eur Spine J. 2008;17(6):822–5.
13. Ding Q, Chen J, Fan J, Li Q, Yin G, Yu L. Effect of zoledronic acid on lumbar spinal fusion in osteoporotic patients. Eur Spine J. 2017;26(11):2969–77.
14. Cho PG, Ji GY, Shin DA, Ha Y, Yoon DH, Kim KN. An effect comparison of teriparatide and bisphosphonate on posterior lumbar interbody fusion in patients with osteoporosis: a prospective cohort study and preliminary data. Eur Spine J. 2017;26(3):691–7.
15. Ohtori S, Orita S, Yamauchi K, Eguchi Y, Ochiai N, Takahashi K. More than 6 months of teriparatide treatment was more effective for bone union than shorter treatment following lumbar posterolateral dusion surgery. Asian Spine J. 2015;9(4):573–80.
16. Rivindra VM, Godzik J, Dailey AT, Schmidt MH, Bisson EF, Hood RS, Cutler A, Ray WZ. Vitamin D Levels and 1-year fusion outcomes in elective spine surgery: a prospective observational study. Spine. 2015;40(19):1536–41.
17. Xu Y, Zhou M, Liu H, Zhang Q, Hu Z, Zhang N, Ren Y. Effect of 1,25 dihydroxyvitamin D3 on posterior transformanial lumbar interbody fusion in patients with osteoporosis and lumbar disc degenerative disease. Zhongguo Xiu Fu Chong Jian Wai Ke Za Zhi. 2014;28(8):969–72.
18. Glassman SD, Alegre G, Carreon L, Dimar JR, Johnson JR. Perioperative comlications of lumbar instrumentation and fusion in patients with diabetes mellitus. Spine J. 2003;3(6):496–501.
19. Lee N, Kim KN, Yi S, Ha Y, Shin DA, Yoon DH, Kim KS. Comparison of outcomes of anterior, posterior and transforaminal lumbar interbody fusionsurgery at a single lumbar level with degenerative spinal disease. World Neurosurg. 2017;101:216–26.
20. Metha VA, McGirt MJ, Garces Ambrossi GL, Parker SL, Sciubba DM, Bydon A, Wolinsky JP, Gokasian ZL, Witham TF. Transforaminal versus posterior lumbar interbody fusion: comparison of surgical morbidity. Neurol Res. 2011;33(1):38–42.

21. Lan T, Hu SY, Zhang YT, Zheng YC, Zhang R, Shen Z, Yang XJ. Comparison between posterior lumbar interbody fusion and transforaminal lumbar interbody fusion fort he treatment of lumbar degenerative diseases: a systematic review and meta-analysis. World Neurosurg. 2018;112:86–93.
22. Aono H, Takenaka S, Nagamoto Y, Tobimatsu H, Yamashita T, Furuya M, Iwasaki M. Fusion rate and clinical outcome in 2-level posterior lumbar interbody fusion. World Neurosurg. 2018;115: 490–502.
23. Yun DJ, Yu JW, Jeon S, Lee HC, Lee SH. Salvage anterior lumbar interbody fusion for pseudarthrosis after posterior or transforaminal lumbar interbody fusion. World Neurosurg. 2018;111:746–55. https://doi.org/10.1016/j.wneu.2017.12.155. Epub 2018 Jan 5.
24. Seaman S, Kerezoudis P, Bvdon M, Torner JC, Hitchon PW. Titanium vs. polyetheretherketone (PEEK) interbody fusion: Meta-analysis and review oft he literature. J Clin Neurosci. 2017;44:23–0.
25. Nemoto O, Asazuma T, Yato Y, Imabavashi H, Yasuoka H, Fujikawa A. Comparison of fusion rates following trandforaminal lumbar interbody fusion using polyetheretherketone cages or titanium cages with transpedicular instrumentation. Eur Spine J. 2014;23:2150–5.
26. Rickert M, Fleege C, Tarhan T, Schreiner S, Makowski MR, Rauschmann M, Arabmotlagh M. Transforaminal lumbar interbody fusion using polyetheretherketone oblique cages with and without a titanium coating: a randomised clinical pilot study. Bone Joint J. 2017;99-B(10):1366–72.
27. Langmantel R, Karantzoulis V, Ebner R, Vazifehdan F. Die postoperative sagittale Instabilität erhöht das Pseudarthroserisiko nach Lumbalfusion. Die Wirbelsäule. 2017;01(01):66–8.
28. Galimberti F, Lubelski D, Healy AT, Wang T, Abdullah KG, Nowacki AS, Benzel EC, Mroz TE. A systematic review of lumbar fusion rates with and without the use of rhBMP-2. Spine. 2015;40(14):1132–9.
29. Kim DH, Lee N, Shin DA, Yi S, Kim KN, Ha Y. Matched comparison of fusion rates between hydroxyapatide demineralized bone matrix and autograft in lumbar interbody fusion. J Korean Neurosurg Soc. 2016;59(4):363–7.

Proximal Junctional Kyphosis Despite Best Efforts in Planning and Execution

77

Caglar Yilgor and R. Emre Acaroglu

77.1 Introduction

Concepts in spinal deformity surgery as well as the instrumentation used to surgically treat spinal deformities has constantly been evolving in the last few decades. The biomechanics of the growing, grown and degenerated spine, and the biomechanical effects of the implants used are not yet fully understood. After instrumented fusion, the interchange between the instrumented and non-instrumented spinal segments are referred to as junctional area.

Patients can develop junctional diseases after instrumentation and fusion; one particular problem being proximal junctional kyphosis (PJK). PJK, first described as a surgical complication after Scheuermann's kyphosis, currently, is a well-recognized postoperative phenomenon that can occur after surgery for any spinal condition. Originally defined as an abnormal kyphotic deformity of the spinal segment proximally adjacent to the instrumentation, more recently, it is recognized that increased junctional stresses may cause soft tissue, ligament, bone, and bone-implant interface to fail. Thus, PJK encompass a spectrum of disease severities both radiographically and clinically.

Radiographically, PJK was defined by Glattes et al [1]. to occur when the postoperative kyphosis angle of the proximal junctional segment is $\geq 10°$ than the preoperative value. The proximal junctional angle (PJA) is measured from the inferior endplate of the upper instrumented vertebra (UIV) to the superior endplate of the second upper adjacent vertebra (UIV +2). As the interpretation of the compensatory mechanisms are better understood, this definition has evolved to refer to PJA changes between early postoperative and follow-up radiographs [2]. This is because compensation is a process in which the change in a given direction is counteracted by another conscious or unconscious change, and angular changes from preoperative to postoperative are recognized as a reciprocal change of the thoracic hypokyphosis that is compensating the lumbar hypolordosis.

On the other hand, proximal junctional failure (PJF), radiographically includes both kyphosis and compromised structural integrity of the vertebral body, facet joints, discs, posterior ligament complex and/or implantation. As such, PJF can be presented as UIV and/or UIV +1 fracture, UIV screw cutout or pullout, hook dislodgement, and/or as sagittal subluxation [3].

Clinically, PJK refers to a simple radiological finding that is associated with no clinical impact. PJF, however; causes adverse impact, and may

C. Yilgor
Acibadem Mehmet Ali Aydinlar
University School of Medicine,
Department of Orthopedics and Traumatology,
Istanbul, Turkey

R. E. Acaroglu (✉)
Ankara Spine Center, Ankara, Turkey

B. Meyer, M. Rauschmann (eds.), *Spine Surgery*, https://doi.org/10.1007/978-3-319-98875-7_77

present with pain, neurological consequences, ambulatory difficulty, social isolation, and/or inability to maintain horizontal gaze due to progressive deterioration of sagittal alignment. Any symptomatic junctional problem requiring any type of revision surgery is also referred to as PJF [4].

In different clinical settings, PJK was reported to occur between 20% and 59% [5], while PJF incidence may be as low as 1–5.6% [4]. Many studies have documented numerous modifiable and non-modifiable risk factors of PJK and PJF. Knowledge of such risk factors are important for minimizing the occurrence of PJK/PJF. Yet, despite recent reports and best efforts in surgical planning proximal junctional problems are still prevalent.

The objective of this case is to demonstrate a case that resulted in PJF and discuss future directions for a step forward in the prevention of this complication. Being able to prevent PJK and PJF may be a key component in providing optimal clinical outcomes after surgery for ASD.

77.2 Case Description

The case was a 75-years-old male patient. In the baseline examination, the patient was 178 cm tall and weighed 80 kg, to yield a BMI of 25.3 kg/m^2. He was retired and residing at home. He was an ex-smoker.

The patient described claudication, accompanied with back and leg pain. He reported to feel weakness in both legs. He started experiencing back pain issues, more than 15 years ago. Leg pain, being the prominent clinical symptom, was present for more than 10 years. The patient denies any history of prior physical therapy, bracing, chiropractic care, injections, narcotic use, and spine surgery. His past medical history reveals hypertension and osteoarthritis and was assessed as ASA I (American Society of Anesthesiologists).

His physical examination revealed a steady gate and intact neurological motor functions. His bone mineral density results showed no signs of osteoporosis with a femoral neck T score of −0.50 and total spine T score of +1.30.

Radiographic analysis revealed no coronal deformity. Pelvic incidence (PI) was measured to be 37°. Pelvic tilt and sacral slope were 25° and 12°, correspondingly. L1-S1 Lumbar Lordosis (LL) Cobb angle was 10°, and L4-S1 Lordosis Cobb angle was 22°. PI minus LL (PI–LL) was 27°. T2–T12 Thoracic kyphosis was 8°. Sagittal Vertical Axis (SVA) was −2.75 cm, T1 Pelvic Angle (TPA) was 16° and Global Tilt (GT) was 18°. (Fig. 77.1).

MRI scans revealed moderate to severe central and lateral recess stenosis at L3-4, L4-5 and L5-S1. There were mild to moderate diffuse disc bulges asymmetric to the left at L5-S1, accompanied by moderate to severe bilateral facet hypertrophy. Mild to moderate neuroforaminal narrowing was present bilaterally at L3-4, L4-5 and L5-S1, most pressure being on the exiting left L5 nerve root.

The patient was operated with a single-stage, posterior-only surgery that lasted 185 min from "knife-to-skin". He was instrumented from T12 to ilium using 16 pedicle screws with a 2.0 implant density per level. Central and foraminal decompression was performed at L3-4, L4-5 and L5-S1. Transforaminal lumbar interbody fusion (TLIF) procedure was applied at L3-4, L4-5 and L5-S1 with the use of autograft and polyetheretherketone (PEEK) cage. A 6 mm cobalt-chrome rod was used on both sides for deformity correction and stabilization. Decortication and local autograft was applied to achieve fusion.

No changes were recorded in the intraoperative neurophysiological monitoring. Estimated surgical blood loss was 1800 ml. Intraoperatively, 1270 ml of blood and 400 ml of fresh frozen plasma were transfused.

Postoperatively, the patient spent 24 h in the intensive care, and consequently was taken to the ward. Total drain output was 1620 ml and no

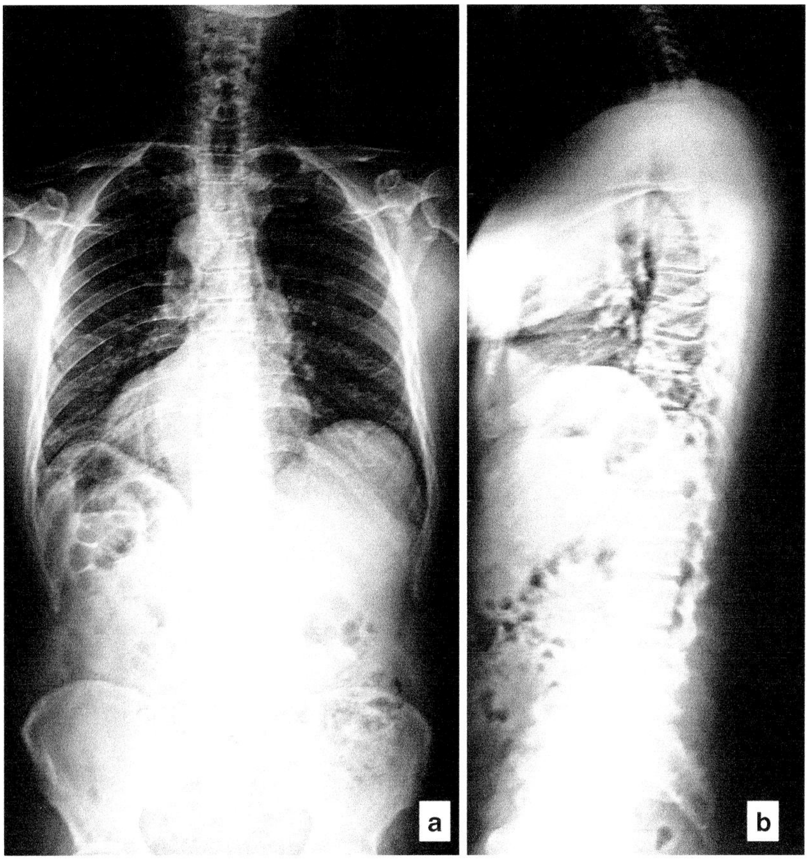

Fig. 77.1 (**a**) Ap and (**b**) Laterals whole-spine standing radiographs before the operation

postoperative transfusions were made. The total course of hospitalization was 11 days.

Early postoperative first-erect radiograph showed no coronal off-balance. Pelvic tilt and sacral slope were 19° and 18°, correspondingly. L1-S1 lordosis was 32°, and L4-S1 lordosis was 26°. PI–LL was 5°. T2-T12 kyphosis was 19°. SVA was −3.1 cm, TPA was 7° and GT was 9°. (Fig. 77.2).

Preoperative and follow-up patient-reported outcome scores are given in Table 77.1. The patient was prescribed and used a custom-made protective full contact brace until 6 months' follow-up. He had a course of 12 months of physiotherapy after which he reported 9/10 pain relief. UIV instrumentation pullout was observed 51 days after surgery at the 6-weeks' postoperative visit. The patient experienced a rod breakage 398 days after surgery. The patient had his last follow-up visit 1128 days after the surgery corresponding to 3-years' postoperative visit. (Fig. 77.3).

77.3 Discussion of the Case

Numerous modifiable and non-modifiable risk factors of PJK/PJF have been identified in the literature [4]. Radiographic risk factors are preoperative hyperkyphosis, greater pelvic incidence and SVA, and non-anatomic restoration of thoracic kyphosis. Patient-related factors are older age, higher BMI, poor bone quality, and preoperative comorbidities. Technical and biomechanical risk factors are posterior approach and disruption of the posterior ligaments and

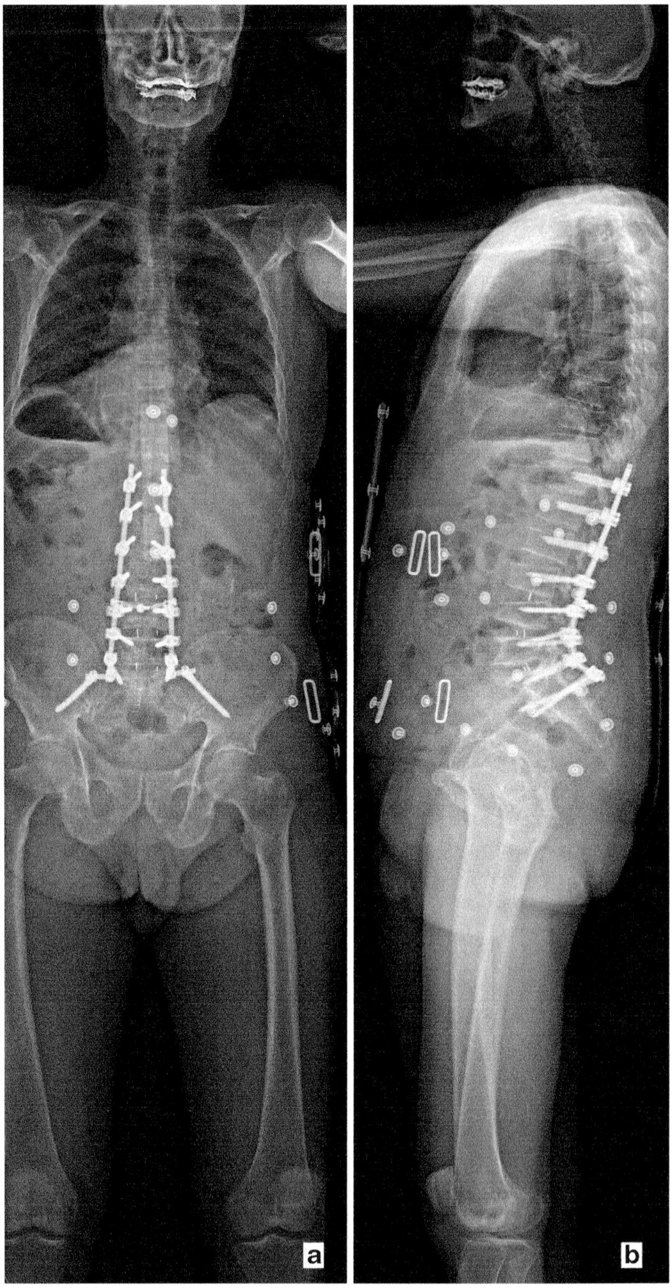

Fig. 77.2 (**a**) Ap and (**b**) Laterals whole-spine standing radiographs before discharge, 10 days after the operation

Table 77.1 Patient-reported outcome scores at preoperative visit and 6 months', 1 year's and 2 years' follow-up

	VAS back	VAS leg	ODI	COMI	SF-36 PCS	SF-36 MCS	SRS-22 function	SRS-22 pain	SRS-22 MH	SRS-22 self-image	SRS-22 subtotal
Pre-op	4	7	24	4.9	39.11	54.79	3.5	3.5	4.2	2.0	3.28
6 month	1	0	18	3.2	39.61	46.18	3.0	4.3	4.2	3.0	3.60
1 year	1	0	9	0.7	44.71	62.04	4.0	4.5	4.6	4.4	4.40
2 years	1	0	14	1.7	36.75	56.36	3.3	4.4	4.2	3.4	3.80

VAS Visual Analog Scale, *ODI* Oswestry Disability Index, *COMI* Core Outcomes Measures Index, *SF*-36 Short Form-36, *PCS* Physical Component Summary, *MCS* Mental Component Summary, *SRS*-22 Scoliosis Research Society-22 spinal deformity questionnaire, *MH* Mental Health

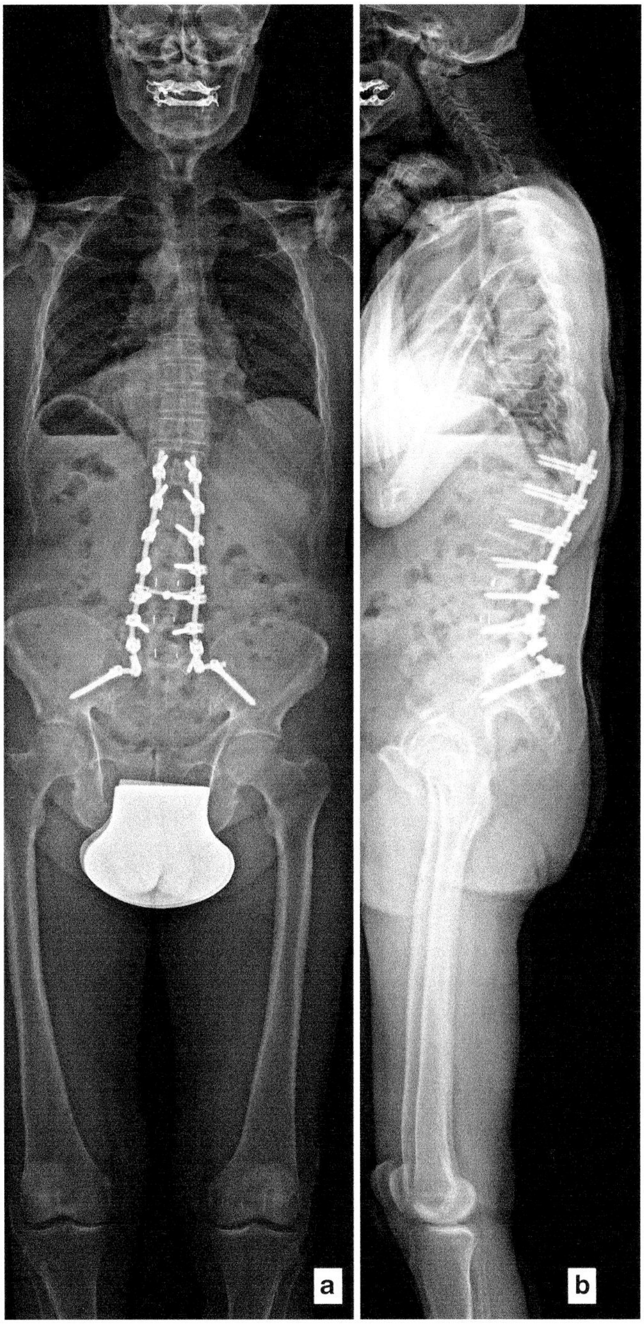

Fig. 77.3 (**a**) Ap and (**b**) Laterals whole-spine standing radiographs in the latest follow-up visit, 3 years after the operation

damage to the paravertebral muscles, the rigidity of the instrumentation, UIV at lower thoracic level, fusion to the lower lumbar vertebra and sacrum, the use of thoracoplasty, the correction forces applied intraoperatively to reduce the thoracic kyphosis or to restore the sagittal balance and/or greater curvature correction or greater change in SVA, and revision surgery [6]. There remains a lack of evidence supporting prevention strategies such as the use of vertebral body cement augmentation and posterior polyester tethers.

Despite all these efforts, retrospective clinical studies of PJK have not been able to isolate a strongly related risk factor that can be used in prevention, and findings were often inconclusive and/or controversial, and included confounding results. Postoperative disability have been largely attributed to inadequate restoration of sagittal alignment. Sagittal plane undercorrection and overcorrection have both been reported to be a main cause of mechanical complications [7]. According to the Scoliosis Research Society (SRS)-Schwab classification, the targets for achieving satisfactory alignment and favorable outcomes are a value of ≤10° for PI–LL, <20° for PT, and a SVA of <4 cm.

In the presented case, preoperatively, PT was 25° classified as '+' indicating moderate retroversion, PI–LL was 27°, classified as '++' indicating severe spinopelvic mismatch, and SVA was −2.75 cm classified as '0' indicating normal global alignment according to SRS-Schwab classification.

Leg pain and claudication being the most prominent clinical symptoms, the main focus of the surgery was on decompression. A subtotal laminectomy preserving the middle third of the lamina was performed on L3, L4 and L5. Bilateral foraminotomies were performed at L3-4, L4-5 and L5-S1. Articular surfaces were widely resected in the preserved joints to complete the decompression into a posterior column osteotomy in order to restore lordosis. Following discectomy, TLIF cages were inserted at L3-4, L4-5 and L5-S1 for anterior column support. The rods were then bent according to the desired contour, and correction was done from distal to proximal focusing on rotating the pelvis and increasing the lordosis.

Postoperatively, PT was 19° classified as '0', PI–LL was 5°, classified as '0', and SVA was −3.1 cm classified as '0' indicating good restoration of all criteria according to SRS-Schwab classification.

It is not uncommon to observe mechanical complications even after ideal correction of all SRS-Schwab sagittal modifiers, as demonstrated in this case. This might be due to some inherent disadvantages of these modifiers [2]. Interpreting numerous studies that have sought to uncover ideal spinal curvatures and alignment, the only reasonable conclusion to draw is that these curvature metrics must be reviewed in light of each other. Thus, using the PT, PI–LL and SVA solely as linear numerical values can be misleading, especially for patients with PI values near the upper-normal and lower-normal limits.

The presented case has a PI of 37°, which is more than 1 standard deviation smaller than reported average normative magnitudes. Therefore, although the surgical goal of pelvic tilt <20° was achieved, this patient, according to his specific anatomical features required even lower PT values. Postoperative 19° of PT, in a patient with 37° of PI, still corresponds to retroversion [8]. PI-adjusted individualized parameter of Relative Pelvic Version (RPV) was −12.8° and was classified as moderate retroversion.

The simplistic criterion of PI–LL within 10° also has limitations when applied to individuals with different PI values. PI–LL is easy to calculate, yet hard to evaluate, since it also needs to be adapted to the intrinsic pelvic morphology of each patient. Therefore, although the surgical goal of PI–LL <10° was achieved, this patient, still had a spinopelvic mismatch [9]. PI-adjusted individualized parameter of Relative Lumbar Lordosis (RLL) was −19.9° and was classified as moderate hypolordosis.

SVA delivers a quick and useful metric to describe trunk's general alignment. SVA can be masked by pelvic retroversion. Therefore, although the surgical goal of SVA <4 cm was achieved almost to a level that can be interpreted as overcorrection, this patient, still had a positive malalignment depicted by TPA and GT. The retroverted pelvis was hiding this positive malalignment well enough to bring C7 over the pelvis in a compensated malalignment. PI-adjusted individualized parameter of Relative Spinopelvic Alignment (RSA) was +6.2° and was classified to be within the limits of 'aligned' as >10° is considered to be positively malaligned [2].

Today, it is crystal clear that pelvic morphology regulates spinal morphology by affecting the magnitude of the curves as well as the shape. Yet, SRS-Schwab sagittal modifiers suggest the same

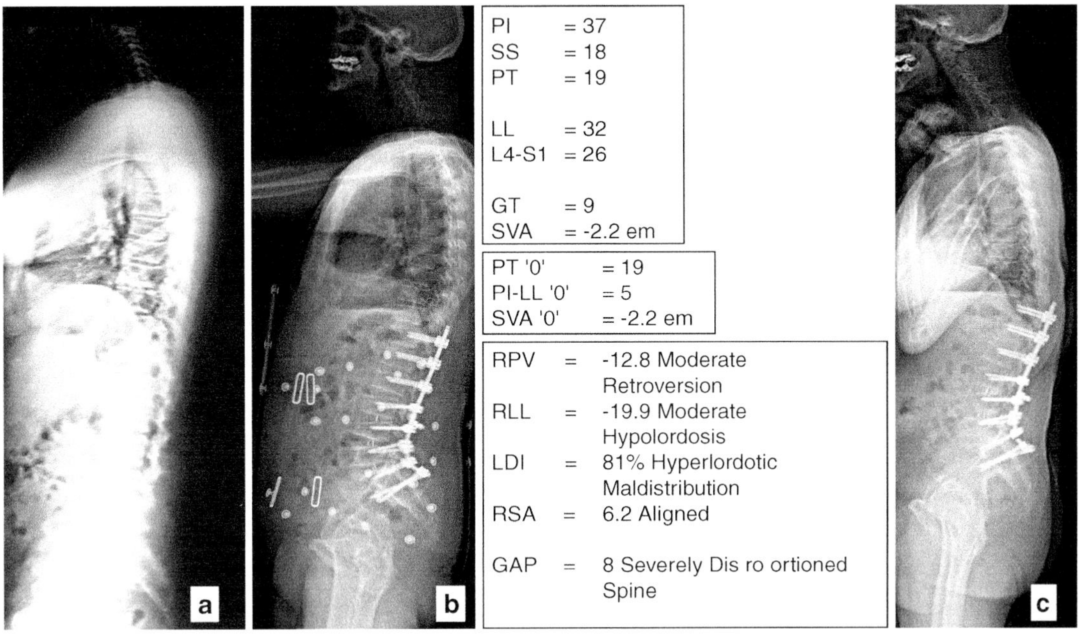

Fig. 77.4 (**a**) Pre-operative, (**b**) First-erect and (**c**) 3-years post-operative lateral whole-spine standing radiographs. Measurements in the first-erect radiograph reveal all three SRS-Schwab sagittal modifiers to be '0'. Using the same measurements to calculate the PI-adjusted individualized parameters, it is demonstrated that the patient is hypolordotic and retroverted. The GAP Score is calculated to be 8, indicating a severely disproportioned spinopelvic state. PJF with implant pullout (at 6 weeks) and double rod breakage (at 1 year) was observed, both of which were not revised. PI Pelvic incidence, SS Sacral Slope, PT Pelvic Tilt, LL L1-S1 Lumbar Lordosis, GT Global Tilt, SVA Sagittal Vertical Axis, RPV Relative Pelvic Version, RLL Relative Lumbar Lordosis, LDI Lordosis Distribution Index, RSA Relative Spinopelvic Alignment, GAP Global Alignment and Proportion Score

rules for every size of PI. More recently, an individualized analysis system was proposed that uses PI-adjusted radiographic parameters to evaluate the pelvic version, magnitude and distribution of lordosis and global spinopelvic alignment [2].

Using the same radiographs and same radiographic measurements of PI, SS, L1-S1 and L4-S1 lordosis and GT, but interpreting them as disproportion compared with the calculated "ideal" based on the specific PI of the given patient, one can easily realize that the patient is still lacking ~20° of lordosis, and compensating >10° from the pelvis only to reach ~5° of positive malalignment. (Fig. 77.4).

It was suggested that the amount of compensatory mechanisms used after instrumented fusion determines the distribution of loads on implants, instrumented vertebrae, adjacent segments, and grafts [2]. Postoperative GAP Score of 8 in the presented case, indicates a severely disproportioned spinopelvic state, representing the extent of the compensation the patient has to use.

77.4 Conclusions and Take Home Message

As opposed to absolute numeric values of SRS-Schwab criteria that are the same for all PI magnitudes, the PI-based individualized parameters of the GAP Score parameters better fit the individual variability of human anatomy [2]. The aim of any instrumented fusion should be to stabilize the patient in a position that would require no or minimum compensation after surgery. PI-adjusted interpretation of the spinopelvic alignment allows the setting of personalized radiographic targets for preoperative planning.

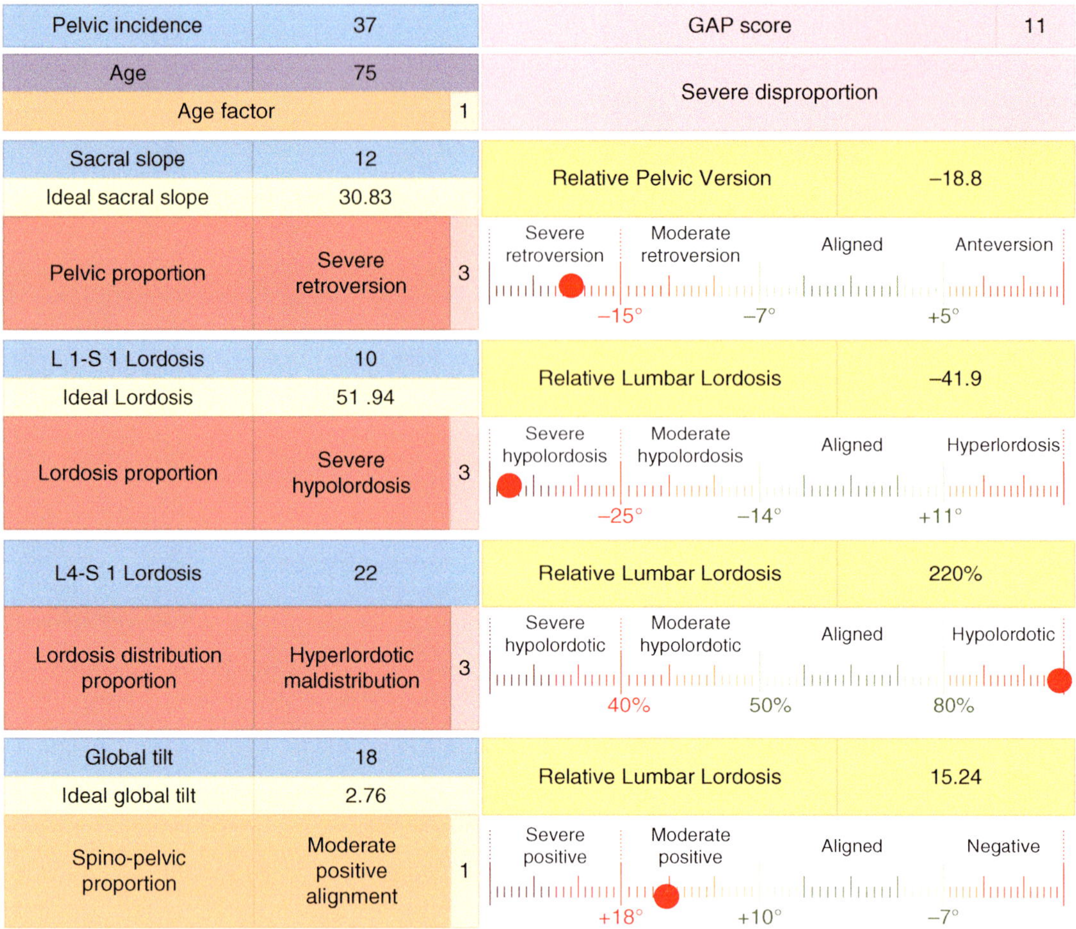

Fig. 77.5 Preoperative GAP Score Analysis of the patient. The use of the PI-based proportional radiographic parameters together with the scales allows for a better interpretation of the individualized pelvic, lordotic and global alignment. Patient's pelvis is 18.8° retroverted than the calculated ideal for a PI of 37. Similarly he lacks 41.9° of lordosis then the individualized ideal

Preoperative analysis of the patient according to GAP score denotes that the patient had a severely retroverted pelvis (despite a PT of 25° indicating moderate retroversion) and that the ideal PT for for this specific patient was as low as 6°. Similarly, the spinopelvic mismatch was as big as ~42° although PI–LL was only calculated to be 27°. (Fig. 77.5) The GAP Score further allows to plan the shape of lordosis using the lordosis distribution index.

Setting surgical goals in the sagittal plane on the basis of the proportional indices reflected by the GAP Score might have allowed reaching the goal of GAP score of ≤2 that reflects a proportioned spinopelvic state. Such a state requires minimum usage of compensatory mechanisms and a more appropriate distribution of loads on implants, instrumented vertebrae, adjacent segments, and grafts. Preoperative planning with the GAP score might be used as a prevention tool for mechanical complications.

References

1. Glattes RC, Bridwell KH, Lenke LG, Kim YJ, Rinella A, Edwards C 2nd. Proximal junctional kyphosis in adult spinal deformity following long instrumented posterior spinal fusion: incidence, outcomes, and risk factor analysis. Spine. 2005;30:1643–9. (EBM Level III).

2. Yilgor C, Sogunmez N, Boissiere L, et al. Global Alignment and Proportion (GAP) Score: development and validation of a new method of analyzing spinopelvic alignment to predict mechanical complications after adult spinal deformity surgery. J Bone Joint Surg Am. 2017;99:1661–72. (EBM Level II).
3. Arlet V, Aebi M. Junctional spinal disorders in operated adult spinal deformities: present understanding and future perspectives. Eur Spine J. 2013;22(Suppl 2):S276–95. (EBM Level III).
4. Lau D, Clark AJ, Scheer JK, et al. Proximal junctional kyphosis and failure after spinal deformity surgery: a systematic review of the literature as a background to classification development. Spine. 2014;39:2093–102. (EBM Level N/A).
5. Kim YJ, Bridwell KH, Lenke LG, Glattes CR, Rhim S, Cheh G. Proximal junctional kyphosis in adult spinal deformity after segmental posterior spinal instrumentation and fusion: minimum five-year follow-up. Spine. 2008;33:2179–84. (EBM Level III).
6. Cammarata M, Aubin CE, Wang X, Mac-Thiong JM. Biomechanical risk factors for proximal junctional kyphosis: a detailed numerical analysis of surgical instrumentation variables. Spine. 2014;39:E500–7. (EBM Level N/A).
7. Bridwell KH, Baldus C, Berven S, et al. Changes in radiographic and clinical outcomes with primary treatment adult spinal deformity surgeries from two years to three- to five-years follow-up. Spine. 2010;35:1849–54. (EBM Level III).
8. Yilgor C, Yavuz Y, Sogunmez N, et al. Relative pelvic version (RPV): an individualized pelvic incidence-based proportional parameter that quantifies pelvic version more precisely than pelvic tilt. Spine J. 2018; https://doi.org/10.1016/j.spinee.2018.03.001. pii: S1529-9430(18)30084-6. (EBM Level II).
9. Yilgor C, Sogunmez N, Yavuz Y, et al. Relative lumbar lordosis and lordosis distribution index: individualized pelvic incidence-based proportional parameters that quantify lumbar lordosis more precisely than the concept of pelvic incidence minus lumbar lordosis. Neurosurg Focus. 2017;43:E5. (EBM Level II).

78 Management of Failure of Osteoporotic Fixation

Andreas Pingel and Frank Kandziora

78.1 Introduction

Especially in osteoporotic spine the rate of implant failures is high. Even experienced spine surgeons often are confronted with implant failures and especially proximal junctional kyphosis (PJK) in the short- to mid-term follow up after surgical correction and stabilization of vertebral fracture in osteoporotic spine. There is very poor scientific evidence how to treat osteoporotic vertebral fractures and how to prevent PJK as a typical complication.

This chapter will describe solutions for the prevention and management of failure of osteoporotic fixation. The presented case outlines typical pitfalls and surgical problems in osteoporotic spine and highlights the problem of PJK in osteoporotic spine and dysbalanced sagittal profile.

78.2 Case Description

A 51 y/o male patient had a fall from 7 stairs while suffering from steroid-induced osteoporosis. Delayed CT scan showed a compression fracture T7 with slight involvement of caudal posterior vertebral wall. A conservative treatment was started including bracing and analgetic drugs. The conservative treatment failed, nine months after the trauma the patient suffered from increasing pain in the midthoracic region and the thoracolumbar junction; he felt instability in standing position.

Because of posttraumatic deformity with significant sagittal dysbalance (bisegmental Cobb-angle 38° T6-T8, Fig. 78.1a, b) and intractable back pain there was the need for surgical correction. Multiple osteotomies according to Ponte were done to reach a posterior shortening and fusion with multilevel pedicle screw stabilization T2- L2 (Fig. 78.2a, b). The corrective result was acceptable, sagittal balance was normalized, the patient felt a good pain relief.

Two months later patient suffered from severe pain in the neck. Radiographies showed a junctional kyphosis with a fixed luxation T1-2 with significant kyphosis (Cobb- angle T1-3: 64°) (Fig. 78.3a) in the cervicothoracic junction with disruption of posterior osseous and ligamentous structures of T2 (Fig. 78.3b). An open reduction with incomplete vertebral column resection T2 and stabilization with pedicle screws C6/7/T1 were performed. Sagittal profile was acceptable after this measurement, stability was reached (Fig. 78.4a, b).

Twelve months after revision surgery patient was admitted with recurrent neck pain, holding his head with both hands. Radiographies detected a rod breakage with a loss of correction

A. Pingel (✉) · F. Kandziora
Zentrum für Wirbelsäulenchirurgie und Neurotraumatologie, Berufsgenossenschaftliche Unfallklinik Frankfurt am Main, Frankfurt, Germany
e-mail: andreas.pingel@bgu-frankfurt.de

B. Meyer, M. Rauschmann (eds.), *Spine Surgery*, https://doi.org/10.1007/978-3-319-98875-7_78

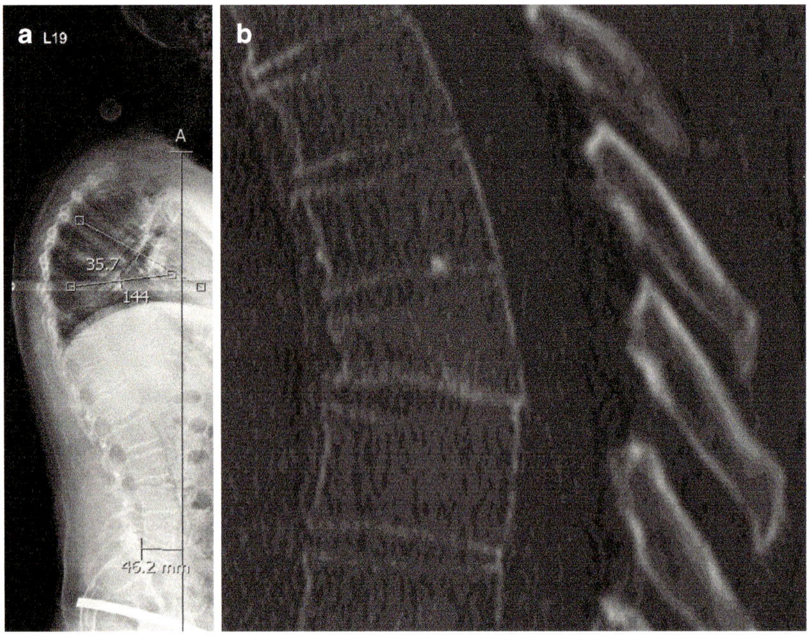

Fig. 78.1 (a, b) 9 months after trauma: Decompensated posttraumatic kyphosis after conservative treated compression fracture T7 (Cobb-angle T 2 to T 12: 90°), bisegmental angle: 37°, T-score: −2, 87

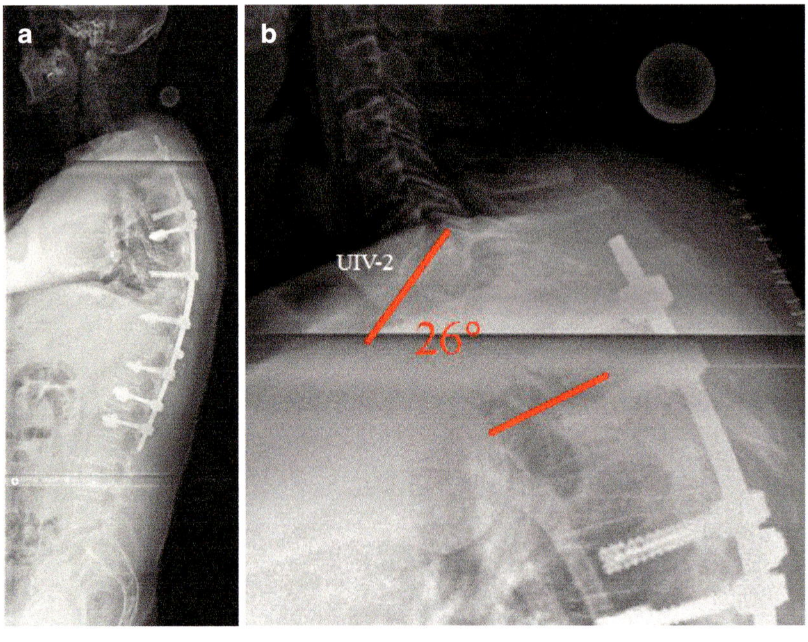

Fig. 78.2 (a, b) postoperative result after first surgical correction T2-L2 1 yr after trauma. Look at the overall good result of correction, the spine is balanced. Nevertheless,the junctional angle between the upper endplate C7 (UIV-2) and the lower endplate T2 is 26° and so there is a predisposition for development of a PJK

C6-T3 with significant kyphosis in the cervicothoracic junction (Cobb- angle C6-T3: 68°, Fig. 78.5a, b). Due to this highly unstable situation with severe dysbalance corrective surgery was urgently indicated. To treat this problem, a vertebral column resection T2 and partial T1 was performed via costotransversectomies of the 1st and 2nd rib (Fig. 78.6a), an expandable cage was implanted to get stability in the anterior column. Cobalt-Chrome-rods were connected to the implants.

After this last revision, the further course was uneventful. Apart from reduced cervical mobility the patient felt not very restricted.

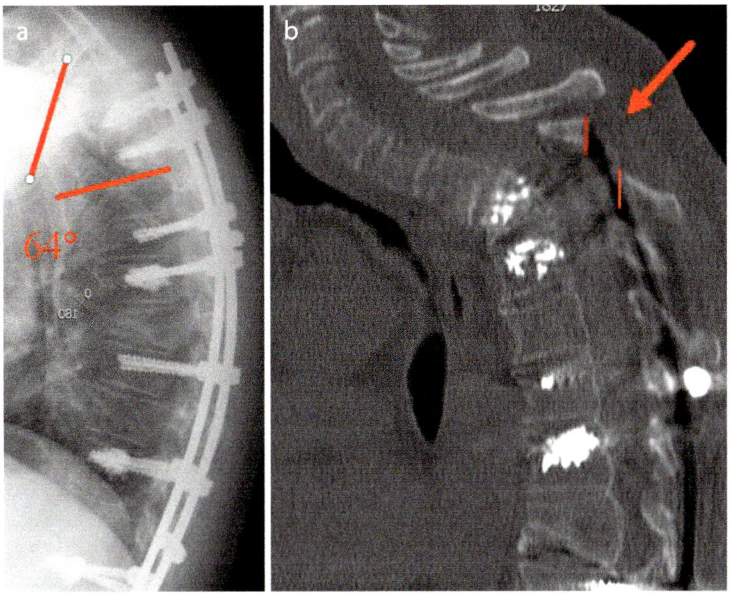

Fig. 78.3 (**a**, **b**) 2 months after surgery there is a PJK with a fixed luxation T1-2 with significant kyphosis (Cobb- angle T1-3: 64°) in the cervicothoracic junction. The red arrow shows disruption of posterior osseous and ligamentous structures of T2

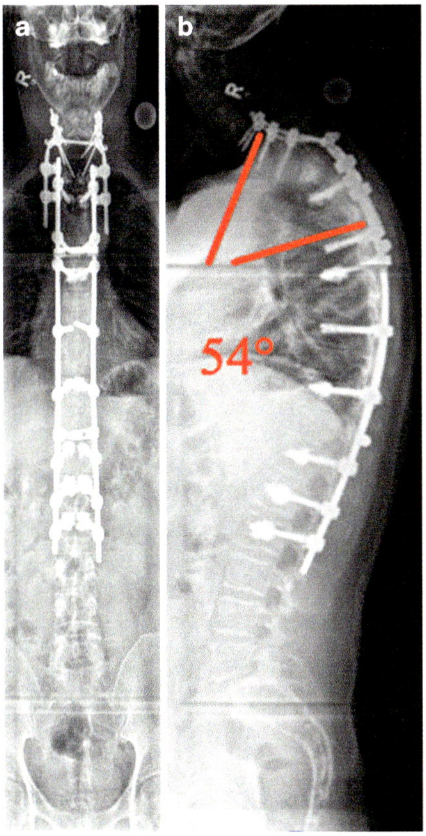

Fig. 78.4 (**a**, **b**) After reduction and neuronavigated stabilization with incomplete VCR T2 with pedicle screws C6/7 to T3

78.3 Discussion of the Case

Conservative treatment of posttraumatic kyphosis could be a choice in cases of mild deformity. However, in the long run success rates are significantly lower in conservative treatment (27%) [3].

In the case of persistant or increasing pain with concomitant kyphotic changes a surgical treatment is recommended. Especially in older people with osteoporotic bone the risk of implant failure and adjacent level problems is crucial.

An important type of postoperative sagittal decompensation, especially after long spinal correction surgery, is the PJK. A uniform definition of the PJK does not exist until today. The most reliable diagnostical method is the measurement of the angle between the lower end plate of the uppermost instrumented vertebra (UIV) and the upper end plate of the vertebra two level above (according to Cobb). (Fig. 78.7) [7, 17, 24, 25].

The reported revision rates due to a PJK range from 13–55% [16]. When operative therapy is required, it usually involves decompression of neural structures, dorsal shortening to restore the spinal alignment and stabilization and fusion. If the spine is flexible, a stable vertebral body

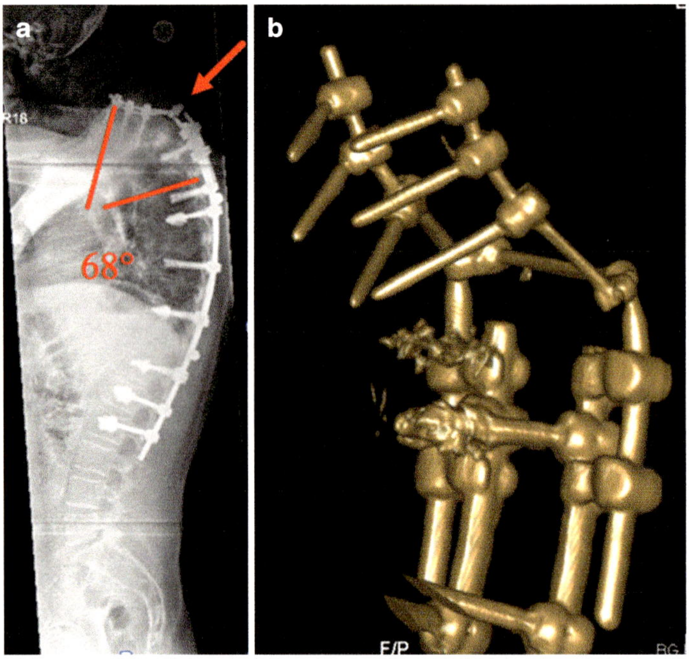

Fig. 78.5 (**a**, **b**) 12 months after revision surgery there is a rod breakage with a loss of correction C6-T3 with significant kyphosis (Cobb- angle C6-T3: 68°). (**b**) shows breakage of the left transition rod

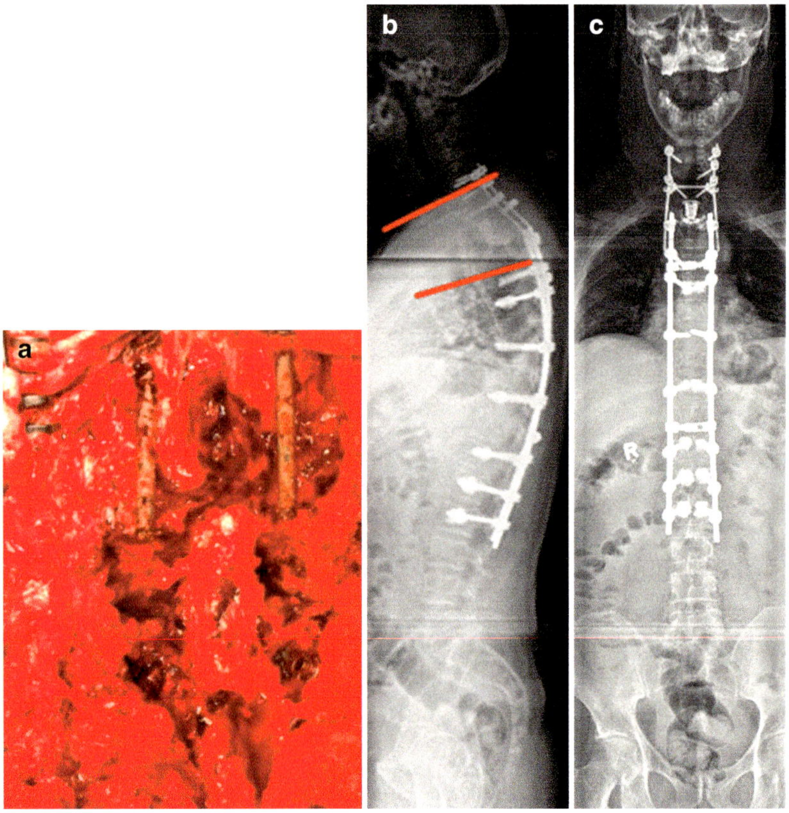

Fig. 78.6 (**a**) Intraoperative situs of vertebral column resection T2 and partial T1, visible are the decompressed dural sac, the CoChr rods and the pedicle screws C6; C7 and T1. (**b, c**) Final result after revision surgery with vertebral column resection T2 and partial resection T1, with costotransversectomies 1st and 2nd rib and additional vertebral body replacement T2 with an extendable titanium cage were performed

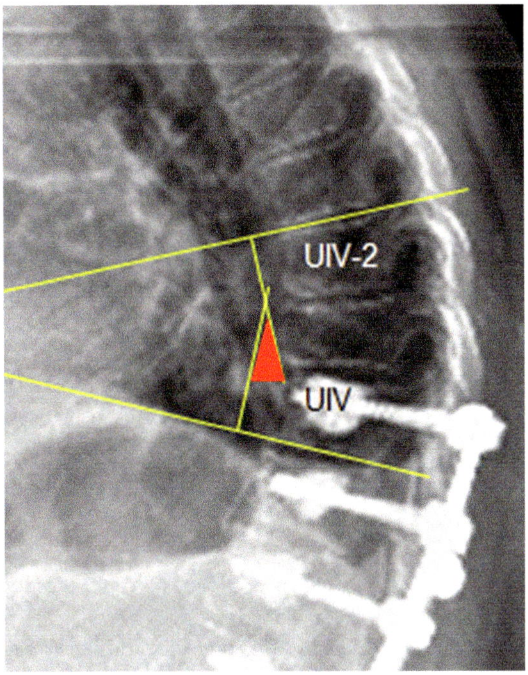

Fig. 78.7 Measurement method for determining the proximal junctional angle (red triangle) from the base plate of the uppermost instrumented vertebra (UIV) to the upper endplate of the 2-segment cranial vertebra (UIV-2). The definition PJK involves the presence of 2 criteria: 1. At least 10 ° kyphosis of the proximal junctional angle, 2. Proximal junctional angle >10 ° greater in comparison to the preoperative measurement

should be found cranial to the upper instrumented vertebra. If the spine is rigid, Ponte's corrective osteotomy or a PSO should be performed to reconstruct the global alignment.

In the literature there are different definitions of a PJK after adolescent deformity correction: varying between at least 10° [4], more than 15° in the 2 vertebrae above the UIV [10] or 20° between UIV2 and UIV [20].

It is generally assumed that PJK usually remains asymptomatic, but a proportion of about 3–4% suffers from symptoms that require follow-up stabilization [18].

Yagi et al. could establish a direct correlation between the extent of PJK (Cobb angle) and pain and an inverse correlation with function [24]. The PJK is a progressive change that usually begins within the first postoperative year and is still detectable 2 years after index surgery. Two thirds of all PJK occur within 3 months of a spinal adult deformity correction [24].

A classification by severity was prepared by the International Spine Study Group (ISSG) and the Hart working group. Six different relevant components were integrated: neurological deficit, local pain, instrumentation problems, changes in kyphosis, integrity of the posterior ligament complex, fracture localization, and the level of UIV [5].

This scoring system (Hart-ISSG PJK Severity Scale) has demonstrated good reliability and reproducibility compared to others. A score of 7 or more leads to the recommendation of a revision operation. One can distinguish surgical, patient-related and radiographic risk factors for the PJK. Patient-dependent risk factors include higher age, reduced mineral salt content of bone, and increased BMI [2, 19]. In all studies uniform correlation with age (> 55 years) [2, 13, 14, 16] and with poor bone quality [24] was found.

Some authors consider patient-dependent unpredictable predisposing factors for PJK to be pre-operative thoracic kyphosis >40° [12, 15].

The type of surgical procedure may correlate with the risk for PJK. Dorsoventral stabilization appears to be associated with an increased rate of PJK. Here, the risk is about 3 times higher to develop a PJK compared to the purely posterior-supplied patient group [11, 12, 23].

Extent of sagittal correction: The more aggressive the correction, the greater the risk of a PJK. Why this happens is unclear. Patients who had a LL closer to PI after their correction had a higher risk to develop a PJK compared to patients whose LL was much lower than PI [14, 15].

The fact that the extent of the correction is associated with the probability of decompensation in the adjacent segment is confirmed by a study by Maruo et al. In his research, he found that a correction of LL by more than 30° was associated with a significantly higher rate of PJK (58% vs 28%). Kim et al. estimated a correction of greater than 40° for PJK risk [12, 15].

The design of thoracic kyphosis in interaction with the LL seems to play a major role in the development of a adjacent level problem. A non-ideal global sagittal alignment (GSA)

(TK + LL + PI>45°) has been reported by Yagi [24] to a 70% risk of a PJK. A complete correction of the spine to a normal level with an SVA = 0 is obviously not ideal for all patients. In particular older people should be corrected more restrained. Examinations of symptom-free volunteers showed that the SVA increases with age [22].

The type of fixation systems (whether pedicle screws or lamina hooks are used) may influence the incidence of PJK. Helgeson compared lamina hooks alone against pedicle screws alone, as well as combinations of both, and found that the highest prevalence of PJK was in the pedicle screw group [9].

Other authors found similar results [8, 15].

The reason for these results could be the more aggressive preparation of the muscles and injury of ligamentous structures, which is necessary for placing pedicle screws. In addition, laminar hook systems appear to have lower stiffness compared to more rigid pedicle screw rod systems. In a biomechanical animal model, the main mobility in pedicle screws takes place directly in the cranially adjacent segment, while this is distributed more widely in laminar hook systems [27]. The stability of the spine in flexion is critically dependent on an intact dorsal ligament complex. Biomechanical studies have shown that resection of the interspinous and supraspinous ligaments significantly reduces flexion stability [28]. Iatrogenic injury to the posterior ligament complex or adjacent facet joints may be one of the possible reasons for PJK [1]. In addition, an affection of the autochthonous muscles at the highest instrumented level may contribute to the development of a PJK. Whether the use of percutaneous screw-rod systems in the upper part of multilevel stabilization lowers the incidence of PJK remains to be worked out. The level of the UIV is another critically discussed point. A significantly higher incidence of PJK is observed when fixation is stopped at T3 compared to T4 (53% vs 12.5%) In addition, instrumentation T2-6 in the upper area of the thoracic spine showed a higher incidence of PJK than instrumentation in the lower thoracic and upper lumbar spine [4]. This may be explained by the fact that more upper fixations are more likely to damage the facets and that predisposing the transition from rigid thoracic to the more mobile cervical spine is a PJK [21]. PJK in the upper thoracic spine is more prone to subluxation and dorsal tension band failure and occurs later, while lower thoracic spine is more likely to have vertebral fractures in an earlier time frame after instrumentation [10, 17]. A cement augmentation of the UIV should prevent compression fractures and implant failure [6]. To date, it is unclear whether the length of the construct plays a role. Both many instrumented vertebrae and short instrumentation were accused of being risk factors [2, 12].

The presence of a previous kyphosis and an increased preoperative proximal junctional angle seems predisposing to the onset of PJK. Most likely it is a multifactorial genesis, with a variety of possible risk factors.

78.4 Conclusions and Take Home Message

Especially older patients after surgical spinal correction frequently develop problems in the proximal adjacent segments. PJK in the upper thoracic spine seems to be mainly a type of subluxation and dorsal tension band failure and occurs later, while lower thoracic spine is more likely to have vertebral fractures in an earlier time frame after instrumentation. There are some strategies for avoiding a PJK. One is the reduction of the construct stiffness, it might be important to use laminar hooks on the upper thoracic vertebrae rather than pedicle screws. In addition one should avoid any damage to the dorsal soft tissues and adjacent facet joints. The upper instrumented vertebra should be chosen carefully, one should try to extend the fusion to segments with segmental kyphosis greater than 5°. It is well known that stopping the fixation in spinal transition zones leads to early PJK. In case of poor bone density, the screw augmentation with bone cement especially in the end vertebrae might be helpful to improve the pull out strength and decrease the rate of implant failure. Another important fact is that an optimal spinal balance and good postoperative alignment should be created in any spinal correction to reduce the risk of adjacent segment problems. It remains unclear, whether this rule ist true for older people with lower SVA as well. Several studies showed a correlation between the extent of correction and the prevalence of PJK.

Pearls

- To prevent implant failure in osteoporotic spine surgery, the use of bone cement for the augmentation of the pedicle screws is useful
- Use screws in suitable diameter and length- at least 80% of pedicle width and anterior third of the vertebral body
- Use more fixation points to improve construct stability
- The uppermost instrumented vertebra should be horizontal; don't stop in a junctional zone, include the apex of the kyphosis
- To lower the risk of PJK, try not to harm adjacent facet joints or ligamentous structures
- Creation of sufficient global balance seems to be an important cofactor in the prevention of PJK
- To reduce tendency of PJK, prevent biomechanical corrective stress to the uppermost pedicle screws

References

1. Anderson AL, McIff TE, Asher MA, Burton TC, Smooth RC. The effect of posterior thoracic spine anatomical structures on motion segment flexion stiffness. Spine. 2009;34:441–6.
2. Bridwell KH, Lenke LG, Cho SK, et al. Proximal junctional kyphosis in primary adult deformity surgery. Neurosurgery. 2013;72:899–906.
3. Farcy JP, Schwab FJ. Management of flatback and related kyphotic decompensation syndromes. Spine. 1997;22(20):2452–7.
4. Glattes RC, Bridwell KH, Lenke LG, Kim YJ, Rinella A, Edwards C II. Proximal junctional kyphosis in adult spinal sdeformity following long instrumented posterior spinal fusion: incidence, outcomes, and risk factor analysis. Spine. 2005;30:1643–9.
5. Hart R, Bess S, Burton DC, et al. Proximal junctional failure (PJF). AFS/CNS section: disorders of the spine and peripheral nerves; 2013a; Phoenix, AZ.
6. Hart RA, Prendergast MA, Roberts WG, Nesbit GM, Barnwell SL. Proximal junctional acute collapse cranial to multi-level lumbar fusion: a cost analysis of prophylactic vertebral augmentation. Spine J. 2008;8:875–81.
7. Hart R, McCarthy I, O'Brien M, et al. Identification of decision criteria for revision surgery among patients with proximal junctional failure following surgical treatment for spinal deformity. Spine. 2013b;38:E1223–7.
8. Hassanzadeh H, Gupta S, Jain A, El Dafrawy MH, Skolasky RL, Kebaish KM. The proximal fusion level has a significant effect on the incidence of proximal junctional kyphosis and outcome in adults after long posterior spinal fusion. Spine Deform. 2013;1:299–305.
9. Helgeson MD, Shah SA, Newton PO, et al. Evaluation of proximal junctional kyphosis in adolescent idiopathic scoliosis following pedicle screw, hook, or hybrid instrumentation. Spine (Phila Pa 1976). 2010;35:177–81.
10. Hostin R, McCarthy I, O'Brien M, et al. Incidence, mode, and location of acute proximal junctional failures after surgical treatment of adult spinal deformity spine. Phila Pa 1976. 2013;38:1008–15.
11. Kim HJ, Yagi M, Nguyen J, Cunningham ME, Boachie-Adjei O. Combined anterior-posterior surgery is the most important risk factor for developing proximal junctional kyphosis in idiopathic scoliosis. Clin Orthop Relat Res. 2012;470:1633–9.
12. Kim YJ, Bridwell KH, Lenke LG, et al. Proximal junctional kyphosis in adolescent idiopathic scoliosis f12. ollowing segmental posterior spinal instrumentation and fusion: minimum 5-year follow-up. Spine. 2005;30:2045–50.
13. Kim YJ, Bridwell KH, Lenke LG, Smooth CR, Rhim S, Cheh G. Proximal junctional kyphosis in adult spinal deformity after segmental posterior spinal instrumentation and fusion: minimum five-year follow-up. Spine (Phila Pa 1976). 2008;33:2179–84.
14. Kim HJ, Bridwell KH, Lenke LG, et al. Patients with proximal junctional repair surgery have higher postoperative lumbar lordosis and larger sagittal balance corrections. Spine (Phila Pa 1976). 2014;39:E576–80.
15. Kim YJ, Lenke LG, Bridwell KH, et al. Proximal junctional kyphosis in adolescent idiopathic scoliosis after 3 different types of posterior segmental spinal instrumentation and fusion: incidence and risk factor analysis of 410 cases. Spine (Phila Pa 1976). 2007;32:2731–8.
16. Lau D, Funao H, Clark AJ, Nicholls F, Smith J, Bess S, Shaffrey C, Schwab FJ, Lafage V, Deviren V, Hart R, Kebaish KM, Ames CP, International Spine Study Group. The Clinical Correlation of the Hart-ISSG Proximal Junctional Kyphosis Severity Scale With

Health-Related Quality-of-Life Outcomes and Need for Surgery Revision. Spine. 2016;41:213–23.
17. Maruo K, Ha Y, Inoue S, et al. Predictive factors for proximal junctional kyphosis in long fusions to the sacrum in adult spinal deformity. Spine. 2013;38:E1469–76.
18. McClendon J Jr, O'Shaughnessy BA, Sugrue PA, et al. Techniques for surgical correction of proximal junctional kyphosis of the upper thoracic spine. Spine (Phila Pa 1976). 2012;37:292–303.
19. O'Leary PT, Bridwell KH, Lenke LG, et al. Risk factors and outcomes for catastrophic failures at the top of long pedicle screw constructs: a matched cohort analysis performed at a single center. Spine. 2009;34:2134–9.
20. O'Shaughnessy BA, Bridwell KH, Lenke LG, et al. Does a long-fusion "T3-sacrum" portend a worse outcome than a short-fusion "T10-sacrum" in primary surgery for adult scoliosis? Spine (Phila Pa 1976). 2012;37:884–90.
21. Smooth RC, Bridwell KH, Lenke LG, Kim YJ, Rinella A, Edwards C II. Proximal junctional kyphosis in adult spinal deformity following long-instrumented posterior spinal fusion: incidence, outcomes, and risk factor analysis. Spine. 2005;30:1643–9.
22. Vedantam R, Lenke LG, Keeney JA, Bridwell KH. Comparison of standing sagittal alignment in asymptomatic adolescents and adults. Spine. 1998;23:211–5.
23. Wang J, Zhao Y, Shen B, et al. Risk factor analysis of proximal junctional kyphosis after posterior fusion in patients with idiopathic scoliosis. Injury. 2010;41:415–20.
24. Yagi M, King AB, Boachie-Adjei O. Incidence, risk factors, and natural course of proximal junctional kyphosis: surgical Outcomes review of adult idiopathic scoliosis: minimum 5 years follow-up. Spine. 2012;37:1479–89.
25. Yagi M, Akilah KB, Boachie-Adjei O. Incidence, risk factors and classification of proximal junctional kyphosis: surgical outcomes review of adult idiopathic scoliosis. Spine. 2011;36:E60–8.
26. Kim HJ, Bridwell KH, Lenke LG, et al. Proximal junctional kyphosis results in inferior SRS pain subscores in adult deformity patients. Spine. 2013;38:896–901.
27. Thawrani DP, Glos DL, Coombs MT, Bylski-Austrow DI, Sturm PF. Transverse process hooks at upper instrumented vertebra provide more gradual motion transition than pedicle screws. Spine. 2014;39(14):E826–32.
28. Cammarata M, Aubin C-É, Wang X, Mac-Thiong J-M. Biomechanical risk factors for proximal junctional kyphosis. Spine. 2014;39(8):E500–7.

Postoperative C5 palsy

79

David Rodríguez-Rubio and Jesús Lafuente

79.1 Introduction

This case will detail postoperative C5 palsy, a decrease of more than one grade of deltoid and/or biceps muscle power measured using the manual muscle test that happens after a cervical surgical procedure [1]. Its occurrence after cervical surgery is well documented, more frequently in posterior than in anterior procedures. Leading not just to muscle weakness, but to brachialgia and numbness of the upper limbs, C5 palsy can add a significant burden upon patients' quality of life and upon healthcare systems during the postoperative recovery period. The period of onset of C5 palsy can varied from immediately to 2 months after surgery.

Recent meta-analyses [2, 3] of C5 palsy after posterior cervical decompression report an estimated incidence around 6%. This value varies depending on the performed technique [4], being less common in laminoplasties (specially in double-door type) than in laminectomies (level of evidence:3).

D. Rodríguez-Rubio (✉) · J. Lafuente
Servicio de Neurocirugía, Hospital del Mar, Universidad de Barcelona, Barcelona, Spain

79.2 Case Description

A 40 y/o male carpenter was referred to the neurosurgery clinics by his general practitioner because of gait impairment progressing during the previous 4 months. He complained of neck pain and told symptoms consistent with urinary urgency during that period of time as well. As significant past medical history he suffered of non-insulin dependent diabetes, hypertension and dyslipidemia, and had a severe head injury 3 years before.

On examination, a broad-based unsteady gait was noticed, drifting towards the right side. Lhermitte and bilateral Hoffmann signs were observed, with tetraspasticity and clonus impairing mainly the right limbs.

MRI of the cervical spine (C-spine, Fig. 79.1) showed severe degenerative spondylotic changes from C2 to C6 segments, more evident at the C3/C4 and C4/C5 levels. The spinal cord was significantly compressed at these two levels, showing myelomalacia. A bilateral reduction of the width at the C3/C4 and C4/C5 foramina (and at the left C5/C6 foramen) was also reported. The radiological pictures showed a loss of the physiological cervical lordosis and a mild scoliotic component as well.

With the diagnosis of cervical spondylotic myelopathy, surgical treatment was proposed and performed in the form of C3 to C5 laminectomy (Bonescalpel/Misonix® was

B. Meyer, M. Rauschmann (eds.), *Spine Surgery*, https://doi.org/10.1007/978-3-319-98875-7_79

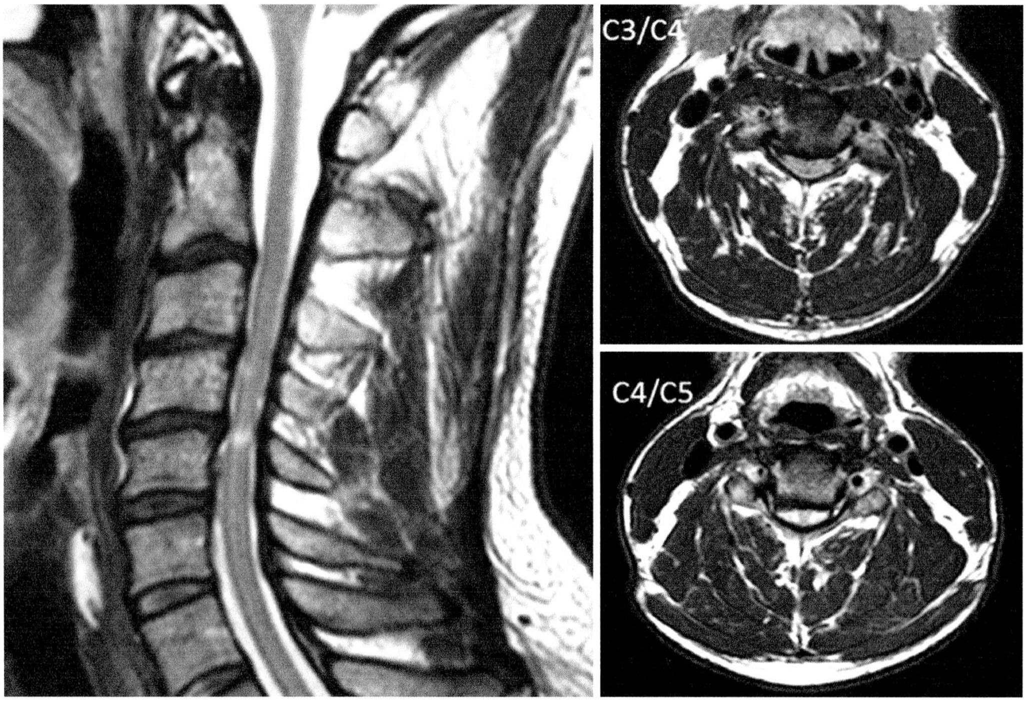

Fig. 79.1 C-spine preoperative MRI: sagital and axial T2 secuences

used to cut at the junction between laminae and lateral masses) with lateral masses screw fixation. During the procedure, intraoperative neurophysiological monitoring showed a significant decrease in the amplitude of the motor evoked potentials (MEP) on both sides (mainly on the right one, where they were almost lost) as the laminectomy was carried out. MEP were recovered on the left side at the end of the intervention, but not on the right one. Evoked somatosensory potentials were normal during the procedure.

On the second postoperative day a 1–2/5 paresis (Medical Research Council scale) on the abduction of both shoulders was noticed. Postoperative C-spine X rays (Fig. 79.2), CT (Fig. 79.3) and MRI (Fig. 79.4) were done, showing satisfactory C3-C5 vertebral canal decompression and position of the fixation implants. Specific muscle strength rehabilitation was started on the patient after postoperative radiological tests and after hospital discharge.

The 3 months follow-up showed an almost complete recovery of the power and tone of the left shoulder, but with 2/5 paresis of the right deltoid muscle and pain in the right C5 dermatome. Electromyogram (EMG) at that time showed bilateral C5 and C6 root lesion with moderate/severe motor axonal degeneration mainly on the right side, where marked signs of acute denervation, and no evidence of reinnervation in the motor units of the right infraspinatus muscle were noticed.

Nearly 18 months after the surgical procedure, the clinical and functional recovery of both shoulders was almost complete. EMG showed then a significant improvement in comparison to the previous one, with signs of reinnervation in all the explored muscles, but still with impairment on both C5 myotomes.

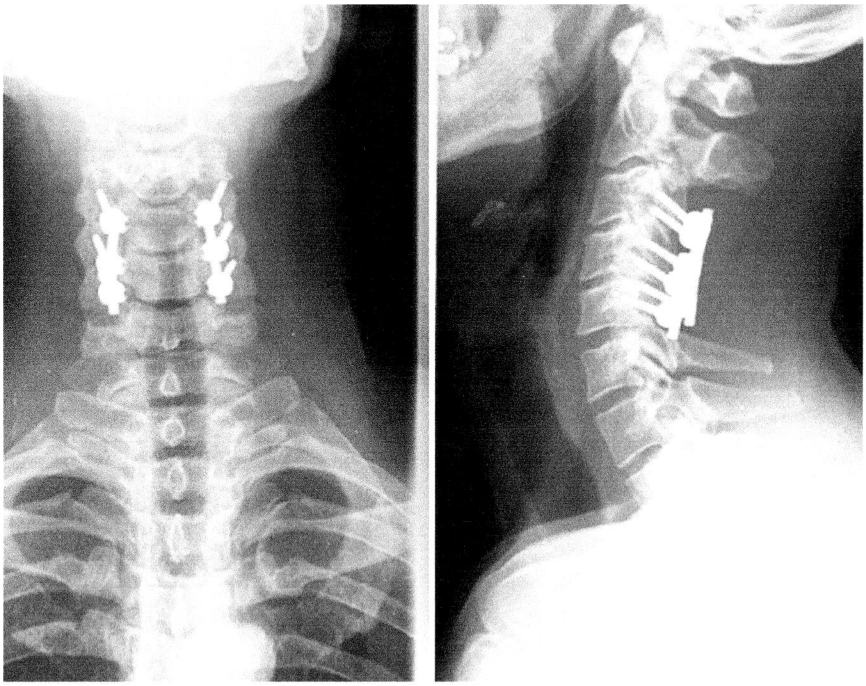

Fig. 79.2 C-spine postoperative Xrays

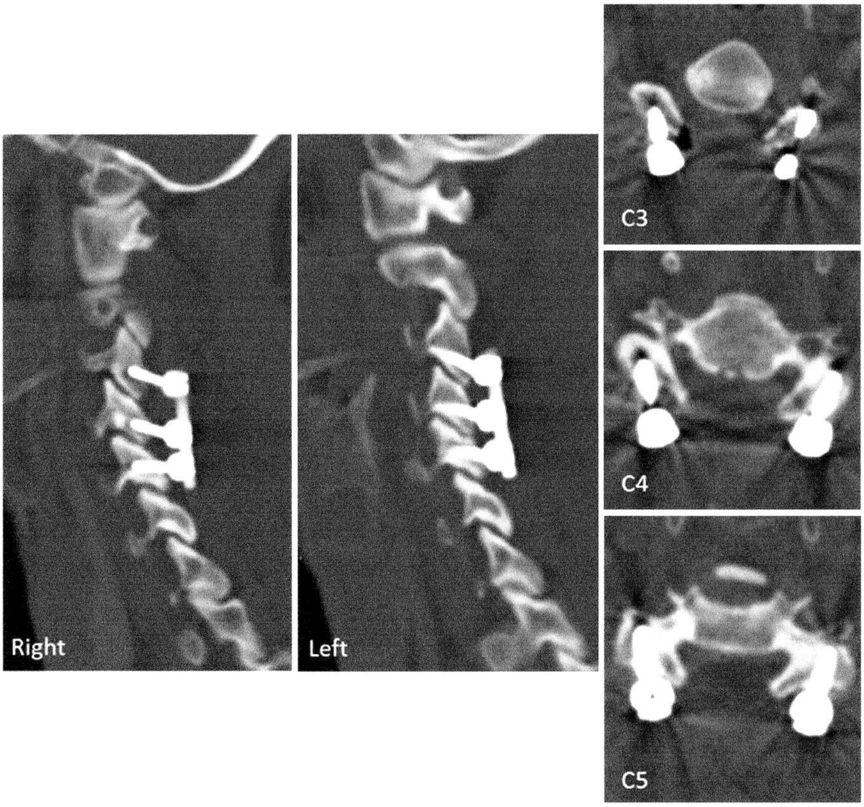

Fig. 79.3 C-spine postoperative CT scan

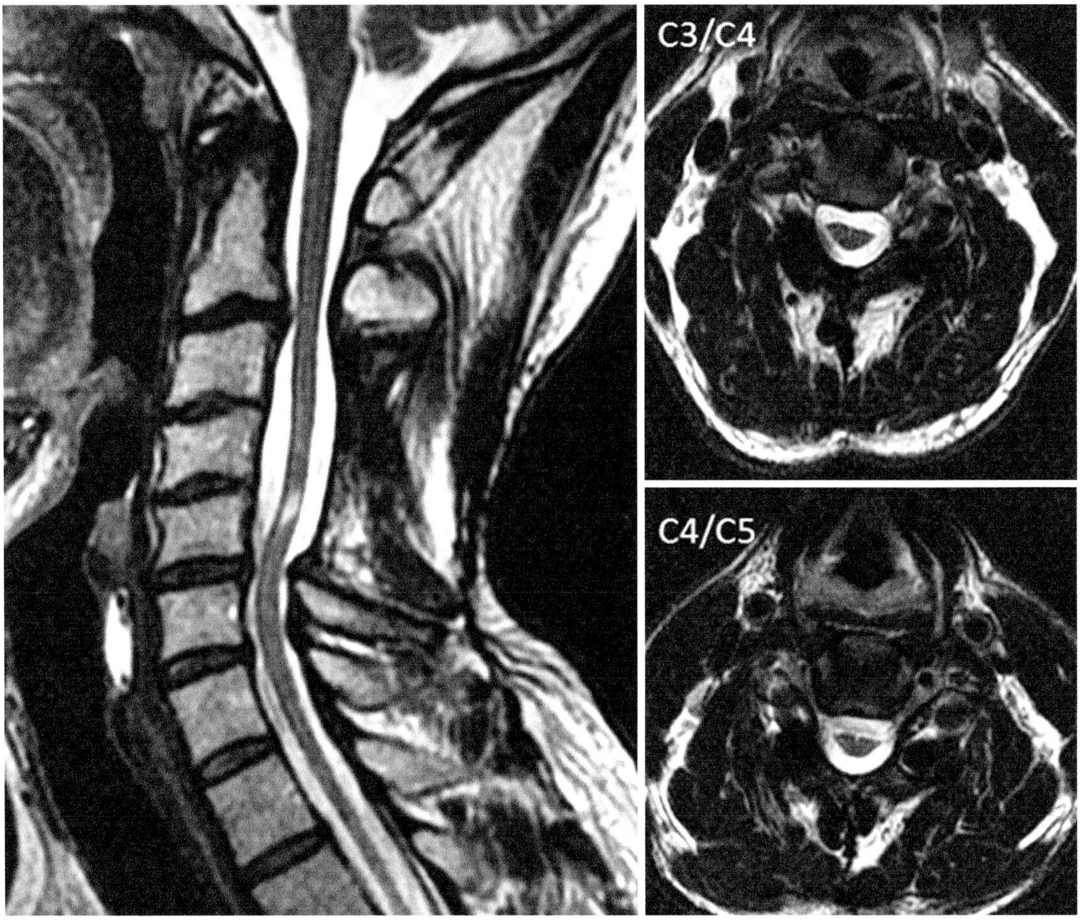

Fig. 79.4 C-spine postoperative MRI. A significant right C4/C5 persistent foraminal stenosis can be noticed on the axial T2 sequence

79.3 Discussion of the Case

The etiology of postoperative C5 palsy is poorly understood, having been suggested several hypothesis, some of them inconclusive or even conflicting. The most possible underlying pathologic mechanisms of this palsy include intraoperative nerve root injury, nerve root traction, segmental spinal cord disorder and ischemia/reperfusion injury of the spinal cord [5]. Nerve root traction (the so called "tethering effect") has been considered the most acceptable of all these proposed mechanism of postoperative C5 palsy. The posterior drift of the spinal cord after posterior cervical decompression occurs at its peak at the C5 vertebral level because C5 is the apex of the cervical lordosis. In addition, the superior articular process of C5 protudes in a more anterior direction, and C5 roots are shorter when compared with other levels, being therefore more sensitive to the tension created by a posterior shift. Systematic reviews have showed that the posterior shift in patients with C5 palsy is significantly larger than that observed in patients without palsy.

79.3.1 Risk Factors

Ossification of the posterior longitudinal ligament (OPLL), narrower intervertebral foramen, laminectomy (vs. open-door laminoplasty), excessive spinal cord drift and male gender have been identified as significant risk factors of C5 palsy [2, 6].

OPLL is a significant risk factor of postoperative C5 palsy compared with cervical spondylotic myelopathy and other cervical degenerative conditions. Presumably, the ossified hypertrophic posterior longitudinal ligament increases the spinal cord shifting and tethering effect on the C5 nerve root.

A significant preexisting foraminal stenosis at C4/C5 has been shown in patients with preoperative C5 palsy. The width of the C5 intervertebral foramen (both on palsy and normal sides) has been noticed significantly smaller in patients with C5 palsy, with also greater anterior protusion of the C5 superior articular process in them. Therefore, several studies have recommended prophylactic bilateral foraminotomy to prevent C5 palsy.

Cervical laminectomy have been compared with laminoplasty in several studies and meta-analyses [2–4]. The results have shown a significant higher incidence of C5 palsy in the laminectomy group. Laminectomy removes the intact posterior arch of the vertebra, thus providing an excessive space for the spinal cord to shift posteriorly. When comparing incidence of C5 palsy in open-door and double-door laminoplasties, it has been pointed that in patients who underwent open-door laminoplasty (especially in those with OPLL), the spinal cord was prone to rotate due to asymmetrical decompression, resulting in tethering of the nerve root on the open side. A pooled incidence of 3.1% of C5 palsy has been reported in double-door laminoplasty, vs. 4.3% in open-door laminoplasty and 11.3% in patients who underwent laminectomy [2]. On the other hand, cervical laminectomy with instrumented fusion achieves wider decompression and avoidance of kyphotic change and axial neck pain, which are common complications of laminoplasty. There are controversies over whether intraoperatively correction of the cervical lordotic alignment through posterior instrumentation (causing iatrogenic foraminal stenosis and excessive posterior shifting of the spinal cord) has an effect on the occurrence of C5 palsy.

Several studies have shown that the posterior shift in patients with C5 palsy is significantly larger than that in patients without palsy. For this reason, it has been suggested a limited decompression to avoid excessive posterior shifting of the spinal cord.

79.4 Conclusions and Take Home Message

79.4.1 Prevention and Treatment

Prophylactic bilateral partial foraminotomy is one of the most reported preventive methods to reduce the incidence of postoperative C5 palsy [7]. Narrowing the width of the laminectomy can also prevent the spinal cord from shifting excessively and reduce this incidence as well [8]. When performing laminoplasties, an open angle between 15° and 30° should be maintained also with this purpose. Some authors have hypothesized that intraoperative damage to the C5 nerve root may be caused by the heat generated by high-speed drills, and suggested therefore standard irrigation with cooled saline during bone drilling as a preventive maneuvre.

To date, the evidence-based treatment for postoperative C5 palsy is very limited. Most patients recover within a week to several months after conservative treatment including rest, muscle strength rehabilitation, hyperbaric oxygen therapy and/or immediate drug therapy with high-dose corticosteroids combined with dehydration therapy. Even further surgery can be required to ease the symptoms [2].

Pearls

- Prophylactic bilateral partial foraminotomy can reduce the incidence of postoperative C5 palsy

Editorial Comment

This chapter elaborates on a frequent and poorly understood complication after cervical spine surgery. I have in part a slightly different opinion than outlined here. I have come to consider the so called "C5 palsy" as a traction injury primarily and the avoidance of it starts with refraining from any traction on the shoulders of the patient. A major trial is recruiting patients to test this hypothesis.

References

1. Nakashima H, Imagama S, Yukawa Y, et al. Multivariate analysis of C5 palsy incidence after cervical posterior fusion with instrumentation. J Neurosurg Spine. 2012;17:103–10.
2. Gu YF, Cao P, Gao R, et al. Incidence and risk factors of C5 palsy following posterior cervical decompression: a systematic review. PLoS One. 2014;9:e101933.
3. Wang T, Wang H, Liu S, et al. Incidence of C5 nerve root after cervical surgery. A meta-analysis for last decade. Medicine (Baltimore). 2017;96(45):e8560.
4. Lee S-H, Suk K-S, Kang K-C, et al. Outcomes and related factors of C5 palsy following cervical laminectomy with instrumented fusion compared with laminoplasty. Spine. 2016;41:E574–9.
5. Sakaura H, Hosono N, Mukai Y, et al. C5 palsy after decompression surgery for cervical myelopathy. Spine. 2003;28:2447–51.
6. Kaneyama S, Sumi M, Kanatani T, et al. Prospective study and multivariate analysis of the incidence of C5 palsy after cervical laminoplasty. Spine. 2010;35:E1553–8.
7. Komagata M, Nishiyama M, Endo K, et al. Prophylaxis of C5 palsy after cervical expansive laminoplasty by bilateral partial foraminotomy. Spine J. 2004;4:650–5.
8. Radcliff KE, Limthongkul W, Kepler CK, Sidhu GDS, et al. Cervical laminectomy width and spinal cord drift are risk factors for postoperative C5 palsy. J Spinal Disord Tech. 2014;27(2):86–92.

Nonspinal Complications

80

Sandro M. Krieg

80.1 Introduction

The spectrum and complexity of spinal procedures vary widely and so does the rate of complications. While we all are well-trained in the management of spinal complications, such as dural tears, secondary hemorrhage, or wound infections, many of us are less experienced and trained in the management of the more infrequent non-spinal complications of spine surgeries. Arterial, venous, esophageal or bowel injury, hernias, ileus, sympathetic dysfunction or even vascular compression along with intraoperative hypoperfusion are complications many spine surgeon only know from courses or textbooks. If they occur, however, we all should be prepared to be able to provide the best management of this unplanned situation. Although quite rare for smaller spinal procedures, such as microdiscectomy, these complications increase in frequency along with the complexity and size of the approach and procedure. While for microdiscectomy these incidents are mostly case reports or such a rare complication, some ALIF series report vascular complications in up to 20% of cases [1]. Vice versa, the risk of misdiagnosing leading to no or improper management can be higher in smaller procedures since the surgeons is not prepared for it. Diagnosis can be delayed, sequelae become more severe, and consequences for the patients can get worse [2]. For instance, the two largest analyses of intraoperative arterial injury during microdiscectomy reported an associated mortality rate of 38% and 61% [3, 4].

Thus, the aim of this chapter is to provide an overview on the potential non-spinal complications, as well as their diagnosis and management. The presented cases provide a practical example of complications which are frequent or – on the other side – hard to imagine in order to prepare the reader for their potential occurrence:

1. Esophageal laceration along with anterior cervical spine surgery
   - Diagnosis & Management
   - Further potential complications of anterior cervical spine surgery
2. Vertebral artery injury during posterior cervical spine surgery
   - Diagnosis & Management
   - Vertebral artery injury during anterior cervical spine surgery
3. Segmental artery injury with pedicle screws
   - Diagnosis & Management
   - Further potential complications of pedicle screw placement
4. Urether injury during anterior lumbar surgery
   - Diagnosis & Management
   - Further potential complications of anterior lumbar surgery

S. M. Krieg (✉)
Department of Neurosurgery, Klinikum rechts der Isar, Technische Universität München, Munich, Germany
e-mail: Sandro.Krieg@tum.de

B. Meyer, M. Rauschmann (eds.), *Spine Surgery*, https://doi.org/10.1007/978-3-319-98875-7_80

5. Bowel injury after lumbar microdiscectomy
   - Diagnosis & Management
   - Further potential complications of lumbar microdiscectomy

80.2 Case Description and Discussion

80.2.1 Case 1: Esophageal Laceration Along with Anterior Cervical Spine Surgery

A 76 y/o male patient had cervical disc replacement in another hospital 2 years ago. He now presented with progressive myelopathy and paresthesia of bilateral C6 and C7 due to spinal and neuroforaminal stenosis C4-T1. Therefore, ACDF C4-T1 with anterior plating was done (Fig. 80.1a). Co-morbidities were osteoporosis, cardiac bypass 2 years ago, cardiac insufficiency NYHA III with CPR 2 years ago, and COPD Gold 3 with chronic steroid medication. Two months later, the patient presented with pain from ventral plate dislocation due to osteoporosis (Fig. 80.1b).

The patient received an anterior VBR C5-6-7 and then dorsal instrumentation. During dorsal instrumentation in prone position patient required CPR, surgery was not finished, After a long ICU stay with cardiac bare metal stenting, 6 weeks Aspirin & Clopidogrel, several medical complications, i.e. pneumonia and tracheotomy the VBR was dislocated (Fig. 80.2).

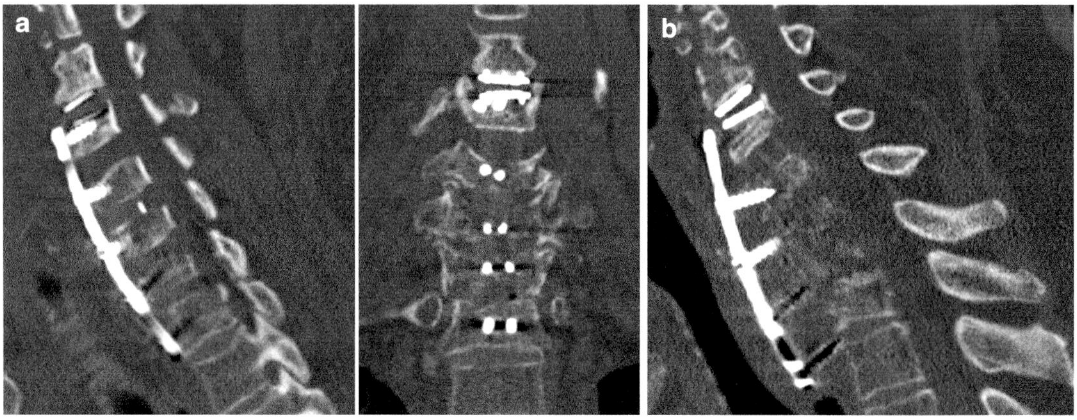

Fig. 80.1 CT scan after 1st surgery. This is the sagittal (**a**) and coronal (**b**) view from the postoperative CT scan after ACDF C4-T1 with anterior plating

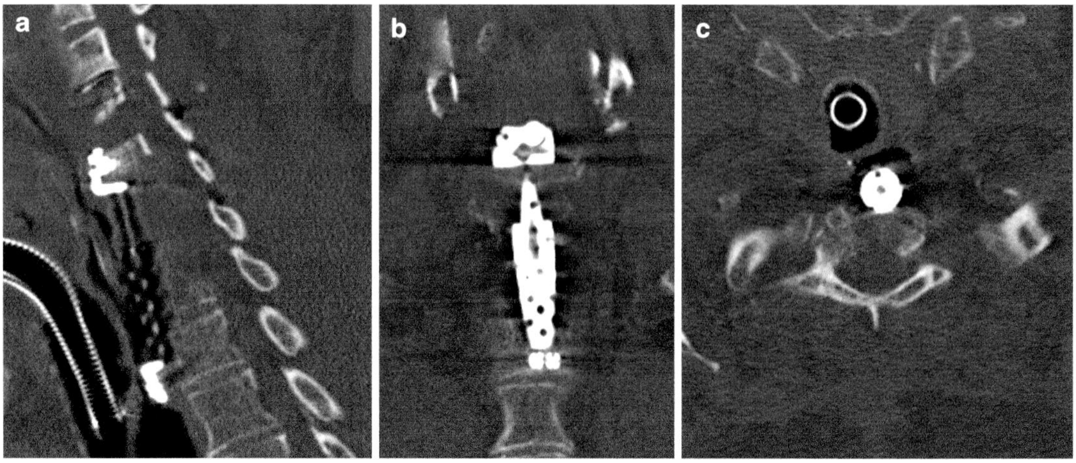

Fig. 80.2 CT scan after 2nd surgery and long-term ICU stay. This is the sagittal (**a**), coronal (**b**), and axial (**c**) view from the preoperative CT scan showing the dislocated VBR

The patient then underwent completion of the dorsal instrumentation and at the same day revision of the VBR (Fig. 80.3) during which an esophagus laceration was observed. The patient was trachotomized so conservative management was decided initially. However, he underwent another septic complication due to mediastinitis originating from the esophagus laceration.

Primary esophageal suture by a general surgeon with an additional sternocleidomastoid flap was performed, hardware was left in place despite anterior infection and long-term antibiotic treatment was done. At discharge, the neurological status was unchanged compared to the preoperative status and the final X-ray examination proved swallowing without any leakage (Fig. 80.4). Tracheostomy was removed during rehabilitation.

80.2.2 Case 1 Discussion

This case offers a large variety of aspects, which can be discussed:

1. Would initial 360°stabilization at first surgery have been indicated due to the comorbidities of the patient? (Please see Chaps. 3, 6, 7, and 87)
2. Would a conservative myelopathy management of the patient have been reasonable considering the comorbidities? (Please see Chap. 6)
3. Should the hardware been removed due to infection or left in place? (Please see Chap. 84)
4. Was the esophageal injury during revision surgery or due to dislocated hardware and just detected instead of caused by the surgeon?
5. How can we ensure early diagnosis of esophageal laceration in general?
6. How do we manage these lacerations?

While the issues of points 1–3 are discussed in other chapters of this book, we will focus on points 4–6.

Whether the esophageal injury was only detected rather than caused by the surgeon cannot be said for sure. Yet, the literature tells us that it is a not that rare complication, which can even be undetected at first. While postoperative dysphagia occurs in 9.5–67% of patients after anterior cervical spine surgery, actual esophageal perforation is reported to have an

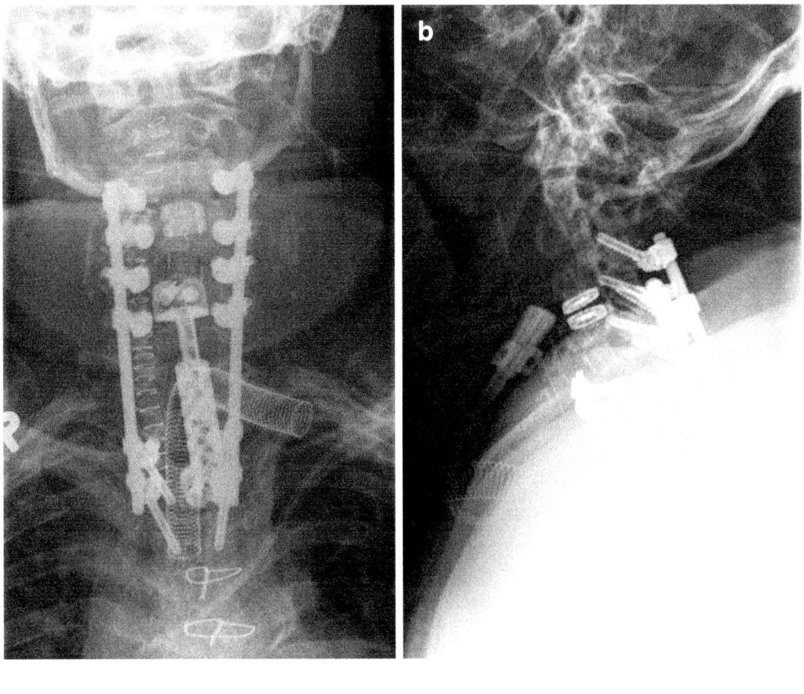

Fig. 80.3 X-rays after 360° fusion. This is the anterior-posterior (**a**) and lateral (**b**) X-ray after final revision with 360° fusion due to the dislocated VBR

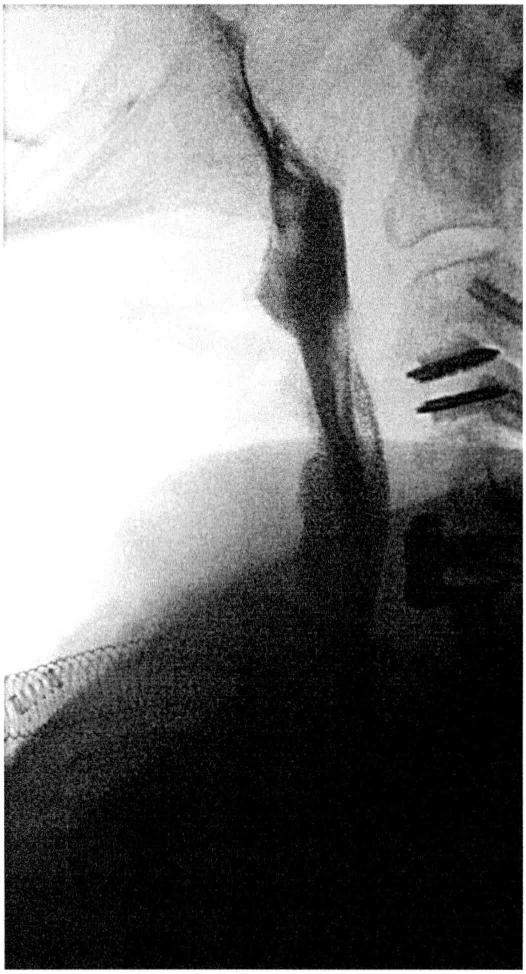

Fig. 80.4 Contrast dye swallow study. This lateral X-ray examination shows proper swallowing without any leakage at discharge. Tracheostomy is still in place

incidence of 0.2–1.52% of cases [5, 6]. If not detected, it can lead not only to dysphagia, but also to local infection, hardware failure, spondylodiscitis, mediastinitis, and sepsis with potentially fatal outcome. The incidence is higher for traumatic spine injury cases. Presenting symptoms are mostly multiple including dysphagia, fever, wound leakage, and swelling of the neck.

One systematic review analyzed 153 cases reported in 65 articles to further elucidate this topic. The authors found that the origin of esophageal damage was specified in 50% of cases. Out of these cases, the most frequent reason of was hardware failure (41%), such as plate or screw migration, or loosened plates or screws, followed by chronic erosion from the hardware (31%), and injury during surgery (19%) [6]. In our case, several of these most common causes were present, making it still hard to judge whether the esophageal damage was before or during revision surgery. The same review actually found the average time from causative surgery to diagnosis of esophageal damage to be 716.6 days (median 44.5 days, range 0 days to 18 years), which was analyzed in 121 patients. Yet, most of the early diagnosed cases (<30 days after surgery) were due to intraoperative injury [6]. Overall mortality rate in this study due to esophageal perforation and its sequelae was 3.9%. As soon as an esophageal perforation is suspected, further investigation is mandatory. The most commonly used modality is the contrast dye swallow study, which can, however, also be combined with a CT scan. Endoscopy is another option usually used when the esophageal therapy is being planned or if no leakage was found on the contrast dye swallow study but still suspected.

Depending on the local settings, esophageal repair is usually done in collaboration with otolaryngology, general, or thoracic surgery. For the further treatment, several options are at hand, varying from conservative treatment to primary suture to muscle flaps. In the recent literature analysis, 11% of cases were managed conservatively, while 34% of cases underwent primary suture and 55% received a muscle flap, most frequently using the sternocleidomastoid muscle (as in our case) but also others, such as pectoral, infrahyoid, omohyoid, latissimus dorsi, radial forearm, or longus colli muscle. Omental flaps and jejunum were also used [6]. In 96 reported patients, an average of 1.54 attempts to repair the laceration were required. 66% of patients (63 pts) only required one attempt. In the remaining, 21 out of 29 patients only showed successful closure after the anterior spinal implants were explanted. Likewise, complications of esophageal repair are quite common summing up to 12.4% including pneumonia, osteomyelitis, sepsis, and mediastinitis. The most common germ found were coagulase-positive Staphylococcus, Streptococcus, Pseudomonas, and Candida species. The published data on reported outcome is surprisingly good; 30 days after esophageal repair patient were capable of oral intake. Conservative treatment averaged to 68 days until oral nutrition.

Coming back to our case and having the long time between laceration and diagnosis in mind, it is crucial during anterior cervical spine surgery to inspect the esophagus at the end of surgery in order to detect any injury as early as possible. When detected, an interdisciplinary management is required. Depending on the size and location of injury, conservative management can be an option, especially when the inner part of the mucosa is still intact. Yet, as seen in our case, it harbors the risk of severe complications making these patients mandatory to be observed on an ICU. The majority of cases can actually be managed without hardware removal. If not successful, this plans needs to be subject of discussion, however. Concerning chronic erosive processes leading to delayed esophageal perforation, many risk factors contribute to this complex complication including nutritional state, hardware mass effect, smoking, diabetes, radiation to the neck, and potentially preexisting infection [6]. As in our case, the reconstruction via a sternocleidomastoid flap is the most standard approach do to its size and proximity to the potential perforation. The whole medial and lateral surface of the muscle is prepared and used as an inferiorly pedicled flap which is then placed between esophagus and cervical spine by suturing it to the contralateral prevertebral tissue [7].

To conclude this part, esophageal perforation is infrequent but quite serious and if detected early linked with a good outcome [6]. Thus, patients presenting with an untypical dysphagia (symptoms or duration) after an anterior cervical spine surgery should undergo a workup ruling out esophageal perforation.

Further potential complications of anterior cervical spine surgery are injuries to the vertebral artery (see case 2), the carotid artery including retracting-associated thrombosis or cerebral ischemia, tracheal injury with tension pneumothorax, mediastinitis, or sepsis, thoracic duct injury (dorsal to the subclavian vein), and injury to the cervical sympathetic chain causing Horner's syndrome.

80.2.3 Case 2: Vertebral Artery Injury During Cervical Spine Surgery

A 75 y/o female patient demonstrated progressive cervical myelopathy which did not get better or stopped progressing after previous laminectomy 1 year ago in another hospital. However, she also suffered from consecutive progressive neck pain. Indication for dorsal instrumentation (lateral mass plus navigated pedicle screws in C7), fusion and decompression of C2-7 was posed and performed. During drilling of right C2 pars screw brisk bleeding from the burr hole occurred and intraoperative laceration of the right vertebral artery at C2 with the drill was suspected. Packing with bone wax could control intraoperative bleeding and the patient underwent a postoperative CT angiography (Fig. 80.5a–c) followed by invasive digital subtraction angiography (DSA) (Fig. 80.5d).

The laceration was treated by a flow diverter and the patient woke up with no new neurological symptoms. 4 days later the patient complaint about a pulse-synchronous noise in the right neck. Another DSA was performed showing an arteriovenous shunt at C2 (Fig. 80.6a) leading to coiling and closure of the right vertebral artery (Fig. 80.6b).

The patient was discharged some days later with no new neurological symptoms but still

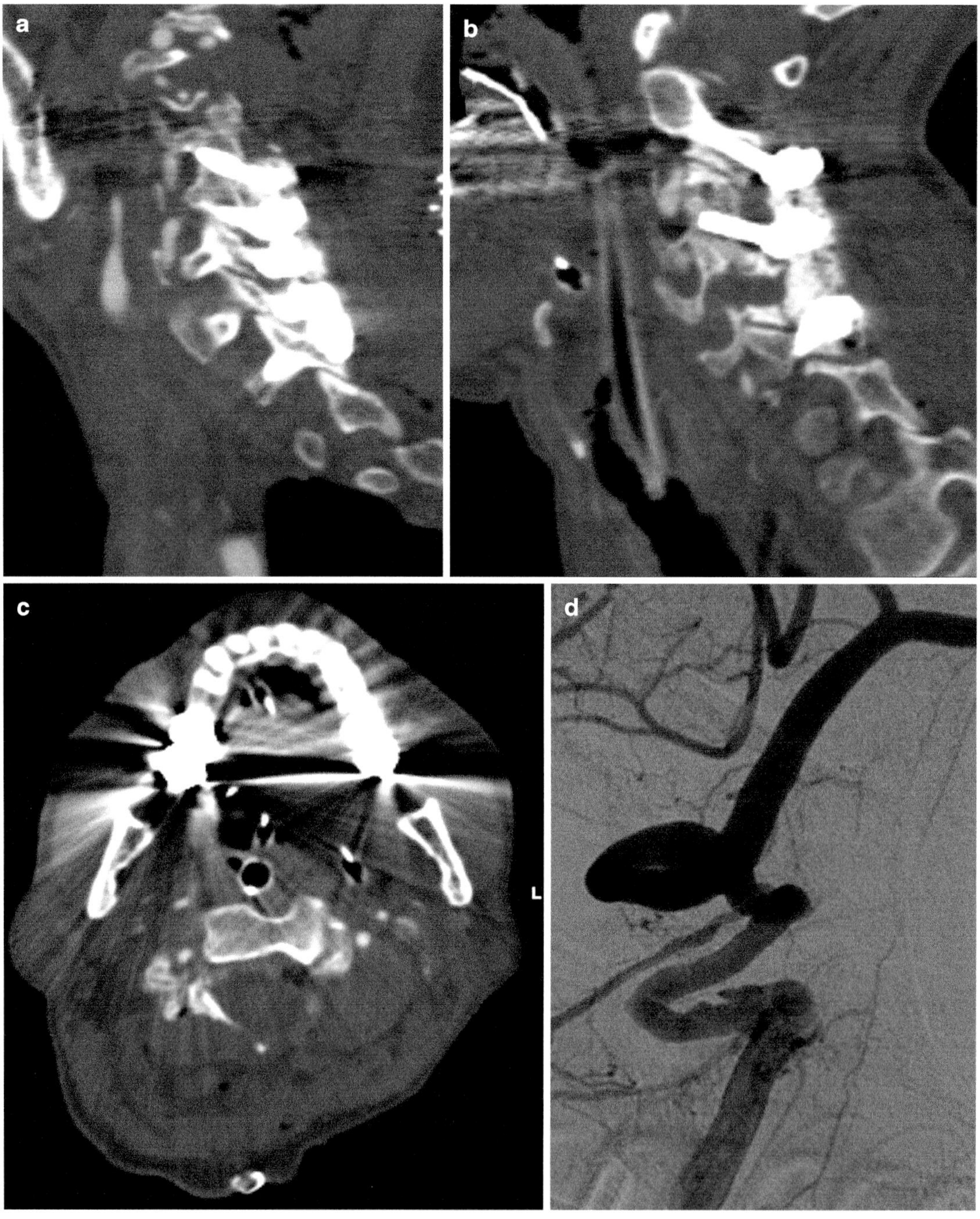

Fig. 80.5 Postoperative imaging of the right-sided VA laceration. These are the sagittal (**a, b**) and axial (**c**) images of the CT angiography plus digital subtraction angiography (**d**) showing the laceration and bleeding of the right-sided vertebral artery

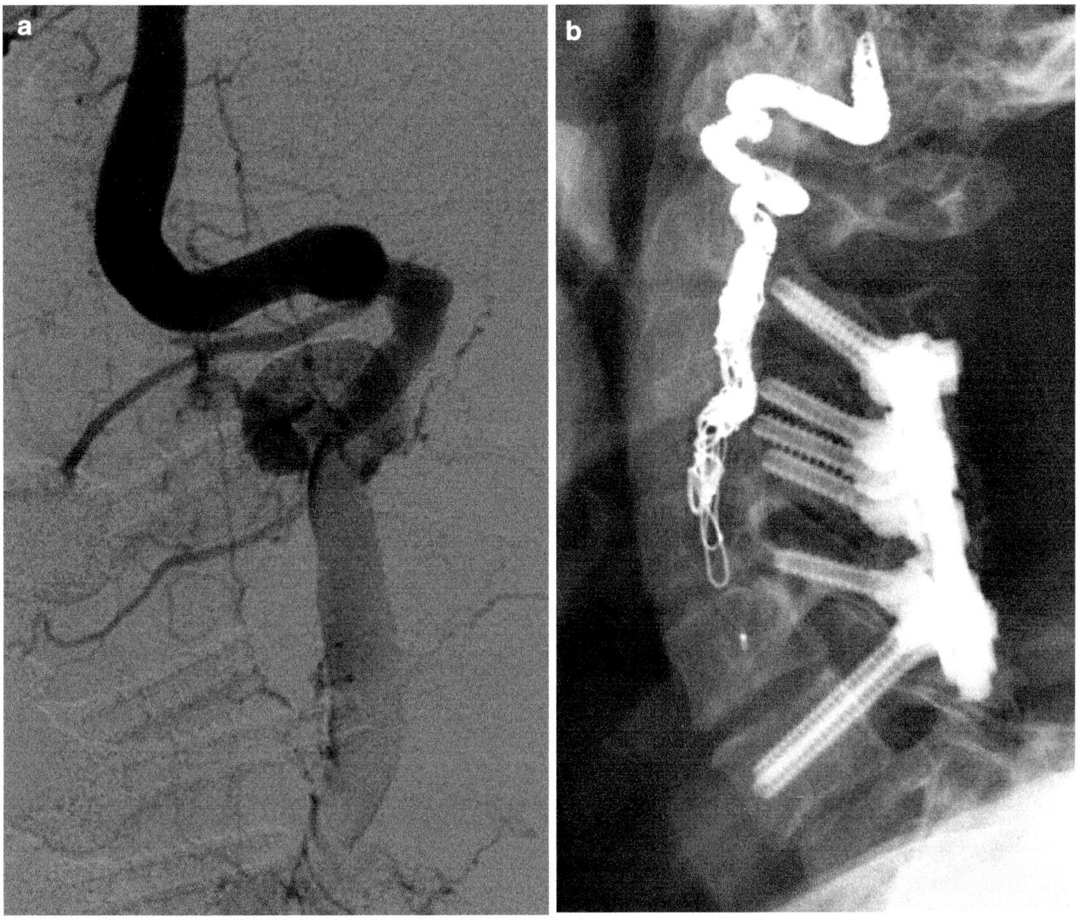

Fig. 80.6 Digital subtraction angiography 4 days later. The digital subtraction angiography performed 4 days later showed an arteriovenous shunt at C2 at the location of the flow diverter (**a**). After consultations, coiling of the right vertebral artery was decided and performed (**b**)

persisting neck pain. Finally, an aneurysm at the right femoral artery due to the angiography access required surgical resection by a vascular surgeon.

80.2.4 Case 2 Discussion

The vertebral artery is the structure most spine surgeons are most respectful of when operating the cervical spine. If vertebral artery injuries are not detected initially or even after treatment as in our case, arteriovenous fistulae and pseudoaneurysms are delayed complications. Most commonly, lacerations of the vertebral artery occur during C1–C2 transarticular screw fixation procedure, which can be in up to 4.1% of cases [8, 9]. This is just due to the proximity of the screw trajectory and the vertebral artery but also due to an irregular course of the vertebral artery at C2 [10]. Yet, most patients overcome this complication without developing any symptoms [9]. In general, the risk for subaxial vertebral artery injury in posterior instrumentation is low for lateral mass as well as pedicle screws (Table 80.1 and 80.2). As in our case, the risk is higher at C1 and C2 [8, 9].

While vertebral artery injury is reported to be significantly higher for cervical pedicle

Table 80.1 Procedural risks for cervical lateral mass and pedicle screws

			Periop complication						Late complication							
Authors & Year	No. of Pts	No. of screws (C3–7)	Nerve root injury	SCI	VA injury	Fx of lateral mass	Facetviolation	Malposition reacquired; removal	Screw loosening	Screw pullout	Screw breakage	Plate/rod breakage	Loss of reduction	Pseudarthrosis	Required Rev Op	ASD Requiring Op
LMS																
Heller et al. [58]	78	654	4 screws, 4 pts	0	0	NR	1 screw	4 screws, 4 pts	7 screws	1 screw, 1 pt	2 screws	1 pt	2 pts	1/71 pts	4 pts	2 pts
Fehlings et al. [56]	44	210	0	0	0	NR	NR	NR	8 screws, 5 pts	NR	NR	NR	3 pts	3/42 pts	3 pts	NR
Graham et al. [57]	21	164	3 screws, 3 pts	0	0	NR	NR	4 screws, 3 pts	0	0	0	0	NR	0	0	NR
Wellman et al. [72]	43	259	0	0	0	NR	NR	0	0	0	0	0	1 pt	1/35 pts	1 pt	1 pt
Sekhon [68]	143	1026	0	0	0	NR	8 screws	0	NR	6 screws, 3 pts	4 screws	1 pt	2 pts	NR	NR	1 pt
Pateder and Carbone [67]	29	198	NR	NR	NR	NR	NR	NR	NR	0	1 pt	0	1 pt	NR	0	NR
Wang and Levi [71]	18	77	0	0	0	NR	NR	NR	NR	0	0	0	NR	0	NR	NR
Wu et al. [73]	115	673	0	0	0	NR	NR	NR	NR	1 pt	0	0	1 pt	NR	0	NR
Katonis et al. [60]	225	1662	3 screws, 3 pts	0	0	27 screws	NR	3 screws, 3 pts	NR	3 pts	0	0	NR	6 pts	9 pts	0
Audat et al. [55]	50	405	0	NR	0	NR	4 screws	1 screw, 1 pt	NR	0	0	0	NR	NR	0	0
CPS																
Abumi et al. [76]	180	595	2 screws, 2 pts	0	1 screw, 1 pt	NR	NR	1 screw, 1 pt	0	0	NR	NR	0	1 pt	NR	NR
Neo et al. [66]	18	70	NR	0	0	NR	NR	NR	NR	NR	2 screws, 2 pts	NR	NR	NR	NR	NR
Kast et al. [59]	24	85	2 screws, 2 pts	NR	0	NR	NR	1 screw, 1 pt	NR	0	0	0	NR	0	NR	NR

Takahashi et al. [69]	13	37	0	0	0	NR	NR	0	NR	0	0	0	0	0	0	NR
Yoshimoto et al. [74]	52	264	0	0	0	NR	NR	NR	NR	NR	NR	NR	NR	NR	NR	NR
Yukawa et al. [75]	144	559	1 screw, 1 pt	0	1 screw, 1 pt	NR	NR	0	NR	1 pt	1 pt	NR	5 pts	NR	NR	NR
Liu et al. [63]	25	150	0	0	0	NR	NR	NR	0	0	0	0	0	NR	NR	NR
Miyamoto and Uno [64]	29	71	0	0	0	NR	NR	NR	NR	NR	NR	NR	NR	NR	NR	NR
Kotil and Ozyuvad [61]	10	70	0	0	0	NR	NR	0	NR	NR	NR	NR	NR	0	NR	NR
Tofuku et al. [70]	32	125	0	0	0	NR	NR	NR	NR	0	0	0	0	0	NR	NR
Lee et al. [62]	50	277	0	NR	0	NR	NR	NR	NR	NR	NR	NR	NR	NR	NR	NR
Nakashima et al. [65]	84	365	3 screws, 3 pts	0	2 screws, 2 pts	NR	NR	3 screws, 3 pts	5 screws, 5 pts	NR	3 screws, 3 pts	NR	2 pts	2 pts	1pt	1 pt

This it Table 3 from Yoshihara et al. [11] showing the review data on articles on the procedural risks associated with lateral mass and pedicle screws for instrumentation of the cervical spine [11]

Fx fracture, *NR* not reported, *rev* revision

Table 80.2 Early and late complications for cervical lateral mass and pedicle screws

Type of Complication	LMS	CPS	p Value
periop			
root injury	**0.19 (10/5130)**	**0.31 (8/2598)**	**0.47**
	1.36 (10/737)	1.24(8/643)	0.96
SCI	0 (0/687)	0 (0/569)	–
VA injury	**0 (0/5328)**	**0.15 (4/2668)**	**0.012**[a]
	0 (0/766)	0.61 (4/661)	0.046[a]
Fx of lateral mass	1.62 (27/1662)	NA	–
facet violation	0.62 (13/2085)	NA	–
malposition requiring postop rev/removal	**0.38 (12/3144)**	**0.29 (5/1711)**	**0.80**
	2.64 (11/417)	1.1 (5/455)	0.15
late			
screw loosening	**1.17 (15/1287)**	**0.45 (5/1110)**	**0.09**
	unknown	1.73 (5/289)	–
screw pullout	1.1 (8/722)	0.24 (1/418)	0.17[a]
screw breakage	unknown	176(6/340)	–
plate/rod breakage	0.28 (2/722)	0 (0/94)	1.00[a]
loss of reduction	2.21 (10/452)	146 (7/478)	0.54
pseudarthrosis	2.67 (11/412)	0 87 (3/343)	0.10[a]
required rev op	2.81 (17/605)	1.03(1/97)	0.49[a]
ASD requiring op	0.74 (4/539)	1.19(1/84)	0.51[a]

This it Table 4 from Yoshihara et al. [11] showing the meta-analysis of early and late complications associated with lateral mass and pedicle screws for instrumentation of the cervical spine [11]
All other percentages are based on the number of patients. *NA* not applicable, unknown = unknown, rate could not be calculated because the number of patients was not given in some articles; — = not done
Data are presented as percentages (event/no.). Complications shown in bold have percentages based on the number of screws
[a]Calculated using the Fisher exact test; the other p values were determined using the chi-square test with the Yates continuous correction

screws, the overall numbers are small (lateral mass 0 vs. pedicle screws 0.15%) while lateral mass screws have significantly higher late complications such as screw loosening/pullout (2.3% vs. 0.7%) or pseudarthrosis (2.67% vs. 0.87%; Table 80.2) [11]. In our case, the vertebral artery did not show an untypical course tough. Hemostasis was possible and the patient did not show any signs of further blood loss. So, continuing the surgery with then directly postoperative imaging was the treatment of choice. However, although the literature does not report cerebellar stroke due to vertebral artery injury, this further sequel should still be kept in mind. Most authors recommend endovascular treatment such as stenting or occlusion despite intraoperative control of the bleeding due to potentially rare sequelae such as arteriovenous fistulas or pseudoaneurysms [8, 9]. And this is also what happened in our case. The neuroradiologist in charge aimed for preservation of the injured vertebral artery, which is worth trying, the patient however, still developed a fistula only a few days later (Fig. 80.6a).

In anterior cervical spine surgery vertebral artery is reported to occur in approximately 0.3–0.5% of cases [12]. While it is extremely rarely reported for standard anterior cervical discectomy and fusion (ACDF), it is much more common in anterior cervical corpectomy [13].

A large meta-analysis showed that vertebral artery injury occurred mostly in surgeries for degenerative disease (64%), tumors (14%), and trauma (9%) and was independent from the side or the approach [13]. The most frequent action leading to vertebral artery injury was drilling (61%), followed by screw placement (16%), and soft tissue retraction (8%). 19% of patients with vertebral artery injury actually showed VA anomalies on preoperative imaging [13]. In most cases intraoperative sudden bleeding is the major symptom but also other, such as delayed hemorrhage with neck swelling due to pseudoaneurysm, hypotension, dyspnea, or pulse-synchronous noise due to arteriovenous fistula occurred [13]. For immediate intraoperative control, pressure and Surgicel® or just screw placement provide sufficient control. Other authors, however, use direct suture of clipping as well. With nowadays endovascular options, this should be regarded as not indicated in most cases [14]. After intraoperative bleeding control, postoperative DSA and stenting/coiling are recommended since especially cases treated with tamponade only showed pseudoaneurysm in 48% of patients [13].

Data on vertebral artery injury are quite extensive. For us this means that vertebral artery injury is still rare but due to the amount of spine surgeries performed, still quite frequent. The reviews, questionnaires, multicentric studies, and meta-analyses presented in this chapter tell us not only how to manage this complication optimally, the also tell us how to avoid it. Extensive drilling, tissue resection, loss of landmarks and loss of the midline orientation are factors reported frequently [13, 14]. It is also of utmost importance to study preoperative imaging accurately with special attention to the vertebral artery. While 19% of patients with intraoperative laceration showing an abnormal course in preoperative imaging and cadaver studies proving an abnormal course of the vertebral artery in 2.7%, we can see that such patients have a 7 times higher chance for vertebral artery injury [13, 15].

Yet, if no vertebral artery injury obviously occurred during surgery, patients with untypical postoperative complaints such as pulse-synchronous noise or new untypical neck pain should undergo further imaging due to the potentially dangerous consequences of undetected vertebral artery injury.

80.2.5 Case 3: Segmental Artery Injury with Pedicle Screw

A 86 y/o male patient with known multiple myeloma presented with osteolysis on L2 and severe axial pain. The tumorboard recommended primary instrumentation that was then performed T11-12-L1-3-4. Intraoperatively, the surgeon observed a lateral misplacement of both L3 screws in the O-Arm® scan (Fig. 80.7), causing her to reposition them optimally.

Postoperative plain radiographs showed the proper placement of all screws. Four days after surgery the patient showed anemia with hemoglobin being 5.4 g/dl resulting in blood transfusions. One day later, he required additional transfusions. After dropping down to hemoglobin of 5.7 g/dl again at the 12th day after surgery, receiving additional transfusion and after finally developing abdominal pain, a CT scan was performed showing a large retroperitoneal hematoma (Fig. 80.8a). DSA showed active bleeding from the right segmental artery of L3 resulting in coiling of this

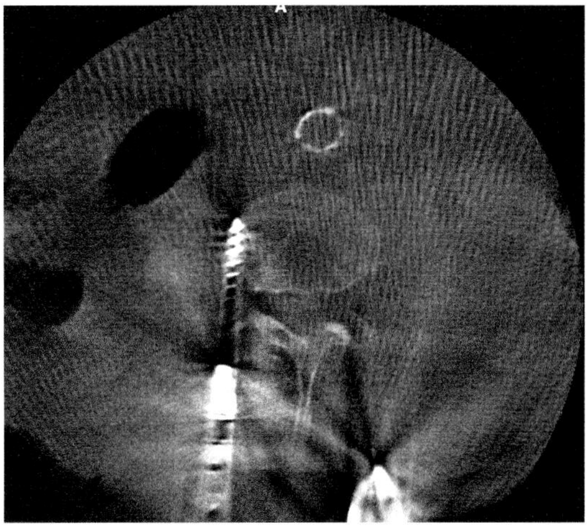

Fig. 80.7 Intraoperative 3D X-ray imaging. This is the axial image of the intraoperatively performed O-Arm® scan showing a lateral misplacement of the right L3 screw

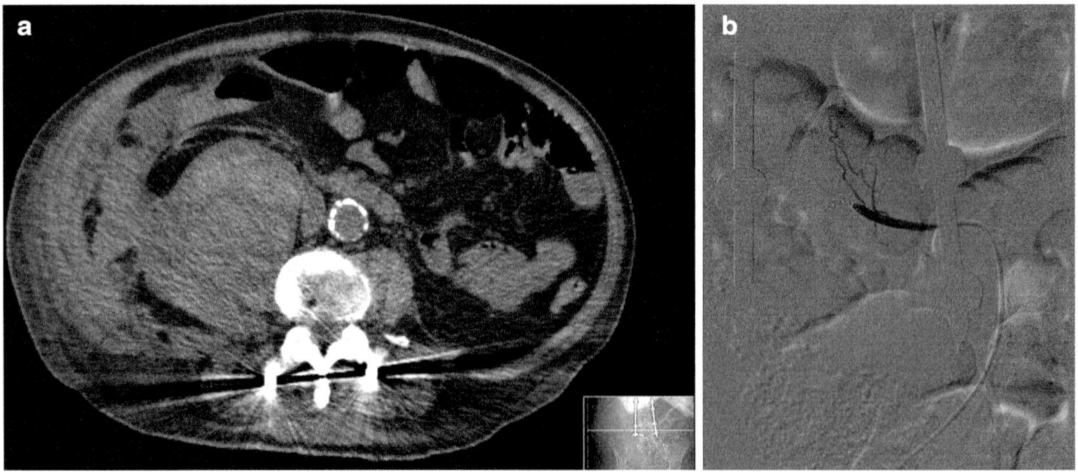

Fig. 80.8 Hematoma and acute bleeding diagnosed at the 12th postoperative day. This is the axial view of the abdominal CT scan (**a**) at level L3 performed after recurrent anemia and abdominal pain showing a large hematoma originating from the right L3 segmental artery, which was then occluded successfully via coiling (**b**)

artery (Fig. 80.8b). The patient recovered well, the hematoma was managed conservatively and the patient was discharged to rehabilitation 21 days after surgery with no sequel.

80.2.6 Case 3 Discussion

Misplacement of lumbar or thoracic pedicle screws cannot only lead to segmental artery injury but also injury to the aorta, inferior vena cava, common iliac artery and common iliac vein. All of those are rare but serious complications. If patients do not develop immediate shock, it might even stay unnoticed during surgery as in the case presented above. Although these injuries by misplaced pedicle screws are rare, the pure number of placed pedicle screws worldwide should provide a considerable number to be reported. Yet, only case reports are available on this topic [16].

Most reports agree that the typical symptoms are immediate vital shock and/or postoperative hemoglobin drop and abdominal pain [16, 17]. So quite the symptoms our presented case suffered from. If vital shock occurs after pedicle screw misplacement, it is usually impossible to repair the injured vessel from a posterior approach. Yet, arterial bleeding might be stopped with pressure and gauze. All authors agree that such arterial injury requires managed by immediate emergency exploratory laparotomy with and direct repair of the bleeding vessel [17]. Depending on the suspected vessel, endovascular treatment and coil embolization can be an option as well, which has recently been advocated to be the first-line treatment nowadays [17, 18]. However, the best option in the situation at hand depends also in the hemodynamic stability of the patient. If the patient is stable, abdominal CT and angiography can be done, whereas an unstable patient requires immediate prevention of further bleeding. If the vascular injury does not cause and intraoperative symptoms, patients can still suffer from postoperative hypotension, anemia or pain. Thus, whenever we observe a laterally or anteriorly misplaced screw or K-wire, we should keep an eye on these patients after surgery. As our case shows impressively, the clinical course including postoperative hemoglobin decline may even occur if there was no intraoperative bleeding. Especially recurrent anemia should by a imminent warning sign.

While the presented case concerns the lumbar spine, the same is true for the thoracis spine. Aortic injury was repeatedly reported from misplaced pedicle screws or K-wires [16]. Yet, misplaced screws do not always cause acute laceration. While some authors reported later pseudoaneurysm others reported no sequelae at all in a large series of cases [19]. Even more than in the lumbar spine, endovascular treatment is favored for thoracic aortic repair [16].

Concerning the published reports, the risk for vascular injury by pedicle screw a similar for degenerative, trauma and scoliosis cases. Regarding anterior scoliosis surgery, segmental vessel ligation is routine. One large series reported several rules which need to be fulfilled in order to minimize the risk for ischemic spinal cord symptoms: only at the convexity of the curve, unilateral vessel ligation, and ligation at the mid-vertebral body level [20]. The value of neuromonitoring to avoid such ischemic complications is controversial, however [20, 21].

In conclusion, for any misplaced screw close to known vascular structures we need to be aware of potential vascular injury despite intraoperative absent symptoms. Moreover, we should be attentive for signs of hypovolemia, e.g. asking the anesthetist for symptoms he / she might not have judged as surgery-related like a transient drop in blood pressure requiring some more vasopressors. Whether symptoms occur during of after surgery, optimal management needs to be immediate and usually requires endovascular stenting or even open vascular reconstruction.

For the sake of completeness, anatomy also tells us that the thoracic duct can be at risk when pedicle screws are misplaced. Actually, Medline only contains one report of thoracic duct laceration due to pedicle screw misplacement resulting in chyluria and chylothorax which resolved after prolonged thoracic drainage and a medium chain triglyceride diet [22].

80.2.7 Case 4: Urether Injury During Anterior Lumbar Surgery

A 69 y/o male patient was refered to us with spondylodiscitis T12 to L5 after a dental abscess. The patient underwent dorsal instrumentation T11-S2, decompression, and discectomy. 9 days later ALIF L5/S1 and partial VBR L4/5 via an extraperitoneal anterior approach. Another 11 days later, the patient also underwent lateral interbody fusion via a lateral retroperitoneal approach L1/2, 2/3 and 3/4 and was discharge to rehabilitation 10 days later. After 2 further days the patient was refered back due to increase in inflammatory blood parameters, such as CRP. After extensive lab work, an abdominal CT scan was performed showing a hypodens formation suspected being due to a lacerated urether (Fig. 80.9a). The patient was

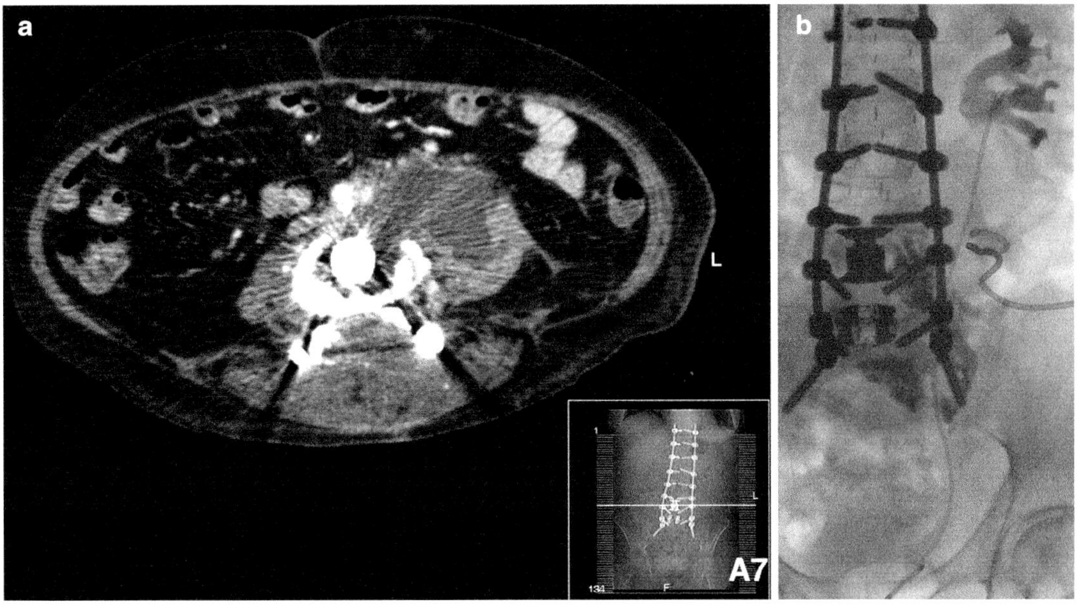

Fig. 80.9 Imaging after re-referal. This axial view of the CT scan (**a**) shows the hypodens formation suspected being due to a lacerated urether. The patient received a pigtail catheter (**b**) to the retroperitoneal mass as well as a retrograde catheter from the bladder to the kidney proving no discontinuation of the urether

referred to the urology department where he received a pigtail catheter to the retroperitoneal mass as well as a retrograde catheter from the bladder to the kidney proving no discontinuation of the urether (Fig. 80.9b). Thus, the urether laceration was managed conservatively and 2 weeks later the patient was discharge to rehabilitation again.

80.2.8 Case 4 Discussion

In the presented case, the urether injury occurred at the level of L4. Whether the anterior approach to L4/5 or the lateral retroperitoneal approach to L3/4 caused the injury cannot be judged for sure. Concerning the literature on ureteral injuries during anterior spinal procedures, the occurrence of this complication is rather small, 0.1% respectively [23]. Regarding lateral interbody fusion, two other large reviews were also not able to identify a reportable number of cases [1, 16]. Yet, one series on anterior lumbar revision surgery reported a rate of 8% of ureteral injuries despite the preoperative placement of a double-J ureteral stent even leading to nephrectomy in one case [24]. Ureteral injuries were however, much more frequently reported as a complication from lumbar discectomy [25]. In conclusion, ureteral injury during anterior lumbar surgery is very rare, is usually not recognized during surgery and can be treated conservatively via double-J stent if not discontinued or via anastomosis. In order to further lower this risk, preoperative stenting via a double-J ureteral stent should be done since nephrectomy can even be the final consequence when ureteral repair is not successful.

Other potential complications of anterior lumbar surgery are much more common, including lumbar plexus injury, lymphocele, abdominal hernia, erectile dysfunction, and retrograde ejaculation [23]. The most common ones, however, are vascular complications of the aortic artery, iliac artery, iliac vein, and vena cava which can all be hemorrhagic or thrombotic, too [1]. Table 80.3 provides an overview.

Recent cohort studies show, however, that this complication rate can be considerable lower when performed in cooperation with a vascular surgeon [26]. As Table 80.3 shows, the complication rate and variety for ALIF procedures is actually large and is mostly linked to the nearby critical anatomy, such as aortic artery, iliac artery, iliac vein, and vena cava which need to be visualized and partially mobilized for this approach. Thus, in recent years most surgeon tend to limit ALIF to L5/S1, sometimes L4/5, and use LLIF, XLIF, or OLIF instead due to the considerably quicker approach and lower complication rates [1].

For the 3 mentioned retroperitoneal approaches, to major risks are also easily understandable by the respective anatomy, such as peritoneum and its contents, the lumbar plexus nerves, segmental vessels and great vessels. Yet, the great vessels are usually not in the direct corridor – with the exception of the OLIF approach. However, compared to ALIF, the vascular complication rates are far less [1]. In most studies, vascular injuries during ALIF ranged from 2% to 6%, but even went up to 20% [27]. Injuries to the bowel are reported to range between 1% and 2% for ALIF but also for TLIF during discectomy [1]. Yet, ileus is much more frequent than actual injury. In a current investigation covering more than 13,000 patients undergoing MIS-LIF, only 0.1% of vascular and 0.08% visceral injuries were observed [1].

If small venous injuries occur, they can usually be managed be compression and a Tachosil® patch, if not, direct suture by a vascular surgeon is indicated. For arterial lacerations, direct suture is the treatment of choice. If further difficulties develop, a vascular surgeon should also be consulted.

Table 80.3 Early and late complications for ALIF procedures

References	Year	Study design	Number of patients studies	Procedure	Complication	Incidence (%)
Acosta et al. [52]	2009	Retrospective chart review	73 patients	ALIF	Wound infection	2.8
Baker et al. [35]	1993	Retrospective chart review	102 patients	ALIF	Vascular injury	15.6
Brau et al. [32]	2002	Retrospective cohort study	684 patients	Mini-open ALIF	Arterial injury	0.8
					Death	0.2
					Hernia	0.3
					Ileus	0.6
					MI	0.2
					RE	0.1
					Venous injury	0.8
					Wound infection	0.4
Brau et al. [45]	2003	Prospective nonrandomized observational study	45 patients	ALIF	Left iliac artery compression causing distal oxygen desaturation	57
Brau et al. [42]	2004	Retrospective review of prospective database	1310 patients	ALIF	Iliac artery thrombosis	0.5
					Venous injury	1.4
Faciszeswki [23]	1995	Retrospective chart review	1233 (contains other anterior thoracolambar cases)	ALIF	Vascular injury	0.3
Fantini et al. [44]	2007	Retrospective chart review	338 patients	ALIF	Aorta injury	0.3
					Common iliac vein injury	2.6
Fantini et al. [36]	2013	Literature review	9 studies	ALIF	Vascular injury	1.6–4.3
Flynn et al. [37]	1984	Survey	4500 patients	ALIF	Impotence	0.44
					RE	0.42
Garg et al. [25]	2010	Retrospective review of prospective database	212 patients	ALIF	Vascular injury	6.1
Hamdan et al. [46]	2008	Retrospective cohort study	480 patients	ALIF	Vascular injury	11
Hrabalek et al. [47]	2012	Retrospective chart review	120 patients	ALIF	Sympathectomy	15.8
Hrabalek et al. [53]	2014	Retrospective chart review	175 patients	Mini-open ALIF	Hernia	2.9
					Sympathetic dysfunction	1.1
					Vaacular injury	1.1
					Wound dehiscence	1.1
Inamasu et al. [16]	2006	Literature review	31 studies 6923 patients	ALIF	Vascular injury	0–20
Jiang et al. [33]	2012	Systematic review	9 studies 948 patients	ALIF	DVT/PU	6.3
					Hernia	0.4

(continued)

Table 80.3 (continued)

References	Year	Study design	Number of patients studies	Procedure	Complication	Incidence (%)
					RE	3.1
					Vascular injury	2.2
					Wound infection/ dehiscence	6.4
Kulkarni et al. [38]	2003	Case–cortrol study	336 patients	ALIF	Arterial injury	2.4
Li et al. [27]	2010	Prospective nonrandomized observational study	112 patients	ALIF	Vascular injury	1.8
					Wound infection	7.1
Lindley et al. [39]	2012	Retrospective cohort study	54 patients	ALIF	RE	7.4
Penta et al. [34]	1997	Retrospective cohort study	103 patients	ALIF	PE	3.9
					Wound infection/ dehiscence	2.8
Quraishi et al. [54]	2013	Retrospective cohort review	304 patients	ALIF	Arterial injury	1.6
				ADR	Venom injury	6.2
					Wound dehiscence	3.9
					Wound infection	4.3
Rajaraman et al. [51]	1999	Retrospective chart review	60 patients	ALIF	Acute pancreatitis	1.7
					Bowel Injury	1.7
					DVT	1.7
					Ileus	5.0
					Sexual dysfunction	5.0
					Sympathetic dysfunction	10.0
					Vascular injury	6.7
					Wound income petence	3.3
Regan et al. [48]	1999	Retrospective chart review	58 patients	ALIF	RE	1.7
					Vascular injury	5.2
Sasso et al. [40]	2003	Multicenter, prospective nonrandomized observational study	146patients	ALIF	RE	4.1[a]
Scaduto et al. [49]	2003	Retrospective cohort review	88 patients	ALIF	Ileus	6
					Vascular injury	2
Wood et al. [41]	2010	Systematic review	40 studies	ALIF	Vascular injury	0–16
Zahradnik et al. [50]	2013	Retrospective cohort review	260 patients	ALIF	Vascular injury	13.8

This it Table 7 from Uribe et al. (2015) showing a review of early and late complications associated with ALIF procedures [1]

ALIF Anterior lumber interbody fusion, *ADR* artificial disc replacement, *DVT* deep vein thrombosis, *MI* myocandial infarction, *PE* pulmonary embolism, *PLIF* posterior lumber interbody fusion, *RE* retrograde ejaculation, *TLIF* transforminal lumbar interbody fusion, *XIJF* extreme lateral interbody fusion

[a]Incidence of RE wav 1.7%; through retroperitoneal approach and 13.3% through transperitoneal approach

80.2.9 Case 5: Bowel Injury After Lumbar Microdiscectomy

A 47 y/o male patient presented with sciatica since 2 years originating from a L5/S1 prolapse on the right side (Fig. 80.10a). The patient was operated via a right-sided L5/S1 interlaminar fenestration. While he felt fine with no further sciatica at the first day, he developed a new right-sided L5 and S1 sciatica including a L5 paresis BMRC 3/5. The patient therefore underwent another MRI scan at the 2nd postoperative day showing an even larger L5/S1 prolapse on the right side (Fig. 80.10b). He was then scheduled for reoperation.

During surgery the L5 foramen was also decompressed on the right side. During decompression and discectomy, the surgeon later said that she was unsure about the actual nature but there was some kind of unusual fluid. Whether

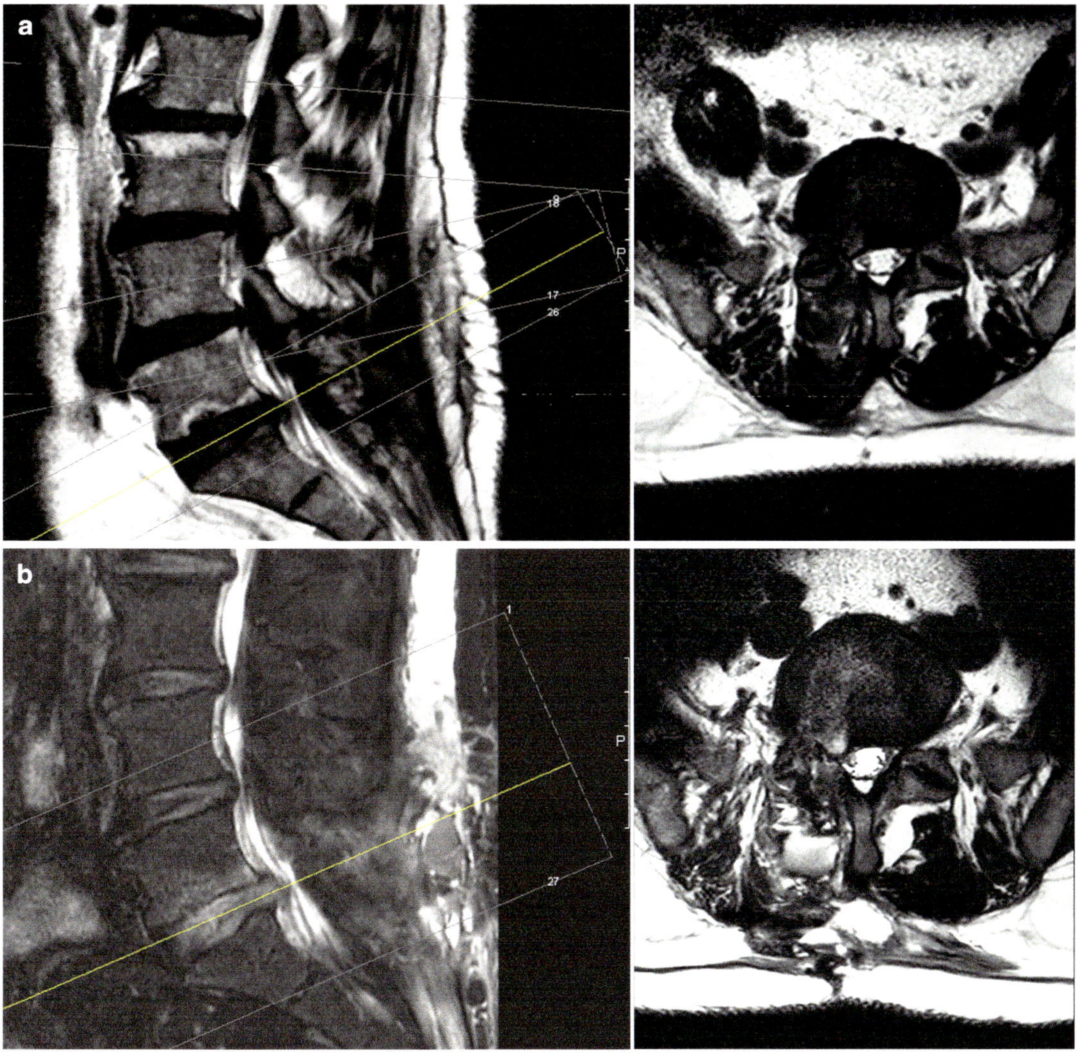

Fig. 80.10 Initial and postoperative MRI scan. These are the sagittal and axial views of the MRI scans at initial presentation (**a**) and at the 2nd postoperative day (**b**) showing a L5/S1 prolapse on the right side

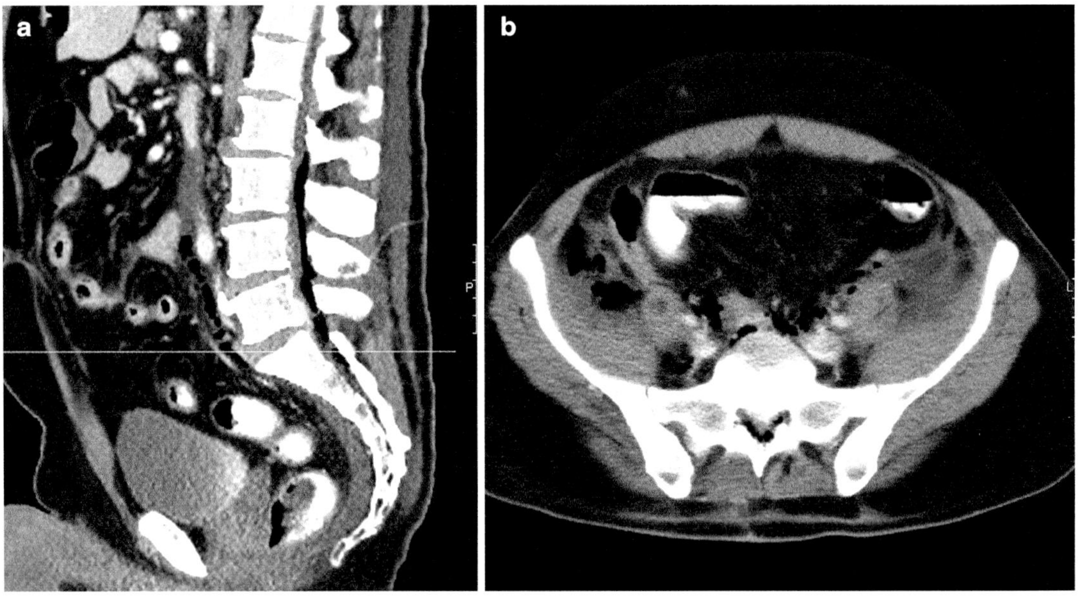

Fig. 80.11 Postoperative abdominal CT scan. Sagittal (**a**) and axial (**b**) views of the postoperative CT scan showing intrabdominal free air. The air can also be seen right anterior of the L5/S1 disc and continues into the spinal canal cranially up to L2/3

this could have been hematoma from the first discectomy or anything from anterior cannot be said for sure. The patient improved neurologically with no sciatica anymore, but the morning after surgery he complaint about severe abdominal pain thus indicating a CT scan (Fig. 80.11).

Abdominal surgeons were then consulted and brought to the OR where he underwent partial ileum resection and end to end anastomosis. The surgeons observed a transmucous hole and beginning peritonitis. The patient recovered well, received antibiotics due to the peritonitis and was observed for several days afterwards in order to face the risk of associated discitis properly.

80.2.10 Case 5 Discussion

Bowel injury associated with lumbar microdiscectomy is rare but not unknown. Eighteen case reports have been published until now [28]. Some authors suggest that a concomitant anterior disc herniation due to perforation of the anterior part of the annulus could be a risk factor for injuries due to anterior breach of the disc space with the rongeur. Most of the reported cases occurred at L5/S1 and affect the small intestine, as in our case. Since discectomy patients are operated in prone position the intestines are compressed towards the lumbosacral disc. Early or even very late detected bowel injury is really rare but if unnoticed associated with considerable morbidity and mortality [28].

Another much more common and potentially life-threatening complication is the intraoperative vascular injury during lumbar discectomy, which occurs in 1.6–4.5 per 10.000 cases and which is associated with a mortality rate of 38–61% [3, 4, 28]. If immediate intraoperative bleeding with hypotension or shock does not occur, late complications by pseudoaneurysms or arteriovenous fistulas (e.g. right common iliac artery and the inferior vena) can also develop. Most commonly, laceration of the left or right common iliac artery occur. Moreover, about 80% of vascular injuries during microdiscectomy occur at the level of L4/5 since the left common iliac artery crosses along the disc space from the right to the left side only separated from the disc space by the anterior spinal ligament. Altogether, the vascular laceration during discectomy is an emergency requiring immediate action such as dorsal control and immediate laparotomy or endovascular treatment if possible [3, 4, 16, 29]. It is also decisive to consider any intraoperative hypotensive episode as a warning sign; even if the anesthetist does not do so, and decide for emergency laparotomy if the patient suspected of vascular injury is becoming unstable [4, 30].

After bowel laceration, Patients generally complain of acute abdomen or abdominal pain. Yet, if there are uncommon symptoms even late after discectomy, any vascular or anterior complication such as arteriovenous fistulas should be kept in mind and further diagnostics are indicated, such as abdominal CT scan with arterial and venous contrast in order to rule are concomitant injury to other ventral structures, e.g. urether, which was reported as well [28, 31]. If diagnosed early, the prognosis of discectomy-associated bowel laceration is quite good compared to vascular incidents [3, 4, 16, 28, 29]. Yet, fatal courses including progressive peritonitis and sepsis are possible [28]. As in our illustrative case, early exploratory laparotomy and repair via primary suture or resection and end-to-end anastomosis are the treatment of choice.

Avoiding such incidences is much better than reaction, however. Thorough imaging studies for anterior annulus breach and proximity or abnormalities of critical anterior structures are mandatory. Especially for younger surgeons, depth markings of rongeurs might be helpful. Likewise, opening the rongeur right when entering the disc space also helps to prevent anterior perforation. If anterior perforation is suspected, filing the disc space with saline can help to confirm: if it escapes quickly through the disc space, anterior perforation of the annulus and anterior spinal ligament is likely.

In our case, the surgeon intraoperatively suspected an anterior problem, asked the anesthetist for hypotension and proceeded with surgery due to unsuspicious further course. However, when the team report at the morning meeting reported abdominal pain, she immediately connected her intraoperative impression with the current complaint and CT imaging was done 30 min later leading to emergency laparotomy. Thus, despite this severe and rare complication, immediate care avoided at least further harm and lead to optimal treatment of the complication.

80.2.11 Accordance with the Literature Guidelines

Concerning these complications, there are no guidelines at hand. Depending on the surgery, patient, risk factors and reoperations, indication and technical nuances can help us to further reduce the rate of complications in spine surgery.

Level of Evidence
C

The available level of data quality concerning complications and their is considerably good but not optimal due to the differing frequencies of occurence.

80.3 Conclusions and Take Home Message

The illustrative cases above shall serve as examples which stay in the mind of the reader in order to connect these sometimes quite unfortunate courses with the potential complications of these mostly routine procedures. Independently from the complication itself, early diagnosis and optimal treatment reduce morbidity and mortality considerably.

Pearls

- When suspecting non-spinal comlications, immediate action is required
- always check for transient or permanent blood pressure drops when suspecting vascular injury
- anterior lacerations of any structure can not only cause acute but also late and diffuse symptoms

References

1. Uribe JS, Deukmedjian AR. Visceral, vascular, and wound complications following over 13,000 lateral interbody fusions: a survey study and literature review. Eur Spine J. 2015;24(Suppl 3):386–96. https://doi.org/10.1007/s00586-015-3806-4.
2. Birkeland IW Jr, Taylor TK. Bowel injuries coincident to lumbar disk surgery: a report of four cases and a review of the literature. J Trauma. 1970;10(2):163–8.
3. Harbison SP. Major vascular complications of intervertebral disc surgery. Ann Surg. 1954;140(3):342–8.
4. Papadoulas S, Konstantinou D, Kourea HP, Kritikos N, Haftouras N, Tsolakis JA. Vascular injury complicating lumbar disc surgery. A systematic review. Eur J Vasc Endovasc Surg. 2002;24(3):189–95.
5. Cheung JP, Luk KD. Complications of anterior and posterior cervical spine surgery. Asian Spine J. 2016;10(2):385–400. https://doi.org/10.4184/asj.2016.10.2.385.
6. Halani SH, Baum GR, Riley JP, Pradilla G, Refai D, Rodts GE Jr, et al. Esophageal perforation after anterior cervical spine surgery: a systematic review of the literature. J Neurosurg Spine. 2016;25(3):285–91. https://doi.org/10.3171/2016.1.SPINE15898.
7. Navarro R, Javahery R, Eismont F, Arnold DJ, Bhatia NN, Vanni S, et al. The role of the sternocleidomastoid muscle flap for esophageal fistula repair in anterior cervical spine surgery. Spine (Phila Pa 1976). 2005;30(20):E617–22.
8. Inamasu J, Guiot BH. Iatrogenic vertebral artery injury. Acta Neurol Scand. 2005;112(6):349–57. https://doi.org/10.1111/j.1600-0404.2005.00497.x.
9. Wright NM, Lauryssen C. Vertebral artery injury in C1-2 transarticular screw fixation: results of a survey of the AANS/CNS section on disorders of the spine and peripheral nerves. American Association of Neurological Surgeons/Congress of Neurological Surgeons. J Neurosurg. 1998;88(4):634–40. https://doi.org/10.3171/jns.1998.88.4.0634.
10. Epstein NE. From the neurointerventional lab... intraoperative cervical vertebral artery injury treated by tamponade and endovascular coiling. Spine J. 2003;3(5):404–5.
11. Yoshihara H, Passias PG, Errico TJ. Screw-related complications in the subaxial cervical spine with the use of lateral mass versus cervical pedicle screws: a systematic review. J Neurosurg Spine. 2013;19(5):614–23. https://doi.org/10.3171/2013.8.SPINE13136.
12. Shen FH, Samartzis D, Khanna N, Goldberg EJ, An HS. Comparison of clinical and radiographic outcome in instrumented anterior cervical discectomy and fusion with or without direct uncovertebral joint decompression. Spine J. 2004;4(6):629–35. https://doi.org/10.1016/j.spinee.2004.04.009.
13. Guan Q, Chen L, Long Y, Xiang Z. Iatrogenic vertebral artery injury during anterior cervical spine surgery: a systematic review. World Neurosurg. 2017;106:715–22. https://doi.org/10.1016/j.wneu.2017.07.027.
14. Hsu WK, Kannan A, Mai HT, Fehlings MG, Smith ZA, Traynelis VC, et al. Epidemiology and outcomes of vertebral artery injury in 16 582 cervical spine surgery patients: an AOSpine North America Multicenter Study. Global Spine J. 2017;7(1 Suppl):21S–7S. https://doi.org/10.1177/2192568216686753.
15. Curylo LJ, Mason HC, Bohlman HH, Yoo JU. Tortuous course of the vertebral artery and anterior cervical decompression: a cadaveric and clinical case study. Spine (Phila Pa 1976). 2000;25(22):2860–4.
16. Inamasu J, Guiot BH. Vascular injury and complication in neurosurgical spine surgery. Acta Neurochir. 2006;148(4):375–87. https://doi.org/10.1007/s00701-005-0669-1.
17. Sugimoto Y, Tanaka M, Gobara H, Misawa H, Kunisada T, Ozaki T. Management of lumbar artery injury related to pedicle screw insertion. Acta Med Okayama. 2013;*67*(2):113–6. https://doi.org/10.18926/AMO/49670.
18. Tong X, Gu P, Yu D, Guo F, Lin X. An endovascular treatment of a thoracic aortic injury caused

by a misplaced pedicle screw: Case report and review of the literature. J Formos Med Assoc. 2015;114(5):464–8. https://doi.org/10.1016/j.jfma.2013.09.014.
19. Foxx KC, Kwak RC, Latzman JM, Samadani U. A retrospective analysis of pedicle screws in contact with the great vessels. J Neurosurg Spine. 2010;13(3):403–6. https://doi.org/10.3171/2010.3.SPINE09657.
20. Winter RB, Lonstein JE, Denis F, Leonard AS, Garamella JJ. Paraplegia resulting from vessel ligation. Spine (Phila Pa 1976). 1996;21(10):1232–3. discussion 1233-1234.
21. Leung YL, Grevitt M, Henderson L, Smith J. Cord monitoring changes and segmental vessel ligation in the "at risk" cord during anterior spinal deformity surgery. Spine (Phila Pa 1976). 2005;30(16):1870–4.
22. Weening AA, Schurink B, Ruurda JP, van Hillegersberg R, Bleys R, Kruyt MC. Chyluria and chylothorax after posterior selective fusion for adolescent idiopathic scoliosis. Eur Spine J. 2017; https://doi.org/10.1007/s00586-017-5066-y.
23. Faciszewski T, Winter RB, Lonstein JE, Denis F, Johnson L. The surgical and medical perioperative complications of anterior spinal fusion surgery in the thoracic and lumbar spine in adults. A review of 1223 procedures. Spine (Phila Pa 1976). 1995;20(14):1592–9.
24. Flouzat-Lachaniette CH, Delblond W, Poignard A, Allain J. Analysis of intraoperative difficulties and management of operative complications in revision anterior exposure of the lumbar spine: a report of 25 consecutive cases. Eur Spine J. 2013;22(4):766–74. https://doi.org/10.1007/s00586-012-2524-4.
25. Garg N, Panwar P, Devana SK, Ravi Mohan SM, Mandal AK. Ureteric injury after lumbosacral microdiscectomy: a case report and review of literature. Urol Ann. 2017;9(2):200–3. https://doi.org/10.4103/0974-7796.204191.
26. Asha MJ, Choksey MS, Shad A, Roberts P, Imray C. The role of the vascular surgeon in anterior lumbar spine surgery. Br J Neurosurg. 2012;26(4):499–503. https://doi.org/10.3109/02688697.2012.680629.
27. Li J, Dumonski ML, Liu Q, Lipman A, Hong J, Yang N, et al. A multicenter study to evaluate the safety and efficacy of a stand-alone anterior carbon I/F Cage for anterior lumbar interbody fusion: two-year results from a Food and Drug Administration investigational device exemption clinical trial. Spine (Phila Pa 1976). 2010;35(26):E1564–70. https://doi.org/10.1097/BRS.0b013e3181ef5c14.
28. Kim D-S, Lee J-K, Moon K-S, Ju J-K, Kim S-H. Small bowel injury as a complication of lumbar microdiscectomy : case report and literature review. J Korean Neurosurg Soc. 2010;47(3):224–7. https://doi.org/10.3340/jkns.2010.47.3.224.
29. Uei H, Tokuhashi Y, Oshima M, Miyake Y. Vascular injury following microendoscopic lumbar discectomy treated with stent graft placement. J Neurosurg Spine. 2014;20(1):67–70. https://doi.org/10.3171/2013.9.SPINE13282.
30. Goodkin R, Laska LL. Vascular and visceral injuries associated with lumbar disc surgery: medicolegal implications. Surg Neurol. 1998;49(4):358–70. discussion 370-352.
31. Fruhwirth J, Koch G, Amann W, Hauser H, Flaschka G. Vascular complications of lumbar disc surgery. Acta Neurochir. 1996;138(8):912–6.
32. Brau SA. Mini-open approach to the spine for anterior lumbar interbody fusion: description of the procedure, results and complications. Spine J. 2002;2:216–23.
33. Jiang SD, Chen JW, Jiang LS. Which procedure is better for lumbar interbody fusion: anterior lumbar interbody fusion or transforaminal lumbar interbody fusion? Arch Orthop Trauma Surg. 2012;132:1259–66.
34. Penta M, Fraser RD. Anterior lumbar interbody fusion. A minimum 10-year follow-up. Spine. 1997;22:2429–34.
35. Baker JK, Reardon PR, Reardon MJ, Heggeness MH. Vascular injury in anterior lumbar surgery. Spine. 1993;18:2227–30.
36. Fantini GA, Pawar AY. Access related complications during anterior exposure of the lumbar spine. World J Orthop. 2013;4:19–23.
37. Flynn JC, Price CT. Sexual complications of anterior fusion of the lumbar spine. Spine. 1984;9:489–92.
38. Kulkarni SS, Lowery GL, Ross RE, Ravi SK, Lykomitros V. Arterial complications following anterior lumbar interbody fusion: report of eight cases. Eur Spine J. 2003;12:48–54.
39. Lindley EM, McBeth ZL, Henry SE, et al. Retrograde ejaculation after anterior lumbar spine surgery. Spine. 2012;37:1785–9.
40. Sasso RC, Kenneth BJ, LeHuec JC. Retrograde ejaculation after anterior lumbar interbody fusion: transperitoneal versus retroperitoneal exposure. Spine. 2003;28:1023–6.
41. Wood KB, Devine J, Fischer D, Dettori JR, Janssen M. Vascular injury in elective anterior lumbosacral surgery. Spine. 2010;35:S66–75.
42. Brau SA, Delamarter RB, Schiffman ML, Williams LA, Watkins RG. Vascular injury during anterior lumbar surgery. Spine J. 2004;4:409–12.
43. Lee P, Fessler RG. Perioperative and postoperative complications of single-level minimally invasive transforaminal lumbar interbody fusion in elderly adults. J Clin Neurosci. 2012;19:111–4.
44. Fantini GA, Pappou IP, Girardi FP, Sandhu HS, Cammisa FP Jr. Major vascular injury during ante-

rior lumbar spinal surgery: incidence, risk factors, and management. Spine. 2007;32:2751–8.
45. Brau SA, Spoonamore MJ, Snyder L, et al. Nerve monitoring changes related to iliac artery compression during anterior lumbar spine surgery. Spine J. 2003;3:351–5.
46. Hamdan AD, Malek JY, Schermerhorn ML, Aulivola B, Blattman SB, Pomposelli FB Jr. Vascular injury during anterior exposure of the spine. J Vasc Surg. 2008;48:650–4.
47. Hrabalek L, Adamus M, Wanek T, Machac J, Tucek P. Surgical complications of the anterior approach to the L5/S1 intervertebral disc. Biomed Pap Med Fac Univ Palacky Olomouc Czech Repub. 2012;156:354–8.
48. Regan JJ, Aronoff RJ, Ohnmeiss DD, Sengupta DK. Laparoscopic approach to L4-L5 for interbody fusion using BAK cages: experience in the first 58 cases. Spine. 1999;24:2171–4.
49. Scaduto AA, Gamradt SC, Yu WD, Huang J, Delamarter RB, Wang JC. Perioperative complications of threaded cylindrical lumbar interbody fusion devices: anterior versus posterior approach. J Spinal Disord Tech. 2003;16:502–7.
50. Zahradnik V, Lubelski D, Abdullah KG, Kelso R, Mroz T, Kashyap VS. Vascular injuries during anterior exposure of the thoracolumbar spine. Ann Vasc Surg. 2013;27:306–13.
51. Rajaraman V, Vingan R, Roth P, Heary RF, Conklin L, Jacobs GB. Visceral and vascular complications resulting from anterior lumbar interbody fusion. J Neurosurg. 1999;91:60–4.
52. Acosta FL, Cloyd JM, Aryan HE, Ames CP. Perioperative complications and clinical outcomes of multilevel circumferential lumbar spinal fusion in the elderly. J Clin Neurosci. 2009;16:69–73.
53. Hrabalek L, Adamus M, Gryga A, Wanek T, Tucek P. A comparison of complication rate between anterior and lateral approaches to the lumbar spine. Biomed Pap Med Fac Univ Palacky Olomouc Czech Repub. 2014;158:127–32.
54. Quraishi NA, Konig M, Booker SJ, et al. Access related complications in anterior lumbar surgery performed by spinal surgeons. Eur Spine J. 2013;22(Suppl 1):S16–20.
55. Audat ZA, Barbarawi MM, Obeidat MM. Posterior cervical decompressive laminectomy and lateral mass screw fixation. Neurosciences (Riyadh). 2011;16:248–52.
56. Fehlings MG, Cooper PR, Errico TJ. Posterior plates in the management of cervical instability: long-term results in 44 patients. J Neurosurg. 1994;81:341–9.
57. Graham AW, Swank ML, Kinard RE, Lowery GL, Dials BE. Posterior cervical arthrodesis and stabilization with a lateral mass plate. Clinical and computed tomographic evaluation of lateral mass screw placement and associated complications. Spine (Phila Pa 1976). 1996;21:323–9.
58. Heller JG, Carlson GD, Abitbol JJ, Garfin SR: Anatomic comparison of the Roy-Camille and Magerl techniques for screw placement in the lower cervical spine. Spine 16 (Phila Pa 1976) (10 Suppl):S552–S557, 1991
59. Kast E, Mohr K, Richter HP, Börm W. Complications of transpedicular screw fixation in the cervical spine. Eur Spine J. 2006;15:327–34.
60. Katonis P, Papadakis SA, Galanakos S, Paskou D, Bano A, Sapkas G, et al. Lateral mass screw complications: analysis of 1662 screws. J Spinal Disord Tech. 2011;24:415–20.
61. Kotil K, Ozyuvaci E. Multilevel decompressive laminectomy and transpedicular instrumented fusion for cervical spondylotic radiculopathy and myelopathy: a minimum follow-up of 3 years. J Craniovertebr Junction Spine. 2011;2:27–31.
62. Lee SH, Kim KT, Abumi K, Suk KS, Lee JH, Park KJ. Cervical pedicle screw placement using the "key slot technique": the feasibility and learning curve. J Spinal Disord Tech. 2012;25:415–21.
63. Liu Y, Hu JH, Yu KY. Pedicle screw fixation for cervical spine instability: clinical efficacy and safety analysis. Chin Med J. 2009;122:1985–9.
64. Miyamoto H, Uno K. Cervical pedicle screw insertion using a computed tomography cutout technique. Technical note. J Neurosurg Spine. 2009;11:681–7.
65. Nakashima H, Yukawa Y, Imagama S, Kanemura T, Kamiya M, Yanase M, et al. Complications of cervical pedicle screw fixation for nontraumatic lesions: a multicenter study of 84 patients. J Neurosurg Spine. 2012;16:238–47.
66. Neo M, Sakamoto T, Fujibayashi S, Nakamura T. The clinical risk of vertebral artery injury from cervical pedicle screws inserted in degenerative vertebrae. Spine (Phila Pa 1976). 2005;30:2800–5.
67. Pateder DB, Carbone JJ. Lateral mass screw fixation for cervical spine trauma: associated complications and efficacy in maintaining alignment. Spine J. 2006;6:40–3.
68. Sekhon LH. Posterior cervical lateral mass screw fixation: analysis of 1026 consecutive screws in 143 patients. J Spinal Disord Tech. 2005;18:297–303.
69. Takahashi J, Shono Y, Nakamura I, Hirabayashi H, Kamimura M, Ebara S, et al. Computer-assisted screw insertion for cervical disorders in rheumatoid arthritis. Eur Spine J. 2007;16:485–94.
70. Tofuku K, Koga H, Komiya S. Cervical pedicle screw insertion using a gutter entry point at the transitional area between the lateral mass and lamina. Eur Spine J. 2012;21:353–8.
71. Wang MY, Levi AD. Minimally invasive lateral mass screw fixation in the cervical spine: initial clinical

experience with long-term follow-up. Neurosurgery. 2006;58:907–12.
72. Wellman BJ, Follett KA, Traynelis VC. Complications of posterior articular mass plate fixation of the subaxial cervical spine in 43 consecutive patients. Spine (Phila Pa 1976). 1998;23:193–200.
73. Wu JC, Huang WC, Chen YC, Shih YH, Cheng H. Stabilization of subaxial cervical spines by lateral mass screw fixation with modified Magerl's technique. Surg Neurol. 2008;70(Suppl 1):S1:25–33.
74. Yoshimoto H, Sato S, Hyakumachi T, Yanagibashi Y, Kanno T, Masuda T. Clinical accuracy of cervical pedicle screw insertion using lateral fluoroscopy: a radiographic analysis of the learning curve. Eur Spine J. 2009;18:1326–34.
75. Yukawa Y, Kato F, Ito K, Horie Y, Hida T, Nakashima H, et al. Placement and complications of cervical pedicle screws in 144 cervical trauma patients using pedicle axis view techniques by fluoroscope. Eur Spine J. 2009;18:1293–9.
76. Abumi K, Shono Y, Ito M, Taneichi H, Kotani Y, Kaneda K. Complications of pedicle screw fixation in reconstructive surgery of the cervical spine. Spine (Phila Pa 1976). 2000;25:962–969.

Management of CSF Fistula

81

John M. Duff and Rodolfo Maduri

81.1 Introduction

Unintentional dural tear with spinal cerebrospinal fluid (CSF) fistula has a prevalence of 1–17% approximately [1]. It is almost certainly underreported and the clinical consequences can carry a significant morbidity [1, 2]. One of the most serious risks of that of meningitis [1, 3]. Additionally, it can lead to further surgeries, prolonged hospitalisation and a significant increase in health care costs [4, 5].

This case illustrates how the seemingly innocuous problem of a small dural tear leading to a leak of CSF can carry significant morbidity. It also illustrates the importance of dealing appropriately with such leaks at the time of occurrence. Several problems will be outlined, including the hazard of "pinhole" leaks, the need to adequately expose the site of dural tear, the difficulties encountered following multi-attempt unsuccessful repairs, and possible salvage operative strategies for dural repair including the use of vascularised local tissue cover to facilitate wound closure.

The goal of this case presentation is to emphasize these potential problems and to highlight the lack of scientific evidence in the treatment of postoperative CSF fistula. This case will highlight the fact that a proactive approach to pseudomeningocele, especially when it is not contained by the deep fascia, is usually the best one, and that this approach should often be a "maximalist" one.

81.2 Case Description

An 84 year old male with a history of coronary artery disease and hypertension complains of typical neurogenic claudication and is limited to 200 metres walking distance. His neurological examination of his lower extremities is normal. He underwent an L2 to L5 posterior decompression. He woke up from surgery with a distal paraparesis. An MRI scan showed a "small" hematoma at L4 which was not explored surgically. He was transferred to a rehabilitation facility.

The patient was re-admitted 8 days later with a large visible and palpable subcutaneous fluid collection compatible with a pseudomeningocele. A blood patch was attempted and was unsuccessful. CSF subsequently began to leak through the wound. At 11 days after the index surgery, the patient was taken back to the operating room and re-explored. A collection of pus was drained, and a dural repair was carried out with a local fascial patch and reinforced with fibrin glue. Wound cultures revealed Escherichia

J. M. Duff (✉) · R. Maduri
Department of Clinical Neurosciences, University Hospital of Lausanne, CHUV, Lausanne, Switzerland

B. Meyer, M. Rauschmann (eds.), *Spine Surgery*, https://doi.org/10.1007/978-3-319-98875-7_81

coli and Serratia marcescens, and the patient was treated with vancomycin and ciproxin. He was subsequently transferred back to rehab. Several days later, a new large subcutaneous fluid collection was noted and the patient was transferred to our institution for evaluation.

On admission, the patient was afebrile. He did not complain of any back or leg pain, but complained of weakness in both legs. On examination, he could walk a few steps with the use of crutches, and he had distal weakness of his foot dorsiflexors, more on the right side than on the left side. There was a very obvious large subcutaneous pseudomeningocele with fluid leaking through the skin incision. His laboratory values showed a normal white blood cell count and a normal C-reactive protein and erythrocyte sedimentation rate through antibiotic coverage. A lumbar MRI scan with gadolinium was done (Fig. 81.1), which revealed a voluminous pseudomeningocele breeching the lumbar fascia as far as the skin. A CT of the lumbar spine (Fig. 81.2) showed a degenerative lumbar scoliosis with resection of the facet joints at multiple lumbar levels. Full spine X-rays (Fig. 81.3) show a compensated lumbar scoliosis with good alignment in the sagittal and coronal planes. It was decided to re-explore the patient to perform a definitive dural closure and to control the wound infection. A decision was taken to defer any surgical fusion to a possible later date.

The patient was placed prone on the operating table following induction of general anesthesia. The whole thoracolumbar region and both lateral thighs were prepped and draped into the field, so access to fascia lata and local muscle flaps was ensured. The previous midline incision was re-opened. A large fluid collection was immediately encountered and drained. A large musculofascial defect was found and the posterior lumbar dura was immediately visible. The remainder of the fascia and muscles was re-opened to expose the entire length of the decompression. Careful examination of the dura with the operating microscope revealed CSF emanating from the left L5 foramen area. Following additional bone removal and removal of epidural inflammatory material, the fistula site was clearly identified, which was pinhole-sized. Sutures were identified on the dura close to the dural defect. Sutures of 6-0 prolene were placed in the dura and a small piece of local muscle was harvested, placed over the defect as a patch and the sutures were tied down. The repair was reinforced with Duraseal®. A vascularised latissimus dorsi flap was harvested by the plastic surgery team using a separate incision and was placed over the dural repair. For the closure, the skin flaps were undermined for

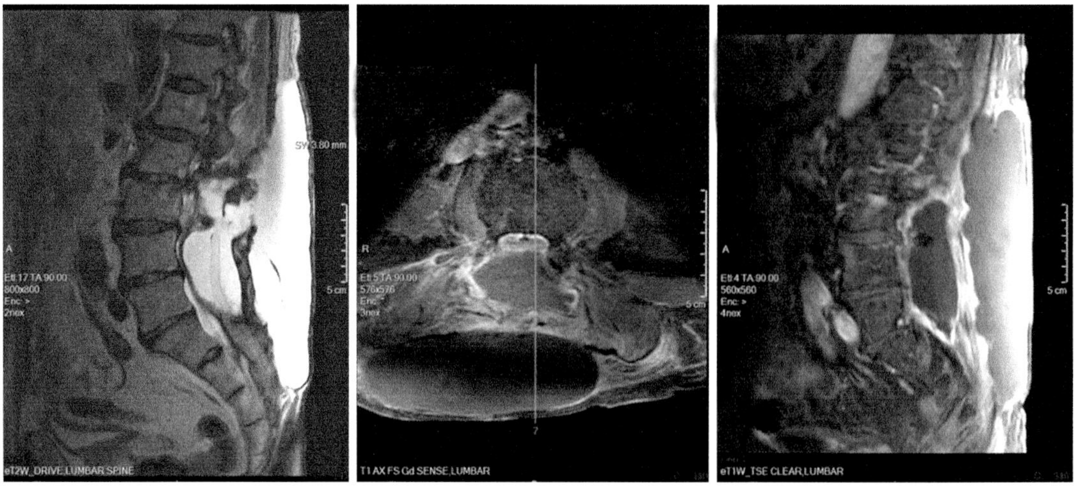

Fig. 81.1 MRI lumbar spine at presentation. The large sub and supra-fascial fluid collection is visible. There is mass effect on the lumbar thecal sac

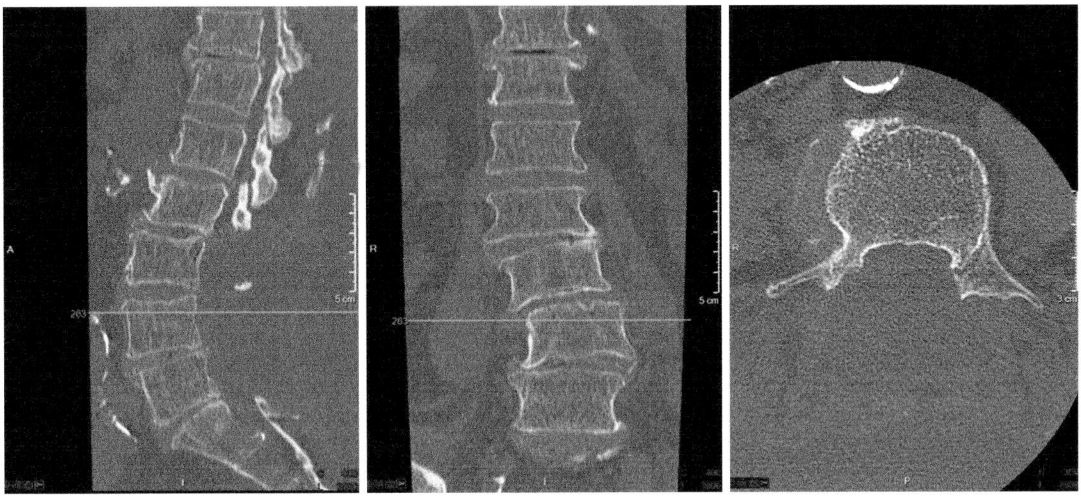

Fig. 81.2 Lumbar CT scan shows a degenerative scoliosis with extensive postoperative posterior element bone resection

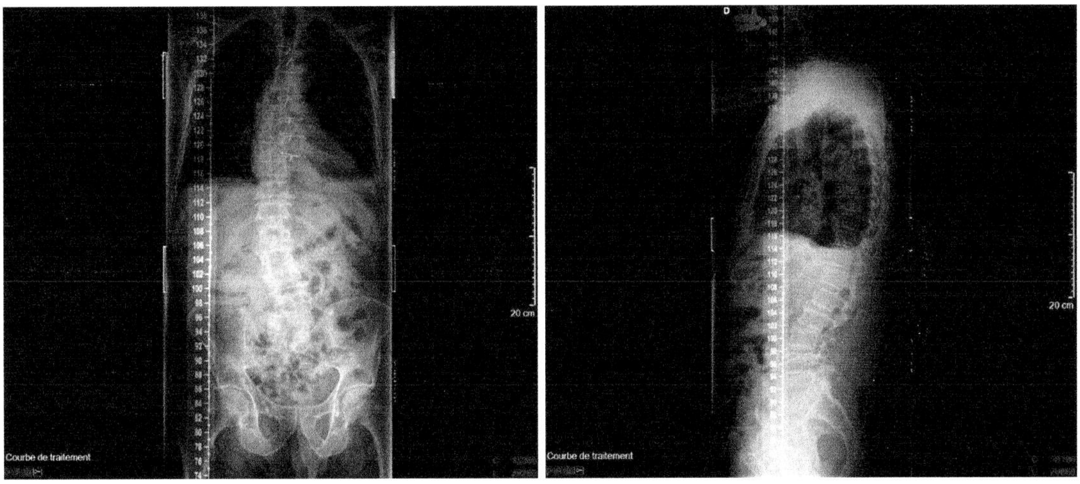

Fig. 81.3 Full spine X-rays at presentation. The degenerative scoliosis is seen and spinal alignment is well compensated

several centimeters on both sides, relaxing incisions were performed in the lateral lumbar fascia to assist in a low tissue tension closure. A subcutaneous drain was placed and the skin was closed.

At 8 months postoperatively, the patient had fully recovered his paraparesis, and his lumbar wound healed, which was confirmed by MRI (Fig. 81.4). At 3 year follow up, the patient had minimal low back pain and no evidence of spinal instability.

81.3 Discussion of the Case

The management of this case is open to discussion. A blood patch had been attempted as has a surgical re-exploration prior to presentation at our institution. The body of literature for postoperative CSF fistulae is small, and as a surgical complication, is likely to be underreported. Furthermore, treatment guidelines are sparse and are largely based on expert opinion, as is the management of this case.

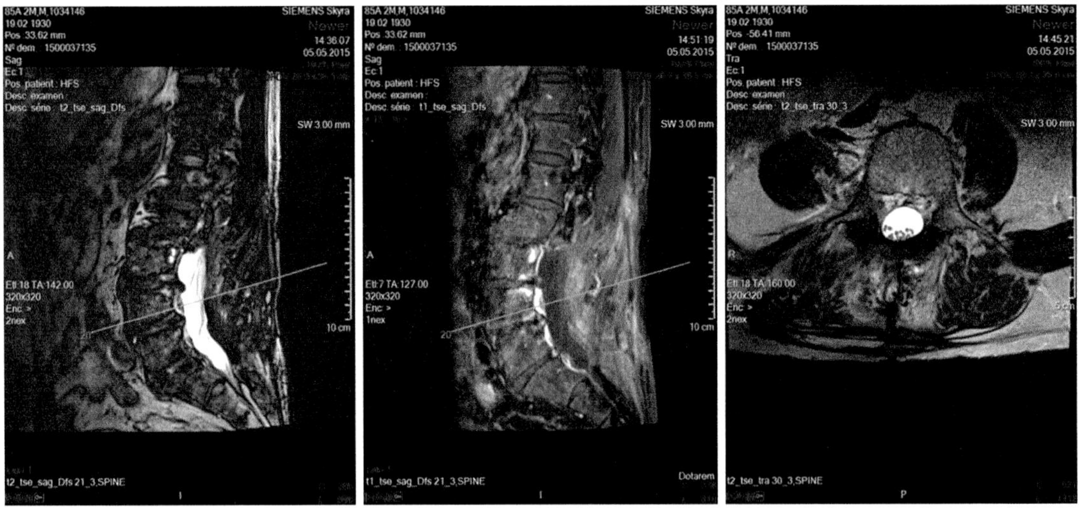

Fig. 81.4 Follow-up MRI showing resolved pseudomeningocele

The first important point is that the decision to perform a blood patch is difficult to justify. Injecting blood into a large fluid filled cavity has a low probability to adhere to the dural defect, particularly in a completely open spinal canal. We would not recommend this strategy.

The second point is that 2 unsuccessful attempts have been made to close the dura, once at the index surgery, and again 11 days later. The dural defect is likely to be small and possibly difficult to access. The hydrodynamics of a very small dural defect means that it operates like a "valve". In other words, CSF flows out and cannot get back in, as it would with a very large dural defect, which has "ebb & flow" and is a low pressure system. Small dural defects therefore can lead to very large pseudomeningoceles, as in this case.

For this case, there is no choice but to revise the wound. The strategy is to find and primarily close the dural defect with some local muscle or fascial patch, unless the dura is robust (highly unlikely in the older ager group, infected, multi-operated). Coverage with healthy vascularised tissue enhances dural healing and closes off some dead space around the defect, and in a complicated dural closure revision should be strongly considered.

The above discussion is purely case-based reasoning/expert opinion, and constitutes level 5 evidence.

81.4 Conclusions and Take Home Message

Postoperative CSF fistulae with fluid leaking out through the skin almost always require a surgical solution. We recommend a thorough exploration, identification and closure of the fistula site. We do not recommend blindly covering a large area of the dura with fibrin glue or dural substitutes in the hope that it will "do the trick". As in this case, further bone removal may be required to adequately identify the fistula site. The use of a vascularised local muscle flap should be considered in multi-operated cases, and interdisciplinary collaboration with plastic surgery colleagues is invaluable here. We caution against underestimating the problem and thus undertreating it. The exact choice of surgical strategy depends on the surgeons experience, however, it requires a clear understanding of the contributing underlying factors, and mandates accurate localization of the fistula.

Pearls

- Postoperative CSF fistulae with fluid leaking out through the skin require a surgical solution
- thorough exploration, identification and closure of the fistula site

- further bone removal may be required to adequately identify the fistula site
- a vascularised local muscle flap should be considered in multi-operated cases
- we caution against underestimating the problem and thus undertreating it

References

1. Guerin P, El Fegoun AB, Obeid I, Gille O, Lelong L, Luc S, et al. Incidental durotomy during spine surgery: incidence, management and complications. A retrospective review. Injury. 2012;43:397–401.
2. Epstein NE. The frequency and etiology of intraoperative dural tears in 110 predominantly geriatric patients undergoing multilevel laminectomy with noninstrumented fusions. J Spinal Disord Tech. 2007;20:380–6.
3. Patel MR, Louie W, Rachlin J. Postoperative cerebrospinal fluid leaks of the lumbosacral spine: management with percutaneous fibrin glue. AJNR Am J Neuroradiol. 1996;17:495–500.
4. Kothe R, Quante M, Engler N, Heider F, Kneissl J, Pirchner S, et al. The effect of incidental dural lesions on outcome after decompression surgery for lumbar spinal stenosis: results of a multi-center study with 800 patients. Eur Spine J. 2017;26:2504–11.
5. Menon SK, Onyia CU. A short review on a complication of lumbar spine surgery: CSF leak. Clin Neurol Neurosurg. 2015;139:248–51.

Index

B. Meyer, M. Rauschmann (eds.), *Spine Surgery*, https://doi.org/10.1007/978-3-319-98875-7

Printed by Printforce, the Netherlands